Meningiomas

Diagnosis, Treatment, and Outcome

Edited by

Joung H. Lee

Brain Tumor & Neuro-Oncology Center/Department of Neurosurgery,
Neurological Institute, The Cleveland Clinic Foundation, Cleveland, OH, USA

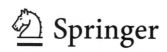 Springer

Editor
Joung H. Lee, MD
Brain Tumor & Neuro-Oncology Center
Department of Neurosurgery, Neurological Institute
Cleveland Clinic Foundation, Cleveland, OH, USA

ISBN 978-1-84628-526-4   e-ISBN 978-1-84628-784-8
DOI: 10.1007/978-1-84628-784-8

Library of Congress Control Number: 2007940436

To all my patients,
Who inspire me to do my very best in their care

Foreword

Joung H. Lee has assembled a masterful volume on the diagnosis, treatment, and outcome of meningiomas. It is complete in that it covers all aspects of this tumor; every location is discussed by acknowledged experts and every technique is described in detail. Basic biology forms an important and up-to-date part of the text. This book will serve as a reference for many years; in particular, Dr. Lee feels surgeons and future patients will benefit. There is little question that these aims will be fulfilled in this important tour de force.

John A. Jane, Sr., MD, PhD
Charlottesville, VA, USA

Foreword

Preface

In planning this book, I had three major goals. The first was to compile and disseminate all the advances and new information relating to meningiomas which became available in the last 15-20 years. In this time frame, there has been a significant increase in our understanding in regards to the meningioma pathologic classification, the natural history and basic science. Dramatic technological advancements have also been made in diagnostic and interventional radiology as well as in surgical and radiation treatments for meningiomas, such as incorporation of the following in the treatment armamentaria: endoscopy, various skull base techniques, computer-assisted surgery and radiosurgery. Additionally, new information regarding surgical outcome and patient selection for surgery are becoming available, all of which are resulting in a significant change in how neurosurgeons treat patients with meningiomas.

The second goal for this book was to teach and stimulate the next generation of neurosurgeons. Because meningiomas can occur anywhere within the intracranial space or along the spine, for an individual neurosurgeon, mastering the surgery of meningiomas allows one to become a master surgeon. In other words, to learn the basics of meningioma surgery – i.e. surgical decision making, positioning, anatomy, approach, exposure and microdissection, tumor removal, hemostasis, closure- is to learn the basics of neurosurgery. Moreover, meningioma surgery is arguably the most rewarding, challenging and, at times, daunting task for neurosurgeons: rewarding, because of the benign nature of most meningiomas, leading to a possible cure following total removal, challenging because of the tumors' common sites of involvement in proximity to critical neurovascular structures especially when involving the central skull base, and daunting due to the tumor's tendency to recur in higher grades of histologic subtypes and to its frequent involvement of the surrounding skull base bone, dura and neurovascular structures making complete removal often risky or impossible. Although meningioma surgery can be enjoyable and rewarding, I wanted young readers to appreciate and respect the challenging and daunting aspects, which will undoubtedly serve as the stimulus for continued learning, refinement and progress in this field in the future.

The third goal, but the most important one, was to give back to our patients. As neurosurgeons or physicians, we are nothing without our patients. Our patients are truly the backbone of our professional livelihood. It is a great privilege to be able to provide care for other human beings. I firmly believe that the best way to show sincere gratitude to our patients is to not only provide the best care possible, but also to learn from each, so that treatment for the subsequent patients is better and improved.

Editing this book was a much greater task than initially anticipated, with 64 chapters contributed by over 110 distinguished authors from 5 different continents. I am truly honored to be given the opportunity to complete this project which could not have been possible without the support of all the contributors and the publisher, Springer-Verlag. My only regret is that I could not possibly include all of the international experts to join me in this project.

I intentionally solicited differing views and approaches when there are multiple reasonable ways of dealing with the same problem. I thought presentation of multiple ways is superior to pre-selected (and, hence biased) single presentation. Moreover, I wanted very much for young readers to appreciate the fact that there is no single best way of treating certain meningiomas. Hopefully, they will appreciate that whatever technique or approach that results in the best long-term patient outcome in their local setting is what really matters, whether it is surgery vs. radiosurgery for cavernous sinus meningiomas, endoscopic surgery vs. microsurgery in anterior skull base meningiomas, total vs. subtotal resection followed by radiosurgery in parasagittal or skull base meningiomas, anterior vs. posterior transpetrosal approach in petroclival meningiomas, aggressive surgery vs. radiation in optic nerve sheath meningiomas, etc.

This book could not be completed without the valuable assistance of Ms. Christine Moore, an editorial assistant in the Department of Neurosurgery, Cleveland Clinic, and Dr. Burak Sade, my former fellow and present colleague. I cannot thank them enough! I am also greatly indebted to all my mentors: as stated above, they include all my patients, in addition to Professors Eve Marder (neurophysiology professor in college), Alain B. Rossier (college senior thesis preceptor) and John A. Jane, Sr. Lastly, I thank my lovely wife, Heeyang, and my dearest sons, Terry, Nick and Ryan, for their constant support, love and inspiration.

As stated earlier, one of the goals of this book was to teach. However, in completing this book, I became the biggest beneficiary, having learned so much. Just like meningioma surgery, editing this book was immensely enjoyable, rewarding and challenging. If through this book, I have stimulated even a small number of young neurosurgeons to learn and make continued progress in the area of meningiomas, so that they in turn can provide better and improved care for their future patients, I have fulfilled my goals.

Joung H. Lee
Cleveland, Ohio, USA

Contents

III. Basic Science

IV. Management and Outcome

V. Adjunct Treatment Modalities

Contributors List

Siviero Agazzi, MD
Department of Neurosurgery, University of South Florida, Tampa, FL, USA

Manzoor Ahmed, MD
Department of Radiology, Cleveland Clinic, Cleveland, OH, USA

Felipe C. Albuquerque, MD
Department of Neurosurgery, Barrow Neurological Institute, Phoenix, AZ, USA

Amro Al-Habib, MD
Hopsita l for Sick Children, Toronto, Ontario, Canada

Ossama Al-Mefty, MD
University of Arkansas, Little Rock, AR, USA

Jorge E. Alvernia, MD
Department of Neurosurgery, Tulane University, New Orleans, LA, USA

David W. Andrews, MD
Thomas Jefferson University Hospital, Philadelphia, PA, USA

Lilyana Angelov, MD, FRCS
Brain Tumor and Neuro-Oncology Center, Neurological Institute, Cleveland Clinic, Cleveland, OH, USA

Khaled A. Aziz, MD, PhD
Department of Neurosurgery, University of Cincinnati College of Medicine. Cincinnati, OH, USA

A. Bacciu, MD, ENT
Department of Neurosurgery, University of Parma, Parma, Italy

Gene H. Barnett, MD
Brain Tumor and Neuro-Oncology Center, Neurological Institute, Cleveland Clinic, Cleveland, OH, USA

Samuel L. Barnett, MD
Department of Neurosurgery, University of Mississippi Medical Center, Jackson, MS, USA

Edward C. Benzel, MD
Center for Spine Health, Neurological Institute, Cleveland Clinic, Cleveland, OH, USA

Luis A.B. Borba, MD
Department of Neurosurgery, Evangelic University Medical School, Curitiba, Parana, Brazil

Jacques Brotchi, MD, PhD
Department of Neurosurgery, Universite Libre de Bruxelles, Bruxelles, Belgium

Ralf M. Buhl, MD, PhD
Department of Neurosrugery, Clemens Hospital, Munster, Germany

John Butler, MD
Center for Spine Health, Neurological Institute, Cleveland Clinic, Cleveland, OH, USA

Paolo Cappabianca, MD
Department of Neurological Sciences, Universita degli Studi di Napoli Federico II, Napoli, Italy

Luigi M. Cavallo, MD, PhD
Department of Neurological Sciences, Universita degli Studi di Napoli Federico II, Napoli, Italy

Albert S. Chang, MD
Department of Radiology and Neuro-Radiology, Cleveland Clinic, Cleveland, OH, USA

Eric L. Chang, MD
Department of Radiation Oncology, MD Anderson Cancer Center, Houston, TX, USA

Han Soo Chang, MD
Department of Neurosurgery, Saitama Medical Center, Saitama, Japan

Kyung Gi Cho, MD, PhD
Department of Neurosurgery, Ajou University School of Medicine, Suwon, South Korea

Benedicto O. Colli, MD
Department of Neurosurgery, University of São Paulo, Ribeirao Preto, São Paulo, Brazil

William T. Couldwell, MD, PhD
Department of Neurosurgery, University of Utah, Salt Lake City, UT, USA

Anthony L. D'Ambrosio, MD
Department of Neurosurgery, University of South Florida, Tampa, FL, USA

Enrcio de Divitiis, MD
Department of Neurological Sciences, Universita degli Studi di Napoli Federico II, Napoli, Italy

G. DeDonato, MD
Gruppo Otologico, Piacenza, Rome, Italy

Johnny B. Delashaw, Jr., MD
Department of Neurosurgery, Oregon Health Sciences University, Portland, OR, USA

Roberto Delfini, MD, PhD
Department of Neurosurgery, University of Roma, Roma, Italy

Vivek R. Deshmukh, MD
Department of Neurosugery, Barrow Neurological Institute, Phoenix, AZ, USA

Nicholas de Tribolet, MD
Department of Neurosurgery, Geneva University Hospital, Geneva, Switzerland

Kadir Erkmen, MD
Department of Neurosurgery, Darthmoth-Hitchcock Medical Center, Lebanon, NH, USA

Felice Esposito, MD, PhD
Department of Neurological Sciences, Universita degli Studi di Napoli Federico II, Napoli, Italy

James J. Evans, MD
Department of Neurological Surgery, Thomas Jefferson University Hospital, Philadelphia, PA, USA

Maurizio Falcioni, MD
Gruppo Otologico, Piacenza, Rome, Italy

David J. Fiorella, MD, PhD
Department of Neurosurgery, Neurological Institute, Cleveland Clinic, Cleveland, OH, USA

Sean Flanagan, MD
Gruppo Otologico, Piacenza, Rome, Italy

Douglas Fox, MD
Department of Neurosurgery, Barrow Neurological Institute, Phoenix, AZ, USA

Shifra Fraifeld, MBA
Department of Neurosurgery, Hadassah - Hebrew University Medical Center, Jerusalem, Israel

William A. Friedman, MD
Department of Neurosugery, University of Florida, Gainesville, FL, USA

Sebastein C. Froelich, MD
Department of Neurosurgery, University of Cincinnati College of Medicine, Cincinnati, OH, USA

Sarah E. Gibson, MD
Department of Anatomic Pathology, Cleveland Clinic, Cleveland, OH, USA

Mladen Golubic, MD, PhD
Brain Tumor and Neuro-Oncology Center, Neurological Institute, Cleveland Clinic, Cleveland, OH, USA

Jorge A. González-Martínez, MD, PhD
Department of Neurosurgery & Epilepsy Center, Neurological Institute, Cleveland Clinic, Cleveland, OH, USA

Takeo Goto, MD
Department of Neurosurgery, Osaka City University, Osaka, Japan

Werner Hassler, MD, PhD
Neurosurgical Clinic, Duisburg, Germany

Gregory A. Helm, MD, PhD
Department of Neurosurgery, University of Virginia, Charlottesville, VA, USA

Seok Ho Hong, MD, PhD
Department of Neurosugery, Asan Medical Center, University of Ulsan, Seoul, South Korea

John A. Jane, Jr. , MD
Department of Neurosurgery, University of Virginia, Charlottesville, VA, USA

Hee Won Jung, MD, PhD
Department of Neurosurgery, Seoul National University College of Medicine, Seoul, South Korea

Nobutaka Kawahara, MD
Department of Neurosurgery, University of Tokyo, Tokyo, Japan

Takeshi Kawase, MD, PhD
Department of Neurosurgery, Keio University School of Medicine, Tokyo, Japan

Andrew H. Kaye, MBBS, MD, FRACS
Department of Neurosurgery, Royal Melbourne Hospital, Melbourne, Australia

Noojan J. Kazemi, MBBS
Department of Neurosurgery, Royal Melbourne Hospital, Melbourne, Australia

Vini G. Khurana, MD, PhD
Department of Neuroscience, Barrow Neurological Institute, Phoenix, AZ, USA

Chae-Yong Kim, MD, PhD
Department of Neurosurgery, Seoul National University College of Medicine, Seoul, South Korea

Chang Jin Kim, MD, PhD
Department of Neurosurgery, Asan Medical Center, University of Ulsan, Seoul, South Korea

Han Kyu Kim, MD, PhD
Department of Neurosurgery, Eulji University, Dae Jeon, South Korea

Gregory Kosmorsky, DO
Department of Neuro-Ophthalmology, Cole Eye Institute, Cleveland Clinic, Cleveland, OH, USA

P. Pradeep Kumar, MD
Department of Radiation-Oncology, James H. Quillen VA Medical Center, Mountain Home, TN, USA

Edward R. Laws, Jr. , MD
Department of Neurosurgery, Brigham &Women's Hospital, Boston, MA, USA

Joung H. Lee, MD
Brain Tumor & Neuro-Oncology Center, Department of Neurosurgery, Neurological Institute, Cleveland Clinic Foundation, Cleveland, OH, USA

Michael J. Link, MD
Department of Neurological Surgery, Mayo Clinic, Rochester, MN, USA

Simon S. Lo, MD
Department of Neuro-Radiation Oncology and Radiosurgery, Ohio State University Medical Center, Columbus, OH, USA

M. Beatriz S. Lopes, MD
Department of Pathology, University of Virginia School of Medicine, Charlottesville, VA, USA

Thomas J. Masaryk, MD, FACR
Department of Neuroradiology, Cleveland Clinic, Cleveland, OH, USA

Cameron G. McDougall, MD
Department of Neurosurgery, Barrow Neurological Institute, Phoenix, AZ, USA

H. Maximilian Mehdorn, MD, PhD
Department of Neurosurgery, University Hospitals of Schleswig-Holstein, Kiel, Germany

Imad M. Najm, MD
Epilepsy Center, Neurological Institute, Cleveland Clinic, Cleveland, OH USA

Sabareesh Kumar Natarajan, MD, MS
Department of Neurosurgery, University of Washington Medical Center, Seattle, WA, USA

Steven A. Newman, MD
Department of Ophthalmology, University of Virginia HSC, Charlottesville, VA, USA

Kenji Ohata, MD
Department of Neurosurgery, Osaka City University Graduate School of Medicine, Osaka, Japan

David O. Okonkwo, MD, PhD
Department of Neurosurgery, University of Pittsburgh, Pittsburgh, PA, USA

Bong Jin Park, MD, PhD
Department of Neurosurgery, Kyung Hee University, Seoul, South Korea

David M. Peereboom, MD
Department of Medical Oncology, Brain Tumor and Neuro-Oncology Center, Cleveland Clinic, Cleveland, OH, USA

Arie Perry, MD
Department of Neuropathology, Washington University School of Medicine, St. Louis, MO, USA

Angelo Pichierri, MD
Department of Neuroscience, University of Rome, Rome, Italy

Benoit J.M. Pirotte, MD, PhD
Department of Neurosurgery, Universite Libre de Bruxelles, Bruxelles, Belgium

Nader Pouratian, MD, PhD
Department of Neurosurgery, University of Virginia HSC, Charlottesville, VA, USA

Svetlana Pravdenkova, MD, PhD
Department of Neurosurgery, University of Arkansas, Little Rock, AR, USA

Richard A. Prayson, MD
Department of Neuropathology, Cleveland Clinic, Cleveland, OH, USA

Ivan Radovanovic, MD
Department of Neurosurgery, Geneva University Hospital, Geneva, Switzerland

Brian T. Ragel, MD
Department of Neurosurgery, University of Utah, Salt Lake City, UT, USA

Guy Rosenthal, MD
Department of Neurosurgery, Hadassah - Hebrew University Medical Center, Jerusalem, Israel

Jeffrey S. Ross, MD
Department of Neuro-Radiology, Barrow Neurological Institute, Phoenix, AZ, USA

James T. Rutka, MD
Department of Neurosurgery, Hospital for Sick Children, Toronto, Ontario, Canada

Burak Sade, MD
Brain Tumor and Neuro-Oncology Center, Neurological Institute, Cleveland Clinic, Cleveland, OH, USA

Mario Sanna, MD
Gruppo Otologico, Piacenza, Rome, Italy

Charles A. Sansur, MD
Department of Neurosurgery, University of Virginia HSC, Charlottesville, VA, USA

Antonio Santoro, MD
Department of Neuroscience, University of Rome, Rome, Italy

Tomio Sasaki, MD
Department of Neurosurgery, Kyushu University Graduate School of Medical Sciences, Fukuoka, Japan

Uta Schick, MD, PhD
Neurosurgical Clinic, Duisburg, Germany

Laligam N. Sekhar, MD, FACS
Department of Neurosurgery, University of Washington Medical Center, Seattle, WA, USA

Jason Sheehan, MD, PhD
Department of Neurosurgery, University of Virginia HSC, Charlottesville, VA, USA

Yigal Shoshan, MD
Department of Neurosurgery, Hadassah - Hebrew University Medical Center, Jerusalem, Israel

Eric H. Sincoff, MD
Deaprtment of Neurosurgery, Oregon Health Sciences University, Portland, OR, USA

Marc P. Sindou, MD, DSc
Department of Neurosurgery, Hospital Neurologique, Lyon, France

Sergey Specktor, MD
Department of Neurosurgery, Hadassah - Hebrew University Medical Center, Jerusalem, Israel

Robert F. Spetzler, MD
Department of Neurosurgery, Barrow Neurological Institute, Phoenix, AZ, USA

Ladislau Steiner, MD, PhD
Department of Neurosurgery and Radiology, University of Virginia HSC, Charlottesville, VA, USA

Glen H.J. Stevens, MD, PhD
Brain Tumor and Neuro-Oncology Center, Neurological Institute, Cleveland Clinic, Cleveland, OH, USA

John H. Suh, MD
Department of Radiation Oncology, Cleveland Clinic, Cleveland, OH, USA

Abdelkader Taibah, MD
Gruppo Otologico, Piacenza, Rome, Italy

John M. Tew, Jr., MD
Department of Neurosurgery, University of Cincinnati College of Medicine, Cincinnati, OH, USA

Philip Theodosopoulos, MD
Department of Neurosurgery, University of Cincinnati College of Medicine, Cincinnati, OH, USA

Tina Thomas, MD
Brain Tumor and Neuro-Oncology Center, Neurological Institute, Cleveland Clinic, Cleveland, OH, USA

Brent A. Tinnel, MD
Department of Radiation Oncology, Walter Reed Army Medical Center, Washington, DC, USA

Jörg-Christian Tonn, MD
Department of Neurosurgery, University of Munich, Munich, Germany

Eve C. Tsai, MD, PhD
Center for Spine Health, Neurological Institute, Cleveland Clinic, Cleveland, OH, USA

Koichi Uchida, MD
Department of Neurosurgery, Keio University School of Medicine, Tokyo, Japan

Felix Umansky, MD
Department of Neurosurgery, Hadassah - Hebrew University Medical Center, Jerusalem, Israel

Harry R. van Loveren, MD
Department of Neurosurgery, University of South Florida, Tampa, FL, USA

Marcus L. Ware, MD, PhD
Department of Neurosurgery, University of Arkansas, Little Rock, AR, USA

Peter A. Winkler, MD, PhD
Department of Neurosurgery, University of Munich, Munich, Germany

Tetsumori Yamashima, MD, PhD
Department of Restorative Neurosurgery, Kanazawa University Graduate School of Medical Science, Kanazawa, Japan

Kazunari Yoshida, MD
Department of Neurosurgery, Keio University School of Medicine, Tokyo, Japan.

I
General Information

1
Meningiomas: Historical Perspective

David O. Okonkwo and Edward R. Laws, Jr.

In 1614, Felix Plater, Professor of Medicine, issued a case report from the University of Basel:[1]

Caspar Bonecurtius, a noble knight, began to lose his mind gradually over a two year period, to such an extent that finally he was completely stupefied and did nothing rationally. He had no desire for food and ate only when forcibly fed. ... Finally after matters had gone on thus for six months, he died.

It is unclear from the historical record whether Plater (Fig. 1-1) met Bonecurtius during life, but Plater did perform his autopsy, which revealed

a round fleshy tumor, like an acorn. It was hard and full of holes and was as large as a medium-sized apple. It was covered with its own membrane and was entwined with veins. However, it was free of all connections with the matter of the brain, so much so that when it was removed by hand, it left behind a remarkable cavity.

Plater's report of the case of Caspar Bonecurtius is the earliest known literary reference to a patient with a lesion that is most compatible with a meningioma.

Meningiomas are benign tumors of the meninges and arise from arachnoidal cap cells. They represent 15% of all primary brain neoplasms. Meningiomas may occur in any location throughout the neuraxis, and location imparts unique clinical, diagnostic, and treatment characteristics. These fascinating lesions generate as much enthusiasm as any specific subset of challenges in neurosurgery. The place of meningiomas in the hearts and minds of neurosurgeons was best described by Cushing when he wrote in 1922,[2] "There is nothing in the whole realm of surgery more gratifying than the successful removal of a meningioma with subsequent perfect functional recovery," a sentiment that persists today.

Meningiomas in Paleopathology

The description by Plater of Caspar Bonecurtius may be the earliest reference to a meningioma on record, but Bonecurtius was by no means the first human to harbor a meningioma.

Because of their tendency to cause an overlying thickening of the bone, meningiomas have left unmistakable traces, in the form of hyperostosis, on human skulls throughout the course of human history. Eleven paleopathologic records of meningiomas, recovered from archeological excavations throughout the world, have been documented (Table 1-1).

The oldest of these specimens was discovered in 1933 in a quarry near Steinheim on the Murr in southern Germany. Seventy years after the initial discovery of the "Steinheim skull," Czarnetzki et al. reexamined the fossil specimen endoscopically and with three-dimensional computed tomography (CT) and described several features consistent with the diagnosis of meningioma.[3] The Steinheim skull, stratigraphically dated at 365,000 years old, is the earliest record in the *Homo erectus* line of the benign leptomeningeal growth now known as meningioma.

The paleopathologic hallmark of the lesion is meningiomatous hyperostosis, and the differentiation between meningiomatous hyperostosis and other causes has become more distinct.[4,5] Prehistoric meningiomatous hyperostotic specimens have been found most often in Incan skulls of the Peruvian Andes, where climate and high-lime content soil, like the quarry in Steinheim, Germany, bestowed good preservation of bones.

The most recent paleopathologic example of meningioma was discovered during the excavation of a cemetery of the Rochester, Canterbury Cathedral in 1990. Anderson described the specimen of a 35- to 50-year-old female who died around 1400 AD.[6] The "patient" had a 6 × 6 × 5 cm sphenoid wing and frontal meningioma producing unilateral exopthalmos and, likely, blindness secondary to obliteration of the optic canal. This specimen was subjected to CT scanning, which confirmed the diagnosis of intra-osseous meningioma.

Pathogenesis

Meningiomas are now known to arise from arachnoidal cap cells of the leptomeninges. Arachnoidal granulations were first

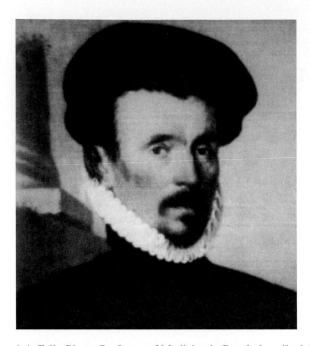

FIG. 1-1. Felix Plater, Professor of Medicine in Basel, described the earliest known case of meningioma in the literature in 1614

TABLE 1-1. Paleopathologic Records of Meningiomas.

Location	Date	Sex	Age (yr)
Steinheim, Germany[3]	363000 BC	F	25–30
Stetten, Germany[42]	32500 BC	?	adult
Chavina, Peru[43]	?	F	Middle age
Paucarcancha, Peru[44]	?	M	Elderly
Chicama, Peru[43]	?	M	Adult
St. Nicholas Island, CA[45]	?	M	Elderly
Helouan, Upper Egypt[46]	3400 BC	M	40–60
Meydun, Upper Egypt[46]	1500 BC	M	50–70
Radley, Oxfordshire[47]	100 AD	F	Adult
Chernovski, Alaska[4]	1000 AD	M	~40
Rochester, Canterbury[6]	1400 AD	F	35–50

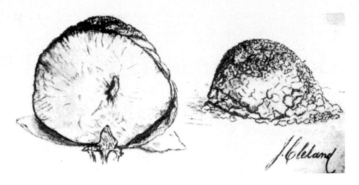

FIG. 1-2. John Cleland's illustration of a "villous tumor of the arachnoid." Cleland was the first to propose that meningiomas arose from pacchionian granulations (From Ref. 25)

described by Antonio Pacchioni in Rome in 1705, believing them to be the nervous system counterpart to lymph glands.[7] In 1846, Rainey suggested that arachnoidal or pacchionian granulations arose from the meninges.[8] This association was confirmed by Luschka in 1852[9] and later by Meyer in 1859.[10]

It was not until John Cleland in 1864, however, that the association between pacchionian granulations and meningeal tumors was drawn.[11] Working in Glasgow, Cleland described two leptomeningeal tumors at autopsy and deemed them "villous tumors of the arachnoid," as he was able to separate the growths from the dura (Fig. 1-2). He hypothesized their origin as from the pacchionian granulations.

Cleland's conclusion was later confirmed by both Robin,[12] who reported from Paris two meningeal tumors as arising from the arachnoid, and Martin Schmidt[13] in Strasbourg, who examined a series of meningeal tumors and reported that the neoplastic cells most closely resembled arachnoidal cap cells.

Contemporaries, however, postulated that meningeal tumors arose from such sources as glia, connective tissue, fibroblasts, and neuro-epithelial cells.[14–16]

Harvey Cushing sided with Cleland in a report in 1915 with Weed from Baltimore that meningeal tumors arose from arachnoidal cap cells.[17] This position was later substantiated by Percival Bailey and Paul Bucy in 1931, when they wrote the definitive histopathologic description of meningiomas:

… the cells of these masses are somewhat elongated and wound around each other to form whorls. The central cells of the whorls undergo a hyaline transformation and become calcified. They cause a gritty noise when the tumor is cut, hence their name of psammoma (sand-like) bodies.[18]

Bailey and Bucy stated the cell of origin of meningiomas as arachnoidal cap cells, and the neurosurgical literature has principally been in agreement since.

Nomenclature

Seven years after concluding that these tumors arise from arachnoid cap cells, Harvey Cushing proposed the term "meningioma" during his Cavendish lecture in Cambridge in 1922.[2] As the term achieved eventual global acceptance, a centuries-old argument on the appropriate moniker for this group of tumors was laid to rest.

The earliest known illustration of a meningioma appeared in 1730 in the publication of the Collegium Naturae Curiosum (the present-day Germany Academy of Natural Sciences Leopoldino). Johann Salzmann (1672–1738) reported the autopsy results of a patient he had followed in life. The case, titled "Exostosis seu excrescentia cranii osseo-spongiosa," was a 43-year-old man who presented with progressive behavioral change, seizures, headaches, and vertigo.[19] The patient eventually died following a seizure in 1727.

At autopsy, Salzmann noted a large left frontoparietal mass with intra- and extracranial components. The tumor was soft, osseo-spongious, and had left an impression in the underlying

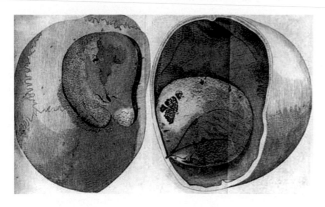

FIG. 1-3. Earliest known illustration of a meningioma, as reported by Johann Salzmann in 1730

brain of exactly the same form as the tumor, but without invasion of dura or brain. Salzmann attributed the man's symptomatology to pressure from the tumor on the brain. Salzmann's illustration is likely the first of a meningioma in the literature (Fig. 1-3).

The first reference to deal exclusively with meningiomas was written by Antoine Louis in 1774. (Louis was also a pioneer of French medical jurisprudence and in 1749 presented a classic discussion of the differential signs of murder and suicide in cases of hanging.) In 1764, Louis was appointed lifetime secretary to the Académie Royale de Chirurgie, a reflection of his esteem among his peers and a reward for his earlier struggles to confirm the field of surgery in the face of the more domineering French medical physicians. It was in his capacity as secretary that he published his personal experience with 20 specimens in the 1774 *Mémoires de l' Académie Royale de Chirurgie* titled, "Sur les Tumeurs fongueses de la Dure-mere."[20] It is likely that at least some of the cases described by Louis were in fact osteosarcomas. Nevertheless, it is interesting to note that Cushing and Eisenhardt begin their 1938 masterpiece, *Meningiomas*, with a quote from Antoine Louis's 1774 treatise, a sign of Cushing's deference to Louis's seminal compilation.

The nomenclature of meningiomas changed repeatedly in the ensuing century. This evolution included the terms *exostosis seu excrescentia cranii osseo-spongiosa* (Salzmann, 1730),[19] *de tumore capitis fungoso* (Heister and Crellius, 1743),[21] fungoid tumor (Bright, 1831),[22] fungus of the dura mater (Pecchioli, 1838),[23] *tumeurs fibro-plastiques* (Lebert, 1851),[24] epithelioma (Meyer, 1859),[10] psammoma (Virchow, 1859),[25] dural sarcoma (Virchow, 1863),[25] dural endothelioma (Golgi, 1869),[25] and fibrosarcoma (Durante, 1885).[26]

Cushing, troubled by the confusion of a multiplicity of names, drew together the group of tumors under a single designation that he intended to be brief and convenient. In his foreword to his monograph with Eisenhardt, Cushing noted that a "place-name," similar to the term "acoustic neuroma," would be insufficient for this diverse group of tumors that occur throughout the neuraxis but have pathologic and embry-

onic commonalities. He also wished to avoid a histiogenic name since the cellular origin of meningiomas had not yet been established in his early series. He first proposed the term meningothelioma in 1922. Later that year, in his Cavendish lecture, Cushing presented his experience of 85 fungating dural tumors to date and proposed the term "meningioma."[2]

Classification Schemata

Virchow made the earliest known attempt to classify the fungating tumors of the dura in 1863. In 1900, Engert described four types: fibromatous, cellular, sarcomatous, and angiomatous.[27] Cushing's initial classification scheme in 1920 was anatomic: frontal, paracentral, parietal, occipital, and temporal. Cushing later adopted a histopathologic classification system with his student, Percival Bailey, who must be considered the greatest of the early pioneers in meningioma classification. Cushing and Bailey listed four variants: meningothelial; fibroblastic; angioblasic; and osteoblastic.

Percival Bailey left his mark on neurosurgery and the study of meningiomas in a number of ways. His serendipitous partnership with Cushing, beginning in 1919, produced many breakthroughs. Bailey's first experiments in Cushing's laboratory at the Peter Bent Brigham Hospital led to the accidental discovery of hypothalamic contributions to pituitary function, a groundbreaking contribution to the budding field of neurosurgery. Bailey also described leptomeningeal spread of medulloblastomas, authored the first significant text on pediatric tumors,[28] coined the term "hemangioblastoma," and was the first to describe brain edema as a complication of cranial irradiation.

But it was Bailey's interest in and dedication to neuropathology for which he is best remembered today. Some of his greatest work came in conjunction with his protégé Paul Bucy while at the University of Chicago, having left Cushing's tutelage in 1928. In addition to their definitive histopathologic description of meningiomas quoted above, Bailey and Bucy expanded the histopathologic classification scheme with such elegance that little changed from their article in 1931[18] to the 2000 WHO classification scheme of Grade I meningiomas[29] (Table 1-2), a feat all the more remarkable when one considers the astonishing revolution in technology, molecular biology, and biochemistry in the intervening seventy years.

Yet, in clinical practice, meningiomas are most commonly classified according to site of origin. It was Jean Cruveilhier (1791–1874) who first classified meningiomas by anatomic site of origin. Working in Paris, Cruveilhier was author of perhaps the most beautiful medical book ever printed, *L'Anatomie Pathologique du Corps Humain*, illustrated with colored lithographs and taken from his extensive collection of specimens as Professor of Pathology.[30] The chapter on meningiomas was titled, "Des Tumeurs Cancereuses des Meninges," a reflection of Cruveilhier's belief that meningiomas were malignant lesions. Cruveilhier was uniquely qualified to

TABLE 1-2. Classification Schemata for Meningiomas.

Bailey and Bucy (1931)	WHO Grade I (2000)
Meningotheliomatous	Meningothelial
Fibroblastic	Fibroblastic
Psammomatous	Psammamotous
Angioblastic	Angiomatous
Mesenchymatous	Metaplastic (mesenchymatous)
Chondroblastic	Secretory
Osteoblastic	Transitional
Melanoblastic	Lymphoplasmocyte-rich
Lipomatous	Microcystic

study meningiomas because he saw patients in the morning at the Charité and Salpetrière hospitals and performed autopsies in the afternoon in his private dissecting room. Thus, he frequently performed autopsies on patients he had followed clinically.

Cruveilhier grouped the tumors in his autopsy series by location and noted several important clinical characteristics distinct to "fungating tumors" in specific locations. He noted epilepsy and lower extremity weakness in falcine meningiomas, anosmia and blindness from olfactory groove lesions, aphasia in temporal fossa lesions, and deafness in petrous ridge lesions. He described the beaten silver appearance of the inner table of the skull resulting from increased intracranial pressure secondary to large tumors. Cruveilhier also described a case of frontal lobe syndrome in a female patient who developed apathy, stupor, and hemiplegia and was found to have a huge frontal meningioma with severe compression of the frontal lobes at autopsy.

Alhough Cruveilhier's *L'Anatomie Pathologique du Corps Humain* contained the first grouping of meningiomas by location, it is in the classification scheme of Cushing and Eisenhardt in their landmark text of 1938 that the modern classification of meningiomas was established. As did Bailey and Bucy with their histopathologic classification, Cushing and Eisenhardt demonstrated notable perspicacity in their classification by site of origin.[25] Cushing's cumulative experience of 313 cases as published in 1938 very closely resembles our contemporary understanding of the frequency of meningiomas by location (Table 1-3).

TABLE 1-3. Frequency of Meningiomas by Location.

Cushing and Eisenhardt (1938)		(2003) Meta-analysis	
Parasagittal/Falcine	23%	25%	Parasagittal/Falcine
Convexity	17%	19%	Convexity
Sphenoidal ridge	17%	17%	Sphenoidal ridge
Olfactory groove	9%	8%	Olfactory groove
Suprasellar	9%	9%	Suprasellar
Cerebellar chamber	7%	4%	Posterior fossa
Tentorial	6%	3%	Tentorial
Spinal	6%	3%	Spinal
Intraventricular	2%	1%	Intraventricular
Meckel's cave	2%	4%	Meckel's cave
Foramen magnum	.3%	1%	Foramen magnum
Orbital/Optic nerve sheath	.3%	1%	Orbital/Optic nerve sheath

Surgical Removal of Meningiomas

Laurence Heister ushered in the era of surgical treatment of meningiomas with an operation in 1743 in Helmstad, Germany.[31] Heister operated on a 34-year-old Prussian soldier who presented with a fungating cranial lesion (Fig. 1-4). Heister applied a caustic of lime; the patient died of postoperative infection. At the autopsy performed by Crellius, the tumor was designated "de tumore capitis fungoso." The case was first reported later that year by Kaufman.

Olaf Acrel, considered the father of Swedish surgery, operated on a patient in 1768 with a pulsating tumor that developed 18 months after a head injury. He explored the lesion with his finger, triggering severe hemorrhage and delayed seizures, followed by death a few days later. He reported the case in his *Chirurgiska Handelser*[32] in 1775 and described the lesion as "Cranii Cerebrique fungus Cancrosus."

Andrea Berlinghieri (1772–1826) published *Trattato di Chirurgi Teorica Practico* in 1813, containing his series of surgical procedures. In one of these operations, Berlinghieri describes the attempted removal of a dural-based mass. The location of the lesion and the outcome of the patient are not known;[33] however, Berlinghieri, in addition to positing trauma as an etiology for dural tumors, put forth the following recommendations for future surgeons for the surgical treatment of these lesions:

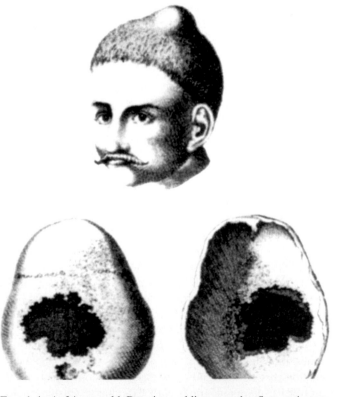

FIG. 1-4. A 34-year-old Prussian soldier was the first patient to undergo surgical treatment of a fungating dural tumor. Laurence Heister, a German physician, applied a caustic of lime to this fungating calvarial lesion, but the patient died of infection (From Ref. 25)

… after craniectomy with five or six burr holes, to cut out the tumor together with the dura mater from which it arose with a knife and tie the cut vessels. If the meningeal artery is damaged during cranial resection, occlude it by bending onto the edge of the bone a lead plate coated with rosin or agaric or keep a small feather pad over the mouth of the vessel.

Early experiences with surgical treatment of meningiomas were not particularly successful, and of the first nine recorded attempts whose outcomes were known, all nine patients died postoperatively. But in 1835, Zanobi Pecchioli (1801–1866) finally broke through. Pecchioli was Professor of Surgery and Operating Medicine at the University of Siena from 1830 to 1851. He performed the first successful removal of an intracranial meningioma in Siena on July 29, 1835.[23] The patient was a 43-year-old with a fungating mass at the right sinciput that developed over the course of 3 years after a head injury. Pecchioli developed a triangular bone flap by drilling three widely placed burr holes. He covered the operative site with cambric soaked in almond oil. The patient recovered, experienced remission of his symptoms, and was noted to be in perfect health and free of recurrence 30 months after his operation. The success of this operation led to Pecchioli's selection for the competition for Chair of Surgery at the University of Paris in 1840, although he remained in Siena.

Sir William Macewen (1848–1924), at age 31, removed a left olfactory groove meningioma from a 14-year-old girl.[34] The patient had exhibited a swelling at her left orbital cavity that was refractory to treatments with iodide and potassium. She was admitted to hospital and witnessed to have recurrent generalized seizures. Macewen diagnosed the child with a brain tumor and operated on July 27, 1849.[35] The patient was discharged from hospital and returned to full employment within a few months of the operation. Macewen went on to become Regius Professor of Surgery at Glasgow at age 44 and was knighted by King Edward VII in 1902 at age 54.[31]

Francesco Durante (1844–1934) studied in Paris with Ranvier and in Berlin with Virchow. Born in Sicily, Durante taught in Rome upon completion of his medical studies and was later chosen as Chair of Clinical Surgery at the Mazzoni Clinic. On June 1, 1885, he successfully removed an apple-sized olfactory groove meningioma.[26] During that operation, he first had the idea of an osteoplastic bone flap. The patient did quite well but experienced a recurrence leading to reoperation 11 years later. The patient was known to remain in good health in 1905, more than 20 years after the initial operation. Durante was nominated Senator of the Kingdom of Italy in 1889.[36]

Robert Fulton Weir (1838–1927) is known more for his contributions as a pioneer in plastic and reconstructive surgery, including the first documented xenograft, using a duck sternum to reconstruct the collapsed nose of a syphilitic man. However, while Professor of Surgery at the College of Physicians and Surgeons in New York City, Weir performed the first attempted removal of a meningioma in the United States on March 9, 1887, in New York City.[37] The patient died due to hemorrhage in the immediate postoperative period.

William W. Keen (1837–1932) was one of the early pioneers in neurosurgery in the United States and was the most prominent American neurosurgeon before the twentieth century.[38] He was a prolific writer, learned scholar, and dedicated teacher. It was perhaps only his advanced age at the time of neurosurgery's maturation as a surgical discipline that limited his influence on the budding field. Keen (Fig. 1-5, top) was valedictorian at Brown University in 1859 and later was graduated from Jefferson Medical College. His medical studies were interrupted by a stint as surgeon in the U.S. Civil War. In 1884, he was appointed Chair of Surgery at Jefferson, where he imported the Gigli saw to American practice in 1898.

Keen is most famous for the first successful removal of a meningioma in the United States in 1887.[39] The patient was a 26-year-old carriage maker who presented with headaches, seizures, and partial blindness (Fig. 1-5, bottom). The patient also had a remote history of head injury at age three. On examination, Keen noted aphasia and right hemiparesis and diagnosed the patient with a brain tumor.

Surgery was performed on December 15, 1887, and elaborate antiseptic measures were taken, including removing the carpet from the operating theatre and cleaning the walls and ceiling. Keen scheduled surgery to begin at 1 p.m. to maximize

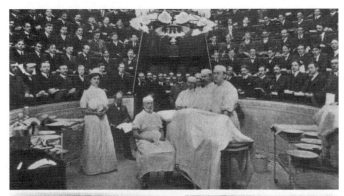
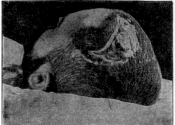
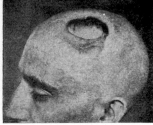

FIG. 1-5. (Top) William W. Keen in theater at Jefferson Medical College in 1903 (photo courtesy of James L Stone). (Bottom) Keen performed the first successful resection of a meningioma in the United States in 1887 on a patient who presented with a fungating calvarial lesion more than 20 years after a head injury. The patient experienced an excellent outcome and survived over 30 years (From Keen WW, Ellis AG. Removal of a brain tumor: report of a case in which the patient survived for more than thirty years. JAMA 1918;70:1905–1909)

natural light. The patient was anesthetized with drop ether and a left frontotemporal incision was made. The tumor was removed in its entirety during the 2-hour operation. The procedure was complicated by poor wound healing and a cerebrospinal fluid leak that persisted for 5 weeks. The patient ultimately recovered and was discharged after a 7-week hospitalization. In gratitude, the patient promised Keen his brain for study and, although he was 30 years the elder, Keen outlived his patient and performed the autopsy following the patient's death in 1918.

Herbert Olivecrona (1891–1980) is considered the father of Swedish neurosurgery and was mentor to Gosta Norlén, Lars Leksell, and many other European pioneers. He received his medical certificate from the Karolinska Institute in 1918. Olivecrona spent the final months of World War I in Leipzig, Germany, assisting general surgeons in treating missile wounds of the brain. He then traveled to Baltimore and worked in the Hunterian laboratory and on the clinical service of William Halsted. Olivecrona had no formal neurosurgical training at Johns Hopkins, but he did observe Walter Dandy's neurosurgical approaches.[40] He returned to Stockholm in 1922, turning down a position in Cushing's program for financial considerations.

In 1935, Olivecrona was appointed Professor of Neurosurgery at the Karolinska. That same year, his second book, *Die Parasagittalen Meningeome*, was published. Cushing and Eisenhardt cite this text as having "forestalled much of our thunder." In 1952 in Chicago, Olivecrona was the first honored guest at the Congress of Neurological Surgeons. Felix Plater may be credited with the earliest literary reference to meningiomas, but every modern discussion of meningiomas must begin with Harvey Cushing. Cushing's first resection of a dural sarcoma (as Virchow called them) or a dural endothelioma (as Golgi referred to them) occurred in 1903. Thirty-five years later, his treatise with Louise Eisenhardt on meningiomas (as Cushing came to call them) was published. It remains the classic description of this group of tumors and continues to fascinate neurosurgeons the world over today. It is an opportunity lost when a young neurosurgeon fails to read the masterpiece, *Menigiomas: Their Classification, Regional Behaviour, Life History, and Surgical End Results*, by Harvey Cushing and Louise Eisenhardt.[25]

Cushing's most famous patient with a meningioma was General Leonard Wood, United States Army. General Wood was Chief of Staff of the U.S. Army and himself a military surgeon. He sustained a head injury from striking his head against a low-lying chandelier in 1898. General Wood later noted exostosis at the site of the previous trauma at the vertex, right of midline. By 1902, he had developed left foot parasthesias followed by epilepsy. His complex partial seizures characteristically began in the left foot and ascended the left leg. In 1905, General Wood underwent removal of the calvarial mass and the epidural portion of the tumor. General Wood's Jacksonian attacks recurred and he was referred to Cushing in 1909. After General Wood failed conservative management, Cushing brought him to theatre in 1910 for two-stage surgery separated by 4 days to remove an intracranial parasagittal meningioma.[41]

General Wood made a complete recovery, going on to serve his country in World War I, expanding his role as a public figure, and nearly securing the Republican nomination for President of the United States in 1920. In fact, General Wood's personal fame undoubtedly helped Cushing secure the post as Surgeon-in-Chief of the new Peter Bent Brigham Hospital and solidify the specialty of neurosurgery in the eyes of the American public.

In August, 1927, General Wood again presented to Cushing, this time in Boston, with left-sided spastic hemiparesis and homonymous hemianopsia. Cushing reoperated for a recurrence without apparent complication during a long procedure. General Wood died unexpectedly a few hours later as a result of hemorrhage that reached the ventricle. Cushing later commented, "I've never lost a patient after operation that so upset me. It was so near to success. He was a great man."

Cushing (Fig. 1-6) established the term meningioma, defined the anatomic classification of these tumors still in use today, and established the field of neurosurgery as a surgical subspecialty. His love affair with meningiomas was described best by his concluding remarks in his Cavendish Lecture in 1922:

There is today nothing in the whole realm of surgery more gratifying than the successful removal of a meningioma with subsequent

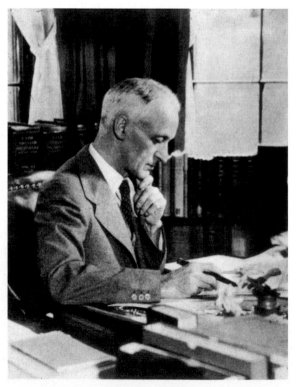

FIG. 1-6. Harvey Cushing (1869–1939) (author's collection)

perfect functional recovery, especially should a correct pathological diagnosis have been previously made. The difficulties are admittedly great, sometimes insurmountable, and though the disappointments still are many, another generation of neurological surgeons will unquestionably see them largely overcome.[2]

Conclusion

Meningiomas have been front and center in the evolution of the discipline of neurosurgery. The current understanding and treatment of meningiomas represent the culmination of centuries of dedication by anatomists, pathologists, neurosurgeons, and others to this ever-intriguing group of tumor. Patients will continue to benefit as contemporary neurosurgeons pursue their craft from the shoulders of the giants before them.

References

1. Plater F. Observationum in hominis affectibus plerisque, corpori et animo, functionum laesione, dolore, aliave, molestia et vitio incommodantibus, libri tres. Ludovici Konig, 1614.
2. Cushing H. The meningiomas (dural endotheliomas): their source and favored seats of origin (Cavendish Lecture). Brain. 1922;45:282–316.
3. Czarnetzki A, Schwaderer E, Pusch CM. Fossil record of meningioma. Lancet. 2003;362:408.
4. Jonsdottir B, Ortner DJ, Frohlich B. Probable destructive meningioma in an archaeological adult male skull from Alaska. Am J Phys Anthropol. 2003;122:232–239.
5. Ortner DJ, Putschar WGJ. Identification of Pathological Conditions in Human Skeletal Remains. Washington, DC: Smithsonian Institution Press, 1985.
6. Anderson T. An example of meningiomatous hyperostosis from medieval Rochester. Med Hist. 1992;36:207–213.
7. Pacchioni A. Dissertatio epistolaris ad Lucam Schroeckium de glandulis conglobatis durae meningis humanae. Francesco Buagni, 1705.
8. Rainey G. On the gangliotic character of the arachnoid membrane of the brain and spinal marrow. Med Chir Trans. 1846;29:85–102.
9. Luschka H. Ueber das Wesen der Pacchionischen Drusen. Arch Anat Physiol (Berlin). 1852;19:101–114.
10. Meyer L. Die Epithelsgranulationen der Arachnoidea. Virchows Arch. 1859;17:209–227.
11. Cleland J. Description of two tumors adherent to the deep surface of the dura mater. Glasgow Med J. 1864;11:148–159.
12. Robin C. Researches anatomiques sur l'epithelioma des sereuses. J Anat (Paris). 1869;6:239–288.
13. Schmidt M. Uber die pachionischen Granulationen und ihr Verhältnis zu den Sarcomen und Psammomen der Dura Mater. Virchows Arch. 1902;170:429–469.
14. Learmonth JR. On leptomeningiomas (endotheliomas) of the spinal cord. Br J Surg. 1927;14:396–476.
15. Oberling C. Les tumeurs des meninges. Bull Assoc Franc Cancer. 1922;11:365–394.
16. Ribbert MW. Uber das endotheliom der dura. Virchows Arch. 1910;200:141–151.
17. Cushing H, Weed LH. Studies on the cerebrospinal fluid and its pathway. IX. Calcarious and ossseous deposits in the arachnoidea. Johns Hopkins Hosp Bull. 1915;26:372.
18. Bailey P, Bucy PC. The origin and nature of meningeal tumors. Am J Cancer. 1931;15:15–54.
19. Salzmann J. Exostosis seu excrescentia cranii osseo-spongiosa. Acta Physico-Medica Academiae Caesareae Leopoldino-Carolinae Naturae Curiosum exhibentia Ephemerides sive Observationes Historias et experimenta a Celeberrimis Germaniae et exterarum regionum viris habita & communicate. 1730;2:225–228.
20. Louis A. Sur les Tumeurs fongueses de la Dure-mere. Mem Acad Roy Chirurg. 1774;5:1–59.
21. Al-Rodhan NR, Laws ER. Meningioma: a historical study of the tumor and its surgical management. Neurosurgery. 1990;26:832–846.
22. Bright R. Reports of medical cases, symptoms and morbid anatomy. In: Bright R, ed. Diseases of the Brain and Nervous System, vol II, part I. London: Longman, 1831:342–347.
23. Pecchioli Z. Storia di un fungo della dura madre operato coll'estirpazione dal professore Zanobi Pecchioli. Nuovo Giorn dei Letterati-Scienze, Pisa. 1838;36:39–44.
24. Lebert H. Ueber Krebs und die mit Krebs verwechselten Geshwulste im Gehirn und seinen Hullen. Virchows Arch. 1851;3:462–569.
25. Cushing H, Eisenhardt L. Menigiomas: Their Classification, Regional Behaviour, Life History, and Surgical End Results. Springfield, IL: Charles C Thomas, 1938.
26. Durante F. Contribution to endocranial surgery. Lancet. 1887;2:654–655.
27. Engert F. Ueber Geschwulste der Dura Mater. Virchows Arch. 1900;160:19–32.
28. Bailey P, Buchanan DN, Bucy PC. Intracranial Tumors of Infancy and Childhood. Chicago: University of Chicago Press, 1939.
29. Kleihues P, Cavanee WK. Pathology and Genetics of Tumours of the Nervous System. Lyon: IARC Press, 2000.
30. Cruveilhier J. L'Anatomie pathologique du Corps humain. Paris: J.B. Baillière, 1829.
31. Al-Rodhan NR, Laws ER. The history of intracranial meningiomas. In: Al-Mefty O, ed. Meningiomas. New York: Raven Press, 1991.
32. Acrel O. Chirurgiska Handelser. Stockholm: H. Fought, 1775.
33. Guidetti B, Giuffre R, Valente V. Italian contribution to the origin of neurosurgery. Surg Neurol. 1983;20:335–346.
34. Jennett B. Sir William Macewen 1848–1924. Pioneer Scottish neurosurgeon. Surg Neurol. 1976;6:57–60.
35. Macewen W. Intracranial lesions, illustrating some points in connection with the localization of cerebral affections and the advantages of antiseptic trephining (III. Tumor of the dura mater). Lancet. 1881;2:581–582.
36. Guidetti B. Francesco Durante. June 29, 1844 to October 2, 1934. Surg Neurol. 1983;20:1–3.
37. Weir B. The American centennial of brain tumor surgery. Neurosurgery. 1988;22:986–993.
38. Stone JL. W. W. Keen: America's pioneer neurological surgeon. Neurosurgery. 1985;17:997–1010.
39. Bingham WF. W. W. Keen and the dawn of American neurosurgery. J Neurosurg. 1986;64:705–712.
40. Horwitz NH. Library: historical perspective. Herbert Olivecrona (1891–1980). Neurosurgery. 1998;43:974–978.
41. Ljunggren B. The case of General Wood. J Neurosurg. 1982;56:471–474.

42. Weber J, Spring A, Czarnetzki A. [Parasagittal meningioma in a skull dated 32500 years before present from southwestern Germany]. Dtsch Med Wochenschr. 2002;127:2757–2760.

43. Moodie RL. Studies in paleopathology XVIII. Tumors of the head among pre-Columbian Peruvians. Ann Med Hist. 1926;8: 394–412.

44. MacCurdy GC. Human skeletal remains from the highlands of Peru. Am J Phys Anthropol. 1923;6:217–330.

45. Abbott KH, Courville CB. Historical notes on the meningiomas. I. A study of the hyperostoses in prehistoric skulls. Bull Los Angeles Neurol Soc. 1939;4:101–113.

46. Lambert R. Meningiomas in Pharaoh's people. Br J Surg. 1949;36:423–424.

47. Brothwell D. The evidence for neoplasms. In: Brothwell D, Sandison AT, eds. Diseases in Antiquity. Springfield, IL: Charles C Thomas, 1967:320–345.

2
Epidemiology

Bong Jin Park, Han Kyu Kim, Burak Sade, and Joung H. Lee

Introduction

Meningiomas constitute 13–25% of primary intracranial neoplasms.[1–3] In one population-based study, these tumors accounted for 40% of all primary intracranial neoplasms when tumors diagnosed incidentally at autopsy or by neuroimaging studies were included.[4] Symptomatic tumors were encountered in 2.0/100,000 of the population and the asymptomatic ones in 5.7/100,000, with an overall incidence of 7.7/100,000. Asymptomatic meningiomas can be found in about 1–2.3% of all autopsies.[5] However, the classical teaching of the past few decades, which may be erroneous, suggests the most common primary intracranial neoplasms are gliomas (50.3%), followed by meningiomas (20.9%), pituitary adenomas (15%) and nerve sheath tumors (8%).[6,7] Such discrepancy in these incidence rates underscores the fact that the majority of meningiomas actually remain asymptomatic and undetected during life.[8] With recent advances in neuroimaging, many asymptomatic meningiomas are being detected today, making the true incidence higher than those previously reported.[9] It has been shown that the incidence for meningiomas increased 3- to 3.9-fold in the post–computed tomography (CT) decade.[10,11]

Gender, Race, and Age

Meningiomas show a higher incidence among women as compared to men in most ethnic groups.[12,13] The male-to-female ratio ranges from 1:1.4 to 2.6.[14–16] In population-based studies, the mean annual crude incidence rates are reported to be 2–7/100,000 for women and 1–5/100,000 for men.[1,3]

In a population-based study performed in Los Angeles County, African Americans showed a higher incidence (3.1/100,000) than Caucasians (2.3/100,000).[12] In this study, Asians living in Los Angeles had the lowest rates. In Caucasians, women are approximately twice as likely to develop meningiomas than men, whereas in African American populations the incidence is evenly distributed between males and females.[1] Two studies have also shown a lower incidence of meningiomas in Asia as compared to western countries,[17,18] whereas Chi et al. reported no significant difference in the incidence of meningiomas in relation to other intracranial tumors, namely, 20.8% in Korea, 18.5% in Japan, and 16.6% in China.[19] Others have also observed no racial differences in incidence rates of meningiomas.[13]

The mean age at presentation is 56.4 years (range 10–85 years) in males and 55.9 years (range 26–86 years) in females, whereas in the subgroup of malignant and atypical meningiomas, the mean age shifts to 63.2 years (range 51–78 years) in males and 53.6 years (range 28–79 years) in females, a difference that is not statistically significant.[20] The incidence of meningiomas increases with age.[21] In patients older than 70 years, they have been reported as the most common brain tumors, with an incidence of 50.6%. This represents an almost 3.5 times higher incidence in this age group as compared to those under the age of 70, and it applies to both sexes.[4,22] The age-specific annual incidence rate increases in the eighth decade to 8.4/100,000.[16]

Histology and Location

The vast majority of meningiomas (92%) have a benign histology, whereas 8% show atypical or malignant features.[23] The most common histopathological subtype is the meningotheliomatous type (63%), followed by transitional (19%), fibrous (13%), and psammomatous (2%) meningiomas.[24] The majority of malignant meningiomas are located over the cerebral convexities. In approximately 73.3–75% of cases these tumors are located in the supratentorial compartment.[8] The ratio of calvarial to basal skull meningiomas was reported as 2.3:1.[25] Extracranial metastases from meningiomas have been considered to be one of the strong indicators of malignancy and have been shown to occur in 11–23% of patients with malignant meningiomas.[6]

The most common locations include parasagittal/falcine 25%, convexity 19%, sphenoid ridge 17%, followed by suprasellar 9%, posterior fossa 8%, olfactory groove 8%, middle fossa/Meckel's cave 4%, tentorial 3%, peri-torcular 3%, lateral ventricle 1–2%, foramen magnum 1–2%, and orbit/optic nerve sheath 1–2%.[10] Among the parasagittal meningiomas, 49% are located over the anterior one third of the falx, with 29% in the middle third, and 22% along the posterior third.[16] Medial sphenoid ridge meningiomas were more common than middle or lateral sphenoid ridge meningiomas. Multiple meningiomas or meningiomatosis is encountered in 2.5% of meningiomas The incidence of ectopic location is 0.4% with the vast majority (73%) occurring inside the orbit, paranasal sinuses, eyelids, parotid gland, temporalis muscle, temporal bone, and zygoma. Distant sites have also been reported, such as the lungs, mediastinum, and the adrenal glands.[6,26]

Recently, Lee et al. demonstrated an association between the histology of the tumor and its site of origin.[24] They showed a predominance of meningothelial meningiomas at the midline skull base and spinal locations. Based on this finding, as well as embryological and molecular features, they suggested that this particular subtype of meningiomas may indeed be unique, contrary to the traditional dogma that all benign meningiomas are identical or homogeneous tumors.

Meningiomas in Children

In children, meningiomas account for only 0.4–4.0% of primary intracranial neoplasms.[1,27–29] The age-adjusted annual incidence was reported to be 1.32/1,000,000.[30] There is a male predominance, with a male-to-female ratio of 1.2 to 1.9:1.[27,30]

The majority of meningiomas in the pediatric age group are located supratentorially (66%), whereas 19% occur in the posterior fossa and 17% present as intraventricular meningiomas.[30] They are usually seen in association with neurofibromatosis type 2 (NF-2) or following radiation therapy and show a significantly higher incidence of tumor calcification.[27,28] In NF-2, it has been estimated that 50% of all patients develop meningiomas, and 30% of these patients have multiple meningiomas.[6]

In children, additional unique features include the significantly increased incidence of atypical (36.4%) and malignant (27.2%) subtypes. In infants, meningiomas are extremely rare and show a higher frequency in males and favor convexity location. On the other hand, there is a smaller incidence of seizure, and dural attachment is less frequently seen on preoperative imaging.[1]

Spinal Meningiomas

In women, meningiomas are by far the most common primary spinal tumor, accounting for 58% of all spinal tumors, whereas in men they are third most common primary spinal tumor following gliomas and nerve sheath tumors.[31] Spinal meningiomas are reported to be more frequent in western countries (25–46%) as compared to Asian countries, for example, 14.1% in China and 8.6% in Thailand.[17,19,32] Thoracic spine is the most common site (55–57.1%).[17,19,32] The male-to-female ratio is 1:4 to 1:5.[33] In females, they are very common in the postmenopausal age group, with the majority (75–87%) occurring over the age of 40.[34,35]

The tumor is located completely intradurally in 83–90%, extradurally in 5–14%, and both intradurally and extradurally in 5% of the cases.[32,35] Extradural meningiomas are reported to be more common in children. In 50–68% of the cases, the tumor is located lateral to the spinal cord, in 18–31% posteriorly, and in 15–19% anteriorly.[32,35]

Histologically, 43.9–56.9% of spinal meningiomas show psammomatous subtype, whereas 28–29.9% are meningothelial, 8–19% transitional, 2.3–5% are fibrous, and 0.6% are malignant meningiomas.[32,35] The incidence of multiple spinal meningiomas is reported as 1–9%. In a recent review of our series, contrary to the above, meningothelial subtype was the most common (80%) in the spine.[24]

Radiation

In a population-based study, the incidence of meningiomas among Hiroshima atomic bomb survivors was 8.7/100,000.[36] When this population was stratified according to the hypocenter to the explosion, the incidence of meningiomas was much higher in patients who had been closer to the site of explosion. Similarly, the incidence of meningiomas was reported as 9.5/100,000 population in the group who had undergone low-dose radiation treatment as children for tinea capitis in Israel.[37]

In the medical or occupational setting, no significant associations were observed for diagnostic studies and increased meningioma incidence, but the use of radiation therapy to head and neck for neoplastic conditions has been shown to be associated with an increase in the incidence of meningiomas.[38]

Radiation-induced meningiomas differ significantly from primary intracranial meningiomas in that their incidence of calvarial location, multiplicity, recurrence rate following complete resection, and malignant histology are higher.[25]

Occupation

Association of increased risk of meningioma incidence has been suggested for various occupations in the literature. There is a huge diversity in the nature of proposed occupations such as dentists, teachers, managers, social workers, workers in the petroleum, rubber and plastics industry, auto body repairers, painters, chemists, carpenters, cooks, woodworkers, glassmakers, machine operators, as well as military workers, motor vehicle drivers, computer specialists, and so on.[12,39,40]

Rajamaran et al. have stated that it might be practical to analyze these occupations in two groups.[40] Groups like teachers, managers, etc., tend to be relatively better educated and would be expected to have a higher awareness of their health status, which would result in the increased detection of tumors in these groups, by earlier recognition of the symptoms, or by stronger willingness of the individual to seek medical care. On the other hand, exposure to some chemical agents or other environmental factors may be more influential in other groups. In this context, lead, tin, cadmium, benzene, and metal dusts and fumes have been suggested as possible contributors.[12,39–41]

Cell Phone Use

Over the years, there has been much debate about the potential role of cell phones as a causative factor in the development of brain tumors because of the microwaves emitted by these devices. In a recent population-based case-control study conducted on 366 glioma and 381 meningioma patients with 1494 controls, no association was found between cell phone use and increased meningioma incidence. However, in this study, increased incidence for glioma occurrence was detected in individuals who had used cell phones for more than 10 years.[42] A similar study in a relatively smaller scale also suggested a low risk for development of high-grade glioma for cell phone users, but the overall results did not show any association for either gliomas or meningiomas.[43] The study conducted by the Swedish Interphone Study Group also found no increase in incidence for gliomas or meningiomas located in the temporal or parietal lobes, regardless of tumor histology, phone type, or amount of phone use.[44]

References

1. Bondy M, Ligon BL. Epidemiology and etiology of intracranial meningiomas: A review. J Neurooncol 1996;29:197–205.
2. Claus EB, Bondy ML, Schildkraut JM, et al. Epidemiology of intracranial meningioma. Neurosurgery 2005;57:1088–95.
3. Longstreth WT Jr, Dennis LK, McGuire VM, et al. Epidemiology of intracranial meningioma. Cancer 1993;72:639–48.
4. Radhakrishnan K, Mokri B, Parisi JE, et al. The trends in incidence of primary brain tumors in the population of Rochester, Minnesota. Ann Neurol 1995;37:67–73.
5. Kurland LT, Schoenberg BS, Annegers JF, et al. The incidence of primary intracranial neoplasms in Rochester, Minnesota, 1935–1977. Ann NY Acad Sci 1982;381:6–16.
6. Evans JJ, Lee JH, Suh J, et al. Meningiomas. In: Newell DW, Moore AJ, ed. Neurosurgery: Principles and Practice. London: Springer-Verlag, 2004;205–32.
7. Hoffman SH, Propp JM, McCarthy BJ. Temporal trends in incidence of primary brain tumors in the United States, 1985–1999. Neurooncology 2006;8:27–37.
8. Elia-Pasquet S, Provost D, Jaffre A, et al. Incidence of central nervous system tumors in Gironde, France. Neuroepidemiology 2004;23:110–7.
9. Klaeboe L, Lonn S, Scheie D, et al. Incidence of intracranial meningiomas in Denmark, Finland, Norway and Sweden, 1986–1997. Int J Cancer 2005;20:996–1001.
10. Christensen HC, Kosteljanetz M, Johansen C. Incidence of gliomas and meningiomas in Denmark, 1943 to 1997. Neurosurgery 2003;52:1327–34.
11. Helseth A. The incidence of primary central nervous system neoplasms before and after computerized tomography availability. J Neurosurg 1995;83:999–1003.
12. Preston-Martin S. Descriptive epidemiology of primary tumors of the brain, cranial nerves and cranial meninges in Los Angeles County. Neuroepidemiology 1989;8:283–95.
13. Surawicz TS, McCarthy BJ, Kupelian V, et al. Descriptive epidemiology of primary brain and CNS tumors: results from the central brain tumor registry of the United States, 1990–1994. Neurooncology 1999;1:14–25.
14. Alessandro GD, Giovanni MD, Iannizzi L, et al. Epidemiology of primary intracranial tumors in the Valle d'Aosta (Italy) during the 6-year period 1986–1991. Neuroepidemiology 1995;14:139–46.
15. Lovaste MG, Ferrari G, Rossi G. Epidemiology of primary intracranial neoplasms: experiment in the Province of Trento (Italy), 1977–1984. Neuroepidemiology 1986;5:220–32.
16. Rohringer M, Sutherland GR, Louw DF, et al. Incidence and clinicopathological features of meningioma. J Neurosurg 1989;71:665–72.
17. Huang WQ, Zheng SJ, Tian QS, et al. Statistical analysis of central nervous system tumors in China. J Neurosurg 1982;56:555–64.
18. Ng HK, Poon WS, South JR, et al. Tumors of the central nervous system in Chinese in Hong Kong: a histological review. Aust NZ J Surg 1988;58:573–8.
19. Chi JG, Khang SK. Central nervous system tumors among Koreans. J Kor Med Sci 1989;4:77–90.
20. Das A, Tang WY, Smith DR. Meningiomas in Singapore: demographic and biological characteristics. J Neurooncol 2000;47:153–60.
21. Kuratsu JI, Ushio Y. Epidemiological study of primary intracranial tumors: a regional survey in Kumamoto prefecture in the southern part of Japan. J Neurosurg 1996;84:946–50.
22. Kuratsu J, Ushio Y. Epidemiological study of primary intracranial tumors in elderly people. J Neurol Neurosurg Psychiatry 1997;63:116–8.
23. Feun LG, Raub WA, Landy HJ, et al. Retrospective epidemiologic analysis of patients diagnosed with intracranial meningioma from 1977 to 1990 at the Jackson memorial hospital, Sylvester comprehensive cancer center: the Jackson memorial hospital tumor registry experience. Cancer Detect Prev 1996;20:166–70.
24. Lee JH, Sade B, Choi E, et al. Midline skull base and spinal meningiomas are predominantly of the meningothelial histological subtype. J Neurosurg 2006:105:60–64.
25. Sadamori N, Shibata S, Mine M, et al. Incidence of intracranial meningiomas in Nagasaki atomic-bomb survivors. Int J Cancer 1996;67:318–22.
26. Staneczek W, Janisch W. Epidemiological data on meningiomas in East Germany 1961–1986: incidence, localization, age and sex distribution. Clin Neuropathol 1992;11:135–41.
27. Baumgartner JE, Sorenson JM. Meningioma in the pediatric population. J Neurooncol 1996;29:223–8.
28. Merten DF, Gooding CA, Newton TH, et al. Meningiomas of childhood and adolescence. J Pediatrics 1974;84:696–700.
29. Schoenberg BS, Schoenberg DG, Christine BW, et al. The epidemiology of primary intracranial neoplasms of childhood: a population study. Mayo Clin Proc 1976;51:51–6.
30. Kuratsu J, Ushio Y. Epidemiological study of primary intracranial tumors in childhood: a population-based survey in Kumamoto prefecture, Japan. Pediatr Neurosurg 1996;25:240–7.

31. Preston-Martin S. Descriptive epidemiology of primary tumors of the spinal cord and spinal meninges in Los Angeles County, 1972–1985. Neuroepidemiology 1990;9:106–11.
32. Cohen-Gadol AA, Zikel OM, Koch CA, et al. Spinal meningiomas in patients younger than 50 years of age: a 21-year experience. J Neurosurg (Spine 3) 2003;98:258–63.
33. Levy WJ Jr, Bay J, Dohn D. Spinal cord meningioma. J Neurosurg 1982;57:804–12.
34. Helseth A, Mork SJ. Primary intraspinal neoplasms in Norway, 1955 to 1986: a population-based suevey of 467 patients. J Neurosurg 1989;71:842–5.
35. Solero CL, Fornari M, Giombini S, et al. Spinal meningiomas: review of 174 operated cases. Neurosurgery 1989;25:153–60.
36. Shintani T, Hayakawa N, Hoshi M, et al. High incidence of meningioma among Hiroshima atomic bomb survivors. J Radiat Res 1999;40:49–57.
37. Ron E, Modan B, Boice JD, et al. Tumors of the brain and nerve system after radiotherapy in childhood. N Engl J Med 1988;319:1033–9.
38. Phillips LE, Frankenfeld CL, Drangsholt M, et al. Intracranial meningioma and ionizing radiation in medical and occupational settings. Neurology 2005;64:350–2.
39. Navas-Acien A, Pollan M, Gustavsson P, et al. Occupation, exposure to chemicals and risk of gliomas and meningiomas in Sweden. Am J Ind Med 2002;42:214–27.
40. Rajaraman P, De Roos AJ, Stewart PA, et al. Occupation and risk of meningioma and acoustic neuroma in the United States. Am J Ind Med 2004;45:395–407.
41. Hu J, Little J, Xu T, et al. Risk factors for meningioma in adults: a case-control study in northeast China. Int J Cancer 1999;83:299–304.
42. Schuz J, Bohler E, Berg G, et al. Cellular phones, cordless phones and the risks of glioma and meningioma (Interphone Study Group, Germany). Am J Epidemiol 2006;163:512–20.
43. Christensen HC, Schuz J, Kosteljanetz M. et al. Cellular telephones and risk for brain tumors: a population based, incident case-control study. Neurology 2005;64:1189–95.
44. Lonn S, Ahlbom A, Hall P, et al. Long-term mobile phone use and brain tumor risk. Am J Epidemiol 2005;161:526–35.

3

Human Meninges: Anatomy and Its Role in Meningioma Pathogenesis

Tetsumori Yamashima

Introduction

In this chapter the functional anatomy of human meninges is described, with particular attention paid to the pathological aspects. The meninges, the intricate and complex coverings of the brain and spinal cord, are basically comprised of three distinct yet closely associated layers: dura mater, arachnoid, and pia mater. Dura mater is thick, while the arachnoid is thin, and the subarachnoid space is of varying thickness. Dura mater is comprised of periosteal dura, meningeal dura, and dural border layer. The arachnoid is comprised of an arachnoid barrier layer and arachnoid trabeculae. For the thorough understanding of the meninges and related structures, not only gross but also light and electron microscopic observations and molecular analyses are indispensable. However, from postmortem analyses it is not possible to determine in situ features of the meninges in the living individual.

Meninges are essentially composed of a series of fibroblasts and/or arachnoid cells, as well as varying amounts of extracellular materials, fibers, and fluid-filled cisterns. Usually considered as a simple protective covering, the meninges are closely related to both physiology and pathology of the central nervous system. Dura mater is a rigid but simple covering of the brain as an internal covering of calvaria. Dura mater forms venous sinuses that drain not only blood but also the cerebrospinal fluid (CSF).

The dural border layer, containing electron-dense cytoplasm, is further characterized by the following: (1) extracellular cisterns containing fuzzy amorphous material, but devoid of connective tissue fibers, (2) a relatively modest number of cell junctions, and (3) an absence of tight junctions. These three factors explain the fragile nature of this layer. Contrary to widespread assertions, the subdural space is not a true but a potential space, since the creation of a large cleft within the innermost dural border layer is the result of artificial or pathological tissue tearing. The subarachnoid space is a real space for the CSF pathway and/or absorption, while the subpial and Virchow-Robin spaces might be potential ones that appear in the pathological conditions or in a postmortem state.

The term arachnoid was designated because the arachnoid trabeculae are present as delicate thin pillars, forming three-dimensional spindly trabeculae resembling a spider web. The arachnoid is always affected by the pulsation of the CSF. The arachnoid, although devoid of vasculature, maintains mechanically strong, flexible, and functional structures, having three distinct roles: (1) a covering of the pulsatile brain, (2) a pathway of the CSF circulation, and (3) an anatomical structure for its absorption. For these purposes, arachnoid cells form numerous morphologically distinct cell junctions, intense cell–cell communications, pinocytotic activity, extracellular cisterns, and specialized segments such as arachnoid villi (granulations). Throughout the meninges, tight junctions are unique to cells of arachnoid barrier layer. The role of the arachnoid barrier layer, separating the subarachnoid space from dura mater, is obscure at present, and whether it contributes to the CSF/blood barrier or, on the contrary, to CSF absorption is unknown.

Meningiomas actually derive from two types of cell related to arachnoid villi: arachnoid cells and dural border cells. The syncytial meningioma is similar to the cap cell cluster, while the fibroblastic meningioma is similar to the fibrous capsule of arachnoid villi. In this chapter we postulate a possible role of the arachnoid villi in meningioma development by highlighting roles of E-cadherin and prostaglandin D synthase (ß-trace). Human arachnoid cells synthesize and secrete this enzyme into the subarachnoid space. With the aid of tannic acid mixed with conventional ultrastructural fixatives, extramembranous multilamellar bodies (presumably certain phenotypes of phospholipids) are seen among and within arachnoid or meningioma cells.

Meningioma tumorigenesis is discussed with particular attention paid to the interactions of two key proteins: calpain and merlin. Either the deletion of the N-terminal domain of merlin due to *NF2* gene mutation or merlin cleavage by activated calpain due to the oxidative stress may induce a transfer of merlin from the plasma membrane to the nucleus. The resultant impairment of signal transduction from the membrane to the nucleus might block the signal pathway necessary for cell adhesion and contact inhibition, which leads to the inactive proliferation of meningioma cells. Dural border cells and arachnoid barrier cells show a marked contrast in cell shape and density, junctions, and extracellular material, all of which are presumably reflected by the histological variation of meningiomas. E-cadherin, merlin, and catenin molecules which the author's group identified in arachnoid and meningioma cells may be closely related to the flexible cell adhesion and CSF absorption in arachnoid villi. Further, functional impairment of these molecules with the aid of genetic disorders or calpain activation in arachnoid cells might lead to the occurrence of meningiomas via an impaired intracellular signal transduction.

Dura Mater

Dura mater is the outermost thick layer of the meninges, also called pachymeninx because of its thickness, while the two inner layers—arachnoid and pia mater, which are thin—are collectively called leptomenix. As dyes injected into the blood or bilirubin pigments during icterus stain dura mater but not arachnoid, arachnoid rather than dura mater is actually a barrier between the circulating blood in dural vessels and the CSF in the subarachnoid space. Dura mater is mainly composed of greater and lesser laminae, which are formed mainly of collagen fibers aligned differently. The outer portion is actually a periosteum, while the inner portion is a reinforcing membrane of arachnoid. Although the cranial dura is directly attached to the inner surface of the calvaria, the spinal dura is separated from the vertebrae by the epidural fat tissue. A small number of elongated, flattened fibrocytes are intermingled with large amounts of extracellular collagen fibrils. These dural cells generally have long, finely branched processes showing few mutual contacts. Although fibrocytes of the dura rarely have cell junctions, the interlacing of closely packed collagen fibrils gives the dura mater great strength.

When compared with the external main portions of the dura or arachnoid barrier layer, the innermost part of dura mater, the dural border layer, is structurally fragile and ultrastructurally appears to be quite electron dense. Not only the nucleus but also the cytoplasm and organelles are dark, showing a remarkable contrast with the underlying, translucent arachnoid barrier layer. The dural border layer is characterized by flattened cells with slender processes and extracellular spaces containing a fuzzy amorphous material [1–3]. This material is distinct from collagen and elastic fibers or microfibrils, being a peculiar feature of the human meninges. The dural border layer is attached to the underlying arachnoid barrier layer by occasional cell junctions. Dural border cells are connected not by tight junctions but by desmosomes, intermediate junctions, and gap junctions. The number of these cell junctions is much less than that of arachnoid barrier layer. Namely, arachnoid barrier cells are connected by extensive cell junctions includ-

ing tight junctions, which actually constitute the blood–CSF barrier mentioned above.

At the point where such dural reflections as the falx cerebri or the tentorium cerebelli originate, one can find numerous arachnoid villi along or within the venous sinus, from which most meningiomas originate. Dura of the anterior and middle cranial fossae are innervated by sensory branches arising from the trigeminal nerve, while that of the posterior fossa is innervated by sensory branches from C1–C3 cervical nerves [4].

Arachnoid

Arachnoid is a thin delicate translucent or whitish membrane, being attached to the inner portion of dura mater. An outer part of the arachnoid is the arachnoid barrier layer, comprised of closely packed cells as an actual covering membrane, while an inner part is the arachnoid trabeculae steeped in the CSF of the subarachnoid space to support the arachnoid barrier layer. Arachnoid barrier cells have a large, polygonal, and electronlucent cytoplasm with an oval nucleus, showing a marked contrast to the long and flattened dural border cells. Under the operating microscope, neurosurgeons can see two distinct portions of the arachnoid (arachnoid barrier layer): a whitish portion is thick, consisting of a cap cell cluster, while a translucent portion is thin, consisting of tiers of flattened arachnoid cells. In cap cell clusters, the cytoplasmic processes are compactly arranged, showing interdigitations, and there are very narrow intercellular spaces.

The arachnoid barrier layer is composed of larger cells with numerous cell junctions, and the presence of many tight junctions serves as a barrier to the CSF. Arachnoid barrier cells are closely apposed to each other and joined by numerous cell junctions with very narrow extracellular space. Arachnoid trabecular cells cross the subarachnoid space in a random manner, being reinforced by extracellular collagen and surrounded by phagocytes. Arachnoid trabecular cells attach to both pia mater and the inner surface of arachnoid barrier layer, and the subarachnoid space is actually bordered by these two structures.

Since arachnoid is actually a brain covering that exists between the rigid calvarium and the pulsatile brain surface, special adhesiveness among arachnoid cells is indispensable to maintain mechanically strong but flexible structures. In this sense, for maintaining strong adhesion, arachnoid cells show widespread membrane specializations, including numerous desmosomes as well as junctional devices such as gap junctions, tight junctions, intermediate junctions, hemidesmosomes, and hemidesmosome-like structures [4,5]. Further, for maintaining flexible adhesion, Ca^{2+}-dependent epithelial cell adhesion molecules designated E-cadherin are localized to the opposing plasma membranes of arachnoid cells, being concentrated at the intermediate junctions.

The vimentin-type intermediate filaments attach to the desmosomal plaques. Gap junctions contribute not only to the intercellular adhesion, but also to the intercellular ionic and molecular transfer for the cell–cell communication. Because the arachnoid lacks vascularization, there should be rich intercellular circulation of certain metabolites and ions through gap junctions. Because of the presence of the large extracellular cisterns, the distribution of the tight junction meshwork is patchy, showing a random distribution compared to the epidermal tissue. Tight junctions seal off the intercellular space and prevent the diffusion of macromolecules from dura mater to the subarachnoid space (blood–CSF barrier). Numerous desmosomes are often surrounded by tight junction strands. Hemidesmosome-like structures are developed especially along the extracellular cisterns. Abundant micropinocytotic vesicles are observed in the arachnoid cell membrane along the larger extracellular cisterns. These micropinocytotic vesicles conceivably contribute to the absorption of certain nutrients, secretion of certain enzymes and growth factors, as well as active transport of some metabolites and CSF [5].

Meningioma cells are thought to be derived from arachnoid cells, since these tumor cells exhibit an almost identical ultrastructures to arachnoid cells, including desmosomes, tight junctions, cistern-like extracellular spaces, and abundant micropinocytotic vesicles.

Pia Mater

Pia mater is a layer of cells with long, flattened processes forming the innermost part of the meninges. Pial cells show similarities with arachnoid trabecular cells and have close contact with their attenuated processes. They are composed of a smooth-surfaced, thin layer of cells joined by desmosomes and gap junctions, but no tight junctions are observed. Natural circular, elliptical, and ovoid perforations are distributed irregularly at the surface of pia mater [6]. It separates the subarachnoid space from the brain, being reflected from arteries and veins onto the surface of the brain [7]. Pia mater forms a continuous sheet that separates the subarachnoid space from the subpial space, the bottom of which is glia limitans of the cerebral cortex. The subpial space should be a physiologically negligible space, because pia mater is closely attached to the basement membrane of the glia limitans on the surface of the cerebral cortex.

For many years it has been generally accepted that the subarachnoid space communicates directly with the perivascular space, called the Virchow-Robin space, between blood vessel and nervous tissue as vessels enter or leave the surface of the cerebral cortex. But Hutchings and Weller [8] found that neither the pia mater nor the subarachnoid space extends into the brain beside blood vessels. The perivascular spaces are in continuity with the subpial space, but both of these spaces are separated from the subarachnoid space by an intact layer of pia mater. In subarachnoid hemorrhage, erythrocytes cannot enter the perivascular space from the subarachnoid space, whereas in purulent leptomeningitis inflammatory

cells readily penetrate the pia mater. This suggests that pia mater is an effective barrier to the passage of particulate matter by its intercellular junctions. If a differential permeability does exist whereby different substances cross the pial barrier at different rates, it may have important implications for therapeutic intrathecal injections [8].

Subdural Space (Dura/Arachnoid Interface)

The so-called subdural space was traditionally believed to be located between dura and arachnoid as a fluid-filled potential cavity existing in an extracellular compartment. Then subdural hematomas or hygromas were thought to be the result of blood or fluid accumulation in the preexisting space. Under physiological conditions, however, there is no evidence of naturally occurring space being extant at the dura/arachnoid interface (Fig. 3-1). Actually, the subdural space is not formed at the border between the dural border layer and the arachnoid barrier layer. Instead, this space occurs within the structurally weakest plane of dura mater, the dural border layer, subsequent to various pathological, traumatic, or mechanical events or processes [1–4].

Schachenmayr and Friede [2] showed that instead of a true subdural space, there is a complex, tight layer of cells: the dura/arachnoid interface layer. This layer is characterized by (1) absence of collagenous reinforcement, (2) presence of

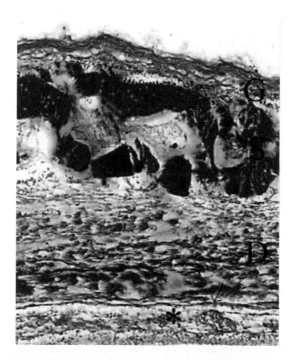

FIG. 3-1. The dura/arachnoid interface in an early infant histologically shows absence of the so-called subdural space. A membranous covering structure consists of galea (G), ossifying skull (S), dura mater (D), arachnoid barrier layer (arrow), subarachnoid space (asterisk) cotaining vessels, and the subpial granular layer underlying the pia mater. Elastica-van Gieson staining

wide extracellular cisterns between dural border cells, and (3) paucity of intercellular contacts. The erroneous macroscopic impression of subdural space results from an extraordinary lack of cohesion. Within a sheet of torn dural border cells, the extracellular space in the dural border layer is enlarged, and cell junctions are separated to form an artificial space. Actually, the "subdural" space occurs within the dura mater (dural border layer), and therefore, the correct term for this space should be the "intradural" space.

An ultrastructural study of outer and inner membranes of chronic subdural hematomas reveals dural border cells in both membranes [9]. An extravasation of blood within dural border layer splits this layer and leaves a few tiers of dural border cells surrounding the hematoma. These cells cover both outer and inner surfaces of the hematoma, proliferate, and, later on, form outer and inner membranes of chronic subdural hematomas.

Subarachnoid Space and CSF

Underneath the arachnoid barrier layer, the arachnoid trabeculae are present as delicate thin pillars, forming a three-dimensional spider web pattern. The arachnoid trabeculae consist of thin cytoplasmic processes of fibroblast being held together by desmosomes and surrounded by bundles of collagen fibrils. Arachnoid trabecular cells attach to the inner surface of arachnoid barrier layer, subarachnoid vessels and pia mater by desmosomes, gap junctions, and some intermediate junctions. The subarachnoid space is located between arachnoid barrier layer and pia mater and is traversed by these trabeculae in a random manner and filled with CSF. A continuous basement membrane covers the inner aspect of arachnoid barrier layer as a roof of the subarachnoid space, while it covers the outer aspect of pia mater as a floor. Blood vessels traverse the subarachnoid space on their way to the brain and spinal cord by penetrating pia mater. The subarachnoid space contains collagen fibrils as well as occasional macrophages, lymphocytes, and mast cells.

Although the subarachnoid space is critically involved in the normal physiology of the CSF circulation as well as in various pathological states such as hydrocephalus, meningitis, subarachnoid hemorrhage, and meningeal dissemination, much remains unknown about this space. The CSF is secreted by the choroid plexuses, flows through the ventricles and the subarachnoid space, and is finally absorbed by arachnoid villi (Figs. 3-2 and 3-3) [10,11]. Spaces where the subarachnoid space is enlarged are called subarachnoid cisterns [4]. For the clinician, dynamic aspects of CSF secretion, flow, and absorption are essential factors with practical consequences in terms of diseases and patient management. The bulk flow of CSF has implications for cell–cell communication by volume transmission, for delivery, distribution, and clearance of nutrient or drug, for the clearance of brain metabolites and β-amyloid deposits, as well as for the migration of neural stem cells and malignant cells.

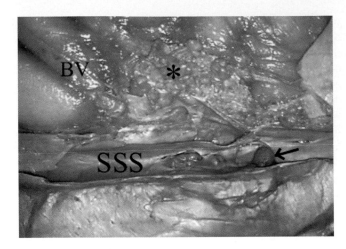

FIG. 3-2. Macroscopic view of the superior sagittal sinus (SSS) containing arachnoid granulations (arrow) and the lateral lacuna (asterisk) containing numerous arachnoid villi. BV, bridging vein

Normal CSF contains approximately 100 proteins, and 1000–3000 leukocytes per milliliter; however, little is known about their function. The cellular composition of CSF, characterized by a predominance of lymphocytes, mononuclear phagocytes, or polymorphonuclear neutrophils, is not a simple reflection of peripheral blood. This suggests a stringently regulated control over cell migration into the subarachnoid space. Multicolor flow cytometry analysis [12] shows that CSF cells predominantly consist of CD4+/CD45RA−/CD27+/CD69+-activated central memory T cells expressing high levels of CCR7 and L-selectin. It is likely that activated memory T cells enter the CSF directly from the systemic circulation to monitor the subarachnoid space.

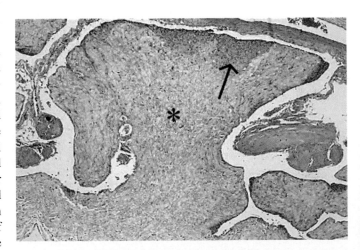

FIG. 3-3. Histological view of an arachnoid villus. The core space (asterisk), being surrounded by the arachnoid cell layer and cap cell clusters (arrow), is in continuity with the cranial subarachnoid space. Hematoxylin-eosin staining

Arachnoid Villi (Granulations)

Arachnoid granulation is a large version of arachnoid villi: arachnoid granulations are small in number and directly protrude into the inner table of the skull by penetrating dura mater (also called Pacchionian granulations) or into the major venous sinus lumen, while arachnoid villi are numerous and mainly protrude into the lateral lacunae of the superior sagittal sinus. In any case, arachnoid villi or granulations are projections of arachnoid barrier layer into the venous sinus and/or its major tributaries (Figs. 3-2 and 3-3). They are closely related not only to the absorption of CSF but also to the occurrence of meningiomas. Especially along the middle third of the superior sagittal sinus, one can find "Pacchionian (arachnoid) granulations" (Fig. 3-2), first described in 1705 by the Italian scientist Antonio Pacchioni. Among his publications, an article entitled "Dissertatio Epistolaris de Glandulis Conglobatis Durae Meningis Humanae" deserves the greatest consideration as the first description of arachnoid granulations [13]. However, it was not until three centuries after Pacchioni's report that the detailed structure of human arachnoid villi was clarified with the aid of electron microscopy [10]. Many questions related to the mechanisms underlying CSF absorption in humans still remain unanswered because of the remarkable differences in the structure of arachnoid villi between humans and experimental animals.

Human arachnoid villi basically consist of four portions: fibrous capsule, arachnoid cell layer, cap cell cluster, and central core (Fig. 3-3). Arachnoid cell layer encompassing the central core is mostly covered by a thin fibrous capsule with an endothelial investment being reflected from the venous sinus lumen. These endothelial cells have numerous micropinocytotic vesicles, microvilli, and some large vacuoles and are joined by desmosomes and tight junctions. The fibrous capsule is composed of connective tissue fibers and reinforced by a layer of electron-dense flattened cells with long processes similar to dural border cells of the neighboring dura. The fibrous capsule is often very thin or negligible, especially at the apical portion of the villus. The arachnoid cell layer abuts directly upon the lumen of lateral lacuna or the sinus. The arachnoid cell layer is found inside the fibrous capsule and is continuous with the arachnoid barrier layer of the neighboring dura. The arachnoid cell layer ultrastructurally consists of outer and inner zones and is thickened in places to form cap cell clusters as a specialized segment. These cap cell clusters are closely packed, polygonal in shape, and show many short interdigitations. Frequently, the center of cap cell clusters shows psammoma body formation, and abundant matrix substances are seen in its vicinity. The cap cells have oval nuclei with peripheral chromatin, and the translucent cytoplasm contains many mitochondria and endoplasmic reticulum. The central core is a drainage route of the CSF and contains an irregular meshwork of arachnoid cells, being intermingled with collagen fibers, and is in continuity with the cranial subarachnoid space (Fig. 3-3) [4,5,10,14]. In the case of severe subarachnoid hemorrhage, the central core and the extracellular cisterns of arachnoid cells are packed with red blood cells to obliterate the CSF pathway.

Arachnoid cells within arachnoid villi (granulations) show widespread membrane specialization such as desmosomes, gap junctions, tight junctions, intermediate junctions, and hemidesmosome-like junctions [4,10,15]. Numerous extracellular cisterns are separated by cytoplasmic bodies or slender processes being joined by junctional complexes. Numerous uncoated and coated vesicles are seen along the surface of extracellular cisterns. Micropinocytotic vesicles are often concentrated in the arachnoid cell cluster up to 40 per μm^2, which is equivalent to their concentration in the brain capillary endothelial cells [5].

On magnetic resonance imaging (MRI), arachnoid granulations are isointense or slightly hyperintense relative to CSF on FLAIR images, which are helpful in differentiating arachnoid granulations from other dural sinus lesions or skull lesions [16]. In autopsy brains after subarachnoid hemorrhage, blood and aseptic inflammatory products are prominent within the arachnoid villi (granulations) during the first week after onset. An abundant mitotic activity is present among cap cluster cells. Further, in the chronic stage, arachnoid cap cell accumulation is seen. Accordingly, Massicotte and Del Bigio [17] postulated that proliferation of arachnoid cells, triggered by the inflammatory reaction or blood clotting products, as well as generalized fibrosis in the subarachnoid space may result in obstruction of the CSF pathway through arachnoid villi.

Expression of E-Cadherin

Ca^{2+}-dependent cell adhesion molecules designated as cadherin are known to play an essential role in embryonic development and morphogenesis. Epithelial (E)-cadherin is detected in almost all epithelial tissues and cancer cells and also in both arachnoid villi (Fig. 3-4) and meningiomas (Fig. 3-5) [14,15].

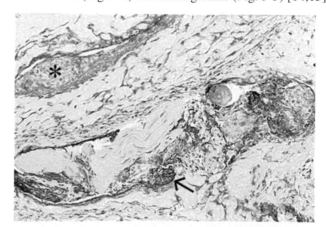

FIG. 3-4. Immunohistochemical staining for E-cadherin in human arachnoid villi, showing intense immunoreactivity in the arachnoid barrier cells (arrow) compared to the cap cell clusters (asterisk). Counterstained with hematoxylin

Because arachnoid cells are known to be pluripotential cells exhibiting both epithelial and mesenchymal properties, it is plausible that arachnoid cells express E-cadherin. Using a monoclonal antibody HECD-1, E-cadherin was identified at the main band of 124 kDa by the immunoblot analysis [18]. By immunocytochemical analysis, it was detected at the cell boundaries (Fig. 3-5) and/or within the cytoplasm (Fig. 3-4). In arachnoid villi (granulations), the expression was usually weak in cap cell cluster, but intense in arachnoid cell layer (Fig. 3-4). E-cadherin is not expressed in the fibrous capsule. Immunoelectron microscopy showed that E-cadherin is localized to the opposing plasma membranes and/or the narrow extracellular cisterns, being concentrated at the intermediate junctions. E-cadherin conceivably plays an important role in the flexible adhesion of arachnoid cells even in the presence of the CSF.

The expression pattern of E-cadherin is quite different between arachnoid villi and meningiomas, as well as among the three histological basic subtypes (syncytial, fibroblastic, and transitional) of meningiomas. E-cadherin was concentrated predominantly at the intermediate junctions in arachnoid villi, while in meningiomas it was diffusely expressed at the cell surface, including the intermediate junctions [14]. It is probable that the concentration of E-cadherin at the cell surface in arachnoid cells might provide stable maintenance of the structure of arachnoid villi; in contrast, the diffuse distribution of E-cadherin in meningiomas might contribute to the labile cell–cell adhesion and the establishment of new contacts [14].

In meningiomas, E-cadherin is expressed in the syncytial and transitional types, but not in the fibroblastic type: it was intensely expressed in the syncytial type, but heterogeneously expressed in the transitional type. Ultrastructurally, both arachnoid and meningioma cells are characterized by interdigitations being connected mechanically by junctional complexes and functionally by E-cadherins. The latter are preferentially localized at the intermediate junctions, which are associated with actin bundles [14]. Membrane–cytoskeleton interactions by means of E-cadherin, merlin, and catenin molecules are thought to be crucial in signal transduction for the contact inhibition of cell growth in normal arachnoid cells. Functional impairment of these molecules in arachnoid villi (granulations) conceivably leads to the occurrence of meningiomas [18].

Expression of PGDS

Glutathione-independent prostaglandin D_2 synthase (PGDS) [EC 5.3.99.2], previously known as β-trace, is the second most abundant protein in the CSF [19–22]. PGDS or β-trace is an enzyme responsible for the biosynthesis of prostaglandin D_2 in the central nervous system and is consistently expressed in both arachnoid and meningioma cells. The immunolocalization of PGDS in the meninges is distinct from portion to portion. In arachnoid, PGDS is mainly expressed in arachnoid barrier cells lining the CSF space rather than arachnoid trabecular cells being steeped in the subarachnoid space (Fig. 3-6). On the contrary, in arachnoid villi it is mainly expressed in the core arachnoid cells within the CSF rather than in cap cell cluster or arachnoid cell layer being reflected from arachnoid barrier layer.

PGDS belongs to the gene superfamily of lipocalins [23], which are transport proteins capable of carrying small lipophilic molecules [21]. PGDS binds retinoids with affinities comparable to other retinoid-transporter proteins in vitro. It is likely that PGDS has a dual function as an enzyme as well as a transporter protein [24]. Prostaglandin D_2 itself is conceivably attached to the enzyme necessary for its synthesis, transferred with the circulating CSF, and then taken up by neurons or glial cells, where it might elicit a function. As the amount of PGDS in the CSF is remarkably increased after subarachnoid hemorrhage, PGDS might be related to the washout of blood breakdown products such as hemoglobin or bilirubin.

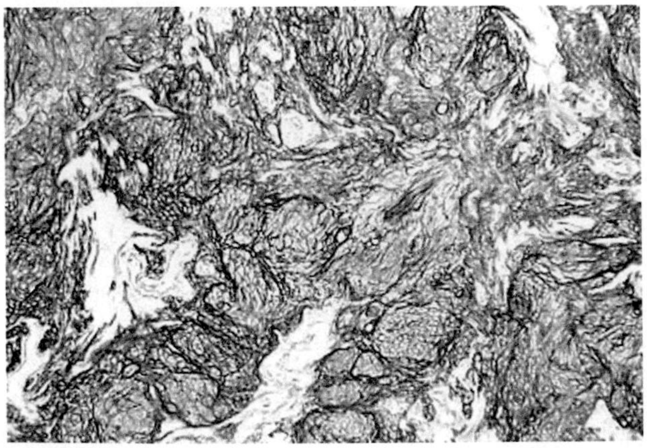

FIG. 3-5. Immunohistochemical staining for E-cadherin in meningioma showing intense immunoreactivity at the cell boundaries

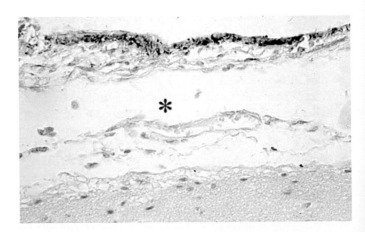

FIG. 3-6. Immunohistochemical staining for PGDS in human arachnoid, showing intense immunoreactivity in the arachnoid barrier cells overlying the subarachnoid space (asterisk). Counterstained with hematoxylin

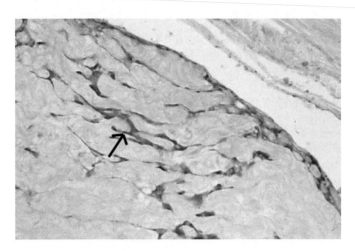

FIG. 3-7. Immunohistochemical staining for PGDS in meningioma of the syncytial type, showing intense immunoreactivity within a syncytium. Note remarkable immunorecativity in certain meningioma cells (arrow). Counterstained with hematoxylin

The roles of PGDS in meningioma cells are unclear at present, but their further characterization might allow a better understanding of these tumors [11]. Although the extent of PGDS protein expression and immunoreactivity (Fig. 3-7) varies from case to case, the PGDS gene is found in all histological subtypes of meningiomas, regardless of benign or malignant character. Meningioma cells show intense immunoreactivity in the perinuclear region, especially at the rough endoplasmic reticulum. Interestingly, the PGDS immunoreactivity in meningiomas is often concentrated within meningocytic whorls containing calcification deposits or at the active calcification/ossification sites around psammoma bodies (Fig. 3-8). Accordingly, it is probable that PGDS and the resultant PGD2 may have some relation to the calcification/ossification processes.

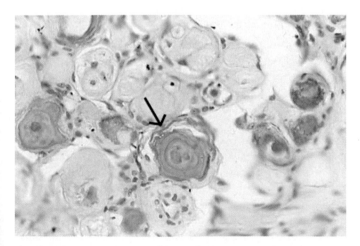

FIG. 3-8. Immunohistochemical staining for PGDS in psammomatous meningioma, showing intense immunoreactivity in the outer aspects of psammoma bodies (arrow). Counterstained with hematoxylin

Not only PGDS but also glutathione-S-transferase are reported to catalyze the conversion of PGH2 to PGD2 [25]. Hara et al. [26] immunohistochemically identified glutathione-S-transferase of the placental type in meningiomas. Accordingly, both PGDS and glutathione-S-transferase can catalyze the reaction to produce PGD2 in meningiomas. PGD2 may play an important role in the growth and differentiation of meningiomas. Because meningioma cells exclusively show abundant PGDS expression, whereas other brain tumors such as malignant astrocytomas, oligodendrogliomas, acoustic schwannomas, ependymomas, pituitary adenomas, craniopharyngiomas, hemangioblastomas, and choroids plexus papillomas show negligible expression, PGDS can be considered a specific cell marker of meningiomas [11].

To clarify the function of PGDS in both arachnoid and meningioma cells, lipophilic candidates as a ligand for this transport enzyme should be determined. The outcome of possible candidates should be studied further, with particular attention paid to the function of arachnoid cells or arachnoid villi, differentiation of meningioma cells, and participation in the calcification or ossification processes. As PGDS and the resultant PGD$_2$ have some relation to the calcification/ossification processes, it is probable that PGDS being secreted from the arachnoid or the tumor is related to the formation and metabolism of the skull [11].

Multilamellar Phospholipids

Cellular and intracellular interfaces are known to contain appreciable quantities of phospholipids that can be microscopically confirmed by Sudan III staining after fixation with potassium dichromate. Chromatographic analyses of meningiomas disclosed the presence of various phospholipids including phosphatidyl ethanolamine, phosphatidyl choline, phosphatidyl serine, sphingomyelin, and phosphatidyl inositol [27]. The ultrastructural fixative glutaraldehyde interacts with phospholipids such as phosphatidyl serine and phosphatidyl ethanolamine by cross-linking at the primary amines in the polar head group. Phosphatidyl choline accounts for over 50% of the total phospholipids present in the membranes of most animal tissues. As the polar heads of phosphatidyl choline lack primary amines, they are unable to react directly with either glutaraldehyde or osmium tetroxide. Then, the main membranous phospholipids may be dissolved through ethanol or acetone dehydration after conventional fixation. Tannic acid interacts with the choline component of phosphatidyl choline or sphingomyelin to form a complex that can be subsequently stabilized by osmium tetroxide.

The conventional ultrastructural fixation with glutaraldehyde and osmium tetroxide fails to retain much of the extramembranous phospholipids. However, both arachnoid and meningioma cells adequately treated with ~0.1% tannic acid

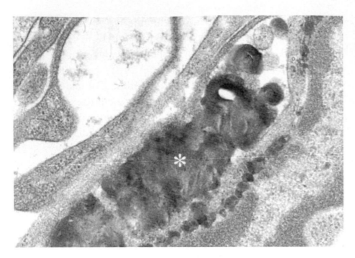

FIG. 3-9. The intercellular space of arachnoid cells in an arachnoid villus contains numerous fingerprint-like multilamellar bodies (asterisk). Ultrastructural fixation by glutaraldehyde mixed with 0.1% tannic acid, before osmication

mixed with 2.5% glutaraldehyde before osmication can retain phospholipids and ultrastructurally disclose highly ordered multilamellar bodies (Figs. 3-9 and 3-10), which could not be observed by the conventional fixation procedure. These multilamellar bodies vary considerably in size and shape, but often show fingerprint-like appearance.

Multilamellar bodies are found in the intercellular space, extracellular cisterns, or within the cytoplasm of arachnoid cells (Fig. 3-9). The number of lamellae in a single lamellar body range from 3 to 20, and the periodical width of the lamellae is approximately 5.0 nm. The outermost lamella sometimes shows a direct continuity with the adjacent plasma membranes

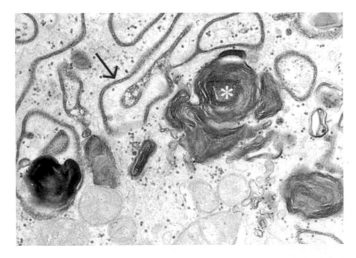

FIG. 3-10. The meningioma cells contain numerous fingerprint-like multilamellar bodies (asterisk) in the cytoplasm, while the intermembranous space appears to be electron-dense (arrow) in spite of no ultrastructural staining. Ultrastructural fixation by glutaraldehyde mixed with 0.1% tannic acid, before osmication

of the cytoplasm or mitochondria. As multilamellar bodies ultrastructurally appear to be quite similar to the pulmonary surfactant, they are assumed to be related to the lubricated flow or absorption of the CSF. Meningioma cells treated with tannic acid also retain phospholipids [27]. They are similarly observed as multilamellar bodies within the cytoplasm, among the plasma membranes, and in the extracellular matrices (Fig. 3-10). It is widely accepted that phospholipids are crucial for calcification at sites of primary mineralization. Precipitation of hydroxyapatite crystals was frequently seen within and outside the multilamellar bodies in both arachnoid villi and meningiomas.

Tumorigenesis: Calpain-Dependent Merlin Proteolysis

Neurofibromatosis type 2 (NF2) is an inherited autosomal dominant disorder affecting approximately 1:40,000 individuals. NF2 is characterized by the development of bilateral vestibular schwannomas as well as multiple meningiomas. The *NF2* gene is identified on chromosome 22q12 and encodes a protein of 595 amino acids, which is called merlin (moesin-ezrin-radixin like protein) [18]. Its sequence is similar to that of the band 4.1 superfamily of proteins, especially ezrin, radixin, and moesin (ERM proteins), which are well known to play an important role in linking the cell membrane and the cytoskeleton. Mutations of the *NF2* gene have been found in 15–35% of sporadic meningiomas. The majority of *NF2* mutations are nonsense or frameshift mutations that result in the premature termination of translation. Then, the resultant deletion of the N-terminal domain of merlin induces transfer of merlin from the plasma membrane to the nucleus. Until now, the mechanism of tumorigenesis has been generally explained only by mutations of oncogenes and/or tumor suppressor genes. Although mutations of *NF2* gene are well known in meningiomas as in schwannomas, they alone cannot explain tumorigenesis of all sporadic meningiomas.

Calcium^{2+}-dependent papain-like neutral cysteine protease (calpain) is found in virtually all vertebrate cells. Calpain is a heterodimer composed of the common 30-kDa regulatory subunit and 80-kDa catalytic subunits. During activation, the 80-kDa catalytic subunit is converted to 76-kDa enzymatically active forms by self-digesting N-terminal 4-kDa domain. Calpain is activated in both the physiological and pathological conditions.

The author's group found that calpain and merlin are both expressed in arachnoid and meningioma cells. Cleavage of the merlin protein by activated calpain was observed to occur in meningiomas [18]. Because ezrin, one of the ERM proteins, is well known to be a good substrate for calpain in vitro, merlin, showing similarity to ERM proteins, might be also cleaved by activated calpain. Both the full-length merlin and activated calpain were localized at the plasma membrane of cultured meningioma cells after oxidative stress. It is widely

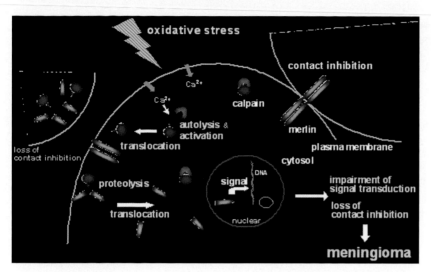

FIG. 3-11. Schematic representation of meningioma tumorigenesis showing an oxidative stress-induced cascade. At first, the oxidative stress, e.g., due to aging, induces Ca^{2+} mobilization, and Ca^{2+} activates calpain. Subsequently, the autolyzed and activated calpain translocates from the cytoplasm to the plasma membrane. Here merlin is cleaved by the activated calpain, and this cleavage product presumably transfers into the nucleus via the perinuclear cytoplasm. Accordingly, the signal pathway for cell adhesion and the contact inhibition may be impaired, leading to development of meningiomas

accepted that genetic mutations cannot explain the occurrence of more than two thirds of sporadic meningiomas. For instance, oxidative stress due to aging, irradiation, or chemicals may induce Ca^{2+} influx in arachnoid cells to induce sustained calpain activation and transfer of activated calpain to the plasma membrane. Although the precise function of a tumor suppressor protein, merlin, is still unknown, the author's group [18] recently found that oxidative stress can induce similar translocation of merlin after cleavage by activated calpain. The impairment of signal transduction from the plasma membrane to the nucleus by merlin proteolysis conceivably blocks the signal pathway necessary for the cell adhesion and the contact inhibition, which may lead to the inactive proliferation of arachnoid cells with the resultant development of meningiomas (Fig. 3-11).

Most meningiomas are benign in biological nature, but some of them are difficult to remove totally when they occur at the skull base. Furthermore, malignant or atypical types of meningiomas often show recurrence even after the total resection. Further analyses concerning calpain activation and inhibition systems in meningioma cells as well as the relation between merlin and calpain are necessary to clarify the pathophysiogenesis of *NF2*-related tumors and to develop a novel therapeutic strategy.

References

1. Haines DE, Harkey HL, al-Mefty O. The "subdural" space: a new look at an outdated concept. Neurosurg 1993; 32:111–20. Review.
2. Schachenmayr W, Friede RL. The origin of subdural neomembranes. I. Fine structure of the dura-arachnoid interface in man. Am J Pathol 1978; 92:53–68.
3. Yamashima T, Friede RL. Light and electron microscopic studies on the subdural space, the subarachnoid space and the arachnoid membrane. Neurol Med Chir (Tokyo) 1984; 24:737–46. (Japanese)
4. Haines DE, Frederickson RG. The meninges. In Meningiomas (Al-Mefty, ed.). Raven Press, New York, 1991.
5. Hasegawa M, Yamashima T, Kida S, Yamashita J. Membranous ultrastructure of human arachnoid cells. J Neuropathol Exp Neurol 1997; 56:1217–27.
6. Reina MA, Lopez Garcia A, de Andres JA. Anatomical description of a natural perforation present in the human lumbar pia mater. Rev Esp Anestesiol Reanim 1998; 45:4–7. (Spanish)
7. Alcolado R, Weller RO, Parrish EP, et al. The cranial arachnoid and pia mater in man: anatomical and ultrastructural observations. Neuropathol Appl Neurobiol 1988; 14:1–17.
8. Hutchings M, Weller RO. Anatomical relationships of the pai mater to cerebral vessels in man. J Neurosurg 1986; 65:316–25.
9. Yamashima T, Yamamoto S. The origin of inner membranes in chronic subdural hematomas. Acta Neuropathol (Berl) 1985; 67:219–25.
10. Yamashima T. Ultrastructural study of the final cerebrospinal fluid pathway in human arachnoid villi. Brain Res 1986; 384:68–76.
11. Yamashima T, Sakuda K, Tohma Y, et al. Prostaglandin D synthase (beta-trace) in human arachnoid and meningioma cells: roles as a cell marker or in cerebrospinal fluid absorption, tumorigenesis, and calcification process. J Neurosci 1997; 17:2376–82.
12. Kivisakk P, Mahad DJ, Callahan MK, et al. Human cerebrospinal fluid central memory CD4+ T cells: evidence for trafficking through choroid plexus and meninges via P-selectin. Proc Natl Acad Sci USA 2003; 100:8389–94.
13. Brunori A, Vagnozzi R, Giuffre R. Antonio Pacchioni (1665–1726): early studies of the dura mater. J Neurosurg 1993; 78:515–8
14. Tohma Y, Yamashima T, Yamashita J. Immunohistochemical localization of cell adhesion molecule epithelial cadherin in human arachnoid villi and meningiomas. Cancer Res 1992; 52:1981–7.
15. Yamashima T, Tohma Y, Yamashita J. Expression of cell adhesion molecule E-cadherin in human arachnoid villi. J Neurosurg 1992; 77:749–56.
16. Ikushima I, Korogi Y, Makita O, et al. MRI of arachnoid granulations within the dural sinuses using a FLAIR pulse sequence. Br J Radiol 1999; 72:1046–51.
17. Massicotte EM, Del Bigio MR. Human arachnoid villi response to subarachnoid hemorrhage: possible relationship to chronic hydrocephalus. J Neurosurg 1999; 91:80–4.

18. Kaneko T, Yamashima T, Tohma Y, et al. Calpain-dependent proteolysis of merlin occurs by oxidative stress in meningiomas: a novel hypothesis of tumorigenesis. Cancer 2001; 92:2662–72.

19. Clausen J. Proteins in normal cerebrospinal fluid not found in serum. Proc Soc Exp Biol Med 1961; 107:170–2.

20. Hoffmann A, Conradt HS, Gross G, et al. Purification and chemical characterization of β-trace protein from human cerebrospinal fluid: its identification as prostaglandin D synthase. J Neurochem 1993; 61:451–6.

21. Pervaiz S, Brew K. Homology and structure-function correlations between 1-acid glycoprotein and serum retinol-binding protein and its relatives. FASEB J 1987; 1:209–214.

22. Zahn M, Mäder M, Schmidt B, et al. Purification and N-terminal sequence of β-trace, a protein abundant in human cerebrospinal fluid. Neurosci Lett 1993; 154:93–5.

23. Nagata A, Suzuki Y, Igarashi M, et al. Human brain prostaglandin D synthase has been evolutionarily differentiated from lipophilic-ligand carrier proteins. Proc Natl Acad Sci USA 1991; 88:4020–4.

24. Urade Y. Dual function of β-trace. Prostaglandins 1996; 51:286.

25. Ujihara M, Urade Y, Eguchi N, et al. Prostaglandin D2 formation and characterization of its synthetases in various tissues of adult rats. Arch Biochem Biophys 1988; 260:521–31.

26. Hara A, Yamada H, Sakai N, et al. Immunohistochemical expression of glutathione S-transferase placental type (GST-), a detoxifying enzyme, in normal arachnoid villi and meningiomas. Virchows Arch [A] 1990; 6:493–6.

27. Yamashima T, Yamashita J. Histological, ultrastructural, and chromatographical discrimination of phospholipids in meningiomas. Acta Neuropathol 1990; 80:255–9.

4
Meninges: Embryology

M. Beatriz S. Lopes

Introduction

The adult central nervous system (CNS) is largely encased by three concentric connective layers named dura mater, arachnoid, and pia mater. They constitute a fibrous envelope, which provides for mechanical protection of the nervous system and participates in formation of the blood-brain barrier. The embryogenesis of the meninges varies across vertebrate species. The human meningeal development is still a matter of great controversy. Although comparative embryologic and anatomic studies have demonstrated that main developmental landmarks are conserved among the species, these findings should be cautiously extrapolated to the human embryonic development (1). Detailed studies on the embryogenesis of the meninges in humans by O'Rahilly and Müller in the late 1980s (2) presented the most comprehensive analysis yet on this complex issue. In this chapter I will provide a review of the development of the cranial and spinal human meninges and their correlation with the morphologic aspects of the adult meninges.

Formation and Development of the Meninges

In the early embryo, the neural tube is enveloped by a mesenchymal layer that will result in the primary meninx. Both mesenchymal and neural crest–derived cells appear to be involved in the formation of the primary meninx that will differentiate during the embryo development and form two different layers: the pachymeninges, or dura mater, and the leptomeninges comprising the arachnoid and the pia mater. The pachymeninges is an external and thick layer of mesenchymal composition while the leptomeninges is a double and thinner layer that contains both mesenchymal and neural crest cells.

Anatomic and embryologic differences exist between the meningeal coverings of the brain and the spinal cord. The encephalic meninges originate from both the mesenchyme and the encephalic neural crest, while the meninges of the spine and caudal regions of the head originate from the paraxial mesenchyme (2). This double origin of the meninges is similar to the avian and mammalian origin of the axial skeletal structures in which the spinal column and the occipital bone are derived from the paraxial mesoderm, whereas the rest of the cranial vault is produced from neural crest-derived and mesodermal cells (3–5).

For understanding of this process, a brief review of the early formation of the embryo is required. During human embryonic development, the primary neural tube closes at approximately 26 postovulatory days, corresponding to embryonic Carnegie stage 12 (6). Thereafter, secondary neurulation occurs with differentiation and canalization of the primary neural tube, which occurs during stages 13 and 20. The neural tube separates from the overlying cutaneous ectoderm by a process of disjunction. The somites migrate to the midline at each side of the neural tube and fuse to form the laminae and spines of the vertebrae. Vertebrae, muscles, and meninges originate from the somites (7). Somites are mesenchymal condensations that first appear around Carnegie stage 9 and develop from the unsegmented paraxial mesoderm. They are the first distinct metameric units of the vertebrate embryo (1). The periodic production of somites and their subsequent patterning occurs in a cranial to caudal fashion under tightly regulated mechanisms. Although these mechanisms of controlling the periodicity of somite formation are not completely understood, *Hox* genes are activated in presomitic mesoderm and appear to be in part responsible for the specification of segmental identity in murines (for review, see Ref. 8). The newly formed somite consists of an epithelial ball of columnar cells encircling mesenchymal cells within a central cavity, the somitocoel. During early maturation, the ventral wall of the somite and the somitocoel cells form the sclerotome, which gives rise to the vertebral column and ribs. The dorsal half of the somite remains epithelial and develops into the dermomyotome, from which the dermis of the back and the skeletal musculature originate.

become visible in the dura (25); during infancy and childhood the villi and granulations increase in number, and they gradually increase in size to become lobulated and more complex in adults (15).

The Meningeal Extracellular Matrix

The contribution of the mesenchyme in the development of the meninges provides to meningothelial cells mesenchymal properties similar to those of fibroblasts. Regardless of their embryologic origin (mesenchyme and/or neural crest), meningothelial cells participate in the formation of the extracellular matrix (ECM) and production of fibrous connective tissues. Collagens are the most abundant ECM structures in human meninges, where the most represented types are I, III, and IV. In addition to collagen, meningothelial cells synthesize non-collagen proteins including fibronectin, laminin, and tenascin (24,26). Montagnani et al. (26) found that differences in structural components of meningeal ECM are present in fetal and adult meninges. During fetal development, both intracranial and spinal meningeal ECM contains an abundance of laminin and tenascin and express β-1 integrin and fibronectin. In the same period, the production of type I collagen is active but accompanied by a large amount of type III fibers as well. Type IV collagen is scarcely present in this period. A difference in the structural components of the meningeal ECM between intracranial and spinal layers is, however, evident in the adult meninges; this change may occur after birth or presumably at early childhood. In intracranial meninges from adults, types I and IV collagen appear prevalent compared to type III. The activity of synthesis of the other ECM components (fibronectin, tenascin, and laminin) is decreased together with the expression of β-1 integrin. On the contrary, fibronectin, tenascin, and laminin activities are constant in the adult spinal meninges, but at a lower level as compared to fetal conditions. In addition, type III collagen is more abundant in the spinal meninges when compared with the intracranial meninges (26).

Plasticity of Embryonal Meningeal Cells

During development, the meninges play an important morphogenetic role on neural structures (3). Experimentally, meninges induce the formation of the superficial glial limitans and stimulate the growth of precursors located in the superficial blastemas of the cerebellum and hippocampus. Destruction of the meninges overlying the cerebellar folia leads to cerebellar hypoplasia, formation of neuronal ectopia and gliosis in the subarachnoid space, fusion of adjacent folia, and reduction of the total number of granular cells (27–31). In the hippocampus, destruction of the meninges may induce secondary malformations of the dentate gyrus (31). These neural malformations are believed to occur due to disorganization of the glia maintenance secondary to the disappearance of the glia limitans. On the other hand, experiments using transgenic mice with a permanent neural crest cell lineage marker (*Wnt1-Cre/R26R*) and exposed to retinoic acid have shown that interaction with the underlying neural crest–derived meninges is crucial for intramembranous ossification of the parietal bones (5).

References

1. Müller F, O'Rahilly R. Segmentation in staged human embryos: the occipiticervical region revisited. J Anat 2003;203:297–315.
2. O'Rahilly R, Müller F. The meninges in human development. J Neuropathol Exp Neurol 1986;45:588–608.
3. Catala M. Embryonic and fetal development of structures associated with the cerebro-spinal fluid in man and other species: Part I: the ventricular system, meninges and choroid plexuses. Arch Anat Cytol Path 1998;46:153–169.
4. Creuzet SE, Martinez S, Le Douarin NM. The cephalic neural crest exerts a critical effect on forebrain and midbrain development. Proc Natl Acad Sci USA 2006;103:14033–14038.
5. Jiang X, Iseki S, Maxson RE, et al. Tissue origins and interactions in the mammalian skull vault. Dev Biol. 2002;241:106–16.
6. O'Rahilly R, Müller F. The Embryonic Human Brain: An Atlas of Developmental Stages. Wiley-Liss, Inc., New York, 1994.
7. Haque M, Ohata K, Takami T, et al. Development of lumbosacral spina bifida: three-dimensional computer graphic study of human embryos at Carnegie stage twelve. Pediatr Neurosurg 2001;35:247–252.
8. Holland PW, Takahashi T. The evolution of homeobox genes: implications for the study of brain development. Brain Res Bull 2005;66:484–490.
9. O'Rahilly R, Müller F. Somites, spinal ganglia, and centra. Cells Tissues Organs 2003;173:75–92.
10. Filly RA, Feldstein VA. Ultrasound evaluation of normal fetal anatomy. In: Callen PW (ed.), Ultrasonography in Obstetrics and Gynecology, 4th ed. W. B. Saunders, Philadelphia, 2000, pp. 221–276.
11. Bagnall KM, Higgins SJ, Sanders EJ. The contribution made by a single somite to the vertebral column: experimental evidence in support of resegmentation using the chick-quail chimaera model. Development 1988;103:69–85.
12. Bagnall KM, Higgins SJ, Sanders EJ. The contribution made by a single somite to tissues within a body segment and assessment of their integration with similar cells from adjacent segments. Development 1989;107:931–943.
13. Bagnall KM. The migration and distribution of somite cells after labeling with the carbocyanine dye, DiI: the relationship of this distribution to segmentation in the vertebrate body. Anat Embryol (Berl) 1992;185:317–324.
14. Patelska-Banaszewska M, Woźniak W. The subarachnoid space develops early in the human embryonic period. Folia Morphol 2005;64:212–216.
15. Weller RO. Microscopic morphology and histology of the human meninges. Morphologie 2005;89:22–34.
16. Weed LH. The development of the cerebro-spinal spaces in pig and man. Contrib Embryol Carnegie Institution 1917;5:5–110.

17. Osaka K, Handa H, Matsumoto S, Yasuda M. Development of the cerebrospinal fluid pathway in the normal and abnormal embryos. Childs Brain 1980;6:26–38.

18. Sensenig EC. The early development of the meninges of the spinal cord in human embryos. In: Contributions to Embryology No. 228. Washington: Carnegie Institution of Washington. Publication 1951;592,34:145–157.

19. Kamiryo T, Orita T, Nishizaki T, Aoki H. Development of the rat meninx: experimental study using bromodeoxyuridine. Anat Rec 1990;227: 207–210.

20. Kuban KCK, Gilles FH. Human telencephalic angiogenesis. Ann Neurol 1985;17:539–548.

21. Kurz H, Horn J, Christ B. Morphogenesis of embryonic CNS vessels. Cancer Treat Res 2004;117:33–50.

22. Marin-Padilla M. Early vascularization of the embryonic cerebral cortex: Golgi and electron microscopic studies. J Comp Neurol 1985;241:237–249.

23. Nelson MD, Gonzalez-Gomez I, Gilles FH. The search for human telencephalic ventriculofugal arteries. AJNR Am J Neuroradiol 1991;12:215–222.

24. Russell DS, Rubinstein JR. Tumors of the meninges and related tissues. In: Pathology of Tumours of the Nervous System, 5th ed. Edward Arnold, England, 1989, pp. 449–532.

25. Gomez DG, Ehrmann JE, Potts DG, et al. The arachnoid granulation of the newborn human: an ultrastructural study. Int J Dev Neurosci 1983;1:139–147.

26. Montagnani S, Castaldo C, Di Meglio F, et al. Extra cellular matrix features in human meninges. It J Anat Embryol 2000;105:167–177.

27. Hartmann D, Schulze M, Sievers J. Meningeal cells stimulate and direct the migration of cerebellar external granule cells in vitro. J Neurocytol 1998;27:395–409.

28. Hartmann D, Ziegenhagen MW, Sievers J. Meningeal cells stimulate neuronal migration and the formation of radial glial fascicles from the cerebellar external granular layer. Neurosci Lett 1998;244:129–132.

29. Sievers J, von Knebel Doeberitz C, Pehlemann FW, Berry M. Meningeal cells influence cerebellar development over a critical period. Anat Embryol (Berl) 1986;175:91–100.

30. Sievers J, Pehlemann FW, Gude S, Berry M. Meningeal cells organize the superficial glia limitans of the cerebellum and produce components of both the interstitial matrix and the basement membrane. J Neurocytol 1994;23:135–149.

31. von Knebel Doeberitz C, Sievers J, Sadler M, Pehlemann FW, Berry M, Halliwell P. Destruction of meningeal cells over the newborn hamster cerebellum with 6-hydroxydopamine prevents foliation and lamination in the rostral cerebellum. Neuroscience 1986;17:409–426.

32. Hartmann D, Sievers J, Pehlemann FW, Berry M. Destruction of meningeal cells over the medial cerebral hemisphere of newborn hamsters prevents the formation of the infrapyramidal blade of the dentate gyrus. J Comp Neurol 1992;320:33–61.

5
Pathology of Meningiomas

Richard A. Prayson

Historical Perspective

The vast majority of meningiomas arise in the meninges from arachnoidal cap cells that are normally present in small nests. Harvey Cushing first introduced the term meningioma in 1922 to designate a group of tumors, which arose from the meninges of the brain and spinal cord [1]. Previous to Cushing, these tumors had been referred to by a variety of designations, including angioendothelioma, arachnoidal fibroblastoma, dural endothelioma, dural sarcoma, endotheliosis of the meninges, meningeal fibroblastoma, meningoblastoma, mesothelioma of the meninges, sarcoma of the dura, and fungus of the dura mater. In 1922, Oberling was one of the first to divide meningiomas into subtypes [2]. This classification was based on the concept of cell structure of the meninges and included three different groups. A few years later, Roussy and Cornil developed a similar three-group classification based on the cytologic structure of these neoplasms [3]. In 1930, del Rio Hortega devised a classification for meningiomas, which was based on structural and architectural features of the tumor [4]. In the following year, the classification began to expand with the recognition of the phenotypic variability of these tumors. Bailey and Bucy devised a classification schema including nine types of meningioma based on these phenotypic differences [5]. Several of the terms coined to describe these types (including meningotheliomatous, psammomatous, osteoblastic, fibroblastic, and angioblastic) are still in current usage today. In 1938, Cushing and Eisenhart's classic work further developed this classification system in recognizing 9 types and 20 subtypes or variants of meningioma [6]. The authors of the first fascicle entitled *Tumors of the Central Nervous System*, in discussing meningiomas, indicated that they used the Bailey-Bucy classification, which was descriptive and allowed for the definition of tumors by means of routine laboratory staining techniques [7]. There was some suggestion in this first fascicle questioning whether angioblastic tumors should be included with meningiomas (a prelude to the recognition that hemangioblastomas and hemangiopericytomas, which were historically considered angioblastic meningiomas, were, in fact, different tumors).

In 1979, the World Health Organization (WHO) classification of tumors of the nervous system as outlined by Zülch recognized seven subtypes of meningioma, including meningotheliomatous, transitional, psammomatous, angiomatous, hemangioblastic, and hemangiopericytic variants [8]. Although there was acknowledgment that hemangioblastomas and hemangiopericytomas existed as distinct entities, there was still reluctance to abandon the notion that certain meningiomas could resemble these tumor types. In addition, WHO also recognized a papillary meningioma and anaplastic or malignant meningioma as higher-grade lesions. In 1982, John Kepes in his monograph on meningiomas outlined and illustrated features of many patterns of meningioma. A number of currently recognized histologic subtypes of meningioma have their origin in this work [9].

In the most recent rendition of the WHO Classification for meningiomas published in 2000 (see Table 5-1) [10], nine low-grade variants (grade I tumors) and three variants each of grade II and grade III meningioma are recognized. The focus of most of the remainder of this chapter will be on the morphologic features of these various subtypes of meningioma.

Gross Features

As previously mentioned, the vast majority of meningiomas arise in superficial locations associated with meninges. Occasional unusual locations for meningioma such as within the ventricular system with a left ventricular preference or in soft tissues in the head and neck region have also been documented [9,11]. Most of those who deal with brain tumors are familiar with the classic gross appearance of an ordinary grade I meningioma. These tumors are often superficially based, round or globular masses, which are firmly attached to the dura and compress the adjacent or subjacent brain tissue (Fig. 5-1). The external aspect of the tumor is often evenly nodular, but is generally smooth and in many cases appears to have a thin capsule.

TABLE 5-1. World Health Organization (WHO) Classification and Grading of Meningiomas of the Central Nervous System

Grade I
  Meningothelial
  Fibrous (fibroblastic)
  Transitional (mixed)
  Psammomatous
  Angiomatous
  Microcystic
  Secretory
  Lymphoplasmocyte-rich
  Metaplastic
Grade II
  Clear cell
  Chordoid
  Atypical
Grade III
  Rhabdoid
  Papillary
  Anaplastic (malignant)
Other Variants (grade not defined by WHO)
  Giant cell
  Meningioma with intracytoplasmic eosinophilic inclusions
  Sclerosing
  Oncocytic

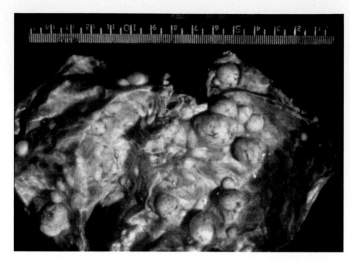

FIG. 5-2. Gross appearance of multiple meningiomas. This is more commonly encountered in the setting of neurofibromatosis types I and II

The tumor is generally easily separated from the adjacent neural tissue. Tumors arising in the falx may have a dumbbell shape. Optic nerve tumors, because of constriction by bone of the optic foramen, may also have a dumbbell-shaped appearance. Multifocality is not uncommon and is particularly noted in the setting of neurofibromatosis I and II (Fig. 5-2). Tumors may grow in a flattened pattern, so-called meningioma en plaque [10]. Some tumors, particularly the en plaque variant growth pattern, may be associated with hyperostosis of the adjacent bone (skull) [12]. Incidence of hyperostosis associated with meningiomas is somewhat uncommon and is probably observed in less than 5% of tumors. At times, the thickened bone is associated with nests of intramedullary tumor cells. Extension of meningioma into contiguous structures including dura and bone is not unusual and is not necessarily indicative of a higher-grade lesion. A small percentage of meningiomas are brain invasive and lack the circumscription that marks the low-grade tumors.

The cut surface appearance of meningioma can be quite variable and correlates with the histologic features of the tumor. The consistency of the lesion may range from soft to quite firm. Some tumors, particularly those with numerous psammoma bodies or extensive osseous metaplasia, may be quite firm and in fact require a decalcification or demineralization procedure in order to process the histologic sections. Typical meningiomas have a light tan or brown coloration on sectioning. This color may be altered by the presence of abundant numbers of lipidized macrophages, which would give the tumor a yellow appearance or areas of hemorrhage, which will lead to a more red appearance. Cystic degenerative changes may occasionally be observed in meningioma and may be grossly evident. Angiomatous meningiomas may have a hemorrhagic appearance due to the presence of prominent numbers of blood vessels.

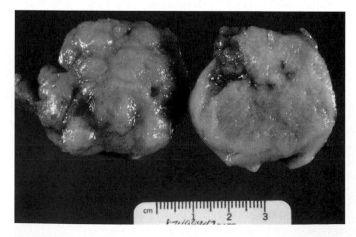

FIG. 5-1. Gross appearance of a fibrous meningioma showing the external aspect on the left and a cross-sectional appearance on the right

Meningothelial Meningioma (WHO Grade I)

The meningothelial variant of meningioma (also known as syncytial or meningotheliomatous meningioma) is perhaps the most common variant of meningioma encountered. Classically, it is marked by the arrangement of tumor cells in lobular nests. These cells are generally polygonal in shape

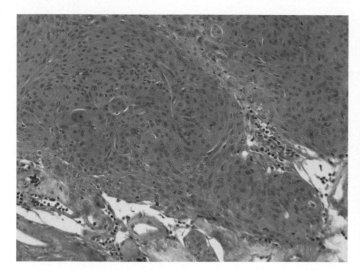

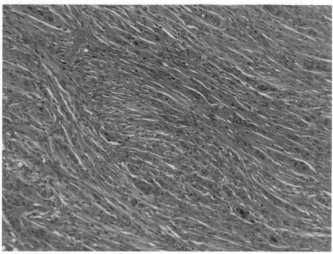

FIG. 5-3. Meningothelial (syncytial) meningioma marked by cells arranged in a syncytium with focal whorling (Hematoxylin and eosin, original magnification 200×)

FIG. 5-4. Fibrous meningioma characterized by spindled cells arranged in interlacing bundles (Hematoxylin and eosin, original magnification 200×)

with poorly defined cytoplasmic borders. Cells are described as being arranged in sheet-like fashion, i.e., in a syncytium, hence the alternate designation "syncytial" (Fig. 5-3). The cytoplasm stains slightly eosinophilic and is fairly homogeneous. The nucleus is generally oval and is centrally placed. Prominent nucleolation is not usually observable. Lobules of tumor cells may be separated by collageneous septa. The cells in this variant most closely resemble the arachnoidal cap cells from whence these tumors arise. A useful diagnostic feature is the occasional presence of prominent numbers of eosinophilic cytoplasmic invaginations into the nucleus (nuclear pseudoinclusions). Sometimes these inclusions may be clear, secondary to increased glycogen accumulation. Although nuclear pleomorphism may be evident focally in some of these tumors, features typically associated with higher grade lesions including increased mitotic activity, prominent nucleolation, necrosis, disordered architectural pattern, and small cell change are not typically observed. Another very typical feature of meningiomas is the presence of whorl formations, with cells that appear to be whorling around a central core. Occasionally, psammoma bodies may be observed in a syncytial meningioma. Other types of cells such as macrophages may also alter the appearance.

Fibrous Meningioma (WHO Grade I)

The fibrous or fibroblastic variant of meningioma, as its name suggests, is a tumor marked by a proliferation of spindled meningothelial cells arranged in interlacing bundles (Fig. 5-4). Cells are arranged against a collagenous or reticulin-rich matrix. The nuclei tend to be narrow and rod-shaped. Occasionally, a palisading of nuclei, reminiscent of the Verocay

bodies observed in schwannomas, may be present. Whorl formations are much less prominent as compared with syncytial meningiomas. Occasional psammoma bodies may also be evident. Interestingly, intraventricular meningiomas are most commonly of the fibrous type [13,14].

Transitional Meningioma (WHO Grade I)

Transitional or mixed meningioma is a tumor marked by both syncytial and fibrous patterns. Areas in which cells are syncytial in appearance merge with those of more spindled cells resembling the fibrous variant. Whorl formations and psammoma bodies may be variably present. Whorl formations are centered around another meningothelial cell, blood vessel, or collagen fibers. The WHO does not provide precise guidelines as to what percentage of a second component must be present in the tumor in order to make this diagnosis [10].

Psammomatous Meningioma (WHO Grade I)

Some view the psammomatous variant of meningioma as a type of transitional meningioma. This variant, however, is still separated from the other types. This particular variant is found almost commonly in the spinal cord region but is not necessarily restricted to that location. These tumors are marked by "abundant psammoma bodies," which in some tumors may become confluent and form calcified and ossified masses (Fig. 5-5). Psammoma bodies themselves are made up primarily of calcium material arranged in a concentric arrangement, collagen fibrils, and small amounts of iron. Again, precise guidelines with respect to how many psammoma bodies one needs

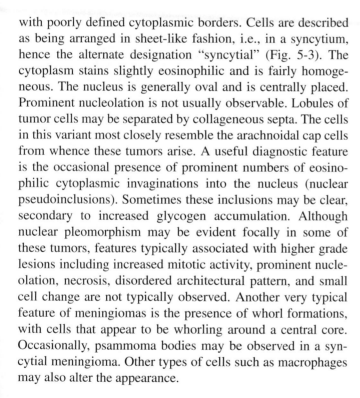

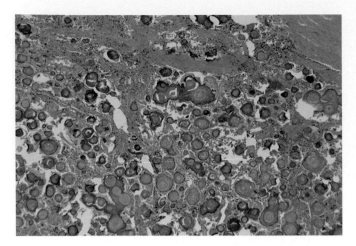

FIG. 5-5. A psammomatous meningioma marked by the presence of numerous calcified psammoma bodies (Hematoxylin and eosin, original magnification 200×)

to see in a given tumor in order to designate the lesion as psammomatous as opposed to meningothelial or transitional are not defined. A variety of hypotheses have been proposed regarding the formation of psammoma bodies, and these have variously included an origin from endothelial cells of obliterated blood vessels, degenerative changes of perivascular collagen, collagenization of the center meningothelial whorls, calcifications of secretory products from arachnoidal cap cells, calcification of necrotic tumor cells, and aberrant attempts at neovascularization [15].

Angiomatous Meningioma (WHO Grade I)

Many meningiomas typically have a rich vascularity. The designation of angiomatous meningioma is specifically used for tumors in which numerous blood vessels are present and appear to represent the predominant background pattern of the tumor (Fig. 5-6). The size of the vessels may be quite variable and ranges from very small capillary-sized vessels to medium-sized vessels. Vascular wall thickening or sclerosis is fairly common. The risk of hemorrhage, despite the increased vascularity, appears to be negligibly increased; spontaneous hemorrhage is most commonly associated with the meningothelial pattern [16]. The old term angioblastic meningioma historically referred to a group of meningiomas with prominent vascularity. This old designation, which should no longer be utilized, included a variety of lesions including what is currently referred to as hemangiopericytoma, hemangioblastoma, and the angiomatous meningioma.

Microcystic Meningioma (WHO Grade 1)

The microcystic variant of meningioma, also known as humid or vacuolated meningioma, is a relatively uncommon variant marked by the presence of cells with elongated processes and a loose mucinous stroma with a microcystic or occasionally grossly cystic appearance [17,18] (Fig. 5-7). The cytoplasm of many of the tumor cells appears to be clear and may be vacuolated. Transition of this pattern to other more conventional-appearing meningothelial or fibrous patterns may also be evident. In many cases, the cystic spaces appear empty; however, the vacuolated cytoplasm may demonstrate evidence of PAS (period acid–Schiff) positivity or oil-red-O positivity indicative of increased glycogen or lipid accumulation. Vessels in these tumors are often sclerotic, and nuclear pleomorphism may, at times, be a striking feature.

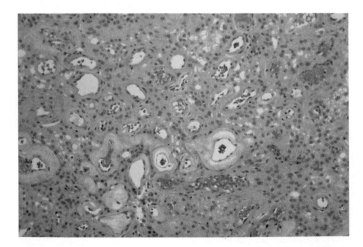

FIG. 5-6. The angiomatous variant of meningioma is characterized by a prominent vascularity (increased numbers of blood vessels) (Hematoxylin and eosin, original magnification 200×)

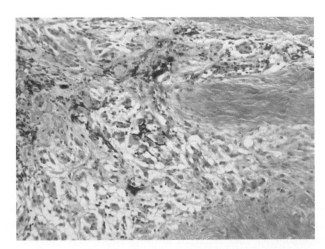

FIG. 5-7. The microcystic meningioma pattern is characterized by a loose, mucinous-type stroma (Hematoxylin and eosin, original magnification 200×)

Secretory Meningioma (WHO Grade I)

Secretory meningioma is a WHO grade I variant marked by the presence of eosinophilic hyaline inclusions in the background of what otherwise appears to be a meningothelial meningioma (Fig. 5-8). These inclusions are strongly PAS positive and may range in size anywhere from 3 to 100 μm in diameter. Inclusions have been shown to demonstrate immunoreactivity to a variety of proteins, including immunoglobulins, α_1-antitrypsin, and carcinoembryonic antigen (CEA) [15]. These inclusions do not calcify or show a tendency toward calcification, hence the former name for this tumor, pseudopsammomatous meningioma, is a bit of a misnomer. Ultrastructurally, these eosinophilic inclusions appear to be principally intercellular [19–21]. Ultrastructural examination has shown these inclusions are localized within cytoplasmic lumens lined by micro villi, which has prompted suggestion that this is a form of glandular metaplasia. It has been suggested that these inclusions represent an active secretory product of meningioma cells rather than degeneration or phagocytic process. A subset of these patients may have elevated serum CEA levels, which normalize after tumor resection [22]. This may have implications clinically in patients who have breast carcinoma. Many of these tumors are also marked by the presence of prominent peritumoral edema [23,24].

Lymphoplasmocyte Rich Meningioma (WHO Grade I)

Occasional meningiomas are marked by the presence of a prominent lymphoplasmacytic infiltrate [25–27] (Fig. 5-9). The background tumor often resembles a meningothelial type

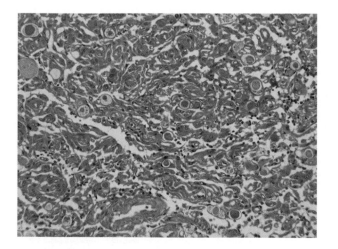

FIG. 5-8. Eosinophilic hyaline inclusions are a salient feature of secretory meningioma (Hematoxylin and eosin, original magnification 200×)

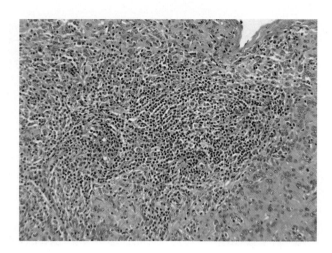

FIG. 5-9. Lymphoplasmacyte-rich meningioma is marked by a prominent chronic inflammatory cell infiltrate (Hematoxylin and eosin, original magnification 200×)

of meningioma. Amyloid material has rarely been described in association with this variant. Increased serum immunoglobulins have also been rarely reported [26]. In tumors with prominent numbers of plasma cells, Russell bodies may be observed. In tumors with a markedly prominent chronic inflammatory cell component, care needs to be taken in order to not overlook the underlying meningioma. This entity has been occasionally associated with sinus histiocytosis with massive lymphadenopathy [15].

Metaplastic Meningioma (WHO Grade I)

Metaplastic meningiomas refer to a group of tumors marked by focal mesenchymal differentiation. The background neoplasm may resemble a meningothelial, fibrous, or transitional meningioma. The mesenchymal differentiation may come in various forms. Patterns of mesenchymal differentiation that have been variously observed in meningiomas include myxomatous or myxoid type (comprised of tumors with stellate multipolar cells distributed against a mucinous background), xanthomatous type (marked by the presence of numerous xanthoma cells with increased lipidized meningothelial cells), lipoblastic or lipomatous meningioma (marked by the presence of adipose tissue), granular cell type (characterized by the presence of cells marked by abundant eosinophilic, finely granular cytoplasm), osseous type (marked by the production of bone) (Fig. 5-10), cartilaginous type (marked by the presence of benign cartilage tissue), and melanotic type (characterized by the presence of melanin pigment) [9, 28–33]. Some of these histologic variants have been historically associated with increased recurrence or more aggressive behavior, although they are, as a group, still designated as grade I tumors. Care needs to be taken with the osseous variant not to misconstrue invasion of tumor into skull as

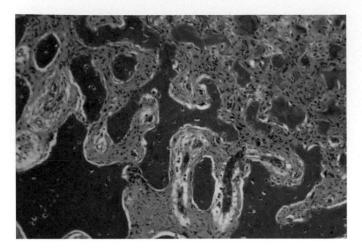

FIG. 5-10. A metaplastic meningioma with prominent bone formation (osseous) (Hematoxylin and eosin, original magnification 200×)

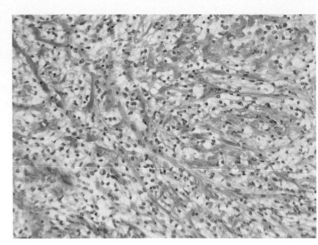

FIG. 5-11. Cells with clear cytoplasm due to increased glycogen material in a clear cell meningioma (Hematoxylin and eosin, original magnification 200×)

representing osseous metaplasia. Many meningiomas that were formerly designated as melanotic have been subsequently reclassified as melanocytomas, which are now recognized as a distinct tumor type.

Other Unusual Variants

Small numbers of other histologic variations of meningioma described in the literature do not currently fit into the WHO classification schema. Since the numbers of these cases is so small, the precise behavior of these tumors has yet to be determined. Among these lesions are tumors with prominent numbers of giant cells [15,34], tumors marked by intracytoplasmic eosinophilic inclusions (distinct from the secretory meningioma) [35,36], sclerosing meningiomas [37], and oncocytic meningiomas [38].

Clear Cell Meningioma (WHO Grade II)

The clear cell meningioma has been recognized since 1995 as a distinct variant of meningioma with an increased propensity to recur locally [39]. As its name suggests, this variant of meningioma is marked by prominence of tumor cells demonstrating abundant clear cytoplasm (Fig. 5-11). Cytoplasmic clearing is related to increased glycogen accumulation (PAS positive) within the cytoplasm. Often, the cells are arranged in a patternless, disordered configuration, making it at times difficult to recognize this tumor for what it is. Of the cases that have been reported in the literature, this variant seems to show a propensity for arising in the cerebellopontine angle and cauda equina regions [40].

Chordoid Meningioma (WHO Grade II)

Chordoid meningioma was described in the late 1980s as another variant of meningioma that appears to behave in a more aggressive fashion [41–43]. This tumor is marked by a prominent myxoid background. Tumor cells are arranged in trabeculae or cords (Fig. 5-12). Cells generally demonstrate eosinophilic and occasionally slightly vacuolated cytoplasm. As the name suggests, the tumor shows features reminiscent of a chordoma. In contrast to chordoma, however, the tumor generally lacks physaliferous or bubble-like cells. It is not unusual for the chordoid pattern of meningioma to be associ-

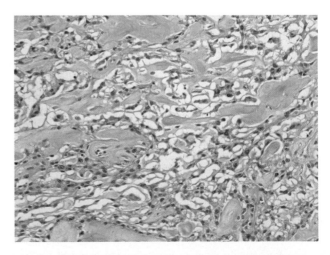

FIG. 5-12. A chordoid meningioma characterized by cords of cells arranged against a myxoid background (Hematoxylin and eosin, original magnification 200×)

ated with other areas of the tumor, which have a more conventional appearance. A lymphoplasmacytic component to the tumor may be observed; this particular feature has been reported in association with Castleman's syndrome, which is marked by hepatosplenomegaly, bone marrow plasmocytosis, dysgammaglobulinemia, iron refractory hypochromic anemia, and delayed sexual development [42].

Atypical Meningioma (Grade II)

Atypical meningioma is a designation used for tumors that are marked by the presence of certain histologic parameters which have been associated with more aggressive behavior, increased association with recurrence, and a small risk of distant metastasis. There is a rather substantial literature that has attempted to delineate histologic features that are associated with more aggressive behavior in meningiomas [9,10,15, 44–51]. Although there are some differences with regard to the relative importance attached to certain histologic features, there seems to be general agreement regarding the relative importance of certain morphologic parameters in predicting more aggressive behavior in these tumors. The most recent rendition of WHO uses the designation of atypical meningioma to delineate tumors that are marked by the presence of four or more mitoses per 10 high-power fields (with a high power field defined as 0.16 mm^2) [10]. Alternatively, atypical meningioma may be characterized by the presence of three or more of the following histologic characteristics: increased cellularity, small cell change, i.e., cells with high nuclear-to-cytoplasmic ratio, prominent nucleolation, and uninterrupted patternless or sheet-like growth pattern, and

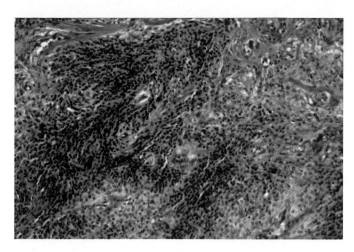

FIG. 5-14. Prominent small cell change (high nuclear to cytoplasmic ratio) in an atypical meningioma (Hematoxylin and eosin, original magnification 200×)

foci of spontaneous or geographic necrosis (Figs. 5-13 to 5-15). Since these tumors may demonstrate these features only regionally, adequate sampling of the tumor is important in arriving at an accurate assessment of the lesion. Although features such as mitosis counts are more specific, some of the other parameters outlined by the WHO are somewhat more vague and open to interpretation. Exactly what constitutes increased cellularity is a somewhat subjective parameter. A special note should be made of the presence of spontaneous or geographic necrosis in a meningioma. Care should be taken not to misconstrue necrosis secondary to embolization of the tumor prior to surgery as carrying the same degree of importance [52] (Fig. 5-16).

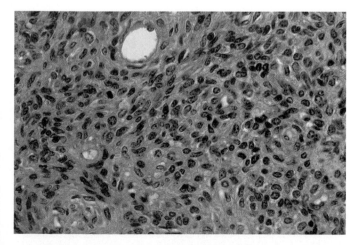

FIG. 5-13. Atypical meningioma marked by a disordered architecture and evidence of mitotic activity (Hematoxylin and eosin, original magnification 200×)

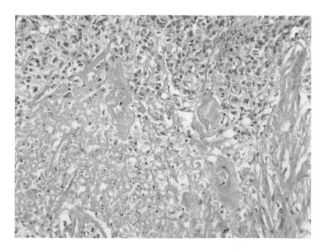

FIG. 5-15. Geographic tumor necrosis in an atypical meningioma (Hematoxylin and eosin, original magnification 200×)

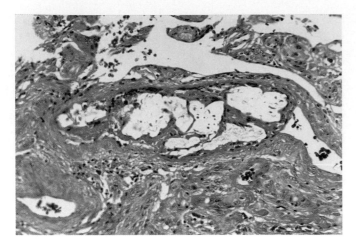

FIG. 5-16. Intraarterial embolization of a meningioma can also result in tumor necrosis (Hematoxylin and eosin, original magnification 200×)

Papillary Meningioma (WHO Grade III)

Papillary meningioma is an uncommon variant that has been recognized since the work of Cushing and Eisenhart in 1938 as a distinct variant [6]. As its name suggests, this tumor is marked by the presence of a focal papillary architectural pattern marked by fibrovascular cores lined by meningothelial cells [53,54] (Fig. 5-17). These tumors frequently demonstrate other morphologic evidence of more aggressive behavior, including other features typically associated with aggressive behavior. These tumors clearly show a propensity to focally recur and to metastasize. Interestingly, this variant of tumor also seems to be more common in children. Care should be taken not to misconstrue pseudopapillary architectural changes associated with microcystic degeneration with true papillary architecture.

Rhabdoid Meningioma (WHO Grade III)

Rhabdoid meningiomas are marked by the presence of tumor cells with an eccentrically placed nucleus, prominent nucleolus, and prominent cytoplasmic eosinophilic inclusions consisting of whorled intermediate molecular weight filaments [55,56] (Fig. 5-18). The cells are often arranged in a sheet-like or haphazard fashion, and frequently these tumors demonstrate other worrisome morphologic features. Histologically, these tumors have cells that resemble rhabdoid tumors arising in other organ systems. Similar to papillary meningiomas, this variant has been associated with increased risk of recurrence and distant metastasis. The significance of a minor rhabdoid component in an otherwise bland appearing meningioma is uncertain.

Anaplastic (Malignant) Meningioma (WHO Grade III)

Anaplastic or malignant meningioma has been clearly associated with poor survival (median survival <2 years). These tumors are defined by WHO as "exhibiting histological features of frank malignancy far in excess of the abnormalities present in a typical meningioma." [10]. WHO further indicates that these features include either obviously malignant cytology (i.e., the tumor has an appearance similar to a carcinoma, melanoma, or sarcoma) or exceedingly high mitotic index (>20 MF/10 HPF) (Fig. 5-19). Interestingly, the gender predominance that is observed with low-grade meningiomas in females is not evident with this grade of tumor.

Historically, brain-invasive meningiomas were generally considered high-grade or malignant tumors [57]. In reality, this probably is the case in the majority of these tumors.

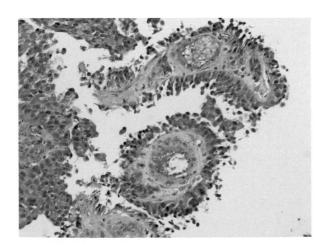

FIG. 5-17. A papillary meningioma marked by papillary fibrovascular cores lined by meningothelial cells (Hematoxylin and eosin, original magnification 200×)

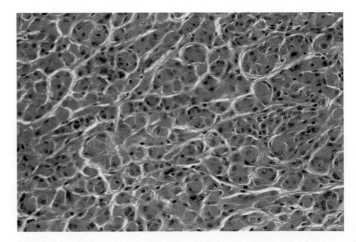

FIG. 5-18. Rhabdoid meningioma comprised of cells with cytoplasmic eosinophilic inclusions (Hematoxylin and eosin, original magnification 200×)

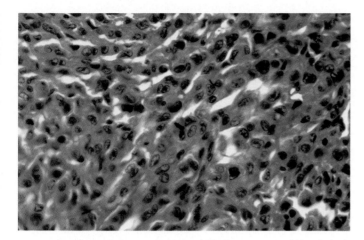

FIG. 5-19. Anaplastic meningioma with prominent mitotic activity and obviously malignant cytology (Hematoxylin and eosin, original magnification 400×)

However, there appears to be a small number of brain-invasive meningiomas that are associated with a more bland histology and better outcome. Some have suggested adding brain invasion to the list of histologic features one evaluates to assess for atypical meningioma [58] (Fig. 5-20). Part of the difficulty that also surrounds the notion of brain invasion is the definition of the lesion. Most believe that one needs to see islands or groups of tumor cells completely surrounded by neural parenchyma in order to make the designation. These tumors are not circumscribed like their lower grade counterparts and are frequently more difficult to excise. Sampling of tissue at the deep aspect of the meningioma, at its interface with brain tissue, is important in order to make this diagnosis.

Similar to brain invasion, metastases also have, for the most part, been associated with anaplastic or malignant meningioma [9,15,57,59,60]. There are rare instances of histologically benign meningiomas that appear to have metastasized,

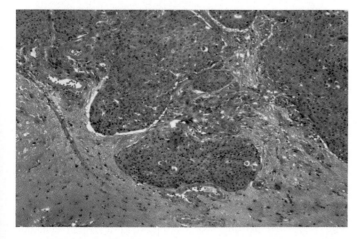

FIG. 5-20. A brain-invasive meningioma lacks the circumscription that marks lower-grade tumors (Hematoxylin and eosin, original magnification 200×)

perhaps by embolism resulting from a surgical procedure. The most common sites of metastasis include lungs, liver, lymph nodes, and bones.

Ultrastructural Features

There has been much work done in describing the electron microscopic features of meningioma [9,61–66]. In general, there is little in the way of ultrastructural appearance that allows one to distinguish a meningothelial versus transitional versus fibroblastic meningioma. Subtle differences or features have been associated with some of the other variants that may be discernable by electron microscopic evaluation. Features that appear to be characteristically present in the majority of meningiomas include the presence of prominent numbers of intermediate molecular weight filaments; this translates into vimentin immunoreactivity in the majority of these tumors. Complex interdigitating cell processes are a notable feature, particularly of the meningothelial variant. Hemidesmosomal zones are also frequently observed. On occasion, these ultrastructural features can be useful in attempting to distinguish between meningioma and other tumors that may resemble a meningioma, particularly when immunohistochemical studies prove to be inconclusive.

Immunohistochemistry

The immunohistochemical profile of meningiomas tends to be fairly nondescript [15]. The majority of meningiomas do stain with antibody to epithelial membrane antigens (EMA). In higher-grade tumors (atypical and anaplastic meningiomas), the immunoreactivity may not be present or may be only focally evident. As previously mentioned, vimentin immunoreactivity is found in almost all meningiomas. Unfortunately, this is a fairly nonspecific marker and not terribly helpful in differentiating meningioma from other tumor types. Immunoreactivity to a variety of other antibodies has been variably observed in meningiomas. In most of these instances, only a minority or subset of the tumors demonstrate immunoreactivity and often in a focal pattern or distribution. A variety of keratin markers may be variably positive in meningioma. S-100 immunoreactivity is observable in a minority of cases. As previously mentioned, CEA immunoreactivity may be evident in the secretory meningioma variant. Staining with a variety of other markers including claudin-1, CD99, bcl-2, and factor XIIIa has also been noted in a subset of these tumors [67]. Immunohistochemical studies have also confirmed the presence of hormonal receptors (estrogen, progesterone, androgen) in these tumors [68,69]. From a practical standpoint, manipulation of meningiomas by drug therapies targeting hormonal status has not been particularly successful. There may be some role in the evaluation of such markers in the setting of pregnant patients or patients with a concomitant breast or gynecologic malignancy in order to assess what effects hormonal manipulation of these tumors potentially have on the meningioma [70].

Cell Proliferation Markers

There is fairly sizable literature that has evaluated the potential role of cell proliferation markers in the assessment of meningiomas [71–80]. Not surprisingly, the rate of cell proliferation tends to correlate with the grade of tumor and the identification of mitotic activity in these lesions. A variety of modalities including flow cytometric studies, radiolabeling studies, as well as immunohistochemical studies have all confirmed this impression.

From a practical standpoint, the application of immunohistochemistry in the evaluation of meningiomas proves to be the most accessible and easily performed methodology. Antibodies such as Ki-67 and MIB-1 have been evaluated in a number of studies and may, under certain circumstances, provide some additional useful information (Fig. 5-21). Among a number of issues one needs to consider in assessing immunostaining with these antibodies in meningiomas is the fact that similar to gliomas, there is some degree of heterogeneity with regard to cell proliferation in meningiomas. The labeling index one observes is, therefore, dependent on the histologic section that is selected for staining and evaluation. There are also differences with regard to methodologies, interpretation of staining results, and determination of labeling indices that make extrapolation of labeling index ranges and cutoffs from one laboratory to the next inappropriate. The routine evaluation of meningiomas using such markers has yet to be substantiated. There may be a role in selected cases that appear histologically borderline with regard to grading. A higher labeling index in this scenario might be indicative of a potentially more aggressive-behaving, rapidly growing tumor. A low labeling index in this scenario is less useful because one is uncertain whether the low labeling index is a true indication of a low rate of cell proliferation in the tumor or whether it is the result of sampling.

Meningothelial Hyperplasia

Although frequently encountered in the setting of autopsy, meningothelial hyperplasia represents a poorly characterized entity and may cause some diagnostic confusion with meningioma [81]. The exact nature of this hyperplasia remains uncertain. There is some evidence to suggest in animals that hyperplasia may represent a precursor lesion to a subset of meningiomas. Such hyperplasias have been reported in a variety of clinical settings in association with increased age, trauma, renal failure, hemorrhage, and adjacent to certain neoplasms. Precise definitions of meningothelial hyperplasia are not available and are debated. Suggested guidelines range anywhere from 3–4 up to 10 cell layers thick. One recent study evaluating meningothelial hyperplasia noted that the immunohistochemical profile is similar to that of normal arachnoidal cap cells, suggesting that the meningothelial hyperplasia is more akin to a reactive process. More data are needed in this area to further assess this.

Meningioangiomatosis

Meningioangiomatosis is a relatively uncommon benign lesion, which is morphologically marked by a proliferation of meningothelial cells and blood vessels involving brain parenchyma and overlying meninges [82–86] (Fig. 5-22). Occasionally, the lesion is associated with an overlying meningioma. The entity was first described in 1915 by Bassoe and Nuzum [87]. The

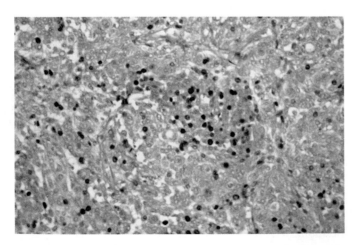

FIG. 5-21. A MIB-1 immunostaining of an anaplastic meningioma shows prominent brown nuclear staining. This tumor had a labeling index of 13.2% (MIB-1 immunostaining, original magnification 400×)

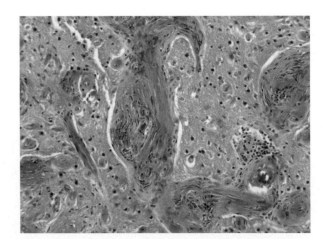

FIG. 5-22. Meningioangiomatosis represents a benign condition marked by an intraparenchymal proliferation of vessels surrounded by meningothelial cells (Hematoxylin and eosin, original magnification 200×)

lesion presents as a plaque-like or nodular mass within the cortex. The intervening brain tissue may show mineralization and gliosis. Mitotic activity, necrosis, and other features associated with a more aggressive behavior in meningiomas are generally not observed in this entity. Of particular note is the association of this lesion with neurofibromatosis type II [86].

Differential Diagnosis

The differential diagnosis, given the phenotypic variability of meningiomas, is quite extensive. Rather than trying to delineate every possible lesion that mimics meningioma, a few general comments are worth making. Since the immunohistochemical profile of meningioma is somewhat nondescript, differentiating other tumors from meningioma may sometimes rest on recognizing certain morphologic features suggestive of the other lesion or demonstrating a particular immunophenotypic characteristic of the other lesion. For example, schwannomas and fibrous meningiomas may be, at times, confused with one another. Both tumors may demonstrate S-100 protein immunoreactivity. The key may rest in recognizing features encountered with schwannoma (such as Verocay bodies) or in the recognition that S-100 immunoreactivity is usually very diffuse and strong in schwannomas, and when present in meningiomas, is often focal. Sometimes a panel of antibodies is required to distinguish one lesion from another, with recognition that a certain constellation of staining findings are more indicative of one tumor type versus another. A recent paper examining cytokeratin markers in separating malignant meningiomas from metastatic carcinoma, suggested that a panel of markers including Ber-EP4, CEA, B72.3, CD15 and vimentin are needed to separate the two [88]. Another paper attempting to distinguish anaplastic meningioma from meningeal hemangiopericytoma suggested evaluating a panel of antibodies including EMA, CD99, bcl-2, and claudin-1 along with certain molecular tests (fluorescent in situ hybridization [FISH] studies of chromosomes 1 p, 14 q, NF2, and 4.1B) [67]. Although tumor location is important, it is not necessarily synonymous with a diagnosis. In other words, not all dural-based tumors are meningiomas. Conversely, not all meningiomas are dural based. Careful attention to morphology will often yield clues that will guide one to the correct classification of the lesion. Where those clues are lacking, judicious use of immunohistochemistry and, on rare occasion, electron microscopy may provide additional help.

References

1. Cushing H. The meningiomas (dural endotheliomas): Their source and favoured seats of origin. Brain 1922; 45:282–316.
2. Oberling C. Les tumeurs des méninges. Bull Assoc Franc l'Etude Cancer 1922; 11:365–394.
3. Roussy G, Cornil L. Les tumeurs méningées. Ann d'Anat Path 1925; 2:63–79.
4. del Río Hortega P. Para el mejor conocimiento histológico de los meningoexoteliomas. Arch Españ Oncol. 1930; 1:477–570.
5. Bailey P, Bucy PC. The origin and nature of meningothelial tumors. Am J Cancer 1931; 15:15–54.
6. Cushing H, Eisenhardt L. Meningiomas: Their Classification, Regional Behavior, Life History and Surgical End Results. Charles C Thomas, Springfield, IL, 1938
7. Kernohan JW, Sayre GP. Tumors of the Central Nervous System. Armed Forces Institute of Pathology Fascicle, Washington, DC, 1952, pp. 97–117.
8. Zülch KJ. Histological Typing of Tumours of the Central Nervous System. World Health Organization, Geneva, 1979.
9. Kepes JJ. Meningiomas. Biology, Pathology and Differential Diagnosis. Masson Publishing, New York, 1982.
10. Louis DN, Scheithauer BW, Budka H, et al. Meningiomas. In: Tumours of the Nervous System (Kleihues P, Cavenee WK, eds.). IARC Press, Lyon, 2000, pp. 176–184.
11. Criscuolo GR, Symon L. Intraventricular meningioma. A review of 10 cases of the National Hospital, Queen Square (1974–1985) with reference to the literature. Acta Neurochirurgica 1986; 83:83–91.
12. Courville CB. Notes on the pathology of cranial tumors; hyperostoses-primary, secondary and neoplastic. Bull Los Angeles Neurol Soc 1947; 12:6–37.
13. Wall AE. Meningiomas within the lateral ventricle. J Neurol Neurosurg Psychiat 1954; 17:91–103.
14. Dunn J Jr, Kernohan JW. Observations on the origin of meningioma from the choroid plexus of the lateral ventricle. Proc Staff Meetings Mayo Clin 1956; 31:25–30.
15. Bruner JM, Tien RD, Enterline DS. Tumors of the meninges and related tissues. In: Russell and Rubinsteins Pathology of Tumors of the Nervous System (Bigner DD, McLendon RE, Bruner JM, eds.). Arnold Press, London, 1998, pp. 69–139.
16. Helle TL, Conley FK. Haemorrhage associated with meningioma: a case report and review of the literature. J Neurol Neurosurg Psychiat 1980; 43:725–729.
17. Kleinman GM, Liszczak T, Tarlov E, et al. Microcystic variant of meningioma. A light microscopic and ultrastructural study. Am J Surg Pathol 1980; 4:383–389.
18. Michard J, Gagné F. Microcystic meningioma. Clinicopathologic report of eight cases. Arch Pathol Lab Med 1983; 107:75–80.
19. Kepes J. The fine structure of hyaline inclusions (pseudopsammoma bodies) in meningiomas. J Neuropathol Exp Neurol 1975; 34:282–289.
20. Alguacil-Garcia A. Pettigrew NM, Sima AAF. Secretory meningioma. A distinct subtype of meningioma. Am J Surg Pathol 1986; 10:102–111.
21. Kubota T, Hirano A, Yamamoto S. The fine structure of hyaline inclusions in meningioma. J Neuropathol Exp Neurol 1982; 41:81–6.
22. Louis DN, Hamilton AJ, Sobel RA, et al. Pseudopsammomatous meningioma with elevated serum carcinoembryonic antigen: a true secretory meningioma. Case report. J Neurosurg 1991; 74:129–132.
23. Buhl R, Huga H-H, Mihajlovic HM. Secretory meningiomas: Clinical and immunohistochemical observations. Neurosurgery 2001; 48:297–302.
24. Philippon J, Foncin JF, Grob R, et al. Cerebral edema associated with meningiomas: possible role of a secretory-excretory phenomenon. Neurosurgery 1984; 14:295–301.

25. Banerjee AK, Blackwood W. A subfrontal tumour with the features of plasmocytoma and meningioma. Acta Neuropathol1971; 18:84–88.

26. Horten BC, Urich H, Stefoski D. Meningiomas with conspicuous plasma cell-lymphocytic components. A report of five cases. Cancer 1979; 43:258–264.

27. Stam FC, van Alphen HAM, Boorsma DM. Meningioma with conspicuous plasma cell components. A histopathological and immunohistochemical study. Acta Neuropathol 1980; 49:241–243.

28. Dahmen HG. Studies on mucous substances in myxomatous meningiomas. Acta Neuropathol 1979; 48:235–237.

29. Kepes JJ. Lipidized meningothelial tumor cells in "xanthomatous" meningioma express macrophage antigen. J Neuropathol Exp Neurol 1994; 53:384–388.

30. Le Roux P, Hope A, Lofton S, et al. Lipomatous meningioma – an uncommon tumor with distinct radiographic findings. Surg Neurol 1989; 32:360–365.

31. Salibi SS, Nauta HJ, Brem H, Epstein JI, Cho KR. Lipomeningioma: report of three cases and review of the literature. Neurosurgery 1989; 25:122–126.

32. Lattes R, Bigotti G. Lipoblastic meningioma: 'Vacuolated meningioma.' Hum Pathol 1991; 22:164–171.

33. Friede RL, Yasargil MG. Suprasellar neoplasm with a granular cell component. J Neuropathol Exp Neurol 1977; 36:769–782.

34. Müller W, Dahmen HG. Iron-induced atypical meningioma cells? Acta Neuropathologica 1979; 48:231–234.

35. Kawasaki K, Takahashi H, Kaneko H, et al. Novel eosinophilic intractyoplasmic inclusions in a meningioma. Cancer 1993; 72:2675–2679.

36. Yamada S, Kawai R, Sano T, et al. Intracytoplasmic granulofilamentous inclusion bodies in a meningioma. Immunohistochemical and ultrastructural studies. Arch Pathol Lab Med 1994; 118:849–851.

37. Rim NR, Im S-H, Chung CK, et al. Sclerosing meningioma: immunohistochemical analysis of five cases. Neuropathol Appl Neurobiol 2004; 30:126–135.

38. Roncaroli F, Riccioni L, Cerati M, et al. Oncocytic meningioma. Am J Surg Pathol 1997; 21:375–382.

39. Zorludemir S, Scheithauer BW, Hirose T, et al. Clear cell meningioma: a clinicopathologic study of a potentially aggressive variant of meningioma. Am J Surg Pathol 1995; 19:493–505.

40. Holtzman RN, Jormark SC. Nondural-based lumbar clear cell meningioma. Case report. J Neurosurg 1996; 84:264–266.

41. Couce ME, Aker FV, Scheithauer BW. Chordoid meningioma. A clinicopathologic study of 42 cases. Am J Surg Pathol 2000; 24:899–905.

42. Kepes JJ, Chen WY, Connors MH, et al. "Chordoid" meningeal tumours in young individuals with peritumoural lymphoplasmacellular infiltrates causing systemic manifestations of the Castleman syndrome. A report of seven cases. Cancer 1988; 62:391–406.

43. Zuppan CW, Liwnicz BH, Weeks DA. Meningioma with chordoid features. Ultrastruct Pathol 1994; 18:29–32.

44. de la Monte SM, Flickinger J, Linggood RM. Histopathologic features predicting recurrence of meningiomas following subtotal resection. Am J Surg Pathol 1986; 10:836–843.

45. Deprez RHL, Riegman PH, von Drunen E, et al. Cytogenetic, molecular genetic and pathological analyses in 126 meningiomas. J Neuropathol Exp Neurol 1995; 54:224–235.

46. Jääskeläinen J. Seemingly complete removal of histologically benign intracranial meningioma: late recurrence rate and factors predicting recurrence in 657 patients. A multivariate analysis. Surg Neurol 1986; 26:461–469.

47. Mahmood A, Caccamo DV, Tomecek FJ, et al. Atypical and malignant meningiomas: a clinicopathological review. Neurosurgery 1993; 33:955–963.

48. Maier H, Ofner D, Hittmair A, et al. Classic, atypical, and anaplastic meningioma: three histopathological subtypes of clinical relevance. J Neurosurg 1992; 77:616–623.

49. Miller DC. Predicting recurrence of intracranial meningiomas. A multivariate clinicopathologic model: interim report of the New York University Medical Center Meningioma Project. Neurosurg Clin North Am 1994; 5:193–200.

50. Perry A, Stafford SL, Scheithauer BW, Suman VJ, Lohse CM. Meningioma grading: an analysis of histologic parameters. Am J Surg Pathol 1997; 21:1455–1465.

51. Skullerud K, Löken AC. The prognosis in meningiomas. Acta Neuropathol (Berl) 1974; 29:337–344.

52. Ng H-K, Poon W-S, Goh K, et al. Histopathology of post-embolized meningioma. Am J Surg Pathol 1996; 20:1224–1230.

53. Ludwin SK, Rubinstein LJ, Russell DS. Papillary meningiomas: a malignant variant of meningioma. Cancer 1975; 36: 1363–1373.

54. Pasquier B, Gasnier F, Pasquier D, et al. Papillary meningioma. Clinicopathologic study of seven cases and review of the literature. Cancer 1986; 58:299–305.

55. Kepes JJ, Moral LA, Wilkinson SB, et al. Rhabdoid transformation of tumor cells in meningiomas: a histologic indication of increased proliferative activity. Report of four cases. Am J Surg Pathol 1998; 22:231–238.

56. Perry A, Stafford SL, Scheithauer BW, et al. "Rhabdoid" meningioma: An aggressive variant. J Neuropathol Exp Neurol 1998; 57:488.

57. Prayson RA. Malignant meningioma. A clinicopathologic study of 23 patients including MIB1 and p53 immunohistochemistry. Am J Clin Pathol 1996; 105:719–726.

58. Perry A, Scheithauer BW, Stafford SL, et al. "Malignancy" in meningiomas. A clinicopathologic study of 116 patients, with grading implications. Cancer 1999; 85:2046–2056.

59. Miller DC, Ojemann RG, Proppe KH, et al. Benign metastasizing meningioma. J Neurosurg 1985; 62:763–766.

60. Stoller JK, Kavuru M, Mehta AC, et al. Intracranial meningioma metastatic to the lung. Cleve Clin J Med 1987; 56:521–527.

61. Napolitano L, Kyle R, Fisher ER. Ultrastructure of meningiomas and their deviation and nature of their cellular components. Cancer 1963; 17:233–241.

62. Humeau C, Vic P, Sentein P, et al. The fine structure of meningiomas: An attempted classification. Virchows Arch A Pathological Anat Histol 1979; 382:201–216.

63. Copeland DD, Bell SW, Shelburne JD. Hemidesmosome-like intercellular specializations in human meningiomas. Cancer 1978; 41:2242–2249.

64. Márquez H, Díaz-Flores L, Caballero T, et al. Histogenesis of hemidesmosome-like intercellular specializations in meningioma. Morfología Normal y Patológica 1979; B3:33–41.

65. Goldman JE, Horoupian DS, Johnson AB. Granulofilamentous inclusions in a meningioma. Cancer 1980; 46:156–161.

66. Robertson DM. Electron microscopic studies of nuclear inclusions in meningiomas. Am J Pathol 1964; 45:835–848.

67. Rajaram V, Brat DJ, Perry A. Anaplastic meningioma versus meningeal hemangiopericytoma: Immunohistochemical and genetic markers. Hum Pathol 2004; 35:1413–1418.

68. Carroll RS, Zhang J, Dashner K, et al. Androgen receptor expression in meningiomas. J Neurosurg 1995; 82:453–460.
69. Khalid H. Immunohistochemical study of estrogen receptor-related antigen, progesterone and estrogen receptors in human intracranial meningiomas. Cancer 1994; 74:679–685.
70. Mehta D, Khatib R, Patel S. Carcinoma of the breast and meningioma. Association and management. Cancer 1983; 51:1937–1940.
71. Abramovich CM, Prayson RA. MIB-1 labeling indices in benign, aggressive, and malignant meningiomas: A study of 90 tumors. Hum Pathol 1998; 29:1420–1427.
72. Hsu DW, Pardo FS, Efird JT, et al. Prognostic significance of proliferative indices in meningiomas. J Neuropathol Exp Neurol 1994; 53:247–255.
73. Iwaki T, Takeshita I, Fukui M, et al. Cell kinetics of the malignant evolution of meningothelial meningiomas. Acta Neuropathol 1987; 74:243–247.
74. Jääskeläinen J, Haltia M, Laasonen E, et al. The growth rate of intracranial meningiomas and its relationship to histology: An analysis of 43 patients. Surg Neurol 1985; 24:165–172.
75. Lanzafame S, Torrisi A, Barbagallo G, et al. Correlation between histological grade, MIB-1, p53, and recurrence in 69 completely resected primary intracranial meningiomas with a 6 year mean follow-up. Pathol Res Pract 2000; 196:483–488.
76. Lee KS, Hoshino T, Rodriguez LA, et al. Bromodeoxyuridine labeling study of intracranial meningiomas: proliferative potential and recurrence. Acta Neuropathol 1990; 80:311–317.
77. Ohta M, Iwaki T, Kitamoto T, et al. MIB1 staining index and scoring of histologic features in meningioma: Indicators for the prediction of biologic potential and postoperative management. Cancer 1994; 74:3176–3189.
78. Salmon I, Kiss R, Levivier M, et al. Characterization of nuclear DNA content, proliferation index, and nuclear size in a series of 181 meningiomas, including benign primary, recurrent, and malignant tumors. Am J Surg Pathol 1993; 17:239–247.
79. Spaar FW, Ahyai A, Blech M. DNA-fluorescence cytometry and prognosis (grading) of meningiomas. A study of 104 surgically removed tumors. Neurosurg Rev 1987; 10:35–39.
80. Zimmer C, Gottschalk J, Cervos-Navarro J, et al. Proliferating cell nuclear antigen (PCNA) in atypical and malignant meningiomas. Path Res Pract 1992; 188:951–958.
81. Perry A, Lusis EA, Gutmann DH. Meningothelial hyperplasia: A detailed clinicopathologic, immunohistochemical and genetic study of 11 cases. Brain Pathol 2005; 15:109–115.
82. Halper J, Scheithauer BW, Okazaki H, et al. Meningio-angiomatosis: A report of six cases with special reference to the occurrence of neurofibrillary tangles. J Neuropath Exp Neurol 1986; 45:426–446.
83. Prayson RA. Meningioangiomatosis. A clinicopathologic study including MIB1 immunoreactivity. Arch Pathol Labl Med 1995; 119:1061–1064.
84. Wiebe S, Munoz DG, Smith S, et al. Meningioangiomatosis. A comprehensive analysis of clinical and laboratory features. Brain 1999; 122:709–726.
85. Sakaki S, Nakagawa K, Nakamura K, et al. Meningioangiomatosis not associated with von Recklinghausen's disease. Neurosurgery 1987; 20:797–801.
86. Stemmer-Rachamimov AO, Horgan MA, Taratuto AL, et al. Meningioangiomatosis is associated with neurofibromatosis 2 but not with somatic alterations of the NF2 gene. J Neuropath Exp Neurol 1997; 56:485–489.
87. Bassoe P, Nuzum F. Report of a case of central and peripheral neurofibromatosis. J Nerv Ment Dis 1915; 42:785–796.
88. Liu Y, Sturgis CD, Bunker M, et al. Expression of cytokeratin by malignant meningiomas: diagnostic pitfall of cytokeratin to separate malignant meningiomas from metastatic carcinoma. Mod Pathol 2004; 17:1129–1133.

6

Natural History, Growth Rates, and Recurrence

Kyung Gi Cho

Introduction

Meningiomas are common intracranial tumors that have been considered benign because of their slow growth rates and the feasibility of surgical cure. Approximately 3% of people older than 60 years of age have been reported to harbor an asymptomatic meningioma at autopsy [1]. Recent advances in neuroimaging and its wider availability, in addition to an increase in the aging population in developed countries, have resulted in the increased incidence of incidental meningiomas. The natural history of untreated meningiomas, however, is not completely clear. In the past, most patients with meningioma presented with neurological symptoms caused by sizable tumors, requiring surgical removal and/or radiation therapy to improve their symptoms and neurological deficits. Understanding the natural history of any disease is critical, as it forms the basis for treatment. The increased detection of incidental meningiomas has provided opportunities to study and better understand the natural history and growth rates of meningiomas.

Natural History of Meningiomas

Most studies of the natural history of meningiomas conducted on patients with incidental tumors have found that the majority of these tumors showed minimal growth, with the majority of patients remaining asymptomatic during the follow-up period [2–6]. For example, in a retrospective study of 60 patients, all 57 who were available for clinical evaluation remained asymptomatic during a mean follow-up period of 32 months [2]. Among the 45 patients who had follow-up imaging, 35 (77.8%) showed no tumor growth during the mean follow-up period of 29 months, while the other 10 patients showed an average tumor growth rate of 2.4 mm/year during the mean follow-up period of 47 months [3]. More recently, 43 of 63 patients (68.3%) with asymptomatic meningiomas showed no increase in tumor size during an average follow-up period of 36.6 months [3]. In a retrospective analysis of the natural history of 51 conservatively treated meningiomas in 43 patients, with a mean follow-up period of 67 months, 2 (4.7%) of these patients became symptomatic and 32 tumors (37%) in 16 patients grew, with a mean growth rate of 4 mm/year.

In most of these studies, the tumor size was calculated by measuring the largest diameter in the anterior-posterior, medio-lateral, or oblique dimension. However, measuring the exact growth rate of benign brain tumors is difficult due to their diverse configurations and directions of growth. To more accurately assess tumor growth, several studies have utilized volumetric measurement methods. For example, in a retrospective study of tumor growth rate in 37 patients, annual growth rates were calculated as the difference in tumor volume between the initial and latest imaging, divided by the time interval (years) between these determinations, with tumor growth defined as an annual increase in tumor volume >1 cm^3/year; in this study, 9 of the 37 patients (24.3%) showed tumor growth [5]. In a study using serial imaging to determine tumor growth of 47 incidental meningiomas, tumor growth rates were calculated as absolute growth rate (cm^3/year), relative growth rate (%/year), and tumor volume doubling time (year) [6]. Among these 47 patients, 6 (12.8%) underwent surgery, and the remaining 41 were managed conservatively, with a mean follow-up period of 43 months. Of the 41 conservatively managed patients, 27 (66%) showed absolute tumor growth rates of <1 cm^3/yr, although the overall absolute growth rates ranged from 0.03 to 2.62 cm^3/year (mean, 0.796 cm^3/year), the relative annual growth rates ranged from 0.48 to 72.8% (mean, 14.6%), and the tumor-doubling time ranged from 1.27 to 143.5 years (mean, 21.6 years). In this same study, what is notable is that all 41 tumors eventually showed varying degrees of growth when followed for up to 105 months.

In addition to understanding the natural history of meningiomas, identification of risk factors that predict tumor growth is important for planning therapeutic strategies. For example, when clinical and radiological characteristics were compared in groups of patients who did or did not experience increases in tumor size during follow-up, the age, tumor size, or all were found not to be important risk factors for growth [3].

However, asymptomatic meningiomas showing calcification on computed tomography (CT) scans and/or hypointensity on T2-weighted magnetic resonance (MR) images appeared to have a slower growth rate [3], a finding supported by two other studies [4,6]. In addition, tumor growth was associated with sphenoid ridge location [4] and with patient age, with the mean growth rate of tumors being higher in patients younger than 60 years when compared to older patients [4,6]. In contrast, another study found no significant correlation between tumor growth and patient age, length of follow-up period, or tumor volume [5]. However, multivariate analysis revealed that the likelihood of tumor growth was independently and significantly higher in younger patients and in those with increased tumor volume at initial diagnosis. Despite many papers suggesting a relatively benign course of incidental meningiomas found in the elderly, a significant percentage of those tumors grow, eventually becoming symptomatic.

For example, in a study of 40 patients (32 women, 8 men) over 70 years old (mean age, 76.1 years; range, 70–95 years) with asymptomatic meningiomas, over a mean follow-up period of 38.4 months, 14 patients (35%) showed tumor growth and 5 became symptomatic [7]. Most of these 14 tumors showed growth 6 months to 2 years after diagnosis. Based on imaging analysis, tumor calcification was associated with lack of growth, and moderate to large size (>30 mm) at initial diagnosis was related to subsequent tumor growth. These findings suggest that elderly patients with asymptomatic meningiomas be kept under careful clinical observation, with repeated imaging studies, because some tumors grew and became symptomatic. When considering surgery for elderly patients, however, the surgeon should be aware of the significantly increased risks of surgery in this group compared to the younger population [8–10].

The above findings suggest that many asymptomatic meningiomas, especially those with calcification and/or hypointense or isointense T2 signals, show only minimal growth and may be kept under clinical and radiological observation without the initial need for surgical intervention. Younger patients, however, should be kept under closer observation due to the higher growth potential of tumors in this group of patients. Although initial tumor size is not a predictive factor for tumor growth per se, patients with large asymptomatic meningiomas should also be kept under close observation. Since some patients, albeit a small number, showed a rapid increase in tumor volume [5], therapeutic strategies should be carefully determined for each individual patient with an incidental meningioma.

Limited data are available on the natural history of skull base meningiomas. A retrospective analysis of 40 patients with meningiomas, predominantly involving the cavernous sinus, anterior clinoid, or petroclival region, who either were never treated or received delayed treatment, found that 11 (27.5%) of these tumors were discovered incidentally during imaging studies performed for other reasons [11]. Radiographically significant brain stem compression was present in 23 patients (57.5%), and the carotid artery was encased in 21 (52.5%) patients and occluded in 3 (7.5%). During a mean clinical follow-up of 83 months, 11 patients (27.5%) experienced neurological progression in the form of new or worsening cranial neuropathy. However, this tumor-related clinical progression was generally mild and in most instances did not change the patient's ability to function. Despite imaging showing alarming brain stem compression at diagnosis, none of the 23 patients developed hemiparesis or long tract signs. During mean radiographic follow-up of 76 months, 7 patients (17.5%) experienced radiographic tumor growth. Of the 40 patients, 16 eventually underwent surgery and/or radiation therapy. The authors concluded that skull base meningiomas that appear very formidable on imaging analysis can be very indolent tumors, often demonstrating no radiographic growth and no progression of symptoms over many years. Although the authors did not advocate that these lesions be left untreated, they did suggest that the indolent behavior of some skull base meningiomas be considered when selecting a treatment plan and when evaluating the potential benefits of surgery and/or radiation.

In a cooperative retrospective study of 21 patients with petroclival meningiomas, 9 (43%) were incidentally diagnosed in the absence of clinical signs, and the remaining 12 (57%) were treated conservatively because of medical contraindications for surgery [12]. During a mean follow-up period of 82 months, 50% of the initially asymptomatic patients developed some kind of cranial nerve deficit. The functional deterioration was mild (10-point change in the Karnofsky index) for 2 patients, moderate (20-point change) for 4 patients, and severe (≥30-point change) for 4 patients, but 11 patients (52%) showed no change in Karnofsky index. During follow-up monitoring, radiological tumor growth was observed in 16 (76%) patients; in these 16, the mean growth rate was 1.16 mm/year in diameter and 1.10 cm^3/year in volume. Ten (62.5%) of the patients with growing tumors showed functional deterioration. Small (maximal tumor diameter <2 cm) to medium-sized (2–3 cm) tumors tended to grow more rapidly than larger tumors, but the difference was not statistically significant. The authors suggested that since most petroclival meningiomas are growing, with small and medium-size tumors being more prone to growth, active treatment of symptomatic patients with small or medium-sized tumors is mandatory.

The two series described above reported very different findings on the natural history of skull base meningiomas. It is difficult to obtain exact measurements of volume or maximal diameter of skull base meningiomas, however, due to their infratentorial location and their irregular configuration. This, in addition to the lack of published data, makes the natural history of skull base meningiomas unclear and suggests that optimal treatment of these tumors should be decided on an individual basis.

Summarizing what is known about the meningioma's natural history, 22–37% of the observed tumors progressed. However, there are several critical limitations in the studies performed to elucidate the natural history. First and foremost, there is a serious selection bias in that only elderly and asymptomatic patients were selected for observation. Additionally, the follow-up period, ranging between 29 and 67 months, is too short to adequately study slow-growing benign tumors such as meningiomas. Moreover, since the patients who were observed had no histological confirmation, not all tumors that were included in these studies may have been true meningiomas. It is important to realize that meningiomas are neoplastic lesions, nonetheless, and given long enough follow-up, most if not all meningiomas will eventually grow.

Growth Rates

Although most meningiomas are slowly growing benign tumors, some show aggressive or malignant behavior. The grading system for meningiomas was recently revised. In the updated World Health Organization (WHO) 2000 classification scheme for the central nervous system tumors, completely benign meningiomas are considered grade I, atypical meningiomas are labeled grade II, and anaplastic or malignant meningiomas are classified as grade III [13]. The criteria for malignancy are hypercellularity, the loss of normal tissue architecture, nuclear pleomorphism, mitotic index, tumor necrosis, and brain invasion. Brain invasion and increased mitotic index are histological predictors of meningioma recurrence. Mean tumor doubling time was found to vary according to the histological grade: 425 days (range, 138–1045 days) for grade I, 178 days (range, 34–551 days) for grade II, and 205 days (range, 30–472 days) for grade III, with the difference between grade I and grades II/III being highly significant [14]. However, these growth rates have wide ranges and there are significant overlaps among the different grades.

Although atypical and anaplastic meningiomas are more prone to progress aggressively and recur [13,15], some benign meningiomas also recur and display unpredictable clinical behavior. Biological behavior indicative of proliferative activity can predict meningioma recurrence. Among the methods used to evaluate proliferative activity are mitotic index, quantitation of proliferative cell nuclear antigen (PCNA), and argyrophilic nucleolar-organizer regions (AgNORs), BUdR labeling index (LI), Ki-67/MIB-1 LI, and flow cytometry.

Mitotic index has been traditionally considered to roughly correlate with tumor growth and recurrence, but it has limited value in predicting tumor doubling time [14]. In addition, the mitosis rate of malignant meningiomas is too low to measure properly, and the distribution of mitotic figures is too inconsistant to provide a basis for a reliable estimate of prognosis.

Evaluation of proliferative activity using BUdR LI is a useful adjunct to conventional histopathology for assessing malignancy and growth rate, as well as predicting recurrence. Tumor doubling time (Td) can be estimated using the formula, $Td = 500 \times Exp(-0.73 \times LI)$, where Exp signifies the natural log base. By predicting meningioma growth rate, the BUdR LI may supplement histopathological diagnosis and improve both the prognosis and the design of treatment modalities in individual patients.

The monoclonal antibody (moAb) Ki-67 recognizes a nuclear antigen that appears in all phases of the cell cycle except G0. The Ki-67 LI has been found to range between 9.3 and 20.5 in anaplastic meningiomas and between 0 and 15.4 in grade I and II meningiomas, indicating that Ki-67 LI increases with increasing histological grade.

Although the BUdR LI is considered the most reliable and predictable index for the growth of brain tumors, it is obtained by intravenous injection of a potentially mutagenic and myelosuppressive agent. In contrast, Ki-67 LI can be obtained without any preoperative treatment, but it must be obtained postoperatively from frozen sections. There is also considerable interobserver and interlaboratory variability in Ki-67 LI. In addition, prolonged storage causes the Ki-67 antigen to degrade, making Ki-67 LI unreliable for retrospectively evaluating proliferation [18,19].

A modification of the Ki-67 LI, using MIB-1 mAb, has proven useful in retrospectively evaluating proliferation using long preserved paraffin sections [20–23]. The immunostaining patterns of Ki-67 and MIB-1 are identical [21,24,25], and the statistically significant correlation between MIB-1 and BUdR measurements [26] indicates that MIB-1 LI can be used instead of BUdR LI to determine the proliferative potential of meningiomas.

MIB-1 LI has been shown to be the most important criterion for distinguishing anaplastic (mean 11%) from atypical (mean 2.1%) meningiomas. A recent MIB-1–labeling study has been used to evaluate the biological activity of meningiomas and to predict their clinical behavior [27–29].

Meningiomas are known to become larger during pregnancy and during the luteal phase of the menstrual cycle, suggesting that their growth may be dependent on female hormones. In addition, Ki-67 expression was found to be inversely correlated with progesterone receptor (PR) concentration, both in paraffin tissues and in cell culture [23,30]. Most malignant meningiomas are PR negative, suggesting a loss of PR during tumor progression [31–33].

Recurrence

Many studies have identified factors predicting meningioma recurrence, including the extent of surgical resection, histopathological grading, and biological potential.

The Extent of Resection and Recurrence

In 1957, Simpson [34] introduced a five-grade classification of surgical removal of meningiomas, which correlated well with tumor recurrence (Table 6-1). The rates of tumor recurrence at 5 years relative to extent of resection were 9% following grade I removal, 19% in grade II, 29% in grade III, and 44% in grade IV, respectively. Subsequent studies have also

TABLE 6-1. Simpson Grade

Grade I	Macroscopically complete tumor removal with excision of the tumor's dural attachment and any abnormal bone
Grade II	Macroscopically complete tumor removal with coagulation of its dural attachment
Grade III	Macroscopically complete removal of the intradural tumor without resection or coagulation of its dural attachment or extradural extensions
Grade IV	Subtotal removal of the tumor
Grade V	Simple decompression of the tumor

Source: From Ref. 34.

found that recurrence rates were dependent on the extent of surgical resection [34,35]. Of 257 surgically resected patients, 57 (22%) experienced tumor recurrence during a mean follow-up of 9 years (range 6 months to 22 years), 11% in patients following grade I resection, 22% in grade II, 50% in grade III, 37% in grade IV, and 100% in grade V, respectively [36].

Clusters of meningioma cells were later observed within the dura mater, at least 3 cm away from the attachment of the meningiomas, suggesting the need for the wide removal of dura mater to at least 4 cm from the dural attachment ("grade 0" surgery) in these patients [37,38]. Of 19 patients with convexity meningiomas, none experienced recurrence 5 years after surgery, suggesting that "grade 0" surgery may be a promising procedure in protecting against tumor recurrence [39].

In addition to wide dural excision, thick arachnoid membranes adjacent to meningiomas may be related to meningioma recurrence [40]. Clusters of meningioma cells were found to be embedded in resected thick arachnoid membranes contiguous to the meningiomas and normal arachnoid membranes. There was a significant difference in recurrence between Simpson's grade 1 surgery with and without extensive removal of surrounding thick arachnoid membranes. In general, therefore, surgical outcome and recurrence of meningiomas are dependent on the degree of resection of the tumor and the surrounding involved dura, arachnoid, and bone.

Tumor Location and Recurrence

Since the report by Simpson [34], most neurosurgeons have taken great care in the treatment of dural and calvarial attachments of meningiomas to reduce the recurrence rates. The degree of resection is practically dependent on the tumor location and, therefore, the accessibility of the tumor and the involved dura and bone [41]. A retrospective study of 225 patients found that tumor sites associated with a high percentage of total excisions had a low recurrence/progression rate [41]. That is, 96% of convexity meningiomas were totally resected, with a 3% recurrence rate at 5 years. In comparison, 58% of parasellar meningiomas were totally excised, with a 5-year recurrence rate of 19%, whereas only 28% of sphenoid ridge meningiomas were totally excised, with a 5-year recurrence rate of 34%.

In a study of 315 patients with cranial base meningiomas, the highest recurrence was observed in patients with medial sphenoid wing/clinoidal meningiomas and with those whose tumors invaded the cavernous sinus [42]. The 10-year recurrence rate in the above was 60–100%. Valuable insights into the behavior of subtotally resected petroclival meningiomas can be gained from a series of 38 tumors [43]. Although tumor progression occurred in 16 (42%) during a mean follow-up period of 47.5 months (range, 6–141 months), the growth rate of residual tumors was low (mean 0.37 cm/yr in diameter and 4.94 cc/year in volume). In 33 (87%) of these 38 patients, Karnofsky performance scale scores at last follow-up were 80 or above. Of 85 patients with petroclival meningiomas during a mean follow-up of 29.8 months (range 6–119 months), 15 (17.6%) experienced radiographic recurrence or progression, and tumor recurrence rates after grossly total resection did not differ significantly from that after near total resection [44].

Neuroradiological Findings and Recurrence

Meningiomas were traditionally regarded as extracerebral capsulated tumors, which separated readily from brain tissue [45]. However, approximately 5–10% of patients experienced tumor recurrence even following a Simpson grade 1 resection. Recurrence is thought to represent the continued proliferation of tumor cells left behind after resection. In about one third of all meningiomas, MR imaging showed thickening of the dura mater around the tumor attachment, the so-called "dural tail" [46–48]. The question arose as to whether this finding represents in vivo existence of the meningioma clusters, but histological studies of the dural tail have not always demonstrated meningioma cells [49–51].

The probability of brain invasion was found to increase by approximately 20% for each centimeter of edema, and the peritumoral edema grade was found to correlate with tumor recurrence after complete resection [52]. These findings suggested that brain invasion causes peritumoral edema and that the invaded brain tissue is the source of residual cells in cases of tumor recurrence after gross-total resection. In addition, peritumoral edema has also been reported to be significantly related to tumor aggressiveness and higher MIB-1 LI [53,54].

In an attempt to preoperatively identify groups of patients at high risk of recurrence, the clinicoradiological features of 101 patients who underwent macroscopically complete removal (Simpson grade I to III) of meningiomas were assessed [55]. Recurrent meningioma was diagnosed in 17 patients (16.8%) during a median follow-up period of 116 months. Multivariate analysis revealed that tumor shape was the only significant predictive factor for recurrence, and that other factors, including tumor size, relation to the major sinuses, calcification, characteristics of the tumor/brain interface, existence of dural tails, and even Simpson grade, were not. Both "mushrooming" and "lobulated" meningiomas were more likely to recur than "round" ones. The median interval for recurrence was 10 months for mushrooming tumors, 82 months for lobulated tumors, and 111 months for round tumors. A large prospective study is required to identify neuroradiological parameters that would predict tumor recurrence.

Histopathological Grade and Recurrence

Aggressive histology according to the histological subtyping (WHO grade II or III) is the second best established predictor of recurrence [52]. These subtypes represent a small proportion of meningiomas (approximately 8%) and are widely believed to carry significantly higher risk of recurrence.

In one study of 936 primary intracranial meningiomas, 94.3% was histologically benign (WHO grade I), 4.7% was atypical (grade II), and 1.0% anaplastic (grade III) [56]. Five years after complete removal, the recurrence rates were 3, 38, and 78%, respectively, and the median times to recurrence were 7.5, 2.4, and 3.5 years, respectively. Of 45 completely removed atypical meningiomas, 19 (42.2%) recurred, and these tumors had increased focal necrosis compared with non-recurrent atypical meningiomas.

To better understand the prognostic difference between atypical and malignant (anaplastic) meningiomas, the long-term prognosis was assessed in 42 patients with atypical meningiomas and 29 with malignant meningiomas [57]. The 3- and 5-year recurrence rates were 35 and 52%, respectively, for atypical meningiomas, and 80 and 84%, respectively, for malignant meningiomas. Recurrence-free survival and median time to recurrence were also significantly longer in patients with atypical than with malignant meningiomas: 11.9 versus 2 years, and 5 versus 2 years, respectively. Thus, most patients with atypical meningiomas had a better prognosis than did those with malignant meningiomas. However, the authors regarded the WHO classification system as inadequate for a minority of patients with atypical meningiomas, who survived only a few years.

Biological Potential and Recurrence

Recurrence is not limited to meningiomas with malignant histological features. Benign meningiomas also recur, especially following incomplete surgical resection. The risk of recurrence in individual patients cannot be predicted by histology alone. Estimation of their proliferative activities is very important for predicting recurrence. High mitotic index is a significant predictor for shorter progression-free interval. For example, the rate of recurrence was increased at least 10-fold when BUdR LI exceeded 1%, regardless of the histological nature of the tumors [58], and the proliferative potential of tumors could be more accurately predicted by BUdR LI than by histopathology [17,59]. In addition, the mean BUdR LI of recurrent tumors was found to be significantly higher than that of nonrecurrent tumors ($3.9 \pm 2.6\%$ vs $1.9 \pm 1.0\%$, $p = 0.005$) [59]. The recurrence rates were 30.6% for tumors with a BUdR LI of 1–5%, 55.6% for a BUdR LI of 3–5%, and 100% for a BUdR LI >5% [59]. In another study [60], the BUdR LI

of recurrent meningiomas ($3.77 \pm 1.22\%$) was significantly higher than that of nonrecurrent meningiomas ($0.77 \pm 0.13\%$), as was the Ki-67 LI ($14.78 \pm 3.17\%$ vs. $4.71 \pm 1.96\%$, respectively). These findings suggested that the clinical behavior of meningiomas may be determined more accurately from BUdR LI, Ki LI and tumor-doubling time than from the current histological criteria.

Although many investigators have shown a correlation between Ki-67 LI and recurrence-free interval [17,28,55,61], others found no correlation between Ki-67 LI and tumor behavior [62]. Because of the variation in Ki-67 LI among different laboratories, presumably due to differences in staining and counting methods and the heterogeneity of Ki-67-positive cells [63], there is no acceptable single cut-off point for Ki-67 LI, making it difficult to interpret its relationship to clinical behavior.

MIB-1 LI, however, showed a strong inverse correlation with log tumor volume doubling time ($p < 0.001$), indicating that proliferative activity, measured using MIB-1 LI, can predict the regrowth potential of a tumor after initial surgery [29].

In an assessment of the prognostic value of DNA flow cytometry, MIB-1 LI (equivalent to Ki-67 LI), and p53 protein expression for tumor recurrence in 425 patients who underwent gross total resection of meningioma, a MIB-1 labeling index (LI) of ≥4.2%, observed in 34 tumors (8%), was strongly associated with decreased recurrence-free survival [64]. Multivariate analysis showed a close association between MIB-1 LI and mitotic index, the latter being the parameter of greatest significance.

Survivin is a newly identified member of the family of proteins that inhibit apoptosis, which contributes to carcinogenesis by prolonging the life span of neoplastic cells. Survivin expression was inversely correlated with apoptotic index and was positively correlated with Ki-67 LI [62]. In addition, correlations among survivin expression, Ki-67 LI, and increased grade of meningiomas suggest that survivin may be an important marker for tumor recurrence or malignant behavior [65].

Mitosin is a 350kDa nuclear phosphoprotein involved in cell division and has been considered a suitable target for evaluating proliferation by immunohistochemistry [66]. It is expressed in the late G1, S, G2, and M phases of cell cycle but is absent in G0. The incidence of recurrence was shown to be higher in tumors with a mitosin LI higher than 3% than in those with a lower mitosin LI ($p = 0.048$) [67]. In a multivariate analysis, mitosin LI ($p = 0.035$) and Ki-67 LI ($p = 0.032$), along with tumor size, were shown to provide independent prognostic information, beyond that obtained by standard clinical and pathological parameters. The prognostic information gained from mitosin LI was superior to that provided by other proliferation markers. In addition, the loss of progesterone expression in nonmalignant meningiomas was found to be an indicator of decreased apoptosis and early tumor recurrence [32].

References

1. Nakasu S, Hirano A, Shimura T, et al. Incidental meningiomas in autopsy study. Surg Neurol 1987;27:319–22.

2. Olivero WC, Lister JR, Elwood PW. The natural history and growth rate of asymptomatic meningiomas: a review of 60 patients. J Neurosurg 1995;83:222–4.

3. Kuratsu JI, Kochi M, Ushio Y. Incidence and clinical features of asymptomatic meningiomas. J Neurosurg 2000;92:766–70.

4. Herscovici Z, Rappaport Z, Sulkes J, et al. Natural history of conservatively treated meningiomas. Neurology 2004;63:1133–4.

5. Yoneoka Y, Fujii Y, Tanaka R. Growth of incidental meningiomas. Acta Neurochir (Wien) 2000;142:507–11.

6. Nakamura M, Roser F, Michel J, et al. The natural history of incidental meningiomas. Neurosurgery 2003;53:62–71.

7. Niiro M, Yatsushiro K, Nakamura K, et al. Natural history of elderly patients with asymptomatic meningiomas. J Neurol Neurosurg Psychiatry 2000;68:25–8.

8. Awad IA, Kalfas I, Hahn JF, et al. Intracranial meningiomas in the aged: surgical outcome in the era of computed tomography. Neurosurgery 1989;24:557–60.

9. Cornu P, Chatellier G, Dagreou F, et al. Intracranial meningiomas in elderly patients. Postoperative morbidity and mortality. Factors predictive of outcome. Acta Neurochir (Wien) 1990; 102:98–102.

10. Gijtenbeek JM, Hop WC, Braakman R, et al. Surgery for intracranial meningiomas in elderly patients. Clin Neurol Neurosurg 1993;95:291–5.

11. Bindal R, Goodman JM, Kawasaki A, et al. The natural history of untreated skull base meningiomas. Surg Neurol 2003;59:87–92.

12. Van Havenbergh T, Carvalho G, Tatagiba M, et al. Natural history of petroclival meningiomas. Neurosurgery 2003;52:55–64.

13. Louis DN, Scheithauer BW. Meningiomas. In: Kleihues P, Cavenee WK (eds.). WHO Classification of Tumor: Pathology and Genetics: Tumors of the Nervous System. Lyon: IARC, 2000:176–84.

14. Jaaskelainen J, Haltia M, Laasonen E, et al. The growth rate of intracranial meningiomas and its relation to histology. An analysis of 43 patients. Surg Neurol 1985;24:165–72.

15. Mahmood A, Caccamo DV, Tomecek FJ, et al. Atypical and malignant meningiomas: a clinicopathological review. Neurosurgery 1993;33:955–63.

16. Cho KG, Hoshino T, Nagashima T, et al. Prediction of tumor doubling time in recurrent meningiomas. Cell kinetics studies with bromodeoxyuridine labeling. J Neurosurg 1986;65:790–4.

17. Roggendorf W, Schuster T, Peiffer J. Proliferative potential of meningiomas determined with the monoclonal antibody Ki-67. Acta Neuropathol (Berl) 1987;73:361–4.

18. Giangaspero F, Doglioni C, Rivano MT, et al. Growth fraction in human brain tumors defined by the monoclonal antibody Ki-67. Acta Neuropathol (Berl) 1987; 4:179–82.

19. Holt PR, Moss SF, Kapetanakis AM, et al. Is Ki-67 a better proliferative marker in the colon than proliferating cell nuclear antigen? Cancer Epidemoid Biomarkers Prev 1997; 6:131–5.

20. Aguiar PH, Tatagiba M, Dankoweit-Timpe E, et al. Proliferative activity of acoustic neurilemomas without neurofibromatosis determined by monoclonal antibody MIB-1. Acta Neurochir (Wien) 1995;134:35–9.

21. Cattoretti G, Becker MHG, Key G, et al. Monoclonal antibodies against recombinant parts of the Ki-67 antigen (MIB 1 and MIB 3) detect proliferating cells in microwave-processed formalin-fixed paraffin sections. J Pathol 1992;168:357–63.

22. Munakata S, Hendricks JB. Effect of fixation time and microwave oven heating time on retrieval of the Ki-67 antigen from paraffin-embedded tissue. J Histochem Cytochem 1993;41:1241–6.

23. Nagashima G, Aoyagi M, Wakimoto H, et al. Immunohistochemical detection of progesterone receptors and the correlation with Ki-67 labelling indices in paraffin-embedded sections of meningiomas. Neurosurgery 1995;37:478–82.

24. Boker DK, Stark HJ. The proliferation rate of intracranial tumors as defined by the monoclonal antibody KI 67. Application of the method to paraffin embedded specimens. Neurosurg Rev 1988;11:267–72.

25. McCormick D, Chong H, Hobbs C, et al. Detection of the Ki-67 antigen in fixed and wax-embedded sections with the monoclonal antibody MIB1. Histopathology 1993;22:355–60.

26. Langford La, Cooksley CS, DeMonte F. Comparison of MIB-1 (Ki-67) antigen and bromodeoxyuridine proliferation indices in meningiomas. Hum Pathol 1996;27:350–4.

27. Ho DM, Hsu CY, Ting LT, et al. Histopathology and MIB-1 labelling index predicted recurrence of meningiomas: a proposal of diagnostic criteria for patents with atypical meningioma. Cancer. 2002;94(5):1538–47.

28. Kalala JP, Caemaert J, De Ridder L. Primary resected meningiomas: relapses and proliferation markers. In Vivo 2004;18:411–6.

29. Nakaguchi H, Fujimaki T, Matsuno A, et al. Postoperative residual growth of meningioma can be predicted by MIB-1 immunohistochemistry. Cancer 1999;85:2249–54.

30. Tonn JC, Ott MM, Bouterfa H, et al. Inverse correlation of cell proliferation and expression of progesterone receptors in tumor spheroids and monolayer cultures of human meningiomas. Neurosurgery 1997;41:1152–9.

31. Hsu DW, Efird JT, Hedley-Whyte ET. Progesterone and estrogen receptors in meningiomas: prognostic considerations. J Neurosurg 1997;86:113–20.

32. Konstantinidou AE, Korkolopoulou P, Mahera H, et al. Hormone receptors in non-malignant meningiomas correlate with apoptosis, cell proliferation and recurrence-free survival. Histopathology 2003;43:280–90.

33. Perry A, Cai DX, Scheithauer BW, et al. Merlin, DAL-1 and progesterone receptor expression in clinicopathologic subsets of meningioma: a correlative immunohistochemical study of 175 cases. J Neuropathol Exp Neurol 2000;59:872–9.

34. Simpson D. The recurrence of intracranial meningiomas after surgical treatment. J Neurol Neurosurg Psychiatry 1957;20: 22–39.

35. Adegbite AB, Khan MI, Paine KWE, et al. The recurrence of intracranial meningiomas after surgical treatment. J Neurosurg 1983;58:51–6.

36. Chan RC, Thompson GB. Morbidity, mortality, and quality of life following surgery for intracranial meningiomas. A retrospective study in 257 cases. J Neurosurg 1984;60:52–60.

37. Borovich B, Doron Y. Recurrence of intracranial meningiomas: the role played by regional multicentricity. J Neurosurg 1986;64:58–63.

38. Borovich B, Doron Y, Braun J, et al. Recurrence of intracranial meningiomas: the role played by regional multicentricity. Part 2: clinical and radiological aspects. J Neurosurg 1986;65:168–71.

39. Kinjo T, Al-Mefty O, Kanaan I. Grade zero removal of supratentorial convexity meningiomas. Neurosurgery 1993;33:394–9.

40. Kamitani H, Masuzawa H, Kanazawa I, et al. Recurrence of convexity meningiomas: tumor cells in the arachnoid membrane. Surg Neurol 2001;56:228–35.

41. Mirimanoff RO, Dosoretz DE, Linggood RM, et al. Meningioma: analysis of recurrence and progression following neurosurgical resection. J Neurosurg 1985;62:18–24.

42. Mathiesen T, Lindquist C, Kihlström L, et al. Recurrence of cranial base meningiomas. Neurosurgery 1996;39:2–9.

43. Jung HW, Yoo H, Paek SH, et al. Long-tern outcome and growth rate of subtotally resected petroclival meningiomas: experience with 38 cases. Neurosurgery 2000;46:567–75.

44. Little KM, Friedman AH, Sampson JH, et al. Surgical management of petroclival meningiomas: defining resection goals based on risk of neurological morbidity and tumor recurrence rates in 137 patients. Neurosurgery 2005;56:546–59.

45. Palma L. Why do meningiomas recur? J Neurosurg Sci 2003;47: 65–8.

46. Aoki S, Sasaki Y, Machida T, et al. Contrast-enhanced MR images in patients with meningioma: importance of enhancement of the dura adjacent to the tumor. AJNR Am J Neuroradiol 1990;11:935–8.

47. Goldsher D, Litt AW, Pinto RS, et al. Dural "tail" associated with meningiomas on Gd-DTPA-enhanced MR images: characteristics, differential diagnostic value, and possible implications for treatment. Radiology 1990;176:447–50.

48. Wilms G, Lammens M, Marchal G, et al. Thickening of dura surrounding meningiomas: MR features. J Comput Assist Tomogr 1989;13:763–8.

49. Nägele T, Peterson D, Klose U, et al. The "dural tail" adjacent to meningiomas studied by dynamic contrast-enhanced MRI: a comparison with histopathology. Neuroradiology 1994;36:303–7.

50. Nakau H, Miyazawa T, Tamai S, et al. Pathologic significance of meningeal enhancement ("flare sign") of meningiomas on MRI. Surg Neurol 1997;48:584–91.

51. Tokumaru A, O'uchi T, Eguchi T, et al. Prominent meningeal enhancement adjacent to meningioma on Gd-DTPA-enhanced MR images: histopathologic correlation. Radiology 1990;175:431–3.

52. Mantle RE, Lach B, Delgado MR, et al. Predicting the probability of meningioma recurrence based on the quantity of peritumoral brain edema on computerized tomography scanning. J Neurosurg 1999;91:375–83.

53. Aguiar PH, Tsanaclis AM, Tella OI Jr, et al. Proliferation rate of intracranial meningiomas as defined by the monoclonal antibody MIB-1: correlation with peritumoural oedema and other clinicoradiological and histoloical characteristics. Neurosurg Rev 2003;26:221–8.

54. Ide M, Jimbo M, Yamamoto M, et al: MIB-1 staining index and peritumoral brain edema of meningiomas. Cancer 1996;78: 133–43.

55. Nakasu S, Nakasu Y, Nakajima M, et al. Preoperative identification of meningiomas that are highly likely to recur. J Neurosurg 1999;90:455–62.

56. Jaaskelainen J, Haltia M, Servo A. Atypical and anaplastic meningiomas: radiology surgery, radiotherapy, and outcome. Surg Neurol 1986;25:233–42.

57. Palma L, Celli P, Franco C, et al. Long-term prognosis for atypical and malignant meningiomas: a study of 71 surgical cases. J Neurosurg 1997;86:793–800.

58. Hoshino T, Nagashima T, Murovic JA, et al. Proliferative potential of human meningiomas of the brain. A cell kinetics study with bromodeoxyuridine. Cancer 1986;58:1466–72.

59. Shibuya M, Hoshino T, Ito S, et al. Meningiomas: clinical implications of a high proliferative potential determined by bromodeoxyuridine labeling. Neurosurgery 1992; 30:494–8.

60. Kakinuma K, Tanaka R, Onda K, et al. Proliferative potential of recurrent intracranial meningiomas as evaluated by labelling indices of BUdR and Ki-67, and tumour doubling time. Acta Neurochir (Wien) 1998;140:26–32.

61. Ohta M, Iwaki T, Kitamoto T, et al. MIB1 staining index and scoring of histologic features in meningioma. Indicators for the prediction of biologic potential and postoperative management. Cancer 1994;74:3176–89.

62. Kawasaki H, Toyoda M, Shinohara H, et al. Expression of survivin correlates with apoptosis, proliferation, and angiogenesis during human colorectal tumorigenesis. Cancer 2001;91: 2026–32.

63. Siegers HP, Zuber P, Hamou MF, et al. The implications of the heterogeneous distribution of Ki-67 labelled cells in meningiomas. Br J Neurosurg 1989;3:101–7.

64. Perry A, Stafford SL, Scheithauer BW, et al. The prognostic significance of MIB-1, p53, and DNA flow cytometry in completely resected primary meningiomas. Cancer 1998;82:2262–9.

65. Kayaselcuk F, Zorludemir S, Bal N, et al. The expression of survivin and Ki-67 in meningiomas: correlation with grade and clinical outcome. J Neurooncol 2004;67:209–14.

66. Zhu X, Mancini MA, Chang KH, et al. Characterization of a novel 350-kilodalton nuclear phosphoprotein that is specifically involved in mitotic-phase progression. Mol Cell Biol 1995;15:5017–29.

67. Konstantinidou AE, Korkolopoulou P, Kavantzas N, et al. Mitosin, a novel marker of cell proliferation and early recurrence in intracranial meningiomas. Histol Histopathol 2003;18:67–74.

II
Diagnostic Considerations

7
Diagnostic Neuroradiology: CT, MRI, fMRI, MRS, PET, and Octreotide SPECT

Albert S. Chang and Jeffrey S. Ross

The majority of meningiomas exhibit highly stereotypic imaging characteristics, which, when combined with their select intracranial dural-adherent localizations, often facilitate their diagnosis without having to resort to invasive diagnostic procedures. Computed tomography (CT) and magnetic resonance imaging (MRI) are the most commonly utilized imaging modalities in such regard. Some intracranial lesions, however, exhibit imaging findings or biologic behavior that are not entirely consistent with benign meningiomas. Such lesions may require additional imaging modalities (e.g., MR spectroscopy, positron emission tomography [PET], or octreotide scintigraphy) as diagnostic problem solvers. This chapter will review the meningioma findings of each of these imaging modalities and, in addition, the potential applicability of spectroscopy and molecular imaging modalities. Meningiomas can also exhibit highly characteristic findings during angiographic examination, which are discussed in detail elsewhere.

Computed Tomography

Meningiomas are usually sharply circumscribed lesions with well-defined tumor/brain interface, which facilitate their identification as extra-axial lesions [1]. They appear as spherical or lobulated masses, or "en plaque" lesions, often surrounded by a cleft of arachnoid with entrapped cerebral spinal fluid (CSF) and vascularity [2]. The overlying dura may be infiltrated by tumor. Tumoral dural attachment can be broad or narrow, giving the tumors either sessile or pedunculated appearance. On nonenhanced CT, meningiomas appear isodense to slightly hyperdense relative to the adjacent brain parenchyma, likely due to microscopic psammomatous calcifications and/or compact cellular matrix [3]. Sometimes dense nodular calcifications are distributed throughout the tumor mass [4]. Examples of meningiomas with hyperdense appearance, or homogeneously dense calcifications, are shown in Figure 7-1.

Dense, homogeneous enhancement is typically seen following intravenous contrast administration [4]. Occasional heterogeneity in the tumor, both before and following contrast administration, is due to presence of blood products, necrosis, fat, or other tissue elements [5]. Peritumoral edema is commonly associated with meningiomas, but highly variable in extent possibly due to angiogenic factors [6].

Some meningiomas can either erode the adjacent bone or induce hyperostotic changes, which can be identified by MRI but are usually better evaluated by CT [7]. Other disease processes can also produce abnormal bony cortical thickening, such as metastatic prostate carcinoma or fibrous dysplasia. Fibrous dysplasia usually produces a "ground glass appearance" on plain films and CT and typically involves an entire bone structure. When involving the calvarium, fibrous dysplasia usually causes a "blistered" appearance due to focal bony expansion around a relatively lucent core [8]. These features are not associated with meningiomas, the hyperostotic foci of which are typically associated with adjacent soft tissue lesions, whereas fibrous dysplasia and metastatic prostate carcinoma are usually confined to the bone [9].

Magnetic Resonance Imaging

Meningiomas are typically isointense to slightly hypointense relative to the adjacent gray matter on nonenhanced T1- and T2-weighted (T1W and T2W) imaging, with a minority of lesions exhibiting slight hyperintensity on T2W imaging [10]. On fluid-attenuated inversion-recovery (FLAIR) pulse sequence, meningiomas are usually mildly hyperintense relative to gray matter [11]. Such signal characteristics are shown in Figure 7-2 for a biopsy-proven meningioma. Signal voids, representing either enlarged vessels or nodular calcifications, are sometimes identified within the tumor mass. Following intravenous gadolinium administration, meningiomas typically enhance in dense and homogeneous fashion. Such enhancement may include the adjoining meninges, giving rise to the linear "dural tail" sign, which reflect either tumor infiltration or elicited inflammation in the adjacent dura [12,13]. This sign has been associated with a variety of intracranial lesions and is therefore not specific for meningiomas [14].

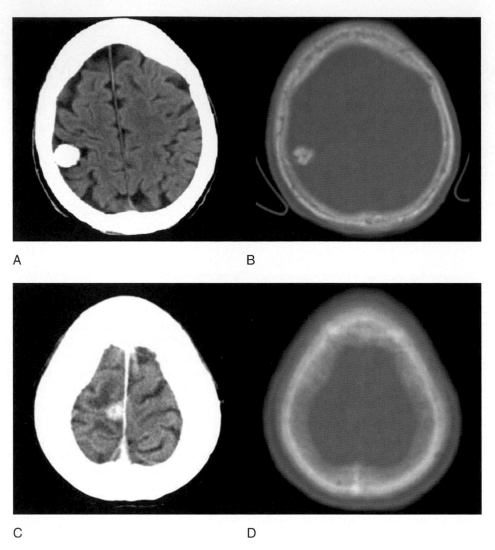

Fig. 7-1. Axial CT images of right frontal convexity meningiomas with dense internal calcification (A and B) and a right parasagittal meningioma with hyperdense appearance but no identifiable internal calcification (C and D). Each meningioma is displayed in brain parenchyma (A or C) and corresponding bone (B or D) windows, respectively, to help define the presence or absence of calcific matrix underlying the hyperdense appearance in both lesions

This MR sign is not readily discerned by contrast-enhanced CT imaging [15].

Meningiomas may extend through the dura and thereby remain extra-axial while moving from one intracranial fossa to another, or infiltrate the adventitia of blood vessels and either encase or narrow the involved vessels. More specifically, tumor invasion and occlusion of the superior sagittal sinus (which can be identified via MR venography, as shown in Fig. 7-3) have important surgical ramifications [16].

Akin to CT findings, tumoral heterogeneities as seen by MR imaging reflect presence of blood products, necrosis, and fat [17]. Cystic meningiomas are rare variants with histologic cystic changes characterized by focal hypointense T1W/hyperintense T2W signals but otherwise imaging features indistinguishable from other meningiomas [18; see Fig. 7-4]. Bony hyperostosis can manifest as increased signal void of the cortical bone (Fig. 7-5), which is better evaluated by CT. Tumoral erosion of the adjacent bone can on rare occasion provide unexpected communication with extracranial tissue space. This is most dramatically demonstrated by pneumatization of the underlying anterior clinoid process in a clinoid meningioma after its erosion into, and subsequent direct communication with, the ethmoid sinus (Fig. 7.6).

In addition to routine MRI pulse sequences, MR perfusion imaging may be useful in the diagnostic assessment of meningiomas. Differential considerations for a homogeneously

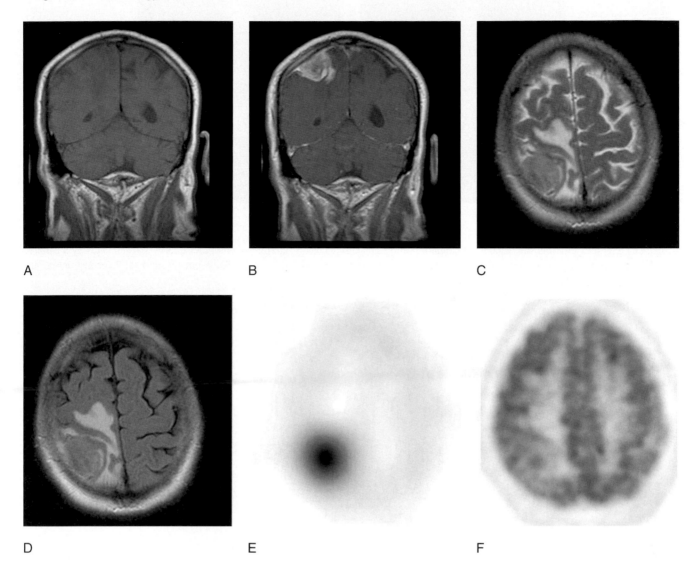

FIG. 7-2. MRI, ^{111}In-octreotide scintigraphy and ^{18}F-FDG PET of a biopsy-proven meningioma in the right frontoparietal convexity [38]. Coronal T1W pre- and postgadolinium (A and B), T2W (C) and FLAIR (D) images demonstrate an extradural lesion with avid gadolinium enhancement. Note the dural tails both medial and lateral to the lesion in (B). Slight internal heterogeneities following gadolinium administration may represent internal necrosis. This lesion is mildly hyperintense on T2 sequence, and iso- to mildly hyperintense on FLAIR sequence, with notable surrounding vasogenic edema on T2W and FLAIR images. Axial SPECT image from ^{111}In-octreotide scintigraphy (E) reveals focal radiotracer accumulation in the right parietal region, which corresponds to the MR findings. Axial ^{18}F-FDG PET image (F), however, demonstrates the isometabolism of this lesion relative to the surrounding grey matter. These imaging/scintigraphic findings are highly characteristic of meningiomas. On histologic analysis, this lesion exhibited local invasion of adjacent brain parenchyma, but such "malignant" behavior is not evident on imaging [38]

enhancing lesion near the cerebellopontine angle include meningioma and schwannoma, which are often indistinct by conventional MRI. Meningiomas typically appear as rapidly perfusing, hypervascular tumors, whereas schwannomas are typically hypovascular or avascular lesions [9]. Differentials in relative cerebral blood volume (rCBV) of a dural-based tumor may also help to distinguish meningiomas from dural metastases [19]. Some initial findings even suggest that differential rCBV may help to distinguish typical from atypical meningiomas [20]. Diffusion-weighted imaging (DWI), on the other hand, is incapable of discriminating meningiomas from intracranial gliomas or metastases [21,22]. DWI, however, may be helpful in differentiating benign from atypical/malignant meningiomas according to a prior study [23].

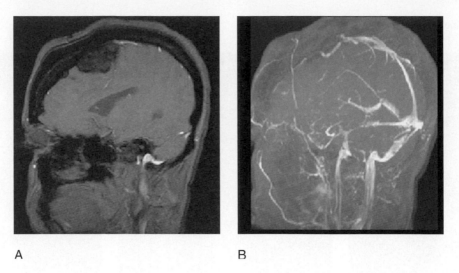

Fig. 7-3. (A) Sagittal view from MR venography, demonstrating stenosis/occlusion anterior aspect of the superior sagittal sinus by a parasagittal/parafalcine meningioma (homogeneously hypointense relative to the brain parenchyma). (B) Three-dimensional MPR reconstruction, in an oblique sagittal plane, of the MR venography shown in (A)

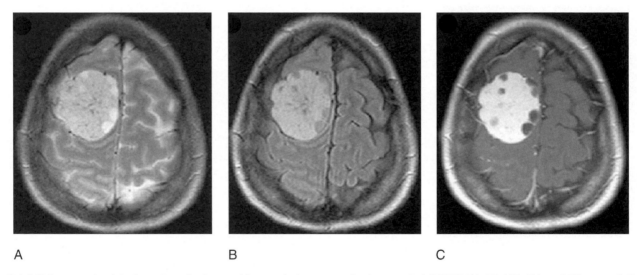

Fig. 7-4. MR images of a right frontal meningioma with vacuolations or cystic changes. Axial T2W (A), FLAIR (B), and T1 postgadolinium (C) images of the meningioma demonstrate multiple vacuoles within the tumor, mostly along the margins of the tumor, and with internal CSF-like signal intensities consistent with cystic changes

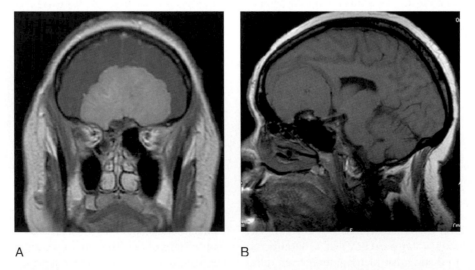

Fig. 7-5. Coronal T1 postgadolinium (A) and sagittal T1 pregadolinium (B) MR images of a large olfactory groove meningioma. This tumor abuts the caudal aspect of the anterior fossa, near the midline with bony hyperostosis in the region of the posterior cribiform plate and planum sphenoidale. There is also significant mass effect on the anterior aspects of the corpus callosum

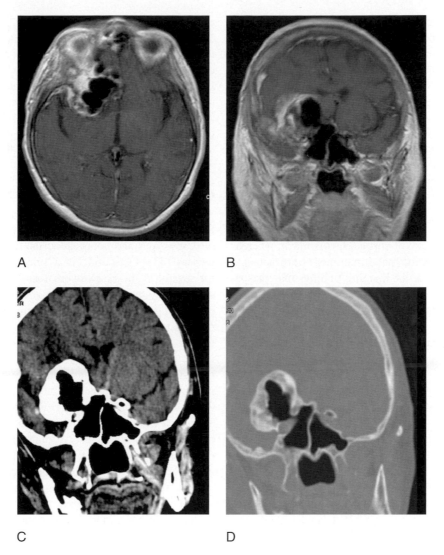

FIG. 7-6. A right clinoidal meningioma with internal pneumatization associated with erosion into the right ethmoid sinus. Axial (A) and coronal (B) T1 postgadolinium MR images demonstrate a crescentic region of intense enhancement around the lateral margin of the pneumatized cavity, which is contiguous with the right ethmoid sinus. Coronal nonenhanced CT images, in brain parenchyma (C) and bone (D) windows, exhibit significant calcification in the meningioma lining the pneumatized cavity

Functional MRI

Resection of some meningiomas may involve irreparable damage to adjacent cortical structures, which are responsible for vital functions. Defining functionally eloquent cortical regions, as well as determining whether surgical or nonsurgical treatment would be optimal for the patients, are therefore central to presurgical planning. One means of identifying vital cortical structures is via functional MRI (fMRI). This method uses blood oxygen level–dependent (BOLD) functional imaging to localize regional cerebral blood flow changes resulting from neural activities elicited by functional paradigms (defined motor, sensory, or cognitive tasks during imaging) performed by the conscious patient [24]. The results reveal the neural substrate(s) subserving each motor or sensory process. Beyond

being a noninvasive method, fMRI also affords adequate spatial resolution for most intracranial mass lesions, as well as epileptic foci, in terms of their surgical planning.

One example of such evaluation is for a left frontal meningioma, situated at the posterior junction of the left middle and inferior frontal gyri. Due to its proximity to the left precentral gyrus, this tumor raised concern for involvement of important language-generation areas (i.e., Broca's and Wernicke areas), the primary sensorimotor cortex, as well as the supplementary and presupplementary motor areas. When performing covert word-generation tasks, this patient exhibited a strong focus of metabolic activation in the left frontal lobe immediately deep to the meningioma. Rhyming tasks, or expressive language paradigms, also elicited a smaller focus of activation deep to the tumor in the left inferior frontal lobe (results not shown). These findings collectively indicated left-sided language dominance in that patient and the importance of cortical regions abutting that tumor in language functions. This patient did not have to undergo an invasive Wada test to establish sidedness of language dominance. Surgical margins for this tumor, if extended beyond the immediate boundaries of the meningioma, could therefore impart irreversible deficits in this patient's language capabilities.

It is important, however, to appreciate some of the limitations of fMRI. One limitation of this technique is that it visualizes blood flow changes particularly in the venous phase, and the results can be inaccurate if venous flow is altered either due to tumoral compression or compensatory activity by the brain tissue surrounding the tumor [25]. Similarly, absence of cortical activation where it is anticipated may signal technical failures rather than true lack of cortical involvement, whereas presence of cortical activation may sometimes be artifactual in etiology [24]. Furthermore, the imaging findings may be spatially separated from the actual site of neural activation by as much as 10–15 mm [26]. One study that correlated intraoperative electrocortical mapping with presurgical fMRI findings indicated that 100% spatial correlation was achieved within 20 mm by the two techniques [27].

MR Spectroscopy

Proton-MR spectroscopy of meningiomas reveals several characteristic features. Their spectra lack detectable *N*-acetyl-aspartate (NAA), a neuronal marker, which is consistent with meningiomas not arising from neural elements as well as neoplastic damage of normal neurons [28]. Additionally, meningiomas have high choline and low to undetectable creatine levels, in contrast to gliomas, which typically exhibit high choline but normal creatine levels [29]. Some meningiomas also have elevated alanine level, which helps to distinguish them from gliomas or metastases [30]. Meningiomas also have elevated glutamate/glutamine levels, which may help to differentiate them from other intracranial neoplasms [31]. Atypical meningiomas may additionally be discernable from benign ones based upon these spectral features [32]. The practical limitation of MR spectroscopy is the requisitely large voxel size, which may obviate adequate assessment of smaller lesions.

Octreotide Scintigraphy

Somatostatin receptor subtypes are present in a wide multitude of tissue types and neuroendocrine tumors, including meningiomas [33]. Octreotide is a selective, high-affinity ligand for several of the known somatostain receptor subtypes, and scintigraphy by using the radiolabeled form of this synthetic peptide (e.g., DTPA chelate of indium-111, or ^{111}In, to [D-Phe[1]]-octreotide) is generally regarded as a sensitive approach toward detecting and localizing neuroendocrine tumors and intracranial meningiomas [34,35; Fig. 2]. Some studies have indicated that radiolabeled octreotide can be used to discern meningiomas from other intracranial neoplasms and for the detection of recurrent meningiomas following resection [36]. There is a widely held notion that positive findings on octreotide scintigraphy can resolve diagnostic dilemmas for intracranial lesions with other imaging or clinical properties that may otherwise be atypical for meningiomas.

However, diverse intracranial lesions such as pituitary adenoma, high-grade glioma, metastasis, lymphoma, osteosarcoma, abscess, angioleiomyoma, chordoma, and hemangiopericytoma have also been identified by ^{111}In-octreotide

TABLE 7-1. Summary of MRI, ^{111}In-Octreotide Scintigraphic, and ^{18}F-FDG PET Findings for Patients with Known Histopathologic Diagnoses for Intracranial Lesions

Patient	Age/Gender	Histopathologic Dx	MRI	Octreotide	PET
1	53 F	Meningioma	Consistent	Consistent	Consistent
2	70 M	Meningioma, "collision tumor"	Consistent	Consistent	Consistent
3	73 M	Meningioma	Consistent	Consistent	Consistent
4	76 F	Meningioma	Consistent	Consistent	Consistent
5	76 F	Meningioma	Consistent	Consistent	
6	51 F	Meningioma, left optic nerve	Consistent	Not consistent	Consistent
7	83 M	Sarcoma, within meningioma resection bed	Consistent	Consistent	
8	22 F	Fibrous dysplasia	Consistent	Consistent	Consistent
9	66 F	Lymphoma, CNS primary	Consistent	Consistent	Not consistent
10	75 F	Metastasis, unknown primary	Consistent	Not consistent	
11	38 F	Pituitary adenoma	Not consistent	Consistent	
12	48 F	Abscess	Not consistent	Consistent	Consistent
13	40 F	Lymphoma, CNS primary	Not consistent	Consistent	Consistent
14	53 F	Metastasis, breast primary	Not consistent	Consistent	Not consistent
15	62 F	Lymphoma, metastatic	Not consistent	Consistent	Not consistent
16	40 F	Hematoma	Not consistent	Not consistent	Consistent
17	74 F	Lymphoma, CNS primary	Not consistent	Not consistent	

All imaging and scintigraphic results were categorized as either "consistent" or "not consistent" with expected findings of benign meningiomas.
Source: From Ref. 38.

scintigraphy [37]. These findings raise concern as to the specificity and utility of radiolabeled octreotide scintigraphy in evaluating meningiomas. To address such concerns, the authors recently completed a retrospective analysis of the utility of ^{111}In-octreotide SPECT versus MRI/ multidetector CT (MDCT) imaging in the diagnosis of intracranial lesions suspected of being meningiomas [38]. We retrospectively compared available histopathologic information, MRI or CT findings, and ^{111}In-octretide SPECT results for patients who presented to our institution for further evaluation of intracranial lesions with imaging or biologic features not entirely consistent with benign meningiomas.

In reviewing records over a 5-year span, we identified 17 such patients who underwent biopsy or resection and thereby had available histopathologic information for their intracra-

nial lesions. The MRI/MDCT, octreotide scintigraphy and FDG PET findings for each lesion were categorized as being "consistent" or "not consistent" with expected findings of benign meningioma. Such findings and the corresponding histopathologic diagnoses are shown in Table 7-1 [38]. Six of these lesions proved to be meningiomas, one of which is "collision tumor" between metastatic renal cell carcinoma and a meningioma [39], and all with MR findings compatible with being meningiomas. All but one of these lesions were intensely accumulated ^{111}In-octreotide by SPECT imaging, the only exception being an optic nerve meningioma possibly due to lack of spatial resolution of SPECT for periorbital lesions. Also, a minority of meningiomas have been shown to not avidly accumulate ^{111}In-octreotide above surrounding background [40,41].

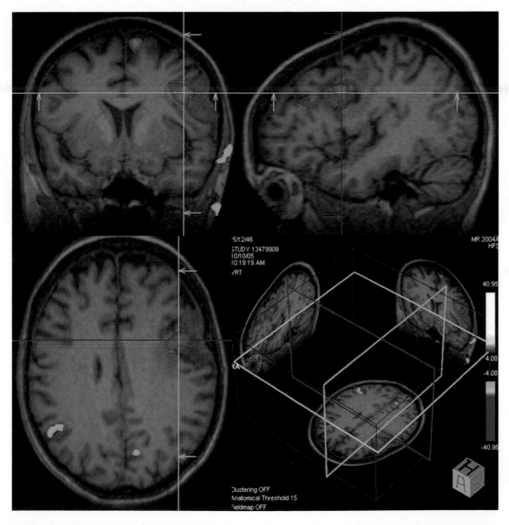

Fig. 7-7. Functional MRI of patient with left frontal meningioma. Blood oxygen level–dependent (BOLD) functional MR images (using a 1.5T MR system), coregistered with T1-weighted images in three orthogonal planes as shown, revealed a focus of strong activation within the left lateral frontal lobe immediately adjacent to the meningioma in response to word-generation tasks by the patient. Additional rhyming tasks demonstrated a smaller focus of activation deep to the tumor in the left inferior frontal lobe (results not shown). These findings demonstrated left-sided language dominance for this patient, and further suggested possible impairment of language capabilities following resection of this meningioma. Receptive speech tasks were assessed in this patient but deemed technically inadequate. Additional simple motor tasks (e.g., bilateral finger tapping) were also performed with expected activation of motor cortical foci in the precentral gyri

The other 11 lesions consisted of lymphoma ($n = 4$), prolactinoma, chronic/resolving hematoma, fibrotic tissue, metastases ($n = 2$), sarcoma (which appeared within the resection bed of a meningioma), and a resolving intracranial abscess. Four of these 11 lesions presented with MR or CT findings consistent with intracranial meningioma, and 3 of the 4 lesions also had positive scintigraphic findings consistent with meningioma. One such lesion was subsequently diagnosed as metastatic lymphoma (Fig. 7.8). The remaining 7 lesions presented with MR or CT findings inconsistent with meningioma, yet among them 5 had positive octreotide findings consistent with meningioma. One such latter lesion, histopathologically shown to be metastatic lymphoma, exhibited MR and scintigraphic features consistent with meningiomas.

These findings indicated that octreotide SPECT had 83% sensitivity, 27% specificity (39% positive predictive value or PPV, 75% negative predictive value or NPV), and 47% overall accuracy in identifying meningioma. By contrast, MRI/MDCT imaging revealed 100% sensitivity, 64% specificity (60% PPV, 100% NPV), and 77% accuracy in identifying meningioma. When combining octreotide scintigraphy with MRI/MDCT imaging, overall sensitivity and specificity of identifying meningioma were not improved upon those of MRI/MDCT imaging alone. These findings indicate that MRI/MDCT imaging and octreotide scintigraphy are both highly sensitive modalities for identifying meningioma, but that octreotide scintigraphy is also highly nonspecific in such regard and will in addition identify a variety of intracranial

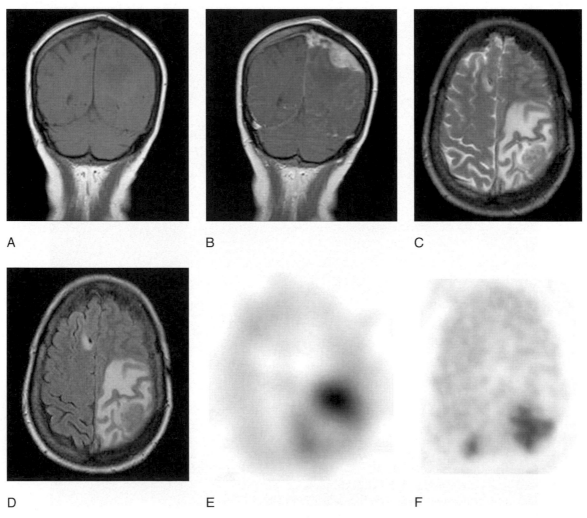

A   B   C

D   E   F

FIG. 7-8. MRI, ^{111}In-octreotide scintigraphy and ^{18}F-FDG PET imaging for a metastatic lymphoma in the left parietal convexity. Coronal T1W pre- and postgadolinium (A and B), axial T2 (C), and FLAIR (D) images demonstrate a dural-based, avidly enhancing lesion with adjacent parenchymal edema in the left parietal lobe, consistent with meningioma. Focal parenchymal encephalomalacia in the right mesial frontal lobe, identified on T2W and FLAIR images, is of unclear etiology and may reflect prior intervention at outside institution. Focally increased ^{111}In-octreotide accumulation is seen corresponding to this lesion (E) as expected of meningioma, but focally increased ^{18}F-FDG accumulation is also seen (F), which is inconsistent with typical presentation of meningioma. Another focus of increased ^{18}F-FDG in the right posterior occipital lobe has no corresponding MRI or scintigraphic abnormality

nonmeningiomatous lesions or pathologies. The apparent high sensitivity and low specificity of octreotide scintigraphy are in accord with other prior studies [37,41,42]. It is noteworthy that a prior study indicated lack of discrimination between meningiomas and other intracranial tumors for lesions smaller than 2.5 cm [40], which may in part contribute to the finding as described.

While the findings from our retrospective analysis need further verification in larger patient cohorts, they are highly suggestive that octreotide scintigraphy must be used with caution as a diagnostic problem solver. This is particularly relevant for intracranial lesions with properties not entirely consistent with benign meningiomas. The reasonably high NPV of octreotide scintigraphy, however, may still warrant inclusion of this imaging modality in the diagnostic regimen, particularly when combined with conventional MRI or MDCT imaging. Moreover, such scintigraphic imaging has proven utility in assessing recurrent or residual meningioma following tumor resection [36].

Positron Emission Tomography

Utility of PET in evaluating meningiomas is not as well established as for other imaging modalities. F-18 fluorodeoxyglucose (^{18}F-FDG) is a widely used metabolic marker for PET imaging. As the majority of meningiomas are benign, they typically exhibit isometabolism on ^{18}F-FDG PET (one example of such is shown in Fig. 7-2). Atypical or malignant meningiomas, however, may exhibit hypermetabolism [43], which may complicate distinction of meningiomas from other intracranial tumors (e.g., metastatic lymphoma, as shown in Fig. 7-7). Postoperative recurrent meningiomas exhibit varying PET responses, with anecdotal reports describing both iso- and hypermetabolic findings [43,44].

In our retrospective analysis of the utility of octreotide scintigraphy in identifying meningioma, 12 of the 17 patients with known histopathologic information also underwent 18F-FDG PET analysis. In that setting, PET imaging had 80% sensitivity, 57% specificity (57% PPV, 80% NPV), and 75% accuracy in identifying meningioma. Thus, FDG PET is highly sensitive but also highly nonspecific in such regard. In this study, there was 75% concordance rate between MRI/MDCT and PET findings. It is, however, noteworthy that ^{18}F-FDG provides the added utility of identifying distant meningiomatous metastases [45].

L-[Methyl-^{11}C]-methionine (^{11}C-Met) is a PET marker for cellular protein synthesis, and provides visualization of meningiomas sometimes not identified by using ^{18}F-FDG. It is usually accumulated by meningiomas in homogeneous fashion and at a level above the surrounding brain parenchyma [46]. PET imaging with ^{11}C-Met can identify meningiomas which are hypo- to isometabolic on FDG PET [47] and without dependency on tumoral malignancy, as has been observed for ^{18}F-FDG [48]. One report indicated that ^{11}C-Met uptake by meningiomas correlated significantly with a histologic marker of proliferative potential, whereas ^{18}F-FDG uptake did not exhibit such cor-

relation [49]. It should be noted that 11C-Met is not specific for meningiomas and is equally avidly accumulated by other intracranial tumors [48]. Several studies have indicated the utility of ^{11}C-Met PET in assessing the efficacy of radiotherapy or interferon-α therapy for postoperative residual, recurrent, and primary inoperable meningiomas [50,51].

Summary

The majority of meningiomas have highly stereotypic imaging findings, particularly as seen by conventional MRI and/or MDCT. Such findings, in combination with preferential intracranial localizations, often facilitate the diagnosis of meningiomas. A minority of meningiomas have atypical or malignant histologic properties, but do not necessarily exhibit imaging characteristics which are readily identifiable. Conversely, imaging characteristics which are not entirely consistent with the stereotypic findings of meningiomas do not necessarily associate with atypical or malignant meningiomas, or even with other intracranial neoplasms. In some instances where conventional MRI or MDCT findings pose diagnostic dilemmas, other imaging modalities (e.g., MR spectroscopy, octreotide scintigraphy, or PET) may have utility in the identification of meningiomas. These latter modalities, while generally sensitive for meningiomas, are nonetheless nonspecific for meningiomas and should only be used as adjuncts to MRI or MDCT imaging, with special care in interpreting their findings. Functional MRI, given its limitations, may provide valuable information for operability and presurgical planning of selected intracranial meningiomas, particularly in minimizing postsurgical neurologic impairment as well as surgical risks.

References

1. Nakasu S, Hirano A, Llena J et al. Interface between the meningioma and the brain. Surg Neurol 1989; 32:206–212.
2. Sheporaitis L, Osborn AG, Smirniotopoulos JG, et al. Radiologic-pathologic correlation intracranial meningioma. AJNR 1992; 13:29–37.
3. Ginsberg LE. Radiology of meningiomas. J Neurooncol 1996; 29:229–238.
4. Kizana E, Lee R, Young M et al. A review of the radiological features of intracranial meningiomas. Australas Radiol 1996; 40:454–462.
5. Russell EJ, George AE, Kricheff II, et al. Atypical computed tomographic features of intracranial meningiomas: Radiological-pathological correlation in a series of 131 consecutive cases. Radiology 1980; 135:673–682.
6. Pistolesi S, Fontanini G, Camacci T, et al. Meningioma-associated brain oedema: The role of angiogenic factors and pial blood supply. J Neurooncol 2002; 60:159–164.
7. Pieper DR, Al-Mefty O, Hanada Y, et al. Hyperostosis associated with meningiomas of the cranial base: Secondary changes or tumor invasion. Neurosurgery 1999; 44:742–746.
8. Chong VF, Khoo JB, Fan YF. Fibrous dysplasia involving the base of the skull. AJR Am J Roentgenol 2002; 178:717–720.

9. Latchaw RE, Rai AT, Branstetter BF, et al. Extra-axial tumors of the head: Diagnostic imaging, physiologic testing, and embolization. In: Latchaw RE, Kucharczyk J, Moseley ME, eds. Imaging of the Nervous System: Diagnostic and Therapeutic Applications. Philadelphia: Elsevior Mosby, 2005:771–851.

10. Latchaw RE, Johnson EW, Kanal E. Primary intracranial tumors: Extra-axial masses and tumors of the skull base and calvarium. In: Latchaw RE, ed. MR and CT Imaging of the Head, Neck and Spine. St. Louis: Mosby-Year Book, 1991:509–560.

11. Tsuchiya K, Mizutani Y, Hachiya J. Preliminary evaluation of fluid-attenuated inversion-recovery MR in the diagnosis of intracranial tumors. AJNR Am J Neuroradiol 1996; 17:1081–1086.

12. Nagele T, Petersen D, Klose U, et al. The "dural tail" adjacent to meningiomas studied by dynamic contrast-enhanced MRI: A comparison with histopathology. Neuroradiology 1994; 36:303–307.

13. Hutzelmann A, Palmie S, Buhl R, et al. Dural invasion of meningiomas adjacent to the tumor margin on Gd-DTPA-enhanced MR images: Histopathologic correlation. Eur Radiol 1998; 8:746–748.

14. Guermazi A, Lafitte F, Miaux Y, et al. The dural tail sign—beyond meningioma. Clin Radiol 2005; 60:171–188.

15. Goldsher D, Litt AW, Pinto RS, et al. Dural "tail" associated with meningiomas on Gd-DTPA-enhanced MR images: Characteristics, differential diagnostic value, and possible implications for treatment. Radiology 1990; 176:447–450.

16. Oka K, Go Y, Kimura H, et al. Obstruction of the superior sagittal sinus caused by parasagittal meningiomas: The role of collateral venous pathways. J Neurosurg 1994; 81:520–524.

17. Murtagh R, Linden C. Neuroimaging of intracranial meningiomas. Neurosurg Clin North Am 1994; 5:217–233.

18. Paek SH, Kim SH, Chang KH, et al. Microcystic meningiomas: Radiological characteristics of 16 cases. Acta Neurochir (Wien) 2005; 147:965–972.

19. Kremer S, Grand S, Remy C, et al. Contribution of dynamic contrast MR imaging to the differentiation between dural metastasis and meningioma. Neuroradiology 2004; 46:642–648.

20. Yang S, Law M, Zagzag D, et al. Dynamic contrast-enhanced perfusion MR imaging measurements of endothelial permeability: Differentiation between atypical and typical meningiomas. AJNR Am J Neuroradiol 2003; 24:1554–1559.

21. Kono K, Inoue Y, Nakayama K, et al. The role of diffusion-weighted imaging in patients with brain tumors. AJNR Am J Neuroradiol 2001; 22:1081–1088.

22. Stadnik TW, Chaskis C, Michotte A, et al. Diffusion-weighted MR imaging of intracerebral masses: Comparison with conventional MR imaging and histologic findings. AJNR Am J Neuroradiol 2001; 22:969–976.

23. Filippi CG, Edgar MA, Ulug AM, et al. Appearance of meningiomas on diffusion-weighted images: Correlating diffusion constants with histopathologic findings. AJNR Am J Neuroradiol 2001; 22:65–72.

24. Moritz C, Haughton V. Functional MR imaging: Paradigms for clinical preoperative mapping. Magn Reson Imaging Clin North Am 2003; 11:529–542.

25. Inoue T, Shimizu H, Nakasato N, et al. Accuracy and limitation of functional magnetic resonance imaging for identification of the central sulcus: Comparison with magnetoencephalography in patients with brain tumors. Neuroimage 1999; 10:738–748.

26. Kober H, Nimsky C, Moller M, et al. Correlation of sensorimotor activation with functional magnetic resonance imaging and magnetoencephalography in presurgical functional imaging: A spatial analysis. Neuroimage 2001; 14:1214–1228.

27. Yetkin FZ, Mueller WM, Morris GL, et al. Functional MR activation correlated with intraoperative cortical mapping. AJNR Am J Neuroradiol 1997; 18:1311–1315.

28. Rand SD, Prost RW, Haughton V. Magnetic resonance spectroscopy in intracranial disease. In: Latchaw RE, Kucharczyk J, Moseley ME, eds. Imaging of the Nervous System: Diagnostic and Therapeutic Applications. Philadelphia: Elsevior Mosby, 2005:125–140.

29. Castillo M, Kwock L. Proton MR spectroscopy of common brain tumors. Neuroimaging Clin North Am 1998; 8:733–752.

30. Kinoshita Y, Kajiwara H, Yokota A, Koga Y. Proton magnetic resonance spectroscopy of brain tumors: An in vitro study. Neurosurg 1994; 35:606–614.

31. Cho YD, Choi GH, Lee SP, et al. (1)H-MRS metabolic patterns for distinguishing between meningiomas and other brain tumors. Magn Reson Imaging 2003; 21:663–672.

32. Majos C, Alonso J, Aguilera C, et al. Utility of proton MR spectroscopy in the diagnosis of radiologically atypical intracranial meningiomas. Neuroradiology 2003; 45:129–136.

33. Schulz S, Pauli SU, Schulz S, et al. Immunohistochemical determination of five somatostatin receptors in meningioma reveals frequent overexpression of somatostatin receptor subtype sst_{2A}. Clin Cancer Res 2000; 6:1865–1874.

34. Krenning EP, Breeman WA, Kooij PPM, et al. Localisation of endocrine-related tumors with radioiodinated analogs of somatostatin. Lancet 1989; Feb 4:242–244.

35. Lamberts SWJ, Krenning EP, Reubi JC. The role of somatostatin and its analogs in the diagnosis and treatment of tumors. Endocrine Rev, 1991; 12:450–482.

36. Klutmann S, Bohuslavizki KH, Brenner W, et al. Somatostatin receptor scintigraphy in postsurgical follow-up examinations of meningioma. J Nucl Med 1998; 39:1913–1917.

37. Schmidt M, Scheidhauer K, Luyken C, et al. Somatostatin receptor imaging in intracranial tumors. Eur J Nucl Med 1998; 25:675–686.

38. Chang AS, Plosker A, Wu G, et al. MRI imaging and [111]indium-octreotide scintigraphy in the diagnosis of intracranial lesions: An institutional experience. Manuscript submitted.

39. Chahlavi A, Staugaitis SM, Yahya R, et al. Intracranial collision tumor mimicking an octreotide-SPECT positive and FDG-PET negative meningioma. J Clin Neurosci 2005; 12:720–723.

40. Bohuslavizki KH, Brenner W, Braunsdorf WE, et al. Somatostatin receptor scintigraphy in the differential diagnosis of meningioma. Nucl Med Commun 1996; 17:302–310.

41. Meewes C, Bohuslavizki KH, Krisch B, et al. Molecular biologic and scintigraphic analyses of somatostatin receptor-negative meningiomas. J Nucl Med 2001; 42:1338–1345.

42. Haldemann AR, Rosler H, Barth A, et al. Somatostatin receptor scintigraphy in central nervous system tumors: Role of blood-brain barrier permeability. J Nucl Med 1995; 36:403–9.

43. Lippitz B, Cremerius U, Mayfrank L, et al. PET-study of intracranial meningiomas: Correlation with histopathology, cellularity and proliferation rate. Acta Neurochir Suppl 1996; 65:108–111.

44. Kado H, Ogawa T, Tatazawa J, et al. Radiation-induced meningioma evaluated with positron emission tomography with fludeoxyglucose F 18. AJNR Am J Neuroradiol 1996; 17: 937–938.

45. Hutchins EB, Graves A, Shelton B. Meningioma metastatic to the lung detected by FDG positron emission tomography. Clin Nucl Med 2004; 29:587–589.
46. Nyberg G, Bergstrom M, Enblad P, et al. PET-methionine of skull base neuromas and meningiomas. Acta Otolaryngol 1997; 117:482–489.
47. Chung JK, Kim YK, Kim SK, et al. Usefulness of 11C-methionine PET in the evaluation of brain lesions that are hypo- or isometabolic on 18F-FDG PET. Eur J Nucl Med Mol Imaging 2002; 29:176–182.
48. Ogawa T, Inugami A, Hatazawa J, et al. Clinical positron emission tomography for brain tumors: Comparison of fludeoxyglucose F 18 and L-methyl-11C-methionine. AJNR Am J Neuroradiol 1996; 17:345–353.
49. Iuchi T, Iwadate Y, Namba H, et al. Glucose and methionine uptake and proliferative activity in meningiomas. Neurol Res 1999; 21:640–644.
50. Gudjonsson O, Blomquist E, Lilja A, et al. Evaluation of the effect of high-energy proton irradiation treatment on meningiomas by means of 11C-L-methionine PET. Eur J Nucl Med 2000; 27:1793–1799.
51. Muhr C, Gudjonsson O, Lilja A, et al. Meningioma treated with interferon-alpha, evaluated with [(11)C]-L-methionine positron emission tomography. Clin Cancer Res 2001; 7:2269–2276.

8
Meningiomas: Imaging Mimics

Manzoor Ahmed, Joung H. Lee, and Thomas J. Masaryk

Introduction

Making a correct neuroradiologic diagnosis is a process akin to assembling a puzzle. Pieces of the puzzle include: patient's age, sex, presenting signs/symptoms, anatomic location, attenuation coefficient (computed tomography [CT]), signal intensity (magnetic resonance imaging [MRI]), and enhancement pattern (CT/MR/angiography). Meningiomas have characteristic imaging features and sites of origin, making diagnosis straightforward in most cases. However, meningiomas can be mimicked by other intracranial tumors and pseudo-tumors [1]. We present a discussion of "meningioma mimics" with emphasis on CT and MRI features.

The Prototypic Meningioma

Meningiomas typically present as an incidental, extra-axial mass lesions or with specific signs and symptoms, often in middle-age females. As such, they may involve the adjacent cranial vault and/or brain but do not possess a blood-brain barrier and therefore enhance vigorously. They may arise, in order of frequency, over the convexity, sphenoid wing/cavernous sinus, tuberculum, clivus/foramen magnum [2]. On CT scan, such lesions are typically iso-dense or hyperdense relative to the adjacent brain parenchyma (Fig. 8-1A), while on MR they are iso-to hypo-intense on T1, iso-to hypo-intense on T2, and enhance on both studies following the intravenous administration of contrast [3] (Fig. 8-1B–D). On MR, there may be an appreciable contiguous dural, linear enhancement, or so-called "dural tail" (Fig. 8-1D), while on angiography there are often enlarged dural feeding vessels, which lead to an intense blush, which appears early and persists well into the venous phase. Changes in adjacent bone may include osseous erosion or hyperostosis [4] (Fig. 8-1D), while involvement of brain parenchyma may be signaled by contiguous vasogenic edema [5].

Specificity of Typical Imaging Features of Meningioma

Hyperdensity

About two thirds of meningiomas are radiographically hyperdense, explained by increased cellularity and diffuse microcalcification, both of which are also responsible for isointensity on T1 and hypointensity on T2. These are suggestive but not very specific features. There are numerous hypercellular, and therefore hyperdense, intracranial tumors, such as lymphoma, ependymoma, primary cerebral neuroblastoma/PNET, astrocytoma, and metastases (e.g., melanoma) (Fig. 8-2A). This group of tumors can pose as mimics of meningiomas provided they share the geographic locations typical for meningiomas.

Calcification

About 25–30% of meningiomas are fully calcified on CT, and the forms of calcification include psammomatous/sand-like, focal, diffuse, and rim calcifications. Tumors that also contain calcification, and thus may resemble meningiomas, include oligodendroglioma (70–90% are calcified) (Fig. 8-3A) and ganglioglioma. Both are typically superficial in location, but fortunately, the incidence and the degree/homogeneity of enhancement is less than is seen in meningiomas [6].

Hyperostosis

An extra-axial mass with skull hyperostosis is highly suggestive of a meningioma, but reactive or invasive changes can be seen with other tumors, such as lymphoma or metastases, in addition to more benign osseous defects such as fibrous dysplasia.

"Dural Tail" Sign

The "dural tail" or "flair" sign is not specific to meningiomas [7,8], as it has been described with a variety of other lesions

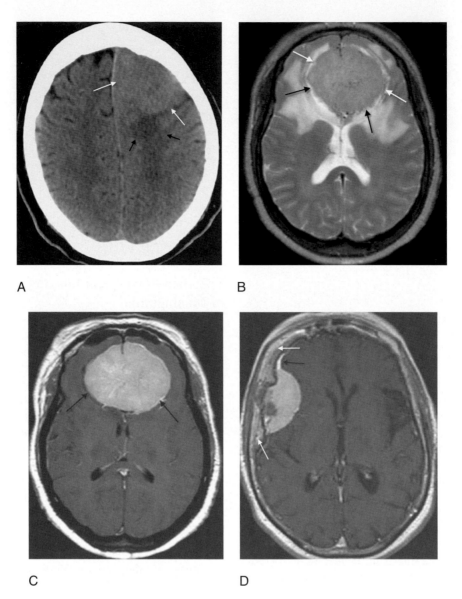

FIG. 8-1. Prototypic meningiomas: Mild hyperdense left frontal mass (white arrows, A) with associated vasogenic edema (dark arrows, A). Another patient with typical large T2 isointense anterior fossa meningioma and intense homogeneous enhancement (B, C)— note the surrounding CSF cleft (dark arrows, C). Axial postcontrast T1 sequence in a different patient showing homogeneously enhancing mass with a dural tail (dark arrow, D) and thickened marrow due to hyperostosis (white arrows, D)

such as metastases [9], glioma [10], acoustic neuroma [11], sarcoidosis [7], pleomorphic xanthoastrocytoma, lymphoma [12], and even giant aneurysm [13] (Fig. 8-4A,B). About 60% of meningiomas manifest a dural tail sign [14]. A broad dural attachment of a tumor with an adjacent dural tail is highly suggestive of a meningioma. Goldsher et al. [14] characterized the "dural tail" in meningiomas by three imaging features: tapered appearance, greater dural enhancement than the tumor, and visualization on two consecutive slices (Fig. 8-1D)

Angiographic Vascular Pattern (Radial "Sunburst" and Prolonged Blush)

Globose, extra-axial mass with radiating linear hypointense signal from the center to periphery in a sunburst pattern on angiography (as well as T2 MR images) and persistent angiographic blush indicate the highly vascular nature of meningioma. Other tumors like choroid plexus papilloma and metastases can demonstrate this appearance, but are much less common neoplasms (Fig. 8-2D).

MR Spectroscopic Profile

Though not specific, the spectroscopic profile in combination with conventional MR features of meningiomas can be helpful in select difficult cases (e.g., schwannoma versus meningioma.). N-Acetylaspartate (NAA) and creatine (Cr) are neuronal markers which, not surprisingly, are significantly reduced in nonneuronal tumors such as a meningioma. But, as with other notably cellular neoplasms, choline (Cho)

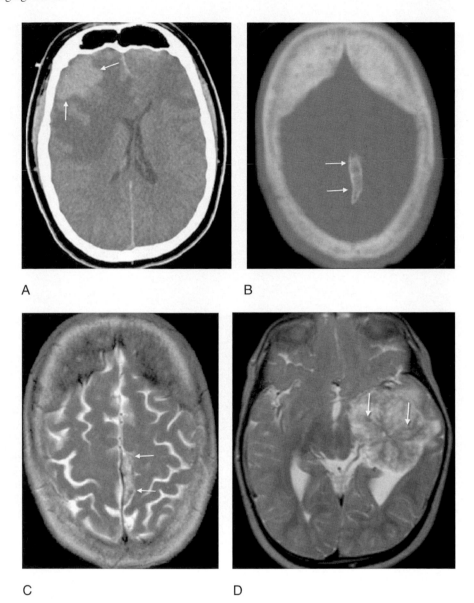

FIG. 8-2. Mimicry of specific imaging features: A hyperdense lymphoma with edema on unenhanced CT abutting the cortex (arrows, A). Dural calcification mimicking as a calcified meningioma (arrows, B, C)— note T2 hypointensity on MRI (arrows, B), laminated outer dense and lucent central attenuation on CT (B). Choroid plexus papilloma with T2 with a "sunburst" T2 appearance (D, arrows)

is increased. Relative specific markers for meningioma are alanine (Ala) and glutamine/glutamate (Glx), which are consistently increased in meningiomas compared to gliomas, schwanommas, and metastases. Meningiomas also show nonspecific peaks of lipids [15].

Beyond X-ray attenuation coefficient and MR signal characteristics, the typical extra-axial location of meningiomas and their inherent vascularity are key features in the differential diagnosis. By virtue of the tumor's involvement of the cranium and subarachnoid space, alternative diagnostic considerations are preferentially given to lesions of bone and hematopoetic tissue of the marrow space as well as vessels and nerves of the adjacent cranial foramena. Beyond these possibilities, dural metastasis or inflammatory disease are also common diagnostic considerations.

Atypical (Nonprototypic) and Malignant Meningiomas

One should remember that about 15% of benign meningiomas have atypical imaging appearance. The triad of these atypical features on CT includes intracranial tumor, osteolysis, and extracranial extension of the mass [16,17]. Markedly irregular tumor margin, presence of irregular nodule, and/or mushrooming pattern and markedly inhomogeneous enhancing pattern on MRI are indicative of nonbenign meningiomas [18]. Malignant meningeal tumors (hemangiopericytomas and sarcomas) and metastases masquerade as atypical and malignant meningiomas by manifesting these features (Fig. 8-5). The differentiation may be very difficult on conventional imaging. However, relative restricted diffusion on diffusion

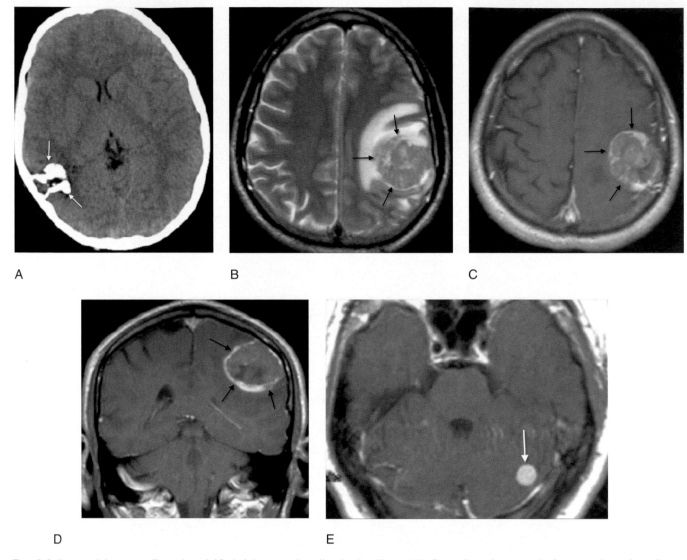

FIG. 8-3. Intra-axial tumors: Densely calcified right posterior oligodendroglioma (A). Parenchymal metastasis from esophageal carcinoma (B–D): intra-axial lesion with T2 hypointensity and surrounding edema (B). Enhancement of the mass (though heterogeneous), abutting the dura, mimicks meningioma (arrows, C, D). Rare case of intra-axial schwannoma (E)

imaging and specific metabolite profile on MR spectroscopy may be helpful in such cases and favor metastases.

Mimics of Meningioma Mass Lesions (by Location)

Lesions of the Convexity and Sphenoid/ Middle Fossa

Convexity, parasagittal, and sphenoid wing meningiomas constitute a large percentage of intracranial meningiomas [19]. Metastases, hematologic disorders, primary brain tumors, vascular lesions, and dystrophic dural calcification represent common mimics at these locations.

Metastatic Disease

Dural metastases, though uncommon, can be difficult to distinguish from meningiomas [20].There are multiple case reports of metastases resembling meningiomas, including breast, lung [20], prostate [21], renal cell, follicular thyroid [22], and adenoid cystic carcinomas [23] (Fig. 8-6). While multiplicity of lesions would indicate a nonprimary tumor (in the absence of neurofibromatosis), dural metastases rarely calcify, a finding much more indicative of meningiomas [24]. Three modes of spread to dura include direct spread from the cranial vault, hematogenous spread, and the rare direct spread from brain parenchyma [24]. Solitary dural-based enhancing metastases are typical meningioma mimics. Factors favoring metastases on conventional MRI include multiplicity, calvarial

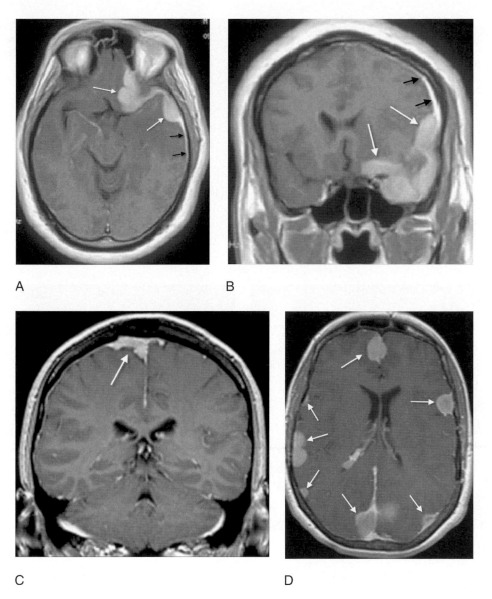

FIG. 8-4. Sarcoidosis: Multifocal lobulated dural-based enhancing masses (white arrows, A, B, C) mimicking multiple meiningiomas (arrows, D). Note dural tail–like appearance adjacent to sarcoid masses (dark arrows, A, B)

infiltration (diploic space T2 hyperintensity and enhancement on MRI), heterogeneous enhancement, and disproportionate vasogenic edema. Atypical or malignant meningioma may not be excluded based on these features. MR spectroscopy may be used to differentiate meningiomas, as discussed previously, and dynamic MR perfusion can suggest metastases by showing low r CBV compared to meningiomas [25].

Parenchymal metastases, such as renal cell carcinoma, thyroid carcinoma, or calcified intra-axial metastases, can be mistaken for meningiomas if they are located peripherally, abutting the cortex or located centrally abutting choroid plexus. Differentiation of the former subset from meningiomas is facilitated by history of a primary tumor and basic imaging features of intra-axial versus

extra-axial location. However, separating meningiomas from others can be difficult in some cases (Fig. 8-3B–D). Although the incidence of intraventricular meningiomas is low [26], metastases to the choroid plexus (e.g., renal cell carcinoma) can be easily confused with meningiomas [27] (Fig. 8-7C).

Hematologic Disorders

Following the basic rule of radiology, which is to look at every image completely, one should always take care to evaluate the sagittal T1-weighted images of the brain to assess the bone marrow signal (typically high on T1 due to Marrow fat). Deviation from this pattern suggests replacement of normal

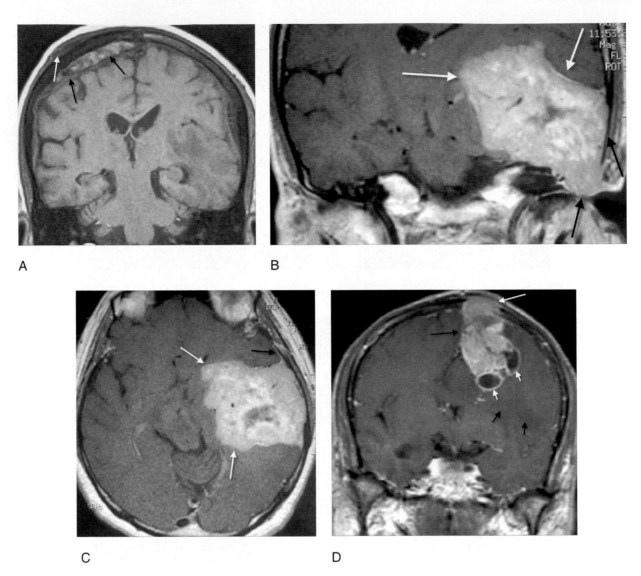

Fig. 8-5. Mimics of atypical meningioma: Dural-based metastases with heterogeneous signal intensity (dark arrows, A) and extracranial soft tissue extension (white arrow, A). Hemangiopericytoma with skull involvement (dark arrow, B) and dural tail (dark arrow, C). Example of atypical meningioma, for comparison, with a complex cystic mass, and transcranial extension (white arrow, D), cystic foci (small white arrows, D), and extensive edema (small dark arrows, D)

marrow lipid by some systemic hematologic disturbance (typically low in signal on T1-weighted scans). Diffuse and multifocal dural involvement are additional key diagnostic features for this group of disorders.

Granulocytic Sarcomatous Masses ("Chloromas")

Extramedullary leukemic tumors, which are typically hypercellular, can present as meningeal chloromas. Their MRI features, consisting of iso- to hypointensity, enhancing brightly with gadolinium, along with their extra-axial location may be confused with typical meningiomas [28] (Fig. 8-8A,B). Imaging characteristics that can be helpful in narrowing the diagnosis of chloromas include associated, diffuse leptomen-

ingeal enhancement, prominent perivascular spaces, and occasional rim enhancement in addition to anticipated changes in the clival marrow [29].

Extramedullary Hematopoeisis

Intracranial extra-axial hematopoesis is a rare manifestation of hematologic disorders which can mimic meningiomas [30]. Distinguished from meningiomas by their multilobulated, often contiguous pattern, these rare "lesions" often have associated skull marrow changes and paranasal soft tissue masses. The histology of these masses is nonneoplastic, consisting of excessively stimulated, hematopoetic marrow, which dramatically extends beyond the bony confines of the marrow space.

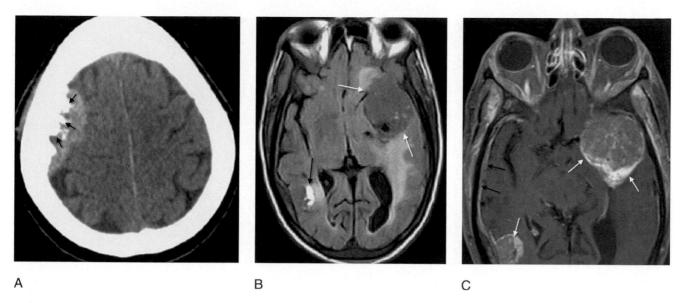

FIG. 8-6. Dural prostatic metastasis: CT apparently shows a calcified mass, which is actually a dural metastasis with associated calvarial involvement rather than calcification (A, small dark arrows). Axial FLAIR image shows left middle cranial fossa and right posterior temporal iso-hyperintense mass, the latter with peripheral small cystic changes (dark arrow, B), moderate enhancement on T1 images (white arrows, C), with associated diffuse dural thickening and enhancement (C, dark arrows)

Plasmacytomas

Cranial plasmacytomas can be diagnosed as solitary extramedullary plasmacytomas or as part of systemic multiple myeloma presenting as extra-axial mass lesions. Having characteristic hypointense signal on T1- and T2-weighted images relative to grey matter and homogeneous gadolinium enhancement, these lesions can mimic meningiomas. CT and plain films are helpful because plasmacytomas primarily involve the skull [31], expanding the diploic space, but, unlike meningiomas,

are lytic with nonsclerotic margins on noncontrast CT. Plasmacytoma, limited to the diploic space, manifests as an expansile soft tissue mass, unlike intraosseous meningiomas, which create a permeative, sclerotic/hyperostotic appearance. Rarely, plasmacytomas can originate from the dura and present as purely enhancing intracranial extra-axial tumors without skull involvement. These solitary plasmacytomas without skull involvement may be much more difficult to distinguish from meningiomas on CT and conventional MRI [31,32].

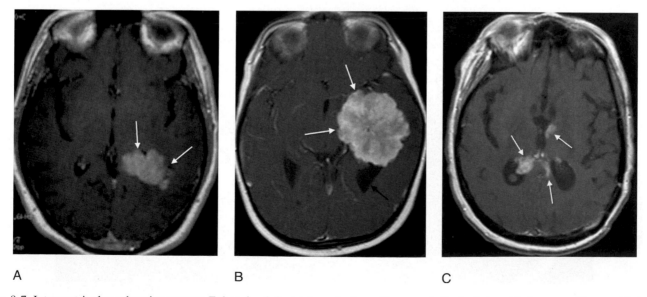

FIG. 8-7. Intraventricular enhancing tumors: Enhancing left atrial meningioma (A, arrows). Typical choroid plexus papilloma with floral pattern on enhanced image (white arrows, B). Note left lateral ventricular mild dilatation (dark arrow, B).Multifocal choroid plexus and subependymal renal cell carcinoma metastases (arrows, C)

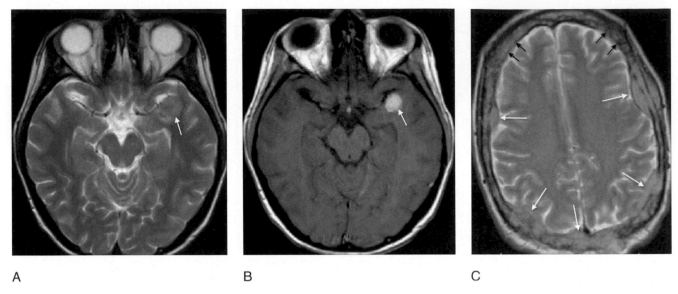

A   B   C

FIG. 8-8. Hematologic tumors: Hypo- to isointense T2 (A) and enhancing (B) extra-axial mass in the left middle cranial fossa due to leukemic extra axial deposit. Multiple isointense T2 dural masses (white arrows, C) with diffuse diploic marrow space replacement (dark arrows, C) in a patient with multiple myeloma

Primary Brain Tumors

Intra-axial primary brain tumors are relatively easy to distinguish from meningiomas with rare exceptions. Broad-based involvement of the cortex with occasional dural reaction, relative homogeneous enhancement, tumor calcification or skull base locations can contribute to diagnostic confusion. Primary brain tumors, notably posterior fossa ependymomas, can have exophytic or infiltrative growth into the cerebrospinal fluid (CSF) space/cerebellopontine angle, giving a false impression of an extra-axial origin (Fig. 8-18E). Addition-

ally, there can be rare examples of intra-axial tumors, which, based on radiographic features, mimic meningioma, such as an intra-axial schwannomas (Fig. 8-3E) or glial sarcomas (discussed below).

Gliomas

Gliomas are generally easy to differentiate from meningiomas unless they are well defined, limited to one or two gyri, superficially located, and show homogeneous enhancement. These features may be seen in low-grade gliomas, but rarely

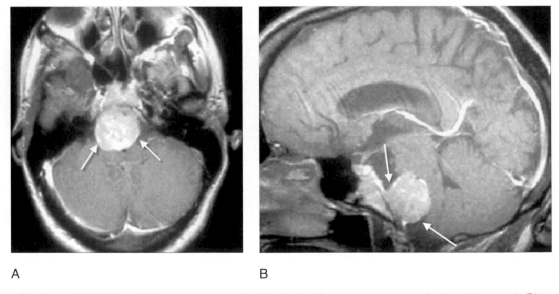

A   B

FIG. 8-9. Example of central skull base clival sarcoma, appearing identical to foramen magnum meningioma (arrows, A, B)

in combination, which would make routine distinction much more difficult. Pleomorphic xanthoastrocytomas (Fig. 8-10A) often favor superficial, almost extra-axial location over the intraparenchymal location but are relatively rare. Occasionally, some examples of large enhancing high-grade gliomas may be difficult to differentiate from meningiomas because of the surrounding edema and mass effect obscuring the cortical sulci, similar to the example of a metastasis in Fig. 8-3B–D. Enhancement pattern, especially a dural tail, is atypical of any glioma [10]. Focal calcification can be seen in low-grade gliomas, especially in oligodendrogliomas. Oligodendrogliomas or oligoastrocytomas demonstrate

some degree of calcification in up to 90% of cases on CT [33] (Fig. 8-3A). The pattern of calcification is less specific in these gliomas relative to the more homogeneous calcification seen in meningiomas [34].

Gliosarcomas

Gliosarcomas represent a subtype of malignant gliomas in which a sarcomatous component is present. Gliosarcomas are typically present along the periphery and may abut the dura [35]. Characteristally, they are hyperdense on CT [36] (Fig. 8-10B,C). However, compared to meningioma, they are more

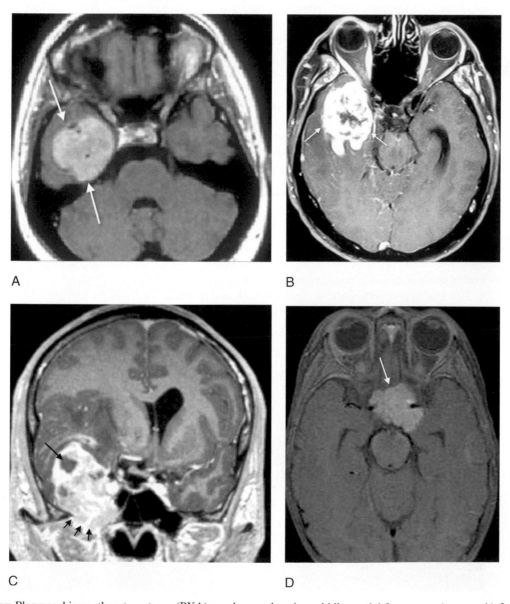

A

B

C

D

FIG. 8-10. Gliomas: Pleomorphic xanthoastrocytoma (PXA) as a large enhancing middle cranial fossa mass (arrows, A). Large right middle cranial fossa enhancing mass with skull base and dural involvement (short dark arrows, C) on postcontrast T1 images (B, C), with cystic foci (long dark arrow, C). Biopsy showed gliosarcoma. Both examples are very difficult to distinguish from meningioma preoperatively. Enhancing chiasmatic glioma (arrow, D)

heterogeneous, have a smaller dural-based attachment, and a much greater degree of parenchymal edema. These aggressive tumors have a tendency to invade the adjacent dural reflections [37].

Vascular Lesions

The resemblance to meningiomas posed by nonaneurysmal vascular lesions such as cavernous malformations and intracranial hemorrhages is generally limited to unenhanced CT images. With the addition of MR imaging, the correct diagnosis is often easily made.

Cavernomas

Dural cavernous malformations are rare, most commonly found in the middle cranial fossa [38]. Interestingly, unlike parenchymal cavernomas, dural subtype shows enhancement that closely resembles that of meningiomas [39] (Fig. 8-11). Like meningiomas, cavernomas are hyperdense on CT and frequently show calcification [40]. Giant cavernomas (>4 cm), often coarsely calcified, can be misinterpreted as a meningioma on noncontrast CT [39]. However, on MR imaging there is often relatively diffuse T2 hyperintensity and hypointense hemosiderin deposits, usually along its periphery [41]. Intra-axial cavernomas have characteristic "popcorn" appearance on MRI. Unlike meningiomas, these lesions show no enhancement [42].

Extra-Axial Hemorrhage

Lentiform or crescent-shaped extra axial acute or subacute hemorrhages as hyperattenuated lesions can mimic meningiomas on unenhanced CTs. The key is the very smooth contours of extra-axial hemorrhages. Not usually a real challenge to experienced eyes, MRI with or without contrast can better characterize the hemorrhage [43] (Fig. 8-12).

Benign Dural Calcifications

Dystrophic, focal dural calcifications along the falx, convexity, and tentorium can mimic densely calcified meningiomas. Differentiation may be difficult in smaller lesions. Large benign dural calcifications may have laminated appearance like calvarium with apparent diploic space (Fig. 8-2B,C).

Lesions of the Cavernous Sinus/Sella, Tentorium, and Anterior Fossa

Mass lesions at these locations include those of the central and anterior skull base (sellar, tuberculum, planum sphenoidale, cavernous sinus, and olfactory groove), which may be confused with meningiomas. Germinomas, as a pineal region mass, are included for the sake of completion. Secondary lymphomas are included here due to their common central skull base, parasellar/cavernous sinus, and anterior fossa / sinonasal locations.

Metastases, lymphoma, and infiltrative pituitary macroadenoma are the typical cavernous sinus lesions that can be easily confused with cavernous sinus meningiomas. All of these enhance, manifest as T2 iso- to hypointense parasellar masses, and encase carotid arteries (Fig. 8-13). Metastases are usually extension from the bones of the skull base. Dominant sphenoid wing, spheno-orbital, cavernous sinus components, or dural tail will favor meningiomas. Adjacent hyperostosis favors the diagnosis of meningioma, especially in tumors arising from the sphenoid bone [44].

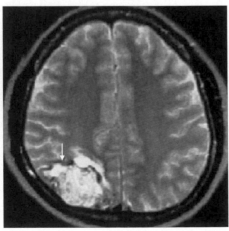
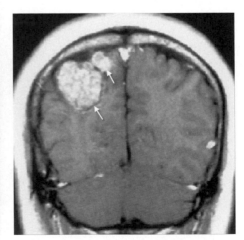

A   B

FIG. 8-11. Vascular malformations: Hyperintense T2 dural cavernoma with hypointensity due to hemosiderin (A, arrow), diffuse enhancement on postcontrast T1 coronal imaging (B, arrows). (From Ref. 40.)

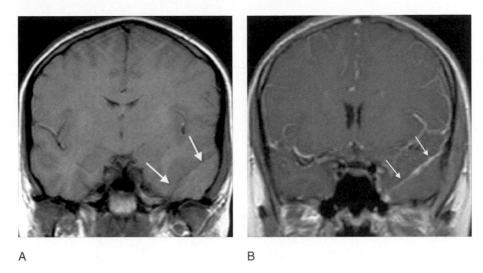

A   B

FIG. 8-12. Epidural hematoma: Mildly hyperintense extra-axial mass in the left middle cranial fossa on precontrast T1 coronal image (arrows, A) with no enhancement. Note reactive dural enhancement (arrows, B)

Pituitary Macroadenomas

Pituitary adenomas occur in sellar, sellar-suprasellar, and suprasellar locations, with pure suprasellar adenomas being rare. Suprasellar (diaphragma sella and sella tuberculum) and parasellar (cavernous sinus) meningiomas can be easily misinterpreted as pituitary macroadenomas if there is intrasellar extension with compression or obscuration of normal pituitary gland [45]. The key is to look for adjacent dural enhancement and discretely visualize pituitary gland from the suprasellar meningioma, which can be facilitated by hypointense separating dural layer of diaphragma sella [45]. Pituitary macroadenomas can also mimic meningiomas because of imaging features such as iso- to hyperdense CT attenuation, dominant suprasellar extension, occasional homogeneous enhancement, cavernous sinus extension, and, rarely, dural tail sign (as discussed above). Distinction between these two tumors is important from a management point of view [46]. The key imaging features to differentiate pituitary macroadenomas from meningiomas include the sellar epicenter of the tumor with sellar expansion, (usually) heterogeneous enhancement, and nonvisualization of the pituitary gland apart from the mass [45] (Fig. 8-14A).

Craniopharyngiomas

The adamantinomatous craniopharyngioma is a pediatric subtype, usually found in sellar and suprasellar locations, whereas the papillary type occurs in the floor of third ventricle, usually in the adult population. The former subtype is commonly mixed solid and cystic, the latter type being mostly solid. Craniopharyngiomas commonly calcify and show enhancement of the solid components, thus resembling meningiomas. Solid enhancing papillary masses may be difficult to distinguish from intraventricular or pineal region meningiomas. The complex cystic suprasellar craniopharyngiomas can mimic cystic meningiomas, usually related to peripherally entrapped CSF.

Primary Benign Tumors of the Cranium

Primary benign calvarial tumors include chondroma, osteochondroma, and osteoma. They can present as dural-based calcified masses on CT, and therefore mimic meningiomas. Intracranial chondroma is a rare lesion, usually showing hyperdense rim and hypodense core with matrix calcification on CT [47], and predominantly hypointense on T1 with heterogeneous hyperintense T2 signal intensity on MRI [48]. Chondromas, unlike meningiomas, are avascular and do not enhance except for its fibrocapsule rim [49]. Osteochondroma (OC) is a common benign tumor but rarely occurs intracranially [50], usually arising from the skull base with mushroom-like intracranial growth. Falx OCs have been described [51]. The similarity to meningioma is due to its calcified/ossified mottled appearance [52]. Intracranial OCs can be sessile or pedunculated. Like extracranial osteochondromas, the key differentiating feature is the continuity of bone marrow in the bone of origin into the tumor and hyperintense T2 cartilagenous cap on MRI. Osteomas of the inner table (OITs)generally appear as hyperdense, mushroom-like masses with well-defined borders attached to the inner table of the skull by a bony stalk or neck. However, sessile osteomas are also commonly seen and may be very difficult to distinguish from densely calcified small meningiomas [53].

Germinomas

Suprasellar and pineal germinomas are less difficult "meningioma mimickers" because of the higher incidence in younger

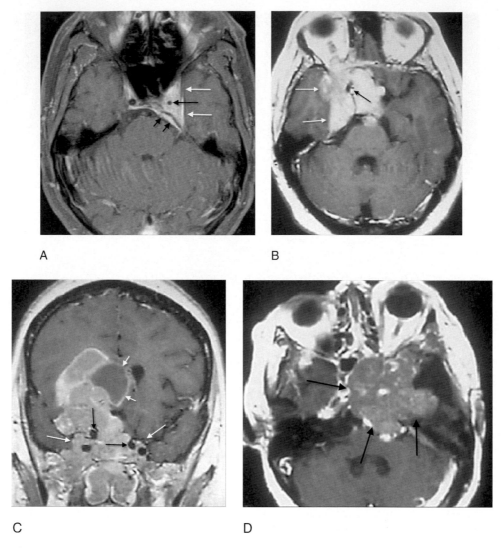

FIG. 8-13. Cavernous sinus and parasellar tumors: (A) Meningioma with expansion of the left cavernous sinus, narrowing of ICA (dark arrow) and associated dural enhancement (small dark arrows) (B, C). Invasive pituitary adenoma with extensive growth, parasellar bulky mass (white arrows, B), and involvement of bilateral cavernous sinuses (white arrows, C) and encasement of ICAs (dark arrow). Note cystic change (small white arrows, C). Skull base neurocytoma—a rare lesion as a meningioma mimic with well-marginated moderately enhancing lobulated mass (arrows, D)

age groups compared to meningiomas. Hyperdense well-marginated suprasellar and pineal masses with engulfment of pineal calcification on CT and iso- to hyperintense on MRI with intense enhancement can simulate suprasellar and pineal /falcotentorial meningiomas (Fig. 8-15) [54]. Pineal meningiomas displace rather than engulf the pineal calcification [55]. Small cystic changes are characteristic for germinomas on MRI. Sometimes it may be the leptomeningeal-enhancing masses related to CSF seeding that mimic meningiomas rather than the primary mass [56].

Sinonasal Tumors

In addition to esthesioneuroblastomas (ENBs), other sinonasal tumors to be considered in the differential diagnosis of anterior skull base meningiomas include sinonasal squamous cell carci-noma, adenocarcinoma, undifferentiated carcinomas, melanoma, and lymphoma. CT attenuation and contrast enhancement of these tumors are generally less intense than seen in meningioma and more heterogeneous in appearance (Fig. 8-16).

Esthesioneuroblastomas

Originating from the olfactory epithelia, large tumor subtypes typically present as dumbbell-shaped intracranial and extra-cranial nasal masses. Anterior fossa ENBs invading through the cribriform plate with homogeneous intense enhancement can appear similar to olfactory groove or extracranial nasal meningiomas (Fig. 8-16B). Significant bone remodeling or destruction can be seen with anterior skull base meningiomas. Peripheral cysts at the tumor brain interface is a characteristic feature of ENB on MRI [57].

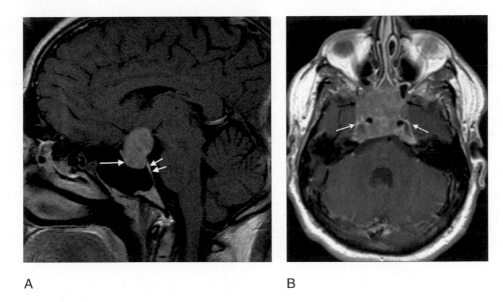

FIG. 8-14. Pituitary adenomas: Sellar and suprasellar pituitary adenoma with homogeneous enhancement, with sellar expansion (long white arrow, A). Note pseudo-dural tail along the clivus due to epidural venous plexus (small white arrows, A). Infiltrating pituitary adenoma involving the planum sphenoidale/anterior cranial fossa (dark arrows, B) and bilateral cavernous sinuses (white arrows, B)

Lymphomas

Secondary intracranial lymphomas commonly involve leptomeninges but rarely manifest as dural-based masses, which by virtue of their hyperdensity on noncontrast CT and intense enhancement on postcontrast imaging can be misinterpreted as meningiomas, particularly the solitary dural-based lesions. Primary lymphoma, particularly of mucosa-associated lymphoid tissue (MALT) type [58], can manifest as dural-based masses, resulting in a false preoperative diagnosis of meningioma [59].

Schwannomas

Trigeminal schwannomas may be confused with meningiomas when their involvement is limited to the cavernous sinus or the Meckel's cave. However, when the posterior fossa extension is present, its characteristic dumbbell shape—in addition to an acute angle the tumor forms with the posterior border of the petrous bone—compared to an obtuse angle in meningiomas easily helps with diagnostic differentiation [60].

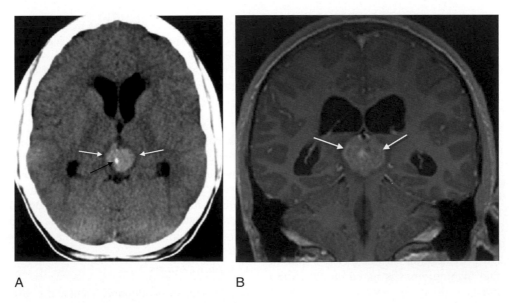

FIG. 8-15. Pineal germinoma: Hyperdense pineal mass, engulfing pineal calcification (dark arrow, A). Coronal image from postcontrast T1 volume acquisition showing enhancement (B)—less intense and homogeneous for a typical meningioma as well as a typical germinoma

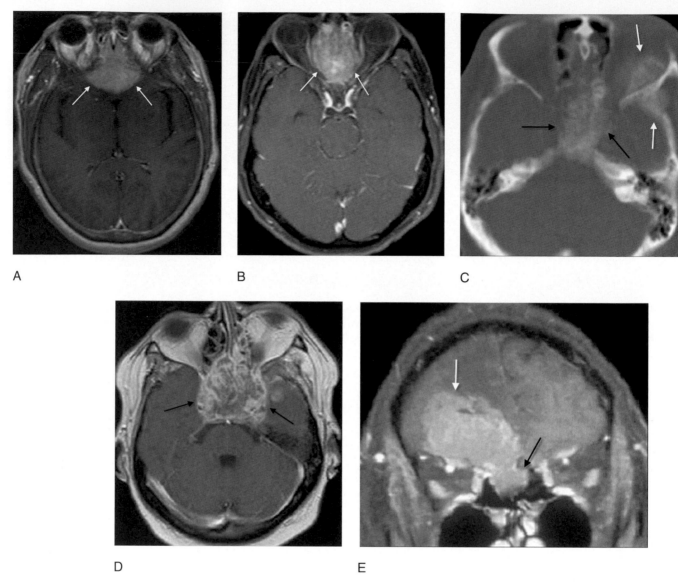

FIG. 8-16. Anterior skull base tumors: Olfactory groove meningioma as typical enhancing tumor along the floor of anterior cranial fossa (arrows, A). A large esthesioneuroblastoma in the anterior fossa (arrows, B), the dominant sinonasal portion (not shown) infiltrated through the cribriform plate. Calcified central skull base (dark arrows, C) and left lateral orbital wall (white arrows, C) masses due to metastasis from osteosarcoma, with heterogeneous enhancement (D, arrows) in contrast to typical homogeneous enhancement of meningiomas. Sinonasal adenocarcinoma as a meningioma mimic. Note ethmoid component (dark arrow, E)

Optic Gliomas

Optic gliomas are three to four times more common than optic nerve sheath meningiomas, with a peak incidence occurring between 2 and 8 years of life, with 90% occurring in the first two decades. Optic gliomas can be categorized into optic nerve gliomas (ONGs), optic chiasm hypothalamic gliomas (OCHGs), and malignant optic nerve gliomas (MONGs), the latter rare subtype occurring in the fifth decade. The imaging distinction between ONGs (orbital and canalicular) and meningiomas is based on the pattern of involvement and growth along the optic nerve sheath complex. ONG causes fusiform thickening and buckling of the nerve, whereas optic sheath meningioma involves optic

nerve sheath manifested as tram-track pattern on postcontrast coronal CT or MRI and stretches the optic nerve without buckling [61]. Both can cause exophthalmos. Optic gliomas are not calcified unless radiated, in contrast to commonly calcified optic nerve sheath meningiomas. Sphenoid wing meningiomas may sometimes extend along the optic nerve sheath. Enhancing chiasmatic gliomas can be confused with suprasellar meningiomas (Fig. 8-10D).

Vascular Lesions

Giant aneurysms commonly occur at the base of the brain, with 43% involving the cavernous segment of the internal carotid artery [62]. On CT, giant aneurysms are homogeneously dense

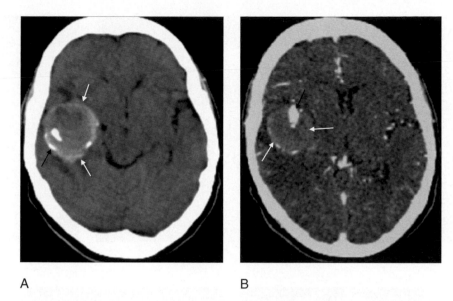

Fig. 8-17. Vascular mimic: Giant MCA aneurysm—large partially calcified rounded hyperdense mass. Note rim calcifications (dark arrow, A) on unenhanced CT, marked luminal thrombosis (white arrows, B) with small residual lumen (black arrow, B) on axial source image of a CTA

in most cases, even without thrombosis. The appearance on pre- and postcontrast CT may be identical to meningioma. However, differentiation can be easily made by using CTA (Fig. 8-17) or MRI and MRA. Rim calcifications on CT and phase-encoding artifact on conventional MRI are helpful for differentiating aneurysms. Giant aneurysm can look more like a tumor as it develops thrombosis with partial to complete loss of flow void characteristics and showing heterogeneous T1 and T2 signals [63]. Small to medium-sized aneurysms can certainly mimic meningiomas, especially when located where meningiomas commonly arise, such as the suprasellar/parasellar regions.

Lesions of the Posterior Fossa/Clivus/Foramen Magnum

Posterior fossa can be host to a variety of mass lesions posing as meningiomas, including vestibular schwannomas and metastases to the cerebellopontine angle and foramen magnum (Fig. 8-18). Among skull base tumors with dominant bone involvement, like chondrosarcomas, chordomas, and metastases, only glomus tumor is discussed due to its hypervascularity and enhancement pattern, commonly resembling meningiomas. Sarcomas involving the skull base are generally heterogeneous, but when calcification is present, these tumors may be confused with meningiomas (Fig. 8-9). Due to the limited space of the posterior fossa, large enhancing cerebellar metastases can be confused with meningiomas due to broader abutment to the posterior fossa walls. Artifacts can look like a mass. The base of skull is a common location for artifacts on both CT and MRI. With CT scanning, this is due to streak artifact from the dense temporal bones, while on MR vascular pulsations from arteries and venous structures at the

base of skull may produce "ghost" or pulsation artifacts in the phase-encoded direction of the image matrix (Fig. 8-19B). Fourth ventricular lesions, though rare in adults, may mimic meningiomas as well.

Schwannomas

A large vestibular schwannoma (VS) can be easily confused with cerebellopontine angle meningioma because of intense enhancement with occasional finding of dural tail sign as well as T2 hypointensity. Intracanalicular component of the tumor, usually with dilatation of the inner ear canal, is a characteristic feature of VS (Fig. 8-18B). However, canalicular extension or even pure intracanalicular meningiomas have been reported [64]. Intracanalicular meningiomas tend to infiltrate into the adjacent bones and inner ear with the irregular medial surface of the tumor. In contrast, VS causes dilatation of the inner ear canal without infiltration, with smooth tumor margins [65].

Glomus Tumors

Glomus jugulare, or glomus jugulo-tympanicum, are hypervascular tumors that are occasionally misdiagnosed as meningiomas. Primary or secondary (extension from other sites) jugular foramen meningiomas complement the differential diagnosis of jugular foramen tumors with glomus tumors, schwannomas, and metastases. "Salt and pepper" appearance on MRI due to T2 hyperintensity and flow voids, intense contrast enhancement, and permeative jugular foraminal margins on CT are typical features of glomus tumors. Arteriography shows early venous filling. Meningiomas, in contrast, generally lack arteriovenous shunting and flow voids, cause sclerotic-permeative destruction of foraminal margins, and show late but persistent venous filling [66].

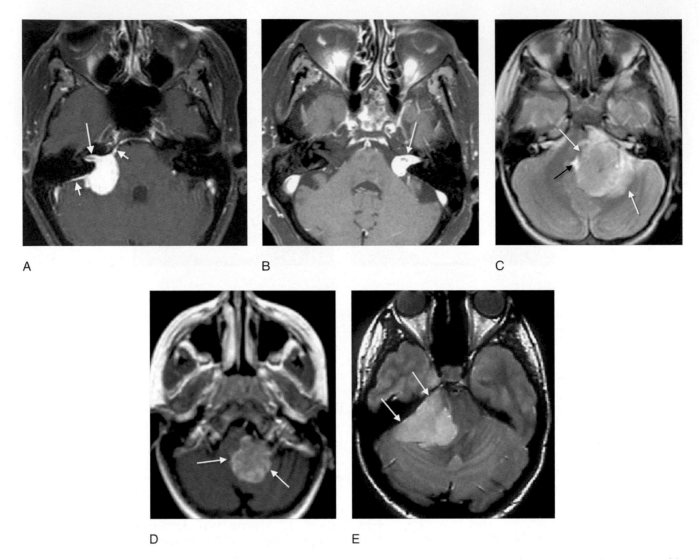

FIG. 8-18. Cerebellopontine angle (CPA) tumors: (A) Example of right CPA meningioma with intense homogeneous enhancement, with a dural tail (short arrows) and intracanalicular extension but without dilatation (long arrow). (B) Typical vestibular schwannoma, with mild IAC expansion (arrow, B). (C, D) Choroid plexus papilloma, with CPA extension from the fourth ventricle (arrows). Note patent 4th ventricle despite the large posterior fossa tumor (dark arrow, C). (E) CPA ependymoma, extension from the fourth ventricle, with an apparent broad dural base along the petrous bone (arrows)

Hemangioblastomas

Solid hemangioblastomas can be confused with meningiomas in the posterior fossa because these show intense homogeneous enhancement [67]. About 40% of hemangioblastomas are purely solid masses [68]. These lesions, occurring along the cerebellar surface or in the fourth ventricle, are difficult to differentiate from meningiomas. However, in large hemangioblastomas, flow voids and prominent draining veins are characteristic diagnostic signs.

Artifacts

Pseudo-masses can be seen due to volume averaging in the recesses of anterior or middle cranial fossa on CT (Fig. 8-19A) and due to pulsation artifacts with apparent mass lesions in the basal cisterns on MRI (typically FLAIR sequence) (Fig.

8-19B). The key is to closely observe the neighboring slices and reproduce the lesion on other sequences or planes. Contrast-enhanced images can be extremely helpful in difficult cases (Fig. 8-19C,D). Dilated veins can appear like dural-based mass but should be reviewed on other sequences and followed on sequential images to avoid misinterpretation (Fig. 8-19E).

Intraventricular Lesions

While intraventricular meningiomas represent a rare subtype, it is nevertheless one of the most common intraventricular tumors in the adult population, especially in the atria of the lateral ventricles [69]. The mimics include choroid plexus papilloma/carcinoma, choroid plexus metastases, ependymoma, oligodendroglioma, astrocytoma, neurocytoma, and lymphoma

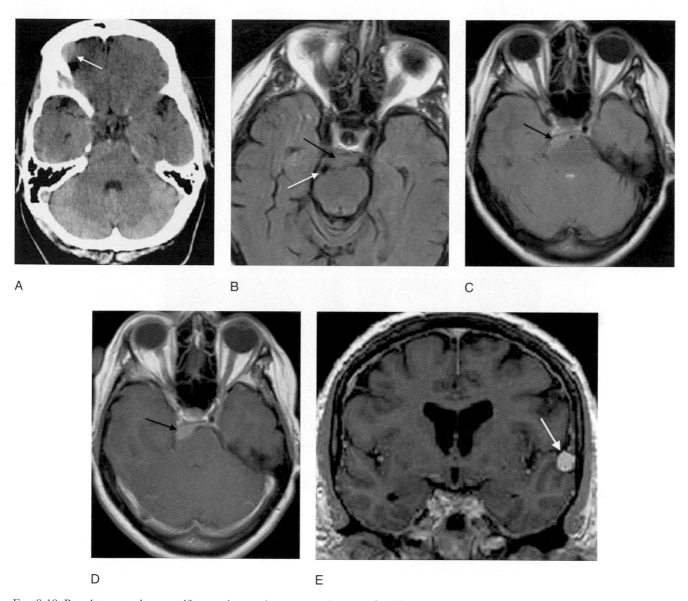

FIG. 8-19. Pseudotumors due to artifacts and normal structures: Apparent focal hyperdense extra-axial mass in the lateral recess of anterior cranial fossa due to volume averaging (arrow, A), commonly observed at the skull base CT images. Pseudo-mass in the prepontine cistern due to pulsation artifact (white arrow, B). Note the adjacent basilar artery flow void (dark arrow, B), which is responsible for the mass effect, further confounding the appearance. A true prepontine mass due to meningioma on FLAIR (arrow, C) showing enhancement (D, arrow). Left-sided apparent enhancing insular mass actually represents a venous varix (arrow, E)

[69] (Fig. 8-7). The key to diagnosis is the age of the patient, with patients in the fourth decade and older favoring meningioma. Imaging features are nonspecific. Preoperative diagnosis is important to determine the surgical approach [26]. MR spectroscopy may also suggest the diagnosis of meningioma.

Intraosseous Lesions

Intraosseous lesions, also termed calvarial meningiomas, are a subtype of primary extradural meningiomas [70]. These typically present as hyperostotic, expansile enhancing masses expanding the diploic space with heterogeneous or sometimes low homogeneous signal intensity on MRI (Fig. 8-20A). Differential diagnosis includes fibrous dysplasia [71], Paget's disease [72], osteoblastic metastases, lymphoma, or less likely hyperdense, intradiploic epidermoid cyst, plasmacytoma [73], and calvarial hemangioma [74] (Fig. 8-20B–D).

Mimics of En Plaque Meningiomas

Granulomatous Disease and Pseudotumors

Basal leptomeningeal nodular enhancement is a typical manifestation of infectous or noninfectious granulomatous disorders. A solitary or dominant dural-based mass can sometimes

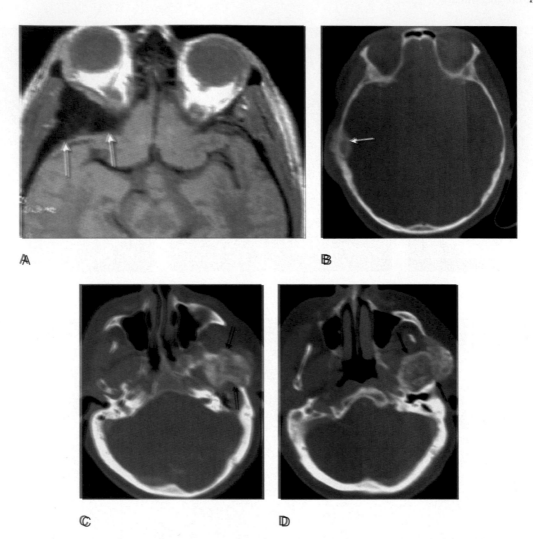

FIG. 8-20. Calvarial meningioma mimics: Note asymmetric hypointense right sphenoid wing expansion (arrows, A) due to calvarial meningioma. Right-side focal sclerotic calvarial expansion due to primary osteosarcoma (arrow, B). Left lateral sphenoid wing and zygomatic exophytic sclerotic lesion due to pseudo-gout (arrows, C, D)

pose a diagnostic challenge [75] by mimicking en plaque meningioma.

Fungal and Tuberculous Granulomatosis

Dural-based inflammatory masses due to fungal infection and tuberculosis are a rare manifestation but can easily resemble meningiomas [76,77]. Clinical information is the key to diagnosis. Intracranial tuberculomas commonly have an isointense or hypointense core with a hyperintense rim on T2-weighted and FLAIR images. Core hypointensity of lesions on these images is related to necrosis and the large number of cells [78].

Sarcoidosis

Neurosarcoidosis, a rare idiopathic inflammatory disease of the CNS, occurs in approximately 5% of patients with sarcoidosis [79]. Intracranial manifestations of neurosarcoidosis includes a spectrum of findings, which include leptomeningeal enhance-

ment and thickening, dural-based masses, and parenchymal lesions. About 5% of cases have solitary extra axial mass [80]. Extra-axial masses as plaque-like dural thickening or discrete dural-based masses can be confused with meningiomas [81]. Increased attenuation on CT, iso- to hypointensity on T1- and T2-weighted images, and homogeneous enhancement can make their distinction from meningioma very difficult (Fig. 8-4).

Idiopathic Hypertrophic Cranial Pachymeningitis

Idiopathic hypertrophic cranial pachymeningitis is a rare inflammatory disorder, the major radiographic finding of which is linear thickening of the falx and tentorium [82]. Focal or diffuse nodularity can simulate a dural mass like meningioma [83]. Rarely, the nodular masses can be very large (Fig. 8-21). To further confuse the distinction from meningioma, the dural sinuses may be involved [82]. Due to dominant fibrous content, the thickened dura is isointense to hypointense on T1

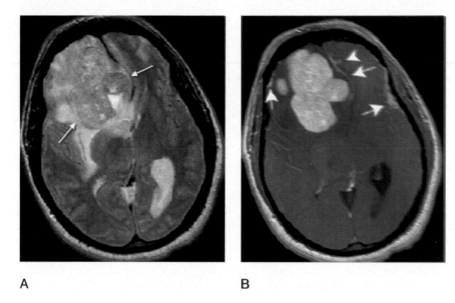

FIG. 8-21. Hypertrophic cranial pachymeningitis: Large right frontal iso- to hypointense T2 mass with edema and mass effect (A, arrows). Homogeneous enhancement of the mass with additional leptomeningeal and pachymeningeal enhancement (B, arrowhead and arrows, respectively) (From Ref. 83.)

and T2 imaging and may show T2 hyperintense rim due to active inflammation [82]. Interestingly, although the nodular dural mass may enhance with intravenous contrast, it is avascular on angiography [83].

Inflammatory Pseudotumor (or Plasma Cell Granuloma)

Intracranial pseudotumor is rare. It can present as a skull base extra-axial enhancing mass, usually parasellar, and may represent an extension of the orbital pseudotumor. Inflammatory pseudotumors are generally iso- to hypointense on T1 and T2 images and may enhance. Flattened growth can mimic en plaque meningiomas [84].

References

1. Rodriguez LE, Rodriguez CY, Cardozo DP, Pena JA, Molina OM, Cardozo JJ. [The classical clinical and neuroimaging features of meningiomas are mimicked by other intracranial, supratentorial expansive lesions]. Rev Neurol 2000;30:907–910.
2. Rohringer M, Sutherland GR, Louw DF, Sima AA. Incidence and clinicopathological features of meningioma. J Neurosurg 1989;71:665–672.
3. Spagnoli MV, Goldberg HI, Grossman RI, et al. Intracranial meningiomas: high-field MR imaging. Radiology 1986;161: 369–375.
4. Sheporaitis LA, Osborn AG, Smirniotopoulos JG, Clunie DA, Howieson J, D'Agostino AN. Intracranial meningioma. AJNR Am J Neuroradiol 1992;13:29–37.
5. Ide M, Jimbo M, Kubo O, Yamamoto M, Takeyama E, Imanaga H. Peritumoral brain edema and cortical damage by meningioma. Acta Neurochir Suppl (Wien) 1994;60:369–372.
6. Koeller KK, Rushing EJ. From the archives of the AFIP: oligodendroglioma and its variants: radiologic-pathologic correlation. Radiographics 2005;25:1669–1688.
7. Tien RD, Yang PJ, Chu PK. "Dural tail sign": a specific MR sign for meningioma? J Comput Assist Tomogr 1991;15:64–66.
8. Guermazi A, Lafitte F, Miaux Y, Adem C, Bonneville JF, Chiras J. The dural tail sign—beyond meningioma. Clin Radiol 2005;60:171–188.
9. Hutzelmann A, Palmie S, Zimmer C, Benz T, Leweke F, Freund M. [The meningeal sign: a new appraisal]. Rofo 1996;164: 314–317.
10. Kuroiwa T, Ohta T. MRI appearances mimicking the dural tail sign: a report of two cases. Neuroradiology 2000;42:199–202.
11. Kutcher TJ, Brown DC, Maurer PK, Ghaed VN. Dural tail adjacent to acoustic neuroma: MR features. J Comput Assist Tomogr 1991;15:669–670.
12. Abdullah S, Morgensztern D, Rosado MF, Lossos IS. Primary lymphoblastic B-cell lymphoma of the cranial dura mater: a case report and review of the literature. Leuk Lymphoma 2005;46:1651–1657.
13. Good CD, Kingsley DP, Taylor WJ, Harkness WF. "Dural tail" adjacent to a giant posterior cerebral artery aneurysm: case report and review of the literature. Neuroradiology 1997;39:577–580.
14. Goldsher D, Litt AW, Pinto RS, Bannon KR, Kricheff II. Dural "tail" associated with meningiomas on Gd-DTPA-enhanced MR images: characteristics, differential diagnostic value, and possible implications for treatment. Radiology 1990;176:447–450.
15. Cho YD, Choi GH, Lee SP, Kim JK. (1)H-MRS metabolic patterns for distinguishing between meningiomas and other brain tumors. Magn Reson Imaging 2003;21:663–672.
16. Younis G, Sawaya R. Intracranial osteolytic malignant meningiomas appearing as extracranial soft-tissue masses. Neurosurgery 1992;30:932–935.

17. Grover SB, Aggarwal A, Uppal PS, Tandon R. The CT triad of malignancy in meningioma—redefinition, with a report of three new cases. Neuroradiology 2003;45:799–803.

18. Tanaka Y, Matsuo M. [Role of MR imaging in the differentiation of benign and nonbenign intracranial meningiomas: the utility of contrast-enhanced T1-weighted images]. Nippon Igaku Hoshasen Gakkai Zasshi 1996;56:1–8.

19. Buetow MP, Buetow PC, Smirniotopoulos JG. Typical, atypical, and misleading features in meningioma. Radiographics 1991;11:1087–1106.

20. Tagle P, Villanueva P, Torrealba G, Huete I. Intracranial metastasis or meningioma? An uncommon clinical diagnostic dilemma. Surg Neurol 2002;58:241–245.

21. Lippman SM, Buzaid AC, Iacono RP, et al. Cranial metastases from prostate cancer simulating meningioma: report of two cases and review of the literature. Neurosurgery 1986;19:820–823.

22. Yodonawa M, Tanaka S, Kohno K, Ishii Z, Tamura M, Ohye C. [Brain metastasis of follicular carcinoma of the thyroid gland. Meningioma-like features demonstrated by CT scan and cerebral angiography—case report]. Neurol Med Chir (Tokyo) 1987;27:995–999.

23. Morioka T, Matsushima T, Ikezaki K, et al. Intracranial adenoid cystic carcinoma mimicking meningioma: report of two cases. Neuroradiology 1993;35:462–465.

24. Umezu H, Sano T, Aiba T, Unakami M. Calcified intracranial metastatic tumor mimicking meningioma—case report. Neurol Med Chir (Tokyo) 1994;34:108–110.

25. Kremer S, Grand S, Remy C, et al. Contribution of dynamic contrast MR imaging to the differentiation between dural metastasis and meningioma. Neuroradiology 2004;46:642–648.

26. Liu M, Wei Y, Liu Y, Zhu S, Li X. Intraventricular meninigiomas: a report of 25 cases. Neurosurg Rev 2006;29:36–40.

27. Quinones-Hinojosa A, Chang EF, Khan SA, Lawton MT, McDermott MW. Renal cell carcinoma metastatic to the choroid mimicking intraventricular meningioma. Can J Neurol Sci 2004;31:115–120.

28. Ahn JY, Choi EW, Kang SH, Kim YR. Isolated meningeal chloroma (granulocytic sarcoma) in a child with acute lymphoblastic leukemia mimicking a falx meningioma. Childs Nerv Syst 2002;18:153–156.

29. Wright DH, Hise JH, Bauserman SC, Naul LG. Intracranial granulocytic sarcoma: CT, MR, and angiography. J Comput Assist Tomogr 1992;16:487–489.

30. Fucharoen S, Suthipongchai S, Poungvarin N, Ladpli S, Sonakul D, Wasi P. Intracranial extramedullary hematopoiesis inducing epilepsy in a patient with beta-thalassemia—hemoglobin E. Arch Intern Med 1985;145:739–742.

31. Atweh GF, Jabbour N. Intracranial solitary extraskeletal plasmacytoma resembling meningioma. Arch Neurol 1982;39:57–59.

32. Provenzale JM, Schaefer P, Traweek ST, et al. Craniocerebral plasmacytoma: MR features. AJNR Am J Neuroradiol 1997;18:389–392.

33. Vonofakos D, Marcu H, Hacker H. Oligodendrogliomas: CT patterns with emphasis on features indicating malignancy. J Comput Assist Tomogr 1979;3:783–788.

34. Becker H, Vonofakos D. [Diagnostic significance of brain tumor calcifications in the computerized tomogram]. Radiologe 1983;23:459–462.

35. Morantz RA, Feigin I, Ransohoff J, III. Clinical and pathological study of 24 cases of gliosarcoma. J Neurosurg 1976;45:398–408.

36. Lee YY, Castillo M, Nauert C, Moser RP. Computed tomography of gliosarcoma. AJNR Am J Neuroradiol 1985;6:527–531.

37. Jack CR, Jr., Bhansali DT, Chason JL, et al. Angiographic features of gliosarcoma. AJNR Am J Neuroradiol 1987;8:117–122.

38. Lewis AI, Tew JM, Jr., Payner TD, Yeh HS. Dural cavernous angiomas outside the middle cranial fossa: a report of two cases. Neurosurgery 1994;35:498–504.

39. Shen WC, Chenn CA, Hsue CT, Lin TY. Dural cavernous angioma mimicking a meningioma and causing facial pain. J Neuroimaging 2000;10:183–185.

40. Vogler R, Castillo M. Dural cavernous angioma: MR features. AJNR Am J Neuroradiol 1995;16:773–775.

41. Rosso D, Lee DH, Ferguson GG, Tailor C, Iskander S, Hammond RR. Dural cavernous angioma: a preoperative diagnostic challenge. Can J Neurol Sci 2003;30:272–277.

42. Rivera PP, Willinsky RA, Porter PJ. Intracranial cavernous malformations. Neuroimaging Clin N Am 2003;13:27–40.

43. Yan HJ, Lin KE, Lee ST, Tzaan WC. Calcified chronic subdural hematoma: case report. Changgeng Yi Xue Za Zhi 1998;21: 521–525.

44. Shrivastava RK, Sen C, Costantino PD, Della RR. Sphenoorbital meningiomas: surgical limitations and lessons learned in their long-term management. J Neurosurg 2005;103:491–497.

45. Cappabianca P, Cirillo S, Alfieri A, et al. Pituitary macroadenoma and diaphragma sellae meningioma: differential diagnosis on MRI. Neuroradiology 1999;41:22–26.

46. Taylor SL, Barakos JA, Harsh GR, Wilson CB. Magnetic resonance imaging of tuberculum sellae meningiomas: preventing preoperative misdiagnosis as pituitary macroadenoma. Neurosurgery 1992;31:621–627.

47. Sebbag M, Schmidt V, Leboucq N, Bitoun J, Castan P, Frerebeau P. [Dura mater chondroma. A case report and review of the literature]. J Radiol 1990;71:495–498.

48. Lacerte D, Gagne F, Copty M. Intracranial chondroma. Report of two cases and review of the literature. Can J Neurol Sci 1996;23:132–137.

49. Brownlee RD, Sevick RJ, Rewcastle NB, Tranmer BI. Intracranial chondroma. AJNR Am J Neuroradiol 1997;18:889–893.

50. Lin WC, Lirng JF, Ho DM, et al. A rare giant intracranial osteochondroma. Zhonghua Yi Xue Za Zhi (Taipei) 2002;65:235–238.

51. Miura FK, De Aguiar PH, Michailowsky C, et al. [Falx osteochondroma: case report and review of the literature]. Arq Neuropsiquiatr 1997;55:618–624.

52. Ikeda Y, Shimura T, Higuchi H, Nakazawa S, Sugisaki Y. [Intracranial osteochondroma—case report (author's transl)]. No Shinkei Geka 1980;8:263–269.

53. Chitkara N, Sharma NK, Goyal N. Osteoma mimicking a partly calcified meningioma. Neurol India 2003;51:287–288.

54. Fujimaki T, Matsutani M, Funada N, et al. CT and MRI features of intracranial germ cell tumors. J Neurooncol 1994;19:217–226.

55. Konovalov AN, Spallone A, Pitzkhelauri DI. Meningioma of the pineal region: a surgical series of 10 cases. J Neurosurg 1996;85:586–590.

56. Yang C, Jagjivan B, Rao K. Germinoma-unusual presentation: a case report. Conn Med 2004;68:617–619.

57. Som PM, Lidov M, Brandwein M, Catalano P, Biller HF. Sinonasal esthesioneuroblastoma with intracranial extension: marginal tumor cysts as a diagnostic MR finding. AJNR Am J Neuroradiol 1994;15:1259–1262.

58. Rottnek M, Strauchen J, Moore F, Morgello S. Primary dural mucosa-associated lymphoid tissue-type lymphoma: case report and review of the literature. J Neurooncol 2004;68:19–23.

59. Kumar S, Kumar D, Kaldjian EP, Bauserman S, Raffeld M, Jaffe ES. Primary low-grade B-cell lymphoma of the dura: a mucosa associated lymphoid tissue-type lymphoma. Am J Surg Pathol 1997;21:81–87.

60. Xu QW, Che XM, Hu J, Yang BJ. Diagnosis and treatment of trigeminal schwannomas extending into both the middle and posterior cranial fossa. Chin Med J (Engl) 2004;117:1876–1879.

61. Kanamalla US. The optic nerve tram-track sign. Radiology 2003;227:718–719.

62. Morley TP, Barr HW. Giant intracranial aneurysms: diagnosis, course, and management. Clin Neurosurg 1969;16:73–94.

63. Bonneville F, Cattin F, Marsot-Dupuch K, Dormont D, Bonneville JF, Chiras J. T1 signal hyperintensity in the sellar region: spectrum of findings. Radiographics 2006;26:93–113.

64. Khaimook W, Hirunpat S, Dejsukum C. Meningioma of the internal auditory canal: a case report. J Med Assoc Thai 2005;88:1707–1711.

65. Asaoka K, Barrs DM, Sampson JH, McElveen JT, Jr., Tucci DL, Fukushima T. Intracanalicular meningioma mimicking vestibular schwannoma. AJNR Am J Neuroradiol 2002;23:1493–1496.

66. Macdonald AJ, Salzman KL, Harnsberger HR, Gilbert E, Shelton C. Primary jugular foramen meningioma: imaging appearance and differentiating features. AJR Am J Roentgenol 2004;182:373–377.

67. Yamada SM, Ikeda Y, Takahashi H, Teramoto A, Yamada S. Hemangioblastomas with blood supply from the dural arteries—two case reports. Neurol Med Chir (Tokyo) 2000;40:69–73.

68. Xie J, Ma Z, Luo S. [Clinical features of hemangioblastomas of the central nervous system]. Zhonghua Yi Xue Za Zhi 1997;77:191–193.

69. Koeller KK, Sandberg GD. From the archives of the AFIP. Cerebral intraventricular neoplasms: radiologic-pathologic correlation. Radiographics 2002;22:1473–1505.

70. Lang FF, Macdonald OK, Fuller GN, DeMonte F. Primary extradural meningiomas: a report on nine cases and review of the literature from the era of computerized tomography scanning. J Neurosurg 2000;93:940–950.

71. Keyaki A, Nabeshima S, Bessho H, et al. [Fibrous dysplasia of the skull presenting interesting neuroradiological findings]. No Shinkei Geka 1999;27:275–279.

72. Jayaraj K, Martinez S, Freeman A, Lyles KW. Intraosseous meningioma—a mimicry of Paget's disease? J Bone Miner Res 2001;16:1154–1156.

73. Nakai Y, Yanaka K, Iguchi M, et al. [A case of multiple myeloma presenting with a subcutaneous mass: significance of "dural tail sign" in the differential diagnosis of the meningeal tumors]. No Shinkei Geka 1999;27:67–71.

74. Politi M, Romeike BF, Papanagiotou P, et al. Intraosseous hemangioma of the skull with dural tail sign: radiologic features with pathologic correlation. AJNR Am J Neuroradiol 2005;26:2049–2052.

75. Lindner A, Schneider C, Hofmann E, Soerensen N, Toyka KV. Isolated meningeal tuberculoma mimicking meningioma: case report. Surg Neurol 1995;43:81–83.

76. Yanardag H, Uygun S, Yumuk V, Caner M, Canbaz B. Cerebral tuberculosis mimicking intracranial tumour. Singapore Med J 2005;46:731–733.

77. Adachi K, Yoshida K, Tomita H, Niimi M, Kawase T. Tuberculoma mimicking falx meningioma—case report. Neurol Med Chir (Tokyo) 2004;44:489–492.

78. Wasay M, Kheleani BA, Moolani MK, et al. Brain CT and MRI findings in 100 consecutive patients with intracranial tuberculoma. J Neuroimaging 2003;13:240–247.

79. Delaney P. Neurologic manifestations in sarcoidosis: review of the literature, with a report of 23 cases. Ann Intern Med 1977;87:336–345.

80. Pickuth D, Heywang-Kobrunner SH. Neurosarcoidosis: evaluation with MRI. J Neuroradiol 2000;27:185–188.

81. Rodriguez F, Link MJ, Driscoll CL, Giannini C. Neurosarcoidosis mimicking meningioma. Arch Neurol 2005;62:148–149.

82. Martin N, Masson C, Henin D, Mompoint D, Marsault C, Nahum H. Hypertrophic cranial pachymeningitis: assessment with CT and MR imaging. AJNR Am J Neuroradiol 1989;10:477–484.

83. Kazem IA, Robinette NL, Roosen N, Schaldenbrand MF, Kim JK. Best cases from the AFIP: idiopathic tumefactive hypertrophic pachymeningitis. Radiographics 2005;25:1075–1080.

84. Narla LD, Newman B, Spottswood SS, Narla S, Kolli R. Inflammatory pseudotumor. Radiographics 2003;23:719–729.

9
Preoperative Embolization of Meningiomas

David J. Fiorella, Vivek R. Deshmukh, Cameron G. McDougall, Robert F. Spetzler, and Felipe C. Albuquerque

Introduction

Surgical excision of hypervascular meningiomas and other central nervous system (CNS) tumors is associated with the potential for significant, sometimes catastrophic, blood loss. The need to mitigate intraoperative tumoral hemorrhage and thereby reduce the morbidity and mortality associated with surgical resection has fostered the refinement of neuroendovascular techniques for the preoperative embolization of tumors. Since these techniques were first described in the early 1970s, the field has matured rapidly with advances in microcatheter technology and ongoing improvements in the design of embolisates. Nonetheless, the tenets fundamental to embolization of tumors, particularly a thorough understanding of the associated neurovascular anatomy, are not novel. This chapter describes embolization techniques, reviews key angioarchitectural features of meningiomas, and offers caveats to minimize complications.

Principles of Embolization

The goal of preoperative embolization is to decrease intraoperative blood loss. Embolization-induced ischemia often softens the meningioma as well, thereby facilitating its resection and reducing the compression exerted on nearby neural structures. Theoretically, tumor resection then becomes safer and more complete. Other purported goals of meningioma embolization are to reduce operating time and to decrease the likelihood of a recurrence.

Preembolization Procedure

As with any neuroendovascular procedure, preoperative planning represents the most important aspect of the entire process. The noninvasive imaging and cerebral angiogram must be reviewed prospectively by the neuroendovascular interventionist and the open neurosurgical team to discuss the utility of preoperative embolization. The operators must agree on the targeted branches

for embolization and upon the degree of aggressiveness required to facilitate safe surgical resection. The targets for embolization are tailored to each patient with the ultimate goal of achieving the lowest risk of morbidity and mortality for the combined procedures of embolization and resection.

Embolization Procedure

Meningioma embolization is most frequently performed via a transfemoral arterial approach. Embolization may be performed in a single session, or it may be staged. Angiography and embolization may be performed under general anesthesia or conscious sedation. We strongly prefer to perform all of these procedures under general anesthesia. While the ability to perform provocative testing is lost under these conditions, the quality of digital subtraction angiography and fluoroscopic road-mapping is tremendously improved by patient paralysis, particularly with prolonged procedures. Even minimal patient movement can obscure critically important vascular anastomoses during superselective angiography. Movement during embolization can impair the detection of embolisate reflux as well as nontarget embolization.

The size of the femoral sheath should be tailored to the surgical goals and attention should be given to the necessity of a balloon delivery system. In the vast majority of cases, the embolization can be performed using a 6F sheath and guiding catheter system. A coaxial Envoy 6F (Cordis, Miami, FL) guiding catheter and UCSF-3 (Cordis, Miami, FL) 4 French catheter are advanced into to the external carotid artery (ECA) or internal carotid artery (ICA). The UCSF-3 catheter is either removed or steered selectively into an ECA branch to provide further support for the microcatheter system.

Once a targeted arterial supply is identified, a microcatheter is advanced coaxially (or tri-axially) through the guiding catheter into the feeding artery with the use of fluoroscopic roadmap guidance. The microcatheter is navigated through the feeding vessel to achieve a catheter position as close to the target as possible. We prefer using the new-generation hydrophilic microcatheters (Renegade; Boston Scientific) and microwires (Transcend or Synchro-14; Boston Scientific). Embolization is typically performed with polyvinyl alcohol (PVA) particles or *n*-butyl cyanoacrylate (NBCA; Cordis) or Onyx (Microtherapeutics) liquid embolisate.

Before embolization begins, several anatomic factors should be carefully assessed with superselective angiography: the presence of extracranial-intracranial (EC-IC) anastomoses, shared arterial supply between tumor and normal structures, the caliber of tumor vessels, the strength of injection required to elicit parent vessel reflux and finally, the potential implications of embolisate reflux (i.e., whether or not the parent vessel supplies a sensitive or eloquent structure). Embolization is most beneficial and has the most favorable risk-benefit profile for tumors primarily supplied by the ECA.[1,2] For particulates, the volume of embolic material that reaches a vascular tumor bed depends on the blood flow to the lesion relative to the blood flow within alternative pathways that are also antegrade to the tip of the microcatheter. Therefore, superselective catheterization of a vessel as proximal as possible to the targeted lesion allows a maximal amount of embolisate to be delivered into the lesion at the lowest risk.

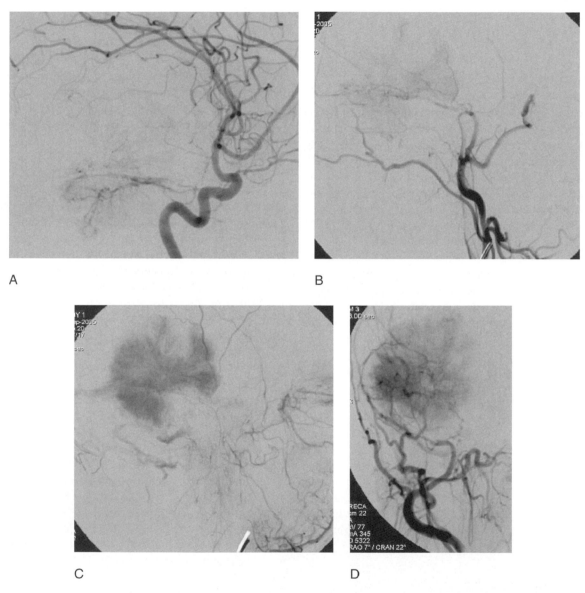

FIG. 9-1. (A) Lateral ICA angiographic injection demonstrates numerous small tortuous arterial feeders arising from the dorsal cavernous ICA providing supply to a large tentorial meningioma. These branches were not accessible to direct catheterization. The risk of a balloon protected embolization from a catheter positioned within the proximal ICA was felt to be of too high a risk. Arterial (B) and capillary (C) phase lateral and (D) RAO ECA angiogram demonstrates arterial supply to the mass arising from the petrous branch of the middle meningeal artery as well as small transmastoid branches of the occipital artery. Both branches were selectively catheterized, and embolization was performed with PVA particles. Care was taken to avoid proximal reflux during embolization of the MMA given the risk of facial nerve paralysis from this catheter position

Occlusion of the proximal feeding arteries only reduces blood flow to the tumor temporarily. Collateral supply quickly develops, and the beneficial effect of the embolization is short-lived. Occlusion of proximal arteries may, however, be considered if access to distal supply is poor. The logical end-point for embolization is an angiographically demonstrated decrease in the vascularity of the tumor with preservation of normal arterial territories. The ideal barometers for efficacy of embolization include MRI-verified tumor infarction, histologic evidence of tumor necrosis, ease of surgical resection, and mitigation of intraoperative blood loss.

The introduction of new-generation variable stiffness and hydrophilic microcatheters has greatly facilitated vascular superselectivity. For tumors with significant blood supply from the cavernous ICA (Fig. 9-1), embolization can rarely be performed via direct microcatheterization of these small branches. If technically infeasible, another option[3,4] (used by the senior author CGM) is occlusion of the distal ICA with a nondetachable balloon and subsequent infusion of embolic material (typically PVA or ethanol) into the segment of the ICA supplying the tumor. Before the balloon is deflated, this region of the ICA must be flushed with at least 20 cc of heparinized saline. A similar volume is withdrawn from the guiding catheter to irrigate the ICA. Theron et al.[4] believe that this balloon-assisted technique may be used for hypervascular lesions supplied by branches of the vertebral artery (i.e., posterior inferior cerebral artery [PICA]) as well. While theoretically attractive, this type of balloon-assisted embolization must be used judiciously due to the significant risk for the distal migration of embolic material upon balloon deflation. Embolization of pial vessels (Fig. 9-2) supplying a meningioma is also relatively hazardous.

These vessels are within the subarachnoid space and are fragile. The negotiation of large ID microcatheters into superselective positions distally within pial vessels is associated with a risk of arterial perforation and intracranial hemorrhage. More importantly, the embolization of pial vessels from a more proximal position presents a significant potential for stroke from nontarget embolization.

When a meningioma is supplied by branches of the ophthalmic artery, embolization may be performed safely if a few principles are followed (Fig. 9-3). First, embolization must be performed only if it is essential and only if the embolized vessel cannot be accessed readily surgically. The central retinal artery and choroidal blush must be visualized. Embolisates must not be allowed to enter the central retinal artery. A lidocaine or Amytal (sodium amobarbital) test may occasionally be useful to verify that occlusion of ophthalmic artery branches will not cause blindness. If the central retinal artery is thought to be at high risk, coils or larger diameter embolisates (>400 μm) may be used. However, their use does not guarantee the integrity of the central retinal artery. Lefkowitz et al.[5] embolized three anterior skull base meningiomas and one nasal angiofibroma via the ophthalmic artery. One patient experienced transient visual deterioration after embolization with PVA (700- to 1000-μm particles).

Intraoperative percutaneous tumor puncture has been advocated for tumors predominantly supplied by the ICA or pial vessels. Patients whose ECA has already been sacrificed are also perhaps better served with direct tumor puncture. Casasco et al.[6] recommended the use of intraoperative fluoroscopy to assist with the embolization. If reflux into the feeding arteries is visualized, embolization should cease.

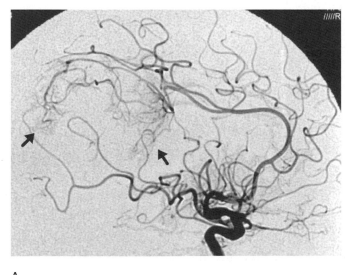 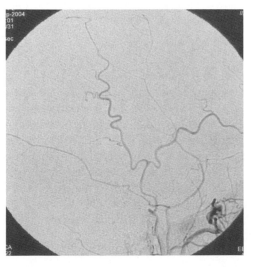

A   B

FIG. 9-2. (A) Lateral ICA injection depicts a falcine meningioma with arterial supply arising solely from the pial (pericallosal branches) vessels. (B) Selective angiography of the ipsilateral ECA demonstrates no supply to the mass. The contralateral ECA demonstrated a similar lack of supply to the tumor

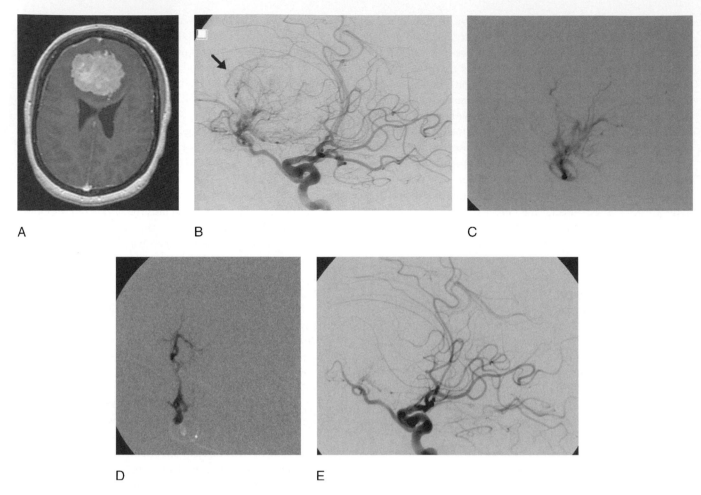

FIG. 9-3. (A) Axial T1 postcontrast MR image depicts a large anterior falcine meningioma. (B) ICA angiogram in the lateral projection demonstrates ethmoidal branches arising from the ophthalmic artery as the dominant vascular supply to the mass (arrow). (C) Superselective angiography (lateral projection) from a microcatheter positioned within a large ethmoidal branch demonstrates flow passing exclusively into the tumor bed with no opacification of the ophthalmic artery or central retinal artery. (D) Fluoroscopic roadmap (in the same projection as the superselective angiogram) depicts a radio-opaque nBCA cast within this branch of the ethmoidal artery. (E) Flow into the tumor bed was markedly reduced following embolization

Postembolization Procedure

After embolization, patients should be monitored in an intensive care unit for 24 hours. Particular attention must be paid to periprocedural stroke, cranial nerve deficits, or intracranial hemorrhage. Corticosteroids are recommended for large tumors associated with significant surrounding edema. Postembolization magnetic resonance imaging (MRI) is often obtained for the purpose of frameless stereotaxy. These images should be reviewed for intracranial hemorrhage or exacerbation of peritumoral edema. Such findings may warrant more urgent surgical excision.

Radiographic Effects of Embolization

Radiographic demonstration of tumor necrosis after particulate embolization appears to be indiscriminate. Terada et al.[7] noted disappearance of tumor flow voids after embolization with gelfoam or PVA. Most tumors showed a decrease in the level of contrast enhancement. Bendszus et al.[8] found that more completely embolized tumors showed less contrast enhancement on postembolization MRI. Wakhloo et al.,[9] however, reported diminished enhancement on contrast MRI in only 2 of 14 patients after embolization with 150- to 300-μm particulates. They theorized that this disappointing radiographic result reflected proximal occlusion of the feeding arteries by larger particulates. Grand et al.[10] described only a minimal decrease in tumor enhancement after embolization and attributed this discrepancy to vasospasm of the embolized vessels. Therefore, smaller particulates may allow embolization of more distal capillaries, increasing the likelihood of tumor necrosis after embolization.

Timing of Embolization

The optimal timing for preoperative embolization is controversial.[11–13] Some authors recommend surgical resection 1–5 days after embolization,[13–15] while others advocate waiting

1–2 weeks. With time, embolization-induced necrosis shrinks and softens the tumor, thereby facilitating surgical resection. Compared to more proximal occlusion, delivering microemboli directly into the tumor maximizes this necrotic effect. The potential for recanalization of embolized vessels and collateral development increases if surgical resection is significantly delayed (>1 week). In contrast, Kai et al.[11] retrospectively reviewed 45 patients with meningiomas embolized with cellulose porous beads. Resectability was greatest in tumors excised 7–9 days after embolization. The consensus remains, however, that the greatest benefit is derived from embolization if surgical resection is performed within a few days of embolization.

Embolisates

The ideal embolic agent should be permanent, easily deployed, and should not encumber tumor resection. Historically, various embolic agents have been used for the preoperative embolization of tumors. These permanent or temporary embolic agents include liquid tissue adhesives such as NBCA, Onyx[13] and silicone rubber and particulates such as silastic beads, lyophilized dura matter, phenytoin, microspheres,[14] microfibrillar collagen,[15] oxidized cellulose, gelatin sponge, PVA,[16] and fibrin glue. Ethanol and detachable coils should also be included in this armamentarium.

PVA

PVA is the most common particulate agent used. It can be used for all tumors, including those associated with high blood flow and arteriovenous shunting. PVA is shaved into precisely sized particles from an original block form.[22–24] The size of particles can range from 50–150 to 500–1200 μm.

Large embolisates do not penetrate deeply into tumor tissue, but they pose less risk of embolizing adjacent normal tissue. Smaller particulates and liquid agents penetrate deeply into the tumor but also have the potential to migrate into normal territory. PVA is delivered until stasis of contrast is noted in the embolized vessel. Should any reflux be visible, embolization should be discontinued.

PVA has several advantages. The particles are inert and water insoluble. They are absorbed slowly and are known to expand to occlude arteries with a diameter larger than the inner diameter of the microcatheter. They produce a vigorous inflammatory reaction. Polymorphonuclear proteins predominate at 2 weeks; a giant cell reaction occurs at 3 months; and an adherent, organized, partially calcified thrombus appears at 9 months. PVA embolisate is long lasting but not permanent. Degradation occurs within several weeks to months. Technically, PVA is easy to deliver. The risk of stroke or cranial nerve palsy with the use of PVA particles diminishes as larger particles are used. PVA, however, has limitations. Early recanalization can occur when thrombus between the particles is dissolved by endogenous physiologic lytic processes. Furthermore, the high friction coefficient of PVA can lead to frequent catheter obstruction.

Tissue Adhesive Embolisate

NBCA glue embolisate is a stable, nonabsorbable, liquid polymerizing agent, which is commonly used to treat arteriovenous malformations (AVMs) or fistulas and, less frequently, tumors. NBCA is mixed with an oil-based contrast agent (ethiodol [ethiodized oil]), usually in a 1:2.5 cc ratio. This formulation polymerizes immediately upon contact with ionic solution or blood and occludes both distal and proximal feeders almost simultaneously.

NBCA is a more permanent agent than PVA, and it immediately obliterates the feeding branch. NBCA, however, is used with tumors less often than PVA because of its tendency to occlude both distal and proximal vessels, which may be associated with a greater likelihood of nontarget embolization, which can result in cranial nerve injury or stroke. The delivery of NBCA has technical constraints that require experience to use it successfully.[13] When used for ophthalmic lesions, NBCA can cause ocular myosits, resulting in ocular pain.[5] If acrylic glue is used for embolization, microcatheters can get caught or break, particularly if the microcatheter is bathed in the glue for an inordinate length of time.[18] These factors are less of an issue with the newer embolic agent ethylene vinyl co-polymer (Onyx, Microtherapeutics, Irvine CA). Onyx may be delivered in a slower and more controlled manner, given its lower likelihood of adhering to the microcatheter. The operator may even perform angiographic runs during the Onyx infusion to assess the progress of the injection.

Cellulose Beads and Microspheres

Cellulose porous beads also have been used for the preoperative embolization of tumors. Their favorable properties include a uniform size, a specific gravity similar to that of blood, and a positive charge that prevents clumping. Hamada et al.[19] performed a prospective clinical trial in which 16 patients, 13 with tumors, underwent embolization with cellulose porous beads measuring 150 or 200 μm. None of the patients suffered complications. Postembolization angiography showed satisfactory stasis in all cases. Histologic analysis of embolized vessels demonstrated no stretching of the embolized vessel and only mild inflammatory reactions. Trisacryl gelatin microspheres (Embospheres, Biosphere Medical, Rockland, MA) are a hydrophilic, nonabsorbable, collagen-coated agent. The size of the particles is calibrated, but the particles are deformable. In addition, the particles tend not to aggregate. Progressively larger embospheres may be used in the course of embolization. Bendszus et al.[20] compared trisacryl gelatin microspheres to PVA particles in achieving distal microembolization and in mitigating intraoperative blood loss. Their most important finding was that the microspheres penetrated more distally within the vascular bed than similarly sized PVA particles. In general, the chosen particulate size should be significantly upsized if embospheres are to be used in the place of PVA. Further investigations are needed to establish the role of cellulose beads and embospheres in this arena.

Alcohol

Alcohol is a powerful sclerotic and cytotoxic agent that allows small caliber arterial feeders to be obliterated. Its capacity to devascularize is potent. It causes anoxic cell damage, protein precipitation, and fibrinoid necrosis of the intimal lining.[21] Because its viscosity is low, alcohol can permeate more distally than other agents and cause sclerosis from within the tumor. The use of ethyl alcohol, however, is associated with a high risk of cranial nerve deficits or normal tissue infarction.[3,16] It also induces a robust inflammatory response that obliterates tissue planes and is directly toxic to both the parent vessel and target tissue. Horowitz et al.[22] embolized a carotid body tumor with ethanol in conjunction with distal balloon occlusion. They circumvented the above limitations by reducing the dosing rate (4×10^{-5} cc/kg/sec) and by resecting the lesions within 24 hours of embolization. Intraoperatively, alcohol injected intratumorally has yielded devascularization. Before alcohol is injected, aspiration is necessary to verify that a large vessel is not receiving this sclerotic agent. Lonser et al.[23] treated three spinal epidural masses and one posterior fossa hemangioblastoma with direct intratumoral injection of ethanol. They avoided exposing normal tissues and used a small needle (28 g) to introduce the embolisate into the tumor. The endpoint was visible blanching of the tumor. They recommended intratumoral injection of ethanol as an inexpensive, universally available method of augmenting preoperative embolization. Ethanol has proven to be a powerful embolisate with a well-defined, albeit limited, role.

Coils

The primary utility of coils in tumor embolization is their ability to augment or facilitate the effects of other embolisates. Liquid or fibered coils are most commonly used for tumor embolization. Liquid coils are soft and injectable. Fibered coils are pushed mechanically through the microcatheter with a coil pusher. Coils may be used to obliterate potentially dangerous EC-IC connections before embolization with particulates. After particulate embolization, they also can be used to obliterate the proximal aspect of a feeding artery to reduce the rate of recanalization.

Gelatin Foam

Gelatin foam particles are typically 40–60 µm. Therefore, their use achieves deep tissue penetration with subsequent necrosis. Gelfoam has the advantage of being easy to use; it is easily delivered through a microcatheter without friction or blockage. However, it is quickly degraded by native proteolytic mechanisms. Embolized vessels therefore recanalize

fairly rapidly. Furthermore, their small caliber increases the risks of embolization of the vaso vasorum of the cranial nerves and of unpredictable embolization via EC-IC collaterals. As with other embolisates, there is a learning curve in avoiding these complications.

Fibrin Glue

Fibrin glue has been used successfully to embolize tumors. The radiopacity of the fibrin glue enables continuous monitoring during embolization. Probst et al. argued that fibrin allows the most distal loading of the vascular bed and decreases the potential for reflux. In their series of 80 patients in whom fibrin glue was used for embolization, two patients suffered permanent neurologic deficits (hypesthesia in the trigeminal nerve distribution and incomplete facial paresis).

Microfibrillar Collagen

Microfibrillar collagen is prepared from purified bovine collagen. It is frequently used as a topical agent during surgery and effectively controls capillary hemorrhage. It promotes platelet aggregation and is effective even in the presence of underlying coagulopathies or heparinization. Kumar et al.[15] contended that the semi-liquid suspension readily passes through microcatheters and that the collagen can penetrate end arteries more effectively than PVA.

Phenytoin

Phenytoin is rarely used as an embolisate. Kasuya et al.[24] demonstrated that phenytoin administered via a microcatheter at a dosage of 250–500 mg resulted in both ischemic and hemorrhagic necrosis with devascularization of meningiomas. They suggested that phenytoin has the added advantages of producing precapillary microthrombosis and more complete devascularization than other agents. They recommended the perioperative administration of steroids as prophylaxis against malignant edema.

Miscellaneous

Kubo et al.[25] used hydroxyapatite ceramic microparticles to embolize meningiomas in 13 patients. They noted excellent biocompatibility, good injection control, and excellent occlusion of the distal capillary bed. No microcatheters became clogged. Histologic analysis revealed mild inflammation with lymphocytic infiltration. No patient suffered a hemorrhage after embolization.

Complications of Embolization

Both minor and major complications can be associated with preoperative embolization. The most common complications of embolization are fever and localized pain.[26]

Potentially more devastating complications include inadvertent delivery of embolisate into the intracranial circulation, intracranial or intratumoral hemorrhage, and cranial nerve injury.

Embolization of ECA branches can be complicated by unrecognized collateral connections with the posterior circulation or ICA, resulting in delivery of embolisate into the intracranial circulation. EC-IC collaterals that warrant particular note include the anastomosis between the ophthalmic artery and the meningolacrimal branch of the middle meningeal artery. Branches of the middle meningeal and accessory meningeal arteries can have reciprocal communications with branches of the cavernous segment of the ICA. The vertebral artery shares collaterals with both the ascending pharyngeal artery and the occipital artery at the odontoid arterial arch and the interspaces of C1-C2, respectively. The internal maxillary artery may have reciprocal connections with branches of the cavernous ICA, namely between the artery of the foramen rotundum and the anterolateral branch of the inferolateral trunk, between the accessory meningeal artery and the posteromedial branch of the inferolateral trunk, and between the middle meningeal artery and the posterolateral branch of the inferolateral trunk.

In the presence of an unrecognized patent foramen ovale, Horowitz et al.[27] showed that particulate embolization may result in paradoxical embolization and subsequent stroke. They recommended the liberal use of neurophysiologic monitoring in patients undergoing general anesthesia and frequent neurologic examinations in sedated patients. Intraoperative monitoring of somatosensory evoked potentials, although cumbersome and expensive, may, in some cases, increase the safety of embolization by enabling the early identification of ischemia.[28]

Embolization can injure cranial nerves by interrupting the vascular supply of the cranial nerves (vaso vasorum), which is often derived from the ECA. A petrous branch of the middle meningeal artery may supply the facial nerve, and the neuromeningeal branch of the ascending pharyngeal artery frequently supplies the spinal accessory and hypoglossal nerves. The potential blood supply of a cranial nerve cannot readily be identified from the dynamic anatomic information provided by angiography. Therefore, provocative testing with lidocaine has been used to determine if a potentially embolizable branch supplies a cranial nerve. Horton and Kerber[29] described 26 patients who underwent the injection of 2% lidocaine mixed in equal volumes with Conray 60 (Mallinckrodt, St. Louis, MO). The injection (30–70cc) was monitored with continuous fluoroscopy to ensure that no reflux occurred into the ICA. Continuous cardiac monitoring was also performed. Patients with heart block did not undergo this lidocaine challenge. Patients underwent embolization with PVA and gelfoam particles, if cranial nerve function remained stable. If the lidocaine test was positive, the catheter was removed from the vessel and the palsy was allowed to resolve. The use of provocative lidocaine testing

for pial arterial branches, which are potential candidates for embolization, is not as widespread given the high rate of false-positive and false-negative results and the associated risk of seizure induction.

Applications of Preoperative Meningioma Embolization

Rates of meningioma recurrence have been estimated at 9–11% if the dural attachment is excised, at 19–22% if the dural attachment is left in place, and at almost 40% if the tumor is excised subtotally.[38–41] Incomplete tumor removal may be related to tumoral hemorrhage during surgery, particularly with hypervascular meningiomas. Angiography allows the arterial supply to the tumor to be determined. It shows the site of dural attachment, the presence of displacement, or the degree of encasement of key vascular structures, including the dural venous sinuses. It also helps determine the vascularity of a tumor.

Vascular Supply

The vascular supply of meningiomas is often both dural and pial. Arterial feeders to the pedicle at the site of attachment and center of the tumor typically arise from branches of the ECA and supply the tumor radially to produce the characteristic "sunburst" appearance on angiography. The apex of the sunburst is usually the site of dural attachment. In some cases, pial arteries supply the meningioma capsule, and this contribution increases as the tumor enlarges. The more common dural pedicle feeders from the ECA include the middle meningeal artery, accessory meningeal artery, neuromeningeal branch of the ascending pharyngeal artery, and stylomastoid branch of the occipital artery. The dural supply from the ICA usually arises from the ethmoidal, cavernous, clival, and tentorial branches. Depending on the location of the meningioma, the primary supply to the meningioma may be from the ICA, ECA, or both. Meningiomas supplied solely by the ICA include diaphragmatic or tuberculum sellae lesions.

Anterior fossa lesions are often supplied by both the ECA and ICA. High-convexity and parasagittal lesions are supplied by the middle meningeal artery and the artery of the falx cerebri. All parasagittal lesions must be examined for contributions from the contralateral middle meningeal artery. Frontal convexity or frontal falcine tumors are supplied by a combination of the meningeal branches of the ethmoidal artery and anterior falcine branches. Bilateral anterior and posterior ethmoidal arteries usually supply olfactory groove meningiomas. Therefore, both the distal ophthalmic and internal maxillary branches as well as the middle meningeal artery must be carefully evaluated.

Middle fossa tumors are supplied by branches from the ECA, including the artery of the foramen rotundum, vidian arteries, and ascending pharyngeal artery. In particular, meningiomas involving the sphenoid wing are supplied by the recurrent meningeal branch of the ophthalmic artery or branches of the middle meningeal artery. Parasellar tumors are frequently fed by branches of the petrous, cavernous, and supraclinoid segments of the ICA; the artery of the foramen rotundum; the artery of the foramen ovale; and the neuromeningeal branch of the ascending pharyngeal artery.

Posterior fossa meningiomas are primarily supplied by the posterior meningeal artery, the middle meningeal artery, and the accessory meningeal artery. The tentorial branch of the meningohypophyseal trunk, the inferolateral trunk, the middle meningeal artery, and the accessory meningeal artery can all supply tentorial meningiomas. These branches also may supply the third through sixth cranial nerves. Consequently, provocative testing may be beneficial. Petroclival meningiomas are supplied by the petrosal, petrosquamosal, and occipital branches of the middle meningeal artery; the transmastoid branches of the occipital and posterior auricular arteries; the subarcuate branch of the anterior inferior cerebellar artery (AICA); and neuromeningeal branches of the ascending pharyngeal artery. The posterior meningeal artery, arising from the vertebral artery or branches of the ascending pharyngeal artery,[1] supplies meningiomas involving the foramen magnum. Posterior fossa tumors share their blood supply with the lower cranial nerves. This point must be recalled when embolizing these tumors. Also, EC-IC anastomoses, specifically between branches of the posterior auricular or occipital artery and the vertebral artery in the high cervical spinolaminar region, may be present.

Angiography is instrumental in determining the patency of the major dural venous sinuses. Meningiomas can invade and occlude a major sinus. Preoperative MR venography or angiography can verify invasion, occlusion, and collateral venous drainage and thereby facilitate surgical decision making. If gross total resection is the goal, preexisting occlusion of a sinus allows more aggressive tumor resection by opening the sinus or resecting the involved segment.

In 1973, Manelfe et al.[30] first described the preoperative embolization of meningiomas. Transcatheter embolization has been advocated to reduce the vascularity of tumors, to facilitate necrosis of the dural attachment site, to mitigate tumoral hemorrhage, and to facilitate tumor resection.[2,12,31,32]

The most commonly used embolisate for meningiomas is PVA. Particles in the range of 150–350 μm are preferred because they can penetrate deeply into the tumor substance. If reflux into the parent artery occurs, embolization should be discontinued. Ideally, the postembolization angiographic goal is obliteration of the tumor blush on injection of the ECA. If embolization obliterates the feeding arteries but the tumor blush remains, the tumor will likely remain hypervascular.

The presence of estrogen and progesterone receptors in many meningiomas introduces the attractive concept of ligand-specific selectivity to preoperative embolization. A report by Suzuki and Komatsu[33] using estrogen to embolize dural AVMS and meningiomas suggests that estrogen or progestins may be used as embolisates for tumors. Although the mechanism of action is unclear, estrogen is thought to injure the vascular endothelium and to increase vascular permeability.

Most meningiomas do not require preoperative embolization because the tumor can be devascularized during surgical resection as a first step. Embolization is valuable for large, hypervascular skull base meningiomas with an arterial supply that is not readily accessible surgically.[34] Embolization should be considered for giant meningiomas (Fig. 9-2), those involving the skull base and middle cranial fossa, falcine or parasagittal meningiomas, and meningiomas at the pineal region. In patients with skull base meningiomas, the vascular pedicle is seldom encountered until a significant portion of the tumor has been resected, making embolization more imperative. To forestall tumor progression, embolization may be considered for patients who are poor surgical candidates.

Embolization of deep arterial feeders such as the meningohypophyseal trunk and inferolateral trunk is technically challenging because their caliber is small and their angle of origin is acute. However, the introduction of variable stiffness and hydrophilic microcatheters and microwires has permitted selective microcatheterization of these vessels. Hirohata et al.[35] described seven patients with large petroclival meningiomas who underwent preoperative embolization with 150- to 250-μm particulates. Branches of the meningohypophyseal trunk and inferolateral trunk (lateral clival, posterior branch, and tentorial branch), which provided the primary blood supply, were catheterized successfully. They did not use lidocaine because of the high reported rates of false-positives and false-negatives and for fear of introducing an epileptogenic agent into the distal territory.[36,37] All tumors were subtotally or completely resected; blood loss was 500 cc or less. Robinson et al.[37] described five patients with skull base meningiomas who underwent successful preoperative embolization of the meningohypophyseal trunk and inferolateral trunk with particulate embolisates. No patient suffered complications, and the tumor blush was obliterated in 80–100% of the cases. The inferolateral trunk, however, must be embolized with caution because it can collateralize with the ophthalmic artery via the deep recurrent ophthalmic artery. Embolization of the inferolateral trunk is therefore associated with the risk of blindness.

Pial and ophthalmic arteries supplying meningiomas are difficult to embolize, and the risk-benefit ratio often precludes an attempt. However, Kaji et al.[38] described two cases in which distal cortical branches of the ICA were successfully and safely embolized with gelfoam before surgical resection. They emphasized that embolization of the pial supply should be attempted only under the following conditions: the tumor is supplied solely by the ICA, the tumor is located in a noneloquent region of the brain, the patient has a negative Amytal test, superselective microcatheterization is performed with the catheter abutting the tumor, and particles are used rather than acrylic glue.[38]

Pineal region meningiomas are typically supplied by meningeal branches of the ECA, the tentorial artery, the medial and lateral posterior choroidal branches, the posterior pericallosal artery, small branches of the posterior cerebral artery, and branches of the superior vermian and superior cerebellar arteries. Meningeal branches may arise from the vertebral artery and PICAs. Sagoh et al.[39] successfully resected a pineal region meningioma after embolizing bilateral middle meningeal arteries with estrogen-alcohol and PVA. Postembolization MRI showed intratumoral necrosis.

Optic nerve meningiomas are seldom amenable to embolization because they are supplied by branches of the ophthalmic artery that concurrently supply the nerve. Terada et al.[40] embolized five hypervascular meningiomas fed primarily by branches of the ophthalmic artery. One patient was blind before embolization, and another patient suffered a visual field deficit after embolization. They contended that this technique is feasible if the microcatheter is distal to the origin of the central retinal artery and emphasized that reflux into this artery must be avoided.

Bendszus et al.[41] prospectively studied the effects of preoperative embolization on the excision of meningiomas at two similar centers. Thirty patients each were enrolled in the embolization and nonembolized groups. One patient in the embolization group suffered a permanent complication (thromboembolic occlusion of the central retinal artery). Overall, there was no significant difference in intraoperative blood loss. Only the subgroup of patients who underwent complete embolization without residual tumor blush had significantly less intraoperative blood loss. They concluded that the value of nonselective preoperative embolization of meningiomas may be limited, especially given the time, expense, and complications associated with embolization.

A retrospective study from the Barrow Neurological Institute examined the utility and risk-benefit profile of 33 appropriately matched embolized and 193 nonembolized meningiomas.[42] Costs of treatment for the two groups were also compared. Preoperative embolization significantly reduced the intraoperative blood loss and need for transfusions associated with large meningiomas. There were no differences between the two groups in terms of cost, length of hospital stay, and rates of major or minor complications. Therefore, embolization may be beneficial for large meningiomas.

Bendszus et al.[43] prospectively followed seven patients who underwent embolization with trisacryl gelatin microspheres (100–300 μm) alone without surgery. At a mean radiographic follow-up of 20 months, the tumors of six of the seven patients were smaller than before treatment. The reduction was most pronounced 6 months after treatment. They contended that embolization alone may be an option for patients who are poor surgical candidates. However, the drawback of this treatment modality is the lack of histologic verification of the diagnosis. Long-term follow-up is also required to determine the efficacy of treatment.

Complications

The overall risk associated with the embolization of meningiomas is low.[12,44] Minor complications include painful trismus, facial pain, or both and may occur in as many as 20–30% of patients.[12] Treatment of these complications includes corticosteroids and analgesic medications. In most patients symptoms resolve within 2–3 days.

Major complications include stroke, blindness, hemorrhage, and cranial nerve palsies. Stroke or blindness is rare but can be the result of unappreciated EC-IC collaterals, or it can be caused by reflux of embolic material. These complications can be avoided by thorough angiographic evaluation, including a superselective examination to delineate anastomoses between the meningeal vessels and the ICA, vertebral artery, or ophthalmic artery.

Seventh cranial nerve palsy results from inadvertent embolization of the petrous branches of the middle meningeal artery, which supplies posterior parasellar and posterior fossa lesions. Lower cranial nerves are at risk when clival or petroclival meningiomas supplied by branches of the ascending pharyngeal artery are to be embolized. The risk of cranial nerve palsies can be mitigated by superselective catheterization of the external branches until the catheter tip is wedged within the vessel supplying the tumor. Cranial nerve damage is also less likely with particle embolization, specifically with larger particulates used. Using particulates larger than 150 μm is thought to prevent inadvertent embolization of the vaso vasorum supplying the cranial nerves. Probst et al. reported cranial nerve deficits in 2 of 80 patients undergoing embolization: temporary in one patient and permanent in the other.

Hieshima et al.[45] reported no permanent neurologic complications in 11 patients undergoing embolization for a meningioma. Richter and Schachenmayr[2] described five patients with transient neurologic deficits and no permanent deficits in 31 patients whose meningiomas were embolized. In a series of 51 patients who underwent embolization, Macpherson[32] described eight patients who experienced scalp necrosis or temporary hemiparesis. Rosen et al.[46] embolized skull base meningiomas in 167 patients, an ostensibly high-risk group for embolization or surgery. Transient neurologic deficit occurred in 12.6%, and 9% had permanent neurologic deficits. In their experience, embolization of the meningohypophyseal trunk, ascending pharyngeal artery, and middle meningeal artery were associated with a high risk of transient and permanent neurologic deficits. Swelling after embolization was readily controlled with intravenous steroids. If swelling persists, emergent surgical resection must be considered. Patients with skull base meningiomas frequently have baseline cranial nerve dysfunction. In this subgroup of patients, embolization may exacerbate this dysfunction, and this possibility should be highlighted during preoperative counseling.[46] Two patients developed monocular blindness after embolization, and neither patient was embolized via the ophthalmic artery.

Subarachnoid, subdural, peritumoral, or intratumoral hemorrhages have followed the embolization of meningiomas.[59–63] Hemorrhage may result from wire perforation or sudden dynamic changes in intracranial blood flow as a result of the embolization. After reviewing the literature on the postembolization risks of intratumoral hemorrhage, Kallmes et al.[47] were unable to discern a correlation between particle size and risk of hemorrhage. They found seven cases of hemorrhage into a meningioma. Eliminating the supply from the ECA to tumors with a significant ICA supply has been reported to increase blood flow from the ICA, exacerbating mass effect and intratumoral hemorrhage.[34,48] This potential complication must be considered when tumors have a significant ICA supply. Intratumoral hemorrhage also may be more common in tumors with cystic components or large necrotic areas than in homogeneous lesions. Barr et al.[49] described an iatrogenic carotid-cavernous sinus fistula that presumably resulted from microwire perforation of the meningohypophyseal artery supplying a skull base meningioma. The fistula was treated with transarterial coil embolization of the venous pouch. Given the risk profile, they concluded that skull base meningiomas must not be embolized indiscriminately.

Scalp necrosis can also follow embolization and surgical resection. Adler et al.[50] described severe scalp necrosis treated with a vascularized free tissue transfer. Both Chan and Thompson[51] and Adler et al.[50] emphasized the need to base the scalp flap on at least one patent supplying artery to prevent this complication. They also recommended maintaining the superficial temporal artery as a potential donor vessel for a free tissue transfer. Scalp necrosis is rare when larger particulates are used as the embolisate.

A potential concern is that embolized meningiomas may be overgraded on histologic examination because of the embolization-induced necrosis and reactive changes.[52,53] Ng et al.[52] suggested that embolization-induced necrosis is characterized by a punched-out outline with confluent areas of necrosis. Embolized meningiomas lack the overall background of anaplasia associated with atypical or aggressive meningiomas. Perry et al.[53] examined 64 embolized meningiomas and concluded that these morphologic changes are uncommon and that current grading schemes rarely overgrade these tumors. They found a higher proportion of atypical meningiomas in patients undergoing embolization but attributed it to selection bias rather than to the effects of embolization.

Conclusion

Preoperative embolization plays an important role in the management of selected giant or skull base meningiomas. Recent advances in microcatheter technology, microembolisates, and neurophysiologic monitoring have improved the safety of preoperative embolization. However, sound endovascular principles and techniques are paramount to prevent major complications such as stroke, blindness, or cranial neuropathy. Preoperative embolization of tumors has become a requisite tool for the neurosurgical team and represents a significant improvement in patient care.

References

1. Choi IS, Tantivatana J. Neuroendovascular management of intracranial and spinal tumors. Neurosurg Clin N Am 2000; 11:167–85.
2. Richter HP, Schachenmayr W. Preoperative embolization of intracranial meningiomas. Neurosurgery 1983;13:261–8.
3. Jungreis CA. Skull-base tumors: ethanol embolization of the cavernous carotid artery. Radiology 1991;181:741–3.
4. Theron J, Cosgrove R, Melanson D, et al. Embolization with temporary balloon occlusion of the internal carotid or vertebral arteries. Neuroradiology 1986;28:246–53.
5. Lefkowitz M, Giannotta SL, Hieshima G, et al. Embolization of neurosurgical lesions involving the ophthalmic artery. Neurosurgery 1998;43:1298–1303.
6. Casasco A, Herbreteau D, Houdart E, et al. Devascularization of craniofacial tumors by percutaneous tumor puncture. AJNR Am J Neuroradiol 1994;15:1233–9.
7. Terada T, Nakamura Y, Tsuura M, et al. MRI changes in embolized meningiomas. Neuroradiology 1992;34:162–7.
8. Bendszus M, Warmuth-Metz M, Klein R, et al. Sequential MRI and MR spectroscopy in embolized meningiomas: correlation with surgical and histopathological findings. Neuroradiology 2002;44:77–82.
9. Wakhloo AK, Juengling FD, Van V, et al. Extended preoperative polyvinyl alcohol microembolization of intracranial meningiomas: assessment of two embolization techniques. AJNR Am J Neuroradiol 1993;14:571–82.
10. Grand C, Bank WO, Baleriaux D, et al. Gadolinium-enhanced MR in the evaluation of preoperative meningioma embolization. AJNR Am J Neuroradiol 1993;14:563–9.
11. Kai Y, Hamada J, Morioka M, et al. Appropriate interval between embolization and surgery in patients with meningioma. AJNR Am J Neuroradiol 2002;23:139–42.
12. Manelfe C, Lasjaunias P, Ruscalleda J. Preoperative embolization of intracranial meningiomas. AJNR Am J Neuroradiol 1986;7:963–72.
13. Kim LJ, Albuquerque FC, Aziz-Sultan A, et al. Low morbidity associated with the use of NBCA liquid adhesive for preoperative transarterial embolization of central nervous system tumors. Neurosurgery 2006; submitted.
14. Flandroy P, Grandfils C, Collignon J, et al. (D,L)Polylactide microspheres as embolic agent. A preliminary study. Neuroradiology 1990;32:311–5.
15. Kumar AJ, Kaufman SL, Patt J, et al. Preoperative embolization of hypervascular head and neck neoplasms using microfibrillar collagen. AJNR Am J Neuroradiol 1982;3:163–8.
16. Latshaw RF, Pearlman RL, Schaitkin BM, et al. Intraarterial ethanol as a long-term occlusive agent in renal, hepatic, and gastrosplenic arteries of pigs. Cardiovasc Intervent Radiol 1985;8:24–30.
17. Kunstlinger F, Brunelle F, Chaumont P, et al. Vascular occlusive agents. AJR Am J Roentgenol 1981;136:151–6.
18. Inci S, Ozcan OE, Benli K, et al. Microsurgical removal of a free segment of microcatheter in the anterior circulation as a complication of embolization. Surg Neurol 1996;46:562–6.
19. Hamada J, Kai Y, Nagahiro S, et al. Embolization with cellulose porous beads, II: Clinical trial. AJNR Am J Neuroradiol 1996;17:1901–6.
20. Bendszus M, Klein R, Burger R, et al. Efficacy of trisacryl gelatin microspheres versus polyvinyl alcohol particles in the

preoperative embolization of meningiomas. AJNR Am J Neuroradiol 2000;21:255–61.

21. Ellman BA, Green CE, Eigenbrodt E, et al. Renal infarction with absolute ethanol. Invest Radiol 1980;15:318–22.

22. Horowitz M, Whisnant RE, Jungreis C, et al. Temporary balloon occlusion and ethanol injection for preoperative embolization of carotid-body tumor. Ear Nose Throat J 2002;81:536–42.

23. Lonser RR, Heiss JD, Oldfield EH. Tumor devascularization by intratumoral ethanol injection during surgery. Technical note. J Neurosurg 1998;88:923–4.

24. Kasuya H, Shimizu T, Sasahara A, et al. Phenytoin as a liquid material for embolisation of tumours. Neuroradiology 1999;41:320–3.

25. Kubo M, Kuwayama N, Hirashima Y, et al. Hydroxyapatite ceramics as a particulate embolic material: report of the clinical experience. AJNR Am J Neuroradiol 2003;24:1545–7.

26. American Society of Interventional and Therapeutic Neuroradiology: Head, neck, and brain tumor embolization. AJNR Am J Neuroradiol 2001;22:S14–5.

27. Horowitz MB, Carrau R, Crammond D, et al. Risks of tumor embolization in the presence of an unrecognized patent foramen ovale: case report. AJNR Am J Neuroradiol 2002;23:982–4.

28. Eskridge JM. Interventional neuroradiology. Radiology 1989;172:991–1006.

29. Horton JA, Kerber CW. Lidocaine injection into external carotid branches: provocative test to preserve cranial nerve function in therapeutic embolization. AJNR Am J Neuroradiol 1986;7:105–8.

30. Manelfe C, Guiraud B, David J, et al. Embolization by catheterization of intracranial meningiomas. Rev Neurol (Paris) 1973;128:339–51.

31. Black PM. Meningiomas. Neurosurgery 1993;32:643–57.

32. Macpherson P. The value of pre-operative embolisation of meningioma estimated subjectively and objectively. Neuroradiology 1991;33:334–7.

33. Suzuki J, Komatsu S. New embolization method using estrogen for dural arteriovenous malformation and meningioma. Surg Neurol 1981;16:438–42.

34. Gruber A, Killer M, Mazal P, et al. Preoperative embolization of intracranial meningiomas: a 17-years single center experience. Minim Invasive Neurosurg 2000;43:18–29.

35. Hirohata M, Abe T, Morimitsu H, et al. Preoperative selective internal carotid artery dural branch embolisation for petroclival meningiomas. Neuroradiology 2003;45:656–60.

36. Halbach VV, Higashida RT, Hieshima GB, et al. Embolization of branches arising from the cavernous portion of the internal carotid artery. AJNR Am J Neuroradiol 1989;10:143–50.

37. Robinson DH, Song JK, Eskridge JM. Embolization of meningohypophyseal and inferolateral branches of the cavernous internal carotid artery. AJNR Am J Neuroradiol 1999;20:1061–7.

38. Kaji T, Hama Y, Iwasaki Y, et al. Preoperative embolization of meningiomas with pial supply: successful treatment of two cases. Surg Neurol 1999;52:270–3.

39. Sagoh M, Onozuka S, Murakami H, et al. Successful removal of meningioma of the pineal region after embolization. Neurol Med Chir (Tokyo) 1997;37:852–5.

40. Terada T, Kinoshita Y, Yokote H, et al. Preoperative embolization of meningiomas fed by ophthalmic branch arteries. Surg Neurol 1996;45:161–6.

41. Bendszus M, Rao G, Burger R, et al. Is there a benefit of preoperative meningioma embolization? Neurosurgery 2000; 47:1306–11.

42. Dean BL, Flom RA, Wallace RC, et al. Efficacy of endovascular treatment of meningiomas: evaluation with matched samples. AJNR Am J Neuroradiol 1994;15:1675–80.

43. Bendszus M, Martin-Schrader I, Schlake HP, et al. Embolisation of intracranial meningiomas without subsequent surgery. Neuroradiology 2003;45:451–5.

44. Ahuja A, Gibbons KJ, Hopkins LN. Endovascular techniques to treat brain tumors. In Youmans Neurological Surgery, 4th Edition, Ahuja A, Gibbons KJ, Hopkins LN (eds), Philadelphia, W.B. Saunders, 1996, pp 2826–40.

45. Hieshima GB, Everhart FR, Mehringer CM, et al. Preoperative embolization of meningiomas. Surg Neurol 1980;14: 119–27.

46. Rosen CL, Ammerman JM, Sekhar LN, et al. Outcome analysis of preoperative embolization in cranial base surgery. Acta Neurochir (Wien) 2002;144:1157–64.

47. Kallmes DF, Evans AJ, Kaptain GJ, et al. Hemorrhagic complications in embolization of a meningioma: case report and review of the literature. Neuroradiology 1997;39:877–80.

48. Teasdale E, Patterson J, McLellan D, et al. Subselective preoperative embolization for meningiomas. A radiological and pathological assessment. J Neurosurg 1984;60:506–11.

49. Barr JD, Mathis JM, Horton JA. Iatrogenic carotid-cavernous fistula occurring after embolization of a cavernous sinus meningioma. AJNR Am J Neuroradiol 1995;16:483–5.

50. Adler JR, Upton J, Wallman J, et al. Management and prevention of necrosis of the scalp after embolization and surgery for meningioma. Surg Neurol 1986;25:357–60.

51. Chan RC, Thompson GB. Ischemic necrosis of the scalp after preoperative embolization of meningeal tumors. Neurosurgery 1984;15:76–81.

52. Ng HK, Poon WS, Goh K, et al. Histopathology of postembolized meningiomas. Am J Surg Pathol 1996;20:1224–30.

53. Perry A, Chicoine MR, Filiput E, et al. Clinicopathologic assessment and grading of embolized meningiomas: a correlative study of 64 patients. Cancer 2001;92:701–11.

10
Neuro-ophthalmic Evaluations in Patients with Meningiomas

Steven A. Newman

Introduction

The shared interests of ophthalmologists and neurosurgeons were voiced by Harvey Cushing in 1938 when he wrote: "in recent years, the ophthalmic surgeon, the earliest surgical specialist, and the neurosurgeon, the latest, have from opposite directions come to meet at the barrier of the optic foramen—each somewhat hesitant to trespass on the other's field of work".[1] Cushing played an additional critical role in recognizing the pathologic manifestations of this common tumor. In his monumental text with Eisenhardt, Cushing set the standard for diagnosis and approach to meningiomas. In the nineteenth century meningiomas were often misdiagnosed. Virchow had recognized psammoma bodies and described these tumors as "sarcomas of the dura." Golgi had coined the term endothelioma in 1869.[2] But it wasn't until 1912 that Hudson made a concerted attempt to separate primary gliomas from endotheliomas and fibromas.[3] Harvey Cushing in 1922 used the term meningioma as a shortened form of meningioendothelioma.[4]

Meningiomas are one of the most common primary intracranial tumors. The visual pathways, both afferent and efferent, are ubiquitous throughout the central nervous system (CNS). The afferent visual pathways account for up to 50% of all sensory input to the CNS. It is thus not unexpected that meningiomas often present with visual system involvement. Involvement of the afferent visual pathways may be appreciated by the patient as decreased vision, visual field defects, or double vision. When meningiomas affect the orbit (either primarily or secondarily), adnexal signs and symptoms include proptosis, dystopia, and lid abnormalities. Even when asymptomatic, a detailed neuro-ophthalmologic examination may detect visual system involvement. In spite of the advent of imaging studies (CT and MRI scanning) detailed quantitative testing remains critical to properly diagnose meningiomas and follow patients with meningiomatous pathology.

Clinical Manifestations

Afferent Involvement

The most common ophthalmic complaint related to meningiomas is visual loss.[5–11] Patients may describe this as blurred, dim, dark vision or simply difficulty seeing. While visual field loss secondary to chiasmal or retrochiasmal pathology may elicit complaints of visual loss,[12–14] in most cases there is involvement of the optic nerve. Unfortunately there may be a considerable delay between the onset of visual loss and the recognition of the meningioma[15] (Fig. 10-1) Optic nerve sheath meningiomas cause optic nerve dysfunction from a combination of direct compression and secondary compromise of the vascular supply to the axons. These tumors may be located intraorbitally, intracanalicularly, or in rare cases eccentrically within the orbit. Transient visual loss has been reported particularly in optic nerve sheath meningiomas.[16] This may be gaze evoked.[6]

Meningiomas arising from the anterior clinoid,[17] the tuberculum sella,[18–21] or the medial sphenoid wing[22,23] may directly affect the optic nerve (Fig. 10-2). Lesions that arise from beneath the optic nerve can elevate the nerve compressing it against the falciform ligament, a fold of dura above the optic nerve as it exits the optic canal. This compression may lead to decreased vision but also to an inferior arcuate visual field defect. Decompressing of the canal may relieve this compression and improve the visual field defect. If a compressive meningioma extends back to involve the anterior chiasm, a junctional syndrome may be produced with an ipsilateral central scotoma and a contralateral superotemporal defect[24] (Fig. 10-3).

Occasionally patients may be aware of difficulty seeing to the side. They may specifically say that they can not see to one side or alternatively may notice that words, objects, or parts of faces may disappear. This usually indicates a lesion affecting the postchiasmal visual pathways[25] (Fig. 10-4). Homonymous defects may also be due to meningiomatous compromise of the vascular system.[26]

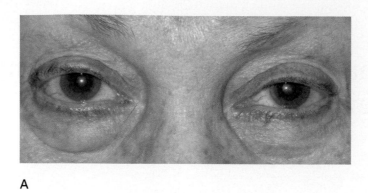

A

Fixation Monitor: Gaze Track   Stimulus: III, White   Pupil Diameter: 5.0 mm   Date: 08-18-2000
Fixation Target: Central   Background: 31.5 ASB   Visual Acuity: 20/20   Time: 10:54 AM
Fixation Losses: 0/0   Strategy: SITA-Standard   RX: +3.50 DS   DC X   Age: 66
False POS Errors: 10 %
False NEG Errors: 3 %
Test Duration: 04:39

Fovea: 37 dB

```
                27  29   28  27
             30  31   29  31  29  27
         31  35  35   33  32  33  33  29
         30  33  32   36  34  32  31  30  28
   30    32   6  32   35  34  33  32  27  25     30
         31  33  32   32  33  36  33  27
             30  32   31  31  31  29
                31  31   28  28
```

```
          1   2  2  1                        -2  -1 -1  -2
       3  3  0  2  2  0 -1                 0   0  -3 -1 -3 -4
    3  6  5  3  1  3  3  1               0   3   2  0 -2  0  0 -2
    1     1  4  2  0  0  1  2           -2     -2  1 -1 -3 -3 -2 -1
    2     1  3  1  1  1 -2 -1           -1     -2  0 -2 -2 -2 -5 -4
    2  3  1  1  1  5  3 -1              -1  0  -2 -2 -2  2  0 -4
       1  1  0  0  0  0                     -2 -2 -3 -3 -3 -3
          2  2 -1  0                         -1 -1 -4 -3
```

GHT
Within normal limits

MD   +1.52 dB
PSD   1.66 dB

Total Deviation   Pattern Deviation

B

FIG. 10-1. This 66-year-old woman presented with a history of double vision and 2 years of progressive decreased visual acuity (A). She had a previously reported negative MRI scan. When evaluated visual acuity was 20/70 and 20/20, with a greater than 1.8 log unit right afferent pupillary defect. Automated static perimetry demonstrated a normal field on the left (B)

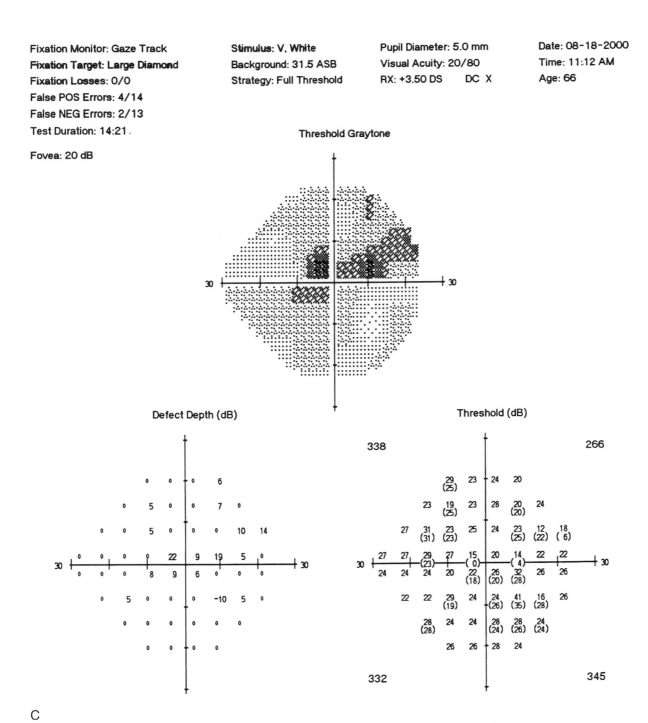

Fixation Monitor: Gaze Track
Fixation Target: Large Diamond
Fixation Losses: 0/0
False POS Errors: 4/14
False NEG Errors: 2/13
Test Duration: 14:21 .

Fovea: 20 dB

Stimulus: V, White
Background: 31.5 ASB
Strategy: Full Threshold

Pupil Diameter: 5.0 mm
Visual Acuity: 20/80
RX: +3.50 DS   DC X

Date: 08-18-2000
Time: 11:12 AM
Age: 66

Threshold Graytone

Defect Depth (dB)

Threshold (dB)

C

FIG. 10-1. (continued) The central scotoma could be better appreciated using a larger test object (C)

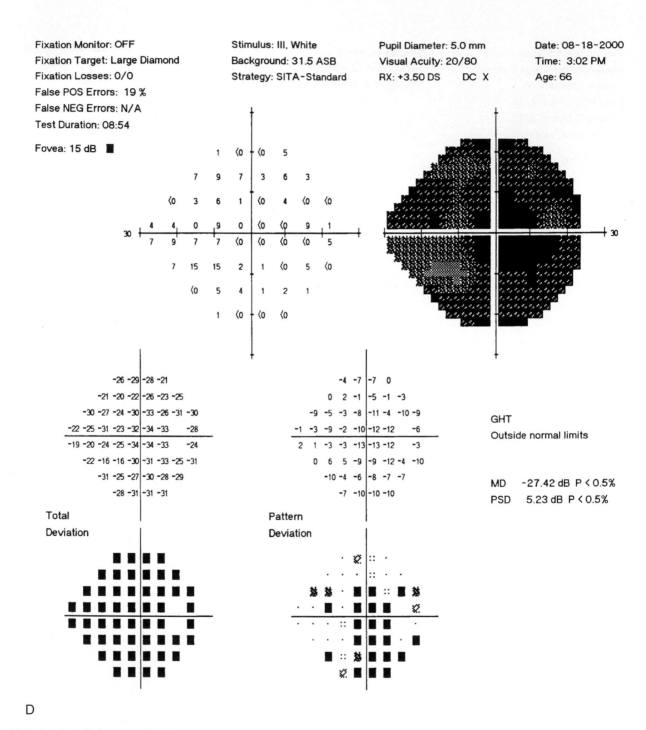

Fixation Monitor: OFF
Fixation Target: Large Diamond
Fixation Losses: 0/0
False POS Errors: 19 %
False NEG Errors: N/A
Test Duration: 08:54

Fovea: 15 dB ■

Stimulus: III, White
Background: 31.5 ASB
Strategy: SITA-Standard

Pupil Diameter: 5.0 mm
Visual Acuity: 20/80
RX: +3.50 DS   DC X

Date: 08-18-2000
Time: 3:02 PM
Age: 66

Total
Deviation

Pattern
Deviation

GHT
Outside normal limits

MD   -27.42 dB P < 0.5%
PSD   5.23 dB P < 0.5%

D

Fig. 10-1. (continued) Automated static perimetry demonstrated a normal field on the left (B) but a central scotoma on the right (D)

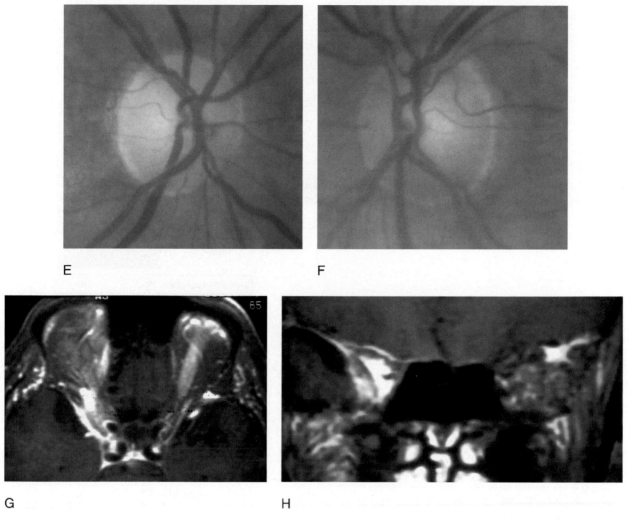

FIG. 10-1. (continued) Her fundoscopic examination revealed clear evidence of optic atrophy on the right (E) and a normal disc on the left (F). A repeat MRI scan confirmed the presence of an apical meningioma affecting the optic nerve (G, H)

Visual impairment may also occur as a result of increased intracranial pressure.[27,28] Patients are often unaware of visual impairment secondary to papilledema (even if they have headaches) since central vision tends to be spared until late in patients with the optic neuropathy of increased intracranial pressure. Patients may complain of visual obscurations (blurring lasting for a few seconds) often precipitated by change in posture such as bending over. Persistent visual changes could also indicate edema extending to the macula.

Positive visual phenomena are unusual with meningiomas but may occur with involvement of the occipital lobe. These may be due to vascular compromise, electrical discharge (occipital seizures), or unrelated migraine.

Involvement of the optic nerve can produce optic disc changes. Direct involvement of the optic nerve can produce disc edema.[29] Very rarely the meningioma may invade the globe.[30–33] The disc edema due to local compression may be indistinguishable from the disc elevation produced by intracranial meningioma induced papilledema. Pressure-induced disc edema (papilledema) is only exceptionally unilateral. Chronic disc edema often demonstrates white spots on the optic nerve head.[16,34] Impairment of venous outflow due to meningiomas of the optic nerve sheath or medial sphenoid meningioma [35–38] can be associated with the development of optociliary shunt vessels (Fig. 10-5).

Optic nerve compromise eventually results in loss of nerve fiber layer, optic disc pallor, and optic atrophy. Unusually the optic cup may increase. Nerve fiber thickness may be measured utilizing the Heidelberg retinal tomograph, the GDx, or optical coherence tomography (OCT) (Fig. 10-1).

Efferent Involvement

Teleologically there are multiple reasons that the eyes move. While it is possible to see abnormal saccades due to frontal lobe pathology and pursuit abnormalities due to pathology

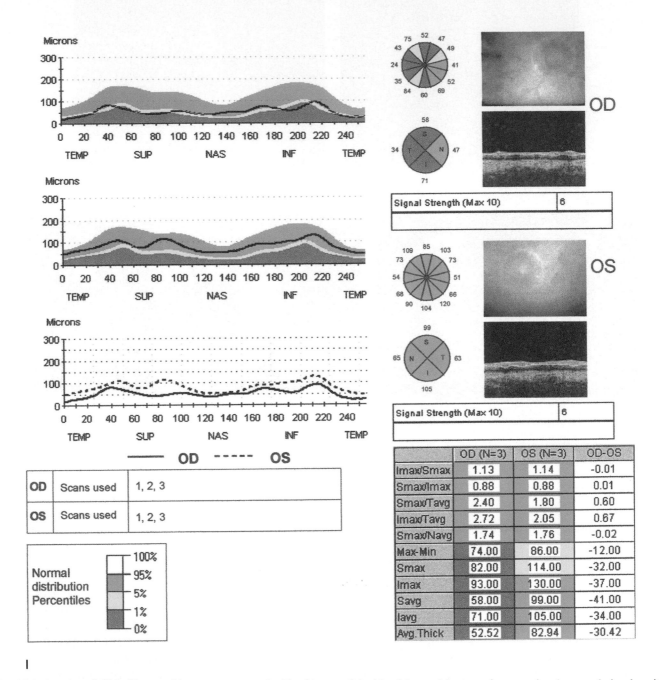

FIG. 10-1. (continued) This 66-year-old woman presented with a history of double vision and 2 years of progressive decreased visual acuity. The amount of optic atrophy could be quantitated with optical coherence tomography demonstrating nerve fiber bundle dropout on the right compared to the left (I)

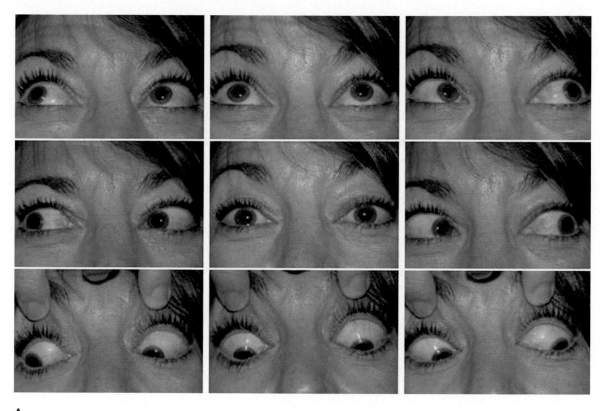

A

FIG. 10-2. This 54-year-old patient was referred with a 2-year history of puffiness around the left eye and tearing (A)

affecting the middle temporal visual area (MT) or the medial superior temporal visual area (MST), this sort of pathology rarely produces symptoms.

Efferent system dysfunction is usually due to pathology within the posterior fossa, the cavernous sinus, or the orbit. A meningioma within the orbit may directly involve the extraocular muscles. This may cause either a paretic or more likely a restrictive problem. An optic nerve sheath meningioma may also produce limitation in motility.

The tonic position of the eyes is determined by input from the vestibular nuclei.[39] Tumors affecting vestibular input (either the vestibular nerves or vestibular nuclei), often in the cerebello-pontine angle, cause asymmetric tonic input. This produces continuous drift of the eyes. Patients may notice oscillopsia. With time the cerebellum will reset the gain, thereafter permitting the eyes to remain stable in primary position. Head shaking will bring out any residual asymmetric gain and thus conjugate eye drift.

Cerebello-pontine angle lesions may also affect the neural integrator (nucleus propositus hypoglossi) by compression of the brain stem at the pontomedullary junction. Although the eyes are stable in primary position, there is inability to maintain eccentric gaze resulting in gaze paretic nystagmus (the eyes drift towards primary position and then beat out toward the direction of eccentric gaze).

Compression at the cervicomedullary junction results in asymmetric involvement of the vertical pathways. This may produce down beat nystagmus or a skew deviation. Patients may complain of blurred vision or, less commonly, oscillopsia. The downbeat nystagmus is typically exacerbated by looking down to either side.

The most common complaint related to involvement of the efferent visual system is double vision. This occurs when the visual axes are out of alignment. While diplopia can be caused by restriction of the extraocular muscles within the orbit, the most common etiology is paresis. Neuromuscular junctional problems and primary weakness in the extraocular muscles (chronic progressive ophthalmoplegia) can also produce paretic strabismus. When related to meningiomas, most paretic strabismus is secondary to cranial nerve palsies. Much less

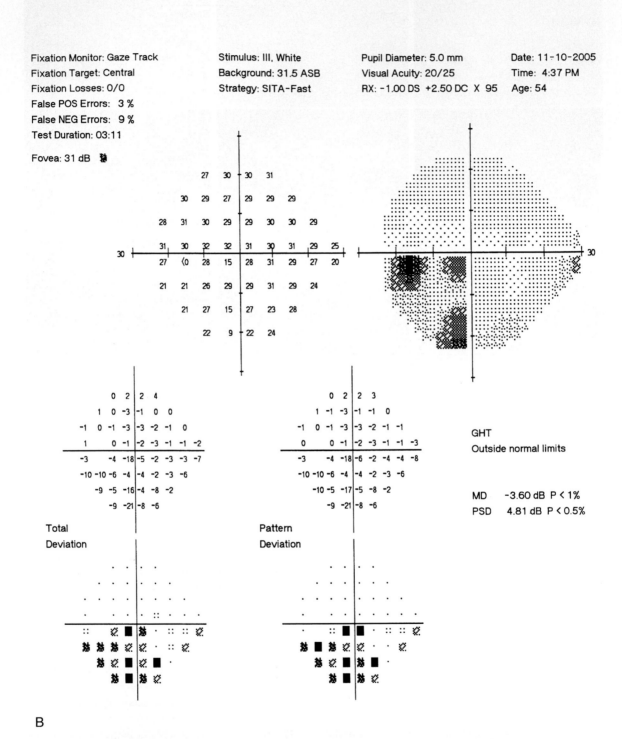

Fixation Monitor: Gaze Track Stimulus: III, White Pupil Diameter: 5.0 mm Date: 11-10-2005
Fixation Target: Central Background: 31.5 ASB Visual Acuity: 20/25 Time: 4:37 PM
Fixation Losses: 0/0 Strategy: SITA-Fast RX: -1.00 DS +2.50 DC X 95 Age: 54
False POS Errors: 3 %
False NEG Errors: 9 %
Test Duration: 03:11

Fovea: 31 dB

```
             27  30    30  31
          30  29  27   29  29  29
       28  31  30  29   29  30  30  29
       31  30  32  32   31  30  31  29  25
   30 ─┼──────────────────────────────┼─ 30
       27  (0  28  15   28  31  29  27  20
          21  21  26  29   29  31  29  24
             21  27  15   27  23  28
                22   9    22  24
```

```
        0   2 | 2   4                    0   2 | 2   3
      1   0  -3 |-1   0   0             1  -1  -3 |-1  -1   0
   -1   0  -1  -3 |-3  -2  -1   0      -1   0  -1  -3 |-3  -2  -1  -1
    1       0  -1 |-2  -3  -1  -1  -2    0       0  -1 |-2  -3  -1  -1  -3
   ─────────────┼───────────────      ─────────────┼───────────────
   -3      -4 -18 |-5  -2  -3  -3  -7   -3      -4 -18 |-6  -2  -4  -4  -8
  -10 -10  -6  -4 |-4  -2  -3  -6      -10 -10  -6  -4 |-4  -2  -3  -6
      -9  -5 -16 |-4  -8  -2               -10  -5 -17 |-5  -8  -2
         -9 -21 |-8  -6                        -9 -21 |-8  -6
```

GHT
Outside normal limits

MD   -3.60 dB P < 1%
PSD   4.81 dB P < 0.5%

Total   Pattern
Deviation   Deviation

FIG. 10-2. (continued) This 54-year-old patient was referred with a 2-year history of puffiness around the left eye and tearing. She had been treated for "allergies" and was unaware of any decrease in vision until 3 months before her referral. On examination visual acuity was 20/15 on the right and 20/25 on the left. She did have 5 mm of relative proptosis on the left side and a 1.2 log unit left afferent pupillary defect. Automated static perimetry in the right eye demonstrates a normal visual field (C) but an inferior arcuate defect with relative paracentral defect on the right (B)

B

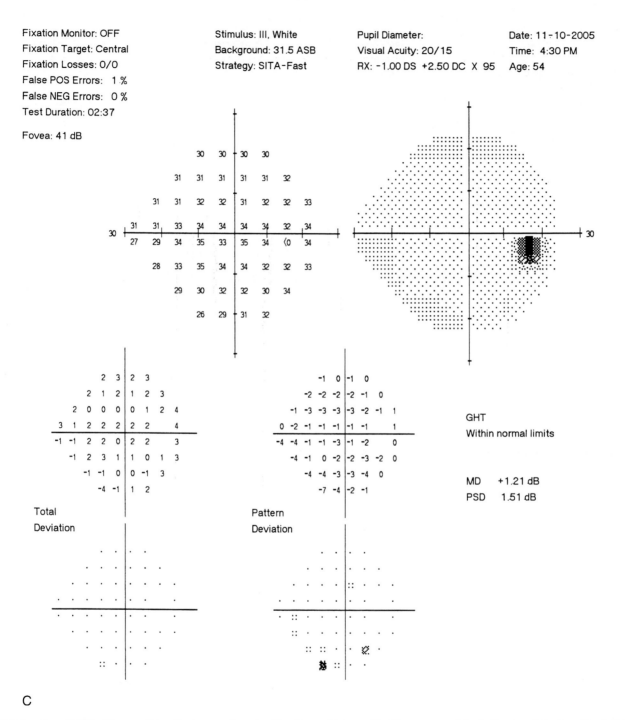

Fixation Monitor: OFF
Fixation Target: Central
Fixation Losses: 0/0
False POS Errors: 1 %
False NEG Errors: 0 %
Test Duration: 02:37

Fovea: 41 dB

Stimulus: III, White
Background: 31.5 ASB
Strategy: SITA-Fast

Pupil Diameter:
Visual Acuity: 20/15
RX: -1.00 DS +2.50 DC X 95

Date: 11-10-2005
Time: 4:30 PM
Age: 54

GHT
Within normal limits

MD   +1.21 dB
PSD   1.51 dB

Total Deviation

Pattern Deviation

C

FIG. 10-2.(continued) This 54-year-old patient was referred with a 2-year history of puffiness around the left eye and tearing. She had been treated for "allergies" and was unaware of any decrease in vision until 3 months before her referral. On examination visual acuity was 20/15 on the right and 20/25 on the left. She did have 5 mm of relative proptosis on the left side and a 1.2 log unit left afferent pupillary defect. Automated static perimetry in the right eye demonstrates a normal visual field (C) but an inferior arcuate defect with relative paracentral defect on the right (B)

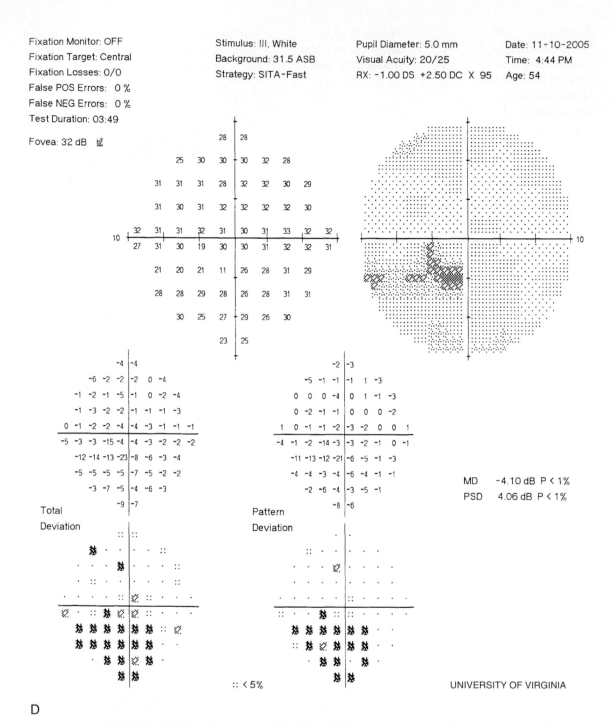

Fixation Monitor: OFF
Fixation Target: Central
Fixation Losses: 0/0
False POS Errors: 0 %
False NEG Errors: 0 %
Test Duration: 03:49

Fovea: 32 dB

Stimulus: III, White
Background: 31.5 ASB
Strategy: SITA-Fast

Pupil Diameter: 5.0 mm
Visual Acuity: 20/25
RX: -1.00 DS +2.50 DC X 95

Date: 11-10-2005
Time: 4:44 PM
Age: 54

MD   -4.10 dB P < 1%
PSD   4.06 dB P < 1%

Total Deviation

Pattern Deviation

:: < 5%

UNIVERSITY OF VIRGINIA

D

FIG. 10-2. (continued) This 54-year-old patient was referred with a 2-year history of puffiness around the left eye and tearing. The relative central and paracentral aspects of this could be better seen on a fine grid program (D)

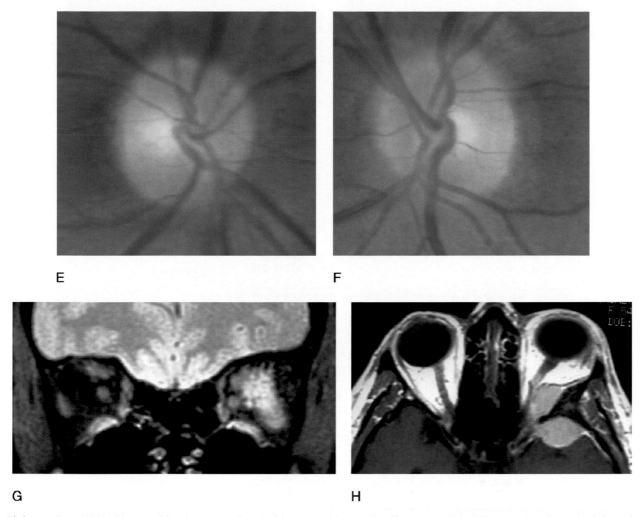

E

F

G

H

FIG. 10-2. (continued) This 54-year-old patient was referred with a 2-year history of puffiness around the left eye and tearing. The right optic disc (E) was normal while her left optic disc (F) confirmed PM bundle dropout and temporal atrophy. Her MRI scan (G, H) confirmed the presence of a meningioma affecting the middle cranial fossa and orbit arising from the greater wing of the sphenoid compressing the optic nerve in the orbital apex

commonly, involvement of the internuclear pathways (medial longitudinal fasciculus or vertical motor pathways) may produce ocular misalignment recognized as double vision.

Ophthalmoplegia is most frequently related to compression within the cavernous sinus involvement. The abducens nerve (VI) is most frequently involved (Fig. 10-6). This produces horizontal diplopia, which is worse on ipsilateral gaze. Oculomotor (III) nerve involvement commonly presents with horizontal or oblique diplopia. Ptosis is very suggestive of third nerve involvement (Fig. 10-7). The pupil may be variably involved. Compression in the area of the cavernous sinus can spare pupillary function (up to 50%). Sometimes following oculomotor dysfunction, recovery of the fibers may be misdirected. If fibers destined for the medial rectus or inferior rectus end up in the levator, the upper lid may elevate when the patient looks in or down. This is the most common sign of aberrant regeneration. Other findings include co-contraction of the superior and inferior rectus muscle, resulting in persistent limitation of vertical gaze and miosis on elevation due to

misdirection of some superior rectus fibers to the pupillary sphincter. In some patients with meningiomas of the cavernous sinus, aberrant regeneration may occur without a previously noted third nerve palsy (primary aberrant regeneration).[40,41] While most third nerve palsies occur with cavernous sinus or orbital apex pathology, rarely posterior fossa meningiomas may affect the oculomotor nerve.[42] Trochlear (IV) neuropathy may be more difficult to diagnose and is very unlikely to occur in isolation.

Two additional findings are strongly suggestive of cavernous sinus pathology. Most common are the sensory abnormalities affecting the trigeminal (V) nerve, particularly the first division (ophthalmic). Less commonly, patients may complain of facial pain related to cavernous sinus involvement. Still less common and often difficult to diagnose is Horner's syndrome due to loss of sympathetic input. This produces mild ptosis and miosis which increases in the dark which may be difficult to recognize especially if there is a partial third nerve dysfunction producing relative mydriasis.

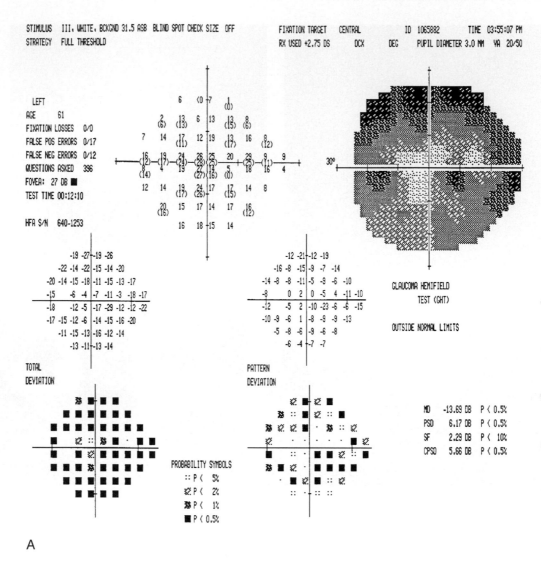

FIG. 10-3. This 61-year-old woman presented with a 3-year history of progressive decrease in vision in the left eye and a year and a half of episodes of trouble with speech. When evaluated, visual acuity was 20/25 and 20/50 with reduced color on the left side and a 2.1 log unit left afferent pupillary defect. Her visual fields demonstrated superior and inferior arcuate defects on the left (A) as well as a relative central scotoma)

The sixth nerve may also be affected by a lesion of the clivus or the petroclival area. This may be bilateral although it is usually asymmetric. Abducens dysfunction producing diplopia may also be seen secondarily related to increased intracranial pressure. This can be seen with large tumors anywhere intracranially.

Lesions affecting the brain stem can asymmetrically involve the vertical motor pathways and produce a skew deviation. Skew deviations may also occur with cerebellar involvement. This vertical deviation may be asymptomatic, produce diplopia, or actually illicit complaints of blurred vision.

Adnexal Involvement

Proptosis is usually a manifestation of sphenoid pathology [43-46] (Fig. 10-8). Hyperostosis is a common manifestation of involvement of the greater wing of the sphenoid.[47,48]

Medial sphenoid wing involvement may precede secondary orbital involvement through the superior orbital fissure. Absence of the orbital roof or lateral wall (usually post surgery) may be associated with pulsatile exophthalmos.

Orbital roof involvement may produce dystopia, eyelid edema, and ptosis[49] (Fig. 10-9). There also may be secondary restrictive strabismus with limited up-gaze. It would be rare for a meningioma to produce problems with up-gaze without associated ptosis. Changes in lid position may occur with anteriorly located meningiomas invading (or rarely originating within the orbit) from above. Ptosis and lid contour changes are possible.

Conjunctival injection may be secondary to several individual abnormalities or more commonly to a combination of them. Proptosis may cause problems with exposure keratopathy, and this may be exacerbated by compromised sensation. Complete loss of sensation can lead to neurotrophic

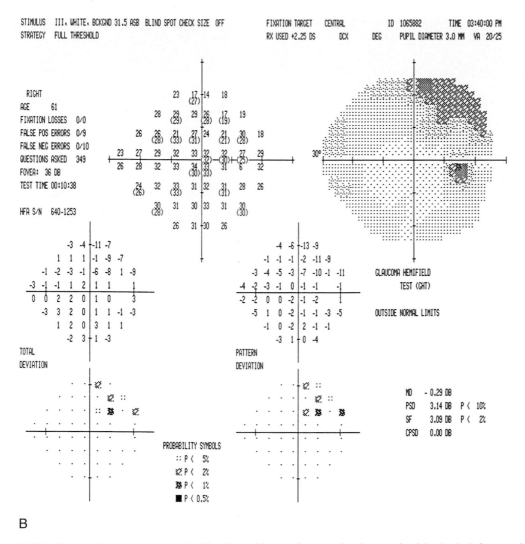

B

Fig. 10-3. (continued) This 61-year-old woman presented with a 3-year history of progressive decrease in vision in the left eye and a year and a half of episodes of trouble with speech. The field on the right eye (B) demonstrates relative superotemporal desaturation

keratitis. Facial nerve palsy may also play a role in conjunctival and corneal abnormalities due to incomplete blinks and exposure. Often chronic exposure is misdiagnosed as infection and unnecessarily treated with antibiotics. Corneal epithelial defects may occur with severe exposure problems and loss of sensation. This can lead to nonhealing epithelial defects, corneal ulceration, corneal melt, vascularization, or even corneal perforation.

Fundus changes commonly accompany optic nerve pathology. The most common finding is optic atrophy,[18,23] but this is not specific (Fig. 10.10). Focal atrophy (in a band pattern) may occur with chiasmal or tract compression. Optic disc edema (elevation, hyperemia, obscuration of the nerve fiber layer, and obscuration of the vessels at the disc margin) may be related to meningiomas that either increase intracranial pressure or directly compress the optic nerve. Optic nerve sheath meningiomas often present with chronic disc edema that may be misdiagnosed as "optic neuritis or papillitis."

Ocular venous outflow obstruction may cause optociliary shunt vessels on the disc surface. These are collaterals that connect the central retinal vein to the choroidal circulation. The most common cause of optociliary shunt vessels is a central retinal vein occlusion but when combined with disc atrophy a meningioma should be suspected (Fig. 10-5).

Neuro-ophthalmic History

Patients with complaints of visual loss should be carefully questioned as to when they first noted problems with their vision. It is also important to distinguish monocular from binocular visual loss. Patients should be questioned as to relative visual field loss. It is also important to obtain a history of progression. Has this been gradual or sudden? Is there any variability? Are there any positive visual phenomena? If so, detailed characterization is helpful including duration, location, and progression.

If there has been a history of double vision, there are several key questions. Does the double vision go away if one eye is occluded? Does the double vision get worse when looking in one

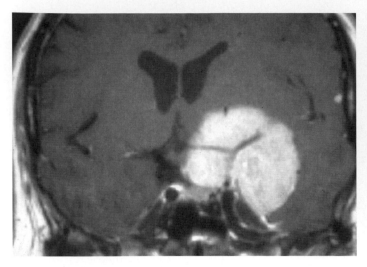

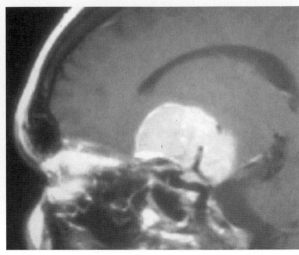

C   D

FIG. 10-3. (continued) This 61-year-old woman presented with a 3-year history of progressive decrease in vision in the left eye and a year and a half of episodes of trouble with speech. This pattern is compatible with a junctional syndrome, indicating a lesion that affects the optic nerve but also impacts the anterior aspect of the chiasm The presence of a clinoidal meningioma was confirmed on MRI scans (C, D)

particular direction? Is the double vision horizontal, vertical, or oblique? Is there anything that makes the double vision worse or better? How long has the double vision been present? Are the images getting further apart or closer together? Does it vary?

One of the most important parts of the history is determining who has seen the patient in the past and getting the old records. Has the patient had previous imaging studies (CT or MRI) and when? Can the scans be sent for review?

Afferent System Evaluation

Understanding the selection of tests of the afferent visual system may be aided by emphasizing the evolutionary development of the mammalian fovea. This specialized portion of the retina has developed maximal spatial resolution. Thus visual acuity (which is a measure of the angular or spatial resolution) is a measure of central retinal (or foveal) function. Extrafoveal function refers to visual sensation outside of foveal alignment. Thus afferent system evaluation is usually divided into central or foveal visual function and extrafoveal assessment.

In 1862 Herman Snellen, working with Donders in Utrecht, Holland, published his quantitative measurement of foveal function.[50] This was based on the description of "optotypes." These optotypes were defined as letters that subtended 5 minutes of visual arc at the distance of their name. Thus a "20" optotype (approximately 9 mm tall) subtended 1 minute of arc for each of the 5 bars at 20 feet. Similarly a "200" optotype would subtend a total of 5 minutes of arc if held at 200 feet. By combining the smallest optotype seen as the denominator of a fraction and the distance at which testing took place as the numerator, Snellen could quantitatively record central resolving power. This was essential in developing refraction. When recording vision it is important to remember that visual acuity should be tested with best correction (patient's glasses or contact lenses).

Over the last three decades a minor modification in the traditional Snellen chart decreased variability by removing some of the more difficult letters, including the same number of letters on each line, spacing the letter size based on a logarthrithmic scale, and placing the letters at proportional spacing. These ETDRS (or Bailey-Lovie) charts are used in multi-institutional studies to maximize accuracy.[51,52] These charts also permit easier translation into "logMAR," which is the most convenient way of comparing acuity change over time. Although the Snellen chart has been adapted for other languages (Cyrilic, Greek, Arabic), the E-game is a more universal solution that is also useful for illiterate or non–English-speaking patients. Other variants include the "Landolt C." In this test the patient is asked to identify the location of the open segment of the C.

Often it is not practical to test patients at 20 feet. A convenient means of assessing foveal visual function is the near card. The near card specifies testing at 14 inches but it is better done (again with appropriate reading correction) at whatever distance is comfortable for the patient. It is of course important to record the distance at which testing took place (a ruler or tape measure is useful). Near acuity may be recorded as J (Eduard Jaeger) print, or better yet, in the point system. Point size is universal; all print size in books, newspapers, and computers is specified in the point system. Near vision has angular resolution that is "equivalent" to distance vision but because it is not the same it is important that near vision should never be recorded as "20/50."

Testing color vision has been a traditional part of the neuro-ophthalmic examination. This is another means of measuring macular function since most cones are located in the fovea. Although congenital red-green color blindness is common

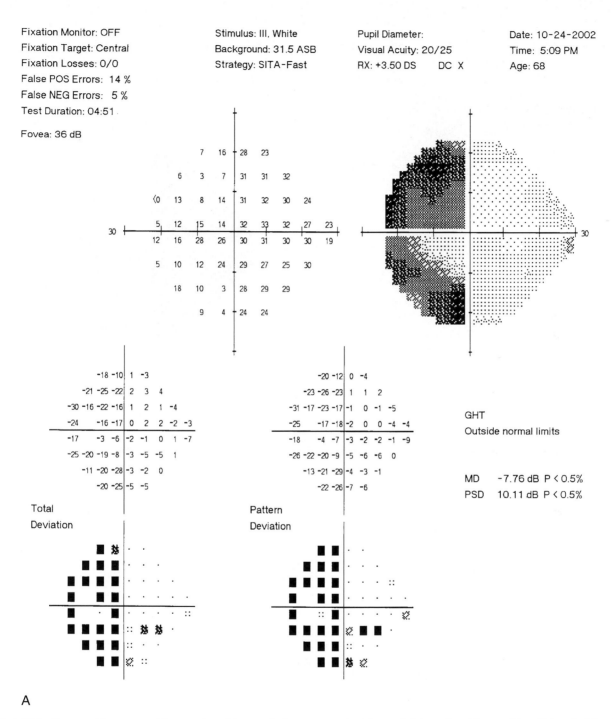

A

FIG. 10-4. This 68-year-old woman with a previous history of glaucoma presented complaining of problems with peripheral vision. Visual acuity was 20/40 and 20/25. She had a 0.3–0.6 log unit right APD and visual fields (A, B) confirmed the presence of a dense left homonymous hemianopsia

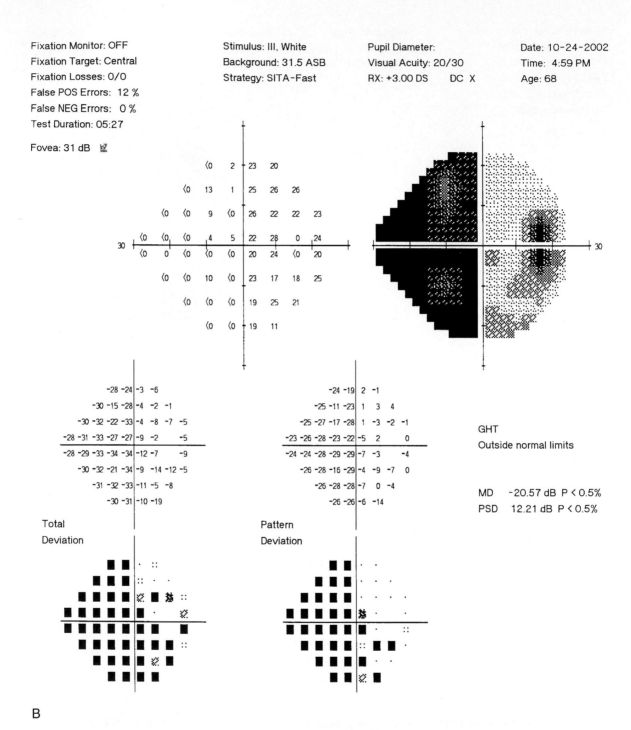

B

FIG. 10-4. (continued) This 68-year-old woman with a previous history of glaucoma presented complaining of problems with peripheral vision. Visual acuity was 20/40 and 20/25. She had a 0.3–0.6 log unit right APD and visual fields (A, B) confirmed the presence of a dense left homonymous hemianopsia

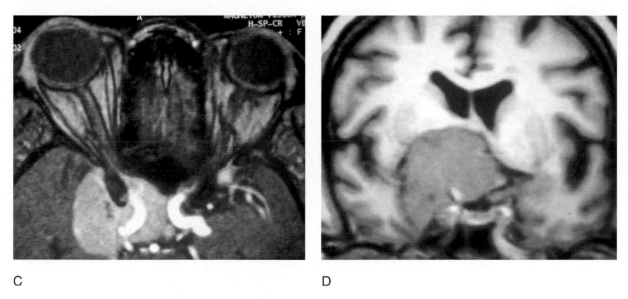

C   D

Fig. 10-4. (continued) This 68-year-old woman with a previous history of glaucoma presented complaining of problems with peripheral vision. An MRI scan confirmed the presence of a large clinoidal meningioma compressing the right optic tract (C, D)

(8% of the male population) and easily detected, acquired color vision deficits are much more difficult to detect and quantitate.[53] The Farnsworth 100 Hue test has been employed to measure color defects, but the findings tend to be non-specific and the testing is of longer duration with a higher variability when compared to Snellen acuity. Color vision testing is therefore considered an adjunctive test and is seldom employed in diagnosing or following patients with meningiomas.

One additional test of central visual function is contrast sensitivity. The supporters of contrast testing rightly point out that we live in a world of contrast, not black and white. Snellen (and even ETDRS) testing is done at high contrast. By lowering the contrast of test letters, much lower acuity measurements may be obtained.[54,55] This is particularly true in patients with recovered optic neuritis.[56] Although optic nerve compromise due to meningiomas may be expected to produce reduction in contrast sensitivity, this additional measurement only occasionally adds to Snellen and near acuity.[57]

Testing acuity should be done one eye at a time. The untested eye should be completely occluded with a patch, tape on the patient's glasses, a tissue behind the glasses keeping the eye closed, or occlusion with the patient's hand. Failure to completely occlude the nontested eye can easily result in a falsely "normal" acuity in the bad eye. Notation should be made of the correction (prescription of the glasses) used including the addition for near vision. If the patient's glasses are old or not available, ideally the patient should be refracted. If this is not available, a pinhole placed in front of the eye often eliminates a large component of the refractive error. Since the pinhole substantially cuts down on the amount of light reaching the retina, a brightly illuminated test screen is essential.

One additional means of testing macular function is stereoacuity. This is done with various commercially available tests including the Titmus test, Randot, or TNO. Normal stereopsis implies good vision in both eyes.[58] A patient that has a history of congenital strabismus even if he or she is not amblyopic (reduced vision due to a lazy eye) will not have normal stereopsis.

Extrafoveal function testing requires perimetry. This may be done qualitatively by confrontation or finger counting.[59] Still qualitative but more sensitive is the comparison of a red test object across the nasal horizontal and vertical midline. Tangent screen testing is a sensitive means of picking up central defects. An Amsler grid (a square of vertical and horizontal lines) is very sensitive to macular pathology.[60,61]

Perimetry may be done kinetically where a target of fixed intensity is moved from a nonseeing area toward fixation until the patient reports seeing it. In static perimetry a location is selected and the intensity of the stimulus is increased until the patient reports seeing it. Quantitative threshold perimetry, although still subjective, is an ideal way of following optic nerve function. Since in threshold determination the patient is expected to see the stimulus only 50% of the time, quantitative static perimetry is quite difficult for the patient. It must be remembered that as all perimetry tasks are subjective, the results are only as good as the patient is willing or able to give you.

Whether done statically or kinetically, the goals of perimetry are twofold. By analyzing the pattern of a visual field defect (abnormalities in Traquair's hill of vision), pathology may be localized along the visual pathways.[62] A second goal is to quantitate the amount of damage. This is a prerequisite for determination of progression or response to treatment.

Older literature emphasizes multiple patterns of visual field defect. Anatomically and teleologically, patterns may be characterized into (1) those that affect the central visual field (Fig. 10-1), (2) arcuate defects due to involvement of the optic nerve (Fig. 10-2), particularly at the disc, (3) bitem-

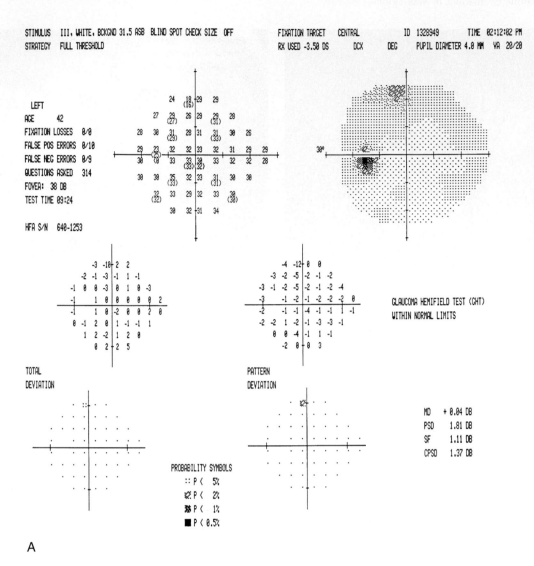

A

FIG. 10-5. This 41-year-old woman presented with a 7-year history of progressive visual loss on the right side. She had had multiple MRI scans and LPs done and was told at one time that she had sinusitis and also a "mild form of optic neuritis." She had been noted to have some swelling of the disc on the right side. When evaluated, visual acuity was 2/200 on the right and 20/20 on the left with a 1.2 log unit right afferent pupillary defect. Visual fields (A, B) confirmed minimal response on the right side and a normal field on the left

poral visual field defects representing chiasmal pathology, or (4) homonymous visual field defects indicating contralateral retrochiasmal pathology (Fig. 10-4). Thus all perimetry should be directed to the central field, testing across the nasal horizontal midline, and testing across the vertical midline.

Interpreting perimetry data emphasizes the anatomic correlates mentioned. A visual field defect in both eyes to the same side that respects the vertical midline strongly suggests retrochiasmal involvement. Similarly, arcuate visual field defects speak to optic nerve involvement. Pattern recognition is aided by the use of probability plots that take into account the age of the patient, the possible contribution of anterior segment or refractive pathology, and the variation of response with increasing eccentricity.

One additional, exceedingly important means of assessing the afferent system is checking for an afferent pupillary

defect.[63] The pretectal nuclei receive input from both eyes via the retina, ganglion cells, optic nerve, chiasm, optic tract, and pupillary tract just anterior to the lateral geniculate. A light source moved rapidly between the two eyes (illuminating the right and left eye) should produce equal reactivity. If one pupil dilates when the light is moved to it from the other eye, this is an indication of asymmetric optic nerve function. This "afferent pupillary defect" may be quantitated by placing neutral density filters in front of the better-reacting eye until there is a balance.[64]

Afferent pupillary defects may be seen with extensive asymmetric retinal disease (retinal detachment, age-related macular degeneration),[65] occasionally with amblyopia[66,67] and contralateral optic tract lesions (Fig. 10-4). They are, however, never seen with cataracts and almost always indicate asymmetric optic nerve function. In the setting of meningiomas,

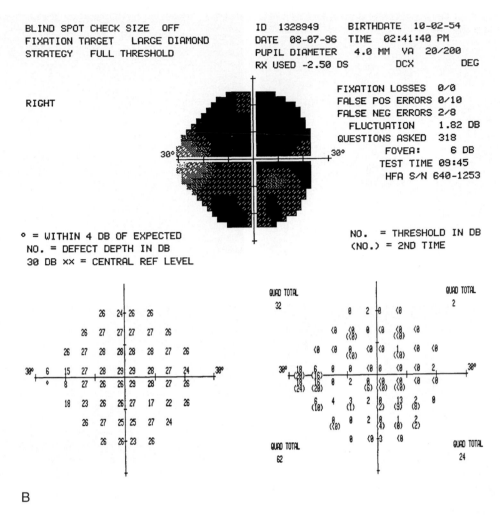

FIG. 10-5. (continued) This 41-year-old woman presented with a 7-year history of progressive visual loss on the right side. She had had multiple MRI scans and LPs done and was told at one time that she had sinusitis and also a "mild form of optic neuritis." She had been noted to have some swelling of the disc on the right side. When evaluated, visual acuity was 2/200 on the right and 20/20 on the left with a 1.2 log unit right afferent pupillary defect. Visual fields (A, B) confirmed minimal response on the right side and a normal field on the left

either direct compression or secondary ischemia can result in decreased acuity, visual field defects, and an afferent pupillary defect.

Electrophysiologic tests can also give information about the function of the afferent visual pathways. Flash visual evoked potentials (VEP) suggests that the visual system to the occipital cortex is grossly intact. Pattern visual evoked potentials attempt to quantitate visual pathway function. Although often variable and subject to artifact, the comparison between the two eyes may be helpful. Recently newer computer techniques have permitted "multifocal VEP" to detect localized pathology affecting the visual pathways[68]. It is hoped that these techniques may afford a more objective assessment of the visual pathways.

Although possibly better included in the discussion of the globe and adnexal structures, the optic disc appearance may give a clue to afferent system dysfunction. The presence of optic disc atrophy indicates evidence of optic nerve dam-

age that is at least 4–6 weeks old. High-tech tests introduced recently also allow us to measure the nerve fiber thickness. This may correlate with damage to the optic nerve or the pregeniculate retrochiasmal pathways. It should be emphasized that there is no data to support a 1:1 correlation between these anatomic measurements and the psychophysical measurement of acuity and visual field. The exact role of these tests remains to be determined.

Efferent System Evaluation

The first part of the ocular motor neuro-ophthalmic examination consists of assessment of stability of each eye first in primary position and then in eccentric gaze. This may be done by direct observation. For more detailed evaluation, Frenzel glasses illuminate and magnify the view of the globe. One very sensitive technique available to all is the use of the direct

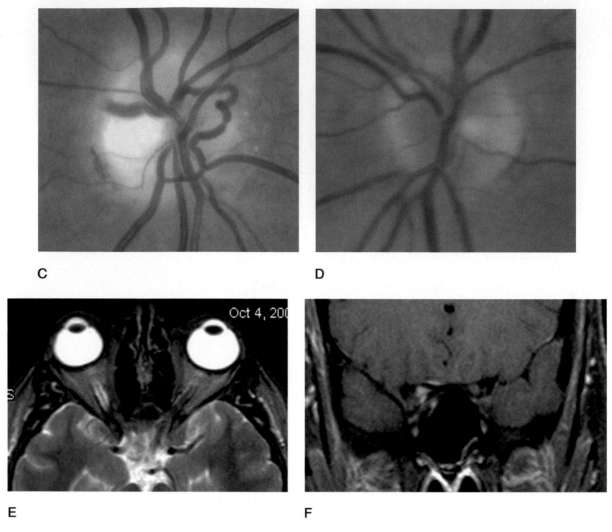

FIG. 10-5.This 41-year-old woman pr sented with a 7-year history of progressive visual loss on the right side. Her fundoscopic examination revealed a normal disc on the left side (D) but optic atrophy with optociliary shunt vessels on the right (C). Her fourth MRI scan confirmed the presence of an optic nerve sheath and canal meningioma (E, F)

ophthalmoscope to view the optic disc. Any subtle tendency to drift will be seen as a drift of the optic disc in the opposite direction. Microsaccadic refixation movements are normal, but when of larger amplitude it may indicate cerebellar dysfunction. Problems with maintaining eccentric gaze may be detected by having the patient look eccentrically while maintaining a view of the optic disc.

Slowed saccades may be a sign of early ophthalmoplegia (third nerve: adducting delay; sixth nerve: abducting delay). Saccades should be evaluated for latency (time to start moving), accuracy (does the eye reach the target or undershoot hypometria), and velocity (the larger the saccade, the greater the peak velocity).[69] Saccadic asymmetry may be brought out with repetitive movements, perhaps best demonstrated with an OKN drum. Adducting saccadic slowing may also be seen with internuclear ophthalmoplegia. This is commonly seen with demyelinating disease in young patients and microvascular disease in older patients. Meningiomas could rarely cause an INO, usually by secondary ischemic changes associated with

basilar compromise. Saccadic slowing can be quantitated with video recording, electro-oculography, infrared tracking, or contact lens coil oculography.[70]

Vestibular ocular response ("doll's eyes") can be tested by asking the patient to read a near card while rotating his or her head.[71] A drop of four lines of vision suggests a vestibular abnormality most commonly seen with vascular disease in older patients and demyelinating disease in young patients. When associated with a meningioma, the tumor is usually in the posterior fossa or cerebello-pontine angle. An additional technique to check vestibular function is to view the optic disc with a direct ophthalmoscope while rotating the patient's head in the dark.[72] Subtle asymmetric abnormalities of vestibular function may be brought out by head shaking and then observing the optic disc for drift. It should be noted that other lesions that affect the vestibular nerves and pathways may also result in reading abnormalities.

Ductions refer to movements of each eye separately. They can be measured with a ruler or with a Goldmann bowl. Recently a cervical range of motion apparatus has been

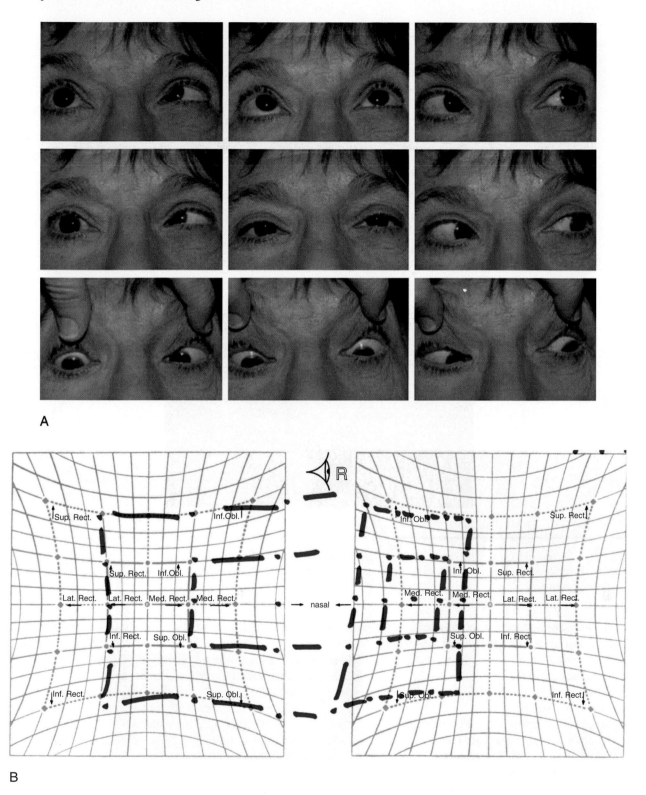

FIG. 10-6. This 55-year-old woman presented with a 4-year history of horizontal diplopia. Visual acuity was 20/20 bilaterally, and there was no evidence of proptosis. Her motility examination, however, demonstrated limitation in abduction on the right side (A). This was confirmed on her Hess screen (B)

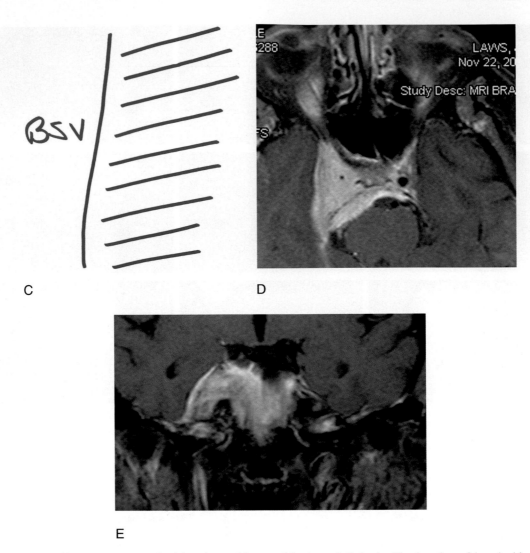

C   D

E

FIG. 10-6. This 55-year-old woman presented with a 4-year history of horizontal diplopia. The location of her double vision could be demonstrated when looking to the right on binocular single vision fields (C). MRI scan confirmed the presence of a cavernous sinus/ petroclival meningioma (D, E)

adapted to measure ductions. Ductions may be reduced by restriction (most commonly thyroid orbitopathy) or paresis (extraocular muscle weakness, myoneural junction deficit, or ophthalmoplegia). Versions refer to movements of the two eyes together. Subtle abnormalities in versions often produce misalignment and thus diplopia.

In most cases of double vision the role of the neuro-ophthalmologist is to detect misalignment. The amount and direction of visual axis misalignment is important in both diagnosis and planning rehabilitation. It is important to realize that tendency to ocular deviation is common. Most of the population has mild exophoria, which is a tendency for the eyes to deviate out. Esophoria (a tendency for the eyes to cross), although less common, can be seen in otherwise normal patients. The tendency for one eye to be higher than the other is the least common and the most likely to be symptomatic. Normally a small tendency to drift is controlled by fusional amplitudes. These are greater for a tendency to drift out and the least for mild hyperdeviations. Fusional amplitudes may vary among individuals. Patients with

congenital cranial nerve palsies (particularly seventh nerve palsy) may have very large fusional amplitudes. Age and illness may reduce fusional amplitudes so that a tendency to deviate becomes manifest and the patient begins to complain of double vision. One clue of motility problems and misalignment is a head turn or tilt. In patients with a seventh nerve palsy the head is typically tilted away from the side of involvement. In a sixth nerve palsy the patient minimizes diplopia by turning the head in the direction of the palsy.

Ocular deviations may be comitant (in which case the deviation is the same in all directions) or incomitant. Incomitant deviations may rarely be due to primary overaction. Most cases of incomitant deviations are due to paretic problems (myoneural conduction problems, extraocular muscle weakness, internuclear connection problems, or most commonly ophthalmoplegia). The distinction between restrictive and paretic strabismus is important. Traditionally this is detected by forced ductions,[73] but may be diagnosed by measuring intraocular pressure in primary and eccentric gaze.[74]

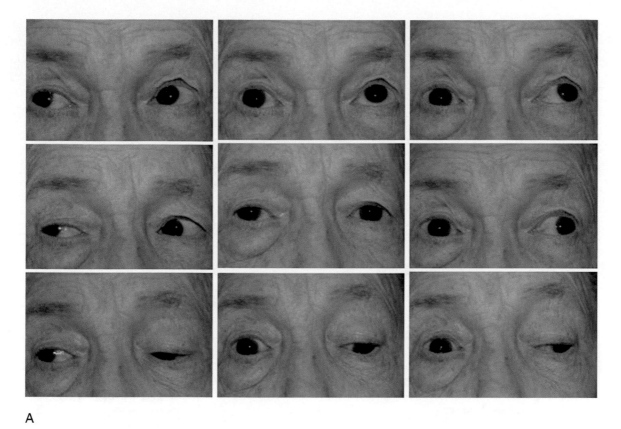

A

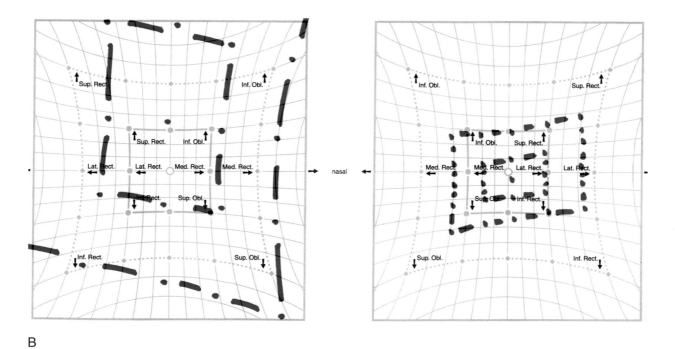

B

FIG. 10-7. This 80-year-old patient was referred for a 6-month history of right lid droop (A). Examination revealed 20/25 and 20/15 vision, but 2 mm of right ptosis. She had limitation of elevation, depression, and adduction on the right side as confirmed by her Hess screen (B)

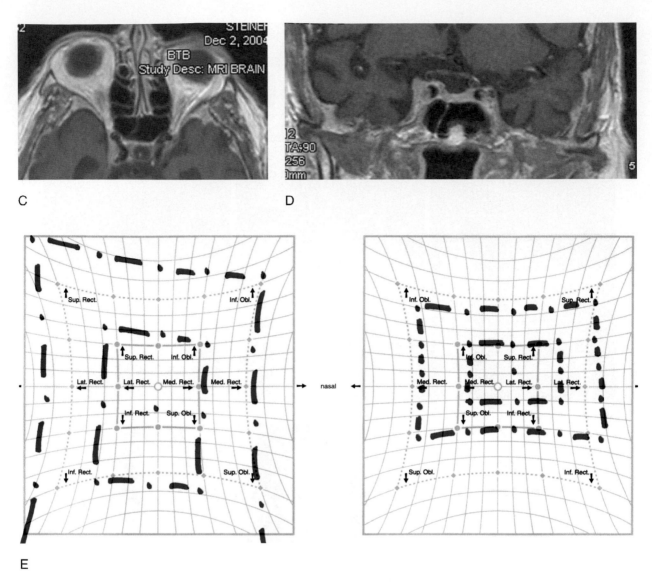

E

FIG. 10-7. (continued) This 80-year-old patient was referred for a 6-month history of right lid droop. An axial MRI scan (C) demonstrates asymmetry in the cavernous sinus. This could be better appreciated on coronals as a lesion involving the superior portion of the right cavernous sinus in the region of the III nerve (D). This was subsequently treated with gamma knife, with stabilization and mild improvement in motility, as confirmed on quantitative Hess screen measurements (E)

Ocular deviation is traditionally detected by cover/uncover and cross-cover testing. If an eye is out of alignment when a cover is placed over the viewing eye, the misaligned eye will shift to take up fixation. This can be measured by placing a filter in front of the deviated eye before covering the fixating eye. It is also important to recognize that the deviation measured when placing a prism in front of one eye is not necessarily the same prism required in front of the other eye. There will be a difference in the setting of an incomitant deviation in which there is either a paretic or restrictive cause of misalignment. Primary deviation is the amount of misalignment measured when the patient fixates with the normal eye, while secondary deviation is the measurement of displacement when the patient fixates with the paretic or restricted eye. The secondary deviation is always greater than the primary deviation due to Hering's law of equal innervation.

Because of the variation of deviation depending on direction of gaze, full evaluation of deviation in a patient with an incomitant deviation requires measurement in all nine positions of gaze (straight, up, down, left, right, up right, up left, down right, and down left). A faster way of at least qualitatively checking motility is the use of the red glass or Maddox rod [75]. In the case of the red glass test, a red lens is placed in front of one eye and a flashlight is moved into all nine positions of gaze. The patient reports the direction of separation between the red and white lights. The patient will report the light in the opposite direction of the eye deviation (if the eye won't abduct as in the sixth nerve palsy, the patient will report the light seen by that eye to be deviated in the direction of the deficient lateral rectus). Thus with an esodeviation the patient will see the lights as uncrossed, while in the case of medial rectus weakness and an exodeviation the lights will look crossed.

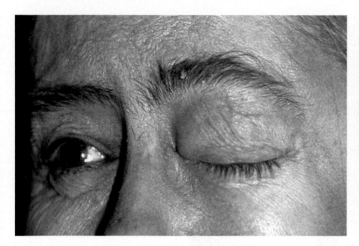
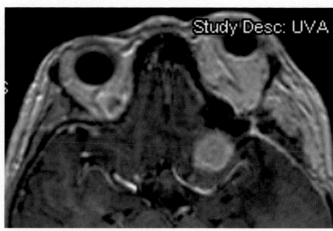

A   B

FIG. 10-8. This 55-year-old patient was initially evaluated in 1987 when she presented with a VI nerve palsy. Workup revealed a meningioma involving the cavernous sinus in Meckel's cave. In spite of several resections, the meningioma continued to grow, producing a complete optic neuropathy and essentially complete ophthalmoplegia (A). The tumor secondarily entered the orbit (B) producing marked proptosis, ptosis, and dystopia

A Maddox rod consists of multiple parallel high-powered half-prisms. When a patient views a light point source through a Maddox rod, he or she will see a line at right angles to the prisms. This, like the red glass, dissociates the two eyes, thus measuring the tendency to deviate (phoria) in addition to any fixed deviation (tropia). Since the deviation seen with a Maddox rod is only perpendicular to the prisms, in order to measure both the vertical and horizontal component, the rod rotation must be changed from vertical to horizontal. While this is "twice" the work by separating out the vertical and horizontal components of a deviation, it actually makes it easier to make a diagnosis. Relative torsion of the two eyes (seen with fourth nerve palsy) may be detected by the use of a double Maddox rod (usually one red and one white).

Deviation detected with a Maddox rod may be quantitated by using a prism. While we normally expect the patient to be fixating the light, since it is easier to place the prism over the eye without the Maddox rod, we are actually measuring the primary deviation of the eye beneath the Maddox rod. The secondary deviation may be checked by moving the Maddox rod to the opposite eye and switching the prism.

More quantitative assessment of misalignment may be obtained with an amblyoscope or haploscope, which presents images separately to the two eyes and measures the deviation. These pieces of equipment also permit measurement of fusional amplitudes.

A very nice semi-quantitative means of recording misalignment is the use of the Hess screen[76] (Fig. 10-6). The patient is instructed to use a green flashlight (or laser pointer) to point at red LEDs on a gray screen while wearing red glass over one eye and a green glass over the other. It is important to fix the distance at which testing takes place and make sure the patient doesn't turn her or his head. In order to detect the primary and secondary deviation, the test must be repeated after switching the lenses. The affected eye is identified by the smaller box. While with a meningioma incomitant deviations are undoubtedly secondary to paretic pathology, the smaller box on the Hess screen may be due to restrictive as well as paretic abnormalites. Occasionally one eye's box may be smaller in vertical movement while the opposite eye is smaller in the horizontal direction. The use of the Hess screen permits (1) recording to present in lectures, (2) quantitative evaluation that may be compared over time (progression or improvement) (Fig. 10-7), and (3) directing the form of surgery that might be most helpful in achieving realignment.[77]

An additional technique involves plotting the visual direction in which the patient has single vision and separating this from the area of diplopia. This is done on a Goldmann bowl usually using a I or III size test object and moving from an area of fusion to an area of diplopia. These binocular single vision fields can be followed and present useful information in tailoring strabismus surgery (Fig. 10-6). Our goals are to maximize binocularity achieving single vision in primary and down reading gaze.

In patients who cannot fixate (mentation changes or severely reduced vision), misalignment may be measured by looking at the reflex on the cornea. Normally this is displaced slightly medially (angle kappa) but should be the same in both eyes. If the light reflex is deviated more medially, that eye is deviated out (exodeviation), displacement of the reflex temporally indicates an esodeviation, and displacement of the reflex inferiorly demonstrates a hyperdeviation. The deviation may be further quantitated by placement of a prism in front of one eye until the reflex is equally centered (Krimsky test) 78 (Fig. 10-10).

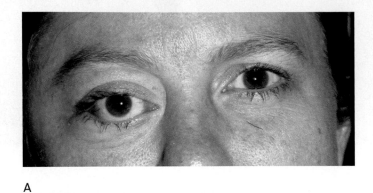

A

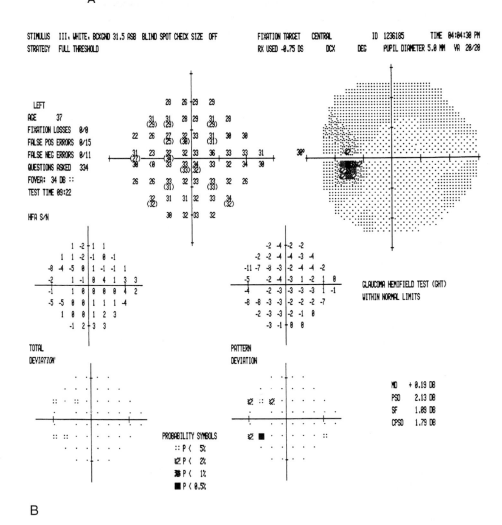

B

FIG. 10-9. (continued) This 37-year-old patient presented with increasing proptosis and significant globe dystopia (A). Although visual acuity was 20/25 bilaterally, she had 8 mm of proptosis, and visual fields (B)

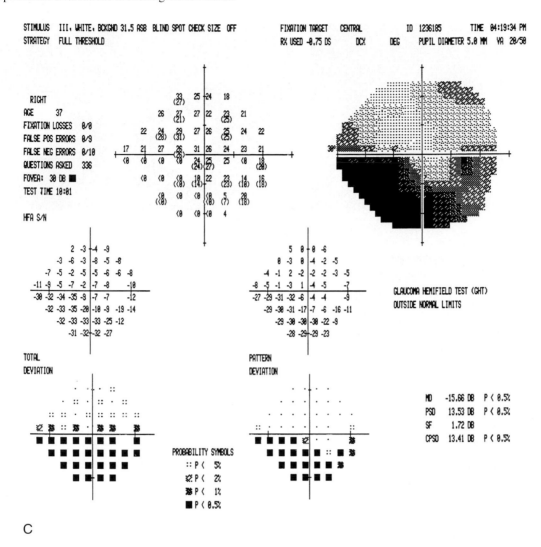

C

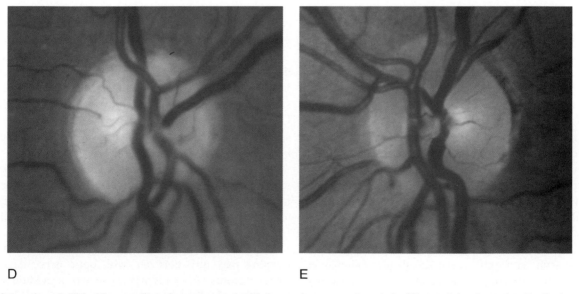

D   E

FIG. 10-9.(continued) This 37-year-old patient presented with increasing proptosis and significant globe dystopia. (B, C) demonstrated an inferior arcuate defect on the right side. Her fundus photos (D, E) confirmed the presence of optic atrophy on the right (D)

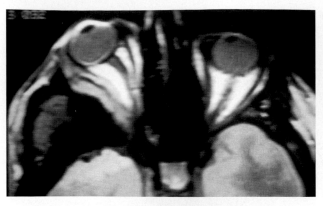

F

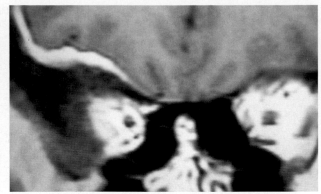

G

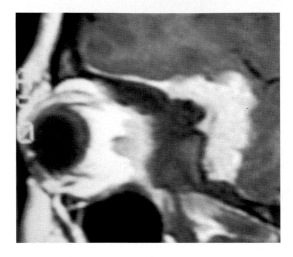

FIG. 10-9. (continued) This 37-year-old patient presented with increasing proptosis and significant globe dystopia. Subsequent imaging studies (F–H) confirmed the presence of an orbitosphenoid meningioma that underwent decompression. Visual field defects can obviously occur, even without evidence of decreased central acuity. In this case, an arcuate defect indicated compression of the optic nerve. The patient also had prominent proptosis and dystopia due to involvement of the orbital roof and greater wing of the sphenoid

H

Adnexal Evaluation

Adnexal evaluation begins with gross observation. Photographs may be helpful in documenting findings. Palpebral fissures should be measured and any asymmetry in the lid contour noted. Upper lid range gives a measure of levator function. Ptosis may be quantitated by measuring the distance from the central corneal light reflex to the upper lid margin.

Dystopia (vertical or horizontal) may be measured as the difference in the height of the two eyes or the distance from the midline to the pupil. Axial displacement is measured relative to the lateral orbital rim using a Hertel apparatus. In patients with previous orbital surgery, this may be misleading, and other techniques are available to measure displacement relative to the cheek or forehead.

Balloting the eyes may indicate asymmetric resistance to retropulsion, which may indicate an active orbital process. This may be seen with optic nerve sheath meningiomas or with meningiomas secondarily affecting the orbit, usually through the greater wing of the sphenoid.

Check for sensory loss should be done in the distribution of the three divisions of the trigeminal nerve. Numbness usually indicates cavernous sinus involvement. A corneal aesthesiometer will give a quantitative assessment of sensory loss to the cornea.

Orbicularis weakness (usually related to facial nerve dysfunction) often leads to problems with lid closure. This lack of closure (lagophthalmos) and secondary corneal exposure and drying may occur with meningiomas affecting the CP angle or the internal auditory meatus. A combination of sensory loss (trigeminal dysfunction) and motor (facial) weakness is a disaster waiting to happen.

Looking for optic disc changes is an important part of the afferent system evaluation. Fundus photography is an important means of recording disc appearance. More recently anatomic measures of the disc appearance include evaluation by Heidelberg ocular tomography.

Nerve fiber layer analysis (GDx or OCT) demonstrating thinning may also correlate with optic nerve dysfunction. These anatomic measures may prove to be an additional objective means of following optic nerve dysfunction (Fig. 10-1).

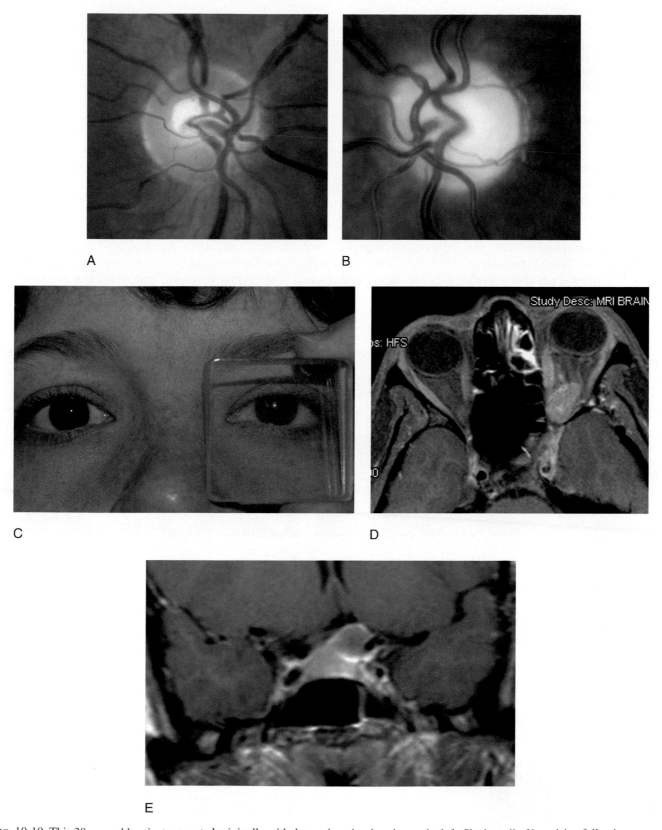

FIG. 10-10. This 38-year-old patient presented originally with decreasing visual acuity on the left. She lost all of her vision following surgery for an orbital apex meningioma. She subsequently developed a left VI nerve palsy and had muscle surgery for realignment. On follow-up examination visual acuity was 20/15 on the right and NLP on the left. Her fundus examination (A, B) confirmed the presence of severe optic atrophy on the left. Her motility examination revealed a residual small angle esotropia in primary position. Because of the loss of vision in that eye, in order to measure the amount of esodeviation, a prism was placed in front of the left eye centering the light reflex (C). Her MRI scan (D, E) confirmed the presence of residual orbital apex meningioma with an extension into the cavernous sinus as well as on to the tuberculum

Adjunctive Evaluation

The clinical examination is being supplemented by new high-tech tests. We have already mentioned the use of optic disc and nerve fiber bundle analysis. In addition, electrophysiologic tests have advanced from flash visual evoked response to pattern VEP and more recently multifocal VEP. This has been an adaptation of advanced computer techniques first used to obtain multifocal electroretinography.[79] It is hoped that multifocal VEP may provide objective assessment of extrafoveal visual function.[68]

Detailed eye movements can be obtained by quantitative infrared tracking or magnetic coil oculography. Infrared tracking is limited in the vertical direction, and coil studies require very specialized equipment.[80,81]

Neuro-ophthalmologists may also help with diagnosis of meningiomas through the use of fine needle aspiration biopsy.[82,83] This is particularly useful when the differential diagnosis can affect treatment options (Fig. 10-11).

Differential Diagnosis

Unfortunately, there are rarely any specific neuro-ophthalmic findings that guarantee the presence of a meningioma.[84] One relative exception is the finding of optociliary shunt vessels on an atrophic optic disc. Other findings involving the optic nerve are quite nonspecific. The slow progression usually seen with meningioma is suggestive, but other lesions, including schwannomas, cavernous hemangiomas, or even aneurysms, can also present with delayed symptoms. Often imaging studies (both CT and MRI) are helpful, but even these are not always adequate to make a diagnosis.[85] The differential diagnosis of lesions of the orbit and the optic nerve include optic nerve gliomas,[86] sarcoidosis,[87–89] and orbital perineuritis.[90,91] Lesions eccentric to the optic nerve include hemangioma,[92] hemangiopericytomas,[93] hemangioblastomas,[94] metastatic disease, leukemic infiltrates,[95] and rarely eosinophilic granulomas (Erdheim

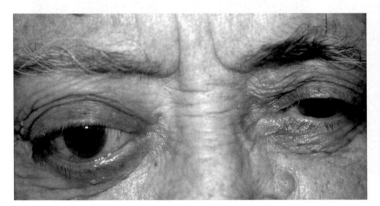

A

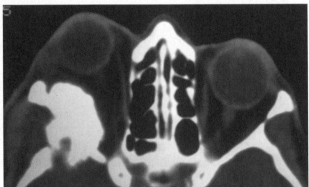

B

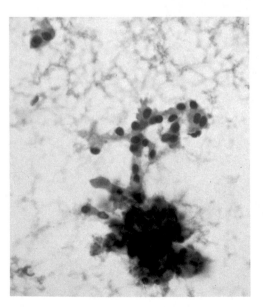

C

FIG. 10-11. An 89-year-old demented patient was referred from a nursing home for 4 months of prominence of the right globe and episodes of spontaneous globe luxation. On examination she had dystopia and 14 mm of proptosis (A). She also had a previous history of breast carcinoma, and the radiologists were worried about atypical features on her CT scan (B); therefore, a fine needle aspiration biopsy was performed, which demonstrated evidence of meningioma (C). In view of her mental status, the patient was treated with a tarsorrhaphy, which stopped the recurrent globe luxation and protected her cornea

Chester).[96] Many of these lesions progress more rapidly than meningiomas.

Visual pathway involvement at the chiasm or tract may be due to meningiomas of the tuberculum, clinoid, dorsal clivus, and parasellar dura. Differential in this area may include craniopharyngioma, pituitary tumor, dysgerminoma, metastatic disease, fibrous dysplasia, and inflammatory lesions, including sarcoidosis. Gliomas usually have a more characteristic appearance. Demyelinating lesions obviously can be distinguished on imaging, but clinically they may produce similar findings.

Ophthalmoplegia related to cavernous sinus lesions may be due to multiple other etiologies.[97] Cavernomas and schwannomas (of the ocular motor nerves and the trigeminal nerves) may be mistaken for meningiomas involving the cavernous sinus. Carotid cavernous aneurysms may enlarge to produce similar ocular motor problems. Pituitary tumors, chordomas, and chondrosarcomas may extend laterally to involve the cavernous sinus.

The differential diagnosis of meningiomas of the dura includes hemangiopericytoma and metastatic disease. Intraventricular tumors causing field defects may include ependymomas and choroid plexus papillomas.

Vestibular schwannomas, epidermoids, aneurysms, and metastatic disease may resemble meningiomas of the cerebello-pontine angle. Acoustic and facial nerve dysfunction may also occur with traumatic and inflammatory lesions of the petrous bone, including meningitis, cholesterol granulomas, and Gradenigo's syndrome.

Clival lesions may include chordomas, chondrosarcomas, lymphoma, and metastatic disease. Pituitary tumors may extend posteriorly. Inflammatory lesions (similar to idiopathic orbital inflammatory disease) can affect the clivus and thus the cranial nerves (particularly the sixth nerve).

Conclusions

In spite of the advent of imaging studies, which form the primary means of diagnosis of meningiomas, quantitative neuro-ophthalmic examination is an indispensable part of the appropriate evaluation of patients with suspected meningiomas. This is not only important in diagnosis, but becomes increasingly important in the assessment of treatment and recognition of natural history. Simple and more sophisticated tests permit both psychophysical and anatomic evaluation of the visual system. These tests will continue to play an essential part in managing patients with meningiomas.

References

1. Cushing H, Eisenhardt L. Meningiomas. Their Classification, Regional Behavior, Life History, and Surgical End Results. Springfield, IL: Charles C Thomas, 1938:283–297.
2. Golgi C. Sulla struttura e sullo svilupper degli psammomi. Morgagni Napoli 1969; 11:874–886.
3. Hudson AC. Primary tumours of the optic nerve. Roy London Ophthalmol Hosp Rep 1912; 18:317–439.
4. Cushing H. The meningiomas (dural endotheliomas): their source, and favoured seats of orgin. Brain 1922; 45:282–316.
5. Walsh RB. Progressive unilateral loss of vision. Criteria indicating neurosurgical intervention. In: Smith JL, ed. Neuro-ophthalmology: Symposium of the University of Miami and the Bascom Palmer Eye Institute, vol 5. Hallandale, FL: Huffman, 1970:1–9.
6. Wright JE. Primary optic nerve meningiomas; clinical presentation and management. Trans Am Acad Ophthalmol Otalaryngol 1977; 83:617–625.
7. Wybar K. Chiasmal compression. Presenting ocular features. Proc Roy Soc Med 1977; 70:307–317.
8. Wilson WB. Meningiomas of the anterior visual system. Surv Ophthalmol 1981; 26:109–127.
9. Anderson D, Khalil M. Meningioma and the ophthalmologist. A review of 80 cases. Ophthalmology 1981; 88:1004–1009.
10. Zevgaridis D, Medele RJ, Muller A. et al. Meningiomas of the sellar region presenting with visual impairment: impact of various prognostic factors on surgical outcome in 62 patients. Acta Neurochirurg 2001; 143(5):471–476.
11. Menke E, Osarovsky E, Reitner A, et al. Functional assessment before and after interventions on the optic chiasm system. Wien Klin Wochenschr 2002; 114(1–2):33–37.
12. Schlezinger NS, Alpers BJ, Weiss BP. Suprasellar meningiomas associated with scotomatous field defects. Arch Ophthalmol 1946; 35:624–642.
13. Mooney AJ, McConnell AA. Visual scotomata with intracranial lesions affecting the optic nerve. J. Neurol Neurosurg Psychiatry 1949; 12:205–218.
14. Chamlin M. Visual field defects due to optic nerve compression by mass lesions. Arch Ophthalmol 1957; 58:37–58.
15. Puchner MJ. Fischer-Lampsatis RC. Herrmann HD et al. Suprasellar meningioma. A disease still frequently diagnosed too late. Dtsch Med Wochenschr 1998; 123(34–35):991–996.
16. Sibony PA, Krauss HR, Kennderdell JS, et al. Optic nerve sheath meningiomas. Clinical manifestations. Ophthalmology 1984; 91:1313–1324.
17. Uihlein A, Weyand RD. Meningiomas of anterior clinoid process as a casue of unilateral loss of vision. Arh Ophthalmol 1953; 49:261–270.
18. Cushing H, Eisenhardt L. Meningiomas arising from the tuberculum sellae. With the syndrome of primary optic atrophy and bitemporal field defects combined with a normal sella turcica in a middle aged person. Arch Ophthalmol 1929; 1:1–41, 168–206.
19. Grant FC, Hedges TR Jr. Ocular findings in meningiomas of the tuberculum sellae. Arch Ophthalmol 1956; 56:163–170.
20. Demailly P, Guiot G. Méningiomes du diaphragme sellaire. Bull Soc D'Ophtalmol Fr 1970; 70:191–196.
21. Finn JE, Mount LA. Meningiomas of the tuberculum sellae and planum spenoidale. A review of 83 cases. Arch Ophthalmol 1974; 92:23–27.
22. Smolin G. Middle cranial fossa meningioma. Causing unilateral loss of visual acuity. Am J Ophthalmol 1966; 61:798–802.
23. Huber A. Eye Signs and Symptoms in Brain Tumors, 3rd ed. St. Louis: CV Mosby, 1976:235–259.
24. Lee AG, Siebert KJ, Sanan A. Radiologic-clinical correlation. Junctional visual field loss. Am J Neuroradiol 1997; 18(6):1171–1174.

25. Komotar RJ, Keswani SC, Wityk RJ. Meningioma presenting as stroke: report of two cases and estimation of incidence. J Neurol Neurosurg Psychiatry 2003; 74(1):136–137.

26. Bejjani GK, Cockerham KP, Kennerdell JS, et al. Visual field deficit caused by vascular compression from a suprasellar meningioma: case report. Neurosurgery 2002; 50(5):1129–1132.

27. Slavin ML. Acute, sever, symmetric visual loss with cecocentral scotomas due to olfactory groove meningioma. J Clin Neuro-ophthalmol 1986; 6:224–227.

28. Thomas DA, Trobe JD, Cornblath WT. Visual loss secondary to increased intracranial pressure in neurofibromatosis type 2. Arch Ophthalmol 1999; 117(12):1650–1653.

29. Spencer WH, Hoyt WF. Chronic disc edema from neoplastic involvement of perioptic meninges. Int Ophthalmol Clin 1971; 11:171–187.

30. Hannesson OB. Primary meningioma of the orbit invading the choroid. Report of a case. Acta Ophthalmol 1971; 49:627–632.

31. Cibis GW, Whittaker CK, Wood WE. Intraocular extension of optic nerve meningiomas in a case of neurofibromatosis. Arch Ophthalmol 1985; 29:239–264.

32. Sammartino A, Cerbella R, Cennamo G, Corriero G. Exophthalmos induced by intracranial meningiomatosis. Orbit 1986; 5:39–44.

33. Schittkowski M, Hingst V, Stropahl G, Guthoff R. Optic nerve sheath meningioma with intraocular invasion—a case report. Klin Monatsbl Augenheilk 1999; 214(4):251–254.

34. Sanders MD. White spots on the optic disc. Trans Ophthalmol Soc UK 1985; 104:70–71.

35. Frisén L, Hoyt WF, Tengroth BM. Optociliary veins, disc pallor and visual loss. A triad of signs indicating spheno-orbital meningioma. Acta Ophthalmol 1973; 51:241–249.

36. Ellenberger C Jr. Perioptic meningiomas. Syndrome of long standing visual loss, pale disc edema, and optociliary veins. Arch Neurol 1976; 33:671–674.

37. Rodriques MM, Savino PJ, Schatz NJ. Spheno-orbital meningiomas with optociliary veins. Am J Ophthalmol 1976; 81:666–670.

38. Tsukahara S, Kobayashi S, Nakagawa F, Sugita K. Optociliary veins associated with meningioma of the optic nerve sheath. Ophthalmologica 1980; 118:188–194.

39. Dieterich M, Brandt T. Vestibulo-oculo reflex. Curr Opin Neurol 1995; 8:83–88.

40. Schatz NJ, Savino PJ, Corbett JJ. Primary aberrant oculomotor regeneration. A sign of intracavernous meningioma. Arch Neurol 1977; 34:29–32.

41. Boghen D, Chartrand J-P, Laflamme P, et al. Primary aberrant third nerve regeneration. Ann Neurol 1979; 6:415–418.

42. Winterkorn JM, Bruno M. Relative pupil-sparing oculomotor nerve palsy as the presenting sign of posterior fossa meningioma. J Neuro-ophthalmol 2001; 21(3):207–209.

43. Elsberg CA, Hare CC, Dyke CG. Unilateral exophthalmos in intracranial tumors with special reference to its occurrence in the meningiomata. Surg Gynecol Obstet 1932; 55:681–699.

44. Kearns TP, Wagener HP. Ophthalmologic diagnosis of meningiomas of the sphenoid ridge. Am J Med Sci 1953; 226:221–228.

45. Birge HL. Meningiomas: an ophthalmic problem. Diagnosis and results of treatment. Am J Ophthalmol 1955; 39:828–838.

46. Bonnal JP, Brotchi J, Born J. Meningiomas of the sphenoid wings. In: Sekhar LN, Schramm VL Jr, eds. Tumors of the Cranial Base: Diagnosis and Treatment. Mount Kisco, NY: Futura, 1987: 373–392.

47. Derome PJ, Guiot G. Bone problems in meningiomas invading the base of the skull. Clin Neurosurg 1978; 25:435–451.

48. Pompili A, Derome, PJ, Visot A, Guiot G. Hyperostosing meningiomas of the sphenoid ridge-clinical features, surgical therapy, and long term observations: review of 49 cases. Surg Neurol 1982; 17:411–416.

49. Reale F, Delfini R, Cintorino M. An intradiploic meningioma of the orbital roof: case report. Ophthalmologica (Basel) 1978; 177:82–87.

50. Snellen H. Probebuchstaben zur Bestimmung der Sehschafe. Utrecht: PW van de Weijer, 1862.

51. Bailey IL, Lovie JE. New design principles for visual acuity letter charts. Am J Optom Physiol Opt 1976; 53:740–745.

52. Ferris FL III, Kassoff A, Bresnick GH, et al. New visual acuity charts for clinical research. Am J Ophthalmol 1983; 94:91–96.

53. Pokorny J, Smith VC, Verriest G, et al., eds. Congenital and Acquired Color Vision Defects. New York: Grune & Stratton, 1979.

54. Regan D, Neima D. Low-contrast letter charts as a test of visual function. Ophthalmology 1983; 90:1192–1200.

55. Pelli DG, Robson JG, Wilkins AJ. The design of a new letter chart for measuring contrast sensitivity. Clin Vision Sci 1988; 2:169–177.

56. Optic Neuritis Study Group. The clinical profile of optic neuritis: Experience of the Optic Neuritis Treatment Trial. Arch Ophthalmol 1991; 109:1673–1678.

57. Kupersmith MJ, Siegel IM, Carr RE. Subtle disturbances of vision with compressive lesions of the anterior visual pathway measured by contrast sensitivity. Ophthalmology 1982; 89:68–72.

58. Donzis PB, Rappazzo JA, Burde RM, Gordon M. Effect of binocular variations of Snellen's visual acuity on Titmus stereoacuity. Arch Ophthalmol 1983; 101:930–932.

59. Trobe JD, Acosta PC, Krischer JP, Trick Gl. Confrontation visual field techniques in the detection of anterior visual pathway lesions. Ann Neurol 1981; 10:28–34.

60. Amsler M. Quantitative and qualitative vision. Trans Ophthalmol Soc UK 1949; 69:397–410.

61. Wall M, May DR. Threshold Amsler grid testing in maculopathies. Ophthalmology 1987; 94:1126–1133.

62. Henson D. Visual Fields. New York: Oxford University Press, 1993.

63. Levatin P. Pupillary escape in disease of the retina or optic nerve. Arch Ophthalmol 1959; 62:768–779.

64. Fineberg E, Thompson HS. Quantitation of the afferent pupillary defect. In: Smith JL, ed. Neuro-ophthalmology Focus 1980. New York: Masson, 1976:25–30.

65. Newsome DA, Milton RC, Fass JDM. Afferent pupillary defect in macular degeneration. Am J Ophthalmol 1966; 62:860–873.

66. Greenwald MJ, Folk ER. Afferent pupillary defects in amblyopia. J Pediar Ophthalmol Strabis 1983; 20:63–67.

67. Portnoy JZ, Thompson HS, Lennarson L, et al. Pupillary defects in amblyopia. Am J Ophthalmol 1983; 96:609–614.

68. Hood DC, Zhang X. Multifocal ERG and VEP responses and visual fields: comparing disease-related changes. Doc Ophthalmol 2000; 100: 115–137.

69. Baloh RW, Sills AW, Kumley WE, et al. Quantitative measurement of saccade amplitude, duration, and velocity. Neurology 1975; 25:1065–1070.

70. Collewijn H, Van Der Mark F, Jansen TC. Precise recording of human eye movements. Vision Res 1975; 15:447–450.

71. Benson AJ, Barnes GR. Vision during angular oscillation: the dynamic interaction of visual and vestibular mechanisms. Aviat Space Environ Med 1978; 49:340–345.

72. Zee DS. Ophthalmoscopy in examination of patiens with vestibular disorders. Ann Neurol 1978; 3:373–374.

73. Oei TH, Verhagen WIM, Horsten GPM. Forced duction test in clinical practice. Ophthalmologica 1983; 186; 87–90.

74. Zappia RJ, Winkelman JZ, Gay AJ. Intraocular pressure change in normal subjects and the adhesive muscle syndrome. Am J Ophthalmol 1971; 71:880–883.
75. Maddox EE. A new test for heterophoria. Ophthalmol Rev 1890; 9:129–133.
76. Hess WR. Ein einfaches messendes Vefahren zur Motilitätsprufung der Augen. Z Augenheilkd 1916; 35:201–219.
77. Zee DS, Chu FC, Optican LM, et al. Graphic analysis of paralytic strabismus with the Lancaster red-green test. Am J Ophthalmol 1984; 97:587–592.
78. Krimsky E. The Management of Binocular Imbalance. Philadelphia: Lea & Febiger, 1948:175 ff.
79. Sutter EE, Tran D. The field topography of ERG components in man I. The photopic luminance response. Vision Res 1992; 32:433–446.
80. Young LR, Sheena D. Survey of eye movement recording models. Behav Res Method Instrum 1975; 7:397–429.
81. Dell'Osso LF, Daroff RB. Eye movement characteristics and recording technique. In: Glaser JS, ed. Neuro-Ophthalmology. Hagerstown, MD: Harper & Row, 1978:185–198.
82. Kennerdell JS, Dekker A, Johnson BL, Dubois PJ. Fine-needle aspiration biopsy. Its use in orbital tumors. Arch Ophthalmol 1979; 97:1315–1317
83. Nguyen GK, Johnson ES, Mielke BW. Cytoloty of meninigiomas and neurilemomas in crush preparations. A useful adjunct to frozen section diagnosis. Acta Cytol 1988; 32:362–366.
84. Lee AG, Lin DJ, Kaufman M, et al. Atypical features prompting neuroimaging in acute optic neuropathy in adults. Can J Ophthalmol 2000; 35(6):325–330
85. Rothfus WE, Curtin HD, Slamovits TL, Kennerdell JS. Optic nerve sheath enlargement. A differential approach based on high resolution CT morphology. Radiology 1984; 150:409–415.
86. Liauw L, Vielvoye GJ, de Keizer RJ, et al. Optic nerve glioma mimicking an optic nerve meningioma. Clin Neurol Neurosurg 1996; 98(3):258–261.
87. Green FD. Optic nerve sarcoidosis: a report of three cases. Trans Ophthalmol Soc UK 1983; 103:551–555.
88. Ing EB, Garrity JA, Cross SA, et al. Sarcoid masquerading as optic nerve sheath meningioma. Mayo Clin Proc 1997; 72(8):791
89. Jennings JW, Rojiani AM, Brem SS, et al. Necrotizing neurosarcoidosis masquerading as a left optic nerve meningioma: case report. Am J Neuroradiol. 2002; 23(4):660–662.
90. Dutton JJ, Anderson RL. Idiopathic inflammatory perioptic neuritis simulating optic nerve sheath meningioma. Am J Ophthalmol 1985; 100:424–430.
91. Zhang TL, Shao SF, Zhang T, et al. Idiopathic inflammation of optic nerve simulating optic nerve sheath meningioma: CT demonstrations. J Comput Assist Tomogr 1987; 11:360–361.
92. Costa e Silva I, Symon L. Cavernous hemangioma of the optic canal. Report of two cases. J Neurosurg 1984; 60:838–841.
93. Boniuk M, Messmer EP, Font RL. Hemangiopericytoma of the meninges of the optic nerve. A clinicopathologic report including electron microscopic observations. Ophthalmology 1985; 92:1780–1787.
94. In S, Miyagi J, Kojho N, Kuramoto S, Uehara M. Intraorbital optic nerve hemangioblastoma with von Hippel-Lindau disease. Case report. J Neurosurg 1982; 56:426–429.
95. Tourje EJ, Gold LHA. Leukemic infiltration of the optic nerves: demonstration by computerized tomography. Comput Tomogr 1977; 1:225–227.
96. Johnson MD, Aulino JP, Jagasia M, et al. Erdheim-chester disease mimicking multiple meningiomas syndrome. Am J Neuroradiol 2004; 25(1):134–137.
97. Trobe JD, Glaser JS, Post JD. Meningiomas and aneurysms of the cavernous sinus. Neuro-ophthalmologic features. Arch Ophthalmol 1978; 96:457–467.

III
Basic Science

11
Meningioma Tumorigenesis: An Overview of Etiologic Factors

Michael J. Link and Arie Perry

Introduction

Almost without fail, one of the first questions a patient with a meningioma asks is, "What caused my tumor?" Many possible etiologic factors have been proposed during the last century. Solid epidemiologic evidence for most of these factors has proven fleeting. The availability and application of molecular biology techniques to investigate meningioma tumorigenesis, however, has revealed many insights into how these tumors develop and progress on the cellular level. Not only will further understanding of meningioma tumorigenesis answer the patient's "first" question, it may also lead to a better molecular classification to complement the current morphologic classification of meningiomas (see Chapter 5) and, of course, hopefully lead to novel therapeutic approaches to treat these tenacious tumors.

Somewhat confounding efforts to elucidate the cause of meningioma is a lack of universal agreement on the cell of origin for all meningiomas. Most meningiomas likely arise from mesodermal arachnoid cap cells normally found at the apex of arachnoid granulations.[1,2] Cleland, in 1846, is credited with first correlating these cells to meningioma formation.[3] They are found adjacent to major venous sinuses where the majority of meningiomas occur, and the normal arachnoid cap cells histologically resemble meningothelial meningiomas. However, meningiomas may occur at unusual sites such as choroid plexus,[4,5] within bone,[6,7] or, very rarely, outside the neural axis.[8] For these tumors a different cell of origin may be possible, or they may arise from heterotopic meningothelial rests.

Incidence, Hormone Receptors and Tumorigenesis

Meningiomas are frequent tumors encountered in any busy neurosurgery/neurooncology/neuropathology practice. Meningiomas have an overall incidence of 2 per 100,000 persons, based on data from the Olmsted County Epidemiology Project.[9] The Central Brain Tumor Registry of the United States revealed a slightly higher incidence of 4.36 per 100,000.[10] In the United States, at least 13,000 cases are expected to be diagnosed in 2006, and over 150,000 persons are believed to be living with meningioma.[10] Hospital-based and community-based incidence studies reveal that meningiomas represent between 13 and 27% of intracranial neoplasms.[11-19] These incidence rates have not changed much over the last 70 years. In 1995, a study reviewing the incidence of primary brain tumors in Rochester, Minnesota, revealed no increase in incidence of meningiomas over a 40-year period (1950–1990.)[9]

The incidence of meningioma increases with advancing age. A Japanese study reported the incidence of meningioma to be 3.5 times higher in patients over 70 years old compared to those under 70.[20] A U.S. epidemiological study also supported increasing incidence with increasing age.[15] This fits well with a multiple-hit hypothesis of tumorigenesis, requiring multiple gene mutations to develop over a lifetime to result in tumor formation. The genes involved are reviewed below, and more detailed coverage is presented elsewhere in this volume.

Meningiomas occur more frequently in women. The female: male ratio of intracranial meningioma is approximately 3:2, and for intraspinal meningioma it is as high as 10:1.[15,16,19] The higher incidence in women raises the possibility of a causative role of female sex hormones. There have been extremely varied reports of the prevalence of estrogen receptors (ER) (0–94%) and progesterone receptors (PR) (40–100%) in meningiomas.[21] While initially thought to be a promising avenue of therapy, current consensus is that ER expression on meningiomas is very rare and of no therapeutic consequence.[22] In contrast, PR expression is common in meningiomas, occurring in 81% of female's and 34% of male's tumors examined in one study.[23] The expression of PR is somewhat associated with a more benign clinical course and better prognosis, although there are many individual exceptions to this rule.[2] Even more interesting is that androgen receptor (AR) expression is also fairly common, but in reverse frequency to PR expression, with 69% of tumors in men and 31% in women expressing AR.[24] A recent study of women in Sweden suggested a positive correlation between the use of female hormone replacement and meningioma development (OR 1.7; 95% CI: 1.0, 2.8).[25] The risk was increased with a history of use of long-acting hormonal delivery systems such as subdermal implants or hormonal intrauterine devices (OR 2.7; 95% CI: 0.9, 7.5).[25] There was no dose-response relationship, however, and there was no association with the use of oral contraceptives—only with hormone replacement.[25] A similar cohort study in 2003 including 1,213,522 person-years of follow-up also found an increased risk of meningioma development in postmenopausal women who had taken hormone replacement (OR 1.86; 95% CI: 1.07,3.24).[26] Similarly, past or current oral contraceptive use was not a risk factor.[26] Inexplicably, later menarche (after age 14 years) had a relative risk of 1.97 (95% CI:1.06,3.66), compared to women whose menarche was age 12 years or younger.[26] However, a definitive role of hormones in meningioma tumorigenesis has yet to be proven, and neither study could provide detailed information on when in time the patients had taken hormones or what types of hormones they had used.[25,26] In fact, in the more recent study, up to two thirds of the women surveyed could not recall the name of the compounds they used.[25] Unfortunately, no clinical trials have proven the effectiveness of antihormonal therapy for selected meningiomas.[2]

Other hormone receptors have also been implicated in meningioma progression and tumorigenesis. Both D_1 and D_2 dopamine receptors or their mRNA have been detected in meningiomas.[27,28] Additionally, prolactin receptors,[28] somatostatin receptors, especially somatostatin type 2a receptors,[29] and growth hormone receptors[30] have all been found to be expressed in meningiomas. Once again, the true functional importance of these receptors, particularly as it may relate to tumorigenesis or tumor growth, is unclear and similar to sex hormones, no solid therapeutic benefit has been determined.[31]

Whether race has any influence on tumor formation is even more controversial. Meningiomas are felt to represent approximately 30% of intracranial tumors in Africans from studies done in the early 1970s in multiple sub-Saharan countries.[32–35] This represents an approximately 10% higher incidence than reported in populations of European descent. Likewise, in Los Angeles County the incidence rates were higher for African Americans (3.1/100,000) than Caucasian Americans (2.3/100,000).[16] One possible confounding factor is that the higher incidence of meningiomas in Africans may be secondary to underreporting of primary gliomas falsely lowering the denominator of the total number of intracranial tumors. Regardless, neither an environmental nor a genetic factor has been discovered to explain the apparent racial difference in meningioma tumorigenesis.

Environmental Factors and Tumorigenesis

Multiple environmental factors have been suggested as possible causes for meningioma development. Probably the oldest purported association is trauma. In their monograph published in 1938, Cushing and Eisenhardt suggested trauma as an etiology for tumor formation because 32% of patients had a history of head trauma.[36] Likewise, more contemporary studies have implicated head trauma, moreso in men than in women, including a recent report from 2002 suggesting an odds ratio of 4.33 (95% CI = 2.06, 9.10) for meningiomas occurring 10–19 years after head trauma.[37,38] A dose-response relationship was present for number, but not severity, of head traumas.[38] However, whether this association is truly causal remains unclear, and multiple studies,[39–42] including a large study from the Mayo Clinic encompassing 29,859 patient-years, found no increase in meningiomas in persons with a history of head trauma.[43]

Similarly, the role of viruses in meningioma tumorigenesis is unclear. Polyomaviruses, a subset of papovaviruses and simian virus 40 (SV40) in particular, have been shown to induce brain tumors in experimentally infected animals.[44–47] Initial reports in the late 1970s and 1980s demonstrated SV40-related tumor antigens (SV40 TAg) in meningioma specimens, suggesting a possible viral involvement in the etiology of these tumors.[48–52] Most alarmingly, a report appeared in 2004 of a 42-year-old laboratory researcher with probable direct exposure to SV40 diagnosed with a 5.5-cm posterior fossa meningioma, whose tumor was positive for viral DNA sequences indistinguishable from those of the laboratory source.[53] However, other studies done more recently, using polymerase chain reaction and immunohistochemistry, have failed to show SV40 TAg, JC virus, or BK virus in a large number of meningiomas.[54–56] Similarly, there was no association of herpes viruses with the development of meningiomas.[57] It remains inconclusive whether these viruses or others have any causative role, and the detection of viral DNA, RNA, or antigens in tumors may just be a result of contamination or latent infection.

One of the most intriguing purported risk factors for meningioma development of late is cellular telephone use (Fig. 11-1). Without question, human exposure to radiofrequency radiation has increased dramatically from widespread use of mobile phones. At the turn of the century it was estimated that 500 million people worldwide had mobile phones.[58] Fueling some of the public's concern, a senior neurosurgeon in Los Angeles suggested in a July 2005 interview with a CNN medical correspondent that famed defense attorney Johnny Cochrane's malignant primary brain tumor could have been caused by cell phone use. As of yet, however, a biologic mechanism that could explain any possible carcinogenic effect from radiofrequency radiation has not been identified.[59]

Several cohort and case-controlled studies in the past decade have failed to find an association between mobile phone use and brain tumors.[60–66] A case-controlled study of cellular telephone use in the United States, encompassing three academic medical centers and 1581 patients, found a relative risk of 0.8 (95% CI = 0.4, 1.3) for the development of a meningioma among regular users.[63] Neither duration of regular use, average daily use, cumulative use, or year use began increased the relative risk of getting a meningioma in this study.[63] Cellular

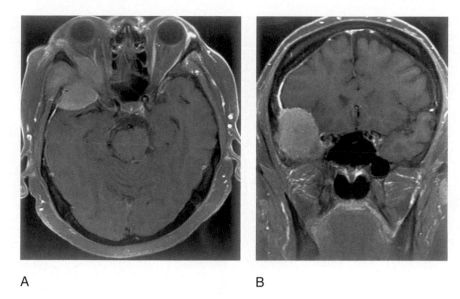

FIG. 11-1. Axial (A) and coronal (B) postgadolinium T1-weighted MRI scan reveals a right sphenoorbital meningioma in a 61-year-old man who stated he was one of the first mobile telephone users in the United States dating back to the late 1980s. He claimed to have used mobile telephones exclusively for daily telecommunications for the previous 20 years and always placed the phone to his right ear. He noted proptosis of the right eye that prompted the MRI scan. Despite the best epidemiologic evidence to the contrary, he is convinced cellular telephone use caused his tumor

telephones were introduced in Sweden in the late 1980s and became ubiquitous relatively quickly, making the Swedish population very suitable to study this issue. The study population in the case-control Swedish Interphone Study included approximately 3.7 million people studied between 2000 and 2002.[66] There was no increased risk of meningioma related to mobile phone use regardless of type of phone (analog vs. digital), frequency of use, duration of regular use, time since first regular use, cumulative hours of use, or cumulative number of calls.[66] Even more specifically, there was no increased risk (OR 0.8, 95% CI = 0.5, 1.1) when controlling for laterality of mobile phone use and the development of meningioma.[66] Admittedly, a latency period of 10 or even 20 years may be necessary to detect a tumorigenic effect.[67] However, if radiofrequency acts as a promoter, an effect could be seen sooner. All of the studies to date which include a large number of long-term mobile phone users do not support an increased risk of meningioma tumorigenesis.[60–66] Most recently, the German Interphone Study Group examined a broader exposure to radiofrequency/microwave electromagnetic fields (RF/MW-EMF) such as might occur in amateur radio operators or military personnel using radar equipment.[68] They found no association between occupational exposure to RF/MW-EMF and the development of meningioma (OR 1.34, 95% CI = 0.64, 2.81).[68]

Direct exposure to ionizing radiation, on the other hand, has been associated with meningioma development (Fig. 11.2).[41,69] The mean latency between radiotherapy and meningioma diagnosis ranges from 34 to 48 years.[70–73] The most convincing evidence and best studied population in this regard is the "tinea capitis cohort."[74] During a 10-year period between 1949 and 1959, more than 20,000 children who immigrated to Israel were treated with radiotherapy for tinea capitis.[75] Approximately 11,000 of these children along with two matched control groups have been followed for more than 35 years.[74] The mean dose to the brain was relatively low, averaging 1.45 Gy (range 1–6 Gy).[76] A previous study found a relative risk of 9.5 (95% CI: 3.5, 25.7) for meningioma development compared to control children who had not undergone any radiotherapy.[77] Patients with meningiomas developing after exposure to low-dose radiation for tinea capitis were diagnosed at a significantly lower age, had a higher prevalence of calvarial tumors, and were associated with a higher proportion of multiple meningiomas compared to control patients with non–radiation-induced meningiomas.[74] There was also a trend for earlier recurrence after treatment compared to non–radiation-induced tumors but it did not reach statistical significance.[74]

One of the most notable aspects of the tinea capitis cohort is that they were all exposed as children and received similar dosing. Atomic bomb survivors include a large proportion of people exposed to varying radiation doses, including a wide range of ages at exposure. Reports in the late 1990s examining the Hiroshima and Nagasaki atomic bomb survivors revealed that the incidence of meningioma was increased in this population.[78,79] Most significantly, there was a correlation between the incidence and dose of radiation to the brain, and thus a high correlation between incidence of meningioma and distance from the epicenter of the bomb.[78,79]

Over the last several decades, it became apparent that ionizing radiation, even at relatively low doses, does appear to be involved in meningioma tumorigenesis. There was also concern about diagnostic and occupational exposure to radiation,

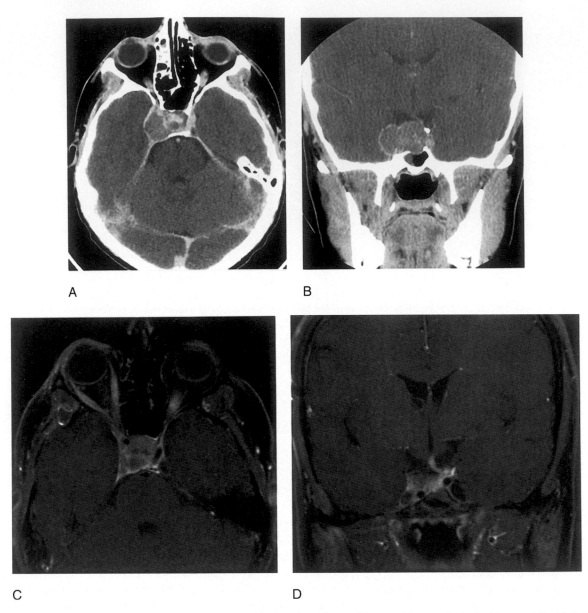

FIG. 11-2. Axial (A) and coronal (B) contrast-enhanced CT scan of the head from a 26-year-old man who had a history of Burkitt's lymphoma 19 years prior to presentation. He was treated with Cytoxan, vincristine, adriamycin, methotrexate, prednisone, and 1500 cGy whole brain radiotherapy. He was considered cured of his lymphoma. In 2003 he developed diplopia and was discovered to have an enhancing mass in the sella, suprasellar cistern, and right cavernous sinus. Treatment included subtotal removal followed by stereotactic radiosurgery. Pathology following subtotal resection was atypical meningothelial meningioma with 4/10 mitoses per high-powered field and focal necrosis. Axial (C) and coronal (D) contrast-enhanced MRI images 3 years after treatment reveal stable residual disease

such as during routine x-rays or computed tomography scans, etc. Initial studies from Los Angeles suggested an increased risk of meningioma development with a history of having undergone repeated full-mouth dental x-rays, especially when exposed before age 20, or before 1945, when higher radiation doses were used.[80] A Swedish study also suggested dental radiography at least once a year after age 25 years increased the risk of meningioma (OR 2.1, 95% CI = 1.0, 4.3).[81] An Australian population-based, case-controlled study found only a possible increased risk for meningioma in males exposed to dental x-rays.[82] A study involving 200 patients from Washington state found an increased risk of meningioma only in participants who had undergone more than six full-mouth series performed 15–40 years ago, when radiation exposure from full-mouth series was much greater than it is now.[83] Conversely, a recent study found no significant association between intracranial meningioma and exposure to ionizing radiation from a wide variety of nondiagnostic medical or occupational settings that might predispose to radiation exposure.[84] However, they did observe an association for prior radiation therapy to head or neck, especially when treatment was given for a neoplastic condition (OR 3.7, 95% CI = 1.5, 9.5).[84]

A few other possible environmental factors have been implicated in meningioma tumorigenesis. Two studies have found an increased risk of smoking and meningioma development in women only.[85,86] Interestingly, an Australian group found a risk for spouses subjected to passive smoking, especially women, but no association to direct smoking.[87] Other studies, however, have failed to discern an association between smoking and development of meningioma.[40,88,89] Occupational exposure to lead, tin, and cadmium among factory workers in China was associated with a significant risk of meningioma development.[86] Excess mortality due to meningioma was observed in young and middle-aged Swedish horticulturists, thought to be secondary to insecticide and/or pesticide exposure.[90] Even the old admonition to eat one's vegetables has come under fire, as one study suggested a vegetarian lifestyle in childhood was associated with the risk of meningioma in adult life,[88] while another study showed the risk of meningioma was reduced in subjects who reported high consumption of fruits and vegetables.[86]

Genetic Factors and Tumorigenesis

Meningiomas may develop in families in association with neurofibromatosis type 2 (NF2), and rarely in Gorlin's syndrome, Cowden's syndrome, Li-Fraumeni syndrome, Turcot's/Gardener's syndrome, and von Hippel-Lindau disease (Fig. 11-3).[91] There are also many reports of familial meningiomas not associated with NF2 or any other known or recognized genetic syndrome.[92–95]

Meningioma was one of the first human solid tumors reported to exhibit a uniform chromosomal aberration. Monosomy or partial loss of chromosome 22 (involving 22q12.2) has been detected in up to 70% of cases with standard karyotypes or modified cytogenetic techniques, and this alteration was originally identified in 1972 using tumor cultures.[96,97] Subsequently, much work has been done using advanced cytogenetic analysis to understand meningioma tumorigenesis as it relates to other abnormalities involving chromosome 22[98–100] and other chromosomes and their specific genes and proteins (recently reviewed in Refs. 2, 91). The discovery of the accumulation of genetic abnormalities with increasing histologic malignancy supports the stepwise theory of tumorigenesis with progressive loss of tumor suppressor genes and activation of oncogenes.

Briefly, the NF2 gene located on chromosome 22 codes for the protein merlin,[101] also called schwannomin.[102] It is a member of the protein 4.1 family of structural proteins that are involved in linking integral membrane proteins to the cytoskeleton and functions as a tumor suppressor.[103] Up to 60% of sporadic meningiomas harbor NF2 gene mutations, varying somewhat by tumor histology.[104–107] Meningioma tumorigenesis appears to be closely linked to the inactivation of one or more of the protein 4.1 family members. Besides NF2 mutations resulting in loss of merlin expression, other protein 4.1 family members are downregulated in meningioma. Loss of

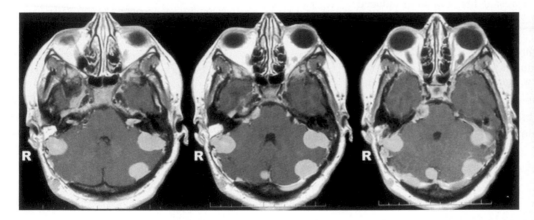

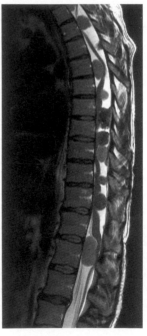

A

B

FIG. 11-3. Axial, postgadolinium T1-weighted MRI of the head (A) and sagittal T2-weighted MRI of the spine (B) reveal multiple meningiomas and bilateral vestibular schwannomas in a 35-year-old woman with high penetrance neurofibromatosis type 2

protein 4.1B (DAL-1) and 4.1R expression is a common finding in sporadic meningiomas.[108,109] Additionally, tumor suppressor in lung cancer–1 (TSLC1), a gene originally identified as important in development of non–small-cell lung cancer and closely interacting with protein 4.1B, has reduced expression in high-grade meningiomas.[110]

A number of cytogenetic alterations are associated with meningioma progression and atypical or anaplastic histology, including the presence of dicentric or ring chromosomes, losses of chromosome arms 1 p, 6 q, 9 p, 10, 14 q, and 18 q, as well as gains/amplifications on 1 q, 9 q, 12 q, 15 q, 17 q, and 20 q.[111–116] Also, there is some evidence that 14 q deletions are more common in benign meningiomas that subsequently recur.[112] The candidate genes responsible for these findings, for the most part, have not been elucidated. However, high-throughput techniques such as gene expression profiling using oligonucleotide microarrays have provided the ability to screen thousands of genes simultaneously yielding additional gene candidates potentially involved in meningioma tumorigenesis.[117]

Meningiomas developing in the pediatric population tend to present with higher frequencies of larger size, cyst formation, lack of dural attachment, higher-grade histology and aggressive behavior.[118,119] Despite these worrisome clinical differences compared to sporadic adult meningiomas, they tend to share similar genetic features. Both sporadic and NF2-associated meningiomas in children have a high incidence of NF2 and Protein 4.1B deletions.[119] Most concerning, pediatric meningiomas frequently have 1 p and 14 q deletions, alterations that are commonly associated with tumor progression.[119]

At least one group has suggested that radiation-induced meningiomas arise from different genetic abnormalities than their sporadic counterparts.[120] Cleveland Clinic reported that NF-2 gene mutations and chromosome 22 q deletions were less common in radiation-induced tumors. Also, allele losses on 1 p, 9 q, 19 q, 22 q, and 18 q were found more commonly compared to sporadic meningiomas, suggesting these sites may be where the damaging effects of ionizing radiation have their impact[120] (see also Chapter 14).

Summary

In addition to advances in imaging, microsurgery, neuropathology and radiation therapy in the past several decades, much has been learned about meningioma tumorigenesis. While meningiomas occur more frequently in women and may express sex hormone and other receptors, an underlying causative factor in this regard is hard to implicate. Multiple environmental risk factors have been proposed over the last almost one hundred years from head trauma to cellular telephones, and only prior exposure to ionizing radiation has emerged as a definitive risk factor. Finally, many chromosomal abnormalities have been reported to have a potential role in meningioma tumorigenesis or progression. Further elucidation of the genes involved and their protein product functions will not only improve our understanding of how meningiomas develop, but hopefully lead to novel treatment strategies and better classifications of meningiomas.

References

1. O'Rahilly R, Muller F. The meninges in human development. J Neuropathol Exp Neurol 1986;45:588–608.
2. Drummond KJ, Zhu JJ, Black PM. Meningiomas: updating basic science, management, and outcome. Neurologist 2004;10: 113–130.
3. Cleland J. Description of two tumours adherent to the deep surface of the dura-mater. Glasgow Med J 1864;11:148–159.
4. Nakamura M, Roser F, Bundschuh O, et al. Intraventricular meningiomas: a review of 16 cases with reference to the literature. Surg Neurol 2003;59:491–504.
5. Criscuolo GR, Symon L. Intraventricular meningioma. A review of 10 cases of the National Hospital, Queen Square (1974–1985) with reference to the literature. Acta Neurochir 1986;83:83–91.
6. Crawford TS, Kleinschmidt-DeMasters BK, Lillehei KO. Primary intraosseous meningioma. Case report. J Neurosurg 1995;83:912–915.
7. Lang FF, Macdonald OK, Fuller GN, DeMonte F. Primary extradural meningiomas: a report on nine cases and review of the literature from the era of computerized tomography scanning. J Neurosurg 2000;93:940–950.
8. Shuangshoti S. Primary meningiomas outside the central nervous system. In: Al Mefty O, ed. Meningiomas. New York: Raven, 1991:107–128.
9. Radhakrishnan K, Mokri B, Parisi JE, et al. The trends in incidence of primary brain tumors in the population of Rochester, Minnesota. Ann Neurol 1995;37:67–73.
10. CBTRUS. Statistical Report: Primary brain tumors in the United States, 1997–2001. Hinsdale, IL: Central Brain Tumor Registry of the United States, 2004.
11. Cushing H. Intracranial Tumors. Notes Upon a Series of Two Thousand Verified Cases. Springfield, IL: Charles C Thomas, 1932.
12. Grant FC. A study of the results of surgical treatment in 2326 consecutive patients with brain tumors: the national survey of intracranial neoplasms. Neurology 1956;32:219–226.
13. Zimmerman HM. Brain tumors: their incidence and classification in man and their experimental production. Ann NY Acad Sci 1969;159:337–359.
14. Schoenberg GS, Christine BW, Whisnant JP. The descriptive epidemiology of primary intracranial neoplasms: The Connecticut experience. Am J Epidemiol 1976;104:499–510.
15. Kurland LT, Schoenberg BS, Annegers JF, et al. The incidence of primary intracranial neoplasms in Rochester, Minnesota, 1935–1977. Ann NY Acad Sci 1982;381:6–16.
16. Preston-Martin S, Henderson BE, Peters JM. Descriptive epidemiology of central nervous system neoplasms in Los Angeles County. Ann NY Acad Sci 1982;381:202–208.
17. Fogelholm R, Uutela T, Murros K. Epidemiology of central nervous system neoplasms: a regional survey in central Finland. Acta Neurol Scand 1984;69:129–136.
18. Walker AE, Robins H, Weinfeld FD. Epidemiology of brain tumors: the national survey of intracranial neoplasms. Neurology 1985;32:219–226.

19. Sutherland GR, Florell R, Louw D, et al. Epidemiology of primary intracranial neoplasms in Manitoba, Canada. Can J Neurol Sci 1987;14:586–592.

20. Kuratsu J, Ushio Y. Epidemiological study of primary intracranial tumors in elderly people. J Neurol Neurosurg Psychiatry 1997;63:116–118.

21. Kirsch M, Santarius T, Black P. Molecular biology of meningiomas and peripheral nerve sheath tumors. In: Raffel C, Harsh G, eds. The Molecular Basis of Neurosurgical Disease. Baltimore: Congress of Neurological Surgeons, 1996:126–145.

22. Goodwin JW, Crowley J, Eyre HJ, et al. A phase II evaluation of tamoxifen in unresectable or refractory meningiomas: a Southwest Oncology Group study. J Neurooncol 1993;15:75–77.

23. Carroll R, Glowacka D, Dashner K, Black P. Progesterone and glucocorticoid receptor activation in meningiomas. Cancer Res 1993;53:1312–1316.

24. Carroll R, Zhang J, Dashner K, et al. Androgen receptor expression in meningiomas. J Neurosurg 1995;82:453–460.

25. Wigertz A, Lonn S, Mathiesen T, et al. Risk of brain tumors associated with exposure to exogenous female sex hormones. Am J Epidemiol 2006;164:629–636.

26. Jhawar BS, Fuchs CS, Colditz GA, Stampfer MJ. Sex steroid hormone exposures and risk for meningioma. J Neurosurg 2003;99:848–853.

27. Schrell U, Fahlbusch R, Adams E, et al. Growth of cultured human cerebral meningiomas is inhibited by dopaminergic agents. Presence of high affinity dopamine-D1 receptors. J Clin Endocrinol Metab 1990;71:1669–1671.

28. Carroll RS, Schrell UM, Zhang J, et al. Dopamine D1, dopamine D2, and prolactin receptor messenger ribnucleic acid expression by the polymerase chain reaction in human meningiomas. Neurosurgery 1996;38:367–375.

29. Schulz S, Pauli SU, Schulz S, et al. Immunohistochemical determination of five somatostatin receptors in meningioma reveals frequent overexpression of somatostatin receptor subtype sst2A. Clin Cancer Res 2000;6:1865–1874.

30. Friend K, Radinsky R, McCutcheon I. Growth hormone receptor expression and function in meningiomas: effect of a specific receptor antagonist. J Neurosurg 1999;91:93–99.

31. Whittle IR, Smith C, Navoo P, Collie D. Meningiomas. Lancet 2004;363:1535–1543.

32. Giordano C, Lamouche M. Meningiomes en Cote D'Ivoire. Afr J Med Sci 1973;4:249–263.

33. Odeku EL, Adeloye A. Cranial meningiomas in the Nigerian Africans. Afr J Med Sci 1973;4:275–287.

34. Manfredonia M. Tumors of the nervous system in the African in Eritrea (Ethiopia). Afr J Med Sci 1973;4:383–387.

35. Levy LF. Brain tumors in Malawi, Rhodesia and Zambia. Afr J Med Sci 1973;4:393–397.

36. Cushing H, Eisenhardt L. Meningiomas: their classification, regional behaviour, life history, and surgical end results. Springfield, IL: Charles C Thomas, 1938.

37. Preston-Martin S, Pogoda JM, Schlehofer B, et al. An international case-control study of adult glioma and meningioma: the role of head trauma. Int J Epidemiol 1998;27:579–586.

38. Phillips LE, Koepsell TD, van Belle G, et al. History of head trauma and risk of intracranial meningioma: population-based case-control study. Neurology 2002;58:1849–1852.

39. Parker H, Kernohan J. The relation of injury and glioma of the brain. J Am Med Assoc 1931;97:535–539.

40. Choi N, Schuma L, Gullen W. Epidemiology of primary central nervous system neoplasms II. Case-control study. Am J Epidemiol 1970;91:467–485.

41. Bondy M, Ligon BL. Epidemiology and etiology of intracranial meningiomas: a review. J Neurooncol 1996;29:197–205.

42. Inskip PD, Mellemkjaer L, Gridley G, Olsen JH. Incidence of intracranial tumors following hospitalization for head injuries (Denmark). Cancer Causes Control 1998;9:109–116.

43. Annegars JF, Laws ER Jr, Kurland LT, Grabow JD. Head trauma and subsequent brain tumors. Neurosurgery 1979;4:203–206.

44. Eddy BE, Borman GS, Grubbs GE, Young RD. Identification of the oncogenic substance in rhesus monkey kidney cell culture as simian virus 40. Virology 1962;17:65–75.

45. Gerber P, Kirschstein RL. SV40-induced ependymomas in newborn hamsters. I. Virus-tumor relationships. Virology 1962;18:582–588.

46. Brinster RL, Chen HY, Messing A, et al. Transgenic mice harboring SV40 T-antigen genes develop characteristic brain tumors. Cell 1984;37:367–379.

47. Pinkert CA, Brinster RL, Palmiter RD, et al. Tumorigenesis in transgenic mice by a nuclear transport-defective SV40 large T-antigen gene. Virology 1987;160:169–175.

48. Weiss AF, Portmann R, Fischer H, et al. Simian virus 40-related antigens in three human meningiomas with defined chromosomal loss. Proc Natl Acad Sci USA 1975;72:609–613.

49. Weiss AF, Zang KD, Birkmayer GD, Miller F. SV40 related papova-viruses in human meningiomas. Acta Neuropathol (Berl) 1976;34:171–174.

50. Scherneck S, Lubbe L, Geissler E, et al. Detection of simian virus 40 related T-antigen in human meningiomas. Zentralbl Neurochir 1979;40:121–130.

51. Zimmermann W, Schernick S, Geissler E, Nisch G. Demonstration of SV 40-related tumour antigen in human meningiomas by different hamster SV 40-T-antisera. Acta Virol 1981;25(4):199–204.

52. Ibelgaufts H, Jones KW. Papovavirus-related RNA sequences in human neurogenic tumours. Acta Neuropathol (Berl) 1982;56:118–122.

53. Arrington AS, Moore MS, Butel JS. SV40-positive brain tumor in scientist with risk of laboratory exposure to the virus. Oncogene 2004;23(12):2231–2235.

54. Weggen S, Bayer TA, von Deimling A, et al. Low frequency of SV40, JC and BK polyomavirus sequences in human medulloblastomas, meningiomas and ependymomas. Brain Pathol 2000;10:85–92.

55. Sabatier J, Uro-Coste E, Benouaich A, et al. Immunodetection of SV40 large T antigen in human central nervous system tumours. J Clin Pathol 2005;58:429–431.

56. Rollison DE, Utaipat U, Ryschkewitsch C, et al. Investigation of human brain tumors for the presence of polyomavirus genome sequences by two independent laboratories. Int J Cancer 2005;113:769–774.

57. Poltermann S, Schlehofer B, Steindorf K, et al. Lack of association of herpesviruses with brain tumors. J Neurovirol 2006;12:90–99.

58. Independent Expert Group on Mobile Phones. Mobile Phones and Health. Chilton: National Radiological Protection Board, 2000.

59. Valberg PA. Radio frequency radiation (RFR): the nature of exposure and carcinogenic potential. Cancer Causes Control 1997;8:323–332.

60. Hardell L, Nasman A, Pahlson A, et al. Use of cellular telephones and the risk of brain tumors: a case-control study. Int J Oncol 1999;15:113–116.

61. Dreyer NA, Loughlin JE, Rothman KJ. Cause-specific mortality in cellular phone users. JAMA 1999;282:1814–1816.

62. Muscat JE, Malkin MG, Thompson S, et al. Handheld cellular telephone use and risk of brain cancer. JAMA 2000;284:3001–3007.

63. Inskip PD, Tarone RE, Hatch EE, et al. Cellular-telephone use and brain tumors. N Engl J Med 2001;344:79–86.

64. Johansen C, Boice JD Jr, McLaughlin JK, Olsen JH. Cellular telephones and cancer—a nationwide cohort study in Denmark. J Natl Cancer Inst 2001;93:203–207.

65. Auvinen A, Hietanen M, Luukkonen R, Koskela R-S. Brain tumors and salivary gland cancers among cellular telephone users. Epidemiology 2002;13:356–359.

66. Lonn S, Ahlbom A, Hall P, et al. Long-term mobile phone use and brain tumor risk. Am J Epidemiol 2005;161:526–535.

67. United Nations Scientific Committee on the effects of atomic radiation (UNSCEAR). Sources and effects of ionizing radiation. UNSCEAR 2000. Report to the General Assembly, with scientific annexes. New York: United Nations, 2000.

68. Berg G, Spallek J, Schuz J, et al. Occupational exposure to radiofrequency/microwave radiation and the risk of brain tumors: Interphone Study Group, Germany. Am J Epidemiol 2006;164:538–548.

69. Longstreth WT Jr, Dennis LK, McGuire VM, et al. Epidemiology of intracranial meningioma. Cancer 1993;72:639–648.

70. Beller AJ, Feinsod M, Sahar A. The possible relationship between small dose irradiation to the scalp and intracranial meningiomas. Neurochirurgia 1972;15:135–143.

71. Giaquinto S, Massi G, Ricolfi A, Vitali S. On six cases of radiation meningiomas from the same community. Ital J Neurol Sci 1984;5:173–175.

72. Harrison MJ, Wolfe DE, Lau TS, et al. Radiation-induced meningiomas: exprience at the Mount Sinai Hospital and review of the literature. J Neurousurg 1991;75:564–574.

73. Soffer D, Pittaluga S, Feiner M, Beller AJ. Intracranial meningiomas following low-dose irradiation to the head. J Neurosurg 1983;59:1048–1053.

74. Sadetzki S, Flint-Richter P, Ben-Tal T, Nass D. Radiation-induced meningioma: a descriptive study of 253 cases. J Neurosurg 2002;97:1078–1082.

75. Modan B, Baidatz D, Mart H, et al. Radiation-induced head and neck tumours. Lancet 1974;1:277–279.

76. Werner A, Modan B, Davidoff D. Doses to brain, skull, and thyroid, following x-ray therapy for Tinea capitis. Phys Med Biol 1968;13:247–258.

77. Ron E, Modan B, Boice JD Jr, et al. Tumors of the brain and nervous system after radiotherapy in childhood. N Engl J Med 1988;319:1033–1039.

78. Sadamori N, Shibata S, Mine M, et al. Incidence of intracranial meningiomas in Nagasaki atomic-bomb survivors. Int J Cancer 1996;67:318–322.

79. Shintani T, Hayakawa N, Hoshi M, et al. High incidence of meningioma among Hiroshima atomic bomb survivors. J Radiat Res (Tokyo) 1999;40:49–57.

80. Preston-Martin S, Henderson BE, Bernstein L. Medical and dental X rays as risk factors for recently diagnosed tumors of the head. Natl Cancer Inst Monogr 1985;69:175–179.

81. Rodvall Y, Ahlbom A, Pershagen G, et al. Dental radiography after age 25 years, amalgam fillings and tumours of the central nervous system. Oral Oncol 1998;34:265–269.

82. Ryan P, Lee MW, North B, McMichael AJ. Amalgam fillings, diagnostic dental X-rays and tumours of the brain and meninges. Eur J Cancer B Oral Oncol 1992;28B:91–95.

83. Longstreth WT Jr, Phillips LE, Drangsholt M, et al. Dental X-rays and the risk of intracranial meningioma. A population-based case-control study. Cancer 2004;100:1026–1034.

84. Phillips LE, Frankenfeld CL, Drangsholt M, et al. Intracranial meningioma and ionizing radiation in medical and occupational settings. Neurology 2005;64:350–352.

85. Preston-Martin S, Paganini-Hill A, Henderson BE, et al. Case-control study of intracranial meningiomas in women in Los Angeles County, California. J Natl Cancer Inst 1980;65:67–73.

86. Hu J, Little J, Xu T, et al. Risk factors for meningioma in adults: a case-control study in northeast China. Int J Cancer 1999;83:299–304.

87. Ryan P, Lee MW, North B, McMichael AJ. Risk factors for tumours of the brain and meninges: results from the Adelaide adult brain tumor study. Int J Cancer 1992;51:20–27.

88. Mills PK, Preston-Martin S, Annegers JF, et al. Risk factors for tumours of the brain and cranial meninges in Seven-Day Adventists. Neuroepidemiology 1989;8:266–275.

89. Schlehofer B, Kunze S, Sachsenheimer W, et al. Occupational risk factors for brain tumours: results from a population-based case-control study in Germany. Cancer Causes Control 1990;1:209–215.

90. Littorin M, Attewell R, Skerfving S, et al. Mortality and tumour morbidity among Swedish market gardeners and orchardists. Int Arch Occup Environ Health 1993;65:163–169.

91. Perry A, Gutmann DH, Reifenberger G. Molecular pathogenesis of meningiomas. J Neurooncol 2004;70:183–202.

92. Ferrante L, Acqui M, Artico M, et al. Familial meningiomas. Report of two cases. J Neurosurg 1987;31:145–151.

93. McDowell JR. Familial meningioma. Neurology 1990;40:312–314.

94. Pulst SM, Rouleau GA, Marineau C, et al. Familial meningioma is not allelic to neurofibromatosis 2. Neurology 1993;43:2096–2098.

95. Maxwell M, Shih SD, Galanopoulos T, et al. Familial meningioma: analysis of expression of neurofibromatosis 2 protein Merlin. Report of two cases. J Neurosurg 1998;88:562–569.

96. Mark J, Levan G, Mitelman F. Identification by fluorescence of the G chromosome lost in human meningiomas. Hereditas 1972;71:163–168.

97. Zankl H, Zang K. Cytological and cytogenetical studies on brain tumors. 4. Identification of the missing G chromosome in human meningiomas as no. 22 by fluorescence technique. Humangenetik 1972;14:167–169.

98. Peyrard M, Fransson I, Xie YG, et al. Characterization of a new member of the human beta-adaptin gene family from chromosome 22q12, a candidate meningioma gene. Human Mol Genet 1994;3:1393–1399.

99. Lekanne Deprez RH, Riegman PH, Groen NA, et al. Cloning and characterization of MN1, a gene from chromosome 22q11, which is disrupted by a balanced translocation in a meningioma. Oncogene 1995;10:1521–1528.

100. Schmitz U, Mueller W, Weber M, et al. INI1 mutations in meningiomas at a potential hotspot in exon 9. Br J Cancer 2001;84:199–201.

101. Trofatter JA, MacCollin MM, Rutter JL, et al. A novel moesin-, ezrin-, radixin-like gene is a candidate for the neurofibromatosis 2 tumor suppressor. Cell 1993;72:791–800.

102. Rouleau GA, Merel P, Lutchman M, et al. Alteration in a new gene encoding a putative membrane-organizing protein causes neuro-fibromatosis type 2. Nature 1993;363:515–521.

103. Gusella JF, Ramesh V, MacCollin M, Jacoby LB. Merlin: the neurofibromatosis 2 tumor suppressor. Biochim Biophys Acta 1999;1423:M29–36.

104. Ruttledge MH, Sarrazin J, Rangaratnam S, et al. Evidence for the complete inactivation of the NF2 gene in the majority of sporadic meningiomas. Nat Genet 1994;6:180–184.

105. Harada T, Irving RM, Xuereb JH, et al. Molecular genetic investigation of the neurofibromatosis type 2 tumor suppressor gene in sporadic meningioma. J Neurosurg 1996;84: 847–851.

106. Papi L, De Vitis LR, Vitelli F, et al. Somatic mutations in the neurofibromatosis type 2 gene in sporadic meningiomas. Hum Genet 1995;95:347–351.

107. Wellenreuther R, Kraus J, Lenartz D, et al. Analysis of the neurofibromatosis 2 gene reveals molecular variants of meningioma. Am J Pathol 1995;146:827–832.

108. Gutmann DH, Donahoe J, Perry A, et al. Loss of DAL-1, a protein 4.1-related tumor suppressor, is an important early event in the pathogenesis of meningiomas. Hum Mol Genet 2000;9:1495–1500.

109. Robb VA, Li W, Gascard P, et al. Identification of a third Protein 4.1 tumor suppressor, Protein 4.1R, in meningioma pathogenesis. Neurobiol Dis 2003;13:191–202.

110. Surace EI, Lusis E, Murakami Y, et al. Loss of tumor suppressor in lung cancer–1 (TSLC-1) expression in meningioma correlates with increased malignancy grade and reduced patient survival. J Neuropathol Exp Neurol 2004;63: 1015–1027.

111. Buschges R, Ichimura K, Weber RG, et al. Allelic gain and amplification on the long arm of chromosome 17 in anaplastic meningiomas. Brain Pathol 2002;12:145–153.

112. Cai DX, Banerjee R, Scheithauer BW, et al. Chromosome 1p and 14q FISH analysis in clinicopathologic subsets of meningioma: diagnostic and prognostic implications. J Neuropathol Exp Neurol 2001;60:628–636.

113. Cai DX, James CD, Scheithauer BW, et al. PS6K amplification characterizes a small subset of anaplastic meningiomas. Am J Clin Pathol 2001;115:213–218.

114. Lamszus K, Kluwe L, Matschke J, et al. Allelic losses at 1p, 9q, 10q, 14q and 22q in the progression of aggressive meningiomas and undifferentiated meningeal sarcomas. Cancer Genet Cytogenet 1999;110:103–110.

115. Ozaki S, Nishizaki T, Ito H, Sasaki K. Comparative genomic hybridization analysis of genetic alterations associated with malignant progression of meningioma. J Neuro-Oncol 1999;41:167–174.

116. Weber RG, Bostrom J, Wolter M, et al. Analysis of genomic alterations in benign, atypical, and anaplastic meningiomas: toward a genetic model of meningioma progression. Proc Natl Acad Sci USA 1997;94:14719–14724.

117. Watson MA, Gutmann DH, Peterson K, et al. Molecular characterization of human meningiomas by gene expression profiling using high-density oligonucleotide microarrays. Am J Pathol 2002;161:665–672.

118. Amirjamshidi A, Mehrazin M, Abbassioun K. Meningiomas of the central nervous system occurring below the age of 17: report of 24 cases not associated with neurofibromatosis and review of literature. Childs Nerv Syst 2000;16:406–416.

119. Perry A, Giannini C, Raghavan R, et al. Aggressive phenotypic and genotypic features in pediatric and NF2-associated meningiomas: a clinicopathologic study of 53 cases. J Neuropathol Exp Neurol 2001;60:994–1003.

120. Shoshan Y, Chernova O, Juen SS, et al. Radiation-induced meningioma: a distinct molecular genetic pattern? J Neuropathol Exp Neurol 2000;59:614–620.

12
Molecular Basis of Meningioma Tumorigenesis and Progression

Lilyana Angelov and Mladen Golubic

Meningiomas are among the earliest and most extensively karyotyped human tumors. Much has been learned over the years regarding the genetic and epigenetic abnormalities integral to meningioma tumor development and progression. With the completion of the Human Genome Project and accumulated knowledge about the genome's function, there is also a growing recognition that environmental changes interacting with genetic predisposition within the host contribute to health, disease, and response to therapies.[1,2] Several genetic conditions that predispose to meningioma development as well as numerous somatic alterations in tumor suppressor genes and oncogenes are documented and molecularly well characterized in this tumor type. In contrast, polymorphisms at loci encoding less penetrant but highly prevalent genetic polymorphisms that influence individual responses to environmental exposures and the nature of these exposures and interactions in meningioma tumorigenesis are poorly understood (Fig. 12-1). This chapter will cover the contribution of these alterations as they relate to meningioma tumorigenesis and progression.

NF2 Gene Mutation and Sporadic Meningiomas

Meningiomas were one of the first solid tumors to be studied for genetic alternations. In the early 1970s, cytogenetic analysis of meningioma primary tumor culture cells revealed that 70% of the cells exhibited either monosomy or partial loss of chromosome 22 (Ch 22).[3,4] This observation has been confirmed with numerous molecular genetic techniques including loss of heterozygosity (LOH) with restricted fragment length polymorphism (RFLP) and microsatellite polymorphic markers, fluorescent in situ hybridization (FISH), single-strand conformational polymorphism (SSCP), automatic sequencing, comparative genomic hybridization (CGH), and spectral karyotyping, with abnormalities in the 22 q locus identified in up to 78% of sporadic meningiomas.[5–13]

Interest in the neurofibromatosis 2 (NF-2) gene (22q12.2) developed quickly after the gene was identified, since meningiomas were found in approximately 50% of patients with NF-2.[14–16] Further inactivating mutations in the gene and loss of its protein product schwannomin/merlin (Moesin-Ezrin-Radixin-like protein) are found in approximately half of all sporadic and nearly all NF-2–associated meningiomas, often associated with loss of the other Ch 22 allele, implicating NF2 as a of tumor suppressor gene important for meningioma pathogenesis.[17–25]

The wild-type NF2 gene spans 110 kb and is comprised of 17 exons.[26,27] Its protein product, schwannoma/merlin, is a 595-amino-acid protein that is part of the band Protein 4.1 family of cytoskeleton-associated proteins, a group of tumor suppressors that also includes Protein 4.1 B (previously knows as DAL-1 or "differentially expressed in adenocarcinoma of the lung") and Protein 4.1 R, which have recently been implicated in meningioma tumorigenesis (discussed later in this chapter).[28–30]

Merlin is mainly expressed in the nervous system, including schwann cells, neurons, astrocytes, and cells in the lens.[31] It is localized underneath the cell membrane in regions of cellular extensions and acts as a link between the cytoskeleton and the plasma membrane.[26,32,33] Inactivation of Merlin through truncating mutations in the NF2 gene results in disruption of the signaling cascade leading to cytoskeletal reorganization, decreased cell adhesion, and meningioma formation.[34,35] Conversely, transfection of the NF2 gene can reverse the Ras-induced malignant phenotype and restore contact inhibition of cell growth,[36] while overexpression of Merlin in human meningioma cells (both NF2-negative and NF2-positive) significantly inhibited proliferation.[35] Merlin is thus a unique type of tumor suppressor with a role in cytoskeleton dynamics, but the exact suppressor mechanism remains to be fully elucidated.

NF2 mutations appear to occur early in tumorigenesis and are common in benign (WHO I) as well as atypical and anaplastic meningiomas (WHO II and III),[37–41] but the individual meningioma subtypes variably express NF2 mutations.

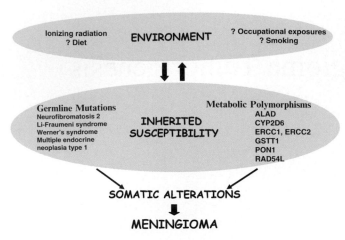

FIG. 12-1. Numerous genetic and environmental predisposing factors have been implicated in the development of meningiomas

Specifically, 70–86% of fibroblastic and transitional meningiomas demonstrate gene mutations, while they are found in less than 30% of meningothelial meningiomas.[42,43] The significance of this is unclear since the various meningioma subtypes are clinically indistinguishable in terms of recurrence or progression.

Meningiomas and Other Protein 4.1 Molecules

Protein 4.1 membrane-associated molecules are known to be important in regulating cellular architecture, and their role in growth regulation has also been studied in meningiomas. These proteins have significant homology to Merlin and have been found to be downregulated in menigioma. Specifically, gene inactivation of *4.1R* (chromosome 1p36) and *4.1B/DAL-1* (chromosome 18p11.3) have both been identified, suggesting that these genes may function as tumor suppressor genes with a role in tumor initiation and progression either alone or in combination with *NF2* mutations.[28,30,44] Hence, meningiomas may develop when one or more Protein 4.1 family members are inactivated.

Other Candidate Genes on Chromosome 22 Implicated in Meningioma Development

While the majority of meningioms have *NF2* mutations, studies have shown that an even more frequent finding is Ch 22 LOH, with deletion mapping demonstrating deletions that are discrete from the *NF2* locus in some meningiomas.[24,45] To this end, within the region near the *NF2* gene, *BAM 22(ADTB1, β-adaptin), RRP22, GAR 22, MN1, hSNF5/INI1 (SMARCB1)*, and *LARGE* have all been studied. However, they have not been found to be consistently mutated in meningiomas, suggesting

that these genes are not the relevant tumor suppressor gene essential for the development of meningiomas.[9,46–50]

Chromosomal Abnormalities

Beyond Ch 22, other karyotypic abnormalities (Fig. 12-2) have been identified and implicated in meningioma development or progression. Specifically, (1) loss of chromosome 1p, 6q, 7, 9p, 10, 14q, 18q, 19, and 20 or (2) gain/amplification of 1q, 9q, 12q, 15q, 17q, or 20q have all been identified.[19,38,41,51–60] Of note, 60% of meningiomas are hypodiploid, 33% diploid, 4.5% hyperdiploid, and 2.5% hypotriploid.[7] Furthermore, aggressive meningiomas have been found to have complex karyotypes including hypodiploidy, ring chromosomes, dicentrics, and double minutes.[61,62] Microsatellite instability has also been identified in meningiomas.[63] Many genes relevant in tumorigenesis have been identified in the abnormal chromosome regions and have been proposed as essential to the development or progression of meningiomas although key target genes have not been consistently identified.

Telomerase

Telomeres have repetitive DNA sequences important in chromosomal stability. Chromosomal arm length/stability is regulated by the reverse transcriptase telomerase (hTERT), a ribonucleoprotein enzyme that functions to replicate telomeric DNA. This enzyme has been found to be reactivated in a number of cancers where it is implicated in tumor growth. Increased mRNA expression of *hTERT* and increased activity of the enzyme have been identified in both benign (0–30%) and malignant meningiomas (up to 75% of atypical meningiomas and 100% of anaplastic meningiomas). Studies further demonstrate that telomerase activity may be a marker of an aggressive tumor and is associated with shorter progression free survival, independent of the tumor grade.[64,65]

Somatic genetic pathways of meningioma tumorigenesis

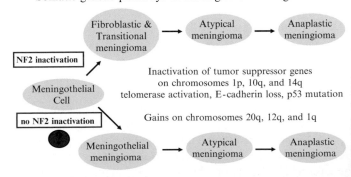

FIG. 12-2. Many karyotypic abnormalities have been identified and implicated in meningioma development and progression (see text for details and more complete discussion)

Growth Factors, Oncogenes, and Meningiomas

Growth factors, their receptors, and downstream pathways have been evaluated in meningiomas and implicated in meningioma growth and progression. The most commonly overexpressed of these are PDGF-BB (platelet-derived growth factor BB) and its receptor PDGFR-β, suggesting that meningioma cell proliferation occurs partially through activation of the Ras-RAF1-MAPKK/MEK1-MAPK/ERK and the PI3K-Akt/PKB signaling pathways.[66,67] Epidermal growth factor receptor (EGFR), while not amplified as extensively as in glioblastomas, is also consistently expressed in meningiomas, but not in normal or reactive meningothelial cells.[68,69] Vascular endothelial growth factor (VEGF) and its receptors have also been identified in meningiomas and are thought to be relevant in modulating vascular permeability (peritumoral edema) and more aggressive behavior.[70,71] Insulin-like growth factors (IGF) have also been implicated in meningioma development or progression, and increased IGF-II has been found to be associated with invasiveness and malignant progression.[72–74]

Increased expression of antigens, DNA, and RNA from oncogenic viruses have been identified in human meningiomas.[7,12,75,76] However, it is currently unclear if these viruses are relevant in meningioma development or are only a contaminant or latent infection.

Meningiomas and Radiation

The criteria for radiation induced tumors were first described by Cahan in 1998[77] and incorporate the following aspects: (1) second tumor within the field of irradiation used to treat the primary disease, (2) tumor not present prior to irradiation and reasonable interval between the radiation and detection of a second tumor (usually several years), (3) histologically different primary and subsequent tumor, and (4) no known genetic or predisposing conditions to secondary malignancy. In the case of radiation-induced meningiomas (in contrast to sporadically arising meningiomas), tumors occur in younger patients, with an equal male-to-female ratio. They are often multiple, higher grade, and tend to recur despite treatment. These tumors are less likely to be associated with Ch 22 LOH or *NF2* gene inactivation and are most frequently associated with Ch 1 p abnormalities.[78,79]

Chromosomes and Genes Involved in Meningioma Progression

NF2 gene mutations are identified at a similar frequency in benign, atypical, and anaplastic meningiomas, suggesting that this is an early event essential for tumor development rather than progression. With progression to higher grades of tumor, more complex and numerous genetic changes are identified (Fig. 12-1). However, the exact mechanism by which these abnormalities result in tumor progression is unknown.

Atypical meningiomas have been found to be associated with 1p, 6q, 10, 14q, and 18q chromosomal losses and gains/amplifications of chromosomes 1q, 9q, 12q, 15q, 17q, and 20q.[80] Significantly, after Ch 22 abnormalities, chromosomal deletions in the short arm of Ch 1 are the second most frequent abnormality found overall in meningiomas, with 70% of atypical and 100% of anaplastic meningiomas showing 1p monosomy.[81–84] This target region on the short arm of Ch 1 encompasses several putative tumor suppressor and cell cycle–regulating genes including *ALPL, TP73, CDKN2C* (encoding p18[INK4C]), and RAD 54L, but abnormalities within these genes have not been consistently identifed.[52,85–88] Recent evidence further suggests that the important mechanism may be silencing of these genes through hypermethylation of the promoter rather than direct gene mutations.[89,90]

With progression to the most aggressive meningiomas, anaplastic meningiomas, even more extensive chromosomal deletions, mutations, or amplifications have been identified, especially involving 6q, 9p, 10, 14q, and 17q23.[18,41,56,91] Of particular interest is the 9p21 deletion, where several genes (*CDKN2A, ARF,* and *CDKN2B*) that are relevant in cell cycle regulation/progression are often lost in anaplastic meningiomas.[52,78] Further, 70% of these anaplastic meningioma patients with 9p21 deletions demonstrated a decreased overall survival and poor prognosis relative to patients with anaplastic meningiomas lacking this deletion.[92]

Meningioma Familial Syndromes

In meningiomas, standardized incidence ratios for familial risk are increased about three- to fourfold.[93] Neurofibromatosis type 2 (NF2), multiple endocrine neoplasia type 1 (MEN1), Werner's, and Li-Fraumeni syndromes are known heritable causes, but other, yet unknown heritable conditions are likely to be present in meningioma families.[94] While the frequency of these inherited genetic abnormalities is relatively low in the general population, their high penetrance results in overt clinical manifestations of meningiomas in a distinctly familial pattern.

The best characterized of these is in families with NF2 where there is a clearly established genetic predisposition to meningiomas. Sporadic meningiomas account for 99% of all meningiomas, with only 1% arising in patients with NF2. However, many (up to 50%) patients with NF2 develop meningiomas within their lifetime, with meningiomas being the second most frequent tumor occurring in these patients after vestibular schwannomas.[95] Their tumors are typically the fibroblastic histologic variant, arise several decades earlier, and are frequently multiple when compared to patients with sporadic meningiomas. They exhibit Ch 22 deletions in nearly 100% of the cases, significantly higher than the rate documented in sporadic meningiomas.[18,21] Meningiomas with *NF2* mutations may have a higher recurrence rate than corresponding patients with meningiomas with no *NF2* mutations.[96,97] However, the majority of studies indicate that the incidence of atypical or anaplastic meningiomas is not increased in NF2-associated tumors relative to those occurring sporadically.[18,96,98,99]

Germ line mutations in the tumor suppressor gene p53 are observed in patients with a rare familial dominantly inherited Li-Fraumeni cancer syndrome, who are predisposed to development of sarcomas, breast cancer, and brain tumors, including meningiomas.[100] A combination of three single nucleotide polymorphisms (SNPs) within the p53 gene (in the promoter region, exon 4, and intron 6) has been associated with an increased risk of meningiomas in a recent case-control study. When the analysis was restricted to controls and patients with a positive family history of cancer, increased risk of meningioma was even greater (more than fivefold).[101]

Multiple endocrine neoplasia type 1 (MEN1) is an autosomal dominant disease with multiple endocrine as well as nonhormonal manifestations of benign and malignant tumors.[102] The results of a recent prospective study show that meningiomas developed in about 8% of patients with MEN1. These tumors had a loss of heterozygosity at MEN1 locus and variety of other loci, but not at the NF2 gene locus, suggesting that the MEN1 gene product called menin may play a role in their tumorigenesis.[103] Menin is a ubiquitously expressed protein that interacts with a variety of proteins that participate in multiple biological functions, including DNA transcription and repair as well as regulation of cytoskeleton functions.[102]

Werner syndrome is another genetic condition associated with meningioma development. Besides meningiomas, this autosomal recessive disorder of premature aging is associated with predisposition to cardiovascular disease and rare cancers, including thyroid carcinoma, melanoma, sarcoma, and myeloid disorders.[104,105] The Werner syndrome protein (WRN) has a strong homology to a class of enzymes called the RecQ helicases, which may play a role in the surveillance of genome integrity, maintenance of telomeres, and control of the cell's response to genotoxic stress by interacting with several partner proteins, including PARP-1 and p53.[106]

Meningiomas and the Environment: The Role of Genetic Polymorphisms

Studies in which genetic and environmental components in brain tumors were assessed suggest that inherited genetic factors account only for about 13% of causation of nervous system tumors and that environment has a principal causative role in these tumors.[107] In addition to high-penetrance genes that occur in a population at a low frequency, genetic susceptibility to meningioma may be conferred, in interaction with environmental exposures, by low-penetrance genes that are highly prevalent and may facilitate tumor formation. Genetic polymorphisms of several genes have been suggested to modulate the susceptibility to meningioma tumorigenesis. No studies, however, were conducted so far to examine the gene–environment interactions, but rather focused on analysis of gene polymorphisms and risk of meningioma.

Polymorphisms in DNA Repair Pathways

Polymorphisms of genes that function in DNA repair pathways have been investigated and found to be associated with meningioma risk. ERCC2 gene functions in nucleotide excision repair of DNA damaged by UV, ionizing radiation, and oxidants and may be relevant for cancer in general and meningioma in particular. ERCC2 K751Q (A to C) polymorphism leading to a change from lysine to glutamine was significantly associated with the risk of meningioma; that is, the presence of the A allele increased the risk compared with the CC genotype.[108] Although K751Q variant is expected to have great functional effects because of the nature of the amino acid change and its critical location, conflicting results have been reported about the efficacy of DNA repair in lymphocytes from people with this ERCC2 variant.

A polymorphism (2290C/T) in the RAD54L gene that is essential in the repair of DNA double-strand breaks by the homologous recombination pathway[109] has also been linked with meningioma risk. The evaluation of distribution of 2290C/T genotype among meningioma patients and matched healthy controls suggested that the rare 2290T allele is associated with an increased risk of meningioma development.[110] Interestingly, this polymorphism is located in the chromosomal region 1p32, an area of frequent loss of heterozygosity in sporadic and hereditary meningiomas, and it could, therefore, be used as a genetic marker for that region.

Polymorphisms Involved in Activation and Detoxification of Chemicals

Serum paraoxonase (PON1) is a calcium-dependent esterase that functions as a part of a free-radical–scavenging system and contributes to detoxification of organophosphorous compounds and carcinogenic products of lipid peroxidation. There is a 10- to 40-fold interindividual variability in serum PON1 that, in part, stems from polymorphisms in PON1 gene.[111] The enzymatic activity of the glutamine-192 (allele A) PON1 isoform has been described to be lower than that of arginine-192 (B allele isoform). It was recently reported that meningioma patients with AA and AB genotypes, but not BB genotype, showed significantly lower serum PON1 activities than controls.[112] It is, however, not known if the lipid peroxidation–scavenging system is less active in AA and AB genotypes and could thus contribute to increased risk of meningioma. There are data that support such an idea, because patients with meningioma were reported to have decreased activities of other antioxidant enzymes, including glutathione reductase and superoxide dismutase in blood or tumor tissue.[113,114] These decreases in antioxidant defenses may, in part, explain the findings of increased oxidative stress in meningiomas.[115]

Exposures to other environmental factors, including occupational exposures to lead, have been associated with increased risk of meningiomas,[116–119] particularly in people who carry a genetic variant for δ-aminolevulinic acid dehydratase (ALAD), an enzyme involved in the synthesis of heme.[120] The most commonly studied polymorphism in this gene contains a G-to-C transversion at position 177 (G177C) and has two codominant alleles: ALAD1 and ALAD2, with an ALAD2 prevalence of about 10%. Interestingly, individuals with ALAD2 allele have higher blood lead levels than do ALAD1 homozygotes, probably due to tighter binding of lead by the ALAD2 enzyme. People who carried ALAD 2 allele, both heterozygotes and homozygotes, had a significantly increased risk of meningioma development.[120] However, the combined effects of exposure to lead and the ALAD2 allele was not examined, and it will hopefully be the focus of future investigations.

Glutathione S-transferases (GST) are enzymes that are involved in metabolism of a variety of chemical compounds and display a spectrum of gene polymorphisms that are associated with their enzymatic activity. Persons with variant alleles for GST genes may differ in their ability to metabolize carcinogenic compounds and, thus, may have altered risk of cancer. For example, GSTT1 and GSTM1 protect against epoxide- and benzene-induced sister chromatide exchange.[121] Individuals with null alleles at these loci are at greater risk of DNA adducts in peripheral leukocytes[122] and thus possibly chromosomal aberrations. Several studies, including two recent meta-analyses, reported that GSTT1-null genotype was significantly associated with almost twofold increased risk of meningioma.[123,124] Nevertheless, larger studies are required to confirm this relationship and to examine the possible interactions with dietary practices.

Higher intake of Brassica vegetables and isothiocyanates (naturally occurring compound of these foods) were associated with reduced risk of lung[125–127] and colon cancer[128] among people with homozygous deletion of GSTM1 and/or GSTT1 compared to those with normal expression levels of these genes. Although knowledge about the role of dietary factors in meningioma tumorigenesis is essentially nonexistent,[129–130] the studies of polymorphisms of genes that may be modulated with dietary exposures are likely to provide an impetus for new studies on diet–gene interactions among patients with meningioma.

Conclusion

After more than four decades, genetic evaluation of meningiomas has led to the characterization of many alterations relevant in tumorigenesis and progression. Our understanding, however, remains incomplete, with many relevant genes still to be identified. In future, array-based high-throughput screening and perhaps in vivo and in vitro models will yield even more information regarding the complex relationships and distinct patterns of gene expression in these tumors, insights that will enhance our understanding of the genetic pathways and biological mechanisms of meningioma initiation and progression. This will be relevant not only for the development of complete diagnostic and prognostic criteria, but also important in the identification of pathways that may be targeted and exploited for the development of novel therapeutic strategies.

References

1. Collins FS: The case for a US prospective cohort study of genes and environment. Nature 429:475–477, 2004.
2. Lai C, Shields PG: The role of interindividual variation in human carcinogenesis. J Nutr 129:552S–555S, 1999.
3. Mark J, Levan G, Mitelman F: Identification by fluorescence of the G chromosome lost in human meningomas. Hereditas 71:163–168, 1972.
4. Zankl H, Zang KD: Cytological and cytogenetical studies on brain tumors. 4. Identification of the missing G chromosome in human meningiomas as no. 22 by fluorescence technique. Humangenetik 14:167–169, 1972.
5. Dumanski JP, Carlbom E, Collins VP, et al.: Deletion mapping of a locus on human chromosome 22 involved in the oncogenesis of meningioma. Proc Natl Acad Sci USA 84:9275–9279, 1987.
6. Dumanski JP, Rouleau GA, Nordenskjold M, et al.: Molecular genetic analysis of chromosome 22 in 81 cases of meningioma. Cancer Res 50:5863–5867, 1990.
7. Mark J: Chromosomal abnormalities and their specificity in human neoplasms: an assessment of recent observations by banding techniques. Adv Cancer Res 24:165–222, 1977.
8. Meese E, Blin N, Zang KD: Loss of heterozygosity and the origin of meningioma. Hum Genet 77:349–351, 1987.
9. Peyrard M, Fransson I, Xie YG, et al.: Characterization of a new member of the human beta-adaptin gene family from chromosome 22q12, a candidate meningioma gene. Hum Mol Genet 3:1393–1399, 1994.
10. Seizinger BR, de la MS, Atkins L, et al.: Molecular genetic approach to human meningioma: loss of genes on chromosome 22. Proc Natl Acad Sci USA 84:5419–5423, 1987.
11. Yamada K, Kondo T, Yoshioka M, et al.: Cytogenetic studies in twenty human brain tumors: association of no. 22 chromosome abnormalities with tumors of the brain. Cancer Genet Cytogenet 2:293–307, 1980.
12. Zang KD: Cytological and cytogenetical studies on human meningioma. Cancer Genet Cytogenet 6:249–274, 1982.
13. Zankl H, Zang KD: Correlations between clinical and cytogenetic data in 180 human meningiomas. Cancer Genet Cytogenet 1:351–356, 1980.
14. Evans DG, Sainio M, Baser ME: Neurofibromatosis type 2. J Med Genet 37:897–904, 2000.
15. Rouleau GA, Merel P, Lutchman M, et al.: Alteration in a new gene encoding a putative membrane-organizing protein causes neuro-fibromatosis type 2. Nature 363:515–521, 1993.
16. Trofatter JA, MacCollin MM, Rutter JL, et al.: A novel moesin-, ezrin-, radixin-like gene is a candidate for the neurofibromatosis 2 tumor suppressor. Cell 75:826, 1993.

17. Gutmann DH, Giordano MJ, Fishback AS, et al.: Loss of merlin expression in sporadic meningiomas, ependymomas and schwannomas. Neurology 49:267–270, 1997.

18. Lamszus K, Vahldiek F, Mautner VF, et al.: Allelic losses in neurofibromatosis 2-associated meningiomas. J Neuropathol Exp Neurol 59:504–512, 2000.

19. Lekanne Deprez RH, Bianchi AB, Groen NA, et al.: Frequent NF2 gene transcript mutations in sporadic meningiomas and vestibular schwannomas. Am J Hum Genet 54:1022–1029, 1994.

20. Lekanne Deprez RH, Riegman PH, van DE, et al.: Cytogenetic, molecular genetic and pathological analyses in 126 meningiomas. J Neuropathol Exp Neurol 54:224–235, 1995.

21. Perry A, Giannini C, Raghavan R, et al.: Aggressive phenotypic and genotypic features in pediatric and NF2-associated meningiomas: a clinicopathologic study of 53 cases. J Neuropathol Exp Neurol 60:994–1003, 2001.

22. Perry A, Scheithauer BW, Stafford SL, et al.: "Malignancy" in meningiomas: a clinicopathologic study of 116 patients, with grading implications. Cancer 85:2046–2056, 1999.

23. Ruttledge MH, Sarrazin J, Rangaratnam S, et al.: Evidence for the complete inactivation of the NF2 gene in the majority of sporadic meningiomas. Nat Genet 6:180–184, 1994.

24. Ruttledge MH, Xie YG, Han FY, et al.: Deletions on chromosome 22 in sporadic meningioma. Genes Chromosomes Cancer 10:122–130, 1994.

25. Ueki K, Wen-Bin C, Narita Y, et al.: Tight association of loss of merlin expression with loss of heterozygosity at chromosome 22q in sporadic meningiomas. Cancer Res 59:5995–5998, 1999.

26. Gusella JF, Ramesh V, MacCollin M, et al.: Merlin: the neurofibromatosis 2 tumor suppressor. Biochim Biophys Acta 1423: M29–M36, 1999.

27. Gutmann DH: Molecular insights into neurofibromatosis 2. Neurobiol Dis 3:247–261, 1997.

28. Gutmann DH, Donahoe J, Perry A, et al.: Loss of DAL-1, a protein 4.1-related tumor suppressor, is an important early event in the pathogenesis of meningiomas. Hum Mol Genet 9:1495–1500, 2000.

29. Gutmann DH, Hirbe AC, Huang ZY, et al.: The protein 4.1 tumor suppressor, DAL-1, impairs cell motility, but regulates proliferation in a cell-type-specific fashion. Neurobiol Dis 8:266–278, 2001.

30. Robb VA, Li W, Gascard P, et al.: Identification of a third Protein 4.1 tumor suppressor, Protein 4.1R, in meningioma pathogenesis. Neurobiol Dis 13:191–202, 2003.

31. Hitotsumatsu T, Iwaki T, Kitamoto T, et al.: Expression of neurofibromatosis 2 protein in human brain tumors: an immunohistochemical study. Acta Neuropathol (Berl) 93:225–232, 1997.

32. Sainio M, Zhao F, Heiska L, et al.: Neurofibromatosis 2 tumor suppressor protein colocalizes with ezrin and CD44 and associates with actin-containing cytoskeleton. J Cell Sci 110 (Pt 18):2249–2260, 1997.

33. Vaheri A, Carpen O, Heiska L, et al.: The ezrin protein family: membrane-cytoskeleton interactions and disease associations. Curr Opin Cell Biol 9:659–666, 1997.

34. Dirven CM, Grill J, Lamfers ML, et al.: Gene therapy for meningioma: improved gene delivery with targeted adenoviruses. J Neurosurg 97:441–449, 2002.

35. Ikeda K, Saeki Y, Gonzalez-Agosti C, et al.: Inhibition of NF2-negative and NF2-positive primary human meningioma cell proliferation by overexpression of merlin due to vector-mediated gene transfer. J Neurosurg 91:85–92, 1999.

36. Tikoo A, Varga M, Ramesh V, et al.: An anti-Ras function of neurofibromatosis type 2 gene product (NF2/Merlin). J Biol Chem 269:23387–23390, 1994.

37. Harada T, Irving RM, Xuereb JH, et al.: Molecular genetic investigation of the neurofibromatosis type 2 tumor suppressor gene in sporadic meningioma. J Neurosurg 84:847–851, 1996.

38. Lamszus K, Kluwe L, Matschke J, et al.: Allelic losses at 1 p, 9 q, 10 q, 14 q, and 22 q in the progression of aggressive meningiomas and undifferentiated meningeal sarcomas. Cancer Genet Cytogenet 110:103–110, 1999.

39. Leone PE, Bello MJ, de Campos JM, et al.: NF2 gene mutations and allelic status of 1 p, 14 q and 22 q in sporadic meningiomas. Oncogene 18:2231–2239, 1999.

40. Menon AG, Rutter JL, von Sattel JP, et al.: Frequent loss of chromosome 14 in atypical and malignant meningioma: identification of a putative 'tumor progression' locus. Oncogene 14:611–616, 1997.

41. Weber RG, Bostrom J, Wolter M, et al.: Analysis of genomic alterations in benign, atypical, and anaplastic meningiomas: toward a genetic model of meningioma progression. Proc Natl Acad Sci U S A 94:14719–14724, 1997.

42. Evans JJ, Jeun SS, Lee JH, et al.: Molecular alterations in the neurofibromatosis type 2 gene and its protein rarely occurring in meningothelial meningiomas. J Neurosurg 94:111–117, 2001.

43. Wellenreuther R, Kraus JA, Lenartz D, et al.: Analysis of the neurofibromatosis 2 gene reveals molecular variants of meningioma. Am J Pathol 146:827–832, 1995.

44. Nunes F, Shen Y, Niida Y, et al.: Inactivation patterns of NF2 and DAL-1/4.1B (EPB41L3) in sporadic meningioma. Cancer Genet Cytogenet 162:135–139, 2005.

45. Lomas J, Bello MJ, Alonso ME, et al.: Loss of chromosome 22 and absence of NF2 gene mutation in a case of multiple meningiomas. Hum Pathol 33:375–378, 2002.

46. Lekanne Deprez RH, Riegman PH, Groen NA, et al.: Cloning and characterization of MN1, a gene from chromosome 22q11, which is disrupted by a balanced translocation in a meningioma. Oncogene 10:1521–1528, 1995.

47. Peyrard M, Pan HQ, Kedra D, et al.: Structure of the promoter and genomic organization of the human beta -adaptin gene (BAM22) from chromosome 22q12. Genomics 36:112–117, 1996.

48. Peyrard M, Seroussi E, Sandberg-Nordqvist AC, et al.: The human LARGE gene from 22q12.3–q13.1 is a new, distinct member of the glycosyltransferase gene family. Proc Natl Acad Sci U S A 96:598–603, 1999.

49. Schmitz U, Mueller W, Weber M, et al.: INI1 mutations in meningiomas at a potential hotspot in exon 9. Br J Cancer 84:199–201, 2001.

50. Zucman-Rossi J, Legoix P, Thomas G: Identification of new members of the Gas2 and Ras families in the 22q12 chromosome region. Genomics 38:247–254, 1996.

51. Al Saadi A, Latimer F, Madercic M, et al.: Cytogenetic studies of human brain tumors and their clinical significance. II. Meningioma. Cancer Genet Cytogenet 26:127–141, 1987.

52. Bostrom J, Meyer-Puttlitz B, Wolter M, et al.: Alterations of the tumor suppressor genes CDKN2A (p16(INK4a)), p14(ARF), CDKN2B (p15(INK4b)), and CDKN2C (p18(INK4c)) in atypical and anaplastic meningiomas. Am J Pathol 159:661–669, 2001.

53. Cai DX, Banerjee R, Scheithauer BW, et al.: Chromosome 1p and 14q FISH analysis in clinicopathologic subsets of meningioma: diagnostic and prognostic implications. J Neuropathol Exp Neurol 60:628–636, 2001.

54. Cai DX, James CD, Scheithauer BW, et al.: PS6K amplification characterizes a small subset of anaplastic meningiomas. Am J Clin Pathol 115:213–218, 2001.

55. Katsuyama J, Papenhausen PR, Herz F, et al.: Chromosome abnormalities in meningiomas. Cancer Genet Cytogenet 22:63–68, 1986.

56. Ozaki S, Nishizaki T, Ito H, et al.: Comparative genomic hybridization analysis of genetic alterations associated with malignant progression of meningioma. J Neurooncol 41:167–174, 1999.

57. Prempree T, Amornmarn R, Faillace WJ, et al.: 1;19 translocation in human meningioma. Cancer 71:2306–2311, 1993.

58. Schneider BF, Shashi V, von Kap-herr C, et al.: Loss of chromosomes 22 and 14 in the malignant progression of meningiomas. A comparative study of fluorescence in situ hybridization (FISH) and standard cytogenetic analysis. Cancer Genet Cytogenet 85:101–104, 1995.

59. Simon M, von DA, Larson JJ, et al.: Allelic losses on chromosomes 14, 10, and 1 in atypical and malignant meningiomas: a genetic model of meningioma progression. Cancer Res 55:4696–4701, 1995.

60. Vagner-Capodano AM, Grisoli F, Gambarelli D, et al.: Correlation between cytogenetic and histopathological findings in 75 human meningiomas. Neurosurgery 32:892–900, 1993.

61. Lopez-Gines C, Cerda-Nicolas M, Barcia-Salorio JL, et al.: Cytogenetical findings of recurrent meningiomas. A study of 10 tumors. Cancer Genet Cytogenet 85:113–117, 1995.

62. Lopez-Gines C, Cerda-Nicolas M, Gil-Benso R, et al.: Loss of 1 p in recurrent meningiomas. a comparative study in successive recurrences by cytogenetics and fluorescence in situ hybridization. Cancer Genet Cytogenet 125:119–124, 2001.

63. Pykett MJ, Murphy M, Harnish PR, et al.: Identification of a microsatellite instability phenotype in meningiomas. Cancer Res 54:6340–6343, 1994.

64. Boldrini L, Pistolesi S, Gisfredi S, et al.: Telomerase in intracranial meningiomas. Int J Mol Med 12:943–947, 2003.

65. Maes L, Lippens E, Kalala JP, et al.: The hTERT-protein and Ki-67 labelling index in recurrent and non-recurrent meningiomas. Cell Prolif 38:3–12, 2005.

66. Johnson MD, Woodard A, Kim P, et al.: Evidence for mitogen-associated protein kinase activation and transduction of mitogenic signals by platelet-derived growth factor in human meningioma cells. J Neurosurg 94:293–300, 2001.

67. Yang SY, Xu GM: Expression of PDGF and its receptor as well as their relationship to proliferating activity and apoptosis of meningiomas in human meningiomas. J Clin Neurosci 8 Suppl 1:49–53, 2001.

68. Perry A, Gutmann DH, Reifenberger G: Molecular pathogenesis of meningiomas. J Neurooncol 70:183–202, 2004.

69. Torp SH, Helseth E, Dalen A, et al.: Expression of epidermal growth factor receptor in human meningiomas and meningeal tissue. APMIS 100:797–802, 1992.

70. Yamasaki F, Yoshioka H, Hama S, et al.: Recurrence of meningiomas. Cancer 89:1102–1110, 2000.

71. Yoshioka H, Hama S, Taniguchi E, et al.: Peritumoral brain edema associated with meningioma: influence of vascular endothelial growth factor expression and vascular blood supply. Cancer 85:936–944, 1999.

72. Nordqvist AC, Mathiesen T: Expression of IGF-II, IGFBP-2, -5, and -6 in meningiomas with different brain invasiveness. J Neurooncol 57:19–26, 2002.

73. Nordqvist AC, Peyrard M, Pettersson H, et al.: A high ratio of insulin-like growth factor II/insulin-like growth factor binding protein 2 messenger RNA as a marker for anaplasia in meningiomas. Cancer Res 57:2611–2614, 1997.

74. Watson MA, Gutmann DH, Peterson K, et al.: Molecular characterization of human meningiomas by gene expression profiling using high-density oligonucleotide microarrays. Am J Pathol 161:665–672, 2002.

75. Ibelgaufts H, Jones KW: Papovavirus-related RNA sequences in human neurogenic tumours. Acta Neuropathol (Berl) 56:118–122, 1982.

76. Ibelgaufts H, Jones KW, Maitland N, et al.: Adenovirus-related RNA sequences in human neurogenic tumours. Acta Neuropathol (Berl) 56:113–117, 1982.

77. Cahan WG: Radiation-induced sarcoma—50 years later. Cancer 82:6–7, 1998.

78. Al-Mefty O, Topsakal C, Pravdenkova S, et al.: Radiation-induced meningiomas: clinical, pathological, cytokinetic, and cytogenetic characteristics. J Neurosurg 100:1002–1013, 2004.

79. Zattara-Cannoni H, Roll P, Figarella-Branger D, et al.: Cytogenetic study of six cases of radiation-induced meningiomas. Cancer Genet Cytogenet 126:81–84, 2001.

80. Riemenschneider MJ, Perry A, Reifenberger G: Histological classification and molecular genetics of meningiomas. Lancet Neurol 5:1045–1054, 2006.

81. Henn W, Cremerius U, Heide G, et al.: Monosomy 1 p is correlated with enhanced in vivo glucose metabolism in meningiomas. Cancer Genet Cytogenet 79:144–148, 1995.

82. Muller P, Henn W, Niedermayer I, et al.: Deletion of chromosome 1 p and loss of expression of alkaline phosphatase indicate progression of meningiomas. Clin Cancer Res 5:3569–3577, 1999.

83. Steudel WI, Feld R, Henn W, et al.: Correlation between cytogenetic and clinical findings in 215 human meningiomas. Acta Neurochir Suppl 65:73–76, 1996.

84. Zang KD: Meningioma: a cytogenetic model of a complex benign human tumor, including data on 394 karyotyped cases. Cytogenet Cell Genet 93:207–220, 2001.

85. Bello MJ, de Campos JM, Vaquero J, et al.: High-resolution analysis of chromosome arm 1 p alterations in meningioma. Cancer Genet Cytogenet 120:30–36, 2000.

86. Lomas J, Bello MJ, Arjona D, et al.: Analysis of p73 gene in meningiomas with deletion at 1 p. Cancer Genet Cytogenet 129:88–91, 2001.

87. Mendiola M, Bello MJ, Alonso J, et al.: Search for mutations of the hRAD54 gene in sporadic meningiomas with deletion at 1p32. Mol Carcinog 24:300–304, 1999.

88. Niedermayer I, Feiden W, Henn W, et al.: Loss of alkaline phosphatase activity in meningiomas: a rapid histochemical technique indicating progression-associated deletion of a putative tumor suppressor gene on the distal part of the short arm of chromosome 1. J Neuropathol Exp Neurol 56:879–886, 1997.

89. Bello MJ, Aminoso C, Lopez-Marin I, et al.: DNA methylation of multiple promoter-associated CpG islands in meningiomas: relationship with the allelic status a 1 p and 22 q. Acta Neuropathol (Berl) 108:413–421, 2004.

90. Lomas J, Aminoso C, Gonzalez-Gomez P, et al.: Methylation status of TP73 in meningiomas. Cancer Genet Cytogenet 148:148–151, 2004.

91. Buschges R, Ichimura K, Weber RG, et al.: Allelic gain and amplification on the long arm of chromosome 17 in anaplastic meningiomas. Brain Pathol 12:145–153, 2002.

92. Perry A, Banerjee R, Lohse CM, et al.: A role for chromosome 9p21 deletions in the malignant progression of meningiomas

and the prognosis of anaplastic meningiomas. Brain Pathol 12:183–190, 2002.

93. Hemminki K, Li X: Familial risks in nervous system tumors. Cancer Epidemiol Biomarkers Prev 12:1137–42, 2003.

94. Melean G, Sestini R, Ammannati F, Papi L: Genetic insights into familial tumors of the nervous system. Am J Med Genet C Semin Med Genet 129:74–84, 2004.

95. Ragel BT, Jensen RL: Molecular genetics of meningiomas. Neurosurg Focus 19:E9, 2005.

96. Antinheimo J, Haapasalo H, Haltia M, et al.: Proliferation potential and histological features in neurofibromatosis 2-associated and sporadic meningiomas. J Neurosurg 87:610–614, 1997.

97. Sanson M, Richard S, Delattre O, et al.: Allelic loss on chromosome 22 correlates with histopathological predictors of recurrence of meningiomas. Int J Cancer 50:391–394, 1992.

98. Lamszus K: Meningioma pathology, genetics, and biology. J Neuropathol Exp Neurol 63:275–286, 2004.

99. Louis DN, Ramesh V, Gusella JF: Neuropathology and molecular genetics of neurofibromatosis 2 and related tumors. Brain Pathol 5:163–172, 1995.

100. Rieske P, Zakrzewska M, Biernat W, Bartkowiak J, Zimmermann A, Liberski PP: Atypical molecular background of glioblastoma and meningioma developed in a patient with Li-Fraumeni syndrome. J Neurooncol 71:27–30, 2005.

101. Malmer B, Feychting M, Lonn S, Ahlbom A, Henriksson R: p53 Genotypes and risk of glioma and meningioma. Cancer Epidemiol Biomarkers Prev 14:2220–3, 2005.

102. Agarwal SK, Kennedy PA, Scacheri PC, Novotny EA, Hickman AB, Cerrato A, Rice TS, Moore JB, Rao S, Ji Y, Mateo C, Libutti SK, Oliver B, Chandrasekharappa SC, Burns AL, Collins FS, Spiegel AM, Marx SJ: Menin molecular interactions: insights into normal functions and tumorigenesis. Horm Metab Res 37:369–74, 2005.

103. Asgharian B, Chen YJ, Patronas NJ, Peghini PL, Reynolds JC, Vortmeyer A, Zhuang Z, Venzon DJ, Gibril F, Jensen RT: Meningiomas may be a component tumor of multiple endocrine neoplasia type 1. Clin Cancer Res 10:869–80, 2004.

104. Goto M, Miller RW, Ishikawa Y, Sugano H: Excess of rare cancers in Werner syndrome (adult progeria). Cancer Epidemiol Biomarkers Prev 5:239–46, 1996.

105. Nakamura Y, Shimizu T, Ohigashi Y, Itou N, Ishikawa Y: Meningioma arising in Werner syndrome confirmed by mutation analysis. J Clin Neurosci 12:503–6, 2005.

106. Comai L, Li B: The Werner syndrome protein at the crossroads of DNA repair and apoptosis. Mech Ageing Dev 125:521–8, 2004.

107. Czene K, Lichtenstein P, Hemminki K: Environmental and heritable causes of cancer among 9.6 million individuals in the Swedish Family-Cancer Database. Int J Cancer 99:260–6, 2002.

108. Sadetzki S, Flint-Richter P, Starinsky S, Novikov I, Lerman Y, Goldman B, Friedman E: Genotyping of patients with sporadic and radiation-associated meningiomas. Cancer Epidemiol Biomarkers Prev 14:969–76, 2005.

109. Peterson CL, Cote J: Cellular machineries for chromosomal DNA repair. Genes Dev 18:602–16, 2004.

110. Leone PE, Mendiola M, Alonso J, Paz-y-Mino C, Pestana A: Implications of a RAD54L polymorphism (2290C/T) in human meningiomas as a risk factor and/or a genetic marker. BMC Cancer 3:6, 2003.

111. Humbert R, Adler DA, Disteche CM, Hassett C, Omiecinski CJ, Furlong CE: The molecular basis of the human serum paraoxonase activity polymorphism. Nat Genet 3:73–6, 1993.

112. Kafadar AM, Ergen A, Zeybek U, Agachan B, Kuday C, Isbir T: Paraoxonase 192 gene polymorphism and serum paraoxonase activity in high grade gliomas and meningiomas. Cell Biochem Funct 2005 Sep 2; [Epub ahead of print DOI: 10.1027/cbf.1284]

113. Pu PY, Lan J, Shan SB, Huang EQ, Bai Y, Guo Y, Jiang DH: Study of the antioxidant enzymes in human brain tumors. J Neurooncol 29:121–8, 1996.

114. Rao GM, Rao AV, Raja A, Rao S, Rao A: Role of antioxidant enzymes in brain tumours. Clin Chim Acta 296:203–12, 2000.

115. Iida T, Furuta A, Kawashima M, Nishida J, Nakabeppu Y, Iwaki T: Accumulation of 8-oxo-2′-deoxyguanosine and increased expression of hMTH1 protein in brain tumors. Neuro-oncology 3:73–81, 2001.

116. Rajaraman P, De Roos A, Stewart P, Linet M, Fine H, Shapiro W, et al. Occupation and risk of meningioma and acoustic neuroma in the United States. Am J Ind Med 45:395–407, 2004.

117. Navas-Acien A, Pollan M, Gustavsson P, Plato N. Occupation, exposure to chemicals and risk of gliomas and meningiomas in Sweden. Am J Ind Med 42:214–227, 2002.

118. Hu J, Little J, Xu T, Zhao X, Guo L, Jia X, et al. Risk factors for meningioma in adults: a case-control study in northeast China. Int J Cancer 83:299–304, 1999.

119. Cocco P, Heineman E, Dosemeci M. Occupational risk factors for cancer of the central nervous system (CNS) among US women. Am J Ind Med,36:70–74, 1999.

120. Rajaraman P, Schwartz BS, Rothman N, Yeager M, Fine HA, Shapiro WR, Selker RG, Black PM, Inskip PD: Delta-aminolevulinic acid dehydratase polymorphism and risk of brain tumors in adults. Environ Health Perspect 113:1209–11, 2005.

121. Xu X, Wiencke JK, Niu T, Wang M, Watanabe H, Kelsey KT, Christiani DC: Benzene exposure, glutathione S-transferase theta homozygous deletion, and sister chromatid axchanges. Am J Ind Med 33:157–163, 1998.

122. Palli D, Vineis P, Russo A, Berrino F, Krogh V, Masala G, Munnia A, Panico S, Taioli E, Tumino R, Garte S, Peluso M: Diet, metabolic polymorphisms and DNA adducts: the EPIC-Italy cross-sectional study. Int J Cancer, 87:444–451, 2000.

123. Liu L, Zhou YH: Review and meta-analysis of glutathione S-transferase polymorphisms and the risk of brain tumors. Neuro-Oncology 6:238, 2004 (abstract).

124. Lai R, Crevier L, Thabane L: Genetic polymorphisms of glutathione S-transferases and the risk of adult brain tumors: a meta-analysis. Cancer Epidemiol Biomarkers Prev 14:1784–90, 2005.

125. Zhao B, Seow A, Lee EJD, Poh W-T, The M, Eng P, Wang Y-T, Tan W-C, Yu MC, Lee H-P: Dietary isothiocyanates, glutathione S-transferase –M1, -T1 polymorphisms and lung cancer risk among Chinese women in Singapore. Cancer Epidemiol Biomarkers Prev 10:1063–1067, 2001.

126. Spitz MR, Duphorne CM, Detry MA, Pillow PC, Amos CK, Lei L, de Adrade M, Gu X, Hong WK, Wu X: Dietary intake of isothiocyanates: evidence of joint effect with glutathione S-transferase polymorphisms in lung cancer risk. Cancer Epidemiol Biomarkers Prev 9:1017–1020, 2000.

127. Brennan P, Hsu CC, Moullan N, Szeszenia-Dabrowska N, Lissowska J, Zaridze D, Rudnai P, Fabianova E, Mates D, Bencko V, Foretova L, Janout V, Gemignani F, Chabrier A, Hall J, Hung RJ, Boffetta P, Canzian F: Effect of cruciferous vegetables on lung cancer in patients stratified by genetic status: a mendelian randomisation approach. Lancet 366:1558–60, 2005.

128. Yeh CC, Hsieh LL, Tang R, Chang-Chieh CR, Sung FC: Vegetable/fruit, smoking, glutathione S-transferase polymorphisms and risk for colorectal cancer in Taiwan. World J Gastroenterol 11:1473–80, 2005.

129. Hu J, La Vecchia C, Negri E, Chatenoud L, Bosetti C, Jia X, Liu R, Huang G, Bi D, Wang C: Diet and brain cancer in adults: a case-control study in northeast China. Int J Cancer 81:20–23, 1999b.

130. Boeing H, Schlehofer B, Blettner M, Wahrendorf J: Dietary carcinogens and the risk for glioma and meningioma in Germany. Int J Cancer 53:561–5, 1993.

13
Meningiomas of the Central Neuraxis: Unique Tumors

Joung H. Lee and Burak Sade

Introduction

Meningiomas are a histologically heterogeneous group of tumors, which have been classified into three grades based on their behavior. Grade I tumors are considered "benign" according to the most recent World Health Organization (WHO) classification for meningiomas in 2000.[1,2] There are nine histologic subtypes included in grade I: meningothelial, fibrous, transitional, psammomatous, angiomatous, microcystic, secretory, lymphoplasmacyte-rich, and metaplastic. Grade II tumors, more aggressive than grade I meningiomas in their behavior, include the clear cell, chordoid, and atypical subtypes. Papillary, rhabdoid, and anaplastic meningiomas are included in the WHO grade III tumors. Histologic grade has been shown to have a significant impact on tumor recurrence rates following aggressive surgical resection: 3–20% of grade I meningiomas recur as compared to 30–40% of grade II and 50–80% of grade III cases.[3–6] The median survival of patients diagnosed with anaplastic meningiomas has been reported to be in the range of 2–7 years.[3,5,7,8]

The prevailing attitude among most neurosurgeons and pathologists is that all benign meningiomas constitute a homogeneous group of tumors and that their wide variation in histologic appearance has no bearing on tumor location or their overall biological behavior.[9] Contrary to these long-held popular views, the findings we present in this chapter suggest that meningiomas arising from the central neuraxis (i.e., the midline skull base) are unique tumors. In particular, we will suggest that meningiomas arising from the midline skull base are predominantly of the meningothelial subtype and that they are rarely aggressive or malignant.

Predominance of Meningothelial Meningiomas in the Midline Skull Base

Shortly after identification and cloning of neurofibromatosis type 2 (NF2) gene,[10,11] our laboratory investigated the expression level of NF2 protein, schwannomin/merlin, in human sporadic meningiomas. Because of the high incidence of meningiomas in NF2 patients, a hypothesis was tested that the NF2 protein level would be reduced in sporadic meningiomas.[12] In the study, 57% of meningiomas analyzed (8/14) showed a significant reduction in NF2 protein levels. The remaining 43% of the meningiomas tested, which showed normal NF2 protein level, was uniformly of the meningothelial subtype. Subsequently, a larger study of NF2 mutational analysis involving 20 meningothelial meningiomas (MM) and 7 non-MM was done, revealing only 5% (1/20) NF2 gene mutation in MM.[13] Similar findings of relatively rare NF2 gene mutations in MM were reported by other investigators.[14–17] These studies suggest that NF2 gene may be a critical tumor suppressor gene involved in the pathogenesis of non-MM such as fibrous, transitional, and other subtypes of meningiomas, while an alternate gene(s) as yet unidentified is involved in the MM tumorigenesis.

In 2001, we encountered an interesting finding while conducting a clinical study of clinoidal meningiomas. Among the 14 benign meningiomas analyzed in the study, upon review of their pathology reports it was surprising to find all 14 tumors to be of the meningothelial subtype.[18] Around the same time, Kros et al. showed an association between meningiomas of the "anterior skull base" locations (olfactory groove and clinoidal) and an intact chromosome 22 in their series of 42 tumors, and the "anterior skull base" tumors were often MM.[19]

Given these interesting observations and other reports[20,21] suggesting that MM may be unique tumors having a predilection for certain locations of origin, we reviewed our series of meningiomas and sought to test the hypothesis that meningiomas of the midline neuraxis, namely the midline skull base (Fig. 13-1) and the spine, are predominantly of the menigothelial histologic subtype.

For this purpose, we reviewed a total of 794 consecutive surgical cases of cranial and spinal meningiomas operated at our institution. The tumor site of origin was determined from operative reports and preoperative magnetic resonance imaging (MRI) scans. Non–skull base (NSB) locations included convexity, parasagittal, falcine, tentorial, cerebellar convexity,

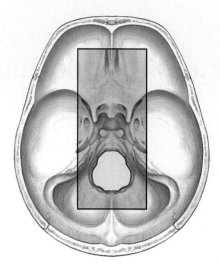

FIG. 13-1. Median/paramedian skull base region is depicted in this drawing by the shaded area inside the square and includes olfactory groove, planum sphenoidale, tuberculum sella, anterior clinoid process, optic sheath/canal, cavernous sinus, cerebello-pontine angle, petroclival, clivus, bony foramina (jugular foramen, hypoglossal canal), and foramen magnum

ventricular, pineal, and scalp. The skull base locations were further divided into the medial and lateral skull base. The medial skull base consisted of olfactory groove, planum sphenoidale, tuberculum sella, anterior clinoid process, optic nerve sheath, cavernous sinus, cerebellopontine angle/ventral petrous, petroclival, clivus, foramen magnum, and neural foramina (jugular foramen and hypoglossal foramen). The lateral skull base included the middle and lateral sphenoid wing, orbitosphenoid, posterior petrous, orbital roof, and temporal fossa floor/temporal bone. Spinal meningiomas were defined as those arising from the meninges caudal to the foramen magnum (Table 13-1).

Overall, among a total of 794 patients with meningiomas initially reviewed, 92.1% (731/794) consisted of the WHO grade I, 5.9% (47/794) grade II, and 2% (16/794) grade III meningiomas.

TABLE 13-1. Classification of Tumor Location in Intracranial Meningiomas.

Skull base		Non–Skull base
Midline	Lateral	
Cavernous sinus	Lateral/ middle sphenoid wing	Convexity
Anterior clinoid	Orbitosphenoid	Parasagittal
Olfactory groove	Posterior petrous	Falcine
Tuberculum sellae	Orbital roof	Cerebellar convexity
Optic sheath	Lateral tentorial temporal bone	Intraventricular
Planum sphenoidale		Pineal
Medial tentorial		
Petroclival		
Foramen magnum		
Bony foramina		

TABLE 13-2. Incidence of Meningothelial Meningiomas According to Location in 731 WHO Grade I Meningiomas.

Site of origin	Incidence of MM
Skull base (n = 279)	**221 (79.2%)**
Midline skull base (n = 219)	*186 (84.9%)*
Cavernous sinus (n = 38)	37 (97.3%)
CPA (n = 30)	23 (76.7%)
Clinoid (n = 30)	25 (83.3%)
Olfactory groove (n = 25)	23 (92%)
Petroclival (n = 25)	21 (84%)
Tuberculum sellae (n = 17)	13 (76.5%)
Foramen magnum (n = 12)	7 (58.3%)
Temporal bone (n = 12)	11 (91.6%)
Optic sheath (n = 12)	11 (91.6%)
Planum sphenoidale (n = 10)	8 (80%)
Other (n = 8)[a]	7 (87.5%)
Lateral skull base (n = 60)	*35 (58.3%)*
Lateral/middle sphenoid wing (n = 32)	24 (75%)
Orbitosphenoid (n = 12)	7 (58.3%)
Posterior petrous (n = 10)	1 (10%)
Orbital roof (n = 6)	3 (50%)
Non–skull base (n = 377)	183 (48.5%)
Spinal (n = 75)	**60 (80%)**
Overall (n = 731)	464 (63.5%)

MM, meningothelial meningiomas; CPA, cerebellopontine angle.
[a] Five clivus menigiomas and two bony foramina meningiomas.

Among the 731 grade I meningiomas, 63.5% (464/731) was MM, 19% (139/731) transitional, 13.5% (99/731) fibrous, 1.8% (13/731) psammomatous, and 2.2% (16/731) consisted of the other miscellaneous histologic subtypes. The tumor sites of origin and the incidence of MM according to these sites are shown in Table 13-2. MM incidence was significantly higher in the midline skull base and spinal locations.

Rarity of Aggressive or Malignant Meningiomas in the Midline Skull Base

There has been a small number of studies in the past showing a predilection for certain locations by aggressive (WHO grade II and III) meningiomas. In an analysis of 9827 meningioma patients of the National Cancer Data Base, McCarthy, et al. reported a small but statistically significant difference in the incidences of atypical or malignant meningiomas between the skull base and non–skull base locations (7.4% in skull base vs 9.7% in non–skull base).[22] Mahmood et al.observed that most atypical and anaplastic meningiomas were located over the cerebral convexities.[23] Maier et al. also reported a higher incidence of atypical or malignant meningiomas in the falcine or convexity locations in their analysis of 1582 patients.[5] To confirm these observations, we also analyzed 63 WHO grade II and III meningiomas and their respective locations of tumor origin.

Among these 63 meningiomas, 47 were grade II and 16 were grade III. The site of origin was the skull base in 10 (15.9%) patients, spine in 1 (1.6%), and non–skull base in the

TABLE 13-3. Incidence of WHO Grade II and Grade III Meningiomas by Site of Origin.

Site	Grade II	Grade III	Grade II + Grade III
Non–skull base ($n = 429$)	39 (9.1%)	13 (3%)	**52 (12.1%)**
Skull base ($n = 289$)	8 (2.8%)	2 (0.7%)	**10 (3.5%)**
Midline ($n = 219$)	6 (2.7%)	2 (0.9%)	8 (3.6%)
Lateral ($n = 70$)	0	2 (2.9%)	2 (2.9%)
Spinal ($n = 76$)	0	1 (1.3%)	**1 (1.3%)**
Total ($n = 794$)	47 (5.9%)	16 (2%)	**63 (7.9%)**

remaining 52 (88.4%). The details regarding the incidence of grade II and grade III histology with regard to the site of origin are shown in Table 13-3

Discussion

In our institutional review, the majority of tumors arising from the midline neuraxis, i.e., the midline skull base and the spine, consisted of WHO grade I meningiomas, and specifically the meningothelial subtype, in contrast to meningiomas arising from non–skull base or the lateral skull base sites. This relative overrepresentation of MM in the midline skull base and the spine suggests that the tumorigenesis of these tumors, and/or the leptomeningeal embryogenesis of the midline neuraxis, may be unique.These results, together with the findings of the previous reports, challenge the traditional notion that meniniomas' wide variation in histologic appearance has no bearing on either the tumor location or their overall biological behavior.[9]

Histologic Subtype vs. Tumor Location

The factors responsible for the differences seen in the histologic characteristics of meningiomas in different locations are largely unknown. However, we believe that a number of mechanisms may be proposed as possible explanations.

Meningioma: The Cells of Origin

The arachnoid membrane constitutes the interface layer between the pachymeninx and the leptomeninx during the meningeal embryogenesis. The outer layers are referred to as the "dural border layer" and are a part of the pachymeninx, whereas the inner layers are referred to as the "arachnoid barrier layer" and are a part of the leptomeninx.[2] The arachnoid cap cells form the outer layer of the arachnoid, whereas the trabecular cells form the inner layers, which are seperated by the basal lamina.[24] Histologically, fibrous and transitional meningioma subtypes have features similar to the fibroblasts found in the deeper layers of the arachnoid close to the subarachnoid space, resembling the cells of the arachnoid trabeculae, while MM resemble the arachnoid cap cells of the outer layers.[19,25,26] The arachnoid cap cells, through an unknown mechanism, may be preferentially transformed to MM in the midline skull base and spinal locations, whereas in other regions this selective transformation of arachnoid cap cells is lost.

Leptomeningeal Embryogenesis

Embryologic studies suggest that meninges covering the brainstem and the spinal cord may have different origins from those of the lateral skull base and convexities. In the early embryo, the primitive mesenchyme around the neural tube condenses to form the primary meninx.[9,27] While the unsegmented mesoderm rostral to the somites contributes to the primary cranial meninx, the somatic counterpart is involved in the formation of the spinal meninges. The neural crest cells combine with the mesenchyme to participate in the development of the hindbrain and spinal pia, whereas the prechordal plate has been offered as having a role in the formation of the tentorium cerebelli. The frontal bone periosteum and the nasal septum cells, both of which are derived from the neural crest cells, contribute to the development of falx cerebri and the adjacent dura.[9,27]

Others have described that the meninges around the brainstem arise from the cephalic mesoderm, whereas the telencephalic meninges likely arise from the neural crest cells.[19,24,28,29] Based on the available information, it is not possible to infer the exact embryogenic source(s) of the leptomeninges of the midline skull base. However, these findings do suggest that the meninges covering the brainstem and spinal cord arise from a clearly different embryologic lineage than the meninges of the cerebral convexity, which may form the basis of the observed predominence of the meningothelial subtype in the central neuraxis. One possibility is that the differential leptomeningeal embryogenesis may result in the predominence of one cell type (cap cells vs. trabecular fibroblasts) in certain locations over the other. The second possibility is that the differential leptomeningeal embryogenesis creates a unique "host" environment, which selectively favors activation of tumorigenesis of MM from activation of the cap cells in the central neuraxis. This view may also be helpful in explaining why meningiomas at certain locations would have a tendency for a more aggressive biological behavior.

Meningioma Tumorigenesis

The development of meningiomas likely results from interactions of genes and environmental factors, such as the NF2 tumor supressor gene, growth factors, Ras signal transduction pathway, telomerase activity, sex hormone receptors, and radiation.[24,30,31] The role of NF2 tumor suppressor gene mutation or protein inactivation has been well demonstrated in all meningiomas, except for the meningothelial subtype.[14–17,24,25,30]

Meningothelial meningiomas have been shown to possess different characteristics at the molecular level in various other studies. For instance, compared to transitional or fibroblastic types, they have significantly higher progesterone receptor (PR) expression.[32] This distinct feature has led Perry et al. to suggest that PR immunohistochemistry may have a diagnostic utility in meningothelial neoplasms.[32] Since PR expression is inversely proportional to the tumor proliferation as well as histologic grade and is, therefore, associated with benign nature,[24,25,33] the increased PR expression in MM may imply a more benign course for this particular subtype than the other grade I tumors. In their recent analysis of 588 patients with WHO grade I meningiomas, Roser et al. also showed a higher PR positivity for MM as compared to fibrous or transitional subtypes.[34] They demonstrated that higher PR status was related to increased time to recurrence and suggested the combined use of PR status and proliferation index as a prognostic tool for benign meningiomas. Sanson et al. have suggested that the loss of chromosome 22 alleles might be a potent genetic marker of the aggresiveness of meningiomas,[35] and since MM show this genetic abnormality very rarely, they may exhibit a more benign phenotype.[31]

In other studies, the expression of matrix metalloproteinases (MMP-2 and MMP-9), which are important mediators of angiogenesis and tumor invasion, is the weakest in MM, as compared to other most common meningioma subtypes.[36] P-glycoprotein (Pgp), a major factor in multidrug resistance, also shows less expression in MM.[37] Interestingly, the expression level of vascular endothelial growth factor (VEGF) has been shown to be higher in MM, however, without any correlation to tumor vascularity or invasiveness.[38] Xenon-enhanced computed tomography studies have shown an increased blood flow in MM as compared to other histologic subtypes, such as fibrous meningiomas,[39] which may have relevance with the increased expression of VEGF in MM. Amplification of INS gene located at the short arm of chromosome 11 and TCL1A gene located at the long arm of chromosome 14 occur more frequently with MM.[36] However, clinical significance of these changes is unknown.

Unique Inherent Characteristics of Skull Base Meningiomas and Their Implications for Tumorigenesis

One possible explanation regarding the lower incidence of aggressive and malignant meningiomas in the skull base could be that skull base meningiomas may be more likely to present with signs and symptoms while tumors are still relatively small, due to their proximity to the cranial nerves and the brain stem. Non–skull base tumors, on the other hand, may remain clinically silent until they reach a large size. This could presumably give the tumor sufficient time to undergo additional molecular alterations resulting in aggressive/malignant transformation. Murphy et al. showed that meningiomas originating at the convexity carry more chromosomal abnormalities than those at the skull base.[40]

Perry et al. have recently reviewed the current knowledge of the genetic changes observed with the histologic progression in meningiomas:[24] Mutation or loss of NF2 gene on chromosome 22 q, loss of 4.1B and 4.1R genes, as well as an increased expression of progesterone receptors are documented in benign meningiomas. In benign but recurrent meningiomas, deletions on 14 q are observed. With progression to atypical histology,

additional deletions (1 p, 6 q, 10, 18 q), gains or amplifications (1 q, 9 q, 12 q, 15 q, 17 q, 20 q), formation of ring or dicentric chromosomes, increase in telomerase activity, overexpression of vascular endothelial growth factor and loss of progesterone receptors are encountered more frequently. Further amplification of 17 q and deletion of 9 p are observed in malignant meningiomas. Lee et al. have reported increased frequency of allelic loss with the progression from grade I to II and III.[41]

Additionally, the natural history of skull base meningiomas may be more benign than for its non–skull base counterparts. The tumor growth rate for asymptomatic meningiomas in all locations has been reported to be 22–32% with follow-up periods of 3 years.[42,43] A similar incidence of 35% has been reported for patients over the age of 70.[44] In another study, with a longer follow-up of 6 years, the tumor progression was detected in 37% of the patients who were initially treated conservatively.[45] Although there is scant information regarding the natural history of meningiomas, in general, as well as for skull base meningiomas, in particular, several recent reports indicate a relatively low growth rate for the tumors of skull base meningiomas, such as optic nerve sheath, cavernous sinus, and petroclival meningiomas.[13,46,47] In a recent study with a mean follow-up of 6 years, only 18% of the patients with petroclival meningiomas showed radiographic progression.[46] Couldwell et al. reported the recurrence incidence as 13% in patients who underwent resection for petroclival meningiomas.[48] In this series, close to one third of the recurrences were histologically malignant. The study of Jung et al. looked at the growth rates and incidences of petroclival meningiomas that initially had a subtotal resection and also revealed a relatively low growth rate for the residual tumors.[49] Analyzing the raw data reported by Nakamura et al., which looked into the patients with incidental meningiomas who were initially followed conservatively, 3 of the 28 (11%) skull base meningiomas progressed and were eventually operated as compared to 3 of the 13 (23%) non–skull base meningiomas.[50] All of the 6 patients who progressed had grade I histology.

In this context, one may assume that this more indolent course of skull base meningiomas may in part be due to (1) the inherent low incidence of aggressive or malignant histologic types in skull base locations and 2) the natural history, which seems more benign than for meningiomas of other locations.

Implications for Past and Future Meningioma Research and Treatment

Treatment strategies precisely targeting the molecular abnormalities underlying tumorigenesis make a promising future treatment modality. In this regard, awareness of a possible different tumorigenic background of MM as compared to the other grade I meningioma subtypes becomes important. In the past, trials have shown no benefit from antiprogesterone drugs in the management of meningiomas. Since PR is significantly more expressed in MM,[32–34] it would be interesting to see the results of new antiprogesterone receptor trials focusing only on MM. Similarly, anti-VEGF agents, which appear to be promising for the treatment of other types of vascular tumors, may be a potential venue to explore in the treatment of MM as well. Significantly lower expression of drug-resistance factors in MM[37] may also imply a more encouraging outcome with future antineoplastic agent trials in the treatment of meningiomas with more specifically defined patient populations.

Finally, meningiomas located in the central skull base, which are predominantly of the meningothelial subtype, are difficult tumors to completely and safely remove. In the future, once the exact mechanism of MM tumorigenesis is fully elucidated and molecular treatment specifically targeting MM is made available, risky surgery may be avoided and the appropriate molecular therapy administered with the confidence level approaching 85%, on average, to 97% for tumors of certain location such as the cavernous sinus (Table 13-2). Surgical indications, especially for the high-risk central skull base meningiomas, therefore, may be re-evaluated and revised in the future.

Summary

Meningiomas of the central neuraxis are predominantly of the meningothelial histologic subtype. The increasing data on genetic and topographic characteristics of MM suggest that meningiomas of the central neuraxis may indeed be a unique subgroup of meningiomas. We believe that future studies focusing on genetic characteristics and treatment of meningiomas should be designed with this new information in mind as opposed to accepting all the histologic subtypes of WHO grade I meningiomas as a homogenous group. Additionally, the WHO grade II and grade III meningiomas are found to be rare in the skull base and spinal locations. This information may support a more conservative management strategy at the skull base, especially when the risk-benefit ratio of aggressive surgery is not so favorable such as in small and/or incidental skull base meningiomas. On the other hand, 12.1% incidence of atypical or anaplastic histology should encourage the surgeon to plan as extensive resection as possible in non–skull base locations.

References

1. Kleihues P, Louis DN, Scheithauer BW, Rorke LB, Reifenberger G, Burger PC, Cavenee WK. The WHO classification of tumors of the nervous system. J Neuropathol Exp Neurol 2002;61:215–25.

2. Louis DN, Scheithauer BW, Budka H, et al: Meningiomas, in Kleihues P, Cavenee WK (eds): Pathology and genetic of tumors of the nervous system. Lyon: IARC Press, 2000.

3. Jaaskelainen J, Haltia M, Servo A. Atypical and anaplastic meningiomas: radiology, surgery, radiotherapy, and outcome. Surg Neurol 1986;25:233–42.

4. Kolles H, Niedermayer I, Schmitt C, Henn W, Feld R, Steudel WI, Zang KD, Feiden W. Triple approach for diagnosis and grading of meningiomas: histology, morphometry of Ki-67/

5. Maier H, Ofner D, Hittmair A, Kitz K, Budka H. Classic, atypical, and anaplastic meningioma: three histopathological subtypes of clinical relevance. J Neurosurg 1992;77:616–23.

6. Perry A, Stafford SL, Scheithauer BW, Suman VJ, Lohse CM. Meningioma grading: an analysis of histologic parameters. Am J Surg Pathol 1997;21:1455–65.

7. Palma L, Celli P, Franco C, Cervoni L, Cantore G. Long-term prognosis for atypical and malignant meningiomas: a study of 71 surgical cases. J Neurosurg 1997;86:793–800.

8. Perry A, Scheithauer BW, Stafford SL, Lohse CM, Wollan PC. "Malignancy" in meningiomas: a clinicopathologic study of 116 patients, with grading implications. Cancer 1999;85:2046–56.

9. Russell D, Rubenstein L. Pathology of Tumours of the Central Nervous System. Baltimore: Williams and Wilkins, 1989:449–532.

10. Rouleau GA, Merel P, Lutchman M, et al. Alteration in a new gene encoding a putative membrane-organizing protein causes neuro-fibromatosis type 2. Nature 1993;363:515–21.

11. Trofatter JA, MacCollin MM, Rutter JL, et al. A novel moesin-, ezrin-, radixin-like gene is a candidate for the neurofibromatosis 2 tumor suppressor. Cell 1993;72:791–800.

12. Lee JH, Sundaram V, Stein DJ, Kinney SE, Stacey DW, Golubic M. Reduced expression of schwannomin/merlin in human sporadic meningiomas. Neurosurgery 1997;40:578–87.

13. Egan RA, Lessell S. A contribution to the natural history of optic nerve sheath meningiomas. Arch Ophthalmol 2002;120:1505–8.

14. Lekanne Deprez RH, Bianchi AB, Groen NA, Seizinger BR, Hagemeijer A, van Drunen E, Bootsma D, Koper JW, Avezaat CJ, Kley N. Frequent NF2 gene transcript mutations in sporadic meningiomas and vestibular schwannomas. Am J Hum Genet 1994;54:1022–9.

15. Papi L, De Vitis LR, Vitelli F, Ammannati F, Mennonna P, Montali E, Bigozzi U. Somatic mutations in the neurofibromatosis type 2 gene in sporadic meningiomas. Hum Genet 1995;95:347–51.

16. Wada K, Maruno M, Suzuki T, Kagawa N, Hashiba T, Fujimoto Y, Hashimoto N, Izumoto S, Yoshimine T, Chromosomal and genetic aberrations differ with meningioma subtype. Brain Tumor Pathol 2004;21:127–33.

17. Wellenreuther R, Kraus JA, Lenartz D, Menon AG, Schramm J, Louis DN, Ramesh V, Gusella JF, Wiestler OD, von Deimling A. Analysis of the neurofibromatosis 2 gene reveals molecular variants of meningioma. Am J Pathol 1995;146:827–32.

18. Lee JH, Jeun SS, Evans J, Kosmorsky G. Surgical management of clinoidal meningiomas. Neurosurgery 2001;48:1012–9.

19. Kros J, de Greve K, van Tilborg A, Hop W, Pieterman H, Avezaat C, Lekanne Dit Deprez R, Zwarthoff W. NF2 status of meningiomas is associated with tumour localization and histology. J Pathol 2001;194:367–72.

20. Horning ED, Kernohan JW. Meningiomas of the sphenoidal ridge: a clinicopathologic study. J Neuropathol Exp Neurol 1950;9:373–84.

21. Jellinger K, Slowik F. Histological subtypes and prognostic problems in meningiomas. J Neurol 1975;208:279–98.

22. McCarthy BJ, Davis FG, Freels S, Surawicz TS, Damek DM, Grutsch J, Menck HR, Laws ER, Jr. Factors associated with survival in patients with meningioma. J Neurosurg 1998;88:831–9.

23. Mahmood A, Caccamo DV, Tomecek FJ, Malik GM. Atypical and malignant meningiomas: a clinicopathological review. Neurosurgery 1993;33:955–63.

Feulgen stainings, and cytogenetics. Acta Neurochir (Wien) 1995;137:174–81.

24. Perry A, Gutmann DH, Reifenberger G. Molecular pathogenesis of meningiomas. J Neurooncol 2004;70:183–202.

25. Evans JJ, Lee JH, Suh J, et al. Meningiomas. In: Moore AJ, Newell DW, editors: Neurosurgery, principles and practice. London: Springer Verlag, 2005:205–33.

26. Kepes JJ. Presidential address: the histopathology of meningiomas. A reflection of origins and expected behavior? J Neuropathol Exp Neurol 1986;45:95–107.

27. O'Rahilly R, Muller F. The meninges in human development. J Neuropathol Exp Neurol 1986;45:588–608.

28 Catala M. Embryonic and fetal development of structures associated with the cerebro-spinal fluid in man and other species. Part I: The ventricular system, meninges and choroid plexuses. Arch Anat Cytol Pathol 1998;46:153–69.

29 Couly GF, Le Douarin NM. Mapping of the early neural primordium in quail-chick chimeras. II. The prosencephalic neural plate and neural folds: implications for the genesis of cephalic human congenital abnormalities. Dev Biol 1987;120:198–214.

30 Evans JJ, Jeun SS, Lee JH, Harwalkar JA, Shoshan Y, Cowell JK, Golubic M. Molecular alterations in the neurofibromatosis type 2 gene and its protein rarely occurring in meningothelial meningiomas. J Neurosurg 2001;94:111–7.

31. Sanson M, Cornu P. Biology of meningiomas. Acta Neurochir (Wien) 2000;142: 493–505.

32. Wolfsberger S, Doostkam S, Boecher-Schwarz HG, Roessler K, van Trotsenburg M, Hainfellner JA, Knosp E. Progesterone-receptor index in meningiomas: correlation with clinico-pathological parameters and review of the literature. Neurosurg Rev 2004;27:238–45.

33. Perry A, Cai DX, Scheithauer BW, Swanson PE, Lohse CM, Newsham IF, Weaver A, Gutmann DH. Merlin, DAL-1, and progesterone receptor expression in clinicopathologic subsets of meningiomas: a correlative immunohistochemical study of 175 cases. J Neuropathol Exp Neurol 2000;59:872–9.

34. Roser F, Nakamura M, Bellinzona M, Rosahl SK, Ostertag H, Samii M. The prognostic value of progesterone receptor status in meningiomas. J Clin Pathol 2004;57:1033–7.

35. Sanson M, Richard S, Delattre O, Poliwka M, Mikol J, Philippon J, Thomas G. Allelic loss on chromosome 22 correlates with histopathological predictors of recurrence of meningiomas. Int J Cancer 1992;50:391–4.

36. Rooprai HK, van Meter TE, Robinson SD, King A, Rucklidge GJ, Pilkington GJ. Expression of MMP-2 and -9 in short term cultures of meningioma: influence of hitological subtype. Int J Mol Med 2003;12:977–81.

37. Andersson U, Malmer B, Bergenheim AT, Brannstrom T, Henriksson H. Heterogeneity in the expression of markers for drug resistance in brain tumors. Clin Neuropathol 2004;23: 21–7.

38. Lamszus K, Lengler U, Schmidt NO, Stavrou D, Ergun S, Westphal M. Vascular endothelial growth factor, hepatocyte growth factor/ scatter factor, basic fribroblast growth factor and placenta growth factor in human meningiomas and their relation to angiogenesis in malignancy. Neurosurgery 2000;46:938–48.

39. Nakatsuka M, Mizuno S. Investigation of blood flow in meningothelial and fibrous meningiomas by xenon-enhanced CT scanning. Neurol Res 2000;22:615–9.

40. Murphy M, Pykett MJ, Harnish P, Zang KD, George DL. Identification and characterization of genes differentially expressed in meningiomas. Cell Growth Differ 1993;4:715–22.

41. Lee JYK, Finkelstein S, Hamilton RL, Rekha R, King JT, Omalu B. Loss of heterozygosity analysis of benign, atypical and anaplastic meningiomas. Neurosurgery 2004;55:1163–73.

42. Kuratsu J, Kochi M, Ushio Y. Incidence and clinical features of asymptomatic meningiomas. J Neurosurg 2000;92:766–70.

43. Olivero WC, Lister JR, Wlwood PW. The natural history and growth rate of asymptomatic meningiomas: a review of 60 patients. J Neurosurg 2004;83:222–4.

44. Niiro M, Yatsushiro K, Nakamura K, et al. Natural history of elderly patients with asymptomatic meningiomas. J Neurol Neurosurg Psychiatry 2000;68:25–8.

45. Herscovici Z, Rappaport Z, Sulkes J, et al. Natural history of conservatively treated meningiomas. Neurology 2004;63:1133–4.

46. Bindal R, Goodman JM, Kawasaki A, Purvin V, Kuzma B. The natural history of untreated skull base meningiomas. Surg Neurol 2003;59:87–92.

47. Saeed P, Rootman J, Nugent RA, White VA, Mackenzie IR, Koornneef L. Optic nerve sheath meningiomas. Ophthalmology 2003;110:2019–30.

48. Couldwell WT, Fukushima T, Giannotta SL, Weiss MH. Petroclival meningiomas: surgical experience in 109 cases. J Neurosurg 1996;84:20–8.

49. Jung HW, Yoo H, Paek SH, Choi KS. Long-term outcome and growth rate of subtotally resected petroclival meningiomas: experience with 38 cases. Neurosurgery 2000;46:567–75.

50. Nakamura M, Roser F, Michel J, Jacobs C, Samii M. The natural hsitory of incidental meningiomas. Neurosurgery 2003;53:62–71.

14
Radiation-Induced Meningioma: Historical Perspective, Presentation, Management, and Genetics

Yigal Shoshan, Sergey Spektor, Guy Rosenthal, Shifra Fraifeld, and Felix Umansky

Historical Perspective

On November 8, 1895, while doing cathode ray research, Wilhelm Conrad Roentgen (1845–1923) discovered the x-ray. By mid-January 1896, scientific and news articles on x-rays appeared in *Lancet*, the *British Medical Journal*, *Nature*, *Science*, and leading newspapers worldwide. Nearly 1000 articles and several textbooks on x-rays and radioactivity were published in 1896.[1]

A few months after Roentgen's breakthrough, Henri Becquerel described the radiation-emitting properties of uranium, and Marie and Pierre Curie discovered polonium and radium—two new radioactive elements. Roentgen, Becquerel, the Curies, and more than 20 other scientists received Nobel Prizes in Physics, Chemistry, or Medicine for groundbreaking research relating to x-rays and radiation during the twentieth century.

The wide-ranging diagnostic and therapeutic value of x-rays was quickly apparent, and for a long time radiation was freely used with almost no protection for patients, physicians, or auxiliary personnel (Fig. 14-1). However, the widespread benefits of x-rays were offset by their harmful effects. The great majority of the diagnostic radiologists of this era suffered hand injuries or developed cancers of the skin or other organs, and many succumbed to leukemia[2]. Precautionary measures were suggested in scholarly journals as early as 1916,[2] and studies describing the harmful effects of radiation appeared in scientific journals before World War II, particularly in German- and French-language medical publications.[3,4] But the general public and a great part of the medical community remained unaware of the dangers of radiation until after atomic bombs were dropped on Hiroshima and Nagasaki in 1945 and were later tested in the atmosphere.[2] Only in the 1950s and 1960s did discussions of risks and constructive suggestions for limiting exposure begin to appear in the lay press.[5–7]

Human neural tissue was long considered relatively resistant to the carcinogenic effects of ionizing radiation by many,[8,9] even though evidence of functional and morphologic changes following irradiation of the brain and spinal cord in patients and experimental animals was in fact recognized in the 1920s, when therapeutic irradiation was first used routinely for cancer treatment.[3,4] The long-term or delayed side effects of irradiation on neural tissue are now known to include visual deterioration, hearing loss, hormonal disturbances, vasculopathy, brain and bone necrosis, atrophy, demyelination, calcification, fatty replacement of bone marrow, and the induction of new central nervous system (CNS) neoplasms.[10] A dose-effect relationship has been documented for many ill effects, including tumor induction.[2,11–15] Radiation-induced changes in neural tissue, bone, and superficial and deep soft tissues are increasingly evident radiologically.[16]

Radiation-Induced Meningioma

Many neoplasms within the CNS have been reported as radiogenic in origin, but radiation-induced meningioma (RIM) is the most common radiation-induced brain neoplasm, and radiation is the only proven cause of meningioma to date.[10] Harrison et al.[17] grouped RIM into three categories: those arising from high-dose radiation (>20 Gy), those from intermediate doses (10–20 Gy), and those secondary to low-dose radiation (<10 Gy). Other authors define doses above 10 Gy as high.[18,19] Average latency between radiation therapy (RT) and tumor occurrence ranges from 19 to 35 years and varies with dose,[17] but RIM has been reported with a latency period of 63 years.[20]

High-Dose RIM

The first report of RIM appeared in 1953 when Mann et al.[21] presented a case report describing a 4-year-old girl who developed a meningioma in the irradiated field of a previously treated optic nerve glioma. Her meningioma eventually became malignant. Several authors have summarized reports of up to 126 cases of high-dose RIM reported in the literature from 1953 to 2002.[18,19,22–26] Radiation doses in these reports range from 22 to 87 Gy. The majority of high-dose RIM patients were irradiated as children, and there is a strong female preponderance. Mean reported latency is approximately 19 years,[18,25] but tends to be

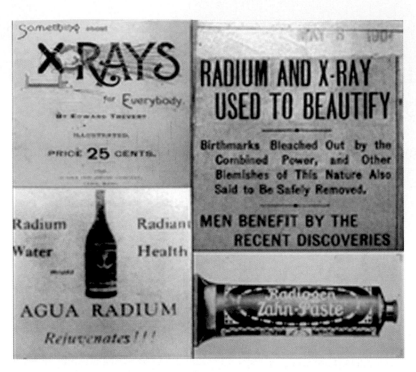

FIG. 14-1. X-rays for everybody—four examples illustrating the free use of x-rays in the first years following Roentgen's discovery, when risks from exposure were unknown

shorter in patients irradiated at younger ages and following higher doses of radiation.[17–19,23] Incidence of high-dose RIM is expected to rise with increasing survival of young brain tumor patients who require RT for their initial disease.[18]

Low-Dose RIM Following Irradiation for Tinea Capitis

Among the early uses of therapeutic radiation was treatment of tinea capitis, most often with the Keinbock-Adamson (KA) technique, which was designed to irradiate the entire scalp as uniformly as possible using exposure of five overlapping treatment areas.[27] Phantom dosimetry studies showed that when this technique was applied conscientiously the radiation dose to the scalp ranged from 5 to 8 Gy, the surface dose to the brain was approximately 1.4–1.5 Gy, and the skull base received an average of 0.7 Gy[28,29] (Fig. 14-2).

Transient somnolence, the first neurologic symptom reported as a consequence of low-dose irradiation for treatment of tinea capitis, was reported in 1929.[30] Additional symptoms and signs, including epilation, atrophic and telangiectatic changes in the scalp, epilepsy, hemiparesis, emotional changes, and dilatation of the ventricles, were described in 1932 and 1935 in two patients who had been irradiated for tinea capitis as young children.[31,32] However, irradiation remained an acceptable treatment for fungal infections of the scalp until the introduction of griseofulvin circa 1960.[33–35]

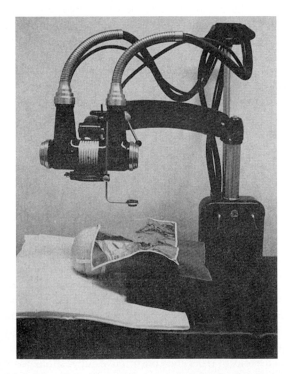

FIG. 14-2. Low-dose therapeutic x-ray machine for the treatment of tinea capitis. The head and x-ray tube are shown arranged for exposure. Most tinea capitis patients were treated using the Adamson-Keinbock technique. Five overlapping areas were exposed to provide uniform irradiation of the scalp

The first large patient series describing harmful side effects related to radiation for tinea capitis was published in 1966, when Albert et al.[28] reported a disproportionate incidence of cancer, mental illness, and permanent damage to the scalp hair among 1908 irradiated patients compared with 1801 nonirradiated controls. Both groups were treated at New York University Hospital between 1940 and 1958. Increased incidence of mental disorders and psychiatric hospitalization, as well as long-term electroencephalographic changes and permanent functional damage to the CNS, were also described in a later report from these authors on irradiated patients.[29] Reports from other institutions followed.[17,36–40] Additional large series of patients who were irradiated for tinea capitis in the former Soviet Union supported this relationship.[41]

Soffer et al.[40] found a significantly higher number of calvarial tumors ($p < 0.001$), a higher proportion of multiple meningiomas, and an increased number of histologically malignant meningiomas ($p < 0.01$) in a group of 42 low-dose RIM patients compared with 84 patients with sporadic meningioma (SM).

The largest body of controlled research on RIM secondary to irradiation for tinea capitis has been published by physicians at the Sheba Medical Center in Tel Aviv, Israel, in a series of reports between 1974 and 2005. A 1974 retrospective cohort study by Modan et al.[42] showed significantly higher risk of malignant and benign head and neck tumors among approximately 11,000 Israeli adults treated during childhood for tinea capitis. In 1988 Ron et al.[43] reported that radiation of only 1–2 Gy received in childhood resulted in a 9.5-fold increase in the incidence of meningiomas (as well as an 18.8 relative risk of vestibular schwannoma) in a follow-up study of the same population.

More recently Sadetzki et al.[13,44,45] published a series of studies based on long-term follow-up of this population more than 30 years after treatment. These studies found that the risk for developing both benign and malignant brain tumors was positively associated with dose. Excess relative risk (ERR) of developing benign meningiomas was 2.64 for doses ≤ 1.2 Gy and rose to 18.82 for doses more than 2.6 Gy.[13] This analysis showed a lower patient age at diagnosis, higher prevalence of calvarial tumors, higher proportion of multiple meningiomas, higher recurrence rates (nonsignificant), and genetic variability among RIM patients in comparison with a cohort of patients presenting with SM. The mean latency period in this tinea capitis low-dose RIM population was approximately 36 years.[44,45]

Low-Dose RIM Due to Dental X-Ray Examination

In 1953, Nolan[46,47] published studies showing surface radiation doses to the face and neck from dental x-ray series of the full mouth. He reported significant blood changes in patients exposed to 1.15–2.8 Gy during full-mouth x-ray examinations. He observed that the full-mouth series delivered lines of radiation that converge near the meninges, producing points of high ionization.

Nearly 30 years later, in 1980, Preston-Martin et al.[48] published a study of women in Los Angeles County diagnosed with meningioma in the years 1972–1975 and a cohort of matched controls showing a strong association between early exposure (age < 20 years) to medical and dental x-rays to the head and neck, and meningioma. The odds ratio for developing meningioma after 1–10 exposures to full-mouth x-rays was 1.8, and for more than 10 exposures the odds ratio rose to 4.9. Risk was higher among individuals who received their first diagnostic dental x-rays as children or teenagers and those who had their first full-mouth dental x-ray series before 1945 when doses were higher. In 15 of 22 patients (68%) with exposure to more than 10 full-mouth x-ray series who developed meningiomas, tumors were located in the tentorial or subtentorial region.

A more recent case-control study in Sweden[49] showed that dental radiography after age 25 years also increases the risk for meningioma development. In 2004 a new population-based case control study in western Washington state[50] reported that a history of ≥ 6 full-mouth dental x-ray series over a lifetime was associated with a significantly increased risk of meningioma several decades later (odds ratio 2.06). Associations were stronger when only women were considered. Evidence for a dose-response relationship and for greater risk from early exposure to x-rays was lacking in this relatively small (200 patients, 400 controls) study.

RIM in Survivors of Atomic Explosions at Hiroshima and Nagasaki

During the first 10 years after atomic bombs were dropped on Hiroshima and Nagasaki in August 1945, an excess number of leukemia cases among survivors was reported and linked to radiation exposure. But the question of whether survivors had a higher risk of developing solid tumors was still being strongly debated in the 1950s.[51] A 1960 tumor registry report by Harada and Ishida[52] was the first study to demonstrate a clear relationship between solid cancer incidence and distance from hypocenter.

In 1994, nearly 50 years after the bombs were dropped, Shibata et al.[53] showed a statistically significant relationship between meningioma incidence and distance from hypocenter in Nagasaki survivors. Subsequent studies confirmed Shibata's findings in survivors from both cities.[12,14] Shintani et al.[14,15] reported incidence of 6.3, 7.6, and 20.0 cases of RIM per 100,000 population among Hiroshima survivors exposed at 1.5–2.0, 1.0–1.5, and <1.0 km from hypocenter, respectively, compared to 3.0 cases per 100,000 among nonexposed individuals in Japan. Incidence among survivors rose earlier for those within 2.5 km of the center and continued to rise for all survivors as the study closed in 1992. Preston et al.[11] found that excess risks were higher for women than for men and for those exposed during childhood than those exposed as adults.

In summary, history shows that even low doses of radiation lead to elevated risk of RIM. There is higher risk of meningioma and shorter latency as radiation dose increases. Irradiation at a younger age appears to increase the risk of developing meningioma and shorten the latency. As is the case with SM, RIM incidence is higher in women than men. RIM location corresponds to the treatment field. RIM is more aggressive and recurs more frequently than sporadic meningioma. Cellular and genetic characteristics also vary.

The purpose of this chapter is to review the unique aspects of presentation and management of patients with RIM.

Clinical Presentation

Meningioma is the most common intracranial neoplasm induced by cranial irradiation.[54,55] RIM differs from SM in age at presentation, aggressiveness, and rate of recurrence.

Patient age at RIM presentation is linked to the age at which exposure to radiation occurred and to radiation dose. Higher-dose RT and earlier exposure result in shorter latency periods, and thus younger age at RIM diagnosis. Mean age at presentation is reported as 29.2–35 years following high-dose RT[17,24,25,38,56,57] and 45– 58 years after low-dose treatment[17,39,40,58]. Meningiomas not associated with radiation commonly arise in the fifth and sixth decades of life[59].

SM typically displays strong female predominance. Female/male incidence approaches 2/1 in most series, and the difference is greatest in older age groups.[60] Some studies have suggested a change in gender incidence for low-dose RIM. Albert et al.[28] reported female/male incidence of 1/6.3 but suggested that these findings be viewed in reference to epidemiologic data, which show that approximately 80% of patients undergoing RT for tinea capitis were male in these studies. Rubinstein et al.[39] and Soffer et al.[40] reported female/male incidence of 0.87/1 and 1.1/1, respectively, in low-dose RIM patients. Sadetzki et al.[44] reported female/male incidence of 1.9/1 in the Israeli low-dose RIM group versus 2.1/1 in SM patients. Since radiation treatment was equally distributed between boys and girls in the Israeli cohort, Sadetzki et al. concluded that any change in gender distribution could not be attributed to differences in exposure.

Sadamori et al.[12] reported female predominance of 3.5/1 in 45 patients operated for meningioma after exposure to the atomic bomb in Nagasaki. There are no large series of RIM patients subsequent to high- or intermediate-dose RT. However Strojan, et al.[19] reported a female predominance of 1.33/1 in a survey of 126 cases of high-dose RIM reported in the literature.

Scanty hair, or alopecia, and an atrophic scalp are hallmarks of irradiation. Although no evidence has been presented in the literature, it is the impression of the authors that the incidence of microcephaly is increased in low-dose RIM patients compared to the general population (Fig 14-3). We assume that microcephaly results from premature closure of the skull sutures secondary to irradiation of the head administered to young children. In addition, patients may have telangiectasia and occasionally keratosis.[39] These findings are striking. When they are present in conjunction with neurologic complaints,

suspicion of meningioma should be raised and appropriate imaging studies ordered. Rubinstein et al.[39] reported that a large percentage of patients (56%) come to clinical attention with seizure disorder. This may reflect in part the large percentage of patients with calvarial location of tumor in that series. Other common findings on neurologic examination include motor or sensory deficits, mental deterioration, and signs of increased intracranial pressure.[39,59]

Latency

The latency period between RT and the clinical diagnosis of meningioma varies with radiation dose and age at initial treatment. Sadetzki et al.[44] reported 36.3 years average latency (range 12–49 years) in the Israeli low-dose cohort study. In a thorough review of the literature, Harrison et al.[17] calculated a mean duration of 35.2 years between low-dose RT (<10 Gy) and clinical diagnosis of meningioma. In patients receiving moderate-dose (10–20 Gy) and high-dose (>20 Gy) RT, the latency period was shorter—26.1 and 19.5 years, respectively.

In a retrospective series of 10 meningiomas induced by high-dose cranial irradiation, Mack and Wilson[61] found a mean latency of 24 years from irradiation to tumor diagnosis. They also noted that age at irradiation was correlated with tumor latency, as patients who were younger at the time of irradiation had shorter intervals to diagnosis. Summarizing 126 reported cases of high-dose RIM, Strojan et al.[19] found average latency of 18.7 years and also noted shorter latency to tumor formation in patients irradiated at younger ages. Ghim et al.[23] found a mean latency of 10.8 years (range 5–15.5) in a literature review of 13 pediatric high-dose RIM patients (mean age at diagnosis 13 years, range 6–18 years) treated for brain tumors at an average age of 2.5 years. A latency period as short as 14 months following high-dose irradiation for a posterior fossa tumor in an 11-year-old boy has been reported.[62]

Location and Mutlipolicity

Several large series from Israel have documented a primarily calvarial location for RIM in patients treated for tinea capitis by the KA technique. In the series of Rubinstein et al.,[39] 51% of tumors were falcine or parasagittal in location, and 44% were on the convexity. Soffer et al.[40] reported 81% of tumors to be calvarial, and Sadetzki et al.[44] reported 59.2% of tumors to be calvarial in location. However, as pointed out by Mack and Wilson,[61] the predominance of calvarial location is not surprising, given that the calvarium is the primary site of radiation exposure in these patients, who were treated by the KA technique for tinea capitis.

Epidemiologic studies of patients receiving full-mouth dental x-ray demonstrated that skull base meningiomas are more common following this type of radiation exposure.[48] When high-dose radiation is given for the treatment of brain

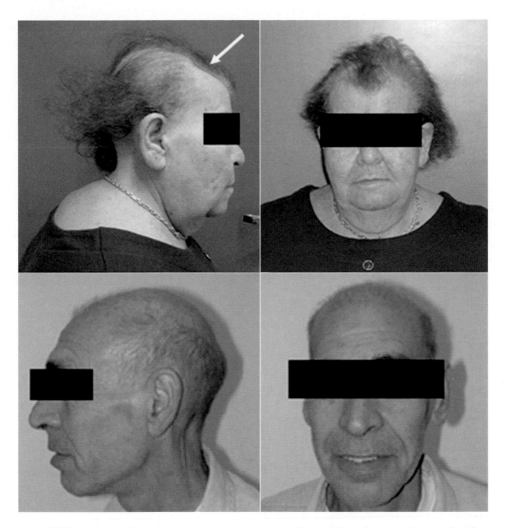

FIG. 14-3. Characteristics of RIM patients. Note scanty hair, or alopecia, as well as relative microcephaly. A defect from craniectomy is seen (arrow) in a patient who has undergone five surgeries to treat recurrent RIM

tumors, meningiomas of the skull base were found in 4–19 % of cases.[25,39,40,63] Ghim et al.[23] found that 11 of 13 pediatric high-dose RIM were located in the calvarial area.

These reports suggest that location of RIM is related primarily to the site of exposure,[48] although referral patterns may also influence data on RIM location. In Al-Mefty's RIM series, and in the authors' experience (unpublished data), a significant proportion of these tumors are located at the skull base. This likely reflects referral patterns to skull-base centers.[22] The authors frequently encounter basal locations among low-dose (tinea capitis) RIM patients treated in their skull base center. Variability in location may also suggest that the KA technique was not consistently applied, and thus irradiated fields and delivered dose varied across patients.

The reported incidence of multiple lesions is elevated in both low- and high-dose RIM patients and ranges from 4.6 to 31.3% of cases[22,39,40] (Fig. 14-4). In comparison, rates of multiplicity in meningiomas not associated with RT are about 1–2%.[64–66]

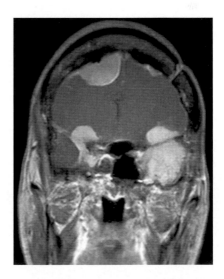

FIG. 14-4 Multiplicity of RIM. Coronal T1-weighted postgadolinium MRI of a patient with multiple radiation-induced meningiomas. Note bilateral sphenoid ridge and temporal fossa meningiomas, as well as bilateral convexity meningiomas

Histopathology

Histologic subtypes of RIM are not different from those for SM, with meningotheliomatous, transitional, and fibroblastic being the most common.[22,40]

Histologic features of RIM have been reviewed by Rubinstein et al.,[39] who reported four distinctive characteristics: (1) a high degree of cellularity; (2) pleomorphic nuclei with great variation in nuclear size, shape, and chromatin density; (3) numerous multinucleated and giant cells; and (4) nuclei with vacuolated inclusions. In addition, they noted frequent mitoses, psammoma bodies, foam cells, and thickened blood vessels that did not stain for amyloid. Soffer et al.[40] noted high cellularity, nuclear pleomorphism, an increased mitotic rate, focal necrosis, bone invasion, and tumor infiltration of the brain in a series of 42 low-dose RIM patients. Louis et al.[67] described RIM as more commonly atypical or aggressive and multifocal, with higher proliferation indices than SM. Musa et al.[18] reported 23% incidence of atypia or malignancy among 79 cases of high-dose RIM (including 69 cases from the literature). This represented a significantly higher incidence of more aggressive histologic subtypes in the high-dose irradiated patients in comparison with 262 SM in this study, and the authors termed the higher overall rate of atypia/anaplasia an important distinguishing feature of high-dose RIM.

In view of the higher rate of atypia and anaplasia, it is not surprising that RIM may demonstrate more aggressive biological and clinical behavior.[17,25,37,39,40,58] These tumors have high rates of recurrence following surgery and radiation therapy and present distinct challenges for the neurosurgeon and neuro-oncologist.

Management of Radiation-Induced Meningioma

Imaging techniques for RIM are comparable to those used for SM, and appearance on MRI and CT is also consistent (Fig. 14-5). Angiography may be considered in some patients for detailed visualization of tumor vascular anatomy.

Surgical removal remains the treatment of choice in most cases of RIM. These tumors often present special problems for the neurosurgeon. Complete and safe excision of these meningiomas often may not be possible because of their aggressive nature, multiplicity, and higher propensity to involve vessels, cranial nerves, and bony structures. These issues need to be considered in the preoperative planning process. Paradoxically, stereotactic radiosurgery (SR) or fractionated stereotactic radiotherapy (FSR) may be appropriate adjuncts to surgery or may take the place of surgery in some high-risk patients in spite of the radiation-related etiology of RIM.

Surgery

The most important point to consider in planning the approach to surgery for RIM is often scalp atrophy. Tumor multiplicity is a second major consideration in many RIM patients.

Planning the skin incision is critical in treating RIM. The scalp is frequently atrophic and poorly vascularized in these patients. Atrophy varies from a slight to very bad, perhaps depending on the dose of radiation received. In some cases the thickness of the entire galeal/skin flap may be only 1.5–2 mm. Careful planning and meticulous surgical technique are required to avoid complications of CSF leak and skin flap dehiscence. Because of the propensity for recurrence of RIM, especially in cases of multiple meningiomas, multiple incisions may be needed, and this fact should be taken into account. It may be appropriate to include a plastic surgeon on the team.

If healthy tissue at the periphery of the atrophic scalp is available it should be used preferentially.[17]

We noticed that maximal skin damage and atrophy occurs in convexity/vertex areas, while in the basal areas (low forehead, low temporal, or occipital areas) tissues are better preserved and better vascularized. In such cases, the incisions may be placed lower than usual, in areas where the skin is healthier. The authors avoid use of hemostatic clamps or coagulation in order to avoid extra skin damage and also to prevent drying and shrinkage of the skin edges. Linear or slightly curved incisions are preferable to horseshoe contours. As always, it is prudent to minimize the size of the surgical flap to the extent possible.

Wound closure may also differ from the routine in other procedures. In some patients the scalp is sufficiently atrophic that it cannot accept additional sutures for multilayer closure, especially in patients with convexity meningiomas. If the scalp is only 1–2 mm thick, the authors do not suture galea aponeurosis with vicryl. Instead we close with a single layer of nylon 3-0 sutures, running with or without locking. On the one hand, it must be understood during closure that this is a single, watertight layer, which must prevent CSF leak. But on the other hand, skin necrosis with dire consequences can result if stitches are closed too tightly. Staples are not suitable in this situation. They provide poor approximation and can easily damage such thin, fragile skin. In addition, staples do not provide hermetic closure. Considering the difficulties of recurrent surgeries in patients with atrophic scalp, we recommend that every effort should be made to reduce the number of potential surgeries by removal of two or even three meningiomas in a single procedure whenever possible in patients with multiple meningiomas.

As discussed previously, a large percentage of RIM are calvarial in location. If these are parasagittal or falcine meningiomas, assessing patency of the superior sagittal sinus prior to surgery is critical for operative planning. In our experience, MRI with MR venography is the examination of choice to assess sinus patency, although in rare cases an angiogram may be required. As with SM, preoperative embolization may be considered for tumors demonstrating a high degree of vascularity.

Obtaining wide resection margins of the involved dura is vital, given the high propensity for recurrence.[68–72] The tumor often involves underlying/overlying bone, and when this occurs resection of the osseous portion of the tumor should be performed,[17,39,40,72,73] as bony invasion has been implicated in

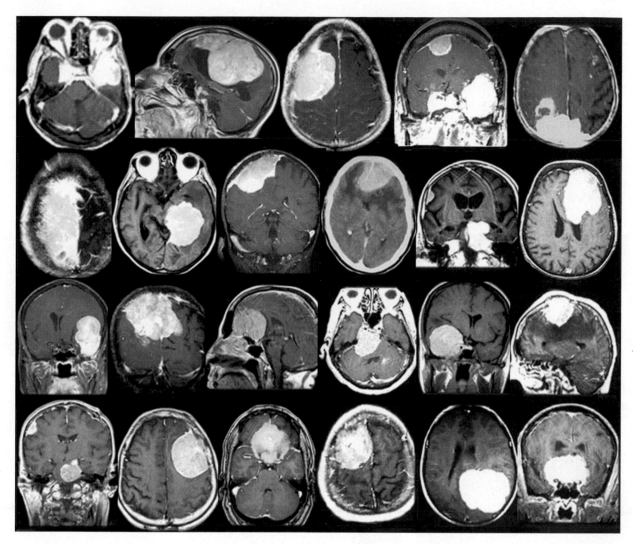

FIG. 14-5. Collage of RIM images—representative images of RIM patients treated at Hadassah–Hebrew University Medical Center in recent years

increasing risk of recurrence.[70,71] When we encounter or suspect bone flap invasion, it has been our practice to autoclave the flap. When the tumor is located in the skull base or involves one of the major cranial sinuses and it is not possible to achieve a wide resection margin, recurrence rates are higher.[59,71,74]

Case Illustration

A 66-year-old woman with a history of childhood RT for tinea capitis was referred to our department by her family physician due to recent onset of cognitive deterioration, memory problems, incontinence, and gait disturbances. On examination, she was in good physical condition and well oriented to time and place. She exhibited mental slowness, anosmia, and ataxic gait. Ophthalmologic examination revealed papilledema. Her scalp evidenced typical postradiation changes of alopecia, atrophy, and keratosis.

MRI revealed multiple lesions, including fused large olfactory groove and right sphenoid ridge meningiomas, a left frontal convexital meningioma, and meningiomatosis (three small fused meningiomas) along the right transverse sinus. Significant brain edema and mass effect with midline shift were seen as a result of the large, fused olfactory groove–sphenoid ridge lesions (Fig. 14-6A).

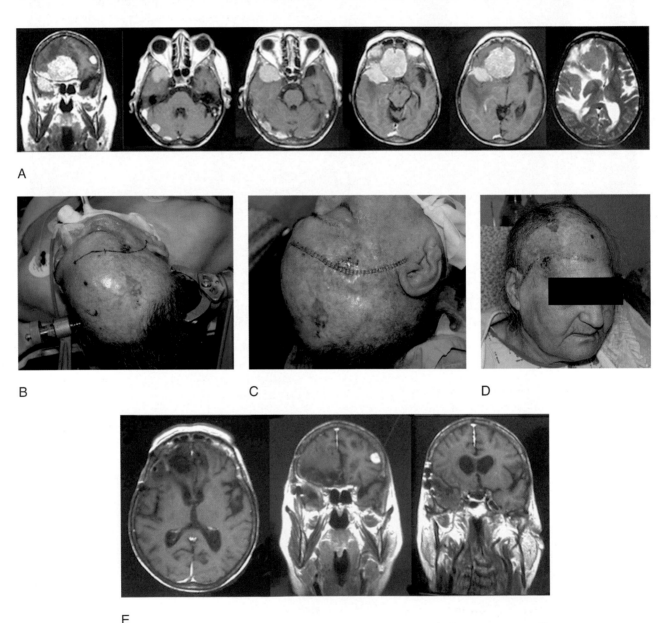

FIG. 14-6. Case illustration of a patient with multiple radiation-induced meningiomas. (A) Preoperative T1-weighted postgadolinium injection and T2-weighted (far right image) MRI depicting multiple meningiomas and significant brain edema. (B) The patient is shown positioned for surgery. Note typical appearance of late postradiation changes in the scalp and unusually low incision line. (C) Scalp closure in a watertight fashion. (D) Wound healing in the early postoperative period. (E) Axial and coronal T1-weighted postgadolinium MR images 3 months postoperative showing fair resection of the olfactory groove–right sphenoid region meningiomas, and remaining small left frontal (convexity) meningioma

Due to the patient's poor skin condition, it was decided to remove the two large meningiomas via a right pterional approach. Skin in the forehead area was less atrophic, and thus the incision was situated lower than usual (Fig. 14-6B). Tumor resection was uneventful, the bone flap was replaced, and the skin was closed in one layer (Fig. 14-6C). The patient recovered, and her wound healed without complications (Fig. 14-6D). Three months after surgery the patient exhibited significant clinical improvement, with fair resection and brain expansion on follow-up MRI (Fig. 14-6E). We are observing the remaining meningiomas with routine MRI and clinical surveillance.

Stereotactic Radiosurgery and Fractionated Stereotactic Radiotherapy

When radical excision is not possible, surgery may be followed by irradiation in patients with prior low-dose irradiation (e.g., for tinea capitis).

In some RIM patients the maximum tolerable dose of radiation has already been administered and conventional radiotherapy is not an option. In these patients, irradiation with fractionated stereotactic radiotherapy (FSR) or stereotactic radiosurgery (SRS) should be considered. When the histopathology is comparable with atypical or anaplastic meningioma (WHO-II or WHO-III, respectively), adjuvant conventional conformal irradiation is generally recommended following surgery/radiosurgery to address viable tumor cells that remain in surrounding brain tissue and along the dura.[68,69,72]

Jensen et al.[75] recently reported that tumor control rates, complications, and outcomes for 16 RIM patients with 20 tumors who were treated with gamma knife radiosurgery correspond well with previously published results of radiosurgery for SM based on a median follow-up of 40 months. In our experience with radiosurgery using the m$_3$® high-resolution micro-multileaf collimater (BrainLAB, Heimstetten, Germany) mounted on a linear accelerator, the response rate to radiation treatment in RIM does not differ from that in SM (unpublished data). Evidence-based data in this regard remain limited.

Treatment planning and dose prescription should be carried out with careful consideration of the original doses and treatment fields in RIM patients.

Recurrence

Rubinstein et al.[39] noted a 26% recurrence rate among RIM patients and a mean time to recurrence of 10.5 years. Soffer et al.[40] reported a rate of 19% in RIM with mean time from surgery to detection of recurrence 6.2 years. Recurrence rates of 18.7–25.6% are reported for RIM in the literature.[25,39,40,58] The rate of multiple recurrence may be higher in RIM than in other meningiomas and may approach 12%.[39] Given the high propensity of RIM for recurrence, more frequent followup with neuroimaging studies is warranted for these tumors as compared to SM.[59]

Genetics of Radiation-Induced Meningiomas

In 40–70% of all SM, genomic alterations are consistent with loss of heterozygosity (LOH) on chromosome 22.[39,48,76,77] The majority of SM with LOH on chromosome 22 carry mutations in the neurofibromatosis type-2 gene (NF2) on 22q12.2, suggesting that NF2 acts as a tumor suppressor gene.[43,77,78] NF2 gene-inactivating mutations have been found in SM of all malignancy grades, suggesting that inactivation of this gene is associated with early tumor formation. More aggressive tumor progression in SM is reported to be frequently associated with LOH on chromosomes 1p, 10q, and 14q.[15,25,40,79] It has been proposed that benign meningiomas might progress to an atypical or anaplastic grade through accumulation of several genetic anomalies, in which LOH on chromosome 22 would represent an early step. Although a significant number of studies have been published describing the genetic characteristics of SM, providing some understanding of the mechanisms for tumor formation and progression, our knowledge of the genetic basis for RIM remains very limited.

Cytogenetics

One cytogenetic study of RIM samples revealed multiple balanced rearrangements and multiple independent clone formations among cell cultures derived from a single tumor.[42] A second cytogenetic study of RIM showed chromosome 22 monosomy.[80] A study of six RIM discovered the same chromosomal abnormality on the region of 1p13, implicating an unknown gene from this region in the pathogenesis of RIM[81] (Fig. 14-7). However, other reports noted no significant differences between RIM and SM regarding the number of genetic changes and the extent and frequency of chromosome 1 and 22 losses using comparative genomic hybridization (CGH) techniques.[82]

Recent studies described cytogenetic alterations in all 16 tumors studied, consistent with frequent aberrations on chromosomes 1p, 6q, and 22. Abnormalities on chromosome 1p were found in 89% of cases, and losses on chromosome 6 were found in 67%.[59]

Molecular Analysis

To understand the molecular mechanism by which low-dose RIM arises, we analyzed DNA from seven RIM and eight sporadic meningioma SM samples.[83] All seven RIM tumors were investigated by single-strand conformation polymorphism analysis (SSCP) of the entire coding region (17 exons) of the NF2 gene and by direct DNA sequencing of the altered fragments. In four out of seven RIM (57.1%), the SSCP studies were followed by Western blot analysis to determine the level of schwannomin/merlin, the NF2 gene product (Fig. 14-8). In addition, LOH analysis of frequently altered genomic areas on

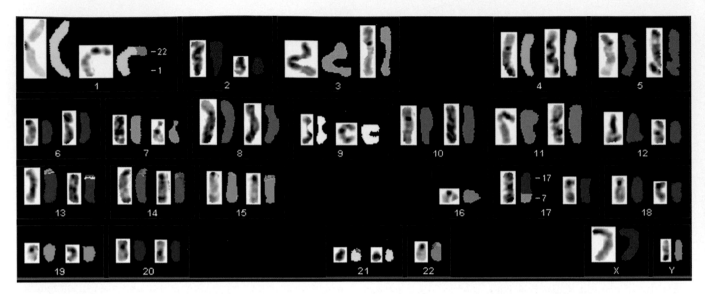

FIG. 14-7. Spectral karyotyping. Note rearrangement between chromosome 1 and chromosome 22, a terminal deletion of a chromosome 7, and a rearrangement between a part of chromosome 7 and chromosome 17. (From Ref. 81.)

chromosomes 1 p, 9 p, 10 p, 10 q, 14 q, 18 q, 19 q, and 22 q was performed in all RIM using 22 polymorphic DNA markers.

We detected inactivating mutations of the NF2 gene in four of eight SM samples (50%). No mutation was found in the NF2 gene in RIM tumor samples. Significant schwannomin/merlin levels were observed in all four RIM tumor sample extracts, suggesting that the NF2 gene structure and function is intact (Fig. 14-1). LOH studies revealed chromosomal deletions on chromosomes 1 p (4/7), 9 p (2/7), 19 q (2/7), 22 q (2/7), and 18 q (1/7) (Fig. 14-9). We concluded that, unlike SM, NF2 gene inactivation and chromosome 22 q deletions do not appear to be associated with meningioma development following low-dose irradiation. LOH on chromosome 1 p, possibly induced by irradiation, may be more important in the development of these tumors. To our knowledge, this was the first study that analyzed a group of radiation-induced solid tumors using molecular genetic tools. These observations were supported by further genetic studies.

Joachim et al.[84] performed comparative analysis of the NF2, TP53, PTEN, KRAS, NRAS, and HRAS genes in 36 SM patients (21 WHO II and 15 WHO III) and 25 patients with RIM (9 WHO I, 5 WHO II, and 11 WHO III). NF2 mutations occurred significantly more often in atypical and anaplastic SM than in RIM. The other genes analyzed in this study did not reveal significant abnormalities in the RIM group.

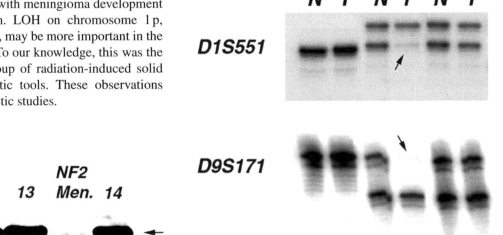

NF2
12   HB   11   13   Men.   14

FIG. 14-8. Immunoblotting of four radiation-induced meningiomas, human brain (HB), and NF2-derived meningioma (NF2-Men). The expression of NF2 protein 66 kDa band, indicated by an arrow at right, was drastically reduced only in NF2-derived meningioma. Four radiation-induced samples expressed high levels of NF2 protein comparable to the level seen in the human brain sample

11   12   13
N T N T N T

D1S551

D9S171

FIG. 14-9. Microsatellite instability and allelic loss detection. LOH is demonstrated on chromosome 1 p (marker D1S551) and 9 p (marker D9S171) for case 12. The faint signals in the tumor lanes might be due to contaminating normal cells or tumor heterogeneity. Note that homozygous alleles are present on loci D1S551 and D9S171 for case 11. Retained heterozygosity is detected for both loci in case 13. N, blood DNA; T, tumor DNA

Rajcan et al.[85] added six cases of RIM and detected an unbalanced genome in five of six cases. Loss of 1 p and 7 p was identified in the majority of RIM with an abnormal karyotype (4/5 cases), whereas loss of 6 q occurred in three of five cases. Only one of five RIM had monosomy for chromosome 22. Loss of 7 p is not frequently reported in SM, and yet it was detected in four of five RIM in this study.

In summary, current studies clearly show that meningiomas in patients who were exposed to therapeutic irradiation may carry distinct chromosomal aberrations compared to SM. Despite the increasing risk of genetic alterations associated with irradiation, the frequency of chromosome 22 q abnormalities and inactivating mutations in the NF2 gene is low in RIM, while a high rate of 1 p deletions in RIM has been constantly observed. A high rate of 1 p deletions has also been noted in high- and low-grade oligodendrogliomas, indicating that this anomaly also occurs at an early step in tumor evolution in this subtype of gliomas.[86] It is possible that two or more tumor suppressor genes located on 1 p are involved in the genesis of these two types of tumors. The meningioma-related tumor suppressor gene on chromosome 1 p may be associated with the formation of RIM, as these tumors tend to be more aggressive than SM in terms of histologic and clinical behavior early in the course of the disease.

Determining the radiation-induced origin of the tumor can be challenging, as clinical, histologic and cytologic criteria cannot provide a definitive answer.[87] Since RIM is clinically and histologically more aggressive than SM, adjustments to routine treatment approaches, clinical follow-up, and prediction of prognosis may be required.[88–90] Identification of markers for the possible tumor etiology in differentiating between tumors that arise as a result of RT and those that arise spontaneously is therefore important.

Conclusions

RIM is a solid tumor arising from cells of the meningeal coverings of the brain following exposure to ionizing radiation. The risk of meningioma increases, and the latent period between radiation exposure and tumor development decreases, with higher doses of radiation, but exposure to even low doses has been shown to significantly increase the risk of meningioma in the treatment field.

As is the case with SM, women are more often at higher risk of developing RIM than men. RIM patients frequently present with multiple tumors. RIM is often more aggressive, with a higher proportion of tumors diagnosed as atypical or anaplastic compared to SM. RIM has a higher recurrence rate than SM. Skin atrophy and devascularization can complicate surgical management. Poor skin condition may necessitate adjustment of the surgical approach and placement of the skin flap in these patients to compensate for the elevated risk of wound infection with resulting CSF leak. Paradoxically, stereotactic radiation (SRS or FSR) may be appropriate to treat RIM patients with nonresectable or residual/recurrent tumors.

Whereas the frequency of chromosome 22 q abnormalities and inactivating mutations in the NF2 gene is high in sporadic meningiomas, LOH studies repeatedly revealed deletions on chromosome 1 p in RIM, with far less frequent observation of deletions on chromosomes 9 p, 19 q, 22 q, and 18 q, leading to the conclusion that RIM may be a distinct genetic entity. The incidence of secondary brain tumors arising as a result of RT and radiosurgery administered for the treatment of a variety of benign and malignant brain tumors will be an increasing problem as treatment protocols improve and patients live longer. A close examination of the elevated risk of RIM for patients exposed to even low doses of irradiation is appropriate when prescribing radiotherapy or radiosurgery to young patients with benign conditions such as arteriovenous malformations, vestibular schwannomas, pituitary adenomas, and skull base meningiomas.

Acknowledgment. The authors wish to thank Efrat Tshopp for her assistance with the preparation of this chapter.

References

1. Morgan RH. The emergence of radiology as a major influence in American medicine. Caldwell Lecture, 1970. Am J Roentgenol Radium Ther Nucl Med 1971;111(3):449–462.
2. Margulis AR. The lessons of radiobiology for diagnostic radiology. Caldwell Lecture, 1972. Am J Roentgenol Radium Ther Nucl Med 1973;117(4):741–756.
3. Davidoff L, Cornelius G, Elsberg C, Tarlov I. The effect of radiation applied directly to the brain and spinal cord. Radiology 1938;31:451–463.
4. Wachowski TJ, Chenault H. Degenerative effffects of large doses of roentgen rays on the human brain. Radiology 1945;45:227–246.
5. X-rays. Consumer Reports. 1961;Sept:493–501.
6. Nader R. Wake up America—unsafe x-rays. Ladies' Home J 1968;85:126–127.
7. Warshofsky F. Warning: x rays may be dangerous to your health. Reader's Digest: Aug. 1972, 1173–1177.
8. National Research Council. Committee on the Biological Effects of Ionizing Radiations. The effects on populations of exposure to low levels of ionizing radiation 1980. Washington, DC: National Academy of Sciences, 1980.
9. Foltz EL, Holyoke JB, Heyl HL. Brain necrosis following X-ray therapy. J Neurosurg 1953;10(4):423–429.
10. Al-Mefty O, Kersh JE, Routh A, Smith RR. The long-term side effects of radiation therapy for benign brain tumors in adults. J Neurosurg 1990;73(4):502–512.
11. Preston DL, Ron E, Yonehara S, et al. Tumors of the nervous system and pituitary gland associated with atomic bomb radiation exposure. J Natl Cancer Inst 2002;94(20):1555–1563.
12. Sadamori N, Shibata S, Mine M, et al. Incidence of intracranial meningiomas in Nagasaki atomic-bomb survivors. Int J Cancer 1996;67(3):318–322.
13. Sadetzki S, Chetrit A, Freedman L, Stovall M, Modan B, Novikov I. Long-term follow-up for brain tumor development after childhood exposure to ionizing radiation for tinea capitis. Radiat Res 2005;163(4):424–432.

14. Shintani T, Hayakawa N, Hoshi M, et al. High incidence of meningioma among Hiroshima atomic bomb survivors. J Radiat Res (Tokyo) 1999;40(1):49–57.

15. Shintani T, Hayakawa N, Kamada N. High incidence of meningioma in survivors of Hiroshima. Lancet 1997;349(9062):1369.

16. Rabin BM, Meyer JR, Berlin JW, Marymount MH, Palka PS, Russell EJ. Radiation-induced changes in the central nervous system and head and neck. Radiographics 1996;16(5):1055–1072.

17. Harrison MJ, Wolfe DE, Lau TS, Mitnick RJ, Sachdev VP. Radiation-induced meningiomas: experience at the Mount Sinai Hospital and review of the literature. J Neurosurg 1991;75(4):564–574.

18. Musa BS, Pople IK, Cummins BH. Intracranial meningiomas following irradiation–a growing problem? Br J Neurosurg 1995;9(5):629–637.

19. Strojan P, Popovic M, Jereb B. Secondary intracranial meningiomas after high-dose cranial irradiation: report of five cases and review of the literature. Int J Radiat Oncol Biol Phys 2000;48(1):65–73.

20. Kleinschmidt-DeMasters BK, Lillehei KO. Radiation-induced meningioma with a 63-year latency period. Case report. J Neurosurg 1995;82(3):487–488.

21. Mann I, Yates PC, Ainslie JP. Unusual case of double primary orbital tumour. Br J Ophthalmol 1953;37(12):758–762.

22. Al-Mefty O, Kadri PA, Pravdenkova S, Sawyer JR, Stangeby C, Husain M. Malignant progression in meningioma: documentation of a series and analysis of cytogenetic findings. J Neurosurg 2004;101(2):210–218.

23. Ghim TT, Seo JJ, O'Brien M, Meacham L, Crocker I, Krawiecki N. Childhood intracranial meningiomas after high-dose irradiation. Cancer 1993;71(12):4091–4095.

24. Salvati M, Cervoni L, Artico M. High-dose radiation-induced meningiomas following acute lymphoblastic leukemia in children. Childs Nerv Syst 1996;12(5):266–269.

25. Salvati M, Cervoni L, Puzzilli F, Bristot R, Delfini R, Gagliardi FM. High-dose radiation-induced meningiomas. Surg Neurol 1997;47(5):435–441; discussion 441–432.

26. Yousaf I, Byrnes DP, Choudhari KA. Meningiomas induced by high dose cranial irradiation. Br J Neurosurg 2003;17(3):219–225.

27. Adamson H. A simplified method of x-ray application for the cure of ringworm of the scalp: Keinbock's method. Lancet 1909;1:1378–1380.

28. Albert RE, Omran AR, Brauer EW, et al. Followup study of patients treated by x-ray for tinea capitis. Am J Pub Health 1966;56:2114–2120.

29. Omran AR, Shore RE, Markoff RA, et al. Follow-up study of patients treated by X-ray epilation for tinea capitis: psychiatric and psychometric evaluation. Am J Pub Health 1978;68(6):561–567.

30. Druckman A. Schlafsucht als Folge der Roentgenbestrahlung. Beitrag zur Strahlenempfindlichkeit des Gehirns. Strahlentherapie 1929;33:382–384. Seen in Wachowski, TJ and Chenault, H. Degenerative effects of large doses of roentgen rays on the human brain. Radiology 345:227–246, 1945.

31. Lorey A, Schaltenbrand G. Pachymeningitis nach Rontgenbestrahlung. Strahlentherapie 1932;44:747–758.

32. Schaltenbrand G. Epilepsie nach Rontgenbestrahlung des Kopfes im Kindsalter. Nervenarzt 1935;8:62–66.

33. Katzenellenbogen I, Sandbank M. [The treatment of tinea capitis and dermatomycosis with griseofulvin. Follow-up of 65 cases.]. Harefuah 1961;60:111–115.

34. Russell B, Frain-Bell W, Stevenson CJ, Riddell RW, Djavahiszwili N, Morrison SL. Chronic ringworm infection of the skin and nails treated with griseofulvin. Report of a therapeutic trial. Lancet 1960;1:1141–1147.

35. Ziprkowski L, Krakowski A, Schewach-Millet M, Btesh S. Griseofulvin in the mass treatment of tinea capitis. Bull World Health Organ 1960;23:803–810.

36. Beller AJ, Feinsod M, Sahar A. The possible relationship between small dose irradiation to the scalp and intracranial meningiomas. Neurochirurgia (Stuttg) 1972;15(4):135–143.

37. Gomori JM, Shaked A. Radiation induced meningiomas. Neuroradiology 1982;23(4):211–212.

38. Munk J, Peyser E, Gruszkiewicz J. Radiation induced head and intracranial meningiomas. Clin Radiol 1969;20:90–94.

39. Rubinstein AB, Shalit MN, Cohen ML, Zandbank U, Reichenthal E. Radiation-induced cerebral meningioma: a recognizable entity. J Neurosurg 1984;61(5):966–971.

40. Soffer D, Pittaluga S, Feiner M, Beller AJ. Intracranial meningiomas following low-dose irradiation to the head. J Neurosurg 1983;59(6):1048–1053.

41. Gabivov G, Kuklina A, Martynov V, et al. [Radiation-induced meningiomas of the brain]. Zh Vopr Neirokhir 1983 (Russian); 6:13–18.

42. Modan B, Baidatz D, Mart H, Steinitz R, Levin SG. Radiation-induced head and neck tumours. Lancet 1974;1(7852):277–279.

43. Ron E, Modan B, Boice JD, Jr., et al. Tumors of the brain and nervous system after radiotherapy in childhood. N Engl J Med 1988;319(16):1033–1039.

44. Sadetzki S, Flint-Richter P, Ben-Tal T, Nass D. Radiation-induced meningioma: a descriptive study of 253 cases. J Neurosurg 2002;97(5):1078–1082.

45. Sadetzki S, Flint-Richter P, Starinsky S, et al. Genotyping of patients with sporadic and radiation-associated meningiomas. Cancer Epidemiol Biomarkers Prev 2005;14(4):969–976.

46. Nolan WE. Radiation hazards to the patient from oral roentgenography. J Am Dent Assoc 1953;47(6):681–684.

47. Nolan WE, Patterson HW. Radiation hazards from the use of dental x-ray units. Radiology 1953;61(4):625–629.

48. Preston-Martin S, Paganini-Hill A, Henderson BE, Pike MC, Wood C. Case-control study of intracranial meningiomas in women in Los Angeles County, California. J Natl Cancer Inst 1980;65(1):67–73.

49. Rodvall Y, Ahlbom A, Pershagen G, Nylander M, Spannare B. Dental radiography after age 25 years, amalgam fillings and tumours of the central nervous system. Oral Oncol 1998;34(4):265–269.

50. Longstreth WT, Jr., Phillips LE, Drangsholt M, et al. Dental X-rays and the risk of intracranial meningioma: a population-based case-control study. Cancer 2004;100(5):1026–1034.

51. Peterson L, Abrahamson S, eds. Effects of Ionizing Radiation: Atomic Bomb Survivors and Their Children (1945–1995). In: Washington, DC, Joseph Henry Press (JHP), The National Academies Press. (Available online http://darwin.nap.edu/books/0309064023/html/117.html); 1998.

52. Harada T, Ishida MI. Neoplasms among A-bomb survivors in Hiroshima: first report of the Research Committee on Tumor

Statistics, Hiroshima City Medical Association, Hiroshima, Japan. J Natl Cancer Inst 1960;25:1253–1264.

53. Shibata S, Sadamori N, Mine M, Sekine I. Intracranial meningiomas among Nagasaki atomic bomb survivors. Lancet 1994;344(8939–8940):1770.

54. Liwnicz BH, Berger TS, Liwnicz RG, Aron BS. Radiation-associated gliomas: a report of four cases and analysis of post-radiation tumors of the central nervous system. Neurosurgery 1985;17(3):436–445.

55. Waga S, Handa H. Radiation-induced meningioma: with review of literature. Surg Neurol 1976;5(4):215–219.

56. Domenicucci M, Artico M, Nucci F, Salvati M, Ferrante L. Meningioma following high-dose radiation therapy. Case report and review of the literature. Clin Neurol Neurosurg 1990;92(4): 349–352.

57. Soffer D, Gomori JM, Siegal T, Shalit MN. Intracranial meningiomas after high-dose irradiation. Cancer 1989;63(8):1514–1519.

58. Pollak L, Walach N, Gur R, Schiffer J. Meningiomas after radiotherapy for tinea capitis–still no history. Tumori 1998;84(1): 65–68.

59. Al-Mefty O, Topsakal C, Pravdenkova S, Sawyer JR, Harrison MJ. Radiation-induced meningiomas: clinical, pathological, cytokinetic, and cytogenetic characteristics. J Neurosurg 2004;100(6):1002–1013.

60. Longstreth WT, Jr., Dennis LK, McGuire VM, Drangsholt MT, Koepsell TD. Epidemiology of intracranial meningioma. Cancer 1993;72(3):639–648.

61. Mack EE, Wilson CB. Meningiomas induced by high-dose cranial irradiation. J Neurosurg 1993;79(1):28–31.

62. Choudhary A, Pradhan S, Huda MF, Mohanty S, Kumar M. Radiation induced meningioma with a short latent period following high dose cranial irradiation - Case report and literature review. J Neurooncol 2005:1–5.

63. Moss SD, Rockswold GL, Chou SN, Yock D, Berger MS. Radiation-induced meningiomas in pediatric patients. Neurosurgery 1988;22(4):758–761.

64. Iacono RP, Apuzzo ML, Davis RL, Tsai FY. Multiple meningiomas following radiation therapy for medulloblastoma. Case report. J Neurosurg 1981;55(2):282–286.

65. Rubinstein L. Pathology of Tumors of the Nervous System. Atlas of Tumor Pathology. Second Series, Fascicle 6. Washington, DC: Armed Forces Institute of Pathology; 1985.

66. Russel D, Rubinstein L. Pathology of Tumors of the Nervous System, 5th ed. Baltimore: Williams & Wilkens, 1989.

67. Louis DN, Scheithauer BW, Budka H, von Deimling A, Kepes JJ. Meningiomas. In: P Kleihues, Cavenee WK, eds. World Health Organization Classification of Tumours Pathology and genetics: tumors of the nervous system. Lyon: International Agency for Research on Cancer (IARC) Press, 2000:176–184.

68. Borovich B, Doron Y. Recurrence of intracranial meningiomas: the role played by regional multicentricity. J Neurosurg 1986;64(1):58–63.

69. Borovich B, Doron Y, Braun J, et al. Recurrence of intracranial meningiomas: the role played by regional multicentricity. Part 2: Clinical and radiological aspects. J Neurosurg 1986;65(2):168–171.

70. Jaaskelainen J. Seemingly complete removal of histologicly benign intracranial meningioma: late recurrence rate and factors predicting recurrence in 657 patients. A multivariate analysis. Surg Neurol 1986;26(5):461–469.

71. Simpson D. The recurrence of intracranial meningiomas after surgical treatment. J Neurol Neurosurg Psychiatry 1957;20(1): 22–39.

72. Wilson CB. Meningiomas: genetics, malignancy, and the role of radiation in induction and treatment. The Richard C. Schneider Lecture. J Neurosurg 1994;81(5):666–675.

73. Stechison MT, Burkhart LE. Radiation-induced meningiomas. J Neurosurg 1994;80(1):177–178.

74. Mirimanoff RO, Dosoretz DE, Linggood RM, Ojemann RG, Martuza RL. Meningioma: analysis of recurrence and progression following neurosurgical resection. J Neurosurg 1985;62(1): 18–24.

75. Jensen AW, Brown PD, Pollock BE, et al. Gamma knife radiosurgery of radiation-induced intracranial tumors: local control, outcomes, and complications. Int J Radiat Oncol Biol Phys 2005;62(1):32–37.

76. Sznajder L, Abrahams C, Parry DM, Gierlowski TC, Shore-Freedman E, Schneider AB. Multiple schwannomas and meningiomas associated with irradiation in childhood. Arch Intern Med 1996;156(16):1873–1878.

77. Weber RG, Bostrom J, Wolter M, et al. Analysis of genomic alterations in benign, atypical, and anaplastic meningiomas: toward a genetic model of meningioma progression. Proc Natl Acad Sci USA 1997;94(26):14719–14724.

78. Lekanne Deprez RH, Riegman PH, van Drunen E, et al. Cytogenetic, molecular genetic and pathological analyses in 126 meningiomas. J Neuropathol Exp Neurol 1995;54(2):224–235.

79. Shore-Freedman E, Abrahams C, Recant W, Schneider AB. Neurilemomas and salivary gland tumors of the head and neck following childhood irradiation. Cancer 1983;51(12): 2159–2163.

80. Shore RE, Albert RE, Pasternack BS. Follow-up study of patients treated by X-ray epilation for Tinea capitis; resurvey of post-treatment illness and mortality experience. Arch Environ Health 1976;31(1):21–28.

81. Zattara-Cannoni H, Roll P, Figarella-Branger D, et al. Cytogenetic study of six cases of radiation-induced meningiomas. Cancer Genet Cytogenet 2001;126(2):81–84.

82. Rienstein S, Loven D, Israeli O, et al. Comparative genomic hybridization analysis of radiation-associated and sporadic meningiomas. Cancer Genet Cytogenet 2001;131(2): 135–140.

83. Shoshan Y, Chernova O, Juen SS, et al. Radiation-induced meningioma: a distinct molecular genetic pattern? J Neuropathol Exp Neurol 2000;59(7):614–620.

84. Joachim T, Ram Z, Rappaport ZH, et al. Comparative analysis of the NF2, TP53, PTEN, KRAS, NRAS and HRAS genes in sporadic and radiation-induced human meningiomas. Int J Cancer 2001;94(2):218–221.

85. Rajcan-Separovic E, Maguire J, Loukianova T, Nisha M, Kalousek D. Loss of 1p and 7p in radiation-induced meningiomas identified by comparative genomic hybridization. Cancer Genet Cytogenet 2003;144(1):6–11.

86. Sulman EP, Dumanski JP, White PS, et al. Identification of a consistent region of allelic loss on 1p32 in meningiomas: correlation with increased morbidity. Cancer Res 1998;58(15): 3226–3230.

87. Bello MJ, Leone PE, Nebreda P, et al. Allelic status of chromosome 1 in neoplasms of the nervous system. Cancer Genet Cytogenet 1995;83(2):160–164.

88. Chauveinc L, Ricoul M, Sabatier L, et al. Dosimetric and cytogenetic studies of multiple radiation-induced meningiomas for a single patient. Radiother Oncol 1997;43(3):285–288.

89. Cowan JM, Beckett MA, Tarbell NJ, Weichselbaum RR. Monosomy 12p in a radiation-induced germ cell tumor. Genes Chromosomes Cancer 1990;2(3):186–190.

90. Tse JY, Ng HK, Lau KM, Lo KW, Poon WS, Huang DP. Loss of heterozygosity of chromosome 14q in low- and high-grade meningiomas. Hum Pathol 1997;28(7):779–785.

15

Emerging Treatment Modalities I: Cyclooxygenase-2 as a Therapeutic Target for Meningioma Tumor Growth

Brian T. Ragel and William T. Couldwell

Introduction

This chapter outlines the rationale and research that supports the treatment of meningiomas with celecoxib, a selective cyclooxygenase-2 (COX-2) inhibitor. Treatments for recurrent or aggressive meningiomas (i.e., atypical or malignant subtypes) are limited, with chemotherapy (e.g., hydroxyurea) and radiation therapy (e.g., stereotactic) modalities offering little benefit. Interest in COX-2 as a therapeutic target for cancer has gained popularity because of the recently observed potential to inhibit this rate-limiting enzyme of prostaglandin synthesis with nonsteroidal anti-inflammatory drugs (NSAIDs) such as ibuprofen and celecoxib. Prostaglandins impart several tumorigenic properties, including angiogenesis, increased cellular proliferation, and anti-apoptotic properties. Treatment with NSAIDs has been shown to curb these pro-tumor properties via both COX-2–dependent and –independent mechanisms. Specifically, treatment of meningiomas with celecoxib in an animal flank model resulted in decreased tumor growth with evidence of decreased COX-2 expression, decreased microvascular density, and increased apoptosis. Finally, celecoxib is well tolerated, making its use as a chronic therapy for meningiomas attractive.

Meningiomas

The term "meningioma" was first coined by Harvey Cushing to describe a benign tumor arising from the central nervous system meninges.[1] The rate of meningioma recurrence is affected by the extent of resection (measured on the overall Simpson resection grade) and the intrinsic tumor biology.[2–4] The World Health Organization recognizes three meningoma grades—benign, atypical, and malignant—with the term "aggressive meningioma" referring to both atypical and malignant grades.[5] Recurrence rates for benign meningiomas 5 years after complete removal are 2–3%, whereas recurrence

rates for atypical and anaplastic meningiomas are 38–50% and 33–78%, respectively.[6,7] The median times to recurrence are 3.1–7.5 years, 2.4–3.3 years, and 3.5–7.7 years, respectively.[6,7] The overall 4- to 5-year survival for patients treated with multimodality treatment (i.e., maximal surgical and medical management) for benign, atypical, and malignant meningiomas are 100%, 59–83%, and 0–59%, respectively.[8–11] Harris et al. reported 10-year survival rates for atypical and malignant meningioma to be 59% and 0%, respectively.[9] These bleak survival statistics underscore the need for new therapies for patients with atypical and malignant meningiomas.

Cyclooxygenase-2

Interest in cyclooxygenase-2 (COX-2) inhibition in meningiomas stems from extensive literature showing COX-2 overexpression in multiple solid tumors, including meningiomas, and our ability to inhibit this rate-limiting enzyme of prostaglandin synthesis with NSAIDs (e.g., ibuprofen, celecoxib). COX-2 expression surges in the setting of inflammation, resulting in prostaglandin synthesis. Prostaglandins have several tumorigenic functions, including angiogenesis, cellular proliferation, and anti-apoptotic activities. A COX-2–meningoma connection is hypothesized because of the causal relationship that has been shown to exist between head trauma and later meningoma development.[12–14] A possible mechanism explaining this head trauma–meningoma relationship involves an inciting inflammatory event followed by neoplastic changes in meningeal tissue caused by healing and the associated release of growth factors.[12–14] In fact, it has been suggested that meningioma formation may occur in the setting of chronic inflammation triggered by head trauma.[15] Recently, the inducible inflammatory enzyme COX-2 has been shown to be upregulated in animal head trauma models.[16,17]

Cyclooxygenase (COX) is the rate-limiting enzyme in the synthesis of prostaglandins from arachidonic acid.[18]

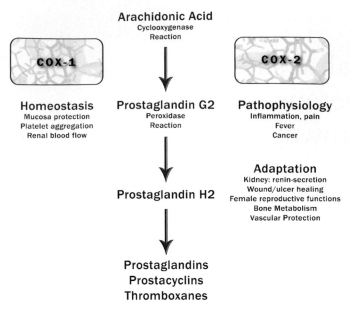

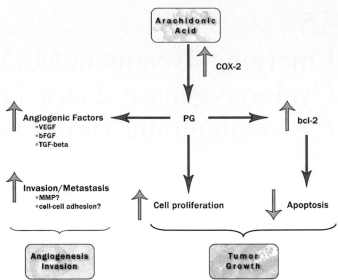

FIG. 15-1. Bifunctional role of cyclooxygenase (COX) enzyme in the synthesis of prostaglandins and thromboxanes. COX has two active sites: (1) a cyclooxygenase site and (2) a peroxidase site. The differences in isozyme physiologic and pathologic roles are outlined

FIG. 15-2. Major effects of COX-2 overexpression in neoplasia are (1) prostaglandin E2 (PGE2) induces the angiogenic factors vascular endothelial factor (VEGF), basic fibroblast growth factor (bFGF), and transforming growth factor-beta (TGF-β); possible pathways also exist with the tumor invasion factors matrix metalloproteinase (MMP) and cell–cell adhesion molecule; (2) increased cell proliferation; and (3) inhibition of apoptosis by PGE2. COX-2 inhibition decreases PGE2 synthesis, which reduces angiogenesis, cell proliferation, and bcl-2 levels. Lack of bcl-2 restores apoptosis and decreases tumor growth

Prostaglandins are a diverse group of autocrine and paracrine hormones that mediate many physiologic and pathologic processes. Physiologically, prostaglandins regulate vascular homeostasis, kidney function, ovulation, and parturition and are equally important as mediators of inflammation, thrombosis, and pain.[19] The formation of prostaglandins requires the catalytic activity of COX, which converts arachidonic acid to the prostaglandin endoperoxide PGH2, from which all other prostaglandins are formed.

Cyclooxygenase is a bifunctional enzyme containing a COX site (converts arachidonic acid to prostaglandin G2) and a prostaglandin peroxidase site (reduces prostaglandin G2 to prostaglandin H2). Two isoforms exist, referred to as COX-1 and COX-2. Although both isoforms catalyze the same enzymatic reactions and have similar K_m and V_{max} values for arachidonic acid, significant differences exist between them (Fig. 15-1).[18] COX-1 is constitutively expressed in most tissues and is thought to serve in general "housekeeping" functions (e.g., cytoprotection of the stomach, platelet aggregation). COX-2 is induced by migratory cells (e.g., macrophages, monocytes, and microglia) responding to proinflammatory stimuli and is considered to be an important mediator of acute and chronic inflammatory states.[20,21] COX-2 expression has a wide range of biologic activities, including angiogenesis, cellular proliferation, and halt of apoptosis (Fig. 15-2).[22] COX-2 expression is ordinarily low at baseline but surges in the context of inflammation or neoplasia.[23] Tight cellular regulation of COX-2 allows for rapid COX-2 upregulation and increased prostaglandin synthesis when necessary.[23]

NSAIDs and Cancer

In 1971, Vane showed that the anti-inflammatory action of NSAIDs rests in their ability to inhibit the activity of the COX enzyme, which in turn results in decreased synthesis of the proinflammatory prostaglandins.[20] The ability of NSAIDs to inhibit the COX enzyme is considered to be their major, but not sole, mode of function.[20] NSAIDs decrease COX activity through nonselective binding, through selective binding to COX-2, or through noncyclooxygenase COX-2 mechanisms (Table 15-1).[20] Celecoxib (Celebrex) and rofecoxib (Vioxx) are specific COX-2 inhibitors that act as slow, time-dependent, irreversible inhibitors of COX-2.[20] From a clinical standpoint, COX-2 inhibition is expected to produce anti-inflammatory and analgesic effects without causing gastric ulcers or platelet dysfunction.

Human cancers of the bladder, breast, uterine cervix, central nervous system, colorectum, esophagus, head and neck, liver, lung, pancreas, prostate, skin, and stomach over express COX-2 and produce more prostaglandins than normal healthy tissues from which they are derived.[24] NSAIDs are important agents for cancer prevention and as possible adjuncts to treatment for the following reasons: (1) COX inhibitors stimulate anticancer effects in vitro; (2) COX inhibitors

TABLE 15-1. Mechanisms of Nonselective, Selective, and Noncyclo-Oxygenase Inhibitors of Cyclooxygenase (COX).

Inhibitor	Action
Nonselective COX inhibitors	
Aspirin	Irreversibly inactivates both COX-1 and COX-2[20]
Ibuprofen	Reversible competitive inhibitor of both COX-1 and COX-2, competes with AA[20]
Flurbiprofen	Reversible inhibition of COX-1 and COX-2, forms salt bridge[20]
Selective COX-2 inhibitors	
Celecoxib	Irreversible inhibitor of COX-2[22]
Rofecoxib	Irreversible inhibitor of COX-2[22]
Noncyclooxygenase inhibitors	
R-flurbiprofen	Inhibits NF-κB and AP1 activation of COX-2 transcription[48]

AA, arachidonic acid; NF-κB, nuclear factor κ-B; AP1, activator binding protein-1.

inhibit carcinogenesis in carcinogen-induced and genetically driven rodent models; (3) COX inhibitors reduce the incidence of colorectal precancerous lesions and colon cancer incidence; and (4) COX inhibitors regress precancerous lesions (e.g., colorectal aberrant crypt foci and adenomas, actinic keratoses of the skin) in genetic and sporadic cancer risk cohorts.[20, 22–28]

Currently, celecoxib is approved by the U.S. Food and Drug Administration for its anti-inflammatory, analgesic, and cancer prevention properties in the treatment of rheumatoid arthritis, osteoarthritis, and familial adenomatous polyposis (FAP), and the National Cancer Institute (NCI) is tracking more than 30 phase I, II, and III cancer trials on COX-2 inhibition with celecoxib in the treatment of colon, prostate, liver, lung, breast, and glioblastoma multiforme (GBM) (NCI cancer database physician's data query at http://www.nci.nih.gov/clinicaltrials/).[20,22]

Research: COX-2 Inhibition in Meningiomas

Meningiomas show extensive immunohistochemical staining for COX-2. The COX-2 enzyme is extensively expressed in meningiomas, with immunohistochemical and Western blot evidence showing localization of this protein to the cytoplasm and nucleus (Fig. 15-3).[29–31] Dura, both normal dura and that adjacent to meningoma tumors, is negative for COX-2 immunohistochemical staining (Fig. 15-3). On the basis of the finding of extensive expression of COX-2 protein in meningiomas, COX-2 inhibition was performed with celecoxib. Celecoxib was chosen because of its FDA approval and evidence of superior antigrowth effects in several cancer cell lines.[32,33] Treatment of meningiomas in vitro and in vivo with celecoxib showed decreased growth. Tumors treated with celecoxib were smaller,

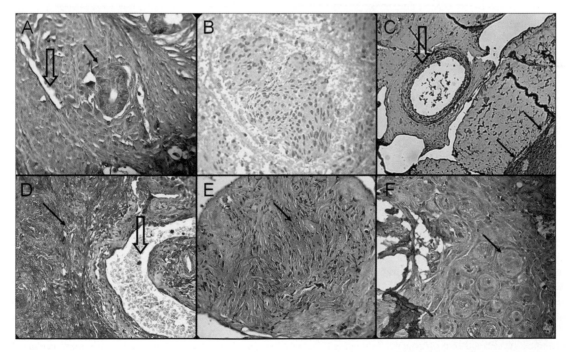

FIG. 15-3. Expression of COX-2 in human colon cancer (A) and human meningiomas (B–F). Positive immunoreactivity appears as reddish-brown staining. Photos taken at 10x magnification. (A) Positive control. Strong COX-2 immunoreactivity seen in the cytoplasm of colonic carcinoma cells (solid arrow), as described previously.[49] Note that vascular endothelium stains positive for COX-2, as described previously (open arrow). (B) Negative control. No staining was noted when slides were incubated with serum only. (C) Normal dura shows staining of vascular endothelium (arrow), as well as meningioma abutting normal dura (arrows). (D–F) Strong COX-2 immunoreactivity noted diffusely throughout cytoplasm of meningioma (solid arrows). Note that monocyte or macrophage within blood vessel stains positive as described previously (open arrow in D) (Modified from Ref. 31)

had less vascular density, and showed increased apoptosis. Finally, removal of treatment resulted in a return of meningioma tumor growth, indicating a growth-suppressive effect.[31,34]

Dose-dependent inhibition of meningioma cell viability by celecoxib was seen in vitro in both a malignant cell line (IOMM-Lee) and in six benign cell lines.[31] In the malignant IOMM-Lee cell line, this correlated with elimination of COX-2 enzymatic activity and a 51% reduction in prostaglandin E2 (PGE2) levels, as well as apoptosis.[31,34] Although the specific in vitro anti-apoptotic mechanisms that COX-2 imparts on tumor cells remain unknown, one possibility is modulation of the BAX-to-bcl-2 ratio, which is key in driving cell apoptosis.[22,24,35] However, Western blot analysis of whole-cell extract showed no change in bcl-2 or BAX expression when the cells were treated with celecoxib.[31] These findings of in vitro growth inhibition of meningoma cells fit with the extensive data on numerous cell lines showing growth inhibi-

tion by selective COX-2 inhibitors.[25,26,31] Specifically, another study on other brain tumors with the COX-2 inhibitor NS-398 showed inhibition of cell proliferation and migration of the glioma cell lines U-87MG and U-251MG.[27,31]

The mouse meningoma flank tumor model was used to demonstrate a statistically significant decrease in meningioma mouse flank tumor sizes with high-dose celecoxib treatment in two of three cell lines, with a final mean tumor volume reduction between 25 and 66% (Fig. 15-4).[34] Prophylactically treating mice with high-dose celecoxib for 6 weeks before induction of IOMM-Lee xenograft tumors resulted in decreased tumor induction rates compared with control, low, and medium-dose groups (80% vs. 100%).[34] Furthermore, removal of drug resulted in the return of tumor growth to baseline tumor growth rates, suggesting a tumor growth suppression of remaining viable cells (Fig. 15-4). These findings agree with those of other in vivo solid tumor studies (e.g., colorectal, prostate, lung, squa-

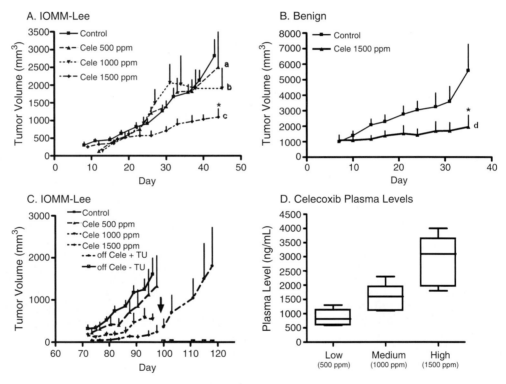

FIG. 15-4. Celecoxib inhibits the growth of meningioma xenograft tumors. (A) IOMM-Lee flank tumors show a dose-dependent growth inhibition with increasing doses of celecoxib. Control mice were fed regular mouse chow. Treated mice were fed low-, medium-, or high-dose celecoxib diets (500, 1000, and 1500 ppm, respectively). No statistically significant difference was found between the control and low (curve a: ANOVA, $p > 0.05$)- or medium (curve b: ANOVA, p greater than 0.05)-dose celecoxib treatment groups, whereas a statistically significant difference between the control and high-dose celecoxib groups was noted by day 43 (curve c: ANOVA, $p < 0.05$). Error bars represent 20, 10, 10, and 15 mice for the control, low-, medium-, and high-celecoxib groups, respectively. (B) Benign meningioma from operative specimen treated with control or high-dose celecoxib. A statistical difference was noted between groups by day 43 (curve d: ANOVA, $p < 0.05$). Error bars represent 5 mice. (C) Effects of prophylactically treating mice with low-, medium-, and high-dose celecoxib for 6 weeks before induction of IOMM-Lee xenograft tumors. A dose-dependent tumor growth inhibition is exhibited between control and pretreatment groups (ANOVA, $p > 0.05$). Error bars represent 5 mice. The high-dose celecoxib group was changed to regular mouse chow 31 days after IOMM-Lee flank injection (arrow) and divided into groups of animals without palpable tumors ($n = 2$, −TU) and animals with flank tumors ($n = 3$, +TU). The animals without palpable tumors remained tumor-free, whereas in animals with tumors, those tumors started to grow at a rate similar to that of control tumors earlier in the study. Error bars after arrow represent at least 2 mice. (D) Celecoxib serum levels in animals fed low-, medium-, and high-dose celecoxib (500, 1000, and 1500 ppm, respectively) mouse chow ad libitum for a minimum of 35 days (i.e., drug levels reflect steady state). Mean celecoxib plasma values (±SD) for low-, medium-, and high-dose celecoxib are 845 (±267), 1540 (±493), and 2869 (±828) ng/mL, respectively (Modified from Ref. 34)

mous cell carcinoma, breast) showing decreased tumor size with celecoxib treatment.[36–42]

Immunohistochemical staining of meningioma flank tumors treated with high-dose celecoxib showed reduced microvascular density by 23–78%, diminished COX-2 and VEGF staining (Fig. 15-5), as well as increased apoptosis.[34] The reduction of COX-2 and VEGF staining suggests that celecoxib ultimately inhibits microvascular proliferation by inhibiting VEGF stimulation. Multiple studies show that COX-2 inhibitors reduce blood vessel formation, probably through direct inhibition of COX-2 and downregulation of VEGF-mediated tumor angiogenesis.[20,25,43–46] Taken together, these results indicate that selective COX-2 inhibitors probably mediate their anti-angiogenic effects via direct inhibition of the COX-2 enzyme (i.e., COX-2–dependent effect).[34]

Celecoxib increased the number of cells undergoing apoptosis in meningoma flank tumors by 36–288%.[34] These findings are consistent with other studies showing that selective COX-2 inhibition promotes apoptosis in numerous cell lines in vivo and in vitro.[22,33,35,44,47]

The recommended dose for celecoxib in the treatment of rheumatoid arthritis, osteoarthritis, and familial adenomatous polyposis ranges from 200 to 800 mg/day, and for clinical trials doses up to 800 mg/day have been reported. The plasma half-life of celecoxib is 13 hours, with steady state reached at 5 days. The mouse plasma levels achieved from the low- and medium-dose celecoxib diets were within reported human ranges.[34] However, the plasma levels of the high-dose celecoxib diet, although achievable in humans, would require ingestion of roughly 3 g of celecoxib daily, which exceeds the recommended dose that would normally be used clinically. Unlike other central nervous system tumors meningiomas derive their blood supply primarily from extracranial blood vessels, thus they are located outside the blood-brain barrier. Therefore, intratumor drug concentrations from systemic therapies should mimic serum levels to a greater extent.

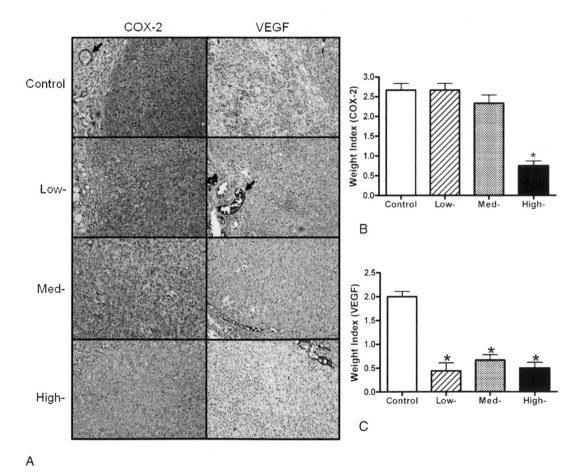

FIG. 15-5. (A) Representative pictures of COX-2 and VEGF immunohistochemical staining of IOMM-Lee xenograft tumors fed low-, medium-, and high-dose celecoxib (500, 1000, and 1500 ppm, respectively) mouse chow ad libitum for 43 days. Magnification is 200X. Decreased COX-2 and VEGF staining intensity was noted as celecoxib dose increased. Arrows identify internal positive controls; both COX-2 and VEGF stain vascular endothelium. (B, C) Weighted index of COX-2 (B) and VEGF (C) staining showing a decrease in score with increasing celecoxib dose. Statistical significance achieved for both COX-2 and VEGF (ANOVA, $*p < 0.001$) (From Ref. 34)

Conclusion

Celecoxib inhibits meningioma growth in vitro and in vivo at therapeutically relevant plasma levels. Overall, celecoxib-treated tumors are less vascular and had increased apoptosis compared to the control with decreased COX-2 and VEGF expression. The meningioma cell lines used in these in vitro and in vivo studies are highly aggressive, perhaps making these findings more applicable to higher-grade tumors. Clinically, we envision using celecoxib in the setting of recurrent or aggressive meningiomas in combination with chemotherapy (e.g., hydroxyurea) or radiation (e.g., stereotactic). Although celecoxib is probably not curative, patient tolerance makes this drug attractive for long-term use. Future studies will focus on the use of other NSAIDs (e.g., aspirin and ibuprofen), as well as a human clinical trial.

Acknowledgments. This work was supported by a grant from the American Association of Neurological Surgeons Neurosurgery Research and Education Foundation to Brian Ragel. We thank Kristin Kraus for her excellent editorial assistance and Kelly Johnson for designing the figures. Finally, without the guidance of Dr. Randy Jensen this research would not have been possible.

References

1. Al-Rodhan RF, Laws ER. The History of Intracranial Meningiomas. In: Al-Mefty O, ed. Meningiomas. New York: Raven Press, Ltd., 1991:1–6.
2. Simpson D. The recurrence of intracranial meningiomas after surgical treatment. J Neurol Neurosurg Psych 1957;20(1): 22–39.
3. Burger PC, Scheithauer BW, Vogel FS, eds. Surgical Pathology of the Nervous System and Its Coverings, 4th ed. Philadelphia: Churchill Livingstone, 2002.
4. Louis DN, Scheithauer BW, Budka H, et al. Meningiomas. In: Kleihues P, Cavenee WK, eds. World Health Organization Classification of Tumours: Pathology and Genetics: Tumours of the Nervous System. Lyon: IARC Press, 2000.
5. Louis DN, Scheithauer BW, Budka H, et al., eds. Meningiomas. Lyon: IARC Press, 2000.
6. Mirimanoff RO, Dosoretz DE, Linggood RM, et al. Meningioma: analysis of recurrence and progression following neurosurgical resection. J Neurosurg 1985;62(1):18–24.
7. Jaaskelainen J, Haltia M, Servo A. Atypical and anaplastic meningiomas: radiology, surgery, radiotherapy, and outcome. Surg Neurol 1986;25(3):233–42.
8. Stafford SL, Pollock BE, Foote RL, et al. Meningioma radiosurgery: tumor control, outcomes, and complications among 190 consecutive patients. Neurosurgery 2001;49(5):1029–37; discussion 37–8.
9. Harris AE, Lee JY, Omalu B, et al. The effect of radiosurgery during management of aggressive meningiomas. Surg Neurol 2003;60(4):298–305.
10. Ware ML, Larson DA, Sneed PK, et al. Surgical resection and permanent brachytherapy for recurrent atypical and malignant meningioma. Neurosurgery 2004;54(1):55–64.
11. Condra KS, Buatti JM, Mendenhall WM, et al. Benign meningiomas: primary treatment selection affects survival. Int J Radiat Oncol Biol, Physics 1997;39(2):427–36.
12. Preston-Martin S, Pogoda JM, Schlehofer B, et al. An international case-control study of adult glioma and meningioma: the role of head trauma. Int J Epidemiol 1998;27(4):579–86.
13. Preston-Martin S, Yu MC, Henderson BE, et al. Risk factors for meningiomas in men in Los Angeles County. J Natl Cancer Inst 1983;70(5):863–6.
14. Phillips LE, Koepsell TD, van Belle G, et al. History of head trauma and risk of intracranial meningioma: population-based case-control study. Neurology 2002;58(12):1849–52.
15. Barnett GH, Chou SM, Bay JW. Posttraumatic intracranial meningioma: a case report and review of the literature. Neurosurgery 1986;18(1):75–8.
16. Koyfman L, Kaplanski J, Artru AA, et al. Inhibition of cyclooxygenase 2 by nimesulide decreases prostaglandin E2 formation but does not alter brain edema or clinical recovery after closed head injury in rats. J Neurosurg Anesthesiol 2000;12(1):44–50.
17. Kunz T, Marklund N, Hillered L, et al. Cyclooxygenase-2, prostaglandin synthases, and prostaglandin H2 metabolism in traumatic brain injury in the rat. J Neurotrauma 2002;19(9):1051–64.
18. Pairet M, Engelhardt G. Distinct isoforms (COX-1 and COX-2) of cyclooxygenase: possible physiological and therapeutic implications. Fundam Clin Pharmacol 1996;10(1):1–17.
19. Meade EA, McIntyre TM, Zimmerman GA, et al. Peroxisome proliferators enhance cyclooxygenase-2 expression in epithelial cells. J Biol Chem 1999;274(12):8328–34.
20. Hinz B, Brune K. Cyclooxygenase-2—10 years later. J Pharmacol Exp Ther 2002;300(2):367–75.
21. Matsuura H, Sakaue M, Subbaramaiah K, et al. Regulation of cyclooxygenase-2 by interferon gamma and transforming growth factor alpha in normal human epidermal keratinocytes and squamous carcinoma cells. Role of mitogen-activated protein kinases. J Biol Chem 1999;274(41):29138–48.
22. Fosslien E. Biochemistry of cyclooxygenase (COX)-2 inhibitors and molecular pathology of COX-2 in neoplasia. Crit Rev Clin Lab Sci 2000;37(5):431–502.
23. Dixon DA, Balch GC, Kedersha N, et al. Regulation of cyclooxygenase-2 expression by the translational silencer TIA-1. J Exp Med 2003;198(3):475–81.
24. Umar A, Viner JL, Anderson WF, et al. Development of COX inhibitors in cancer prevention and therapy. Am J Clin Oncol 2003;26(4):S48–57.
25. Tsujii M, Kawano S, Tsuji S, et al. Cyclooxygenase regulates angiogenesis induced by colon cancer cells. Cell 1998;93(5):705–16.
26. King JG, Jr., Khalili K. Inhibition of human brain tumor cell growth by the anti-inflammatory drug, flurbiprofen. Oncogene 2001;20(47):6864–70.
27. Joki T, Heese O, Nikas DC, et al. Expression of cyclooxygenase 2 (COX-2) in human glioma and in vitro inhibition by a specific COX-2 inhibitor, NS-398. Cancer Res 2000;60(17):4926–31.
28. Cao Y, Pearman AT, Zimmerman GA, et al. Intracellular unesterified arachidonic acid signals apoptosis. Proc Natl Acad Sci USA 2000;97(21):11280–5.
29. Lin CC, Kenyon L, Hyslop T, et al. Cyclooxygenase-2 (COX-2) expression in human meningioma as a function of tumor grade. Am J Clin Oncol 2003;26(4):S98–102.
30. Matsuo M, Yonemitsu N, Zaitsu M, et al. Expression of prostaglandin H synthase-2 in human brain tumors. Acta Neuropathol (Berl) 2001;102(2):181–7.

31. Ragel BT, Jensen RL, Gillespie DL, et al. Ubiquitous expression of cyclooxygenase-2 in meningiomas and decrease in cell growth following in vitro treatment with the inhibitor celecoxib: potential therapeutic application. J Neurosurg 2005;103(3):508–17.

32. Kardosh A, Blumenthal M, Wang WJ, et al. Differential effects of selective COX-2 inhibitors on cell cycle regulation and proliferation of glioblastoma cell lines. Cancer Biol Ther 2004;3(1):55–62.

33. Yamazaki R, Kusunoki N, Matsuzaki T, et al. Selective cyclooxygenase-2 inhibitors show a differential ability to inhibit proliferation and induce apoptosis of colon adenocarcinoma cells. FEBS Lett 2002;531(2):278–84.

34. Ragel BT, Jensen RL, Gillespie DL, et al. Celecoxib inhibits meningioma tumor growth in a mouse xenograft model. Cancer 2006;109(3):588–97.

35. Cui W, Yu CH, Hu KQ. In vitro and in vivo effects and mechanisms of celecoxib-induced growth inhibition of human hepatocellular carcinoma cells. Clin Cancer Res 2005;11(22):8213–21.

36. Fife RS, Stott B, Carr RE. Effects of a selective cyclooxygenase-2 inhibitor on cancer cells in vitro. Cancer Biol Ther 2004;3(2):228–32.

37. Hsu AL, Ching TT, Wang DS, et al. The cyclooxygenase-2 inhibitor celecoxib induces apoptosis by blocking Akt activation in human prostate cancer cells independently of Bcl-2. J Biol Chem 2000;275(15):11397–403.

38. Klenke FM, Gebhard MM, Ewerbeck V, et al. The selective Cox-2 inhibitor Celecoxib suppresses angiogenesis and growth of secondary bone tumors: an intravital microscopy study in mice. BMC Cancer 2006;6:9.

39. Kundu N, Fulton AM. Selective cyclooxygenase (COX)-1 or COX-2 inhibitors control metastatic disease in a murine model of breast cancer. Cancer Res 2002;62(8):2343–6.

40. Sinicrope FA, Gill S. Role of cyclooxygenase-2 in colorectal cancer. Cancer Metastasis Rev 2004;23(1–2):63–75.

41. Srinath P, Rao PN, Knaus EE, et al. Effect of cyclooxygenase-2 (COX-2) inhibitors on prostate cancer cell proliferation. Anticancer Res 2003;23(5A):3923–8.

42. Zhang X, Chen ZG, Choe MS, et al. Tumor growth inhibition by simultaneously blocking epidermal growth factor receptor and cyclooxygenase-2 in a xenograft model. Clin Cancer Res 2005;11(17):6261–9.

43. Liu XH, Kirschenbaum A, Yao S, et al. Inhibition of cyclooxygenase-2 suppresses angiogenesis and the growth of prostate cancer in vivo. J Urol 2000;164(3 Pt 1):820–5.

44. Williams CS, Tsujii M, Reese J, et al. Host cyclooxygenase-2 modulates carcinoma growth. J Clin Invest 2000;105(11):1589–94.

45. Narayanan BA, Narayanan NK, Pittman B, et al. Regression of mouse prostatic intraepithelial neoplasia by nonsteroidal anti-inflammatory drugs in the transgenic adenocarcinoma mouse prostate model. Clin Cancer Res 2004;10(22):7727–37.

46. Ferrandina G, Ranelletti FO, Legge F, et al. Celecoxib modulates the expression of cyclooxygenase-2, ki67, apoptosis-related marker, and microvessel density in human cervical cancer: a pilot study. Clin Cancer Res 2003;9(12):4324–31.

47. Kern MA, Schubert D, Sahi D, et al. Proapoptotic and antiproliferative potential of selective cyclooxygenase-2 inhibitors in human liver tumor cells. Hepatology 2002;36(4 pt 1):885–94.

48. Tegeder I, Niederberger E, Israr E, et al. Inhibition of NF-kappaB and AP-1 activation by R- and S-flurbiprofen. FASEB J 2001;15(3):595–7.

49. Maihofner C, Charalambous MP, Bhambra U, et al. Expression of cyclooxygenase-2 parallels expression of interleukin-1beta, interleukin-6 and NF-kappaB in human colorectal cancer. Carcinogenesis 2003;24(4):665–71.

16
Emerging Treatment Modalities II: Gene Therapy for Meningiomas

Nader Pouratian, Charles A. Sansur, John A. Jane, Jr., and Gregory A. Helm

Introduction

Recent surgical advances for approaching the cranial base, described throughout this book, permit more aggressive resection of skull base tumors that have historically been deemed unresectable. Despite these advances, gross total resections, especially in the case of skull based meningiomas, tumors involving venous sinuses, and tumors with entwined cranial nerves, cannot always be accomplished without placing the patient at significant risk of morbidity and mortality. The goal of surgery should always be to preserve the quality of the patient's life even if it means leaving residual tumor. Options for treatment of residual disease include chemotherapy, brachytherapy, conventional radiation, and radiosurgery, each having distinct indications, advantages, and limitations (discussed elsewhere in this book).

Despite the numerous treatment modalities, a place remains for a minimally invasive, yet effective, treatment for meningiomas. Gene therapy may offer such a modality in the future. Although most previous preclinical and clinical studies of gene therapy have been performed on malignant tumors,[1–10] gene therapy applications are also being explored to treat histologically benign tumors like meningiomas. Gene therapy investigations focus on two distinct, yet intimately related, areas of research: (1) development of targeted gene delivery mechanisms with minimal toxicity to normal tissue and (2) development of transgene strategies, or the identification of candidate genes that induce tumor stability or regression when expressed by tumor cells. Both areas of investigation are briefly reviewed in this chapter and the possible applications to meningiomas are discussed.

Gene Delivery Mechanisms

Gene delivery mechanisms should result in targeted, specific, and sufficient gene expression (both quantitatively and temporally) in the tissue of interest with minimal toxicity to normal tissue and organ systems. Gene delivery systems, or vectors, can be broadly divided into biological and nonbiological systems. Biological systems are composed of viruses and, more recently, bacteria and stem cells.[11,12] These biological systems are modified in the laboratory to eliminate their pathogenecity but to retain, or even enhance, their infectivity and gene transfer efficiency. Nonbiological systems include liposomes, cationic polymers, cationic peptides, and the technique of electroporation.[13] We briefly discuss the various vectors, including each technique's advantages and limitations with respect to issues such as transfection rates, duration of gene expression, ease of production, immunogenecity, and toxicity. Vector selection ultimately depends on the gene therapy strategy being employed. If the goal of therapy is tumor destruction, a vector that yields high yet transient gene expression may be preferable. On the other hand, if the goal of therapy is chronic tumor suppression, a vector that produces lifelong gene expression may be more appropriate. Strategies for improving the specificity of gene transfection and expression are discussed in the section "Targeting Strategies."

Biological Vectors

Adenovirus

Adenoviruses are double-stranded DNA viruses which enter cells by endocytosis and whose contents are then released into the cytoplasm.[14] Advantages of the adenoviral vector include the ability to generate high viral titers, its low neurotoxicity, its extrachromosomal life cycle (thereby avoiding the possibility of insertional mutagenesis), its high-level heterologous gene expression, and its ability to transduce a wide variety of cells.[15–17] The virus can accommodate up to 8 kb of foreign DNA. Most adenoviral vectors studied to date for the treatment of central nervous system (CNS) tumors are derived from the adenovirus serotype-5, which is rendered replication defective by deleting "early genes" involved in viral replication. Its disadvantages stem in part from its advantages. Because the viral genome does not integrate into the cellular genome, therapeutic genes are not passed to the progeny of transduced cells. Also, several early studies demonstrated that adenoviral vector injections into the normal brain can induce marked neurotoxicity, most likely related to host immune responses directed against expressed viral antigens on infected cells.[18,19] No systemic toxicity was reported. Although early versions of adenoviruses showed such toxic side effects, newer adenovirus vectors with further deletions of viral genes have resulted in significant improvements in the targeting profile.[20]

Herpes Simplex Virus

Herpes simplex viruses (HSV) are double-stranded DNA viruses that can cause significant pathology, including cold sores and encephalitis in humans, but are usually dormant after infection without causing disease. Most gene therapy studies utilizing HSV vectors have focused on HSV type 1 (HSV-1). In the normal life cycle of these viruses, the virion fuses with the cell membrane and is transported to the nucleus where, after several phases of gene transcription, the cell lyses and releases progeny viral particles. HSV is notable for being able to accommodate up to 40 kb of foreign DNA (potentially allowing delivery of multiple genes within a single vector),[21,22] its ability to infect both proliferating and quiescent cells, a natural neurotropism, and its latent phase of the life cycle, allowing the viral genome to remain in the cell nucleus for the lifetime of the host organism.[16] This latter characteristic makes this vector most attractive in situations where the goal of gene therapy is lifelong transgene expression. Other advantages of HSV vectors include their high infectivity and requirement of low multiplicity. Yazaki and colleagues described the use of a replication-competent HSV-1 to infect and kill malignant meningioma cells in vitro and in vivo in a xenograft model, resulting in decreased tumor growth and/or cure without associated neurological dysfunction nor pathological changes in the adjacent brain.[23] The original pathologic nature of these viruses may at times limit their therapeutic use.[24]

Retrovirus and Lentiviruses

Retroviruses are RNA viruses which, after entering cells via interactions between viral envelope proteins and cell surface glycoproteins, make a double-stranded DNA copy of the viral genome using reverse transcriptase that integrates into the host genome during mitosis. Because the DNA is integrated into the genome, progeny cells carry the transgene. Retroviral gene therapy is associated with little or no systemic toxicity when injected intracerebrally.[25–27] Retroviruses were originally considered attractive because they can accommodate a relatively large gene inserts (8 kb), and they generally only integrate their genetic material into proliferating cells, thereby sparing and limiting the toxicity to the normal brain parenchyma, which is relatively quiescent.[28] Unfortunately, this benefit proves to be a limitation because it limits the infectivity of retroviral

vectors and most, if not all, tumors contain nondividing cells that would be resistant to retroviral gene therapy. Lentiviruses, a subset of retroviruses that includes the human immunodeficiency virus (HIV), can infect nondividing cells and therefore can achieve more efficient transfection rates but may be less specific in their targeting.[29,30] Safety concerns relating to the origin from HIV-related viruses has limited clinical trials using lentiviruses at the present time. Other limitations of retroviral gene therapy relate to the instability of the virion and challenges associated with producing high viral titers. To circumvent this, retroviral vectors are typically introduced using vector producing cells (VPC), which can transiently produce large quantities of virus and improve transfection rates. VPC increase transfection rates in animals, but the efficacy in humans is questionable.[26] Moreover, although generally safe, serious adverse events in up to 50% of patients treated with direct intracranial infusion of VPC-mediated retroviral gene therapy have been reported.[8] Recognizing this limitation, Kasahara and colleagues have reported improved transfection rates and transgene expression and stability using replication-competent retroviruses that express a suicide gene in a multifocal gliomas model.[31,32] Despite reports of retroviral gene therapy in other brain tumor models, applications in meningiomas have been limited [33]

Adeno-Associated Virus

Adeno-associated virus (AAV) is a single-stranded DNA virus that is part of the parvovirus family. AAV is an attractive vector because it does not cause any natural pathology in humans. Like adenovirus, AAV infects a variety of both dividing and quiescent cells. Unlike adenovirus, however, the viral genome integrates into the host genome. The integration does not cause insertional mutagenesis, as can occur with retroviruses, because the insertion consistently occurs in a specific part of chromosome 19.[34] Because the viral genome integrates, transgene expression is usually long -term, although some suspect it may be more transient.[35] The major limitation of AAV as a vector is the limited capacity to carry DNA (<5 kb) and decreased transfection rates compared to other viruses, such as adenovirus.[36] Moreover, in most cases, AAV need helper viruses (i.e., adenovirus or HSV) for AAV production, which may result in contamination of viral stocks.[37] When carrying the thymidine kinase, angiostatin, or interferon (IFN)-β gene, AAV-mediated gene therapy has inhibited glioma growth and increased survival with minimal systemic toxicity.[38–42] No human brain tumor trials have yet been reported.

Poxvirus and Alphavirus

Poxvirus is a double-stranded DNA virus than can infect both dividing and nondividing cells and can accommodate up to 35 kb of transgenic DNA that does not integrate into the host genome. It has been used extensively for vaccine development.

Studies have largely focused on using poxvirus for delivery of immunotherapy since the virus itself induces a T-cell–mediated immune reaction. Applications for immunotherapy for brain tumors have been explored by Fodor's group, who have transfected interleukin (IL)-2 and IL-12 into gliomas using poxvirus and shown tumor growth inhibition.[43,44] CNS applications have otherwise been limited.

The alphaviruses are enveloped single-stranded RNA viruses that include the Semliki Forest virus (SFV), Sindbis virus, and Venezuelan equine encephalitis virus. Alphaviruses have a broad host range, offer rapid high-titer production, have a natural neural tropism, and have demonstrated significant biosafety, but their transgene expression is transient. Like poxviruses, alphaviruses are immunogenic, inducing cytotoxic T-cell responses that may enhance their efficacy. Recently, dendritic cells isolated from bone marrow were transduced with SFV–IL-12 to treat mice with brain tumors, resulting in prolonged survival.[45,46] Glioma growth inhibition has also been reported with direct intratumoral infusion of SFV-endostatin in an animal model.[47] Ren and colleagues reported a protocol for a phase I/II clinical trial using liposome encapsulated SFV-IL-12 for recurrent GBM, the results of which are pending.[48]

Bactofection

Bactofection is the technique of using transformed bacteria to deliver genes (localized on plasmids) into or adjacent to cells. The plasmid must not only encode for the gene of interest, but also contain sequences needed for transcription and translation. In most scenarios, the bacteria contain a suicide gene that allows controlled bacterial destruction once it is within the cell and thereby deliver the plasmid to the nucleus. Alternatively, the bacteria can take residence adjacent to the cells of interest and create the gene product in situ for local delivery. The primary advantages of bactofection are noted to be its simplicity, the selectivity of gene transfer and the potential to deliver a larger amount of DNA to the target.[12] Although the bacteria used for this type of gene therapy are genetically modified to eliminate their pathogenicity and significant efforts are focused on reducing the antigenicity of these vectors, the major limitation of bactofection remains unwanted host–bacteria interactions. Numerous strains of bacteria have been used, including Listeria monocytogenes, Salmonella typhimurium, Salmonella choleraesuis, and Bifidobacterium longum.[49–52] Bactofection has been used in several neoplastic gene therapy models, including lymphomas, various carcinomas, and melanomas to express genes such as IL-12, IFN-γ, and cytosine deaminase.[51,53,54] No brain tumor applications have yet been described.

Neural Stem Cells

Neural stem cells (NSC) have also been studied as a vector for gene delivery, particularly in gliomas, for which

they have a natural tropism.[11,55–58] Ehtesham and colleagues used adenoviral vectors carrying the genes for either IL-12 or tumor necrosis factor-related apoptosis-inducing ligand (TRAIL) to deliver these genes to NSC in vitro before inoculating the transfected cells into athymic nude mice carrying glioma xenografts.[11,56] In both cases the authors were able to demonstrate significant inhibition of tumor growth. Further studies are warranted to further characterize the utility and toxicity of this gene delivery mechanism. The use of NSC as a vector for meningiomas is as of yet unclear, although no natural tropism has been demonstrated.

Nonbiological Vactors

Cationic Nonbiological Vectors

Nonbiological vectors present a theoretically safer alternative to biological vectors. Advantages include a potentially unlimited clone capacity, presumed decreased toxicity and immunogenecity, and increased potential for repeated applications. Cationic complexes of lipids, proteins, and polymers (e.g., poly(L-lysine)[PLL], poly(ethylenimine)[PEI]) have been devised to protect naked DNA from undesirable degradation and to facilitate entry across the cellular membrane. Cationic complexes are used because they naturally create complexes with negatively charged DNA and because they naturally interact with the negatively charged cell membrane promoting endocytosis of the cationic complex.[59] The precise mechanisms of endocytosis and delivery of DNA to the nucleus is not yet well understood. Transfection rates using such nonbiological vectors depend on the size of the polymer, the size of the DNA being transfected, the ability of DNA to be released from the complex and the lysosome after being endocytosed, and finally the transfer of DNA to the nucleus, which relies on the nuclear pore complex (NPC) binding with a "nuclear localization signal.[60] Similar to biological vectors, these cationic nonbiological vectors can be modified to promote adherence to target-specific ligands and to prevent nonspecific uptake.[61–64] Zhang and colleagues used systemically administered antisense RNA to a segment of the endothelial growth factor receptor (EGFR) mRNA transcript encapsulated within an immunoliposome (associated with receptor-specific monoclonal antibodies) to neutralize EGFR activity in a glioma xenograft model, thereby increasing host animal survival by 88%.[61] A phase I clinical trial studying the toxicity of these nonbiological vectors found minimal toxicity when HSV thymidine kinase (discussed below) was delivered via convection-enhanced delivery to patients with recurrent glioblastoma multiforme.[65,66] Although these nonbiological vectors have been used to investigate gene therapy possibilities in gliomas and brain metasastes, their use has not yet been explored in meningiomas.[61,67]

Electroporation and Gene Guns

For electroporation, short electric impulses produce small pores in cellular membranes enabling DNA entry into the cell.[68] Every tissue is different so a uniform protocol for electroporation is not available. Ultimately, successful transfection will depend upon the amplitude and duration of electrical impulses as well as the amount and concentration of DNA used.[60] In vivo applications involve injecting naked DNA followed by electric impulses delivered to the tissue of interest. It has been used successfully in multiple organ systems, including the brain.[69,70] Gene gun delivery involves using gold particles coated with plasmid containing the gene of interest. The gold particles are then propelled toward the tissue of interest. Although intriguing, gene gun gene therapy has only been demonstrated once in vivo in the brain in a study by Zhang and Selzer, who demonstrated long-term (6-week) β-galactosidase expression in the floor of the fourth ventricle and through anterograde tracts.[71] While the possibility of electroporation has been explored for brain tumor gene therapy applications, the applicability of gene gun technology to brain tumor therapy remains undefined.

Targeting Strategies

The ability to target gene therapy is critical for limiting toxicity to surrounding tissues, especially when applying toxic gene therapies within the CNS. Several targeting strategies have been devised to promote both specific gene delivery to the tissue of interest and tissue-specific gene expression. These strategies include various routes of administration, vector surface modifications, the development of oncolytic viral vectors, and the use of tissue-specific promoters. Although each is described separately, the different strategies are often combined to produce a synergistic effect.

Routes of Administration

Like pharmacologic agents, the route of administration of vectors alters their distribution and bioavailability. The various routes of administration for CNS gene therapy (in order of increased specificity) include systemic administration (relying on other targeting strategies to achieve tissue specificity), selective intra-arterial vector administration,[72] or direct intraparenchymal infusion (either intraoperatively or minimally invasively).[65,73,74] With respect to intraparenchymal infusion, the extracellular channels within the CNS are large enough to convey virus-sized particles such that vector size is not a critical determinant of vector distribution.[74] Instead, surface characteristics are more important in determining distribution characteristics.[74]

Vector Surface Modification

Although some vectors have natural tropisms for neural tissue (e.g., HSV), in most cases additional strategies are employed to more specifically target gene delivery to the tissue of interest. Vector targeting can be accomplished with virtually any type of vector (biological or nonbiological) and uses either antibody-mediated recognition of desired targets or structural modification of the vector itself so that it binds target-specific receptors. Gerritsen's group has reported using both techniques with an adenoviral vector to increase transfection efficiency in meningiomas.[75] EGFR and α_v integrin expression are significantly higher in meningiomas compared with normal brain tissue, whereas the normal receptor for adenovirus (coxsackie-adenovirus receptor [CAR]) is variably expressed in these tumors. Redirecting adenoviral vectors to EGFR and α_v integrins (using bispecific single-chain antibodies and modification of the adenoviral genome to encode for an integrin-targeting peptide on the viral capsid, respectively) increased gene transfer rates up to 123-fold.[75,76] The bispecific antibody, 425-S11, recognizes EGFR on one side and a viral capsid structure on the other. The same group has shown that eliminating the native tropism of the virus for CAR and α_v integrins (by inserting specific mutations in the fiber and penton base genes to eliminate binding) improves transfection rates and specificity of gene transfection.[76] Other groups have also reported genome modification to increase the specificity of infection. For example, lentiviruses have been pseudotyped with lymphocytic choriomeningitis virus glycoproteins resulting in efficient and specific transfection of gliomas, sparing the normal brain.[77]

Replication-Restricted and Oncolytic Vectors

Replication-restricted viruses are designed to propagate in tumor cells but are replication incompetent in normal tissues. Some have argued the failure of some clinical trials may be attributed to nonreplicating viral vector gene therapy strategy.[78] By selectively replicating in tumor cells, they selectively induce cell lysis and cell death of tumors. They have the advantage of increasing viral concentrations in the tumor, which increases transfection efficiency and imparts the capacity to propagate through solid tumors, improving vector penetration. One approach for creating replication-specific vectors is to modify the viral genome such that viral replication genes are under the control of tumor-specific promoter/enhancer regions. Rodriguez and colleagues[79] and Yu and colleagues[80] have utilized the human prostate specific antigen and kallikrein 2 promoters to produce a prostate attenuated replication competent adenovirus, which demonstrates up to fourfold prostate tumor cell specificity between PSA(+)

and PSA(−) controls. Yu and colleagues subsequently demonstrated that the addition of the E3 region to the vector enhances tumor killing, apparently by expressing proteins that play a role in virus release.[81] Since the E3 region also encodes proteins that attenuate the immune response, this region may prove useful for human applications. For meningioma gene therapy, our laboratory has reported modifying the adenovirus so that the E1 region is under the control of the osteocalcin promoter, resulting in tumor-specific oncolytic gene therapy when appropriate concentrations of virus are administered[82] (Fig. 16-1).

A second approach is to genetically engineer viruses to have specific mutations such that their replication is dependent on the expression of tumor-specific genes, rendering them replication incompetent in normal tissue. For exam-

ple, Bischoff and colleagues have constructed an adenoviral mutant that replicates specifically in tumor cells lacking or containing mutated p53.[83] Unfortunately, the majority of human brain tumors do not carry p53 mutations or deletions. Other groups are also studying a genetically modified HSV-1, which selectively replicates and lyses brain tumor cells, but which has limited virulence and toxicity in the normal brain.[73,84,85] In order to achieve this replication selectivity, the HSV vectors contain mutations or deletions in genes, which are typically expressed by proliferating cells, but not in quiescent cells (e.g., thymidine kinase, ribonucleotide reductase, γ_1 34.5 gene).[73,84–87] Although these replication restricted vectors can markedly increase cellular transfection rates in malignant tumors, applications in benign tumors may prove to be more difficult.

A

Temporal Lobe Culture

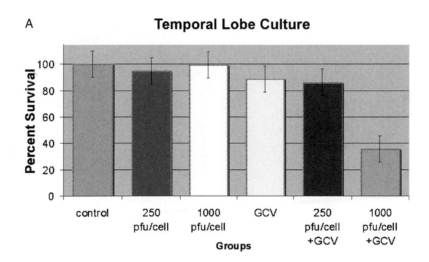

B

Meningioma Culture

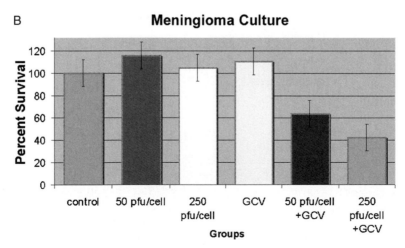

FIG. 16-1. Meningioma-specific oncolytic gene therapy using Ad-OC-E1a, a modified adenovirus made conditionally replication competent by reinserting the E1a gene under the control of the osteocalcin promoter. (A) Dose response of normal temporal lobe tissue to administration of the modifived adenovirus. (B) Dose response of meningioma culture to administration of the modified adenovirus. The difference in dose-response curves provides a therapeutic index for treatment of meningiomas (From Ref. 82)

Tissue-Specific Promoters

The regulatory sequences that control these tumor-specific proteins (i.e., tissue specific promoters) can be exploited to limit transgene expression to tumor cells. This strategy has been used in multiple tumor models. Adenovirus-mediated thymidine kinase (TK) expression using the HKII promoter can effectively kill breast and non–small cell lung carcinoma cells in vitro with a 100-fold therapeutic index relative to normal human epithelial cells.[88] Using the α-fetoprotein (AFP) promoter, plasmids bearing diphtheria toxin-A showed selective cytotoxicity to AFP positive cells in vitro.[89] Systemic administration of adenoviral vector carrying TK under control of the osteocalcin promoter reduced pulmonary osteosarcoma metastases and prolonged survival in nude mice.[90]

Promoters more germane to the CNS have also been investigated. Adenoviral vectors using either the growth hormone or α-subunit promoters were used to drive the synthesis of TK in pituitary tumors.[91] Both exhibited tumor-specific cytotoxicity in vitro and tumorcidal effects in vivo in nude mice with gancyclovir administration. Neuronal and glial specific expression has also been demonstrated using an adenoviral vector with neuronal-specific enolase (NSE) and glial fibrillary acidic protein (GFAP) promoters, respectively, driving expression of the Fas ligand.[92] GFAP promoter driving expression of HSV-TK is also capable of inducing cytotoxicity of glioma cells.[93] When given systemically, these tissue-specific constructs have resulted in lower systemic toxicity compared to vectors containing universal promoters. Our laboratory has explored using meningioma-specific promoters, including the vimentin and osteocalcin promoters, to drive expression of TK in meningiomas. In vitro studies have confirmed that osteocalcin-driven TK expression induces tumor-specific cell lysis and death with no cytotoxic effect on the brain[82,94] (Fig. 16-2A,B).

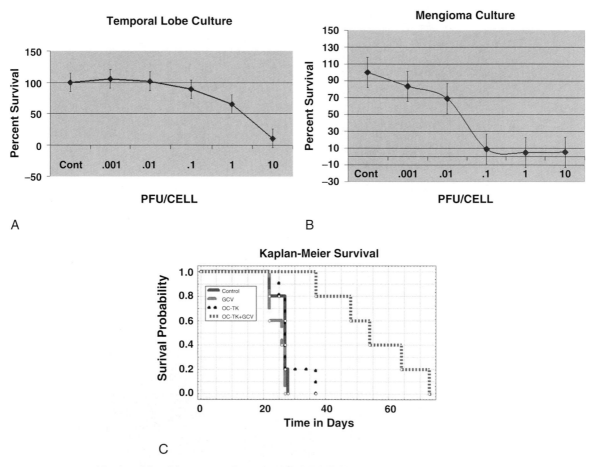

FIG. 16-2. Meningioma-specific thymidine kinase gene therapy using Ad-OC-TK, a replication-defective adenovirus containing the suicide gene thymidine kinase under the control of the osteocalcin promoter. (A) Response of normal temporal lobe culture to administration of Ad-OC-TK. Note that while at a dose of 1000 pfu/cell, the virus is toxic to normal tissue, there is minimal toxicity at a dose of 250 pfu/cell. (B) Response of meningioma culture to administration of Ad-OC-TK. Note that a dose of 250 pfu/cell, which is not toxic to normal temporal lobe, produces significant toxicity to the meningioma culture. (C) In vivo intratumoral administration of this virus to animals implanted with malignant meningiomas produces a distinct survival advantage (From Refs. 82, 94)

In vivoexperiments confirmed in vitro findings, confirming that intratumor infusion of adenovirus carrying osteocalcin-driven TK into malignant meningiomas improves survival in animals treated with gancyclovir[82,94] (Fig. 16-2C).

Transgene Strategies

Successful gene therapy requires not only targeted gene delivery, but an appropriate gene therapy strategy (i.e., gene selection). Gene therapy approaches broadly include (1) direct killing of tumor cells, (2) corrective approaches (i.e., restoring defective tumor suppressor genes), (3) suppression of angiogenesis, (4) immunotherapy, and (5) conferral of drug resistance to hematopoietic cells allowing intensified chemotherapy.[10] The best approach for gene therapy of meningiomas will rely in part on developing a better understanding of the molecular biology of meningiomas.

Killing of Tumor Cells

HSV Thymidine Kinase

HSV thymidine kinase (HSV-TK) is the most widely used suicide gene. HSV-TK, an enzyme that phosphorylates gancyclovir (GCV) or acyclovir (ACV), confers a selective sensitivity to those cells infected with the virus. When these drugs are administered and phosphorylated, first by HSV-TK and then by cellular kinases, the triphosphorylated GCV or ACV can bind to and terminate an elongating DNA chain.[95] The phosphorylated drug can diffuse and kill neighboring, untransfected cells via gap junctions, resulting in a significant "bystander effect."[96,97] In fact, primary brain tumors expressing connexins (which make up gap junctions) have increased bystander killing, suggesting brain tumors should have increased susceptibility to TK gene therapy.[98] Because normal brain tissue does not actively undergo DNA synthesis, it should be relatively unharmed by HSV-TK therapy.[9]

HSV-TK gene therapy has been studied in several glioma models. Ram reported improved survival in rats implanted with 9L gliosarcoma cells and treated with intratumoral injection of retrovirus bearing HSV-TK.[99] Using a HSV vector, Miyatake also found a significant tumorocidal benefit in a subcutaneous GL261 glioma model in mice.[86] The efficacy of HSV-TK has also been studied in clinical trials. Ram and colleagues reported the first clinical trial, in which 15 patients with recurrent glioblastoma were treated with direct intratumoral injection of retrovirus carrying HSV-TK.[100] Although only four patients had radiographic responses (including one who was disease-free 50 months after treatment), the study did show proof of principle for gene therapy for CNS neoplasms. Several other clinical trials have been reported, but the largest to date was reported by Rainov, in which 248 patients were assigned to either surgical resection and radiotherapy

with or without adjuvant retroviral-mediated HSV-TK administration.[3] HSV-TK did not change progression-free, median, or 12-month survival, largely resulting in the abandonment of the VPC-mediated retroviral approach for HSV-TK administration,[10] Adenoviral-mediated HSV-TK therapy has been more successful, highlighting the importance of vector selection.[101] Sandmair and colleagues reported a significant improvement in survival when using adenovirus as a HSV-TK vector compared to using retrovirus as a vector (median survival: 15 vs 7.4 months, p < 0.012).[101] Immonen and colleagues, in a randomized trial, later demonstrated that adjuvant adenovirus-mediated HSV-TK administration resulted in significantly longer mean survival (70.6 weeks) compared to patients who received standard care (39.0 weeks, p < 0.001).[1] Our laboratory has reported successful tumor-specific gene therapy in vitro and in an in vivo animal model of malignant meningiomas using adenoviral-mediated osteocalcin-driven TK expression (described earlier; Fig. 16-2).[82,94] Human trials have not yet been proposed for meningiomas.

Cytosine Deaminase

Cytosine deaminase (CD) is an enzyme that converts 5-flourocytosine (5-FC) to 5-flourouracil (5-FU). 5-FU in turn disrupts both DNA and RNA synthesis and should be cytotoxic to both dividing and nondividing cells, as opposed to TK, which is only toxic to dividing cells. CD may therefore be useful for treatment of benign as well as malignant tumors.

CD has been shown to have marked cytotoxicity and tumorocidal effects in both C6 glioma and 9L gliosarcoma models.[102–104] Bourbeau and colleagues report that susceptibility to CD gene therapy may be related to p53 status, suggesting that gene therapies may be modulated by the genetic status of the target tissue.[105] CD and TK have also been used in combination as a fusion gene and have been shown to significantly improve survival in a rat glioma model.[106–108] CD has also been delivered to tumors using NSC and resulted in tumor mass decrease in a rodent C6 glioma model.[58]

Corrective Approaches

Characterizing the exact mutations associated with meningothelial neoplasms will provide further targets for gene therapy. In general, neoplasms are thought to arise from a combination of activating mutations in oncogenes, which normally promote cell cycling, and/or disruption of tumor suppressor genes, or anti-oncogenes, which normally inhibit cell division. Oncogene gene therapy relies primarily on introducing antisense copies of mutated oncogenes into tumor cells to eliminate expression of the mutant oncogene protein. Although a number of oncogenes have been associated with CNS malignancies, aside from erbB, no single or common oncogene alteration has been found in the majority of tumors.[109] Recent studies identified a possible candidate for antisense gene therapy, noting overexpression of survivin, an anti-apoptotic protein, in the majority of meningiomas.[110,111] Although survivin has been looked at as a potential target for gene therapy in other systems, CNS applications have not been reported.

Gene therapy using tumor suppressor genes provides normal copies of the mutated tumor suppressor gene and restores its normal antioncogenic function. The most widely studied tumor suppressor gene is p53, which normally causes cell cycle arrest and promotes apoptosis. p53 gene therapy application for meningiomas, however, is likely limited since p53 is rarely mutated in meningiomas (even though it may be overexpressed).[112] Nevertheless, p53 gene therapy is briefly reviewed as a model of tumor suppressor gene therapy. The efficacy of p53 gene therapy has been reported in numerous non–CNS tumor models, including lung, pancreatic, prostate, colorectal, ovarian, cervical, and breast carcinoma models.[113-119] Adenoviral-mediated transfer of wild type p53 into several different glioblastoma cell lines has been shown to inhibit growth in vitro and has demonstrated a significant tumorocidal benefit, decreased tumor volumes, and prolonged survival in in vivo models.[120-122] When combined with radiotherapy, rats had significantly improved survival compared to wild-type gene therapy alone.[123] A chemosensitizing effect of transducing glioblastoma cells with wild-type p53 has also been reported in a rodent glioblastoma model using cisplatin therapy.[124] In 2003, Lang and colleagues reported the first and only phase I trial of adenoviral mediated p53 gene therapy for brain tumors, in which 15 patients' tumors were stereotactically injected with the vector. The patients then underwent surgical resection and re-injection of the tumor margins with the vector.[7] Minimal clinical toxicity was noted, and no systemic dissemination of the vector was reported.

Identification of other tumor suppressor gene mutations in meningiomas may provide further opportunities for interventions in meningiomas. Candidate mutations that may be corrected include CDKN2A, p14(ARF), and CDKN2B, which are often deleted or mutated in atypical and anaplastic meningiomas.[125]

Suppression of Angiogenesis

Several factors are known to be angiogenic, including IL-8, vascular endothelial growth factor (VEGF), and bFGF. These angiogenic factors are upregulated by tumor hypoxia and are crucial for tumor angiogenesis.[126] Inhibiting angiogenesis may decrease tumor growth.

Vascular Endothelial Growth Factor and Fibroblast Growth Factor

VEGF expression is known to be increased in glioblastoma[127,128] and, although not upregulated, is a potential angiogenic target in meningiomas.[128-131] VEGF, also known as vascular permeability factor (VPF), is believed to induce vascular permeability and allow plasma proteins to enter the tumor bed, laying down an extracellular matrix for tumor growth.[132,133] The newly formed blood vessels may act as conduits for metastatic spread. VEGF may also prevent maturation of antigen presenting cells, such as dendritic cells, allowing tumors to evade the host immune system.[134]

Using an adenoviral vector carrying antisense VEGF, Im and colleagues showed effective inhibition of U87 malignant glioma cell growth in an in vivo rodent model.[135] Transfection of glioma cells with a mutant nonfunctioning VEGF receptor also prolonged rat survival by competitive inhibition.[136] No clinical trials have been reported targeting VEGF in brain tumors.

While the central portions of large tumors express VEGF, the leading edge of large tumors and small tumors express basic fibroblast growth factor (bFGF), which acts both as a potent angiogenic signal and a tumor mitogen.[137-139] In vitro, C6 glioma cells infected with antisense bFGF show inhibited proliferation, although it is unclear whether this is a direct response on the tumor cells or whether it is secondary to a decreased neovascularity.[140]

Angiostatic Hormones

A number of angiostatic hormones have also been identified, including platelet factor 4 (PF-4), immune protein 10 (IP-10), monokine induced by IFN-γ (MIG), angiostatin, endostatin, and IFN-α_1.[137,141-143] Using both a retroviral and adenoviral vector carrying a gene for a secretable form of PF-4, Tanaka showed glioma growth inhibition both in vitro and in vivo and prolonged survival in the in vivo model.[144] IP-10 and MIG are thought to inhibit angiogenesis, and their recombinant forms have been shown to have antitumoral effects in vivo in rodent non–CNS tumor models.[145,146] No gene therapy studies have specifically targeted IP-10 or MIG in CNS neoplasms, but one report indicated that adenoviral E3 gene expression blocks tumor necrosis factor (TNF)-α–mediated increases in IP-10 in astrocytes.[147] Transfection with either a retroviral or adenoviral vector carrying cDNA for angiostatin has also been shown to effectively inhibit endothelial cell growth in vitro and glioma growth in vivo.[148] Comparing angiostatin, endostatin, and IFN-α_1, De Bouard concluded that IFN-α_1 demonstrated the most potent antiangiogenic effect and found that survival increased significantly when as little as 1% of implanted glioblastomas expressed IFN-α_1.[149] No brain tumor clinical trials have yet to be reported using angiostatic hormones.

Immunotherapy

The immune system is capable of eliminating tumors. This is exemplified by the fact that malignant xenografts do not result in tumor formation in immunocompetent hosts. The mechanism of tumor evasion of immune surveillance is not well understood. Some postulate that tumor-associated antigens have low immunogenicity. In addition, many tumors produce cytokines that either blunt or prevent an immune response.[150] Immune therapy for tumors is centered on the concept that tumors bear tumor specific markers that can be recognized by the stimulated immune system.[151–153] Immunotherapy for brain tumors includes two strategies: (1) blocking immunosuppressive cytokines and (2) expression of immunostimulatory cytokines.

Antisense Prevention of Tumor Evasion

IGF-1, produced by CNS tumors (including meningiomas),[154,155] is thought to either help tumors evade immune surveillance[156–158] or act as a pro-proliferative cytokine.[155,159] Blocking IGF-1 action by delivery of an antisense IGF-1 gene or antisense IGF-1 receptor gene results in decreased tumorogenicity. Trojan and colleagues have shown that antisense IGF-1 gene expression results in a tumor-specific immune response involving CD8+ lymphocytes and is accompanied by increased levels of MHC-1 and the co-signaling molecule B7.[158,160] Transfected cells demonstrated increased apoptosis and interrupted tumor growth in most experiments.[160,160]

Transforming growth factor (TGF)-β inhibits the activation of cytotoxic T cells and is thought to promote tumor evasion of the immune system.[161] Rats implanted with transfected C6 glioma cells with the antisense of TGF-β had significantly improved survival compared to controls.[70] Complete tumor eradication was noted in all rats in whom 9L gliosarcoma cells were transfected with antisense TGF-β.[162] Although no clinical trials have been reported using TGF-β for meningiomas, it likely plays a significant role in meningioma pathophysiology and may therefore provide a possible target for gene therapy.[163,164]

Pro-inflammatory Cytokines

It is also possible to introduce genes whose products increase immune surveillance and response.[142] Immunostimulatory cytokines include IFN-γ., GM-CSF, TNF, IL-1, IL-2, IL-4, IL-10, and IL-12. The results of cytokine gene therapy studies have been mixed. GM-CSF, IL-2, IL-4, AND IFN-γ significantly improved survival of rats implanted with C6 glioma cells modified to secrete these cytokines.[165,166] Mice implanted with gliomas and treated with intratumoral injection of fibroblasts modified to secrete IL-2 have also been reported to have improved survival.[167] Immunostimulatory gene therapy (IL-12) of a tumor has been shown to confer a benefit to other tumors that are separated in space (e.g., contralateral) and/or time (e.g., secondary tumor implantation) from the original tumor in multiple animal tumor models.[168–172] Coadministration of various immunos-

timulatory genes has also been found to be synergistic in some cases. Despite these successes, in a murine glioma model, no therapeutic benefit was found with HSV carrying the gene for IL-10.[173] Cytokine gene therapy clinical trials for CNS neoplasms have been limited and have only included patients with malignant gliomas.[4,48,174,175]

Protection from Toxic Chemotherapy

Gene therapy may also be used to confer hematopoietic stem cells with protection from the toxicity of chemotherapy by transducing them with the multiple drug resistance gene (MDR-1) or other drug resistance genes.[9] Transducing both human and murine hematopoietic stem cells with cDNA for human MDR1 has been shown to provide these cells with resistance to several common chemotherapeutic agents.[176,177] The same authors have also used retrovirus to transduce stem cells with a mutant of the enzyme, dihydrofolate reductase (L22Y), thereby providing these cells with protection from the chemotoxicity of methotrexate.[176] As chemotherapy plays a small role in meningioma management, this gene therapy approach may be limited for meningiomas.

Conclusions

Gene therapy potentially offers a minimally invasive approach to treat selected meningiomas which have an unacceptably high risk of surgical morbidity and mortality. Although the majority of investigations (and all clinical trials) have focused on malignant gliomas, the knowledge attained through these investigations will be essential for the development of meningioma gene therapies. Continued development of vectors, delivery methods, and transgene therapies are essential for the successful application of gene therapy for meningiomas in the future.

References

1. Immonen A, Vapalahti M, Tyynela K, et al. AdvHSV-tk gene therapy with intravenous ganciclovir improves survival in human malignant glioma: a randomised, controlled study. Mol Ther 2004;10(5):967–72.
2. Chiocca EA, Abbed KM, Tatter S, et al. A phase I open-label, dose-escalation, multi-institutional trial of injection with an E1B-Attenuated adenovirus, ONYX-015, into the peritumoral region of recurrent malignant gliomas, in the adjuvant setting. Mol Ther 2004;10(5):958–66.
3. Rainov NG. A phase III clinical evaluation of herpes simplex virus type 1 thymidine kinase and ganciclovir gene therapy as an adjuvant to surgical resection and radiation in adults with previously untreated glioblastoma multiforme. Hum Gene Ther 2000;11(17):2389–401.
4. Eck SL, Alavi JB, Judy K, et al. Treatment of recurrent or progressive malignant glioma with a recombinant adenovirus expressing

human interferon-beta (H5.010CMVhIFN-beta): a phase I trial. Hum Gene Ther 2001;12(1):97–113.

5. Eck SL, Alavi JB, Alavi A, et al. Treatment of advanced CNS malignancies with the recombinant adenovirus H5.010RSVTK: a phase I trial. Hum Gene Ther 1996;7(12):1465–82.

6. Smitt PS, Driesse M, Wolbers J, et al. Treatment of relapsed malignant glioma with an adenoviral vector containing the herpes simplex thymidine kinase gene followed by ganciclovir. Mol Ther 2003;7(6):851–8.

7. Lang FF, Bruner JM, Fuller GN, et al. Phase I trial of adenovirus-mediated p53 gene therapy for recurrent glioma: biological and clinical results. J Clin Oncol 2003;21(13):2508–18.

8. Prados MD, McDermott M, Chang SM, et al. Treatment of progressive or recurrent glioblastoma multiforme in adults with herpes simplex virus thymidine kinase gene vector-producer cells followed by intravenous ganciclovir administration: a phase I/II multi-institutional trial. J Neurooncol 2003;65(3):269–78.

9. Culver KW. Gene therapy for malignant neoplasms of the CNS. Bone Marrow Transplant 1996;18 Suppl 3:S6–9.

10. Pulkkanen KJ, Yla-Herttuala S. Gene therapy for malignant glioma: current clinical status. Mol Ther 2005;12(4):585–98.

11. Ehtesham M, Kabos P, Gutierrez MA, et al. Induction of glioblastoma apoptosis using neural stem cell-mediated delivery of tumor necrosis factor-related apoptosis-inducing ligand. Cancer Res 2002;62(24):7170–4.

12. Palffy R, Gardlik R, Hodosy J, et al. Bacteria in gene therapy: bactofection versus alternative gene therapy. Gene Ther 2006; 13(2): 101–105.

13. El-Aneed A. Current strategies in cancer gene therapy. Eur J Pharmacol 2004;498(1–3):1–8.

14. Seth P, Willingham MC, Pastan I. Adenovirus-dependent release of 51Cr from KB cells at an acidic pH. J Biol Chem 1984;259(23):14350–3.

15. Le Gal La Salle G, Robert JJ, Berrard S, et al. An adenovirus vector for gene transfer into neurons and glia in the brain. Science 1993;259(5097):988–90.

16. Lundstrom K. Latest development in viral vectors for gene therapy. Trends Biotechnol 2003;21(3):117–22.

17. Kramm CM, Sena-Esteves M, Barnett FH, et al. Gene therapy for brain tumors. Brain Pathol 1995;5(4):345–81.

18. Smith JG, Raper SE, Wheeldon EB, et al. Intracranial administration of adenovirus expressing HSV-TK in combination with ganciclovir produces a dose-dependent, self-limiting inflammatory response. Hum Gene Ther 1997;8(8):943–54.

19. Shine HD, Wyde PR, Aguilar-Cordova E, et al. Neurotoxicity of intracerebral injection of a replication-defective adenoviral vector in a semipermissive species (cotton rat). Gene Ther 1997;4(4):275–9.

20. O'Neal WK, Zhou H, Morral N, et al. Toxicity associated with repeated administration of first-generation adenovirus vectors does not occur with a helper-dependent vector. Mol Med 2000;6(3):179–95.

21. Moriuchi S, Glorioso JC, Maruno M, et al. Combination gene therapy for glioblastoma involving herpes simplex virus vector-mediated codelivery of mutant IkappaBalpha and HSV thymidine kinase. Cancer Gene Ther 2005;12(5):487–96.

22. Moriuchi S, Wolfe D, Tamura M, et al. Double suicide gene therapy using a replication defective herpes simplex virus vector reveals reciprocal interference in a malignant glioma model. Gene Ther 2002;9(9):584–91.

23. Yazaki T, Manz HJ, Rabkin SD, Martuza RL. Treatment of human malignant meningiomas by G207, a replication-competent multimutated herpes simplex virus 1. Cancer Res 1995;55(21):4752–6.

24. Hunter WD, Martuza RL, Feigenbaum F, et al. Attenuated, replication-competent herpes simplex virus type 1 mutant G207: safety evaluation of intracerebral injection in nonhuman primates. J Virol 1999;73(8):6319–26.

25. Oldfield EH, Ram Z, Culver KW, et al. Gene therapy for the treatment of brain tumors using intra-tumoral transduction with the thymidine kinase gene and intravenous ganciclovir. Hum Gene Ther 1993;4(1):39–69.

26. Ram Z, Culver KW, Walbridge S, et al. Toxicity studies of retroviral-mediated gene transfer for the treatment of brain tumors. J Neurosurg 1993;79(3):400–7.

27. Culver KW, Ram Z, Wallbridge S, et al. In vivo gene transfer with retroviral vector-producer cells for treatment of experimental brain tumors. Science 1992;256(5063):1550–2.

28. Miller DG, Adam MA, Miller AD. Gene transfer by retrovirus vectors occurs only in cells that are actively replicating at the time of infection. Mol Cell Biol 1990;10(8):4239–42.

29. Naldini L, Blomer U, Gage FH, et al. Efficient transfer, integration, and sustained long-term expression of the transgene in adult rat brains injected with a lentiviral vector. Proc Natl Acad Sci USA 1996;93(21):11382–8.

30. Indraccolo S, Habeler W, Tisato V, et al. Gene transfer in ovarian cancer cells: a comparison between retroviral and lentiviral vectors. Cancer Res 2002;62(21):6099–107.

31. Tai CK, Wang WJ, Chen TC, Kasahara N. Single-shot, multicycle suicide gene therapy by replication-competent retrovirus vectors achieves long-term survival benefit in experimental glioma. Mol Ther 2005;12(5):842–51.

32. Wang WJ, Tai CK, Kasahara N, Chen TC. Highly efficient and tumor-restricted gene transfer to malignant gliomas by replication-competent retroviral vectors. Hum Gene Ther 2003;14(2):117–27.

33. Ikeda K, Saeki Y, Gonzalez-Agosti C, et al. Inhibition of NF2-negative and NF2-positive primary human meningioma cell proliferation by overexpression of merlin due to vector-mediated gene transfer. J Neurosurg 1999;91(1):85–92.

34. Kotin RM, Siniscalco M, Samulski RJ, et al. Site-specific integration by adeno-associated virus. Proc Natl Acad Sci USA 1990;87(6):2211–5.

35. Lo WD, Qu G, Sferra TJ, et al. Adeno-associated virus-mediated gene transfer to the brain: duration and modulation of expression. Hum Gene Ther 1999;10(2):201–13.

36. Vermeij J, Zeinoun Z, Neyns B, et al. Transduction of ovarian cancer cells: a recombinant adeno-associated viral vector compared to an adenoviral vector. Br J Cancer 2001;85(10):1592–9.

37. Janik JE, Huston MM, Cho K, Rose JA. Efficient synthesis of adeno-associated virus structural proteins requires both adenovirus DNA binding protein and VA I RNA. Virology 1989;168(2):320–9.

38. Huszthy PC, Svendsen A, Wilson JM, et al. Widespread dispersion of adeno-associated virus serotype 1 and adeno-associated virus serotype 6 vectors in the rat central nervous system and in human glioblastoma multiforme xenografts. Hum Gene Ther 2005;16(3):381–92.

39. Yoshida J, Mizuno M, Nakahara N, Colosi P. Antitumor effect of an adeno-associated virus vector containing the human interferon-

beta gene on experimental intracranial human glioma. Jpn J Cancer Res 2002;93(2):223–8.

40. Ma HI, Lin SZ, Chiang YH, et al. Intratumoral gene therapy of malignant brain tumor in a rat model with angiostatin delivered by adeno-associated viral (AAV) vector. Gene Ther 2002;9(1):2–11.

41. Mizuno M, Yoshida J, Colosi P, Kurtzman G. Adeno-associated virus vector containing the herpes simplex virus thymidine kinase gene causes complete regression of intracerebrally implanted human gliomas in mice, in conjunction with ganciclovir administration. Jpn J Cancer Res 1998;89(1):76–80.

42. Okada H, Miyamura K, Itoh T, et al. Gene therapy against an experimental glioma using adeno-associated virus vectors. Gene Ther 1996;3(11):957–64.

43. Chen B, Timiryasova TM, Andres ML, et al. Evaluation of combined vaccinia virus-mediated antitumor gene therapy with p53, IL-2, and IL-12 in a glioma model. Cancer Gene Ther 2000;7(11):1437–47.

44. Timiryasova TM, Li J, Chen B, et al. Antitumor effect of vaccinia virus in glioma model. Oncol Res 1999;11(3):133–44.

45. Yamanaka R, Zullo SA, Ramsey J, et al. Marked enhancement of antitumor immune responses in mouse brain tumor models by genetically modified dendritic cells producing Semliki Forest virus-mediated interleukin-12. J Neurosurg 2002;97(3):611–8.

46. Yamanaka R, Zullo SA, Tanaka R, et al. Enhancement of antitumor immune response in glioma models in mice by genetically modified dendritic cells pulsed with Semliki forest virus-mediated complementary DNA. J Neurosurg 2001;94(3):474–81.

47. Yamanaka R, Zullo SA, Ramsey J, et al. Induction of therapeutic antitumor antiangiogenesis by intratumoral injection of genetically engineered endostatin-producing Semliki Forest virus. Cancer Gene Ther 2001;8(10):796–802.

48. Ren H, Boulikas T, Lundstrom K, et al. Immunogene therapy of recurrent glioblastoma multiforme with a liposomally encapsulated replication-incompetent Semliki forest virus vector carrying the human interleukin-12 gene–a phase I/II clinical protocol. J Neurooncol 2003;64(1–2):147–54.

49. Fu GF, Li X, Hou YY, et al. Bifidobacterium longum as an oral delivery system of endostatin for gene therapy on solid liver cancer. Cancer Gene Ther 2005;12(2):133–40.

50. Niethammer AG, Xiang R, Becker JC, et al. A DNA vaccine against VEGF receptor 2 prevents effective angiogenesis and inhibits tumor growth. Nat Med 2002;8(12):1369–75.

51. Shen H, Kanoh M, Liu F, et al. Modulation of the immune system by Listeria monocytogenes-mediated gene transfer into mammalian cells. Microbiol Immunol 2004;48(4):329–37.

52. Lee CH, Wu CL, Shiau AL. Systemic administration of attenuated Salmonella choleraesuis carrying thrombospondin-1 gene leads to tumor-specific transgene expression, delayed tumor growth and prolonged survival in the murine melanoma model. Cancer Gene Ther 2005;12(2):175–84.

53. Nemunaitis J, Cunningham C, Senzer N, et al. Pilot trial of genetically modified, attenuated Salmonella expressing the E. coli cytosine deaminase gene in refractory cancer patients. Cancer Gene Ther 2003;10(10):737–44.

54. Paglia P, Terrazzini N, Schulze K, et al. In vivo correction of genetic defects of monocyte/macrophages using attenuated Salmonella as oral vectors for targeted gene delivery. Gene Ther 2000;7(20):1725–30.

55. Aboody KS, Brown A, Rainov NG, et al. Neural stem cells display extensive tropism for pathology in adult brain: evidence from intracranial gliomas. Proc Natl Acad Sci USA 2000;97(23):12846–51.

56. Ehtesham M, Kabos P, Kabosova A, et al. The use of interleukin 12-secreting neural stem cells for the treatment of intracranial glioma. Cancer Res 2002;62(20):5657–63.

57. Li S, Tokuyama T, Yamamoto J, et al. Bystander effect-mediated gene therapy of gliomas using genetically engineered neural stem cells. Cancer Gene Ther 2005;12(7):600–7.

58. Barresi V, Belluardo N, Sipione S, et al. Transplantation of prodrug-converting neural progenitor cells for brain tumor therapy. Cancer Gene Ther 2003;10(5):396–402.

59. Behr JP. Gene transfer with synthetic cationic amphiphiles: prospects for gene therapy. Bioconjug Chem 1994;5(5):382–9.

60. Gardlik R, Palffy R, Hodosy J, et al. Vectors and delivery systems in gene therapy. Med Sci Monit 2005;11(4):RA110–21.

61. Zhang Y, Zhang YF, Bryant J, et al. Intravenous RNA interference gene therapy targeting the human epidermal growth factor receptor prolongs survival in intracranial brain cancer. Clin Cancer Res 2004;10(11):3667–77.

62. Shi N, Zhang Y, Zhu C, et al. Brain-specific expression of an exogenous gene after i.v. administration. Proc Natl Acad Sci USA 2001;98(22):12754–9.

63. Zhang Y, Zhu C, Pardridge WM. Antisense gene therapy of brain cancer with an artificial virus gene delivery system. Mol Ther 2002;6(1):67–72.

64. Gunther M, Wagner E, Ogris M. Specific targets in tumor tissue for the delivery of therapeutic genes. Curr Med Chem Anti-Canc Agents 2005;5(2):157–71.

65. Reszka RC, Jacobs A, Voges J. Liposome-mediated suicide gene therapy in humans. Methods Enzymol 2005;391:200–8.

66. Voges J, Reszka R, Gossmann A, et al. Imaging-guided convection-enhanced delivery and gene therapy of glioblastoma. Ann Neurol 2003;54(4):479–87.

67. Oga M, Takenaga K, Sato Y, et al. Inhibition of metastatic brain tumor growth by intramuscular administration of the endostatin gene. Int J Oncol 2003;23(1):73–9.

68. Mir LM, Moller PH, Andre F, Gehl J. Electric Pulse-Mediated Gene Delivery to Various Animal Tissues. Advances in Genetics 2005;54:83–114.

69. Yoshizato K, Nishi T, Goto T, et al. Gene delivery with optimized electroporation parameters shows potential for treatment of gliomas. Int J Oncol 2000;16(5):899–905.

70. Liau LM, Fakhrai H, Black KL. Prolonged survival of rats with intracranial C6 gliomas by treatment with TGF-beta antisense gene. Neurol Res 1998;20(8):742–7.

71. Zhang G, Selzer ME. In vivo transfection of lamprey brain neurons by gene gun delivery of DNA. Exp Neurol 2001;167(2):304–11.

72. Chauvet AE, Kesava PP, Goh CS, Badie B. Selective intraarterial gene delivery into a canine meningioma. J Neurosurg 1998;88(5):870–3.

73. Harrow S, Papanastassiou V, Harland J, et al. HSV1716 injection into the brain adjacent to tumour following surgical resection of high-grade glioma: safety data and long-term survival. Gene Ther 2004;11(22):1648–58.

74. Chen MY, Hoffer A, Morrison PF, et al. Surface properties, more than size, limiting convective distribution of virus-sized particles and viruses in the central nervous system. J Neurosurg 2005;103(2):311–9.

75. Dirven CM, Grill J, Lamfers ML, et al. Gene therapy for meningioma: improved gene delivery with targeted adenoviruses. J Neurosurg 2002;97(2):441–9.

76. van Beusechem VW, Grill J, Mastenbroek DC, et al. Efficient and selective gene transfer into primary human brain tumors by using single-chain antibody-targeted adenoviral vectors with native tropism abolished. J Virol 2002;76(6):2753–62.

77. Miletic H, Fischer YH, Neumann H, et al. Selective transduction of malignant glioma by lentiviral vectors pseudotyped with lymphocytic choriomeningitis virus glycoproteins. Hum Gene Ther 2004;15(11):1091–100.

78. Rainov NG, Ren H. Clinical trials with retrovirus mediated gene therapy–what have we learned? J Neurooncol 2003;65(3):227–36.

79. Rodriguez R, Schuur ER, Lim HY, et al. Prostate attenuated replication competent adenovirus (ARCA) CN706: a selective cytotoxic for prostate-specific antigen-positive prostate cancer cells. Cancer Res 1997;57(13):2559–63.

80. Yu DC, Sakamoto GT, Henderson DR. Identification of the transcriptional regulatory sequences of human kallikrein 2 and their use in the construction of calydon virus 764, an attenuated replication competent adenovirus for prostate cancer therapy. Cancer Res 1999;59(7):1498–504.

81. Yu DC, Chen Y, Seng M, et al. The addition of adenovirus type 5 region E3 enables calydon virus 787 to eliminate distant prostate tumor xenografts. Cancer Res 1999;59(17):4200–3.

82. Jane Jr JA, Alden TD, Meek A, et al. Tumor specific gene therapy for benign skull base tumors: an in vitro study. In: Toronto: American Association of Neurological Surgeons, 2001.

83. Bischoff JR, Kirn DH, Williams A, et al. An adenovirus mutant that replicates selectively in p53-deficient human tumor cells. Science 1996;274(5286):373–6.

84. Papanastassiou V, Rampling R, Fraser M, et al. The potential for efficacy of the modified (ICP 34.5(-)) herpes simplex virus HSV1716 following intratumoural injection into human malignant glioma: a proof of principle study. Gene Ther 2002;9(6):398–406.

85. Rampling R, Cruickshank G, Papanastassiou V, et al. Toxicity evaluation of replication-competent herpes simplex virus (ICP 34.5 null mutant 1716) in patients with recurrent malignant glioma. Gene Ther 2000;7(10):859–66.

86. Miyatake S, Martuza RL, Rabkin SD. Defective herpes simplex virus vectors expressing thymidine kinase for the treatment of malignant glioma. Cancer Gene Ther 1997;4(4):222–8.

87. Andreansky S, Soroceanu L, Flotte ER, et al. Evaluation of genetically engineered herpes simplex viruses as oncolytic agents for human malignant brain tumors. Cancer Res 1997;57(8):1502–9.

88. Katabi MM, Chan HL, Karp SE, Batist G. Hexokinase type II: a novel tumor-specific promoter for gene-targeted therapy differentially expressed and regulated in human cancer cells. Hum Gene Ther 1999;10(2):155–64.

89. Murayama Y, Tadakuma T, Kunitomi M, et al. Cell-specific expression of the diphtheria toxin A-chain coding sequence under the control of the upstream region of the human alpha-fetoprotein gene. J Surg Oncol 1999;70(3):145–9.

90. Shirakawa T, Ko SC, Gardner TA, et al. In vivo suppression of osteosarcoma pulmonary metastasis with intravenous osteocalcin promoter-based toxic gene therapy. Cancer Gene Ther 1998;5(5):274–80.

91. Lee EJ, Anderson LM, Thimmapaya B, Jameson JL. Targeted expression of toxic genes directed by pituitary hormone promoters: a potential strategy for adenovirus-mediated gene therapy of pituitary tumors. J Clin Endocrinol Metab 1999;84(2):786–94.

92. Morelli AE, Larregina AT, Smith-Arica J, et al. Neuronal and glial cell type-specific promoters within adenovirus recombinants restrict the expression of the apoptosis-inducing molecule Fas ligand to predetermined brain cell types, and abolish peripheral liver toxicity. J Gen Virol 1999;80(pt 3):571–83.

93. Vandier D, Rixe O, Brenner M, et al. Selective killing of glioma cell lines using an astrocyte-specific expression of the herpes simplex virus-thymidine kinase gene. Cancer Res 1998;58(20):4577–80.

94. Jane Jr JA, Alden TD, Ko SC, et al. Tumor specific treatment of malignant meningiomas using osteocalcin promoter based suicide gene therapy. In: San Diego, CA: Congress of Neurological Surgeons, 2001.

95. Moolten FL. Tumor chemosensitivity conferred by inserted herpes thymidine kinase genes: paradigm for a prospective cancer control strategy. Cancer Res 1986;46(10):5276–81.

96. Asklund T, Appelskog IB, Ammerpohl O, et al. Gap junction-mediated bystander effect in primary cultures of human malignant gliomas with recombinant expression of the HSVtk gene. Exp Cell Res 2003;284(2):185–95.

97. Andrade-Rozental AF, Rozental R, Hopperstad MG, et al. Gap junctions: the "kiss of death" and the "kiss of life." Brain Res Brain Res Rev 2000;32(1):308–15.

98. Estin D, Li M, Spray D, Wu JK. Connexins are expressed in primary brain tumors and enhance the bystander effect in gene therapy. Neurosurgery 1999;44(2):361–8; discussion 8–9.

99. Ram Z, Culver KW, Walbridge S, et al. In situ retroviral-mediated gene transfer for the treatment of brain tumors in rats. Cancer Res 1993;53(1):83–8.

100. Ram Z, Culver KW, Oshiro EM, et al. Therapy of malignant brain tumors by intratumoral implantation of retroviral vector-producing cells. Nat Med 1997;3(12):1354–61.

101. Sandmair AM, Loimas S, Puranen P, et al. Thymidine kinase gene therapy for human malignant glioma, using replication-deficient retroviruses or adenoviruses. Hum Gene Ther 2000;11(16):2197–205.

102. Ge K, Xu L, Zheng Z, et al. Transduction of cytosine deaminase gene makes rat glioma cells highly sensitive to 5-fluorocytosine. Int J Cancer 1997;71(4):675–9.

103. Xu LF, Ge K, Zheng ZC, et al. [Experimental treatment of brain tumor cells using CD suicide gene]. Shi Yan Sheng Wu Xue Bao 1996;29(4):385–93.

104. Dong Y, Wen P, Manome Y, et al. In vivo replication-deficient adenovirus vector-mediated transduction of the cytosine deaminase gene sensitizes glioma cells to 5-fluorocytosine. Hum Gene Ther 1996;7(6):713–20.

105. Bourbeau D, Lavoie G, Nalbantoglu J, Massie B. Suicide gene therapy with an adenovirus expressing the fusion gene CD::UPRT in human glioblastomas: different sensitivities correlate with p53 status. J Gene Med 2004;6(12):1320–32.

106. Wang ZH, Zagzag D, Zeng B, Kolodny EH. In vivo and in vitro glioma cell killing induced by an adenovirus expressing both cytosine deaminase and thymidine kinase and its

association with interferon-alpha. J Neuropathol Exp Neurol 1999;58(8):847–58.

107. Kim JH, Kolozsvary A, Rogulski K, et al. Selective radiosensitization of 9 L glioma in the brain transduced with double suicide fusion gene. Cancer J Sci Am 1998;4(6):364–9.

108. Chang JW, Lee H, Kim E, et al. Combined antitumor effects of an adenoviral cytosine deaminase/thymidine kinase fusion gene in rat C6 glioma. Neurosurgery 2000;47(4):931–8; discussion 8–9.

109. Shapiro WR, Shapiro JR. Biology and treatment of malignant glioma. Oncology (Williston Park) 1998;12(2):233–40; discussion 40, 46.

110. Das A, Tan WL, Smith DR. Expression of the inhibitor of apoptosis protein survivin in benign meningiomas. Cancer Lett 2003;193(2):217–23.

111. Sasaki T, Lopes MB, Hankins GR, Helm GA. Expression of survivin, an inhibitor of apoptosis protein, in tumors of the nervous system. Acta Neuropathol (Berl) 2002;104(1):105–9.

112. Nagashima G, Aoyagi M, Yamamoto M, et al. P53 overexpression and proliferative potential in malignant meningiomas. Acta Neurochir (Wien) 1999;141(1):53–61; discussion 0–1.

113. Zou Y, Zong G, Ling YH, et al. Effective treatment of early endobronchial cancer with regional administration of liposome-p53 complexes. J Natl Cancer Inst 1998;90(15):1130–7.

114. Nguyen DM, Wiehle SA, Koch PE, et al. Delivery of the p53 tumor suppressor gene into lung cancer cells by an adenovirus/DNA complex. Cancer Gene Ther 1997;4(3):191–8.

115. Bouvet M, Bold RJ, Lee J, et al. Adenovirus-mediated wild-type p53 tumor suppressor gene therapy induces apoptosis and suppresses growth of human pancreatic cancer [seecomments]. Ann Surg Oncol 1998;5(8):681–8.

116. Asgari K, Sesterhenn IA, McLeod DG, et al. Inhibition of the growth of pre-established subcutaneous tumor nodules of human prostate cancer cells by single injection of the recombinant adenovirus p53 expression vector. Int J Cancer 1997;71(3):377–82.

117. Spitz FR, Nguyen D, Skibber JM, et al. In vivo adenovirus-mediated p53 tumor suppressor gene therapy for colorectal cancer. Anticancer Res 1996;16(6B):3415–22.

118. Mujoo K, Maneval DC, Anderson SC, Gutterman JU. Adenoviral-mediated p53 tumor suppressor gene therapy of human ovarian carcinoma. Oncogene 1996;12(8):1617–23.

119. Lesoon-Wood LA, Kim WH, Kleinman HK, et al. Systemic gene therapy with p53 reduces growth and metastases of a malignant human breast cancer in nude mice. Hum Gene Ther 1995;6(4):395–405.

120. Badie B, Drazan KE, Kramar MH, et al. Adenovirus-mediated p53 gene delivery inhibits 9 L glioma growth in rats. Neurol Res 1995;17(3):209–16.

121. Kock H, Harris MP, Anderson SC, et al. Adenovirus-mediated p53 gene transfer suppresses growth of human glioblastoma cells in vitro and in vivo. Int J Cancer 1996;67(6):808–15.

122. Li H, Alonso-Vanegas M, Colicos MA, et al. Intracerebral adenovirus-mediated p53 tumor suppressor gene therapy for experimental human glioma. Clin Cancer Res 1999;5(3):637–42.

123. Badie B, Goh CS, Klaver J, et al. Combined radiation and p53 gene therapy of malignant glioma cells. Cancer Gene Ther 1999;6(2):155–62.

124. Dorigo O, Turla ST, Lebedeva S, Gjerset RA. Sensitization of rat glioblastoma multiforme to cisplatin in vivo following resto-ration of wild-type p53 function. J Neurosurg 1998;88(3):535–40.

125. Bostrom J, Meyer-Puttlitz B, Wolter M, et al. Alterations of the tumor suppressor genes CDKN2A (p16(INK4a)), p14(ARF), CDKN2B (p15(INK4b)), and CDKN2C (p18(INK4c)) in atypical and anaplastic meningiomas. Am J Pathol 2001;159(2):661–9.

126. Michelson S, Leith JT. Positive feedback and angiogenesis in tumor growth control. Bull Math Biol 1997;59(2):233–54.

127. Berkman RA, Merrill MJ, Reinhold WC, et al. Expression of the vascular permeability factor/vascular endothelial growth factor gene in central nervous system neoplasms. J Clin Invest 1993;91(1):153–9.

128. Samoto K, Ikezaki K, Ono M, et al. Expression of vascular endothelial growth factor and its possible relation with neovascularization in human brain tumors. Cancer Res 1995;55(5):1189–93.

129. Provias J, Claffey K, delAguila L, et al. Meningiomas: role of vascular endothelial growth factor/vascular permeability factor in angiogenesis and peritumoral edema. Neurosurgery 1997;40(5):1016–26.

130. Bitzer M, Opitz H, Popp J, et al. Angiogenesis and brain oedema in intracranial meningiomas: influence of vascular endothelial growth factor. Acta Neurochir (Wien) 1998;140(4):333–40.

131. Lamszus K, Lengler U, Schmidt NO, et al. Vascular endothelial growth factor, hepatocyte growth factor/scatter factor, basic fibroblast growth factor, and placenta growth factor in human meningiomas and their relation to angiogenesis and malignancy. Neurosurgery 2000;46(4):938–47; discussion 47–8.

132. Brown LF, Guidi AJ, Schnitt SJ, et al. Vascular stroma formation in carcinoma in situ, invasive carcinoma, and metastatic carcinoma of the breast. Clin Cancer Res 1999;5(5):1041–56.

133. Dvorak HF, Nagy JA, Feng D, et al. Vascular permeability factor/vascular endothelial growth factor and the significance of microvascular hyperpermeability in angiogenesis. Curr Top Microbiol Immunol 1999;237:97–132.

134. Gabrilovich DI, Chen HL, Girgis KR, et al. Production of vascular endothelial growth factor by human tumors inhibits the functional maturation of dendritic cells. Nat Med 1996;2(10):1096–103.

135. Im SA, Gomez-Manzano C, Fueyo J, et al. Antiangiogenesis treatment for gliomas: transfer of antisense-vascular endothelial growth factor inhibits tumor growth in vivo. Cancer Res 1999;59(4):895–900.

136. Machein MR, Risau W, Plate KH. Antiangiogenic gene therapy in a rat glioma model using a dominant-negative vascular endothelial growth factor receptor 2. Hum Gene Ther 1999;10(7):1117–28.

137. Szabo S, Sandor Z. The diagnostic and prognostic value of tumor angiogenesis. Eur J Surg Suppl 1998(582):99–103.

138. Kurimoto M, Endo S, Hirashima Y, et al. Elevated plasma basic fibroblast growth factor in brain tumor patients. Neurol Med Chir (Tokyo) 1996;36(12):865–8; discussion 9.

139. Kumar R, Kuniyasu H, Bucana CD, et al. Spatial and temporal expression of angiogenic molecules during tumor growth and progression. Oncol Res 1998;10(6):301–11.

140. Redekop GJ, Naus CC. Transfection with bFGF sense and antisense cDNA resulting in modification of malignant glioma growth. J Neurosurg 1995;82(1):83–90.

141. Voest EE. Inhibitors of angiogenesis in a clinical perspective. Anticancer Drugs 1996;7(7):723–7.
142. Oppenheim J, Fujiwara H. The role of cytokines in cancer. Cytokine Growth Factor Rev 1996;7(3):279–88.
143. Rege TA, Fears CY, Gladson CL. Endogenous inhibitors of angiogenesis in malignant gliomas: nature's antiangiogenic therapy. Neuro-oncol 2005;7(2):106–21.
144. Tanaka T, Manome Y, Wen P, et al. Viral vector-mediated transduction of a modified platelet factor 4 cDNA inhibits angiogenesis and tumor growth. Nat Med 1997;3(4):437–42.
145. Sgadari C, Farber JM, Angiolillo AL, et al. Mig, the monokine induced by interferon-gamma, promotes tumor necrosis in vivo. Blood 1997;89(8):2635–43.
146. Kanegane C, Sgadari C, Kanegane H, et al. Contribution of the CXC chemokines IP-10 and Mig to the antitumor effects of IL-12. J Leukoc Biol 1998;64(3):384–92.
147. Lesokhin AM, Delgado-Lopez F, Horwitz MS. Inhibition of chemokine expression by adenovirus early region three (E3) genes. J Virol 2002;76(16):8236–43.
148. Tanaka T, Cao Y, Folkman J, Fine HA. Viral vector-targeted antiangiogenic gene therapy utilizing an angiostatin complementary DNA. Cancer Res 1998;58(15):3362–9.
149. De Bouard S, Guillamo JS, Christov C, et al. Antiangiogenic therapy against experimental glioblastoma using genetically engineered cells producing interferon-alpha, angiostatin, or endostatin. Hum Gene Ther 2003;14(9):883–95.
150. Lord EM, Frelinger JG. Tumor immunotherapy: cytokines and antigen presentation. Cancer Immunol Immunother 1998;46(2):75–81.
151. Stavrou D, Bilzer T, Hulten M, et al. Immunological aspects of experimental brain tumors (review). Anticancer Res 1982;2(3):151–5.
152. Sikorski CW, Lesniak MS. Immunotherapy for malignant glioma: current approaches and future directions. Neurol Res 2005;27(7):703–16.
153. Khan-Farooqi HR, Prins RM, Liau LM. Tumor immunology, immunomics and targeted immunotherapy for central nervous system malignancies. Neurol Res 2005;27(7):692–702.
154. Antoniades HN, Galanopoulos T, Neville-Golden J, Maxwell M. Expression of insulin-like growth factors I and II and their receptor mRNAs in primary human astrocytomas and meningiomas; in vivo studies using in situ hybridization and immunocytochemistry. Int J Cancer 1992;50(2):215–22.
155. Sandberg-Nordqvist AC, Stahlbom PA, Reinecke M, et al. Characterization of insulin-like growth factor 1 in human primary brain tumors. Cancer Res 1993;53(11):2475–8.
156. Trojan J, Johnson TR, Rudin SD, et al. Treatment and prevention of rat glioblastoma by immunogenic C6 cells expressing antisense insulin-like growth factor I RNA. Science 1993;259(5091):94–7.
157. Ly A, Bouchaud C, Henin D, et al. Expression of insulin-like growth factor-I in rat glioma cells is associated with change in both immunogenicity and apoptosis. Neurosci Lett 2000;281(1):13–6.
158. Trojan J, Duc HT, Upegui-Gonzalez LC, et al. Presence of MHC-I and B-7 molecules in rat and human glioma cells expressing antisense IGF-I mRNA. Neurosci Lett 1996;212(1):9–12.
159. Resnicoff M, Sell C, Rubini M, et al. Rat glioblastoma cells expressing an antisense RNA to the insulin-like growth factor-1 (IGF-1) receptor are nontumorigenic and induce regression of wild-type tumors. Cancer Res 1994;54(8):2218–22.
160. Trojan LA, Kopinski P, Mazurek A, et al. IGF-I triple helix gene therapy of rat and human gliomas. Rocz Akad Med Bialymst 2003;48:18–27.
161. Ruscetti FW, Palladino MA. Transforming growth factor-beta and the immune system. Prog Growth Factor Res 1991;3(2):159–75.
162. Fakhrai H, Dorigo O, Shawler DL, et al. Eradication of established intracranial rat gliomas by transforming growth factor beta antisense gene therapy. Proc Natl Acad Sci USA 1996;93(7):2909–14.
163. Nitta T, Sato K, Okumura K. Transforming growth factor (TGF)-beta like activity of intracranial meningioma and its effect on cell growth. J Neurol Sci 1991;101(1):19–23.
164. Johnson M, Toms S. Mitogenic signal transduction pathways in meningiomas: novel targets for meningioma chemotherapy? J Neuropathol Exp Neurol 2005;64(12):1029–36.
165. Tseng SH, Hwang LH, Lin SM. Induction of antitumor immunity by intracerebrally implanted rat C6 glioma cells genetically engineered to secrete cytokines. J Immunother 1997;20(5):334–42.
166. Fathallah-Shaykh HM, Gao W, Cho M, Herrera MA. Priming in the brain, an immunologically privileged organ, elicits antitumor immunity. Int J Cancer 1998;75(2):266–76.
167. Glick RP, Lichtor T, Mogharbel A, et al. Intracerebral versus subcutaneous immunization with allogeneic fibroblasts genetically engineered to secrete interleukin-2 in the treatment of central nervous system glioma and melanoma. Neurosurgery 1997;41(4):898–906; discussion -7.
168. Addison CL, Bramson JL, Hitt MM, et al. Intratumoral coinjection of adenoviral vectors expressing IL-2 and IL-12 results in enhanced frequency of regression of injected and untreated distal tumors. Gene Ther 1998;5(10):1400–9.
169. Lode HN, Dreier T, Xiang R, et al. Gene therapy with a single chain interleukin 12 fusion protein induces T cell-dependent protective immunity in a syngeneic model of murine neuroblastoma. Proc Natl Acad Sci USA 1998;95(5):2475–80.
170. Myers JN, Mank-Seymour A, Zitvogel L, et al. Interleukin-12 gene therapy prevents establishment of SCC VII squamous cell carcinomas, inhibits tumor growth, and elicits long-term antitumor immunity in syngeneic C3H mice. Laryngoscope 1998;108(2):261–8.
171. Chen PW, Geer DC, Podack ER, Ksander BR. Tumor cells transfected with B7-1 and interleukin-12 cDNA induce protective immunity. Ann NY Acad Sci 1996;795:325–7.
172. Tahara H, Lotze MT. Antitumor effects of interleukin-12 (IL-2): applications for the immunotherapy and gene therapy of cancer. Gene Ther 1995;2(2):96–106.
173. Andreansky S, He B, van Cott J, et al. Treatment of intracranial gliomas in immunocompetent mice using herpes simplex viruses that express murine interleukins. Gene Ther 1998;5(1):121–30.
174. Okada H, Pollack IF, Lotze MT, et al. Gene therapy of malignant gliomas: a phase I study of IL-4-HSV-TK gene-modified autologous tumor to elicit an immune response. Hum Gene Ther 2000;11(4):637–53.
175. Okada H, Pollack IF, Lieberman F, et al. Gene therapy of malignant gliomas: a pilot study of vaccination with irradiated

autologous glioma and dendritic cells admixed with IL-4 trans-duced fibroblasts to elicit an immune response. Hum Gene Ther 2001;12(5):575–95.

176. Galipeau J, Benaim E, Spencer HT, et al. A bicistronic ret-roviral vector for protecting hematopoietic cells against anti-folates and P-glycoprotein effluxed drugs. Hum Gene Ther 1997;8(15):1773–83.

177. Sorrentino BP, Brandt SJ, Bodine D, et al. Selection of drug-resistant bone marrow cells in vivo after retroviral transfer of human MDR1. Science 1992;257(5066):99–103.

IV
Management and Outcome

17
Management Options and Surgical Principles: An Overview

Joung H. Lee and Burak Sade

Management Options

In general, management options for patients with meningiomas include observation, surgery, and radiation alone or as an adjuvant therapy following surgery. To date, no definitively effective chemotherapeutic agent has been identified or developed. As meningiomas are mostly benign and slowly progressive tumors, immediate intervention is usually not required. Final treatment plans must be individualized for each patient based on the age, overall condition of the patient, tumor location and size, neurologic symptoms and deficits caused by the tumor, and the patient's personal wish after a thorough discussion of all available options.

Observation

Surgery is not necessary for every patient with a meningioma. At our institution, we currently evaluate approximately 200 new patients with meningiomas annually, among whom only about 100 undergo surgical intervention. Observation alone, with periodic (usually yearly) follow-up neurologic and magnetic resonance (MR) evaluations, is reasonable for elderly patients, especially if they have minimal or no symptoms caused by the tumor. As people are living healthier and longer lives today, the age at which a person is considered "elderly" is debatable. The patient's absolute age is no longer important in the decision-making process in the management of meningiomas; however, it may be reasonable to consider those with less than 10–15 years of remaining life expectancy (due to various reasons such as other co-morbidities that ultimately determine the overall health status) to be "elderly." In addition, observation may be an appropriate option for the following people regardless of their age: (1) patients with certain skull base meningiomas with minimal or no symptoms (e.g., cavernous sinus or petroclival meningioma causing mild facial tingling or numbness, optic nerve sheath meningioma with minimal or no visual deficit), (2) patients with incidental small tumors with no surrounding edema, and (3) patients who insist on nonintervention after a thorough discussion of all treatment options. However, these patients must be compliant with the necessary radiographic and neurological follow-up evaluations.

As with other brain tumors, the risks of surgery may vary in direct proportion to the tumor size, while the chances of total resection vary inversely proportional to the size of meningioma in most locations. For example, it is quite obvious that removal of parasagittal tumors prior to involvement of the superior sagittal sinus (SSS) would be easier compared to larger tumors intimately involving the SSS. The same may be said of small to medium-sized clinoidal or tuberculum sellae meningiomas before causing optic nerve and internal carotid artery (ICA) involvement or petrous meningiomas prior to reaching a large size that would encase the basilar artery and compress the brainstem and cranial nerves. Therefore, the initial recommendation of observation must be decided upon carefully, especially in younger patients, taking into consideration the increased potential risks posed in the future by further growth in the tumor size and involvement of nearby critical neurovascular structures.

Surgery

General Principles

Surgery is the treatment of choice for most patients with meningiomas. In patients with benign meningiomas, which comprise approximately 92% of all meningiomas,[1] the tumor location largely dictates the extent of resection, which, in turn, determines the tumor recurrence and, ultimately, the patient's survival.[2–4] Primary goals of surgery include: (1) total resection of the tumor and the involved surrounding bone and dura when feasible, thereby possibly providing cure or significantly altering the natural history of the disease process, and (2) reversal or improvement in neurologic deficits/symptoms caused by the tumor. In meningiomas of certain locations, such as the cavernous sinus or petroclival regions where complete resection is not always possible, additional surgical goals may include confirmation of tissue diagnosis and tumor reduction (to less than 3 cm maximum diameter) in preparation for radiosurgery. Given the benign nature of meningiomas and the established efficacy of adjuvant radiation, the goal of total removal must be balanced by the physician's basic credo to "do no harm." When total removal carries a significant risk of morbidity, a small piece of tumor may be left, with further plans of observation followed by reoperation or radiation when the tumor is noted to be growing or causing new symptoms.

Surgical Technique

Meningiomas of different locations require varying surgical approaches that are primarily dictated by anatomic considerations inherent to each particular location. Surgical procedures of different anatomic regions are discussed in detail in the later chapters of this book. Furthermore, an abundance of excellent descriptions of "standard" techniques and approaches for meningioma surgery is available. This chapter is written not to replace, but to supplement, those previous important writings on the topic. Several key concepts and principles deemed important are reiterated, and new insights and lessons learned by the senior author, based on his personal surgical experience with over 700 meningioma patients, are summarized and presented.

In meningioma surgery, approaches may vary, depending on the tumor location and size, as well as the surgeon's personal experience and preference. However, the following basic principles hold for meningioma surgery of most locations:

1. Optimal patient positioning, incision, and exposure
2. Early tumor devascularization
3. Internal decompression and extracapsular dissection
4. Early localization and preservation of adherent or adjacent neurovasculature
5. Removal of involved bone and dura

Positioning, Incision and Exposure

Patient positioning, appropriate incision placement, and selection of the optimal approach for tumor exposure are the critical elements of successful meningioma surgery. The patient is positioned in such a way that his or her safety is maximized. Moreover, the ideal position must allow for an approach that provides complete exposure of the tumor and the involved surrounding bone and dura. At the same time, maximal brain relaxation must be achieved by use of gravity and uncompromised venous drainage. The head should be no lower than the level of the heart, regardless of the position selected, and undue severe neck rotation or flexion must be avoided. In addition, the surgeon's comfort for the duration of surgery must be maintained. The sitting position, preferred by some neurosurgeons for tumors of the pineal and select posterior fossa locations, places the patient at a higher risk of developing air embolism and the surgeon at an increased level of discom-

fort. When considering the sitting position for the aforementioned lesions, preoperative sagittal MRI should be reviewed carefully to appreciate the relative size of the posterior fossa and the steepness of the tentorial angle. Patients with a small posterior fossa usually have a low-lying posterior tentorial attachment because of the inferior location of the torcular and inion. This anatomic variation leads to a very steep, nearly vertical tentorial angle, making the infratentorial/supracerebellar approach with the patient seated extremely difficult. Other approaches to be considered in this situation include the transoccipital/transtentorial approach with the patient in the prone position or the infratentorial/supracerebellar approach with the patient in the modified park-bench (the "Concorde") position.

For superficial tumors (e.g., convexity or parasagittal), the planned scalp flap should contain the tumor in the center, and the patient is positioned so that the tumor is at the highest point. Importantly, the incision must be planned to avoid any visible cosmetic defect or significant compromise to the scalp vascular supply. If a horseshoe-shaped incision is planned, the depth must not exceed the width of the flap. Again, for superficial tumors, the size of the scalp and bone flaps must be sufficiently large so as to allow for maximal exposure of the tumor, the involved bone and dura, as well as the limits of the dural tail as noted on preoperative MRI scans. With the availability of frameless stereotactic image-guidance systems, the exact extent of the tumor and the dural tail may be fully delineated before surgery. This aids in optimal positioning and placement of incision and craniotomy.

An optimal approach should provide the shortest and most direct route to the tumor without "sacrificing" any normal brain tissue or creating undue brain damage by retraction. The need for retraction is minimized by taking advantage of gravity. For example, for surgery of an olfactory groove meningioma the head can be slightly hyperextended, and for a cerebello-pontine-angle lesion the patient may be placed in the lateral position. For large, deep, falcine tumors, the patient's head may be placed with the side of the tumor down and the direction of the sagittal sinus parallel to the operating room floor. In all of these examples, the brain falls away from the tumor and its attachment. In deep-seated tumors, brain retraction may be minimized by use of cerebrospinal fluid (CSF) drainage via either a ventricular drain (in patients with obstructive hydrocephalus) or a lumbar drain. Furthermore, many of the skull base approaches developed over the last two decades, which convert the deep basal meningiomas to more superficial "convexity" lesions by reducing the working distance to the tumor, may minimize or obviate the need for brain retraction.

An optimal surgical approach also facilitates surgery by maximizing exposure of the tumor and surrounding structures, thereby minimizing risks of injury to the adjacent neurovasculature. For example, in surgery of large clinoidal or tuberculum sellae meningiomas, complete removal of the anterior clinoid process (ACP) provides improved access and exposure of the regions surrounding the optic nerve, optic chiasm, ICA, and sella turcica.[5-7] Additionally, by opening the optic sheath as an extension of the dural incision following anterior clinoidectomy, the optic nerve can be decompressed and visualized early and mobilized safely during surgery, thereby reducing the risk of intraoperative injury to the nerve.[8] This maneuver also expands operative windows, particularly the optico-carotid triangle, facilitating access to tumors in the suprasellar and subchiasmatic regions.

In most situations, there exist a number of options for selecting the patient's position, surgical approach, and exposure. The final selection must be based on what is best for the patient and the surgeon, based on the surgeon's knowledge, past experience, and preference.

Tumor Devascularization

Many meningiomas can be quite vascular. In addition to utilization of preoperative embolization when appropriate, early operative devascularization of the tumor reduces blood loss and makes surgery easier. In superficial tumors, upon dural exposure prior to opening the dura, extra time should be expended to coagulate all the dural feeding vessels—most commonly the branches or the main trunk of the middle meningeal artery. In olfactory groove meningiomas, bifrontal craniotomy, preferred by many surgeons, provides early access to the main tumor feeders, i.e., ethmoidal arteries, as they enter the medial anterior fossa floor. In large sphenoid wing meningiomas, which receive siginificant transdural blood supply, utilizing the extradural skull base technique of orbitosphenoid bone removal obliterates many dural feeders prior to dural opening. Similarly, in petroclival meningiomas, the transpetrosal approach allows the exposed petrous dura and tentorium to be aggressively coagulated, and may significantly devascularize the tumor. In falcine or tentorial meningiomas, wide exposure and coagulation of the surrounding falx and tentorium reduce tumor vascularity. Yasargil advocates initial transtumoral devascularization of basal meningiomas by working through a small "window" created in the tumor to reach the blood supply coming through the base.[9] However, this technique may not be suitable for an inexperienced surgeon as there may be a significant risk of injury to unexposed neurovascular structures that may be located on the other side of the tumor.

Internal Decompression and Extracapsular Dissection

Although small meningiomas may be removed "en bloc," internal decompression is a key initial step in actual tumor removal for most meningiomas following adequate exposure and initial devascularization. Internal debulking is carried out until a thin rim of exposed portion of the tumor is remaining. This internal debulking minimizes brain retraction and facilitates extracapsular dissection. Following initial internal decompression, extracapsular dissection is initiated by identifying a layer of arachnoid (maintained in most meningiomas) at the brain–tumor interface. As surgery progresses, rather than increasing brain retraction to expose more of the tumor hidden under the brain, the thinned capsule is pulled towards the center of decompression. Cottonoid patties are placed in the brain–tumor interface as the capsule is being pulled away from the brain, while maintaining the arachnoidal layer intact between the brain and the tumor. As patties are being placed sequentially around the tumor, they are used to gently strip the arachnoid from the tumor capsule, simultaneously covering the brain and arachnoid together, thereby protecting the brain from surgical trauma. As the remaining tumor capsule is brought into the surgeon's view, any adjacent neurovascular structures are carefully dissected, and exposed blood vessels on the capsule surface are thoroughly inspected. Only tumor-feeding vessels are obliterated, preserving and dissecting free those transit vessels that are either passing through the depth of tumor or adherent to the tumor surface. Portions of tumor capsule thus devascularized and completely dissected from the surrounding neurovasculature are further removed in segments. These alternating sequential steps of internal decompression, extracapsular dissection, and removal of devascularized capsule are repeated until the entire tumor is removed.

For meningiomas in the clival, petroclival, or cerebello-pontine-angle regions, the surgeon must analyze the preoperative MRI scan carefully. First, evidence of surrounding edema in the brainstem noted on T2-weighted scan must be appreciated prior to surgery as this indicates disruption of the arachnoidal layer and the blood-brain barrier.[10] This implies that the surgical plane between the brainstem and tumor may have been obliterated and, therefore, aggressive resection off the brainstem should be avoided. Second, the basilar artery location in relation to the tumor and brainstem must be noted. Although rare, if the tumor is located between the brainstem and basilar artery or completely encases the artery, this indicates that all the perforating branches of the basilar artery are stretched and course through the tumor. In this situation, an attempt at aggressive tumor removal is likely to result in a brainstem infarct. When the basilar artery is abutting directly on the brainstem, aggressive tumor removal off the brainstem is possible.

During extracapsular dissection, as a rule, no artery or arterial branch is sacrificed except when the vessel is definitely confirmed to be a tumor feeder. Commonly, loops of vessels may be encased by the tumor or may course onto the capsule surface and become adherent. In these situations, the surgeon may initially misinterpret these vessels as tumor feeders. Before concluding that a vessel is a tumor feeder and therefore amenable to obliteration, the afferent and efferent course of the vessel must be fully appreciated. It is very rare for meningiomas to have feeders directly from main intracranial arterial trunks. Therefore, no vessels coming directly off the ICA (in tuberculum sellae or clinoidal tumors), basilar artery (in petroclival- and cerebellopontine-angle tumors), or vertebral artery (in foramen magnum meningiomas) should be coagulated. If any appreciable vasospasm occurs while dissecting tumor off arteries, small pieces of gelfoam soaked in papaverine applied directly onto the vessel readily reverse the spasm.

In removing the tumor from cranial nerves, especially the optic nerve, fine vessels feeding the nerves must be preserved. The optic chiasm and intradural optic nerve have main feeders on the inferior surface, and therefore removal of large tumors involving the subchiasmatic and suboptic space must be done carefully so as to preserve these fine vessels. Again, the preserved arachnoid around the cranial nerves facilitates tumor removal and reduces risks of intraoperative neurovascular injury.

Early Localization and Preservation of Adjacent Neurovasculature

Whenever possible, any adjacent or nearby normal neurovasculature (e.g., a cranial nerve or a vessel) should be identified and dissection carried out following this structure into the tumor. For example, in large clinoidal tumors encasing the optic nerve and the ICA, the conventional technique for removal has been first to identify the distal middle cerebral artery branches and follow these vessels proximally toward the ICA with subsequent tumor removal and dissection. However, until the ICA and eventually the intradural optic nerve are located, surgery progresses slowly. More importantly, the risk of intraoperative neurovascular injury persists during surgery as the exact location of the optic nerve and ICA remains unknown to the surgeon, and the optic nerve remains compressed. During this time, any minor surgical trauma caused by retraction, dissection, or tumor manipulation may exacerbate compression of the optic nerve, especially against the falciform ligament. To circumvent these critical problems, the optic nerve can be exposed and simultaneously decompressed early in the surgery by unroofing the optic canal, followed by anterior clinoidectomy and opening of the optic sheath. The location of the optic canal, and therefore the intracanalicular segment of the optic nerve, is fairly constant; only the intradural cisternal segment of the optic nerve varies in location, depending on how the tumor causes nerve displacement during its growth. The exposed optic nerve can then be followed from the optic canal proximally, toward the tumor in the intradural location. As tumor resection progresses further, the ICA can be readily found adjacent to the exposed distal intradural segment of the optic nerve. Complete optic sheath opening, along the length of the nerve within the optic canal to the anulus of Zinn, relieves any focal circumferential pressure on the optic nerve contributed by the falciform ligament. Optic nerve decompression thus achieved also leads to reduced intraoperative injury to the nerve, because the force of retraction is then dispersed over a much larger surface area. Moreover, if the tumor eventually recurs, the patient's impending visual deterioration may be delayed as the optic nerve is already decompressed from the surrounding falciform ligament and optic canal. In the senior author's personal experience utilizing the described technique in over 50 patients with presenting clinoidal meningiomas, 73% experienced significant improvement in their vision postoperatively.

Whenever possible, no cortical vein or dural sinus is "sacrificed." Although the anterior third of the sagittal sinus is traditionally said to be amenable to obliteration without any significant sequelae, there is a risk of developing significant venous infarcts. Therefore, even in large olfactory groove or planum sphenoidale tumors, rather than routine anterior sagittal sinus obliteration following a bifrontal craniotomy, either a unilateral pterional or a bilateral interhemispheric approach with preservation of sagittal sinus is used whenever possible in the senior author's practice. In parasagittal meningiomas, the tumor is removed aggressively, along with the involved segment of sagittal sinus, only when the sinus is completely occluded by the tumor. Otherwise, every effort is made to preserve the sagittal sinus integrity and patency while removing as much tumor as possible. Nearby prominent cortical veins, especially in the posterior two thirds along the sinus, are preserved as well.

Removal of the Involved Bone and Dura

Following complete tumor removal, the site of tumor origin is carefully inspected. If possible, the involved dura and bone are removed. In tumors of basal locations, the involved bone is drilled using a diamond burr, which is also quite effective in achieving hemostasis from tumor feeders arising directly from the base of the skull. Involved bone adjacent to paranasal sinuses is aggressively drilled, short of entering the sinus space. Inadvertent opening into paranasal sinuses or mastoid air cells must be recognized and appropriately sealed with muscle or fat graft and/or bone wax.

In 1983, Dolenc introduced an extensive extradural skull base technique to gain safe entry into the cavernous sinus.[11] The critical steps of this technique, following a routine frontotemporal craniotomy and drilling of the lateral sphenoid wing, include complete bone removal around the superior orbital fissure (SOF), posterior orbitotomy, optic canal unroofing, extradural removal of the ACP, and removal of bone around the foramen rotundum and ovale. Meningiomas of the posterior orbital roof, cavernous sinus (CS), sphenoid wing, or orbitosphenoid regions frequently cause hyperostosis of the orbital roof, and the greater and lesser sphenoid wing, including the ACP. For these tumors, the Dolenc approach, with modifications tailored to removal of only the involved bone, is an ideal technique.

In addition, the extensive sphenoid bone removal of the Dolenc approach, when coupled with the extradural exposure of the CS, facilitates removal of the involved dura, especially the portion of temporal dura covering the medial greater sphenoid wing, which simultaneously forms the outer lateral wall of CS. Following extradural bone removal as summarized above, the dural fold at the superolateral aspect of the SOF is sharply cut with microscissors tangential to the temporal dura. The temporal dura forming the outer lateral CS wall is then "peeled" off the underlying inner CS lateral wall. This process of separating the two-layered CS lateral wall is continued laterally and posteriorly until all three divisions of the trigeminal nerve and the gasserian ganglion are exposed. In this manner, the lateral aspect of the CS is exposed entirely extradurally, freeing up the dura of medial temporal pole for removal as necessary, which would not have been possible to resect otherwise. This maneuver is particularly helpful in orbitosphenoid, CS, and sphenoid wing meningiomas, which frequently involve the temporal polar dura.

Postoperative Management

Follow-up evaluations consist of careful neurologic examination and MRI scans with and without gadolinium. For patients with preoperative diplopia and changes in vision, detailed neuro-ophthalmologic evaluations are a critical part of follow-up management. Similarly, patients with posterior fossa meningiomas presenting with hearing loss, or those patients whose surgery involved dissection of the cranial nerve complex VII–VIII, should have thorough audiologic evaluations as part of their postoperative management. Following resection of all meningiomas, a postoperative baseline MRI scan is obtained on day 1 or 2 after surgery. For benign tumors, following confirmation of total removal on postoperative MRI, further follow-up evaluation with imaging studies is performed every 1–3 years, depending on whether Simpson grade I or II removal was achieved. Following a subtotal removal, subsequent follow-up with MRI is done every year, with plans of adjuvant radiation if and when there is clinical or radiographic progression of the residual tumor. If the tumor is noted to be clinically and radiographically stable for a few years after initial surgery, the frequency of follow-up may be decreased to every 2–3 years. For atypical meningiomas, after initial postoperative MRI following either subtotal or total removal, subsequent evaluations with MRI are performed every 6 months for the first 2 years. As with benign tumors, radiation is considered in the presence of documented clinical or radiographic progression of the residual tumor. With malignant meningiomas, adjuvant radiation is administered shortly after surgery regardless of the extent of resection. However, if there is any reversible postoperative neurologic deficit from brain swelling or cranial nerve manipulation, the timing of radiation therapy should be delayed to allow for adequate recovery. Depending on the extent of resection, follow-up MRI scans are performed every 3–6 months.

References

1. Lee JH, Sade B, Choi E, et al. Meningothelioma as the predominant histological subtype of midline skull base and spinal meningioma. J Neurosurg 2006;105:60–4.
2. De Monte F, Al Mefty O. Meningiomas. In: Kaye AH, Laws ER Jr, eds. Brain Tumors. New York: Churchill Livingstone, 1995:675–704.
3. Mirimanoff RO, Dosoretz DE, Linggood RM, et al. Meningioma: analysis of recurrence and progression following neurosurgical resection. J Neurosurg 1985;62:18–24.
4. Simpson D. The recurrence of intracranial meningiomas after surgical treatment. J Neurol Neurosurg Psychiatry 1957;20:22–39.
5. Evans JJ, Hwang YS, Lee JH. Pre- versus post-anterior clinoidectomy measurements of the optic nerve, internal carotid artery, and opticocarotid triangle: a cadaveric morphometric study. Neurosurgery 2000;46:1018–23.
6. Sade B, Kweon CY, Evans JJ, et al. Enhanced exposure of the carotico-oculomotor triangle following extradural anterior clinoidectomy: a comparative anatomical study. Skull Base 2005;15:157–62.
7. Yonekawa Y, Ogata N, Imhof HG, et al. Selective extradural anterior clinoidectomy for supra- and parasellar processes. Technical note. J Neurosurg 1997;87:636–42.
8. Lee JH, Jeun SS, Evans J, et al. Surgical management of clinoidal meningiomas. Neurosurgery 2001;48:1012–21.
9. Yasargil MG. Meningiomas. In: Yasargil MG, ed. Microneurosurgery, Vol 4B. New York: Thieme, 1996:134–85.
10. Carvalho GA, Mathies C, Tatagiba M, et al. Impact of computed tomographic and magnetic resonance imaging findings on surgical outcome in petroclival meningiomas. Neurosurgery 2000;47:1287–95.
11. Dolenc V. Direct microsurgical repair of intracavernous vascular lesions. J Neurosurg 1983;58:824–31.

18
Operative Outcome Following Meningioma Surgery: A Personal Experience of 600 Cases

Joung H. Lee and Burak Sade

Introduction

It has been well discussed in the medical literature that higher patient volume in a given medical center is associated with a more favorable outcome for surgical patients. In the study of Flood and colleagues in the 1980s, a study of 550,000 patients treated in over 1200 hospitals in 15 surgical and 2 medical (nonsurgical) categories, strong and consistent evidence was found suggesting that high patient volume was associated with a better outcome for surgical patients, although the evidence for the medical patients was not as strong [1]. Recently, volume-outcome association has been of interest to scholars from the neurosurgical community as well. Long and colleagues studied the outcome and the cost of tumor-related craniotomies in high- and low-volume medical centers [2]. In this study, the cutoff point for defining low and high volume centers was 50 craniotomies/year. Their results showed the mortality rates in high-volume centers as half of those at low-volume ones. In a more specific patient population, Curry and colleagues looked at the relationship between outcome and case volume in craniotomies for intracranial meningiomas [3]. In that study the cutoff for high and low-volume centers and high and low-volume surgeons was 24 cases/year/institution and 8 cases/year/surgeon, respectively. Their results showed lower mortality and morbidity rates for the high-volume hospitals.

However, although there are growing data in the literature suggesting a more favorable outcome in high-volume centers for various neurosurgical pathologies, there has not been much discussion and data on how to quantify experience throughout the carreer of any given surgeon. As Black points out in his comment for the study of Long and colleagues, the results favoring the outcomes in higher volume centers would not mean that the surgeons working in these centers are "better" than those working in lower volume centers or that these data do not define how many patients are truly necessary to provide surgeons with optimal experience [4]. The data available in the literature on surgical outcomes are mainly institutional, at times multi-institutional, but rarely reflective of the experience of a single surgeon.

In this context, we believe that analysis of the surgical outcome of a particular neurosurgical problem, in this case intracranial meningioma in the experience of a single surgeon, throughout his or her carreer would provide important information. This chapter focuses on the operative experience of the senior author with 600 consecutive cases of intracranial meningiomas over a 13-year period.

Methods

Medical records of 600 patients who were operated by the senior author between July 1993 and December 2006 were reviewed retrospectively. The overall outcome was reported using the Glasgow Outcome Scale (GOS) [5] at 6 weeks and at 1 year. Favorable and unfavorable outcomes were defined as GOS 4 and 5 and GOS 1–3, respectively. In addition, postoperative surgical (major neurologic, minor neurologic, nonneurologic) and medical complications within the first postoperative month were recorded. The impact of the surgeon's experience on the outcome was assessed by stratifying the patients into three groups of 200 successive patients each. Group I consisted of the first 200 patients, Group II the latter 200 patients, and Group III the most recent 200 patients.

Major neurologic complications consisted of new deficits of the following cranial nerves: 2, 3, 5 (V1 division), 7, 9, 10, as well as worsened level of consciousness, motor deficits, aphasia and pituitary insufficiency.

Minor neurologic complications consisted of new deficits involving the cranial nerves 4, 5 (Divisions V2, V3), 6, 8, 11, 12, as well as focal sensory deficits.

Nonneurologic complications included surgical complications such as meningitis, cerebrospinal fluid (CSF) leak either from the wound or in the form of rhinorrhea, wound dehiscence, and infection.

Results

At 6 weeks, 95.2% of the 600 patients had a favorable out-come (85.8% GOS 5, and 9.8% GOS 4) (Fig. 18-1): 92% of Group III patients had GOS 5, as compared to 83.5% of Group I and 82% of Group II ($p = 0.01$) (Fig. 18-2). Overall mortality was 0.6%. Data for 342 patients were available for 1-year review (Fig. 18-3). Of these, 95.9% showed a favorable outcome (92.7% GOS 5, and 3.2% GOS 4).

Early Outcome vs. Late Outcome

Of the 6 patients with a GOS of 2 at 6 weeks, 1-year follow-up was possible in 4. Of these, 3 died, and the remaining one patient had a GOS of 3.

Of the 19 patients with a GOS of 3 at 6 weeks, 13 patients had 1 year follow-up. Of these patients, 4 (30.7%) died, 4 (30.7%) remained at GOS 3, whereas 1 (7.7%) improved to GOS 4, and 5 (38.4%) improved to GOS 5.

Of the 56 patients with a GOS of 4 at 6 weeks, 30 patients had a 1-year follow-up. Of these, 6 (20%) remained the same, whereas 24 (80%) improved to a GOS of 5.

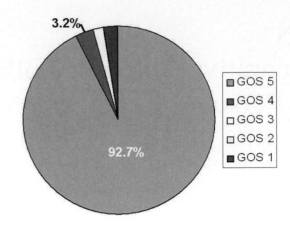

FIG. 18-3. Operative outcome in 342 patients at 1 year. GOS, Glasgow Outcome Score

Of the 294 patients, who had an early GOS of 5, and whose information was available for 1-year follow-up, 292 (99.4%) had still a GOS of 5, whereas 2 (0.6%) were dead at 1 year (1 late ischemic stroke, and 1 late pulmonary embolus).

Complications

Surgical complications were encountered in 17.7% of 600 patients: 22% in Group I, 18% in Group II, and 13.5% in Group III (Fig. 18-4). Medical complications were seen in 9.3%: 12% in Group I, 6.5% in Group II, and 9.5% in Group III (Fig. 18-4).

Further analysis of patients with surgical complications showed that major neurologic complications occurred in 12.5%, 11%, and 4%; minor neurologic complications in 7%, 4.5%, and 2.5%; and nonneurologic complications were seen in 2.5%, 2.5%, and 6.5% of Groups I, II, and II, respectively (Fig. 18-5).

Of the 333 patients whose 1-year following information was available, 31 had major and 18 had minor neurologic complications at their 6-week follow-up. The outcome of these complications during their 1-year follow-up is shown in Table 18-1.

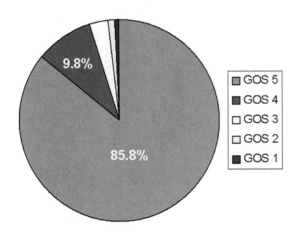

FIG. 18-1. Operative outcome in 600 meningiomas at 6 weeks. GOS, Glasgow Outcome Score

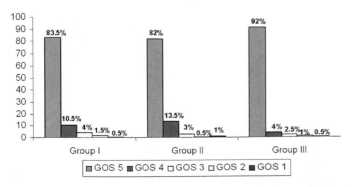

FIG. 18-2. Percentage of operative outcome at 6 weeks according to surgeon's experience in 600 patients. GOS, Glasgow Outcome Score

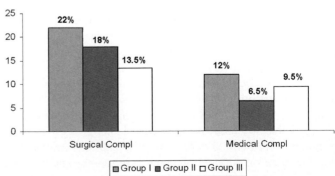

FIG. 18-4. Percentage of surgical and medical complications

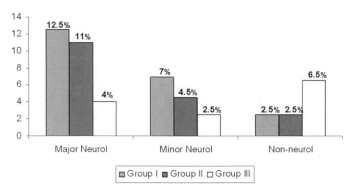

FIG. 18-5. Percentage of surgical complication subgroups

Composition of the Groups

The average patient age was 55 ± 14 for Group I, 56 ± 13 for Group II, and 54 ± 13 for Group III. Average tumor size was 36.5 ± 16.5 mm for Group I, 37.1 ± 18.7 for Group II, and 37.4 ± 18.2 for Group III. There was no difference among the groups with regards to the patient age or tumor size.

The composition of the groups with regards to the patient co-morbidities as defined by the American Society of Anesthesiology (ASA) [6], tumor location classified as high, moderate, or low risk as defined by the CLASS algorithmic scale (please refer to Chapter 20), as well as presence and severity of symptoms are detailed in Tables 18-2, 18-3, and 18-4, respectively.

Discussion

In the experience of the senior author, 85.8% of the patients had a GOS of 5 and 9.8% had a GOS of 4 at 6 weeks. Of the 600 patients, 342 patients were available for 1-year follow-up, and of these, 92.7% had a GOS of 5 and 3.2% had a GOS of 4. Patients who remained with a GOS of 2 or 3, or patients

TABLE 18-1. Outcome of Neurologic Complications at 1 Year.

Complication at 6 weeks	Outcome at 1 year	
	Improved	Not improved
Decreased LOC ($n = 6$)	6 (100%)	—
Hemiparesis ($n = 6$)	4 (67%)	2 (33%)
Cranial nerves		
CNIII ($n = 5$)	3 (60%)	2 (40%)
CNV ($n = 10$)	2 (20%)	8 (80%)
V1 ($n = 8$)	2 (25%)	6 (75%)
V2-3 ($n = 8$)	2 (25%)	6 (75%)
CNVI ($n = 10$)	5 (50%)	5 (50%)
CNVII ($n = 8$)	5 (63%)	3 (37%)
CNVIII ($n = 9$)	—	9 (100%)
CNIX-X ($n = 8$)	3 (37%)	5 (63%)
Other ($n = 8$)	1 (13%)	7 (87%)

LOC, level of consciousness; CN, crania nerve.

TABLE 18-2. Medical Co-morbidity of Patients in Each Group Stratified According to the American Society of Anesthesiology (ASA) Scale.

	ASA I	ASA II	ASA III- IV
Group I ($n = 200$)	92 (46%)	84 (42%)	24 (12%)
Group II ($n = 200$)	88 (44%)	95 (47.5%)	17 (8.5%)
Group III ($n = 200$)	82 (41%)	93 (46.5%)	25 (12.5%)

who were dead at 1 year, were mainly among the patients who had a GOS of 2 or 3 at 6 weeks. It was interesting to note that almost half of the patients (46.1%) who had a GOS of 3 at 6 weeks improved to GOS of 4 or 5. In the group of patients with a GOS of 4 at 6 weeks, 80% improved to GOS 5.

When the outcome was stratified according to the groups as outlined above, the overall favorable outcome was similar in all groups, but the incidence of GOS 5 (92%) was significantly higher in the most recent 200 patients (Group III) as compared to the first 400.

With regard to the types of complications, the incidence of major neurologic complications was significantly lower in Group III (4% in Group III vs. 12.5% in Group I and 11% in Group II). The incidence of minor complications also showed a constant decrease over the years (7% in Group I, 4.5% in Group II, and 2.5% in Group III). It was surprising to see that surgery-related nonneurologic complications such as CSF leak or infection showed an increase in Group III (6.5% in Group III vs 2.5% each for Groups I and II) and was the most common subgroup of surgical complications in this group.

The incidence of patients with meningiomas at high-risk locations was higher in Group I (38.5%) compared to 29.5% in Group II and 28% in Group III, which might have some role in the relatively higher neurologic complication rate in this group. The relatively lower incidence of high-risk location meningiomas in the latter 400 patients as compared to the first 200 can be attributed to the evolution in the management paradigm for such tumors, such as the more widespread use of adjuvant or primary radiation treatment, or to stringht patient selection criteria for surgery in there high-risk patients.

In the subgroup of 49 patients who initially had a neurologic complication at 6 weeks and with available follow-up at 1 year, outcomes of the neurologic functions were diverse. All of the patients who suffered from decreased level of consciousness and two thirds of the patients with hemiparesis improved.

TABLE 18-3. Tumor Location in Each Group According to the CLASS Algorithmic Scale.

	Low risk	Moderate risk	High risk
Group I ($n = 200$)	52 (26%)	71 (30.5%)	77 (38.5%)
Group II ($n = 200$)	55 (27.5%)	86 (43%)	59 (29.5%)
Group III ($n = 200$)	54 (27%)	90 (45%)	56 (28%)

TABLE 18-4. Presence of Symptoms in Each Group.

	Asymptomatic	Mild	Severe
Group I (*n* = 200)	48 (24%)	50 (25%)	102 (51%)
Group II (*n* = 200)	83 (41.5%)	39 (19.5%)	78 (39%)
Group III (*n* = **200**)	76 (38%)	25 (12.5%)	99 (49.5%)

Among the cranial nerve deficits, facial, oculomotor and abducens nerves had the highest incidence of subsequent improvement (63%, 60%, and 50%, respectively). None of the patients with postoperative hearing loss improved at 1 year.

The incidence of medical complications were slightly less in Group II (12% in Group I, 6.5% in Group II, and 9.5% Group III), which may be a reflection of the patient population, since the incidence of high risk (ASA III-IV) patients were also relatively less in Group II (8.5% vs. 12% in Group I and 12.5% in Group III).

In the study of Curry and colleagues, in which they retrospectively reviewed the Nationwide Inpatient Sample for the period of 1988–2000, mortality and adverse hospital discharge rates for resection of intracranial meningiomas were significantly lower for high-volume hospitals and surgeons [3]. Interestingly, the number of coded neurologic complications was higher in these groups also. As the authors also point out, these can result from dealing with higher-risk tumors in high-volume centers. This may also result from the fact that the definition of highest volume quintile was only ≥24 intracranial meningioma cases/year for hospitals and ≥8 cases/year for surgeons in their study. In addition, the annual number of craniotomies for meningioma ranged between 1 and 39, with a median of 3 for the surgeons. In this context, it would be questionable whether 8 cases of intracranial meningiomas per year is a high enough number for a single surgeon to be regarded as a "high-volume" surgeon.

Summary

In the experience of the senior author with over 600 intracranial meningiomas, the incidence of favorable outcome increased and postoperative complications decreased over time. The heterogeneity and varying degrees of complexity of intracranial meningiomas constitute a challenge for the surgeon wishing to master the principles of surgical management of these interesting tumors. Our data clearly demonstrate the existence of a learning curve of at least 400 operative cases in meningioma surgery in achieving optimal outcome with minimal surgical complications further, many patients with immediate postoperative neurologic deficits at 6 weeks showed subsequent improvement at 1 year postoperative follow-up.

References

1. Flood AB, Scott WR, Ewy W. Does practice make perfect? Part I: The relation between hospital volume and outcomes for selected diagnostic categories. Med Care 1984;22:98–114.
2. Long DM, Gordon T, Bowman H, Etzel A, Burleyson G, Betchen S, Garonzik IM, Brem H. Outcome and cost of craniotomy performed to treat tumors in regional academic referral centers. Neurosurgery 2003;52:1056–65.
3. Curry WT, McDermott MW, Carter BS, Barker FG II. Craniotomy for meningioma in the United States between 1998 and 2000: decreasing grate of mortality and the effect of provider caseload. J Neurosurg 2005;102:977–86.
4. Black PM. Outcome and cost of craniotomy performed to treat tumors in regional academic center. [Comment]. Neurosurgery 2003;52:1063–4.
5. Teasdale G, Jennett B. Assessment of coma and impaired consciousness. A practical scale. Lancet 1974;2:81–4.
6. Owens WD, Felts JA, Spitznagel EL Jr. ASA physical status classification. Anesthesiology 1978;49:239–43.

19
Factors Influencing Outcome in Meningioma Surgery

Burak Sade and Joung H. Lee

Introduction

The overall incidence of meningiomas is increasing due to a widespread use of improved neuroimaging techniques for closed head injuries, nonspecific neurologic symptoms (such as headache and dizziness), or paranasal sinus problems. In addition, the aging population is growing. Therefore, neurosurgeons are increasingly experiencing management dilemmas for certain group of patients such as those with incidental meningiomas in all age groups, patients with significant comorbidities, young patients with small tumors, elderly patients with large tumors, and elderly patients with mild symptoms.

For any given disease, the treatment and when it should be administered are determined by the following three factors: (1) a thorough knowledge of the natural history of the disease, (2) benefits of the treatment, and (3) risks of the particular treatment.

Natural History of Meningiomas

The natural history of meningiomas, the knowledge of which is critical in formulating management plans, is poorly understood. The majority of the limited literature on meningiomas' natural history focuses on the elderly population, which results in a significant selection bias. In general, the sample sizes in these studies are relatively small, and the follow-up period is short. In addition, there is a considerable variability in the growth rates among meningiomas.

Kuratsu and colleagues reviewed the incidence and clinical features of asymptomatic meningiomas [1]. They defined 196 patients (39% of their series) as asymptomatic in their series. The incidence was significantly higher in patients over the age of 70. Of these, 63 were conservatively treated and had a follow-up of more than 1 year. Tumor growth was detected in 32% of these patients with an average follow-up of 28 months. Patients with calcification on computed tomography (CT) and/or with hypointensity on T2-weighted magnetic resonance imaging (MRI) appeared to grow at a slower rate. In the series of Yoneoka and colleagues, 24% of the 37 patients with incidental meningiomas showed growth during a mean follow-up of 4 years [2]. They found that younger patients and a larger initial tumor size increased the incidence of tumor growth. The study of Nakamura and colleagues revealed similar findings [3]. In their series of 41 patients with incidental meningiomas, who were managed conservatively, the mean absolute and relative annual growth rates were reported as 0.8 cc and 14.6%, respectively. They also found that these values were higher in younger patients, but their data did not show any correlation with the initial size of the tumor. In this study, when patients were followed for up to 8 years, all incidental meningiomas showed some growth. Olivero and colleagues looked at the growth pattern of 45 patients with incidental meningiomas [4]. Of these patients 22% showed growth, with an average follow-up of 29 months for the stable group and 47 months for the group that showed growth. Their average annual tumor growth rate was 0.24 cc. Niiro and colleagues analyzed their series of 40 patients who were over the age of 70 and had incidental meningiomas with an average follow-up of 38 months [5]. In their series the incidence of tumor growth was 35%. They found that presence of calcification on imaging studies lowered the incidence of growth, whereas a larger tumor size was an unfavorable factor. Nakasu and colleagues analyzed the changes of growth pattern in meningiomas in 31 tumors with a median follow-up of 10 years [6]. They found that atypical meningiomas showed an exponential tumor growth, whereas benign meningiomas were likely to show either exponential or linear growth or no growth. No growth was correlated with the presence of calcification.

It is important to note that the incidence of tumor growth increases in studies with a longer follow-up. Bindal and colleagues reviewed their series of 40 patients with skull base meningiomas whose tumors were managed conservatively [7]. Mean follow-up was 76 months. Tumor growth was detected in none at 1-year, 3% at 2-year, 20% at 5-year, and 58% at 10-year follow-ups. Van Havenbergh and colleagues analyzed their series of 21 patients with conservatively managed petroclival meningiomas [8]. In this study, the average follow-up was 82 months. Tumor growth was detected in 76% of patients, 63% of which was associated with functional deterioration. Jung and colleagues looked at the long-term growth rates of subtotally resected petroclival meningiomas [9]. With an average follow-up of 48 months, they detected the progression-free survival period and 5-year progression-free survival rate as 66 months and 60%, respectively. The annual growth rate of the residual tumor was 5 cc.

Benefits of Meningioma Surgery

Benefits of meningioma surgery are not as readily quantifiable as risks. However, there are two basic benefits of meningioma surgery, which are conceptual in nature: (1) alteration of the natural history, with a chance to cure when Simpson grade 1 resection is performed, and (2) reversal or improvement of neurologic signs and deficits.

In this context, we consider the tumor size and neurologic signs/symptoms as benefit factors for the patient. The larger the tumor, the greater is the benefit for the patient following surgery. Similarly, when the patient presents with neurologic signs and symptoms, there is a potential for reversal, improvement, or stabilization of symptoms following surgery. The more severe or reversible the symptoms are, the greater the benefit would be for the patient.

Risk Factors in the Surgical Management of Meningiomas

Similar to the reports on the natural history of meningiomas, the majority of the studies on the surgical outcome of meningiomas and assessment of risk factors also focus on the elderly population. Meixensberger and colleagues reviewed their results of 385 patients with intracranial meningiomas and analyzed the factors influencing the outcome [10]. Among the factors that are known to the surgeon preoperatively, age, preoperative co-morbidity as assessed by the American Society of Anesthesiology (ASA) score [18], and medial sphenoid wing location were found to be related to an unfavorable outcome. McCarthy and colleagues used the 9827 meningioma cases from the National Cancer Database [11]. In that study, they looked at factors associated with survival in patients with meningiomas. The factors which influenced the 5-year survival, and which were available to the surgeon to guide in the preoperative decision-making process, were tumor size and patient age. Buhl and colleagues reviewed their series of 66 patients over the age of 70 [12]. Their results suggested that tumor location (convexity), lack of significant medical co-morbidity, and smaller tumor size along with less peritumoral edema were associated with a more favorable outcome. Cornu and colleagues also found the preoperative ASA and Karnofsky scores as well as skull base or posterior fossa location as

unfavorable factors affecting outcome in this age group [13]. Caroli and colleagues developed a scale to predict the outcome in the elderly population using clinical and radiologic data [14]. In the literature, the data on the outcome of meningioma surgery in the elderly population are controversial. For example, the study of D'Andrea and colleagues suggest that surgery in this group of patients is relatively safe when their preoperative ASA score and overall Karnofsky score are favorable [15]. On the contrary, the review of the Nationwide Patient Sample Database by Bateman and colleagues suggests caution when considering surgery in the elderly patients with meningiomas [16].

In general, the most common factors associated with outcome following meningioma surgery include the co-morbidity and age of the patient, size and location of the tumor, and the presence and severity of neurological signs and symptoms. However, there is ambiguity regarding what constitutes a "significant" co-morbidity, a "complex" location, "old" age, "large" size, or which signs or symptoms are "significant." Therefore, the current surgical decision-making process is more "art" than "science," based on the surgeon's "gut feeling" due to the lack of systematic evidence-based guideline.

Risk Factors in Personal Series

In light of the limited information available in the literature, we decided to analyze a single surgeon's (senior author) experience to determine the factors (such as co-morbidity, location, age, size, symptoms) influencing the outcome of patients undergoing surgery for intracranial meningiomas. In addition, we included the history of previous surgery at the same operative site, as well as radiation treatment in the analysis. A retrospective analysis was performed on 300 consecutive patients who had resection of intracranial meningioma by the senior author between January 2000 and December 2004. This group represents the second half of the approximately 600 patients treated surgically by the senior author, and this latter group was selected for analysis to remove the effect of the learning curve in the surgical outcome of meningioma patients. Outcome at 6 weeks was assessed using the Glasgow Outcome Scale (GOS) [17]. A GOS of 4 and 5 were accepted as favorable outcome. Postoperative neurologic and medical morbidities were also recorded.

Results

There were 69 males and 231 females with an average age of 55 (range 23–83). There were 126 patients (42%) in the ASA I, 144 (48%) in the ASA II and 30 patients (10%) in the ASA III groups. The tumor was in the "low-risk"/simple location in 94 patients (31.3%), "moderate-risk" in 115 (38.4%), and "high-risk" in 91 patients (30.3%). Age was 60 or below in 187 patients (62.3%), 61–70 in 69 (23%), and 71 or above in 44 patients (14.7%). Tumor size was 2 cm or smaller in 65

TABLE 19.1. Significant Risk Factors Associated with Outcome at 6 Weeks.

Risk factors	Outcome			p-value
	GOS 5	GOS 4	GOS 1–3	
Co-morbidity				
ASA I (n = 126)	115 (91.3%)	11 (8.7%)	—	
ASA II (n = 144)	120 (83.3%)	16 (11.1%)	8 (5.6%)	
ASA III (n = 30)	16 (53.3%)	8 (26.7%)	6 (20%)	<0.001
Age				
<61 yr (n = 187)	170 (90.9%)	16 (8.6%)	1 (0.5%)	<0.001
61–70 yr (n = 69)	48 (69.6%)	12 (17.4%)	9 (13%)	
>71 yr (n = 44)	33 (75%)	7 (15.9%)	4 (9.1%)	
Size				
<2.1 cm (n = 65)	64 (98.5%)	1 (1.5%)	—	<0.001
2.1–4 cm (n = 115)	98 (85.2%)	13 (11.3%)	4 (3.5%)	
>4.1 cm (n = 120)	89 (74.2%)	21 (17.5%)	10 (8.3%)	
Symptoms/ Signs				
Asymptomatic (n = 110)102 (92.7%)	6 (5.5%)	2 (1.8%)	0.009	
Mild (n = 60)	44 (73.3%)	10 (16.7%)	6 (10%)	
Severe (n = 130)	105 (80.8%)	19 (14.6%)	6 (4.6%)	
Previous surgery				
Yes (n = 40)	24 (60%)	10 (25%)	6 (15%)	<0.001
No (n = 260)	227 (87.3%)	25 (9.6%)	8 (3.1%)	
Previous radiation treatment				
Yes (n = 15)	9 (60%)	3 (20%)	3 (20%)	0.012
No (n = 285)	242 (84.9%)	32 (11.2%)	11 (3.9%)	

patients (21.7%), 2.1–4 cm in 115 patients (38.3%), and 4.1 cm or above in 120 patients (40%). One hundred and ten patients (36.7%) were asymptomatic, 60 (20%) had mild symptoms, and 130 (43.3%) had severe symptoms. Forty patients (13.3%) were operated previously on the same location and 15 patients (5%) had prior radiation treatment.

At 6 weeks, the GOS was 5 in 251 patients (83.7%), 4 in 35 (11.7%), and 3 in 10 patients (3.3%). No patient had a GOS of 2 at 6 weeks. The mortality rate (GOS 1) was 1.3% (4/300). The factors found to affect the outcome are listed in Table 19-1. With multivariate analysis, co-morbidity and age showed a stronger impact (Table 19-2).

Postoperative neurologic and medical complications were encountered in 41 (13.7%) and 16 patients (5.3%), respectively, the most frequent being cranial nerve deficits (18) for neurologic and deep venous thrombosis (9) for medical

TABLE 19.2. Odds of Having Unfavorable Outcome (GOS 1–3) at 6 Weeks.

Factor	Odds ratio	95% Confidence interval
Co-morbidity[a]		
Per risk level decrease	0.13	0.04–0.43
Age[b]		
Per risk level decrease	0.40	0.17–0.92

[a] With one risk level decrease, unfavorable outcome decreases 87%.
[b] With one risk level decrease, unfavorable outcome decreases 60%.

TABLE 19.3. Significant Risk Factors Associated with Postoperative Complications.

Risk factors	Yes	No	p-value
Neurologic complications			
Location*			
Simple (n = 94)	6 (6.4%)	88 (93.6%)	
Moderate (n = 115)	12 (10.4%)	105 (89.6%)	
Complex (n = 91)	23 (25.3%%)	66 (74.7%)	<0.001
Medical complications			
Co-morbidity			
ASA I (n = 126)	2 (1.6%)	124 (98.4%)	0.018
ASA II (n = 144)	10 (6.9%)	134 (93.1%)	
ASA III (n = 30)	4 (13.3%)	26 (86.7%)	
Location			
Simple (n = 94)	1 (1.1%)	93 (98.9%)	0.08
Moderate (n = 115)	8 (7%)	108 (93%)	
Complex (n = 91)	7 (7.7%)	84 (92.3%)	

*For definition of simple, moderate and complex locations, please see Chapter 20.

complications. Tumor location significantly associated with both neurologic and medical complications, and existing medical co-morbidity showed association with medical complications (Tables 19-3 and 19-4).

Among the risk factors that were assessed, medical co-morbidity, age, size, presenting symptoms and signs, as well as a history of previous surgery and radiation treatment were found to be influencing the early outcome at 6 weeks following surgery. With one risk level decrease in medical co-morbidity and age, the risk of unfavorable outcome decreased by 87% and 60%, respectively. Tumor location, on the other hand, was found to be a strong determinant of postoperative neurologic complications. One risk level decrease in tumor location decreased the risk of neurologic complication by 63%. In summary, our results supported the available data in the literature, which suggest that medical co-morbidity, tumor location, age, tumor size, presenting symptoms/signs, as well as prior history of surgery and radiation treatment are indeed significant factors that influence the operative outcome in meningioma surgery.

TABLE 19.4. Odds of Having Neurologic and Medical Complications.

Factor	Odds ratio	95% Confidence interval
Neurologic complications		
Location[a]		
Per risk level decrease	0.37	0.22–0.62
Medical complications		
Co-morbidity[b]		
Per risk level decrease	0.35	0.15–0.85
Location[c]		
Per risk level decrease	0.43	0.20–0.95

[a] With one risk level decrease, neurologic complications decrease 63%.
[b] With one risk level decrease, medical complications decrease 65%.
[c] With one risk level decrease, medical complications decrease 57%.

Acknowledgments. We would like to thank Tao Jin, M.S. from the Department of Biostatistics, Cancer Center, Cleveland Clinic, for his assistance in the statistical analysis of the data.

References

1. Kuratsu J, Kochi M,Ushio Y. Incidence and clinical features of asymptomatic meningiomas. J Neurosurg 2000;92:766–70.

2. Yoneoka Y, Fujii Y, Tanaka R. Growth of incidental meningiomas. Acta Neurochir (Wien) 2000;142:507–11.

3. Nakamura M, Roser F, Michel J, Jacobs C, Samii M. The natural history of incidental meningiomas. Neurosurgery 2003;53:62–71.

4. Olivero WC, Lister JR, Elwood PL. The natural history and growth rate of asymptomatic meningiomas: a review of 60 patients. J Neurosurg 1995;83:222–4.

5. Niiro M, Yatsushiro K, Nakamura K, Kawahara Y, Kuratsu J. Natural history of elderly patients with asumptomatic meningiomas. J Neurol Neurosurg Psychiatry 2000;68:25–8.

6. Nakasu S, Fukami T, Nakajima M, Watanabe K, Ichikawa M, Matsuda M. Growth pattern changes of meningiomas: long-term analysis. Neurosurgery 2005;56:946–55.

7. Bindal R, Goodman JM, Kawasaki A, Purvin V, Kuzma B. The natural history of untreated skull base meningomas. Surg Neurol 2003;59:87–92.

8. Van Havenbergh T, Carvalho G, Tatagiba M, Plets C, Samii M. Natural history of petroclival meningiomas. Neurosurgery 2003;52:55–64

9. Jung HW, Yoo H, Paek SH, Choi KS. Long-term outcome and growth rate of subtotally resected petroclival meningiomas: experience with 38 cases. Neurosurgery 2000;46:567–75.

10. Meixensberger J, Meister T, Janka B, Haubitz B, Bushe KA, Roosen K. Factors influencing morbidity and mortality after cranial meningioma surgery—a multivariate analysis. Acta Neurochir (Wien) 1996; Suppl 65:99–101.

11. McCarthy BJ, Davis FG, Freels S, Surawicz TS, Damek DM, Grutsch J, Menck HR, Laws ER Jr. Factors associated with survival in patients with meningioma. J Neurosurg 1998;88:831–39.

11. Buhl R, Hasan A, Behnke A, Mehdorn HM. Results in the operative treatment of elderly patients with intracranial meningiomas. Neurosurg Rev 2000;23:25–9.

12. Cornu P, Chatellier G, Dagreou F, Clemenceau S, Foncin JV, Rivierez M, Philippon J. Intracranial meningiomas in elderly patients. Postoperative morbidity and mortality. Factors predictive of outcome. Acta Neurochir (Wien) 1990;102: 98–102.

13. Caroli M, Locatelli M, Prada F, Beretta F, Martinelli-Boneschi F, Campanella R, Arienta C. Surgery for intracranial meningiomas in the elderly: a clinical-radiological grading system as a predictor of outcome. J Neurosurg 2005;102:290–4.

14. D'Andrea G, Roperto R, Emanuela C, Crispo F, Ferrante L. Thirty seven cases of intracranial meningiomas in the ninth decade of life: our experience and review of the literature. Neurosurgery 2005;56:956–61.

15. Bateman BT, Pile-Spellman J, Gutin PH, Berman MF. Meningioma resection in the elderly: nationwide inpatient sample, 1998–2002.

16. Teasdale G, Jennett B. Assessment of coma and impaired consciousness. A practical scale. Lancet 1974;2:81–4.

17. Owens WD, Felts JA, Spitznagel EL Jr. ASA physical status classification. Anesthesiology 1978;49:239–43.

18. Owens WD, Felts JA, Spitznagel EL Jr. ASA physical status classification. Anesthesiology 1978;49:239–43.

20

The Novel "CLASS" Algorithmic Scale for Patient Selection in Meningioma Surgery

Joung H. Lee and Burak Sade

Introduction

The very basic tenet of medicine is that a treatment is given if the treatment's benefits far outweigh the risks. In the previous chapter, both benefit and risk factors for meningioma surgery were described and reviewed. To briefly reiterate, the risk factors associated with outcome following meningioma surgery include the following: patient's preoperative co-morbidity (C), tumor location (L), patient's age (A), tumor size (S), and the symptoms/signs (S) caused by the tumor. Additionally, a history of prior surgery and radiation were also found to be significant risk factors. The benefit factors, which are largely conceptual and difficult to quantify, include alteration of the natural history, with a chance to cure when Simpson grade 1 resection is performed, and reversal or improvement of neurologic signs and symptoms. Tumor size and neurologic signs/symptoms, although significant risk factors, simultaneously represent only two benefit factors in meningioma surgery. The larger the tumor, the greater is the potential benefit for the patient following surgery. Similarly, when patients present with neurologic symptoms or deficits, there is potential for reversal, improvement, or stabilization of symptoms following surgery. The more severe or reversible the symptoms or deficits are, the greater the benefit would be for the patient.

Based on the previous chapter's data relating to the factors influencing outcome following meningioma surgery, we aimed to develop a novel and simple standardized guideline to help select patients for meningioma surgery. Following the basic principle of medicine described above, this scale simply weighs and assesses the risks and benefits of surgery for an individual patient with meningioma.

The novel "CLASS" algorithm is based on balancing the risks against benefits of surgery (Fig. 20-1). Co-morbidity (C), tumor location (L), and patient age (A) are included as risk factors, whereas tumor size (S) and neurologic signs and symptoms (S) are included as benefit factors. A score is assigned to each factor: risk factors are graded from −2 to 0 while benefit factors are graded from 0 to +2. A score of +1 was added to the total score in the presence of radiographic progression and −1 for previous history of surgery and/or radiation therapy.

Co-morbidity: Co-morbidity was graded using the widely used American Society of Anesthesiologists (ASA) preoperative patient assessment scale [1]. A score of 0 was assigned for ASA Grade I patients, −1 for Grade II, and −2 for Grade III patients. Since ASA grade IV or V patients are most often not considered for meningioma surgery, these groups were not included.

Location: Tumor location was classified based on the experience of the senior author. "Low-risk" locations included convexity and lateral skull base (lateral and middle sphenoid wing, posterior petrous) and were given a score of 0. Olfactory groove, planum sphenoidale, tentorial (lateral/paramedian), parasagittal, intraventricular, cerebellopontine angle, falcine, posterior/lateral foramen magnum as well as para-sigmoid and para-transverse sinus locations constituted the "moderate risk" group and were assigned a score of −1. The "high-risk" locations included clinoidal, cavernous sinus, tuberculum sellae, tentorial (medial/incisural), ventral petrous, petroclival and anterior/anterolateral foramen magnum, for which a score of −2 was given.

Age: A score of 0 was assigned for patients who are 60 years of age or younger, −1 for 61–70 years and −2 for 71 years or older.

Size: A score of 0 was given if the maximum tumor size was 2 cm or less, +1 for between 2.1 and 4 cm, and +2 for tumors larger than 4.1 cm.

Signs and symptoms: A score of 0 was assigned for incidental tumors and +1 for mild symptoms or irreversible neurologic deficits. A score of +2 was assigned for severe symptoms or reversible neurologic deficits.

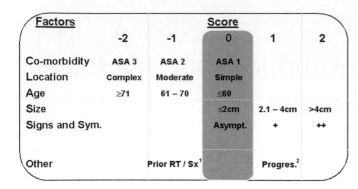

FIG. 20-1. The CLASS algorithmic scale
[1] Sx = surgery
[2] Progres. = radiographic progression

Validity of the CLASS Algorithmic Scale

The following study was conducted to test the validity of this scale by assessing the outcome with respect to the preoperative CLASS score. For all 300 patients who had been reviewed for the assessment of the risk factors, the total CLASS score was calculated and divided into three groups: Group I patients had a total score of +1 or above, Group II 0 or −1, and Group III −2 or below. Early outcome at 6 weeks was assessed using the Glasgow outcome scale (GOS) [2], and postoperative neurologic and medical complications were recorded.

Chi-square and Fisher's exact test were used for the comparison of the groups. A logistic regression model was built to compare each group in terms of the odds of having "bad" GOS (GOS 1–3) and neurologic/medical complications. A p-value of 0.05 and below was accepted as statistically significant.

Results

One hundred and nine patients (36.3%) had a CLASS score of 1 or above (Group I), 154 (51.4%) had a score of 0 or −1 (Group II), and 37 patients (12.3%) had a score of −2 or below (Group III).

Poor outcome (GOS 1-3) was seen in 1.8% (2/109) in Group I, 3.9% (6/154) in Group II, and 16.2% (6/37) in Group III patients (Fig. 20-2). The odds of poor outcome was 936% higher for Group III than that for Group I patients ($p < 0.05$) (Table 20-1). There was no statistically significant difference in outcome between Groups I and II.

Neurologic complications were encountered in 7.3% (8/109) in Group I, 15.6% (24/154) in Group II, and 24.3% (9/37) in Group III. Both Groups II and III had significantly higher odds for having neurologic complications than Group I ($p = 0.021$). Medical complications were 1.8% (2/109) for Group I, 6.5% (10/154) for Group II, and 10.8% (4/37) for Group III. Similarly, Groups II and III had significantly higher odds for having medical complications as compared to Group I ($p = 0.015$) (Fig. 20-3, Table 20-2).

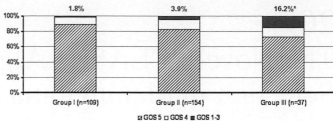

FIG. 20-2. GOS at 6 weeks according to CLASS score ($^*p = 0.016$)

TABLE 20-1. Odds of Having Unfavorable Outcome According to the CLASS Score.

Factor	Odds ratio	95% Confidence interval
Total CLASS score		
Group III vs. Group I[a]	10.36	1.99–53.89
Group II vs. Group I[b]	2.17	0.43–10.95

[a] Odds of having an unfavorable outcome for Group III is 936% higher than Group I.
[b] No significant difference between Groups I and II.

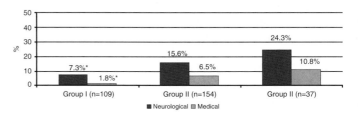

FIG. 20-3. Neurologic and medical complications according to the CLASS score ($^*p = 0.021$ and 0.015, respectively).

TABLE 20-2. Odds of Having Neurologic or Medical Complications According to the CLASS Score.

Factor	Odds ratio	95% Confidence interval
Neurologic complications		
Group III vs. Group I[a]	4.06	1.43–11.48
Group II vs. Group I[a]	2.33	1.101–5.41
Medical complications		
Group III vs. Group I[a]	6.48	1.14–37.01
Group II vs. Group I[a]	3.71	0.80–7.31

[a] Odds of having a neurologic or medical complication are significantly higher in Groups II and III, as compared to Group I.

Utility of the CLASS Algorithmic Scale

In order to assess the utility of the proposed algorithm, 236 new consecutive patients with meningiomas were prospectively evaluated in the outpatient setting between September 2004 and March 2006. Each patient was blindly assessed, and assigned to an appropriate CLASS group (I, II, or III). The decision regarding the surgical management of the patient was made by the senior author, who did not know to which group the patient was assigned.

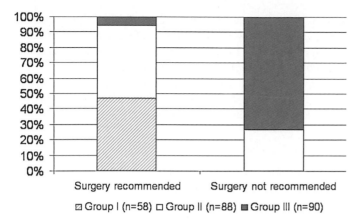

FIG. 20-4. Distribution of patients into "surgery recommended" and "surgery not recommended" groups vs. "CLASS" scores

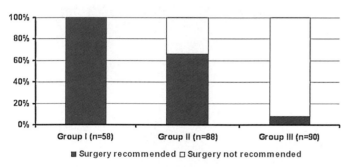

FIG. 20-5. Eligibility of patients for surgery according to CLASS groups

There were 58 patients (24.6%) in Group I, 88 (37.3%) in Group II, and 90 (38.1%) in Group III. Surgery was recommended to 123 patients (52.1%). Of these patients, 47.2% were in Group I, 47.2% in Group II, and 5.6% in Group III. Of the 113 patients for whom surgery was not deemed warranted, 26.5% were in Group II and 73.5% in Group III (Fig. 20-4). All patients in Group I and 58 (65.9%) in Group II were recommended surgery, as compared to only 7 (7.8%) in Group III (Fig. 20-5).

The high correlation of the "CLASS" scores with our decision making demonstrated the reliability and utility of this algorithm in our practice. It is important to note that all of Group I patients were recommended surgery. Only 7 patients (5.6%) in Group III were recommended surgery, all of whom had presented with progressive visual deterioration.

Case Examples

Case 1

A 58-year-old woman presented with an incidental diagnosis of a 10-mm left ventral petrous meningioma (Fig. 20-6). Her medical history was significant for a controlled hypertension, mitral valve prolapse, and a past Guillain-Barré disease. Neu-

rologic exam was completely within normal limits. She had a total CLASS score of −3 [C:−1, L:-2, A:0, S:0, S:0]. She was managed conservatively, since the risks of the surgery exceeded its potential benefits.

Case 2

A 57-year-old woman presented with right-sided hearing loss and facial numbness. Her MRI revealed a 24-mm superior petrous meningioma on the right (Fig. 20-7). Her medical history was unremarkable. Neurologic exam confirmed a partial hearing loss on the right. Her total CLASS score was 1 [C:0, L:-1, A:0, S:1, S:1], and surgery was recommended. Note the score of

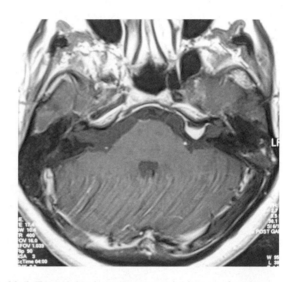

FIG. 20-6. T1-weighted postcontrast axial image of a 10-mm ventral petrous meningioma on the left

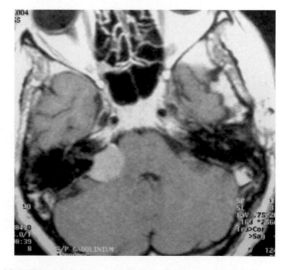

FIG. 20-7. T1-weighted postcontrast axial image of a 24-mm superior petrous meningioma on the right

symptoms of +1, since partial hearing loss on one side is generally perceived as a mild symptom, and is usually irreversible.

Case 3

A 52-year-old man presented with an incidental diagnosis of a 20-mm right antero-lateral foramen magnum meningioma (Fig. 20-8A, B). His medical history was remarkable for a controlled type 2 diabetes mellitus. His neurologic exam was completely within normal limits. His initial total CLASS score was 3[C:-1, L:-2, A:0, S:0, S:0]. The risks of the surgery exceeded the benefits and therefore he was managed conservatively.

The same patient came for his routine 6-month follow-up visit. By that time he had developed a recent onset of right-sided occipital headache and neck pain. His neurologic exam was still within normal limits, but his new MRI revealed the

growth of the tumor from 20 to 28 mm (Fig. 20-8C, D). His new CLASS score was 1 [C:-1, L:-2, A:O, S:1, S:2, (O:1)]. This time the benefits of the surgery exceeded the risks, and he was recommended surgery. Note that the headache described by the patient was severe, new onset, was attributable to the tumor, and was highly likely to be reversible with its removal. Because of these features, a symptom score of +2 was assigned.

Case 4

A 78-year-old woman presented with recent onset of word-finding difficulty and a right fronto-temporal headache. Her tumor was diagnosed elsewhere, and she was managed conservatively. She presented to our clinic with her follow-up MRI, which showed a 40-mm middle sphenoid wing meningioma on the right (Fig. 20-9), which demonstrated that the tumor had grown.

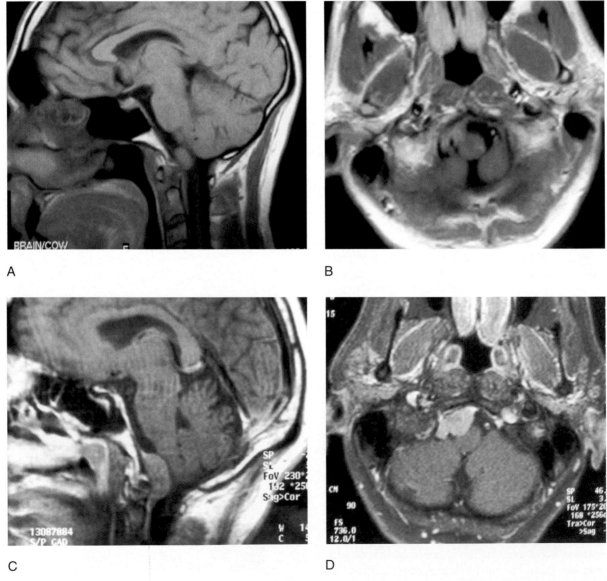

A

B

C

D

FIG. 20-8. T1-weighted (A) sagittal and (B) postcontrast axial image of a 20-mm antero-lateral foramen magnum meningioma on the right. (C) Postcontrast sagittal and (D) axial views of the same patient with the tumor reaching 28 mm in size

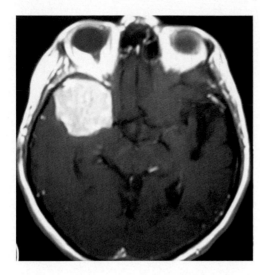

FIG. 20-9. T1-weighted postcontrast axial view of a 40-mm middle sphenoid wing meningioma on the right

Her medical history was unremarkable. Neurologic exam was normal, except for some short-term memory impairment. Her total CLASS score was 1 [C:0, L:0, A:-2, S:1, S:1, (O:1)], and she was offered surgery. It was not certain whether her memory problem was reversible or not. Therefore, her symptom score was +1. It is important to note that despite her advanced age, she was still in the lowest risk group for surgery and had an excellent postoperative outcome.

Conclusion

This simple algorithm is based on the basic tenet of surgery, which is to recommend surgery only if the benefits of the procedure far exceed the risks. It is helpful in selecting meningioma patients for surgery in incidental tumors in all age groups, patients with significant medical illnesses, young patients with small tumors, elderly patients with large tumors, as well as elderly patients with mild symptoms.

This scale is simple in its design and application. In addition to its applicability, simplicity and practicality were two of the major priorities in developing this scale. Therefore, similar to the Spetzler-Martin grading of arteriovenous malformations [3], we simply assigned a score of equal weight for each factor and avoided any further mathematical equations, which would have rendered the scale impractical and difficult to remember.

In summary, surgery is recommended for CLASS Group I and no surgery for Group III patients. For Group II patients, surgery may be considered with caution, knowing that the risks of postoperative complications and unfavorable outcome are higher than in Group I. For Group III patients, surgery can still be recommended if the circumstances of the individual case warrant surgical management (i.e., significant reversible deficit, patient preference), with the knowledge that risks of postoperative complications and unfavorable outcome are significantly higher than the other two groups.

Acknowledgments. We would like to thank Tao Jin, M.S., from the Department of Biostatistics, Cancer Center, Cleveland Clinic, for his assistance in the statistical analysis of the data.

References

1. Owens WD, Felts JA, Spitznagel EL Jr. ASA physical status classification. Anesthesiology 1978;49:239–43.
2. Teasdale G, Jennett B. Assessment of coma and impaired consciousness. A practical scale. Lancet 1974;2:81–4.
3. Spetzler RF, Marin NA. A proposed grading system for arteriovenous malformations. J Neurosurg 1986;65:476–83.

21
Endoscopy in Meningioma Surgery: Basic Principles, Applications, and Indications

Paolo Cappabianca, Luigi M. Cavallo, Felice Esposito, and Enrico de Divitiis

Introduction

No doubt surgery of benign intracranial lesions is among the most exciting and satisfying aspects of everyday neurosurgical practice, because the precise, elegant, safe, and effective surgical deed can give the patient back his or her normal life. As a matter of fact, meningioma surgery follows a general principle: the complete removal of an intracranial meningioma often means cure for the patient. Several exceptions to this rule exist: even though surgery of brain convexity meningiomas is considered something not particularly difficult to be done, surgery of skull base meningiomas or other deeply located lesions could be particularly challenging and requires a particular technical expertise.

The evolution of surgical techniques, with the advent of the operating microscope and the concept of microdissection, has resulted in the last decades in a progressive reduction of invasiveness, with a dramatic improvement in the morbidity and mortality rates. Consequently, the whole concept of daily surgical practice in the field of neurosurgery changed greatly and led to the arousal of the new concept of microneurosurgery. With it, neurosurgeons became able to explore areas that had not been accessed before, define intraoperative pathologic tissues much more accurately, and refine their surgical procedures and approaches, with the end result of decreasing both morbidity and mortality. Technological advances through the years added more and more to the surgical microscopic capabilities and led to complete dependence of the neurosurgeons on it in virtually every discipline of neurosurgical practice. Furthermore, after the introduction of the concept of minimalism in the whole field of surgery, specifically neurosurgery, surgeons became more dependent on it. Now neurosurgical microscopic techniques constitute a fundamental part of any neurosurgical training program.

More or less parallel to the introduction of the surgical microscope, endoscopes have also been introduced. They have been used in a limited way for treatment of hydrocephalus or for attaining tumor biopsies. The endoscope has not gained the same popularity in neurosurgery as the surgical microscope due to technological drawbacks and the far poorer quality of surgical field images. It was not until the last decade—with the many different technological advancements of telescopes, light sources, and digital video cameras leading to an overall improvement of endoscopy—that the endoscope has enjoyed increased acceptance and popularity. This technology assisted many other neurosurgical fields,[1–3] first as an adjunct to the surgical microscope, then as the sole viewing tool in the whole procedure with the advent of the new concept of endoneurosurgery. The development of modern endoscopes with their great illuminating power, wider viewing angle, and the possibility to look around the corners with angled scopes made these instruments useful tools in modern neurologic surgery. The extensive use of endoscopy in neurosurgery in the last several years has helped transform neurosurgical thinking about the possibilities of surgery for deep-located lesions—among them, meningiomas.[1,3]

Although many surgeons around the world use endoscopic techniques both in cranial and spinal procedures, it is worth considering that, so far, endoscopic techniques in neurosurgery have not gained the same wide acceptance and popularity as microscopic ones. The following causes have led to the relatively limited or slower shift of surgeons from microscopic to endoscopic techniques:

- Steep learning curve of the endoscopic techniques
- Two-dimensional nonbinocular views of the surgical field attained by the endoscope
- Limited availability of dedicated surgical instruments
- Initial false impression of insecurity in managing the surgical complications during an endoscopic surgical procedure
- Inherent psychological element of fear in dealing with a new technique/technology
- Bias against a new and unfamiliar technique and simultaneous reluctance in giving up a familiar technique which is proven effective and widely practiced
- High cost of building up a new range of surgical instruments and endoscopic equipment

The advancements of preoperative and intraoperative neuroradiologic studies and the advent of the image-guided surgery coupled with the use of the endoscope itself have led to increased knowledge of the anatomic details, the type of lesion, its extension and the involvement of critical neurovascular structures with a progressive narrowing of the approaches, as well as to improved precision of the operation, the diminution of complications, and the improved outcome of the patient.[4-6] Over the years, neurosurgeons have achieved progressive reduction in the size of craniotomies, resulting in the advent of keyhole surgery to avoid unnecessary manipulations and exposures during a given approach. This concept has been made possible only with the aid of the endoscope, and keyhole surgery became widely accepted in modern microneurosurgery.[1-3,7] Today, a number of different transcranial keyhole approaches are available, each one giving a different angle of maneuverability and vision so that the surgeon can tailor the appropriate approach for the patient.

The Endoscope

The endoscope in meningioma surgery offers three main advantages: (1) improvement of the illumination, because the endoscope has a light source that brings the light in the surgical field where it is needed; (2) better definition of the anatomic details, because of the use of high-definition lenses and the closer position of the scope, which allows an augmented definition of the details at the tumor-tissue interface; and (3) marked increase in the angles of visualization with the use of angled lenses, allowing one to see in areas otherwise hidden to the microsurgical vision and giving a different perception of the anatomy. As a matter of fact, one of the current limitations of the modern endoscope is that it provides a two-dimensional image, which is inferior to the stereoscopic view of the operating microscopes. Nevertheless, the lack of stereoscopy can be overcome with training, multiangled vision, the fine understanding of all the lights and shadows of the image, with fixing the multiple landmarks during the operation, and the knowledge of the surgical anatomy that the endoscope has provided.[8] The endoscope can increase the precision of surgery and permit the surgeon to differentiate different tissues, so that selective removal of the lesion can be achieved.

Currently, different types of endoscope exist, which are classified either as fiber optic endoscopes (fiberscopes) or rod-lens endoscopes. The endoscopes specifically designed for neuroendoscopy can be classified into four types: (1) rigid fiberscopes, (2) rigid rod-lens endoscopes, (3) flexible fiberscopes, and (4) steerable fiberscopes. These different endoscopes have different diameters, lengths, optical quality and number of working channels. The choice among them should be made on the basis of the surgical indication and personal preference of the surgeon. Indeed, for endoscopic meningioma surgery the best endoscopes are the rigid rod-lens scopes, whose better quality of vision is the main advantage. They allow surgeons to remain oriented, thanks to the panoramic view, and permit the other instruments to be inserted alongside it.

Rod-lens endoscopes consist of three main parts: (1) a mechanical shaft, (2) glass fiber bundles for light illumination, and (3) optics (objective, eyepiece, relay system).[9]

The angle of view of rod-lens endoscopes ranges from 0° to 120°, according to the objective, but angled objectives more than 30° are only for diagnostic or visualizing purposes.[9,10] The most frequently used angles are 0°, 30°, and 45°. The 0° objective provides a frontal view of the surgical field and minimizes the risk of disorientation[11] and is generally used during the majority of the operation. The 30° objective offers certain advantages. Rotating the lens 360° increases the surface area of the field of view to twice the size as that obtained with the 0° objective. Visualization of the instruments is improved since they converge towards the center of the image (directed at 30°). With the 0° objective, the instruments remain in the periphery of the image.[10] The major disadvantage of angled scopes is that the indirect image may cause disorientation for unskilled surgeons.[11]

The rod-lens rigid endoscope is commonly used through a sheath, connected to a cleaning-irrigation system, which permits cleaning and defogging of the distal lens, thus avoiding repeated entrances and exits from the surgical field. Preferably, the scopes used are without any working channel (diagnostic endoscopes) and the other instruments are inserted sliding alongside the sheath and using the latter as a guide for the correct direction. The diameter of rod-lens endoscope varies between 1.9 and 10 mm, but for endo-neurosurgery, usually endoscopes with a diameter of 2.7–4 mm are used. It is not advisable to use smaller endoscopes because the smaller the diameter of the lens, the less is the light that can be transmitted. It has been estimated that for each 10% of increase in diameter there is a 46% increase in light transmitted,[9] but endoscopes larger than 2.7 mm can be too bulky, requiring larger approaches. For instance, large-diameter endoscopes are not advisable when performing an endoscopic extended endonasal transsphenoidal surgery for meningiomas of the anterior midline skull base.

Endoscopic Instrumentation

Surgical Instruments

For endoscope-assisted microsurgical techniques, the bayonet-shaped microsurgical instruments designed to avoid any interference with the direct coaxial vision of the surgical field are still good for a safe and effective operation. However, they are not useful for "pure" endoscopic technique. For the endoscopic approach, the instruments need to be inserted along the same axis as the endoscope, with the same position maintained with respect to the endoscope for their entire length. For this reason they need to be straight and not bayoneted. While the microscope produces magnification from a distant lens and light is transmitted from the lamp of the microscope to the surgical field (so that the surgeon can follow the entrance of the instruments from the outside), the vision provided by the endoscope is maintained completely inside the surgical field, beyond the distal lens of the endoscope. The instruments are inserted blindly into the surgical field with the associated risk of injury to the neurovascular structures until the tip of the instrument passes beyond the distal lens to become visible, unless the endoscope is removed and inserted every time a different instrument is used.

Since the introduction of the endoscopic approaches, new instruments have been designed that meet the following criteria:[9,12,13]

Easy and safe in a limited surgical corridor
Well-balanced and ergonomic design for safe handling, while avoiding any conflict among the surgeon's hands, the endoscope, and other instruments that may be present in the same corridor
Capability allowing the surgeon to work in every visible zone of the surgical field provided by the endoscope

Endoscopic instruments are usually 15–25 cm long and can be either straight curettes, hooks, and dissectors, with various tips and diameters, differently angled on the frontal and sagittal planes, or forceps, scissors, etc., which are straight in their part inserted alongside the endoscope while the handle is angled 120° on the horizontal plane.

Several important design modifications have been made for some instruments, such as the blades, to avoid the of risk of injury to the neurovascular or other structures while they are inserted without direct visual control: the lancet has an extractable blade that is protected within a sheath.[9,12,13] It is extracted when it becomes visible to the endoscope, thus avoiding accidental damage to previously encountered structures. Furthermore, angled suction cannulas, with lateral fenestration or with angled tips for the suctioning in the zones of the surgical field visible only by the angled endoscopes and not otherwise reachable with the regular cannulas, have been developed.

Bleeding Control

One of the most difficult and common problems of endoscopic surgery is the control of bleeding. Furthermore, the basic principle of meningioma surgery is devascularization of the lesion, usually achievable with bipolar or even monopolar cautery.

Monopolar coagulation is usually easy to obtain. However, bipolar coagulation is preferable, either alone or in association with hemostatic agents. The use of the microsurgical bipolar forceps, developed for the microscope, is usually feasible with the endoscope, although not easy every time, such as in the case of transsphenoidal approach to the skull base or other limited-exposure approaches. Consequently, different cylindric bipolar forceps have been designed, with various diameters and lengths, which have proven to be quite effective in bleeding control.

Recently, radiofrequency technology for monopolar and bipolar coagulation has been introduced to neurosurgery. Radiofrequency instruments have two main advantages over electric ones: (1) the spatial energy dispersion with radiofrequency is minimal, with consequent minimal risk of injury to the surrounding neurovascular structures, and (2) radiofrequency bipolar forceps do not need to be used with irrigation or to be cleaned every time.

Video Camera and Monitor

In order to properly maneuver the instruments under fine control, the endoscope is connected to a dedicated video camera and the endoscopic images are projected onto a monitor placed in front of the surgeon. Additional monitors can be placed in varying locations in the operating room, as well as outside in the hallways or adjacent rooms, to permit other members of the team to watch the surgery.

Several types of endoscopic video cameras are available, the most common of which utilizes a 3-CCD (charge coupled device) sensor. While the 1-CCD cameras process all three fundamental colors in one chip, the 3-CCD ones have a separate chip for each color (red, blue, green) and provide better color separation, more brilliant colors, and a sharper image with higher contrast.[14] Buttons located on the camera control the focus and the zoom. Optical zoom is preferable because it enlarges the image using the same number of pixels, while the electronic zoom increases the size of each pixel, which degrades the definition of the image. Most modern endoscopic cameras are analog. This means that the signal is transmitted to a central processing unit (CPU), which outputs the signals in RGB, S-video, or composite video formats. Today, digital 3-CCD endoscope cameras are available, which produce the highest quality images that can be directly connected to video recorders for high-quality video reproduction.

The images produced by the endoscope camera are displayed on one or more monitors. These need to have a high-resolution screen to support the signal quality arising from the camera. The monitors most commonly used in endoscopic surgery have a minimum horizontal resolution of 750 lines in order to visualize all the details of the endoscopic images.

A further improvement of the resolution of both the video cameras and the monitors is provided by the high definition technology (HDTV), which is ready for future 3-D endoscopes.

Light Source

The endoscope transmits cold light, which arises from a source inside the surgical field through a connecting cable made of glass fibers. Currently, in endoscopic surgery Xenon light sources are used. They have spectral characteristics similar to the sunlight, with a color temperature of approximately 6000, which is "whiter" than the classic halogen light (3400 K). The power of the unit is commonly 300 W. The flexible connecting cable is made of a bundle of glass fibers that brings the light to the endoscope, virtually without dispersion of visible light. Furthermore, the heat (composed of infrared light) is poorly transmitted by the glass fibers, thus reducing the risk of burning the tissues.

Video Documentation

Documentation and storage of intraoperative images and movie clips is of increasing importance for education and documentation. Although video recording is not mandatory, having the possibility to document either still images or video clips of the surgical procedure is quite important for a series of reasons: (1) to review the operation and, if any mistakes are made, learn how to avoid them in the future; (2) to obtain pictures for publication or produce videoclips to teach residents, course attendees, etc.; (3) to store in an electronic library; and (4) to use the material for legal purposes.

Several systems are available to document endoscopic surgical operations. Any one of a number of film or digital cameras, analog or digital VCRs, mass memory, CD or DVD-based systems can store and even improve the images coming from the video camera. Such systems can be connected to dedicated devices and route the pictures and/or the videos for a complete digital exchange, for computer or video streaming or teleconferencing, for e-learning, e-teaching, or tele-counseling. Furthermore, it is possible for modern integrated operating rooms, such as the OR1® (Karl Storz GmBH, Tuttlingen, Germany) that we use, to share digital images and video by simply pressing a touch screen, which can even be done by the surgeon while operating.

Other Instruments

Modern neurosurgery with microsurgical and/or endoscopic techniques uses special instruments and devices that are quite helpful even if not absolutely needed.

Image-guided neuronavigation systems are very useful for intraoperative identification of the limits of the lesion and of the bony, vascular, and nervous structures, especially if they are encased by tumor. This is especially true in cases of distorted anatomy due to a particular growth pattern of the meningioma, which causes the classic landmarks to not be easily identifiable. In such cases, neuronavigation can help to maintain the surgeon's orientation. High-speed, low-profile drills may be very helpful for opening the bony structures to gain access to the dural space while working in narrow surgical corridors, such as in the endonasal transsphenoidal approach for the removal of anteriorly placed cranial base meningiomas.[15,16] They are specifically designed for endonasal use and have some special characteristics: they are low profile and also long enough but not too bulky, so that they can be easily used together with the endoscope. Furthermore, they have proven to be effective and time-saving during the extended approaches to the skull base, especially for access to the suprasellar or retroclival meningiomas.

Prior to performing sharp dissections or incisions and whenever the surgeon thinks it is appropriate (especially while working very close to vascular structures), it is of utmost importance to use the microDoppler probe to identify the major arteries.[15–18] The use of such a device should be recommended every time a sharp dissection is made to minimize the risk of injury to the major arteries.

Preoperative Planning

Preoperative radiologic investigations for endoscopic meningioma surgery are the same for microsurgical approaches. They include magnetic resonance imaging (MRI), computed tomography (CT), angiography, etc. These evaluations provide the neurosurgeon information about the peculiar anatomic conditions concerning the tumor itself and either the bone and neurovascular structures involved in the approach.

Such studies are important for the planning of the approach and the removal strategy to be used with the image-guided surgery systems (namely, the neuronavigator).

Endoscopic Techniques

Endoscope-Assisted Microsurgery

Endoscope-assisted microsurgery (Fig. 21-1) is the simplest method for using the endoscope. The entire surgical procedure is done under microscopic vision, but the surgeon has the possibility to switch to the endoscope and observe the anatomy with endoscopic images whenever necessary. Then the procedure continues with the microscope. This system is inexpensive and helpful for gaining confidence with the endoscopic view: the surgeon has to continuously change the vision of the surgical field, passing from the microscope to the endoscopic monitor and vice versa. This may cause loss of concentration and may be time-consuming.

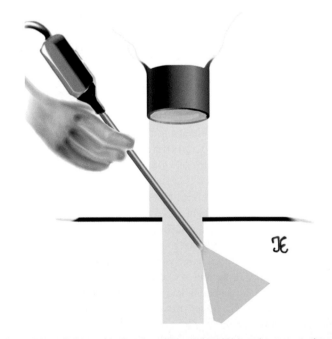

Fig. 21-1. Schematic drawing illustrating the endoscope-assisted microsurgical technique. The procedure and dissection maneuvers are done with the operating microscope and the endoscope is used as an adjunct tool only to see "around the corners"

Endoscope-Guided Microsurgery

Endoscope-guided microsurgery (Fig. 21-2) involves working simultaneously under microscopic and endoscopic vision. The surgeon uses the microscope and microsurgical instruments for the tumor dissection while the endoscope is in place. The endoscopic images can be seen (1) on an endoscopic monitor, with subsequent necessity to continuously move the eyes from the microscope to the monitor; (2) on LCD visors mounted on the surgeon's head, where the movements of the eyes are minimal; or (3) looking in the eyepieces of the microscope with a picture-in-picture system, which allows the surgeon to see the endoscopic images as well. The third method may be a good solution because the surgery is done in the classic way with the microscope and is possible to have the endoscopic vision without moving the eyes.

The first two methods combine the advantages of both the microscope and the endoscope. As a matter of fact, while the microscope provides a high-resolution stereoscopic view, there is a considerable decrease in light intensity provided by microscope for lesions located in the depth distal to narrow surgical corridors. The endoscope brings the surgeon's eye close to the region of interest and provides optimal illumination in depth and has a wide angle of view (30°, 45°, 70°, 120°), as well as a large focus range. With angled scopes, areas that are not visible in a straight line can be inspected and managed using dedicated instruments without drilling or retraction. Care should be taken in prolonged dissections under endo-

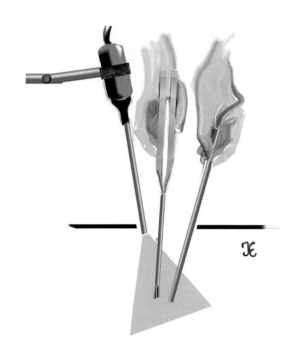

FIG. 21-3. Schematic drawing illustrating the pure endoscopic technique. The procedure and dissection maneuvers are done using the endoscope as the sole visualizing instrument during the entire operation

scopic view, because the tip of the scope may become hot, with a subsequent risk of thermal injury to the surrounding neurovascular structures.

"Pure" Endoscopic Technique

"Pure" endoscopic technique (Fig. 21-3) assumes that the entire procedure is done with the endoscope as the sole visualizing tool. This technique, in some centers and institutions, is among the procedure of choice for the treatment of meningiomas and related lesions of the midline skull base, via endonasal, supraorbital, or transglabellar approaches.[19–23]

The endoscope is better used through a sheath, connected to a cleaning-irrigation system. Such a system permits cleaning and defogging of the distal lens, thus avoiding repeated entrances and exits from the surgical field. The scopes used are usually without any working channel (diagnostic endoscopes), and the other instruments are inserted alongside the sheath. The diameter of a rod-lens endoscope varies between 1.9 and 10 mm, but for most of the time, endoscopes with a diameter of 2.7 mm are used.

The endoscope can be fixed to a scope holder or used freehand. The endoscope can be kept in place with the aid of different endoscopic holders. Many authors prefer to hold the endoscope with a mechanical holder to keep it stable in the surgical field and minimize the danger of injury of the nervous structures. By using the mechanical holder, both of the surgeon's hands are free to use two instruments. The disadvantage is that it gives a static view, while a dynamic view would be preferred. Other systems to hold the endoscope exist: with

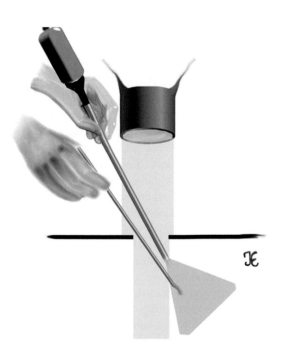

FIG. 21-2. Schematic drawing illustrating the endoscope-guided microsurgical technique. The procedure and dissection maneuvers are done with either the operating microscope or the endoscope. The surgeon can continuously switch between the two visions

steerable and extensible arms, with rigid and jointed arms, both straight and curved, pneumatic, and robotic arms. Nevertheless, the presence of the holder may obstruct the surgeon's movements in the surgical field, already encumbered with autostatic retractors and other instruments.

With the freehand variant the surgeon can dynamically handle the various instruments and continuously receive feedback regarding the anatomy and depth of the operative field, based on the in-and-out movements of the scope. Such a variant could be more versatile, especially during the fine dissection of the tumor. The advantages are the absence of the holder and the dynamic use of the endoscope, which gives more information on the anatomic details. The main limit of this method is that the freehand use of the endoscope involves one hand of the surgeon. Another possibility is to have the endoscope held by an assistant. With this method the dynamic movements of the scope are preserved and, at the same time, the surgeon can simultaneously use two instruments. The realization of such a technique requires the perfect cooperation of two surgeons: the first holds the endoscope and can be considered a sort of "navigator"; the second (the "pilot") moves with both hands two surgical instruments inside the surgical field, following the same principles of the microsurgical technique. An important aspect of the technique is that the "navigator" should constantly have in his or her visual control the instruments moved by the other surgeon, which have to remain under direct endoscopic view. This is the "dynamicity" of the procedure: the endoscope constantly follows the in-and-out movements of the instruments in the surgical field, minimizing the risks of injury to the neurovascular structures during their movements. Different from microsurgery, in which the microscope remains outside and the increasing magnification narrows correspondingly to the visual field, with the endoscope the "pilot" (assisted by able cooperation of the navigator) continuously passes between the close-up view and a panoramic view of the surgical field and the surrounding neurovascular structures.

The Chopstick Technique

The chopstick technique (Fig. 21-4) is an advancement of the pure endoscopic technique and may represent the near future of the endoscopic surgery.

The scope is a rigid fiberscope of different lengths contained in a rigid cylinder, which constitutes a sort of irrigation sheath, together with a small suction cannula, which slides inside the cylinder. The surgeon, via a button, can advance or retract the suction cannula with the sole movement of one finger (either the thumb or the index-finger). Attached to the proximal side of the cylinder is a cable that contains the cleaning system, the suction tube attached to the cannula, the optic fibers bringing the light to the scope from the light source, and the fiberoptic bundle, which brings the light and images from the surgical field and is connected to the videocamera. Such cable is long enough to be far from the surgeon's hands, rendering the cylinder quite light, which is held and

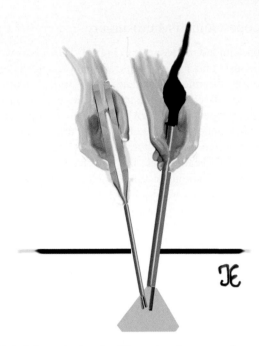

FIG. 21-4. Schematic drawing illustrating the pure endoscopic technique with the chopstick variant. The surgeon holds the fiberscope with built-in suction cannula as a pen during the fine dissection maneuvers

moved by the surgeon as if it were a pen. With the chopstick endoscope the surgeon has in one hand the visualizing tool and the suction cannula and in the other hand another instrument for tumor dissection or coagulation, etc. This technically allows surgeons to use three instruments with two hands.

Current Applications of Endoscopy in Meningioma Surgery

In tumor surgery, particularly for meningiomas, the utility of the endoscope is in seeing hidden and dark areas, where it is important to know if there are important structures before performing dangerous maneuvers. Indeed, the endoscope can be used, either alone or in combination with the operating microscope, for the removal of meningiomas wherever they are deeply located, or when its superior optical qualities are required.

It is employed in cerebellopontine angle tumor surgery, where it can be used effectively to remove the tumor while preserving all the important cranial nerves and vessels located in such narrow anatomic areas, using the different corridors existing between those neurovascular structures[24] or created by the presence of the meningioma itself.

The endoscope is used in anterior skull base surgery, where the coexistence of several neurovascular structures makes the anatomic dissection and tumor removal more difficult. In this field, several clinical studies have been reported.[25–29] In such cases, the endoscope has brought a fundamental contribution in expanding the role of the transsphenoidal approach and other minimally invasive routes to the entire skull base.[30] The selection of cases for the different endoneurosurgical approaches is not strictly defined for the time being, since this topic can be considered "in progress" and in constant reinterpretation, and therefore no definite conclusions should be drawn. What must be stressed is that these minimally invasive approaches require perfect knowledge of anatomy, very good endoscopic surgical skills, up-to-date instrumentation, and a flexible (not dogmatic) way of thinking.

Future Perspectives

The future of the neuroendoscopy, and particularly that of the endoscopic surgery of meningiomas, is certainly promising within neurologic surgery. Further technological advancements and the education of young neurosurgeons with the endoscopic techniques will surely contribute to the expansion of boundaries of the current techniques and indications. 3-D endoscopes are available but are still too poorly used and, for several approaches, still too bulky to be used (e.g., intranasal use.)

Neuroendoscopy is here to stay. However, in meningioma surgery, this new and important technology is currently encountering varying degrees of active resistance, passive resistance, passive acceptance, and lastly active acceptance, as with any other new idea or approach in medicine.[30]

Acknowledgments. We wish to thank Dr. Isabella Esposito, resident in neurosurgery at our institution, for the drawings.

References

1. Cappabianca P, Cavallo LM, de Divitiis O, Esposito F: Keyhole surgery in the treatment of sellar region tumors. Clin Neurosurg 2005;52:116–119.
2. Cinalli G, Cappabianca P, de Falco R, et al.: Current state and future development of intracranial neuroendoscopic surgery. Expert Rev Med Devices 2005;2:351–373.
3. Perneczky A, Muller-Forell W, van Lindert E, Fries G: Keyhole concept in neurosurgery. Thieme, New York, 1999.
4. Apuzzo ML, Heifetz MD, Weiss MH, Kurze T: Neurosurgical endoscopy using the side-viewing telescope. J Neurosurg 1977;46:398–400.
5. Grotenhuis JA: Endoscope-assisted craniotomy. Techniques Neurosurg 1996;1:201–212.
6. Perneczky A, Fries G: Endoscope-assisted brain surgery: part 1—evolution, basic concept, and current technique. Neurosurgery 1998;42:219–224; discussion 224–215.
7. Kaptain GJ, Vincent DA, Sheehan JP, et al.: Transsphenoidal approaches for the extracapsular resection of midline suprasellar and anterior cranial base lesions. Neurosurgery 2001;49:94–100; discussion 100–101.
8. Cappabianca P, de Divitiis E: Endoscopy and transsphenoidal surgery. Neurosurgery 2004:54:1043–1048; discussion 1048–1050.
9. Leonhard M, Cappabianca P, de Divitiis E: The endoscope, endoscopic equiment and instrumentation. In: de Divitiis E, Cappabi-anca P (eds.). Endoscopic Endonasal Transsphenoidal Surgery. Springer, New York, 2003:9–19.
10. Decq P: Endoscopic anatomy of the ventricles. In: Cinalli G, Maixner WJ, Saint-Rose C (eds.). Pediatric Hydrocephalus. Springer, Milan, 2004:351–359.
11. Siomin V, Constantini S: Basic principles and equipment in neuroendoscopy. Neurosurg Clin N Am 2004;15:19–31.
12. Cappabianca P, Alfieri A, Thermes S, et al.: Instruments for endoscopic endonasal transsphenoidal surgery. Neurosurgery 1999; 45:392–395; discussion 395–396.
13. Cappabianca P, Cavallo LM, Esposito F, de Divitiis E: Endoscopic endonasal transsphenoidal surgery: procedure, endoscopic equipment and instrumentation. Childs Nerv Syst 2004:20:796–801.
14. Tasman AJ, Feldhusen F, Kolling GH, Hosemann W: Video-endoscope versus endoscope for paranasal sinus surgery: influence on visual acuity and color discrimination. Am J Rhinol 1999;13:7–10.
15. Dusick JR, Esposito F, Kelly DF, et al.: The extended direct endonasal transsphenoidal approach for nonadenomatous suprasellar tumors. J Neurosurg 2005;102:832–841.
16. Esposito F, Becker DP, Villablanca JP, Kelly DF: Endonasal transsphenoidal transclival removal of prepontine epidermoid tumors: technical note. Neurosurgery 2005;56:E443; discussion E443.
17. Arita K, Kurisu K, Tominaga A, et al: Trans-sellar color Doppler ultrasonography during transsphenoidal surgery. Neurosurgery 1998;42:81–85; discussion 86.
18. Yamasaki T, Moritake K, Hatta J, Nagai H: Intraoperative monitoring with pulse Doppler ultrasonography in transsphenoidal surgery: technique application. Neurosurgery 1996;38:95–97; discussion 97–98.
19. Cappabianca P, Frank G, Pasquini E, et al: Extended endoscopic endonasal transsphenoidal approaches to the suprasellar region, planum sphenoidale & clivus. In: Cappabianca P, de Divitiis E (eds.). Endoscopic Endonasal Transsphenoidal Surgery. Springer-Verlag, New York, 2003:176–187.
20. Cavallo LM, Messina A, Cappabianca P, et al.: Endoscopic endonasal surgery of the midline skull base: anatomical study and clinical considerations. Neurosurg Focus 2005;19:E2.
21. Jho HD: The expanding role of endoscopy in skull-base surgery. Indications and instruments. Clin Neurosurg 2001;48:287–305.
22. Kassam AB, Gardner P, Snyderman C, et al.: Expanded endonasal approach: fully endoscopic, completely transnasal approach to the middle third of the clivus, petrous bone, middle cranial fossa, and infratemporal fossa. Neurosurg Focus 2005;19:E6.
23. Yuguang L, Chengyuan W, Meng L, et al.: Neuroendoscopic anatomy and surgery of the cerebellopontine angle. J Clin Neurosci 2005;12:256–260.
24. Cappabianca P, Cavallo LM, Esposito F: Endoscopic examination of the cerebellar pontine angle. Clin Neurol Neurosurg 2002:104:387–391.
25. Cook SW, Smith Z, Kelly DF: Endonasal transsphenoidal removal of tuberculum sellae meningiomas: technical note. Neurosurgery 2004;55:239–244; discussion 244–236.
26. Couldwell WT, Weiss MH et al.: Variations on the standard transsphenoidal approach to the sellar region, with emphasis on the extended approaches and parasellar approaches: surgical experience in 105 cases. Neurosurgery 2004;55:539–547; discussion 547–550.

27. de Divitiis E, Cappabianca P, Cavallo LM: Endoscopic trans-sphenoidal approach: adaptability of the procedure to different sellar lesions. Neurosurgery 2002;51:699–705; discussion 705–697.

28. Jane JA, Dumont AS, Vance ML, Laws ER: The transsphenoidal transtuberculum sellae approach for suprasellar meningiomas (abstr). In: American Association of Neurological Surgeons, Orlando, FL, 2004.

29. Jho HD, Alfieri A: Endoscopic glabellar approach to the anterior skull base: a technical note. Minim Invasive Neurosurg 2002;45:185–188.

30. Maroon JC: Skull base surgery: past, present, and future trends. Neurosurg Focus 2005;19:E1.

22
Image-Guided Surgery for Meningiomas

Tina Thomas and Gene H. Barnett

Introduction

The primary surgical goals of neuro-oncology are to target and remove lesions while leaving functional brain tissue and vasculature intact, in order to preserve neurologic function (1). The attainment of these goals requires a clear three-dimensional (3-D) understanding and conceptualization of brain and tumor anatomy on the surgeon's part. Significant challenges for planning and actual surgery in oncology are the distortion, envelopment, invasion, and obscuration of normal and pathologic structures by the tumor.

Stereotactic image-guidance techniques aim to assist the surgeon by virtually linking imaging data and in vivo anatomy. They allow the surgeon to transpose 3-D spatial information from diagnostic images onto the live anatomy of the patient, thus providing interactive 3-D localization and orientation (2,3).

Frame-based stereotaxy was initially developed for glial and metastatic tumors. Its main applications in these contexts were for minimally invasive procedures such as biopsy or catheter placement, and for localization of deep lesions (4–6). Frameless image-guided surgery (IGS) techniques were developed later. They were considered advantageous because they entailed less patient discomfort, had easier logistics, and were less cumbersome for surgeons, who no longer had to maneuver around a frame or arc (7–12). The advent of these more surgeon- and patient-"friendly" techniques favored a widespread adoption of stereotactic technology. Software has been developed that provides much more useful 3-D information (7,13,14). Accuracy has progressively improved, and is now generally on the order of approximately 2 mm (9,10,15–20). This progress has opened up the use of IGS for more varied applications such as spinal surgery and other types of intracranial tumors such as meningiomas.

Surgical approaches to meningiomas are primarily determined by their locations; accordingly, this chapter will discuss the uses of image-guidance systems for meningiomas involving various intracranial locations including convexity, falcine, parasagittal, and the skull base.

Principles of IGS Use in Meningioma Surgery

The main goals of meningioma surgery, as with other types of brain tumors, are resection or decompression of the lesion with simultaneous preservation of neurovascular structures. The use of IGS in meningioma surgery bears many similarities to its use in other applications with regard to planning of the approach and tailoring of minimal or "optimal access" craniotomies (4). IGS helps the surgeon to localize the lesion more precisely, to delineate neurovascular relationships, and to establish the most direct route permitting complete removal (9). This allows more accurate head positioning and placement of the incision and craniotomy (9). Optimal access craniotomies have been shown to reduce neurologic and wound complications, operative time, and patient discomfort (15,21–25). Specifically for skull base meningiomas, IGS assists in localization of bony landmarks, determination of the extent of bone removal, and tumor relationship to hidden neurovascular structures, as well as estimation of the extent of residual tumor.

Certain factors set meningioma surgery apart from surgery for gliomas or metastases. First, image guidance is not needed to define the tumor–brain interface. Second, the lesion is tethered in place by its attachments to the dura and to the skull, and therefore "brain shift" has a smaller impact on accuracy (26). As a result, diuretics, cerebrospinal fluid (CSF) drainage, hyperventilation, and diuresis may be used freely, as needed.

Meningiomas: Convexity, Falcine, and Parasagittal

Estimation of Surgical Risk

An accessory function of IGS for convexity, falcine, and parasagittal meningiomas is the use of reformatted images to assess relationships to cerebral surface anatomy. More rarely, fusion with physiologic imaging (PET or functional MR) may be used to estimate the risk of postoperative neurologic deficit (7).

Minimal Access Craniotomies and Incision Planning

As mentioned above, IGS systems can demonstrate the precise location of a lesion with respect to the actual patient's surface anatomy, as well as delineate cortical and vascular relationships to the planned approach (Fig. 22-1) (15). It is important to note that classic triplanar views obtained at the scalp or outer table level may provide a misleading conceptualization of the flap, with a resultant small or displaced opening. On the other hand, oblique or trajectory displays allow the surgeon to point the wand perpendicular to the curvature of the skull. This approximates the actual orientation of the craniotome for precise placement and sizing of the bone flap (7). It is important to plan a craniotomy that is about 1.5 cm larger than the maximum diameter of the dural attachment at the convexity (26–28). On the other hand, limiting the size of the craniotomy to the minimum necessary protects the unexposed uninvolved brain tissue (29). Generally, the incision will be linear or S-shaped.

Special consideration must be given to lesions on or approaching the midline. For falcine lesions, attention must be made to plan the incision and bony opening to allow for control and reconstruction if the superior sagittal sinus is lacerated (26). In the case of parasagittal lesions, placement of an S-shaped incision in the coronal plane allows for lengthening of the incision and extension of the craniotomy if access is needed to control bleeding from the superior sagittal sinus (26).

Optimization of Craniotomy Size and Location ("Tailored Craniotomies")

Many factors must be considered in fashioning the ideal bone flap. The dural tail must be reached in order to attain an optimal Simpson grade resection. Thus, it is especially important in convexity and parasagittal lesions to expose more than the diameter of the tumor attachment (7,30). Localization of underlying venous structures is an even more critical consideration. Cortical and parasagittal vascular structures often appear as nonspecific spots of high intensity on triplanar displays (21). In order to facilitate the task, planning at our institution is done directly on oblique displays (26). These are perpendicular views that both contain the wand axis. One is parallel to the wand and perpendicular to skull, as is the desired surgical trajectory. The other is perpendicular to this plane at a user-selectable depth and allows a systematic visualization of potentially traversed structures including vascular and cortical anatomy (21). This allows projection or simulation of many different trajectory options and selection of the one that best minimizes risk to structures (4,7,31). It also favors precise centering and sizing of the craniotomy.

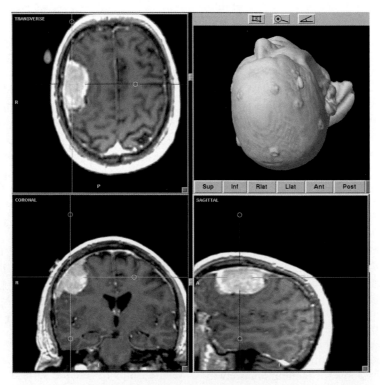

FIG. 22-1. Convexity meningioma: IGS is used here to optimize the cranial and dural openings as well as to help determine the relationship of tumor to cortical anatomy. In this case, tumor appears to be just anterior to precentral gyrus

Consequently, the smallest favorable craniotomy possible minimizes blood loss, while undue brain retraction can be avoided by not making it too small. This can be a significant factor in convexity meningiomas, where the size of the bone flap is known to be an important determinant of blood loss (7). In selected cases, particularly for large or falcine lesions, fusion with MR venography can help in this aspect of planning (21,32).

The patient's head is secured in the fixation device, while taking care to avoid displacement of the reference fiducials.

As explained previously, the superior sagittal sinus (SSS) is exposed as needed. The relationship of adjacent veins draining into the SSS is also studied in order to plan a corridor between them. It is important to maximize the size of the surgical corridor, even if it is not the shortest route to tumor; this may entail a larger craniotomy in certain cases (21).

Dural Opening and Tumor Resection

The dural opening is planned with respect to cortical veins draining the adjacent parenchyma (7,26,27). It is typically begun peripherally, in areas free of large draining veins and continued under direct visualization into areas with underlying veins (21).

The image-guidance system has a more limited role in the actual resection of these tumors. Some potential uses include the demonstration of subjacent veins. If large veins underlie the tumor it is safer to dissect and expose the tumor from proximal to distal along these (21). Otherwise, dissection may proceed from lateral to medial direction. IGS can also be used to define the limits of SSS resection when it is occluded (Fig. 22-2A). In these cases, fusion of magnetic resonance venography (MRV), especially contrast-enhanced MRV (which is more reliable than phase-contrast) may prove useful (32). In addition, some authors have cited the use of IGS for reoperation in recurrent meningiomas to differentiate tumor from surrounding scar tissue or gliosis (33).

Results

IGS can be useful in the surgery of convexity, falcine, and parasagittal meningiomas for the planning of craniotomies and surgical corridors, as well as for decreasing the risk of venous infarction. It may also aid in obtaining complete resections, especially for parasagittal meningiomas, where the SSS may be invaded and occluded, thus decreasing the risk of recurrence.

Meningiomas: Tentorial

Craniotomy and Dural Opening

In approaches to tentorial meningiomas, IGS can first of all assist in ascertaining the location of the transverse sinus (TS) in order to avoid damage to it during the craniotomy (Fig. 22-2B).

It can also pinpoint the location of temporal venous anatomy, including the vein of Labbé, and help to preserve it during the supratentorial dural opening (34). If the interhemispheric approach is chosen, the location of occipital lobe draining veins can be demonstrated with the IGS; aggregations of closely spaced veins may dictate the fashioning of a larger bony opening or even the selection of an alternative approach.

Approach

During the subtemporal approach, as mentioned in the previous section, attention to the location of temporal venous anatomy and to deep venous structures is crucial to their preservation and subsequent avoidance of venous infarction (4,26,34).

If an interhemispheric approach is selected, the bridging veins to the SSS become a crucial concern. These are also a relevant consideration for pineal region meningiomas; in these cases, the deep venous anatomy may also dictate the choice of approach (4,35). IGS is less important for the definition of arterial anatomy in tentorial meningiomas, since there are usually no large arteries behind the lesion. Furthermore, the posterior cerebral and superior cerebellar arteries are small and not reliably identified with current imaging techniques (23).

Meningiomas: Skull Base

Rationale

Skull base approaches require deep exposures, which result in limited visibility around and behind the targeted lesion (31,36). In addition, there is an increased density of surrounding critical neurovascular structures in these areas (37). These approaches were developed and "standardized" before the advent of IGS and thus do not necessitate its use. However, IGS techniques can be complementary in selected cases for orientation, 3-D conceptualization and selection of the optimal approach (4,7,38,39). They may also help to minimize the morbidity inherent to these approaches in several ways (4,7,40–43). Optimal placement of the craniotomy favors minimal brain retraction, which increases safety. Also, tailored (as opposed to standardized) approaches at the skull base attempt to limit bony removal to a minimum, in order to decrease the risks inherent to these approaches (4,7). IGS can also increase safety by identifying hidden neurovascular structures, thus potentially speeding up the learning curve for novice skull base surgeons and shortening surgical time in individual cases (4,44).

In addition to these potential advantages, skull base lesions, which are attached to dura and/or bone, are ideal targets because they remain fixed in space with respect to the skull, and subsequently to the fiducial landmarks and the tracker (44). Thus, they are minimally affected by gravity, retraction, hyperventilation, CSF loss or drainage, and mannitol administration (36). Furthermore, the anatomic landmarks of the skull base provide a good correlation for navigation systems (31,44).

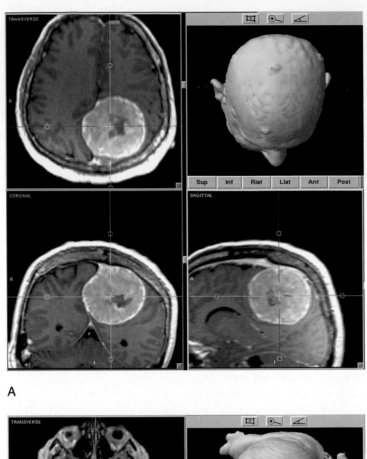

A

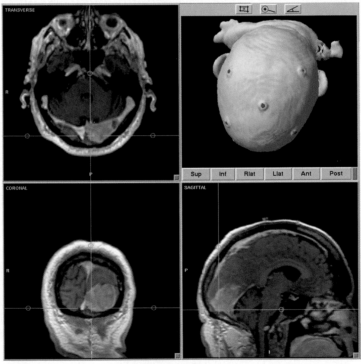

B

FIG. 22-2. Venous sinus patency: IGS can aid in the determination of sinus occlusion when planning the approach to a tumor of the (A) falx or (B) of the tentorium. Here, image fusion can allow a magnetic resonance venogram to be superimposed on the images

Incision and Craniotomy

IGS can be useful from the initial step of incision planning for skull base lesions by favoring a more precise placement. This helps to ensure an adequate exposure of the surface of the skull despite interpersonal anatomic variations (36).

Again, it can also assist in planning the size and location of the craniotomy flap. For example, in retrosigmoid approaches, image guidance can aid in the critical placement of the incision and of the first burr hole, which are not always accurate by surface landmarks, even in experienced hands (45,46). Another example is that of combined middle-posterior fossa craniotomies. In these cases, the surgeon can verify the locations of the vein of Labbé, the transverse sinus (TS), and the sigmoid sinus (SS) prior to placement of the burr holes and passage of the drill, instead of relying solely on skull landmarks. This maximizes exposure while improving safety (4,34,36).

Identification of Skull Base Landmarks and Extent of Bone Resection

Identification of bony skull base landmarks is a vital component of these approaches. This step is essential in order to determine the extent of bone resection at the skull base. It also assists in the tracing of crucial neurovascular structures back from their skull base entry or exit points. This may be an invaluable help to localization when these are obscured or displaced by tumor. In addition, IGS can help the surgeon to pinpoint these more quickly and subsequently shorten surgical time. For example, in anterior approaches, structures that can be localized by IGS include the sphenoid and ethmoid sinuses, the superior orbital fissure, the optic foramen, the anterior clinoid process, and the foraminae ovale, spinosum, and rotundum. This is especially valuable when these structures are eroded or distorted by invasive tumors of the skull base, such as aggressive meningiomas. In transpetrosal approaches it is useful to find the mastoid air cells, the antrum, the semicircular canals, the petrous internal carotid artery (ICA), the petrous apex, and the internal auditory canal (IAC), where the VII–VIII nerve complex will be found (Fig. 22-3)(7). In posterior approaches, it can be helpful to localize the transverse foramen of C1 and the occipital condyle (4). As previously mentioned, precise orientation to the bony anatomy reduces the amount of drilling necessary once the desired trajectory is obtained and confirmed by IGS. Limited drilling may favor the preservation of vital structures, such as the vestibulocochlear and facial nerves in transpetrosal approaches, and may also allow maintenance of craniocervical stability in the far lateral transcondylar approach (4,7,36). Thus, these "tailored" skull base approaches can increase safety and reduce the intrinsic morbidity of skull-base approaches (4).

Orientation Within Lesions

Internal debulking is usually required for the safe resection of skull base lesions. However, with this technique, there is often

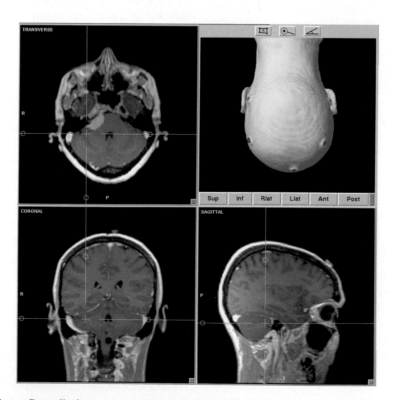

FIG. 22-3. Petroclival meningioma: Petroclival tumors can obscure the VII–VIII nerve complex. Large tumors also displace the basilar artery, which will be in contact with the tumor capsule at the far end of the approach and is at risk if the capsule is inadvertently perforated in its vicinity

uncertainty with respect to the amount of tumor remaining at the distant side (31,36). In this situation, IGS provides helpful cues as to the location of important structures beyond the surgeon's visual perspective (31). It serves as a type of "x-ray vision," which provides a visual warning when these structures are approached (31,37). This helps to avoid inadvertent transgression beyond the limits of tumor, which can lead to serious injury to vital structures (31,36). An example of this would be the case of a clival meningioma, where the basilar artery may border the medial side (Fig. 22-3).

Choice of Imaging Modality

A combination of imaging modalities may be the best choice for navigation in skull base lesions, even more than for other types of lesions. CT is best for bony skull landmarks, for example, during the initial exposure, but it has the weakness of beam-hardening artifact at the skull base. Also, imaging planes other than axial must be reconstructed rather than directly imaged with CT. If the lesion is well shown on CT, the same images may be used for the resection portion of the procedure.

MRI is a better modality for soft tissue components, but does not delineate bone well and has the weakness of paramagnetic susceptibility artifact in certain regions, such as near the mouth in patients with dental work (31). In addition, MRI has a greater inherent spatial infidelity than CT. Thus, the mean accuracy (which may be defined as a smaller difference between the actual position of the wand in space and its predicted position by the IGS computer) is better for registration with CT as opposed to MR images (15,31,47). On the other hand, coronal, sagittal, or in-line views are more distinct on MRI than on reconstructed CT images (48).

Overall, for meningiomas of the skull base (as opposed to true lesions of the bony skull base or craniovertebral junction), MRI is the most useful technique for visualizing tumor relationships to other soft tissue components (48). Alternatively, fusion of MRI and CT images, while introducing a new source of error from the computerized transformation process, may provide the best option for all phases of the operation (7,31,36). Image fusion techniques may also compensate for sources of error of each of these techniques when used separately (31).

Meningiomas of Anterior and Middle Fossae

In planning approaches to these lesions, the craniotomy can be outlined directly with oblique displays, as explained previously. The frontal air sinuses can be precisely located in order to avoid opening them if possible, as there are no reliable surface anatomic landmarks for these (36,48,49). This avoids potential CSF leak and infection, and also saves the operative time required for cranialization of an inadvertently opened sinus.

When choosing a surgical trajectory, it is useful to locate the ICA, the proximal ACA, and the proximal MCA, as well as the *de passage* vessels (Fig. 22-4A). Fusion with magnetic resonance angiography (MRA) may be of use in certain cases. Localization of the optic nerves is also a consideration when planning a surgical corridor to these lesions (Fig. 22-4B).

One of the most practical uses of navigation for skull base lesions is to give an indication of one's location within tumor during debulking. In the case of anterior and middle fossa lesions, nerves and vascular structures which may be obscured by the bulk of the tumor during the initial approach include the internal carotid artery, the proximal ACA and MCA, and the optic nerves (27,30,31). Thus, when removing large olfactory groove, clinoidal, or tuberculum sellae meningiomas, which displace or hide the optic nerves, the optic canal serves as an excellent fixed reference point that is easily located by the IGS (33). This technique can also aid in the identification of a displaced ICA, which will be found just lateral to the intradural segment of the optic nerve in these cases. These additional clues to orientation are particularly invaluable if the posterior portion of tumor abuts the aforementioned vascular or nervous structures, where inadvertent transgression of the posterior wall during internal debulking can have grave consequences (Fig. 22-4A). IGS can also indicate the intralesional location of *de passage* vessels, which can help in their preservation during this phase of the operation.

Meningiomas of Middle and Posterior Fossae

Sphenoid wing lesions are generally accessed through pterional approaches without the need for image guidance. IGS may be of assistance in extradural approaches to anterior clinoidectomy and unroofing of the optic canal, where the ethmoid and sphenoid sinuses should not be transgressed (33). For large or mesial tumors (e.g., those of the cavernous sinus), the locations of major vascular structures (such as a displaced or encased ICA) in relation to the tumor may be appreciated (4,26). Accuracy is usually preserved for mesial structures during debulking until most of the basal attachments are severed.

In the case of petroclival tumors, IGS can help to place the craniotomy or dural opening with respect to the nearby venous sinuses (TS, SS). This is crucial (as with tentorial lesions), as it allows a more accurate placement of the burr holes, facilitates drilling, and can avoid unduly extensive bone removal. IGS can help to define the location of internal auditory canal (IAC) when the seventh and eighth cranial nerves are hidden from view by the tumor (Fig. 22-3). Here again, IGS is most useful for defining one's location within a large tumor in order to avoid inadvertent perforation of the deep capsule and entry into neurovascular structures such as the basilar artery (31,36,50–53).

For large foramen magnum lesions, IGS can help to protect the vertebral artery by locating it at its dural entry point (33). Navigation can also occasionally help to identify hidden lobules of tumor (e.g., in the case of a large tumor at the petrous apex) (31,36). Conversely, it can also confirm that the distal

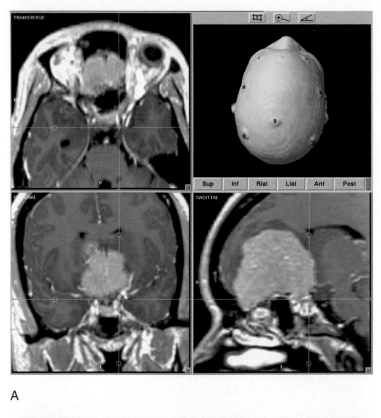

A

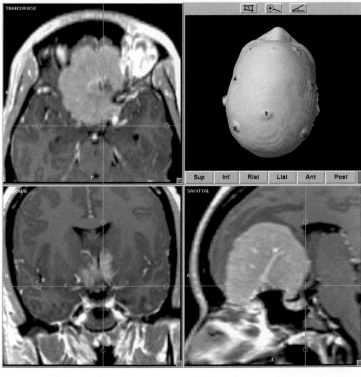

B

FIG. 22-4. Olfactory groove meningioma: In the case of a large olfactory groove meningioma, IGS can assist the surgeon to determine the extent of resection and proximity to the optic apparatus. It also defines relationships to critical vascular structures such as the anterior cerebral and internal carotid arteries that are often displaced or, at least, hidden behind the tumor. (A) Cross-hairs on left internal carotid artery; (B) on optic nerve

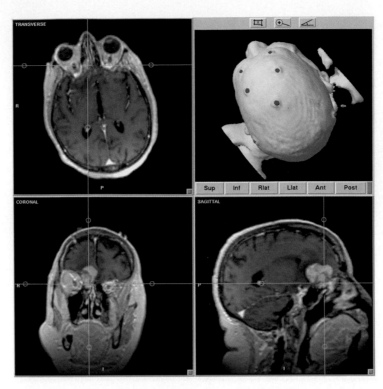

FIG. 22-5. Planned incomplete resection: In some elderly or high-surgical-risk patients (such as this case of olfactory groove menigioma with extension beyond the cribriform plate), the surgical goal is simple decompression in order to avoid exposing the patient to the risks of an attempted gross total resection. In these cases, IGS can provide a more accurate assessment of the amount of tumor resected than visual assessment alone, allowing the surgeon to stop when a volume amenable to stereotactic radiosurgery is attained. Here, the cross-hairs represent the intended inferior extent of resection

extremity of a deep tumor has been reached and thus avoid unnecessary dissection and risk of injury to neural structures (36). In addition, IGS can assist in planned subtotal resections (e.g., brainstem decompression in elderly patient), where it may help the surgeon to estimate the amount of tumor removed (Fig. 22-5) (31,36). Finally, navigation systems can be particularly valuable for invasive tumors and for repeat operations, where anatomy is distorted, or where there is extensive scarring, which may complicate the identification of normal anatomic landmarks (31,36,37,48).

Shortcomings of IGS Systems for Skull Base Surgery

There are certain drawbacks to the use of current navigation systems for skull base lesions. These are mostly related to the depth of the target lesion combined with the use of the operating microscope. In this context, physical constraints can render the use of pointing devices cumbersome. First, the microscope can physically obstruct the placement of the wand. Second, it can block the line of sight between the camera and the wand and/or reference. These difficulties may be alleviated through use of the bipolar forceps with a diode-possessing adapter as an alternative pointing device (36). Also, the microscope can be calibrated with attached diodes and used as a virtual pointing device.

Another drawback to current navigation systems in skull base surgery is that the surgeon must stop operating in order to look up at the television display, which interrupts the flow of the procedure. This was partially alleviated by the creation of a "heads-up display" within the microscope's field of view that shows the tumor outline as defined preoperatively, and the pointer tip with respect to it (9,10,54,55). However, the practical usefulness of this technique has been limited due to the fact that this display does not show the classic three-plane view with the landmark selected by probe. Consequently, the surgeon remains obliged to periodically look away to the television screen in order to ascertain these (36).

The utility of IGS for the protection of cranial nerves is also limited, especially in the case of the smaller ones (e.g., lower cranial nerves in petroclival lesions). This is because they are usually not visualized on CT and are not reliably seen on standard MRIs. Thus, IGS cannot help to locate them except where they pass through visible structures, such as the superior orbital fissure. In fact, even larger cranial nerves (e.g., the optic nerve) can be nonvisualized when they are thinly stretched over a tumor mass or atrophied. In these cases, preserving the integrity of structures relies more on meticulous microsurgical technique and electrophysiologic monitoring (when available) than on the use of IGS itself (7,26).

Brachytherapy

Brachytherapy entails the surgical implantation of radioactive isotopes into a tumor, which delivers high doses to it with a rapid dose fall-off, thus minimizing radiation delivery to the surrounding brain (56,57). It has been used for meningiomas in patients who are considered poor surgical risks for resection due to advanced age or poor health, as well as in patients with unresectable or recurrent tumors (57). These patients must have stable, minimal, or no symptomatology (such as medically controlled seizures) (26). Planning is done for a stereotactic biopsy using imaging with fiducials and a planning computer for locations and angles of approach. The dose given is between 7000 and 17,000 cGy, with dose rate of 5–10 cGy per hour. The number (usually 1–5) and location of the permanently implantable I-125 seeds is decided in collaboration with the radiation oncologist. The target(s) and entry point(s) are decided on the IGS system. The head is shaved and prepped as for a stereotactic biopsy. The scalp is punctured and a twist drill hole is made. Using the IGS, a cannula is then advanced just short of the target to account for the length of the seed. A modified obturator advances the seed to the target site. The cannula is then withdrawn and closure done as usual. Finally, seed placement is verified with radiographs (26).

A Cleveland Clinic series of 13 patients showed stabilization or reduction in volume in 12 of 13 meningiomas treated with the above brachytherapy protocol (56,57). One lesion progressed outside of the implantation zone. There were no acute complications, and the only long-term complication was radiation necrosis in one patient. However, in the subgroup that received doses over 10,000 cGy, all patients had vasogenic edema and/or radiation necrosis.

Use of brachytherapy has been limited to date because of the success of less invasive stereotactic radiosurgery techniques.

Caveats

Despite the sense of reassurance that IGS can provide in surgery, it would be wise for the surgeon to avoid becoming too complacent. Navigation systems, despite their increasing sophistication, do not replace a surgeon's thorough knowledge and 3-D understanding of the anatomy of the approaches (37,41–43). Moreover, they cannot substitute for clinical judgment during the case.

There are several reasons to remain vigilant while using these IGS systems. One is that the systems have a variable application accuracy, which is determined by a variety of system- and user-related factors. In addition, even for skull base tumors (where we generally consider tissue shift to be insignificant), once tumor debulking has been performed, there is an inevitable collapse of the capsule with a real potential for movement of tumor-displaced vessels or cranial nerves (58–62). Blind reliance on preoperative images produced by the IGS comprises a true hazard in this situation.

Nevertheless, the dangers of system malfunction or of loss of accuracy in this situation can be compensated by the aware surgeon. Reality checks may be performed at each stage of the operation. At the surface, accuracy can be visually estimated by comparing actual cortical landmarks (i.e., gyri, sulci, and visible tumor boundaries) with the displayed image-guidance data (2,58,59). At the skull base, bony landmarks may be used for the reality check or for reregistration, if needed (31). The surgeon can also employ various techniques to maintain accuracy for as long as possible and to cope with the inevitable loss of accuracy, especially during critical portions of the surgery. For example, dangerous areas may be approached early on in the surgery, while system accuracy is at its best.

Future Directions

Improvements that will increase the everyday utility of image-guidance systems include progress in image fusion techniques which accurately integrate angiographic and functional data from CT angiography, MR angiography, MR venography, functional MRI, and digital subtraction angiography. Further advances in neuronavigation will permit actual 3-D reconstructions of lesions, as well as of the surrounding nerves, vessels and fiber tracts (4,38). These displays could be even more useful for trajectory simulation and for nuances of positioning, particularly in approaches to skull base lesions (4,35,38). Furthermore, improved dynamic intraoperative imaging using ultrasound, CT, or MRI will produce updated images to permit adjustment of navigation parameters, with minimal or no interruption in the flow of surgery (7,12,58,59,63–68). Certain groups have studied models of deformation based on "predictable" brain shifts during tumor resection (59,69–71). For the moment, these are relatively impractical and expensive (5,58, 65). They will require further development before widespread adoption.

Conclusions

Image-guidance techniques can prove a useful adjunct in meningioma surgery. As opposed to other applications, localization of the tumor is not their primary use in this setting, with the possible exception of small convexity lesions. Nevertheless, IGS systems can complement many phases of the surgery ranging from preoperative planning to intraoperative stages.

IGS is most useful for seven main steps in intracranial meningioma surgery:

1. Preoperative trajectory planning and choice of approach
2. Incision mapping
3. Optimization of bone and dural openings to minimize morbidity related to brain retraction or to avoid excessive bony removal
4. Delineation of lesion and aid to complete resection (rarely)

5. Localization of adjacent arterial and venous structures in order to decrease bleeding/transfusion requirements and the risk of venous infarction (31)
6. Localization of adjacent neural structures (31)
7. Localization within a large tumor devoid of landmarks

These advantages may result in decreased cost to the patient as well as to health care systems through reduced surgical time (subject to the initial learning curve), decreased transfusion rate, shortened hospital and ICU stay/rehabilitation, minimized morbidity, and improved functional outcome and survival (7,44). One study showed a 61% decreased mortality for meningioma surgery between 1988 and 2000, which was more marked at high-volume centers, and which they hypothesized to have been partly due to the use of advanced intraoperative technology (72). This may be more of a concern in skull base lesions, since most contemporary series of convexity and parasagittal meningiomas show a mortality rate approaching zero and morbidity less than 10% for these, compared to 8–12% and over 46%, respectively, for skull base lesions (7). Use of IGS may also aid in obtaining ideal Simpson-grade resections, with subsequent decreased need for reoperations and risk of recurrence (7,31,73,74).

We believe that IGS is particularly useful for small superficial lesions, tumors with a significant dural tail, and for skull base meningiomas with displaced and/or encased neurovasculature or destruction of bony landmarks.

Promising avenues for IGS in the future include the placement of radioactive seed brachytherapy implants in unresectable lesions or for poor-risk cases. In addition, improvements in IGS techniques, with better visualization and more seamless integration into the surgical flow, will likely result in a more widespread adoption of these techniques for meningioma surgery.

References

1. Jolesz FA. Neurosurgical suite of the future II. Neuroimaging Clin N Am 2001;11:581–592.
2. Spetzger U, Hubbe U, Struffert T, et al. Error analysis in cranial neuronavigation. Minimally invasive neurosurgery 2002;45:60–70.
3. Adler JR. Surgical guidance now and in the future: the next generation of instrumentation. Clin Neurosurg 2002;49:105–114.
4. Rohde V, Spangenberg P, Mayfrank L, et al. Advanced neuronavigation in skull base tumors and vascular lesions. Minim Invas Neurosurg 2005;48:13–18.
5. Kelly PJ, Kall BA, Goerss SJ. Results of computed tomography-based computer-assisted stereotactic resection of metastatic intracranial tumors. Neurosurgery 1988;22:7–17.
6. Moore MR, Black PM, Ellenbogen R, et al. Stereotactic craniotomy: methods and results using the Brown-Roberts-Wells stereotactic frame. Neurosurgery 1989;25:572–577.
7. Paleologos T, Wadley J, Kitchen N, et al. Clinical utility and cost-effectiveness of interactive image-guided craniotomy: clinical comparison between conventional and image-guided meningioma surgery. Neurosurgery 2000;47:40–47.
8. Hassenbusch SJ, Anderson JS, Pillay PK. Brain tumor resection aided with markers placed using stereotaxis guided by magnetic resonance imaging and computed tomography. Neurosurgery 1991;28:801–806.
9. Kleinpeter G, Lothaller C. Frameless neuronavigationn using the ISG-system in practice: from craniotomy to delineation of lesion. Minim Invas Neurosurg 2003;46:257–264.
10. Roberts DW, Strohbehn JW, Hatch JF et al. A frameless stereotactic integration of computerized tomographic imaging and the operating microscope. J Neurosurg 1986;65:545–549.
11. Linskey ME. Tha changing role of stereotaxis in surgical neuro-oncology. J Neuro-Oncol 2004;69:35–54.
12. Lindseth F, Kaspersen JH, Ommedal S, et al. Multimodal image fusion in ultrasound-based neuronavigation: Improving overview and interpretation by integrating preoperative MRI with intraoperative 3-D ultrasound. Comput Aided Surg 2003;8:49–69.
13. Barnett GH, McKenzie RL, Ramos L, et al. Nonvolumetric stereotaxy-assisted craniotomy: results in 50 cases. Stereotact Funct Neurosurg 1993;61:80–95.
14. Kelly PJ. Computer-assisted stereotaxis: new approaches for the management of intracranial intra-axial tumors. Neurology 1986;36:535–541.
15. Barnett GH, Kormos, DW, Steiner CP, Weisenberger J. Use of a frameless, armless stereotactic wand for brain tumor localization with two-dimensional and three-dimensional neuroimaging. Neurosurgery 1993;33:674–678.
16. Barnett GH, Kormos DW, Steiner CP, et al. Intraoperative localization using an armless, frameless stereotactic wand. Technical note. J Neurosurg 1993;78:510–154.
17. Galloway RL, Macuimas RJ, Latimer JW. The accuracies of four stereotactic frame systems: an independent assessment. Biomed Instrum Technol 1991;25:457–460.
18. Roessler K, Ungersboeck K, Dietrich W, et al. Frameless stereotactic guided neurosurgery: clinical experience with an infrared based pointer device navigation system. Acta Neurochir 1997;139:551–559.
19. Sipos EP, Tebo SA, Zinreich SJ et al. In vivo accuracy testing and clinical experience with the ISG viewing wand. Neuorsurgery 1996;39:194–204.
20. Spetzger U, Laborde G, Gilsbach JM. Frameless neuronavigation in modern neurosurgery. Minim Invas Neurosurg 1995;38:163–166.
21. Barnett GH. Minimal Access Craniotomy. In: Barnett GH, Roberts DW, Maciunas RJ, eds. Image-Guided Neurosurgery: Clinical Applications of Surgical Navigation. St. Louis, MO: Quality Medical Publishing Inc., 1998:63–71.
22. Barnett GH. Stereotactic techniques in the management of brain tumors. Contemp Neurosurg 1997;19:1–9.
23. Kelly PJ. Volumetric stereotactic surgical resection of intra-axial brain mass lesions. Mayo Clin Proc 1988;63:1186–1198.
24. Kelly PJ, Kall BA, Goerss S, Earnest F IV. Computer-assisted stereotactic laser resection of intra-axial brain neoplasms. J Neurosurg 1986;64: 427–439.
25. Smith KR, Frank KJ, Buchholz RD. The NeuroStation- A highly accurate, minimally invasive solution to frameless stereotactic neurosurgery. Comput Med Imaging Graph 1994;24718:–256.
26. Barnett GH, Kaakaji W. Intracranial Meningiomas. In: Barnett GH, Roberts DW, Maciunas RJ, eds. Image-Guided Neurosurgery: Clinical Applications of Surgical Navigation. St. Louis, MO: Quality Medical Publishing Inc., 1998:87–100.

27. Barnett GH, Steiner CP, Kormos DW, Weisenberger J. Intracranial meningioma resection using interactive frameless stereotaxy-assistance. J Image-Guided Surgery, 1995;1:46–52.

28. Ransohoff J. Removal of convexity, parasagittal, and falcine meningiomas. Neurosurg Clin N Am 1994;5:293–297.

29. Gildenberg PL, Woo SY. Multimodality program involving stereotactic surgery in brain tumor management. Stereotact Funct Neurosurg 2000;75:147–152.

30. Barnett GH, Steiner CP, Weisenberger J. Adaptation of personal projection television to a helmet-mounted display for intraoperative viewing of neuroimaging. J Image Guided Surg 1995;1:109–112.

31. Robinson JR, Golfinos JG, Spetzler RF. Skull base tumors: a critical appraisal and clinical series employing image guidance. Neurosurg Clin N Am 1996;7:297–311.

32. Bozzao A, Finocchi V, Romano A, et al. Role of contrast-enhanced MR venography in the preoperative evaluation of parasagittal meningiomas. Eur Radiol 2005;15:1790–1796.

33. Lee JH, Krishnaney AA, Steinmetz MP, et al. Intracranial meningiomas. In: Barnett GH, Maciunas RJ, Roberts DW, eds. Computer-Assisted Neurosurgery. New York: Taylor and Francis, 2006:195–207.

34. Miabi Z, Midia R, Rohrer SE, et al. Delineation of lateral tentorial sinus with contrast-enhanced MR imaging and its surgical implications. Am J Neuroradiol 2004;25:1181–1188.

35. Suzuki Y, Masateru N, Ikeda H, Takumi A. Three-dimensional computed tomography angiography of the Galenic system for the occipital transtentorial approach. Neurol Med Chir (Tokyo) 2005;45:387–394.

36. Payner TD. Skull base neurosurgery. In: Barnett GH, Roberts DW, Maciunas RJ, eds. Image-Guided Neurosurgery: Clinical Applications of Surgical Navigation. St. Louis, MO: Quality Medical Publishing Inc., 1998:163–177.

37. Kurtsoy A, Menku A, Tucer B, et al. Transbasal approaches: surgical details, pitfalls and avoidances. Neurosurg Rev 2004;27:267–273.

38. Kikinis R, Gleason PL, Moriarty TM, et al. Computer-assisted interactive three-dimensional planning for neurosurgical procedures (technique and application). Neurosurgery 1996;38:640–651.

39. Sekhar LN, Babu RP, Wright DC. Surgical resection of cranial base meningiomas. Neurosurg Clin N Am 1994;5:299–330.

40. Deschler DG, Gutin PH, Mamelak AN, et al. Complications of anterior skull base surgery. Skull Base Surg 1996;6:113–118.

41. VanDijk JM, THomeer TW. Control of complications in the mid-frontobasal approach. Acta Neurochir 1997;139:355–358.

42. Lang DA, Honeybul D, Neil-Dwyer G, et al. The extended transbasal approach: clinical applications and complications. Acta Neurochir 1999;141:579–585.

43. Sekhar LN, Nanda A, Sen CN et al. The extended frontal approach to tumors of the anterior, middle, and posterior skull base. J Neurosurg 1992;76:198–206.

44. Wong GK, Poon WS, Lam MK. The impact of an armless frameless neuronavigation system on routine brain tumour surgery: a prospective analysis of 51 cases. Minim Invas Neurosurg 2001;44:99–103.

45. Day JD, Kellog JX, Tschabitscher M, Fukushima T. Surface and superficial surgical anatomy of the posterolateral cranial base: significance for surgical planning and approach. Neurosurgery 1996;38:1079–1084.

46. Lang J, Samii A. Retrosigmoid approach to the posterior cranial fossa: An anatomical study. Acta Neurochir 1991;111:147–153.

47. Golfinos JG, Fitzpatrick BC, Smith LR, et al. Clinical use of a frameless stereotactic arm: results of 325 cases. J Neurosurg 1995;83: 197–205.

48. McDermott MW, Gutin PH. Image-guided surgery for skull base neoplasms using the ISG wiewing wand: anatomic and and technical considerations. Neurosurg Clin N Am 1996;7:285–295.

49. Carrau RL, Curtin HD, Snyderman, et al. Practical applications of image-guided navigation during anterior cranio-facial resection. Skull Base Surgery 1995;5:51–55.

50. Hwang SK, Gwak HS, Paek SH, et al. Guidelines for the ligation of the sigmoid or transverse sinus during large petroclival meningioma surgery. Skull Base 2004;14:21–29.

51. Miller CG, VanLoveren HR, Keller JT, et al. Transpetrosal approach: surgical anatomy and technique. Neurosurgery 1993;33:461–469.

52. Sekhar LN, Wright, DC, Richardson R, et al. Petroclival and foramen magnum meningiomas: surgical approaches and pitfalls. J Neurooncol 1996;29:249–259.

53. Sakata K, Al-Mefty O, Yamamoto I. Venous consideration in petrosal approach: microsurgical anatomy of the temporal bridging vein. Neurosurgery 2000;47:153–161.

54. Pillay PK. Image-guided stereotactic neurosurgery with the multicoordinate manipulator microscope. Surg Neurol 1997;47:171–177.

55. Westermann B, Trippel M, Reinhart H. Optically-navigable operating microscope for image-guided surgery. Minim Invas Neurosurg 1995;38:112–116.

56. Obasi PC, Barnett GH, Suh JH. Brachytherapy for intracranial meningioma using a permanently implanted iodine-125 seed. Stereotact Funct Neurosurg 2002;79:33–43.

57. Suh JH, Barnett GH. Brachtherapy for brain tumor. Hematol Oncol Clin North Am 1999;13:635–650.

58. Nimsky C, Ganslandt O, Cerny S, et al. Quantification of, visualization of, and compensation for brain shift using intraoperative magnetic resonance imaging. Neurosurgery 2000;47:1070–1079.

59. Nabavi A, Black PM, Gering DT, et al. Serial intraoperative magnetic resonance imaging of brain shift. Neurosurgery 2001;48:787–797.

60. Ferrant M, Nabavi A, Macq B, et al. Serial registration of intraoperative MR images of the brain. Med Image Anal 2002;6: 337–359.

61. Maciunas RJ. Pitfalls. In: Barnett GH, Roberts DW, Maciunas RJ, eds. Image-Guided Neurosurgery: Clinical Applications of Surgical Navigation. St. Louis, : Quality Medical Publishing Inc., 1998:43–60.

62. Jolesz FA, Kikinis RK, Talos IF. Neuronavigation in interventional MR imaging: frameless stereotaxy. NeuroimagClin N Am 2001;11:685–693.

63. Tummala RP, Chu RM, Liu H, et al. Optimizing brain tumor resection. High-field interventional imaging. Neuroimag Clin N Am 2001;11:673–683.

64. Unsgaard G, Gronningsaeter A, Ommedal S, et al. Brain operations guided by real-time two-dimensional ultrasound: new possibilities as a result of improved image quality. Neurosurgery 2002;51:402–411.

65. Unsgaard G, Ommedal S, Muller T, et al. Neuronavigation by intraoperative three-dimensional ultrasound: initial experience during brain tumor resection. Neurosurgery 2002;50:804–812.

66. Moriarty TM, Kikinis R, Jolesz FA, et al. Magnetic resonance imaging therapy: intraoperative MR imaging. Neurosurg Clin North Am 1996;7:323–331.

67. Wirtz CR, Bonsanto MM, Knauth M, et al. Intraoperative magnetic resonance imaging to update interactive navigation in neurosurgery: method and preliminary experience. Comput Aided Surg 1997;2:172–179.

68. Nakao N, Nakai K, Itakura T. Updating of neuronavigation based on images intraoperatively acquired with a mobile computerized computerized tomographic scanner: technical note. Min Invas Neurosurg 203;46:117–120.

69. Nimsky C, Ganslandt O, Hastreiter P, et al. Intraoperative compensation for brain shift. Surg Neurol 2001;56:357–365.

70. Unsgaard G, Ommedal S, Muller T, et al. Neuronavigation by intraoperative three-dimensional ultrasound: initial experience during brain tumor resection. Neurosurgery 2002;50: 804–812.

71. Dorward NL, Alberi O, Velani B, et al. Postimaging brain distortion: magnitude, correlates, and impact on neuronavigation. J Neurosurg 1998;88:656–662.

72. Curry WT, McDermott MW, Carter BS, Barker FG. Craniotomy for meningioma in the United States between 1988 and 2000: decreasing rate of mortality and the effect of provider caseload. J Neursurg 1005;102:977–986.

73. Barnett GH. Surgical management of convexity and falcine meningiomas using interactive image-guided surgery systems. Neuorosurg Clin N Am 7: 279–284.

74. Drummond KJ, Zhu JJ, Black PM. Meningiomas: updating basic science, management, and outcome. Neurologist 2004;10: 113–130.

23
Meningiomas and Epilepsy

Jorge A. González-Martínez and Imad M. Najm

Introduction

Seizures have been recognized for over a century as a symptom of primary and secondary intracerebral tumors.[1,2] These seizures may be very distressing to the patient and resistant to various antiepileptic medications.[3] To date there is a lack of understanding of the pathophysiological, molecular, and cellular mechanisms of tumor-induced epileptogenicity. Some of the previously suggested mechanisms for tumor-induced epileptogenicity include focal cortical hypoxia, direct mass effect, peritumor brain edema, perilesional cortical architectural, and cellular disorganizations,[4] and altered levels of excitatory amino acids (increased extracellular glutamate secondary to decreased glial-based clearance mechanisms).[5,6]

Epilepsy could be the final common neurophysiological pathway in the course of development of various types of lesions (including tumors) that affect the cortical structures (either neocortex or archicortex). Seizures are often the first symptom of intracranial tumor, including meningiomas.[1] Epilepsy may predate the appearance of other neurologic symptoms or tumor diagnosis by many years.[1,7] In this chapter, the incidence, prognosis, and influencing factors in the expression of epilepsy in association with meningiomas will be discussed.

Meningiomas and Epilepsy: An Overview

The incidence of epilepsy as the initial presentation of intracranial meningiomas is reported to be 20–50%.[7–12] In a recent study done by Lieu et al.,[13] epilepsy was the most common clinical presentation in 26.6% of the patients. Although the ratio of female to male patients with intracranial meningiomas is 2:1, Lieu et al. reported no significant gender differences in the occurrence of preoperative epilepsy. In addition, the same study reported a trend toward the occurrence of meningioma-related seizures in the fifth and sixth decades of life.

There is no difference in the occurrence of preoperative epilepsy between left and right hemispheric meningiomas.

Only one study[14] showed a statistically significant greater chance for seizure development with left hemispheric meningiomas. This could be in part explained by the left hemisphere dominance in the majority of patients, and therefore epileptic activity arising from that side may be symptomatic more frequently. Convexity meningiomas are more commonly associated with epilepsy as compared to meningiomas located in other brain locations.[7,13] Previous studies have reported that parietal lobe meningiomas present with a significantly higher incidence of postoperative epilepsy than others.[8,15,16] The reason(s) behind this occurrence remain unclear.

While some studies suggested a higher incidence of epilepsy in patients with fibroblastic[17] or angioblastic[13] meningiomas, others found no significant correlation between the various pathologic meningioma subtypes and the development of epileptic seizures.[7]

Pathogenesis of Meningioma-Associated Epilepsy

In tumor-associated epilepsy, the causative neoplasm somehow acts as a generator to produce an epileptogenic focus in peritumoral brain. The mechanisms of epileptogenesis must vary for different tumors, since some are intracerebral/ intraparenchymal (gliomas) while others are extracerebral/extraparenchymal (meningiomas). Some tumors such as meningiomas distort the cortical structures, which are believed to be the generator areas for focal epilepsies, while others such as gliomas infiltrate. Additionally, there are also significant variations in seizure frequency within the same histologic tumor subtype. This may suggest that the etiology of the seizure disorder is multifactorial, involving both host and tumoral factors.

In 1940, Penfield suggested that tumor-associated epilepsy arises as a result of impaired vascularization and ischemic change in the surrounding cortex.[1] Local peritumoral ischemia induced by the mass effect of the tumor could impair local microcirculation by reducing cerebral perfusion pressure.

Peritumoral brain ischemia could provide one causative mechanism shared by meningiomas, but if this mechanism was to be the only cause of focal epileptogenicity, one would expect the occurrence of seizures to be correlated with the degree of mass effect, cerebral edema and necrosis, which is clearly not the case.[18,19]

Echlin et al.[20] proposed a theory of denervation hypersensitivity related to partial isolation and deafferentation of regions of cerebral cortex. This suggestion cannot explain why in some cases seizures either return or appear for the first time following excision of a tumor.

Meningiomas can also distort rather than disconnect areas of the cortex.[21] If the theory of denervation hypersensitivity is valid, then the tendency of seizures will depend on the location of the areas of isolated cortex, their remaining connections, the degree of remaining functional integrity, and the proportion of active inhibitory neurons.

Recent experimental evidence also raises the possibility that neuronal, axonal, and synaptic plasticity in perilesional regions also contribute to epileptogenesis.[22,23] This concept invokes sprouting of axon collaterals, neosynaptogenesis, and/or generation of neurons in the perilesional brain in addition to modifications of physiological functions in the existing circuitry.[24] Hippocampal CA3 cell axons will sprout from pyramidal cells to the ipsilateral section of Schaffer cell collaterals and lead to hyperexcitability and prolonged postsynaptic potentials.[22]

In addition to possible structural changes, other putative mechanisms of meningioma-associated epilepsy invoke dysequilibrium of levels, or ratios of compounds that alter the membrane potential of neurons in the peritumoral brain regions. Such compounds include the cortical inhibitory (GABA, taurine) and excitatory (aspartate, glutamate) amino acid neurotransmitters[25,26] and electrolytes (magnesium and iron). Decreased extracellular concentrations of Mg^{2+} can also lead to the appearance of spontaneous epileptiform discharges and spreading depression that can be specifically blocked by NMDA receptor antagonists.[27] Increased peritumoral brain extracellular levels of iron ions (Fe^{3+}) may also predispose to seizures since experimental Fe^{3+}-induced perioxidative injury to neural plasma membranes is related to the development of paroxysmal epileptiform activity.[28] How disequilibrium between these compounds could occur in perimeningioma brain is still under investigation.

Levels of amino acids in the tumor interstitium may also modulate peritumoral brain activity.[6] Other tumor-related and potentially pro-epileptogenic compounds could be released into the tumor interstitium and then diffuse into peritumoral brain or could be directly released from tumor cells infiltrating the peritumoral brain. Such mechanisms could explain why tumor-associated epilepsy can occur in both extracerebral tumors such as meningiomas and infiltrative tumors such as gliomas. It is, therefore, likely that there are multiple complex biochemical interactions in the peritumoral brain.

Morphological Changes in Peritumoral Brain

Several patterns of histologic change have been observed in the peritumoral brains of patients with meningioma-associated epilepsy. How these histologic changes relate to epilepsy is unclear due to a lack of adequate epileptic tissue studies. Ideally the peritumoral epileptic focus would be identified electrophysiologically through direct cortical electrical recordings, resected, and its neuropathology studied. However, this is not commonly done, and often the epileptic focus or foci are not contiguous with the tumor.[19]

Some histopathologic changes in the peritumoral tissue include the presence of persistent neurons in the white matter. This might indicate a developmental disorder or inefficiency of neuronal migration, which could be related to the origin of the tumor or could constitute a predisposing factor to seizures in those patients with brain tumors.[29,30] Comparison of the ultrastructure of the peritumoral cortex in patients with and without epilepsy[31] has demonstrated statistically significant changes in the form, size, distribution, and number of presynaptic vesicles. These changes are suggestive of a higher ability of presynaptic structures in releasing neurotransmitters such as the excitatory amino acid glutamate with subsequent increase in postsynaptic excitability.

Treatment and Postsurgical Seizure Outcome in Patients with Meningiomas and Epilepsy

Seizures associated with meningiomas are treated with anticonvulsants. The choice of a particular anticonvulsant would depend on the patient's age, gender, associated medical condition(s), and concurrent treatment with other medications. Double or even triple agent therapy may be required. The response to drug treatment is unpredictable, and some patients develop pharmacoresistance to antiepileptic drugs (AEDs).

Occasional unsatisfactory response to AEDs following tumor resection suggests that there are long-term and permanent focal neocortical changes that dictate the response to AEDs. Schnabel et al.[32] examined carbamazepine concentrations in the tumor tissue and peritumoral brain of carbamazepine-responsive and unresponsive cases of tumor-associated epilepsy, but no difference was observed. This study suggested that the pharmacoresistance in these cases is not due to a lack of in situ drug bioavailability but other factors contribute to this phenomenon.

Penfield originally observed that surgical excision of a tumor can result in a good seizure outcome, without significant neurologic deficit;[1] and this has also been documented in more recent studies.[29,33] Cascino et al.[34] reported on a series of 16 patients with epileptogenic neoplastic lesions, 11 of which were refractory to medical treatment. Of these 11, 9 were initially seizure free for a mean follow-up period of 25 months. Of the 5 patients whose seizures were medically controlled preoperatively, all were seizure-free for a mean follow-up period of 19 months.

In general, the reponse of tumor-associated epilepsy to resective or cytoreductive surgery is good, but other factors may affect the postoperative seizure outcome. These include the lesion location, its histopathologic characteristics, the preoperative and intraoperative electroencephalographic (EEG) findings, and the extent of tumor resection.

Previous studies reported seizure-free outcome following meningioma resection in up to 63.5% of patients with preoperative epilepsy.[7,9,10,16,35,36] Outcome studies showed that the occurrence of early postoperative seizures (within 48 hours of the resection) is a strong predictor of persistent seizures. Almost two thirds of patients with persistent postoperative seizures exhibit their first postresective seizure within the first 48 hours.[13,38]

Factors that have been associated with the development of postoperative epilepsy following intracranial meningioma resection include potential effect of intraoperative brain retraction, interruption of cortical veins, arterial damage, history of preoperative epilepsy, extent of tumor removal, postoperative hydrocephalus, and parietal location.[7–9,16,35,36]

Lieu et al.[13] observed that a history of preoperative epilepsy, evidence of peritumoral edema, and cerebral swelling at the operative site play significant roles in the development of postoperative epilepsy. More than a third of patients with a history of preoperative epilepsy continued to have seizures postoperatively, making it a significant contributing factor to postoperative epilepsy ($p = 0.025$). The success in controlling seizures following meningioma resection in epileptic patients is similar to (or even better than) the outcome following resection of other epileptic lesions.[39,40] The presence of severe peritumoral edema was also found to be an influencing factor for the development of early postoperative seizures, epilepsy, or the persistence of seizures postoperatively. Other factors may play a role in the development of early postoperative seizures, including operative site hematoma, hydrocephalus, and the subtotal resection of the tumor.[13,16]

In addition, the anatomic location of the tumor may be another risk factor for the development of postoperative seizures, as patients with parietal tumors appear to be more susceptible to the development of new-onset postoperative seizures.[8,16]

Conclusion

Although epilepsy occurs in a large number patients with meningiomas, it is extremely important to confirm the diagnosis of epilepsy and the link between the epilepsy and the tumor through prolonged video-EEG recordings as patients may have either nonepileptic seizures, idiopathic generalized epilepsy, or focal epilepsy due to another brain pathology.

The physiopathologic, molecular, and cellular mechanisms underlying this association remain unclear. Changes in the peritumoral brain tissue, brain edema, and other factors in situ can contribute to the generation and perpetuation of the focal epileptic activity.

References

1. Penfield W, Erickson TC, Tarlov I. Relation of intracranial tumors and symptomatic epilepsy. Arch Neurol Psychiatry 1940; 44:300–315.
2. Hoefer PFA, Schlesinger EB, Pennes HH. Seizures in patients with brain tumors. Res Pub Assoc Res Nerv Ment Dis 1947; 26:50–58 (cited in Chan et al., 1979).
3. Kwan P, Brodie MJ. Early identification of refractory epilepsy. N Engl J Med 2000; 342 (5):464–468.
4. Prayson RA, Estes ML. Cortical dysplasia: a histopathologic study of 52 cases of partial lobectomy in patients with epilepsy. Hum Pathol 1995; 26(5):493–500.
5. Chan PH, Fishman RA, Lee JL, Candelise L. Effects of excitatory neurotransmitter amino acid on edema induction in rat brain cortical slices. J Neurochem 1979; 33:1309–1315.
6. Bateman DE, Hardy JA, McDermott JR, Parker DS. Amino acid transmitter levels in gliomas and their relationship to the incidence of epilepsy. Neurol Res 1988; 10:112–114.
7. Chow SY, His MS, Tang LM, Fong VH. Epilepsy and intracranial meningiomas. Chin Med J (Taipei) 1995; 55:151–155.
8. Ramamurthi B, Ravi R, Ramachandran V. Convulsions with meningiomas: incidence and significance. Surg Neurol 1980; 14:415–416.
9. Chan RC, Thompson GB. Morbidity, mortality and quality of life following surgery for intracranial meningiomas. A retrospective study in 257 cases. J Neurosurg 1984; 60:52–60.
10. Giombini S, Solero CL, Lasio G, Morello G. Immediate and late outcome of operations for parasagittal and falx meningiomas. Report of 342 cases. Surg Neurol 1984; 21:427–435.
11. Rohringer M, Sutherland GR, Louw DF, Sima AAF. Incidence and clinical pathological features of meningioma. J Neurosurg 1989; 71:665–672.
12. Yao YT. Clinicopathologic analysis of 615 cases of meningioma with special reference to recurrence. J Formos Med Assoc 1994; 93:145–152.
13. Lieu AS. Intracranial meningiomas and epilepsy: incidence, prognosis and influencing fators. Epi Res 2000; 38:45–52.
14. Scott DF. Left and right cerebral hemisphere differences in the occurrence of epilepsy. Br J Med Psychol 1985; 58:189–192.
15. Flyger G. Epilepsy following radical removal of parasagittal and convexity meningiomas. Acta Psychiatr Scand 1956; 30:245–255.
16. Chozick BS, Reinert SE, Greenblatt SH. Incidence of seizures after surgery for supratentorial meningiomas: a modern analysis. J Neurosurg 1996; 84:382–386.
17. Kawaguchi T, Kameyama S, Tanaka R. Peritumoral edema and seizure in patients with cerebral convexity and parasagittal meningiomas. Neurol Med-Chir (Tokyo) 1995; 35:568–574.
18. Gastaut JL, Sabet Hansan MS, Bianchi CL, Gastaut H. Electroencephalography in brain edema (127 cases of brain tumor investigated by cranial computerized tomography). Electroencephalog Clin Neurophysiol 1979; 46:239–255.

19. Whittle IR, Clarke M, Gregori A, et al. Intersticial white matter brain edema does not alter the electroencephalogram. Br J Neurosurg 1992; 6:433–437.

20. Echlin FA. The supersensitivity of chronically "isolated" cerebral cortex as a mechanism in focal epilepsy. Electroencephalog Clin Neurophysiol 1959; 11:697–732.

21. Nakasu S, Hirono A, Llena JF, et al. Interface between meningioma and the brain. Surg Neurol 1989; 32:206–212.

22. McKinney RA, Debanne D, Gahwiler BH, et al. Lesion induced axonial sprouting and hyperexcitability in the hippocampus in vitro. Inplications for the genesis of post-traumatic epilepsy. Nat Med 1997; 3:990–996.

23. Gray WP, Sundtrom LE. Kainic acid increases the proliferation of granule cells progenitors in the dentate gyrus of the rat. Brain Res 1998; 790:52–59.

24. Prince DA. Epilepsy and the too-well-connected brain. Nat Med 1997; 3(9):957–958.

25. Goldstein DS, Nadi NS, Stull R, et al. Levels of catechols in epileptogenic and non-epileptogenic regions of the human brain. J Neurochem 1988; 50:225–229.

26. Kish SJ, Dixon LM, Sherwin AL. Aspartic acid amino-tranferase activity in increased in activily spiking compared with non-spiking cortex. J Neurol Neurosurg Psychiatry 1988; 51:552–556.

27. Avoli M, Drapeau C, Pumain R, et al. Epileptiform activity induced by low extracellular magnesium in the human cortex maintained in vivo. Ann Neurol 1991; 330:589–596.

28. Singh R, Pathak DN. Lipid peroxidation and gluthatine peroxidase, gluthatione reductase, superoxide dismutase, catalase and glucose-6-phosphate dehydrogenese activities in FeCl3 induced epileptogenic foci in the rat brain. Epilepsia 1990; 31:15–26.

29. Goldring S, Rich KM, Picker S. Experience with gliomas in patients presenting with a chronic seizure disorder. Clin Neurosurg 1986; 33:15–42.

30. Bancaud J, Sallou C. Familial epilepsy and tumoral epilepsy. Epilepsia 1969; 10:83–86.

31. Chubinidze AI, Gobechiia ZV, Abramichivili, Chubinidze MA. Morphological characteristics of cortical synapses in patients with epilepsy. Zh Nevrol Psikhiatr Im S S Karsakova 1985; 89:23–26.

32. Schnabel R, Rambeck B, May TW, et al. Concentrations of carbamazepine and carbamazepine-10 1-epoxide in serum, brain tumors and paratumorous cortex: a prospective study of 37 neurosurgically treated epileptic patients. Eur Neurol 1994; 34:213–220.

33. Drake J, Hoffman HJ, Kobayashi J, et al. Surgical management of children with temporal lobe epilepsy and mass lesions. Neurosurgery 1987; 21:792–797.

34. Cascino G, Kelly P, Hischorn K, et al. Stereotactic resection of intra-axial cerebral lesions in partial epilepsy. Mayo Clin Proc 1990; 65:1053–1060.

35. Logue V. Surgery of supratentorial meningiomas: a modern series. J Neurol Neurosurg Psychiatry 1974; 37:1277 (abstr).

36. Foy PM, Copeland GP, Shaw MDM. The incidence of postoperative seizures. Acta Neurochir 1981; 55:253–264.

37. Giombini S, Solero CL, Morello G. Late outcome of operations for supratentorial convexity meningiomas. Report on 207 cases. Surg Neurol 1984; 21:588–594.

38. Pasquet EG, Pietra M, Iniguez A. Epileptic seizures as an early complication of neurosurgery. Acta Neurol 1976; 22:144–151.

39. Jeha L, Najm I, Bingaman W, et al. Predictors of outcome after temporal lobectomy for the treatment of intractable epilepsy. Neurology 2006; 66:1938–40.

40. Jeha LE, Najm I, Bingaman W, et al. Surgical outcome and prognostic factors of frontal lobe epilepsy surgery. Brain 2007; 130:574–84.

24
Surgical Correction of Postoperative Strabismus

Gregory Kosmorsky

When faced with a patient who has sustained a cranial nerve paresis in the setting of a brain tumor or as a complication of the treatment of that brain tumor, the same surgical principles that underlie all strabismus applies. That is, in order to realign the ocular axes, the extraocular muscles need to be repositioned on one or both globes so that the mechanical plant of the orbit is altered to align both eyes simultaneously on the target of regard. In the case of a meningioma or its treatment, this almost always implies an incomitant strabismus. An incomitant strabismus means that the relative position of the eyes in space changes constantly as a function of position in space. In contrast, a comitant strabismus means that the angle of misalignment is constant in all fields of gaze. A constant misalignment is much more amenable to surgical therapy as it is easier to devise a surgery on the extraocular muscles in order to reestablish ocular alignment. For instance, if a child is born with an esotropia (an inward deviation of the eyes) of 20 diopters, the typical therapy would be to recess both medial recti approximately 5 mm. Because the deviation is comitant, this maneuver would be expected to realign the ocular axes in all positions of gaze. Should, however, the esotropic deviation be incomitant, such as would be found in a sixth nerve paresis, merely recessing both medical recti for the esotropia might only correct the deviation in the primary position and produce misalignment in eccentric gaze positions. Therefore, the treatment of incomitant deviations in the setting of a brain tumor presents a particular challenge to the strabismus surgeon. Typically, the goal of surgery for cranial nerve palsies of 3, 4, and 6 is to attempt to align the eyes only for the primary position and inform the patient that realignment in all positions of gaze is usually not possible.

The timing of surgery for cranial nerve palsies depends to some extent on the situation. In the case of a meningioma, if the surgeon is certain that the nerve was not cut, a period of observation of approximately 6 months is recommended before proceeding with any sort of surgery. If, on the other hand, any of the cranial nerves were cut during a procedure, then a shorter waiting time might be indicated. For meningiomas that are radiated without surgery, most surgeons will wait approximately a year before planning any sort of strabismus surgery in order to judge the effects of the radiation therapy.

In this chapter we will review the options for surgically and nonsurgically addressing the meningioma patient with postoperative diplopia.

Orbital Oculomotor Plant

Treatment of incomitant cranial nerve pareses is complicated by the fact that the orbital muscles are contained within a superstructure of collagenous tissue collectively referred to as Tenon's tissue.[1–3] The posterior two thirds of the extraocular muscles (EOMs) are fixed within this collagenous matrix and are therefore not available for transferring a force to the globe to produce an ocular rotation. In essence, the posterior two thirds of the muscle is unavailable to move the globe, and the Tenon's tissue acts as a joint so as to create a lever arm for movement of the globe. The Tenon's tissue is not entirely rigid, and various types of surgery may modify its position in space. Because of this anatomy, the predicted amount of correction based on models of the arc of contact of the EOMs on the globe is less than would be expected. This difference in the predicted amount of available correction and the amount actually achievable means that there is less ability to correct ocular deviations than would be predicted based on the length of the EOMs and their arc of contact.[4] Magnetic resonance imaging (MRI) has helped to clarify the precise paths that the EOMs take during their normal translations and especially helps to define the unique inflections of these muscle after surgical manipulation.[4]

Assessment of Patients with Diplopia

A patient with cranial nerve palsy in the setting of a meningioma will experience diplopia secondary to the misalignment of the ocular axes. The most common way of assessing the ocular misalignment is to utilize prisms to neutralize the defect in all nine cardinal positions. These cardinal positions are the primary position (straight ahead gaze), right, left, up, down, up and right, up and left, down and right, and down and left. The deviation at near (30 cm) is also recorded. Bar prisms are typically utilized, but individual prisms may also be used.

Binocularity may be assessed by the use of a Goldman perimeter. Instead of one eye being tested at a time, both eyes are tested simultaneously, and patients report when they see double as they follow the target around the sphere. The technician then plots the area where binocularity is achieved so that this may be used to compare the results of surgery with the preoperative testing. More sophisticated instruments such as cervical range of motion device have been reported by Kushner and may be used to accurately assess the range of single binocular vision, but this device is impractical for most practitioners.[5]

Oculomotor Palsies

This is the most difficult of the pareses to address as the third nerve controls four of six of the extraocular muscles, the upper lid, and the pupil. Treatment with prisms is often of little or no use, and the patient will either have to learn to adapt to diplopia (via suppression), wear a patch to eliminate diplopia, or undergo some form of strabismus surgery to partially correct the misalignment. As with all cranial nerve palsies, the treatment depends upon the amount of residual motion of the affected globe. Complete third nerve palsies are not amenable to achieving complete binocularity, and the goal of surgery in these cases is to achieve acceptable cosmesis. The most common surgery undertaken in these circumstances is a large resection of the medial rectus combined with a large recession of the ipsilateral lateral rectus. Although children are usually not affected by meningiomas, acceptable alignment with brain tumors in children may sometimes be achieved, as reported by Mudgil and Repka.[6] One approach to dealing with the hypotropia encountered in third nerve palsies is to superiorly displace both the lateral and medial recti at the time of the recession/ resection procedure on the horizontal rectus muscles.[7, 8] The large recession/resection procedure leads to many undercorrections with complete third nerve palsies.[9] Therefore, other methods have been devised to maintain the eye in the central position. These include anterior transposition of the superior oblique tendon, as reported by Young et al.[10] In this procedure, the oblique tendon is cut and placed at the medial border of the superior rectus muscle, effectively changing the action of the superior oblique muscle to adduction and elevation (as opposed to depression, adduction, and intorsion). Solares et al. described using the patients' own superior oblique tendon to fix the globe to the nasal periosteum.[11] They amputated 12–14 mm of the tendon, fixing one end to the globe and the other end to the nasal periosteum, and combined that procedure with a lateral rectus muscle recession and medial rectus resection of the involved eye. Autogenous and alloplastic materials, including fascia lata, silicone bands, and sutures have been used to fix the globe into the central position. These materials place the patient at risk for infection, foreign body reactions, and extrusion of the implants. Goldberg et al. have advocated the use of an autogenous orbital periosteal flap that is harvested in the affected eye, the base of which is near the orbital apex.[12] The anterior end is freed from the periosteum and sewn to the globe over the medial rectus muscle. Being a vascularized and autogenous flap, this form of therapy holds some promise for severely affected patients.

Because the lateral rectus is not affected by a third cranial nerve palsy, it must always be recessed or otherwise weakened when attempting a surgical correction of a third nerve paresis. Alternatives to recession include suturing the muscle to the lateral wall of the orbit or myectomy.

Selective paresis of the inferior division of the third nerve most commonly occurs as a result of incomplete healing of complete third nerve palsy. Other causes include aneurysm, vasculitis, demyelination, trauma, ophthalmoplegic migraine, and orbital disease. Knapp devised a procedure wherein the superior rectus is transposed toward the insertion of the medial rectus muscle and transposition of the lateral rectus to the temporal border of the inferior rectus muscle combined with a superior oblique tenectomy.[13] His patients were able to fuse in primary position and had some expansion of the diplopia-free visual fields.

Sixth Nerve Palsy

The choices for treatment of a sixth nerve palsy are greater simply because only one muscle is affected. Treatment strategies include patching, prisms, botulinum toxin or surgical repair.

Patching is used when the duration of the sixth nerve palsy is expected to be short and full recovery is expected. Prisms have a similar use as they may be used to temporize a patient with short-term diplopia, although they can be used in patients with chronic sixth nerve palsies. The amount of misalignment that can be accommodated by prism depends on the type of prism being utilized. Fresnel prisms are plastic prisms that are generally used for short-term palsies. These prisms come in many powers and can be cut and placed onto the back surface of the lens of a pair of glasses to eliminate diplopia in the primary position. In this way, generally up to 40 diopters of deviation can be accommodated with this lens system. If ground-in prisms are to be utilized, only about 14 diopters may be accommodated (7 diopters per lens) without the lens edge thickness becoming such that weight, appearance, and optical distortions become a problem.

Botulinum has been used during the acute phase of a sixth nerve palsy.[14,15] It is injected into the antagonist medial rectus muscle to straighten the eye. Although it was initially believed that this method would ultimately provide a better alignment of the eye, subsequent studies have not confirmed that suspicion and controversy still surrounds this form of therapy. In general, patients with a smaller deviation and a shorter interval between the onset of strabismus and botulinum toxin injection tended to achieve a better outcome. Complications include ptosis, abnormal extraocular motility, and subconjunctival hemorrhages; all of which are temporary. Theoretically, globe penetration or perforation could be the result of a misdirected needle used to inject the botulinum. Kerr and Hoehn used botulinum toxin in children with sixth nerve palsies secondary to brain tumors.[16] They concluded that treatment does not improve the ultimate ocular alignment in children with sixth nerve palsies secondary to brain tumors.

The amount of residual function of the lateral rectus determines how well a patient will do with strabismus surgery. In general, if the deviation is small—generally 10 diopters or less—prism therapy is desirable. If the deviation is larger than 10 diopters, consideration may be given to surgical therapy. A recession/resection procedure may suffice for many deviations of a chronic nature with measurements between 10 and 25 diopters.[14, 15] In some cases a combined resection and recession of a single rectus muscle may suffice. Bock et al. described a procedure of this sort that primarily weakens the muscle in its field of action without affecting the alignment in the primary position.[17] When the deviation is large secondary to significant dysfunction of the lateral rectus, some sort of transposition surgery becomes necessary, usually combined with a recession of the ipsilateral medial rectus. The typical procedure in this instance is the Hummelscheim procedure, where the temporal halves of the superior and inferior rectus muscle are placed at the superior and inferior border of the lateral rectus muscle.[15] It is critical in this procedure to split the superior and inferior recti in the middle and to carry that splitting as far back as possible along the axis of the muscle before these pieces are secured to the lateral rectus and, in so doing, preserve the blood supply of the nasal half of the vertical recti. This procedure carries some risk for inducing a vertical misalignment.[18] It is also important to remember to leave the lateral rectus alone so as not to compromise its blood supply to the anterior segment. Brooks et al. described an augmented Hummelscheim procedure in which the temporal halves of the muscles are resected 4–8 mm before fixing them to the tendon of the lateral rectus. This resection increases the abducting force of the half-tendon transpostion.[19] Another modification of the Hummelscheim involves suturing the transposed pieces directly to the lateral rectus muscle and each other as opposed to the sclera as described by Neugebauer so as to increase the effectiveness of the procedure.[20]

Rosenbaum et al. transposed the entire superior and inferior recti to the insertion of the lateral rectus and injected the medial rectus with botulinum to preserve its contribution to the blood supply of the anterior segment.[21] Laby and Rosenbaum utilized adjustable sutures on each of the vertical muscle segments in an attempt to modify a vertical misalignment.[18] Foster modified the transposition surgery of Hummelscheim by placing a posterior fixation suture 8 mm posterior to the lateral rectus

muscle insertion.[22] This procedure connects the transposed segments of the vertical recti to the lateral rectus muscle, adding to the effect of the surgery. He achieved alignment in 19 of 23 patients treated in this fashion, with an average of 20 diopters of fusion in abduction. This modification was also utilized for bilateral sixth nerve palsies, Duane retraction syndrome, and gaze palsies, and it was effective regardless of the preoperative deviation and in patients with positive forced ductions (indicating contracture of the ipsilateral medial rectus). Clark and Demer have investigated the effects of transposition surgeries with and without posterior fixation of the transposed pieces of muscle.[23] They demonstrated that posterior fixation of transposed muscles resulted in a shift of the rectus pulleys posteriorly and in the direction of the transposed extraocular tendons, while translating the globe center in the opposite direction of the transposition. Thus, a posterior fixation of the transposed muscle seems to increase the effectiveness of the duction by shifting the pulley more in line with the axis of rotation making it more effective.

Fourth Nerve Palsy

When paralyzed, the patient with a fourth nerve paresis presents with a hyperdeviation of the affected eye that increases in contralateral gaze and ipsilateral head tilt.[24] A fourth nerve palsy is the most common cause of a vertical misalignment and can result from many causes, including a tumor. Other causes include abnormal tendon length or abnormal insertion of the tendon. Sato, utilizing MRI, was able to demonstrate that in patients with anomalies of the superior oblique tendon, the muscle was also abnormal suggesting a congenital abnormality of innervation.[25, 26] The surgical treatment of this palsy is complicated by the fact that the induced vertical and torsional abnormalities result in an incomitant strabismus.

Several approaches are available to address a fourth nerve palsy. The most direct approach is to tuck the superior oblique tendon. This procedure involves accessing the tendon and using a specialized "tucker" that folds the tendon over upon itself so that it may be fixed at the base of the tool with a nonabsorbable suture. This approach resolves the vertical deviation but may not address the torsional anomaly. Because the superior oblique tendon is functionally divided into a posterior aspect that mediates depression and an anterior aspect that mediates torsion, the tendon may be split into halves to differentially address the torsional and vertical components of a superior oblique palsy. In this instance a Harada-Ito procedure may be necessary.[27] This procedure splits the tendon down its longitudinal axis, and the anterior portion is transposed to the lateral rectus in order to rid the patient of the torsional anomaly. This may also be combined with a tuck of the posterior portion to address the vertical paresis.[28] Many patients with an oblique palsy develop overaction of the antagonist inferior oblique muscle, requiring weakening of this muscle. Mulvihill et al. examined disinsertion of the inferior oblique muscle in 52 patients with longstanding ipsilateral superior oblique muscle paresis and inferior oblique muscle overaction, and symptomatic relief was achieved in all patients.[29] Patients with superior oblique palsy may develop contracture of the ipsilateral superior rectus muscle, recognized by the deficiency of depression of the involved eye with a positive forced duction in the involved eye. In such cases, spread of comitance of the vertical deviation with similar vertical deviations on ipsilateral and contralateral gaze may ensue. Aseff et al. recommend that a superior rectus recession be required in these circumstances.[30] An alternative procedure in fourth nerve palsy is to transpose the insertion of the inferior oblique to the nasal border of the inferior rectus muscle insertion, converting the inferior oblique muscle from an extorter and elevator of the globe to an intorter and depressor as described by Stager.[31]

References

1. Demer JL, Miller JM, Poukens V. Surgical implications of the rectus extraocular muscle pulleys. J Pediatr Ophthalmol Strabismus 1996;33:208–18.

2. Demer JL, Miller JM, Poukens V, Vinters HV, Glasgow BJ. Evidence for fibromuscular pulleys of the recti extraocular muscles. Invest Ophthalmol Vis Sci 1995;36:1125–36.

3. Porter JD, Poukens V, Baker RS, Demer JL. Structure-function correlations in the human medial rectus extraocular muscle pulleys. Invest Ophthalmol Vis Sci 1996;37:468–72.

4. Miller JM, Demer JL, Rosenbaum AL. Effect of transposition surgery on rectus muscle paths by magnetic resonance imaging. Ophthalmology 1993;100:475–87.

5. Kushner BJ. The usefulness of the cervical range of motion device in the ocular motility examination. Arch Ophthalmol 2000;118:946–50.

6. Mudgil AV, Repka MX. Ophthalmologic outcome after third cranial nerve palsy or paresis in childhood. J Aapos 1999;3:2–8.

7. Schumacher-Feero LA, Yoo KW, Solari FM, Biglan AW. Results following treatment of third cranial nerve palsy in children. Trans Am Ophthalmol Soc 1998;96:455–72; discussion 472–4.

8. Schumacher-Feero LA, Yoo KW, Solari FM, Biglan AW. Third cranial nerve palsy in children. Am J Ophthalmol 1999;128:216–21.

9. Mazow M. Third Cranial Nerve Palsy: Diagnosis and Management Strategies. Philadelphia: W.B. Saunders Company, 1999:251–8.

10. Young TL, Conahan BM, Summers CG, Egbert JE. Anterior transposition of the superior oblique tendon in the treatment of oculomotor nerve palsy and its influence on postoperative hypertropia. J Pediatr Ophthalmol Strabismus 2000;37:149–55.

11. Villasenor Solares J, Riemann BI, Romanelli Zuazo AC, Riemann CD. Ocular fixation to nasal periosteum with a superior oblique tendon in patients with third nerve palsy. J Pediatr Ophthalmol Strabismus 2000;37:260–5.

12. Goldberg RA, Rosenbaum AL, Tong JT. Use of apically based periosteal flaps as globe tethers in severe paretic strabismus. Arch Ophthalmol 2000;118:431–7.

13. Knapp P. Paretic Squints. Transactions of the New Orleans Academy of Ophthalmology. New Orleans: Mosby, 1978:350–7.

14. Holmes J. Surgical management of abduction deficits. Am Orghopt J 2000;50:36–41.

15. Santiago A. Sixth Cranial Nerve Palsy. Philadelphia: W.B. Saunders Company, 1999:259–71.

16. Kerr NC, Hoehn MB. Botulinum toxin for sixth nerve palsies in children with brain tumors. J Aapos 2001;5:21–5.

17. Bock CJ, Jr., Buckley EG, Freedman SF. Combined resection and recession of a single rectus muscle for the treatment of incomitant strabismus. J Aapos 1999;3:263–8.

18. Laby DM, Rosenbaum AL. Adjustable vertical rectus muscle transposition surgery. J Pediatr Ophthalmol Strabismus 1994;31:75–8.

19. Brooks SE, Olitsky SE, de BRG. Augmented Hummelsheim procedure for paralytic strabismus. J Pediatr Ophthalmol Strabismus 2000;37:189–95; quiz 226–7.

20. Neugebauer A, Fricke J, Kirsch A, Russmann W. Modified transposition procedure of the vertical recti in sixth nerve palsy. Am J Ophthalmol 2001;131:359–63.

21. Rosenbaum AL, Kushner BJ, Kirschen D. Vertical rectus muscle transposition and botulinum toxin (Oculinum) to medial rectus for abducens palsy. Arch Ophthalmol 1989;107:820–3.

22. Foster RS. Vertical muscle transposition augmented with lateral fixation. J Aapos 1997;1:20–30.

23. Clark RA, Demer JL. Rectus extraocular muscle pulley displacement after surgical transposition and posterior fixation for treatment of paralytic strabismus. Am J Ophthalmol 2002;133:119–28.

24. Plager D. Superior Oblique Palsy and Superior Oblique Myokymia. Philadelphia: .B. Saunders Company, 1999:219–29.

25. Sato M. Magnetic resonance imaging and tendon anomaly associated with congenital superior oblique palsy. Am J Ophthalmol 1999;127:379–87.

26. Sato M, Yagasaki T, Kora T, Awaya S. Comparison of muscle volume between congenital and acquired superior oblique palsies by magnetic resonance imaging. Jpn J Ophthalmol 1998;42:466–70.

27. Helveston EM, Mora JS, Lipsky SN, et al. Surgical treatment of superior oblique palsy. Trans Am Ophthalmol Soc 1996;94:315–28; discussion 328–34.

28. Simons BD, Saunders TG, Siatkowski RM, et al. Outcome of surgical management of superior oblique palsy: a study of 123 cases. Binocul Vis Strabismus Q 1998;13:273–82.

29. Mulvihill A, Murphy M, Lee JP. Disinsertion of the inferior oblique muscle for treatment of superior oblique paresis. J Pediatr Ophthalmol Strabismus 2000;37:279–82.

30. Aseff AJ, Munoz M. Outcome of surgery for superior oblique palsy with contracture of ipsilateral superior rectus treated by superior rectus recession. Binocul Vis Strabismus Q 1998;13:177–80.

31. Stager DR, Sr., Beauchamp GR, Stager DR, Jr. Anterior and nasal transposition of the inferior oblique muscle: a preliminary case report on a new procedure. Binocul Vis Strabismus Q 2001;16:43–4.

V
Adjunct Treatment Modalities

25
Recent Advances in Therapeutic Radiation: An Overview

Simon S. Lo, Eric L. Chang, and John H. Suh

Introduction

Meningiomas account for about 20% of intracranial tumors. They are generally well-circumscribed and slow-growing tumors. Between 90 and 95% of meningiomas are benign, and the remaining are atypical or malignant. They can present as small, indolent, and asymptomatic convexity lesions to skull base tumors encasing major blood vessels, cranial nerves, optic pathways, or compressing vital structures of the brain. For benign meningiomas, complete surgical resection remains the best treatment option. Unfortunately, in many instances tumors in skull base locations such as the cavernous sinus, petroclival region, or the orbit cannot be completely resected because of unacceptable risks of morbidity.[1,2] For incompletely resected or unresectable benign meningiomas, postoperative radiation therapy is frequently employed to reduce the risk of progression. In a surgical series from the Massachusetts General Hospital, the cumulative risk of progression was 37, 55, and 91% at 5, 10, and 15 years, respectively.[2] Several retrospective series have demonstrated that radiotherapy decreases the rate of local failure or progression of benign meningiomas after subtotal resection to less than 20%.[3–7] Atypical and malignant meningiomas, when compared with benign meningiomas, have a higher and more rapid propensity to recur locally.[8,9] Even after complete resection, postoperative radiation therapy is indicated to reduce the risk of recurrence or progression.

For optic nerve sheath meningiomas, surgery often results in postoperative blindness in the involved eye and has been abandoned as a treatment option for some patients.[10] With observation alone, tumor progression can occur resulting in progressive visual impairment, eventually leading to blindness. Radiation therapy can be used to prevent tumor progression and vision stabilization.

Data from retrospective series in the literature have suggested a significant risk of 20% or more of normal tissue complications.[3,4,11] Furthermore, there is a small but real risk of development of radiation-induced tumors or cancer.[12] High-precision radiotherapy techniques such as stereotactic radiosurgery (SRS), fractionated stereotactic radiotherapy (FSRT), intensity-modulated radiotherapy (IMRT), and proton beam radiotherapy (PBT) have been developed in recent years, and the early results appear to be promising. Meningiomas are suitable targets for these high-precision techniques because they are usually sharply delineated, almost never infiltrate normal brain tissue, frequently have complex and irregular shapes, and are often located in close proximity to various sensitive structures such as the optic pathway. This chapter focuses on advanced radiation therapy techniques for the treatment of meningiomas. SRS will be discussed in two other chapters in this book.

Advanced Radiation Therapy Techniques

The common characteristic of these techniques is the steep dose gradient beyond the target volume. Because of this characteristic, accurate target delineation is crucial. Although meningiomas can easily be seen on computed tomography (CT), magnetic resonance imaging (MRI) allows for better target definition and is in most cases fused with treatment planning CT. MRI also helps delineate the critical structures not well visualized on CT (e.g., the optic chiasm).

The gross tumor volume (GTV) is usually defined as the contrast-enhanced tumor on CT or preferably MRI. For benign meningiomas, because of the sharp delineation between the tumor and the normal brain parenchyma, no or minimal margin expansion from the GTV is used to generate a clinical target volume (CTV). However, a margin expansion around the GTV may be used to generate a CTV for atypical or malignant meningiomas. The amount of margin needed for expansion from CTV to planning treatment volume (PTV) depends on the technique of immobilization. The prescription dose is usually in the range of 50–54 Gy in conventional fractionation for benign tumors and 59.4–60 Gy for atypical and malignant tumors. The critical structures to be spared include the optic apparatus, brain stem, cranial nerves, eyes, lacrimal gland, pituitary gland, and cochlea, depending on the clinical scenario. If one or more of those critical structures are within the target volume, none of these advanced techniques can spare those structures. In such circumstances, the prescribed dose has to be lowered or one will have to accept a higher risk of injury to those structures.

This section summarizes the clinical treatment outcomes of fractionated stereotactic radiotherapy, intensity-modulated radiation therapy, and proton beam radiation therapy for meningiomas.

Fractionated Stereotactic Radiotherapy

Although stereotactic radiosurgery (SRS) is an effective treatment for meningiomas, it is in general not suitable for tumors 3–4 cm or larger in diameter or immediately adjacent to eloquent structures such as the optic apparatus. Fractionated stereotactic radiotherapy (FSRT) combines the precision of stereotactic positioning with the radiobiologic advantages of fractionation, allowing higher total doses and safe target coverage. The treatment-planning process is similar to that of linear accelerator-based SRS except for the margin needed for PTV expansion from the GTV to account for daily set-up variation associated with the use of relocatable immobilization device.

Data is emerging in the literature on the use of FSRT for the treatment of meningioma. In the series of 24 patients from Royal Marsden Hospital treated with stereotactically guided conformal radiotherapy for mostly skull base meningiomas, the reported 1-year progression-free survival and overall survival rates were both 100% with a median follow-up of 13 months. The radiation dose ranged from 50 to 55 Gy.[13] Tumor shrinkage occurred in 3 patients (12.5%). Seven of 15 patients with initial neurologic symptoms had symptomatic improvement after treatment. Two patients developed late complications. A subsequent report from the same hospital showed 1- and 3-year tumor control rates of 100% with a median follow-up of 21 months.[14] Four patients developed late complications. Colleagues from University of Minnesota reported a 3-year tumor control rate of 93.3% in 18 patients with meningioma, which was not significantly different from patients treated with SRS in the same series.[15] The median radiation dose was 54 Gy. One patient (6%) developed visual deterioration as late complication.

The group from Heidelberg reported the preliminary results of the FSRT series of 189 patients for skull base meningioma. The mean radiation dose used was 56.8 Gy in conventional fractionation, and the median target volume was 52.5 cm^3 (range 5.2–370 cm^3). The median follow-up time was 35 months. The tumor growth control was 98.3%.[16] A volume reduction of 50% was seen in 14% of patients. The complication rate was 1.6%. In a follow-up series of 317 patients by the same group, 22 patients (6.9%) had local tumor progression on MRI at a median of 4.5 years after FSRT.[17] The median follow-up time was 5.7 years. Of these patients, 8.2% developed worsening of their preexisting neurologic symptoms after FSRT.

In the study from University of California, Los Angeles (UCLA), with a median follow-up of 36 months, the 3-year progression-free survival for the 45 patients treated with FSRT for cavernous sinus meningioma was 97.4%.[18] The prescribed dose ranged from 42.5 to 54 Gy. The median conformality index was 2.2. Preexisting neurologic complaints improved in 20% of patients and were stable in the remainder.[18] One patient developed a late complication. The group from Barcelona reported the outcomes of 30 patients treated with FSRT for cavernous sinus meningiomas. The radiation dose was 52 Gy in 2 Gy fractions. The 4-year progression-free survival rate was 93% with a median follow-up of 50 months.[19] Among the 28 patients with clinical symptoms at the time of treatment, 50% exhibited improvement of their clinical status and 6.6% had neurologic deterioration after treatment.[19] Two patients (6.6%) developed late radiation-induced toxicity.

Similar results were observed with optic nerve sheath meningiomas.[20–23] Apart from tumor control, preservation of vision is another goal of treatment. In one of the largest series of 30 patients with 33 optic nerve sheath meningioma treated with FSRT at Thomas Jefferson University, with a median follow-up of 89 weeks, there was no evidence of tumor progression in all patients. Out of the 22 optic nerves with vision before FSRT, 20 nerves (92%) demonstrated preserved vision, and 42% manifested improvement in visual acuity and/or visual field at follow-up.[20] The prescribed dose ranged from 50.4 to 54 Gy in conventional fractionation to the isodose surface encompassing the target volume. The group from New York Medical College reported similar results on the five patients treated with FSRT to a dose of 45–54 Gy for optic nerve sheath meningiomas. There was a 100% visual preservation rate, with 80% of the patients experiencing improvement of their vision after treatment.[21] None of the patients developed tumor progression or complications related to treatment with follow-up times ranging from 1 to 7 years. Other studies showed similar findings.[22,23]

The preliminary data suggest that FSRT is effective for the treatment of meningioma in various locations such as the skull base and the optic nerve sheath. The tumor control rate is over 90%, and the complication rate is typically low. Table 25-1

TABLE 25-1. Treatment Outcomes of Fractionated Stereotactic Radiation Therapy for Meningiomas.

Ref. no.	No. of patients	Site	Dose (Gy)	Med FU	TC (yr)	Complications (%)
13	24	Mostly SB	50–55	13 mo	100% (1)	8
14	41	Mostly SB	50–55	21 mo	100% (3)	10
15	18	All locations	54	31 mo	93% (3)	6
16	189	SB	56.8	35 mo	98% (NA)	2
17	317	SB	57.6	57 mo	93% (NA)	3
18	45	CS	42.5–54	36 mo	97%[a] (3)	2
19	30	CS	52	50 mo	93%[a] (4)	7
20	30	ONS	50.4–54	89 wk	100% (NA)	8
21	5	ONS	45–54	1–7 yr	100% (NA)	0
22	15	ONS	54	37 mo	100% (NA)	0

Abbreviations: Med FU, median follow-up; TC, tumor control; SB, skull base; CS, cavernous sinus; ONS, optic nerve sheath; NA, not available.
[a] Progression-free survival.

summarizes the treatment outcomes of selected FSRT series. One note of caution: most meningiomas are indolent tumors and late progression can occur. Furthermore, late complications, including second tumor or cancer, can occur several years after treatment. The follow-up times for these series are too short for a firm conclusion to be drawn regarding the long-term efficacy and safety of FSRT for meningioma.

Intensity-Modulated Radiation Therapy

Intensity-modulated radiation therapy (IMRT) is an advanced form of three-dimensional conformal radiotherapy (3DCRT), which can produce highly conformal isodose distribution for complex target volumes while minimizing dose to surrounding critical structures or organs. IMRT involves inverse planning, which entails a process whereby the computer planning system, after being given the desired outcome by the radiation oncologist, determines a combination of beams and beam intensity distribution, which will cause the best compromise of radiation dose to tumor and normal tissues. Because of the typical steep dose gradient across the target volume/brain parenchyma interface, sparing of critical structures surrounding target volume is possible. Figure 25-1 shows the computer plan of a patient with a left sphenoid wing meningioma treated with IMRT.

In recent years, a few academic institutions have reported their experience with IMRT for the treatment of meningiomas predominantly in skull base locations.[24] Colleagues from Baylor College of Medicine treated 40 patients with IMRT for subtotally resected, recurrent, or unresected meningioma. Thirty-two patients had tumors in skull base locations. A Peacock system from NOMOS Corporation (Sewickley, PA) was used for treatment planning and delivery. The prescribed dose ranged from 40 to 56 Gy (median 50.4 Gy) in conventional fractionation. With a median follow-up of 30 months, out of

the 37 patients with follow-up with imaging studies, 9 had tumor regression, 20 had stable disease, and 1 had tumor progression.[24] The patient who failed locally was confirmed to have malignant meningioma at recurrence. The 5-year cumulative local control was 93% for the entire group of patients, and 93% for the 37 with imaging studies.[24] One patient developed grade 3 or higher acute central nervous system toxicity. There was no late optic pathway toxicity. Two patients developed late complications (one with brain stem necrosis and one with peritumoral brain edema).

In the study from University of Heidelberg, 20 patients with skull base meningiomas were treated with IMRT. The inverse planning systems used were KonRad (MRC Systems, Heidelberg, Germany) and CORVUS 2.4 (Nomos Corporation, Sewickley, PA). Dose restrictions to the critical structures were as follows: maximum dose of 54 Gy for optic nerves and chiasm, 32 Gy for the lacrimal glands, 10 Gy for the lenses, and 54 Gy for the brain stem.[25] The prescribed dose was 57.6 Gy in 1.8 Gy fractions. With a median follow-up of 36 months, preexisting neurologic symptoms improved in 12 (60%), remained stable in 7 (35%), and worsened in 1 (5%) out of 20 patients.[25] The majority of these symptomatic improvements occurred 6 weeks after the course of IMRT. Five patients (25%) had tumor shrinkage, while the remaining 15 patients (75%) had stable findings on repeat imaging studies.[25] Acute eye complications including conjunctivitis and increased tearing occurred in 65% of the patients, and this was most likely related to the equidistant beam arrangements with some portion of the beam entering through part of the eye or lacrimal gland.[25] In terms of late complications, one patient developed visual deterioration and another developed pituitary deficiency after IMRT.

A recent study from Cleveland Clinic Foundation also demonstrated similar findings. A Peacock System from NOMOS was used.[26] Thirty-five patients with 37 meningiomas (2 atypical histology) were treated with IMRT either after prior local treatments (surgery or SRS) or primarily after radiologic diagnosis. The majority of the patients had tumors in skull base locations. A reinforced immobilization technique was used to allow a repositioning accuracy of 2 mm.[26] The median IMRT dose was 50.4 Gy (range 27–57.6 Gy) prescribed to the 87% isodose line (median; range 82–91%). Fraction sizes ranged from 1.7 to 2 Gy, depending on the distance of the tumor from the optic apparatus. Out of the 37 tumors treated, 3 showed evidence of progression, and 8 (21%) showed some volume reduction with a median follow-up of 19.1 months.[26] The 3-year actuarial local control was 97%. The Karnofsky Performance Status improved, remained stable, and worsened in 19, 57, and 24% of the patients, respectively.[26] No late complications were observed.

As a result of the steep dose gradient associated with IMRT, the importance of very accurate patient immobilization and localization cannot be overemphasized. Any set-up deviation beyond the limits accounted for in the PTV expansion will result in a geographic miss of tumor volume, which may com-

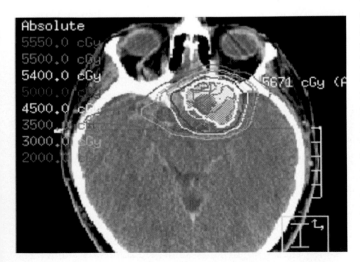

FIG. 25-1. Intensity-modulated radiation therapy plan for a left sphenoid wing meningioma treated to a dose of 54 Gy in 30 fractions

promise tumor control.[25] Furthermore, if the tumor volume is very close to any critical structures, a slight set-up deviation can sometimes cause those structures to shift into the high-dose zone or hot spot, resulting in an increased risk of serious late neural complications. It is crucial that the treating radiation oncologist be familiar with the scenario of the patient being treated, so a decision can be made as to whether a set-up is acceptable or not. Because of inverse planning process, only the structures that are contoured will be recognized by the inverse treatment planning system and can have their doses controlled by the optimizer.[25] The Heidelberg group observed an interesting finding of acute eye complications as a result of some of the beams passing through the eye or the lacrimal gland.[25] Caution should be exercised to avoid any beams passing through those structures.

Preliminary data available in the literature are promising in terms of tumor control and normal tissue complications. However, as in the case of FSRT, the follow-up is too short for any firm conclusion to be made. There is frequently a spread of the low-dose zone over a large area of normal tissue in IMRT plans. This results in a higher nontarget integral dose, which may increase the area at risk for secondary tumors or malignancies. Due to the long latency of radiation tumorigenesis, a much longer follow-up period is required to determine the impact of the increased nontarget integral dose on the risk of secondary tumor or malignancies.

Proton Beam Radiation Therapy

Proton beam radiation therapy (PBRT) can be used to precisely deliver dose to the intracranial target volume while sparing normal brain tissue and other critical structures, such as the optic apparatus, brain stem, and pituitary gland. Protons have the advantage of being more conformal and homogeneous, as compared to photon radiotherapy, as a result of dose deposition in a modulated narrow zone called the Bragg peak.[27] The use of protons decreases the integral nontarget dose when compared to photon beam therapy.[27–30] This may be very important, especially in patients with benign meningiomas, who typically have long life expectancies because higher integral dose may increase the risk of development of secondary tumors or malignancies, which typically have a long latency.

Protons can be used alone or combined with photons for the treatment of meningiomas. In the series from Harvard University, 46 patients with partially resected, biopsied, or recurrent meningiomas were treated with combined photon and proton beam radiation therapy.[31] The energy of the proton beams used was 160 MeV. The median fraction numbers for proton and photon beam were 25 and 6, respectively. The median prescription dose to the tumor was 59 Cobalt Gray Equivalent (CGE = proton Gray X 1.1). With a median follow-up of 53 months and an average follow-up of 73 months, the 5- and 10-year overall survival rates were 93 and 77%, respectively.[31] The recurrence-free survival rates were 100 and 88% at 5 and 10 years, respectively.[31] Out of the 46 patients

treated, 3 had evidence of tumor progression at 61, 95, and 125 months, respectively. Five patients developed severe acute toxicities, including skin desquamation, fibrinous mucositis, and otitis. Eight patients developed one or more grade 3 or 4 late complications, and ophthalmic, neurologic, and otologic complications were observed in four, four, and two patients, respectively. All four patients with ophthalmic complications received doses between 56.4 and 62 CGE to their optic chiasms. Brain stem and temporal lobe doses exceeded the subsequently reduced tolerance levels in 2 of the 4 patients with neurologic injury. The survival rates without long-term complications at 5 and 10 years were both 80%.[31] The relatively higher rate of complications is most likely due to the use of higher tolerance levels in the earlier days. In the study from Centre de Protontherapie d'Orsay, 17 patients received proton beam therapy as a component of treatment for the treatment of meningioma.[32] The median tumor dose was 61 CGE. One third of the radiation dose was delivered by protons. With a median follow-up of 37 months, the 4-year local control and overall survival rates were 87.5 and 88.9%, respectively.[32] One patient failed locally within the tumor volume. Most patients experienced complete or partial clinical improvement. Colleagues from Institut Curie treated 51 patients with skull base meningioma with a combination of photons and protons.[33] The prescribed dose was 60.6 CGE. With a median follow-up of 25.4 months, the 4-year local control rate was 98%.[33] Stabilization, tumor shrinkage, and intratumoral necrosis occurred in 72, 20, and 6% of the cases, respectively. Approximately two thirds of the eye-related symptoms and two thirds of other symptoms improved after treatment. Out of the 51 patients treated, two developed grade 3 complications.[33]

The Swiss Proton User Group reported the treatment outcomes of the 16 patients treated with spot-scanning proton radiation therapy for recurrent, residual, or untreated intracranial meningiomas.[34] The median prescribed dose was 56 CGE. The cumulative 3-year local control, progression-free survival, and overall survival rates were 91.7, 91.7, and 92.7, respectively, with a median follow-up of 34.1 months.[34] One of the 16 patients developed tumor progression. Radiologic response and stable disease were documented in 3 and 12 patients, respectively. The 3-year toxicity-free survival rate was 76.2%.[34] Two patients developed ophthalmic complications, including retinopathy and optic nerve deficits, and one developed symptomatic brain necrosis.

The South African group treated 23 patients with skull base meningiomas with either hypofractionated stereotactic proton beam radiation therapy or stereotactic proton beam radiation therapy to doses of 31.5 CGE in 3 fractions and 54 CGE in 27 fractions to 61.6 CGE in 16 fractions, respectively.[35] The mean clinical and radiologic follow-up times were 40 and 31 months, respectively. For the patients treated with hypofractionated stereotactic proton beam radiation therapy, 89% of the patients improved or remained clinically stable. The 5-year radiologic control rate was 88%. Complete radiologic response, partial radiologic response, and stable findings were observed in 23, 6, and 59% of those patients, respectively.[35] All of the patients treated with stereotactic proton beam radiation therapy had their tumors controlled. Eleven percent of patients who received hypofractionated stereotactic proton beam radiation therapy developed transient cranial nerve deficits, and the same percentage of patients developed late neurologic complications. No acute toxicity was observed in patients who received stereotactic proton beam radiation therapy, and one of the five patients treated developed short-term memory problems.

Investigators from Massachusetts General Hospital reported no difference in overall survival and local control between the dose levels of 55.8 CGE (in 31 fractions) and 63 CGE (in 35 fractions) in a randomized dose escalation trial in patients with recurrent or incompletely resected benign meningiomas treated with proton-photon irradiation (approximately 80% protons).[36] With a median follow-up of 62 months, none of the patients developed local recurrence. Five percent of patients in each arm had increased symptoms after treatment.

The treatment outcomes of proton beam radiation therapy appear to be similar to those for FSRT and IMRT. The dosimetric characteristics of proton beam radiation therapy lead to the decrement in nontarget integral dose, which in turn should translate into a decreased risk of development of secondary cancer or malignancy. However, because of the long latency of this process, long-term follow-up is needed to confirm the gain in therapeutic ratio.

Selection of Advanced Treatment Modality

The dosimetric characteristics of protons render proton beam radiation therapy a more superior treatment modality than FSRT or IMRT.[27–30] Proton beam radiation therapy is associated with superior target dose coverage and sparing of normal structures and a lower nontarget integral dose as a result of the Bragg peak.[28,29] However, due to limited availability, especially in the United States, it is not realistic to offer this treatment to most patients with meningiomas. Currently, there are only three proton beam centers (Loma Linda University, Harvard University, and Midwest Proton Radiotherapy Institute) across the nation actively treating patients. The high cost of the treatment is also a barrier to its widespread use. A few more proton beam centers will open in the next few years, which will improve the availability to patients. Currently, if proton beam radiation therapy is not available, both FSRT and IMRT are suitable treatments for patients with meningiomas, although FSRT is usually more subject to size limitation than IMRT.

Future Directions

Protons are low-LET (linear energy transfer) radiation, the relative biological effectiveness of which is 1.1. Carbon ions are high- LET radiation and combines the advantages of neu-

trons and protons.[37] The combination of superior dosimetric characteristics and increased biological effectiveness may improve the therapeutic ratio. Research on carbon ion therapy is currently underway.

References

1. Stafford SL, Perry A, Suman VJ, et al. Primarily resected meningiomas: outcome and prognostic factors in 581 Mayo Clinic patients, 1978 through 1988. Mayo Clin Proc 1998;73:936–942.
2. Mirimanoff RO, Dosoretz DE, Linggood RM, et al. Meningioma: analysis of recurrence and progression following neurosurgical resection. J Neurosurg 1985;62:18–24.
3. Nutting C, Brada M, Brazil L, et al. Radiotherapy in the treatment of benign meningioma of the skull base. J Neurosurg 1999;90:823–827.
4. Miralbell R, Linggood RM, de la Monte S, et al. The role of radiotherapy in the treatment of subtotally resected benign meningiomas. J Neurooncol 1992;13:157–164.
5. Goldsmith BJ, Wara WM, Wilson CB, et al. Postoperative irradiation for subtotally resected meningiomas. A retrospective analysis of 140 patients treated from 1967 to 1990. J Neurosurg 1994;80:195–201.
6. Glaholm J, Bloom HJ, Crow JH. The role of radiotherapy in the management of intracranial meningiomas: the Royal Marsden Hospital experience with 186 patients. Int J Radiat Oncol Biol Phys 1990;18:755–761.
7. Pourel N, Auque J, Bracard S, et al. Efficacy of external fractionated radiation therapy in the treatment of meningiomas: a 20-year experience. Radiother Oncol 2001;61:65–70.
8. Milosevic MF, Frost PJ, Laperriere NJ, et al. Radiotherapy for atypical or malignant intracranial meningioma. Int J Radiat Oncol Biol Phys 1996;34:817–822.
9. Hug EB, Devries A, Thornton AF, et al. Management of atypical and malignant meningiomas: role of high-dose, 3D-conformal radiation therapy. J Neurooncol 2000;48:151–160.
10. Melian E, Jay WM. Primary radiotherapy for optic nerve sheath meningioma. Semin Ophthalmol 2004;19:130–140.
11. Mathiesen T, Kihlstrom L, Karlsson B, et al. Potential complications following radiotherapy for meningiomas. Surg Neurol 2003;60:193–198; discussion 199–200.
12. Loeffler JS, Niemierko A, Chapman PH. Second tumors after radiosurgery: tip of the iceberg or a bump in the road? Neurosurgery 2003;52:1436–1440; discussion 1440–1432.
13. Alheit H, Saran FH, Warrington AP, et al. Stereotactically guided conformal radiotherapy for meningiomas. Radiother Oncol 1999;50:145–150.
14. Jalali R, Loughrey C, Baumert B, et al. High precision focused irradiation in the form of fractionated stereotactic conformal radiotherapy (SCRT) for benign meningiomas predominantly in the skull base location. Clin Oncol (R Coll Radiol) 2002;14:103–109.
15. Lo SS, Cho KH, Hall WA, et al. Single dose versus fractionated stereotactic radiotherapy for meningiomas. Can J Neurol Sci 2002;29:240–248.
16. Debus J, Wuendrich M, Pirzkall A, et al. High efficacy of fractionated stereotactic radiotherapy of large base-of-skull meningiomas: long-term results. J Clin Oncol 2001;19:3547–3553.

17. Milker-Zabel S, Zabel A, Schulz-Ertner D, et al. Fractionated stereotactic radiotherapy in patients with benign or atypical intracranial meningioma: long-term experience and prognostic factors. Int J Radiat Oncol Biol Phys 2005;61:809–816.

18. Selch MT, Ahn E, Laskari A, et al. Stereotactic radiotherapy for treatment of cavernous sinus meningiomas. Int J Radiat Oncol Biol Phys 2004;59:101–111.

19. Brell M, Villa S, Teixidor P, et al. Fractionated stereotactic radiotherapy in the treatment of exclusive cavernous sinus meningioma: functional outcome, local control, and tolerance. Surg Neurol 2006;65:28–33; discussion 33–34.

20. Andrews DW, Faroozan R, Yang BP, et al. Fractionated stereotactic radiotherapy for the treatment of optic nerve sheath meningiomas: preliminary observations of 33 optic nerves in 30 patients with historical comparison to observation with or without prior surgery. Neurosurgery 2002;51:890–902; discussion 903.

21. Liu JK, Forman S, Hershewe GL, et al. Optic nerve sheath meningiomas: visual improvement after stereotactic radiotherapy. Neurosurgery 2002;50:950–955; discussion 955–957.

22. Pitz S, Becker G, Schiefer U, et al. Stereotactic fractionated irradiation of optic nerve sheath meningioma: a new treatment alternative. Br J Ophthalmol 2002;86:1265–1268.

23. Paridaens AD, van Ruyven RL, Eijkenboom WM, et al. Stereotactic irradiation of biopsy proved optic nerve sheath meningioma. Br J Ophthalmol 2003;87:246–247.

24. Uy NW, Woo SY, Teh BS, et al. Intensity-modulated radiation therapy (IMRT) for meningioma. Int J Radiat Oncol Biol Phys 2002;53:1265–1270.

25. Pirzkall A, Debus J, Haering P, et al. Intensity modulated radiotherapy (IMRT) for recurrent, residual, or untreated skull-base meningiomas: preliminary clinical experience. Int J Radiat Oncol Biol Phys 2003;55:362–372.

26. Sajja R, Barnett GH, Lee SY, et al. Intensity-modulated radiation therapy (IMRT) for newly diagnosed and recurrent intracranial meningiomas: preliminary results. Technol Cancer Res Treat 2005;4:675–682.

27. Cozzi L, Fogliata A, Lomax A, et al. A treatment planning comparison of 3D conformal therapy, intensity modulated photon therapy and proton therapy for treatment of advanced head and neck tumours. Radiother Oncol 2001;61:287–297.

28. Miralbell R, Cella L, Weber D, et al. Optimizing radiotherapy of orbital and paraorbital tumors: intensity-modulated X-ray beams vs. intensity-modulated proton beams. Int J Radiat Oncol Biol Phys 2000;47:1111–1119.

29. Lomax AJ, Cella L, Weber D, et al. Potential role of intensity-modulated photons and protons in the treatment of the breast and regional nodes. Int J Radiat Oncol Biol Phys 2003;55:785–792.

30. Lomax AJ, Bortfeld T, Goitein G, et al. A treatment planning inter-comparison of proton and intensity modulated photon radiotherapy. Radiother Oncol 1999;51:257–271.

31. Wenkel E, Thornton AF, Finkelstein D, et al. Benign meningioma: partially resected, biopsied, and recurrent intracranial tumors treated with combined proton and photon radiotherapy. Int J Radiat Oncol Biol Phys 2000;48:1363–1370.

32. Noel G, Habrand JL, Mammar H, et al. Highly conformal therapy using proton component in the management of meningiomas. Preliminary experience of the Centre de Protontherapie d'Orsay. Strahlenther Onkol 2002;178:480–485.

33. Noel G, Bollet MA, Calugaru V, et al. Functional outcome of patients with benign meningioma treated by 3D conformal irradiation with a combination of photons and protons. Int J Radiat Oncol Biol Phys 2005;62:1412–1422.

34. Weber DC, Lomax AJ, Rutz HP, et al. Spot-scanning proton radiation therapy for recurrent, residual or untreated intracranial meningiomas. Radiother Oncol 2004;71:251–258.

35. Vernimmen FJ, Harris JK, Wilson JA, et al. Stereotactic proton beam therapy of skull base meningiomas. Int J Radiat Oncol Biol Phys 2001;49:99–105.

36. Lopes VV, Chan A, Loeffler J, et al. A randomized radiation dose escalation trial in patients with recurrent or incompletely resected benign meningiomas treated with proton-photon irradiation. Int J Radiat Oncol Biol Phys 2003;57 Suppl :S323–324.

37. Mazeron JJ, Noel G, Feuvret L, et al. Clinical complementarities between proton and carbon therapies. Radiother Oncol 2004;73 Suppl 2:S50–52.

26
Conventional Radiation for Meningiomas

Simon S. Lo, Brent A. Tinnel, and John H. Suh

Introduction

Complete surgical resection is the standard treatment for meningioma and is compatible with long-term progression-free survival (PFS).[1–3] However, about one third of the meningiomas are not amenable to complete resection secondary to the location, large size, and proximity to critical structures.[2] Complete resection of skull base meningiomas can only be achieved in approximately half of the patients.[2,4] Subtotal resection without any adjuvant treatment is regarded as inadequate therapy and is associated with inferior PFS.[2,5–8] Postoperative radiation therapy is frequently employed after subtotal resection of meningiomas and can significantly improve the PFS with relatively low toxicity. In patients with unresectable meningiomas or patients with poor pretreatment factors for surgery, radiation therapy alone has been demonstrated to be effective in terms of long-term PFS.[3,9–12] Radiation therapy is also given to patients who have unirradiated recurrent meningiomas.[6–8] The management of optic nerve sheath meningiomas has been controversial. Surgical resection is indicated for aggressive tumors with intracranial extension. However, this can result in blindness. Observation alone will eventually lead to blindness as a result of tumor progression. Radiation therapy is often given to enhance local control and is regarded as a potentially vision-sparing procedure.[13] For patients with atypical (grade 2) and anaplastic (grade 3) meningiomas, there is an increased risk of tumor recurrence even after complete surgical resection,[9,14,15] and postoperative radiation therapy is frequently given to reduce the risk of recurrence.

This chapter summarizes the data concerning conventional radiation therapy for meningiomas in different settings. Advanced radiation techniques for meningiomas is discussed in the preceding chapter.

Postoperative Radiation Therapy After Subtotal Resection

Abundant retrospective data exist in the literature to support the use of postoperative radiation therapy for subtotally resected meningiomas. Glaholm et al. reported the treatment results of 186 patients who received treatment for meningioma at the Royal Marsden Hospital in England.[9] Tumors were classified as benign ($n = 117$), aggressive benign ($n = 28$), malignant ($n = 9$), and not otherwise specified ($n = 17$) based on the Royal Marsden Hospital legacy system. Eighty-two patients had subtotal resection with minimal residual disease, and 46 had bulky residual disease. Those patients received postoperative radiation to the preoperative treatment volume with a 2–4 cm margin, and a dose of 50–55 Gy was given over 6–6.5 weeks. The corresponding 5-, 10-, and 15-year disease-free survival (DFS) rates for the two groups of patients were 78, 67, and 56% and 81, 68, and 61%, respectively. On the examination of prognostic factors using multivariate analysis, tumor grade, extent of surgery, and Karnofsky Performance Status (KPS) predicted cause-specific survival (CSS).[9] Nutting et al. from the same institution limited the analysis to the 82 patients with skull base benign meningiomas in a subsequent report. Out of the 82 patients, 62 received postoperative radiation therapy upfront after macroscopic resection, subtotal resection, biopsy, and undetermined surgery; the other 20 patients were treated with radiation therapy after salvage surgery for recurrence. Megavoltage radiation therapy was used and a dose of 55–60 Gy in conventional fractionation was given to the preoperative tumor volume with a 2- to 3-cm margin. The PFS rates were 92 and 83% at 5 and 10 years, respectively.[16]

In an updated series from University of California, San Francisco (UCSF), Goldsmith et al. reported the outcomes of 140 patients treated with subtotal resection and postoperative radiation therapy. One hundred and seventeen patients had benign meningiomas. A median dose of 54 Gy was given. A 1- to 2-cm margin was placed around the postoperative residual tumor. The overall survival at 5 years was 85% for patients with benign meningiomas; the corresponding 5-year progression-free survival was 89%.[17] Taylor et al. from University of Florida showed that patients who received postoperative radiation therapy after subtotal resection had equivalent local control and determinate survival compared to those who had complete tumor resection and had better local

TABLE 26-1. Selected Studies Comparing Postoperative Radiation Therapy and Surgery Alone (Complete or Subtotal Resection) for Meningioma.

Ref. no.	No. of patients			Endpoint	Local control		
	GTR	STR	STR + RT		GTR	STR	STR + RT
13	0	0	117	5-/10-yr PFS	N/A	N/A	89%/77%
14	0	0	82 (m) 46 (b)	5-/10-/15-yr DFS	N/A	N/A	78%/65%/ 56% 81%/ 68%/61%
18	174	55	17	15-yr LC	76%	30%	87%
22	0	79	17	8-yr PFS	N/A	48%	88%
30	0	0	82	5-/10-yr PFS	N/A	N/A	92%/83%
31	48	32	12	5-yr PFS	77%	38%	82%

Abbreviations: GTR, gross total resection; STR, subtotal resection; STR + RT, subtotal resection with radiation therapy; PFS, progression-free survival; DFS, disease-free survival; LC, local control; NA, not available; m, minimal residuum; b, bulky residuum.

control and determinate survival compared to those who had subtotal resection alone.[6] The local control rates for patients who underwent subtotal excision alone, subtotal excision plus postoperative radiation therapy, and total excision alone were 18, 82, and 77%, respectively, at 10 years. The corresponding 10-year survival rates were 49, 81, and 93%, respectively. The authors also found that for patients treated at the time of the first recurrence, postoperative radiation therapy after salvage surgery could improve local control. Condra et al. from the same institution subsequently reported the outcomes of 17 patients who were treated with radiation therapy for subtotally resected benign meningioma. A median dose of 53.3 Gy was given to the tumor bed with a 2-cm margin.

The 5-, 10-, and 15-year local control rates were 87, 87, and 87%, respectively; these results were comparable to those of patients in the same series that had complete tumor resection and were significantly better than those of patients who had subtotal resection without postoperative radiation therapy.[3]

Miralbell et al. reported the results of 17 patients with benign meningioma treated with radiation therapy after subtotal resection. They were treated either with megavoltage photons or with combined photons and protons. Radiation therapy in addition to subtotal resection resulted in an 8-year PFS of 88% compared to 48% in patients treated with subtotal resection alone during the same time period ($p = 0.05$) despite the higher percentage of high-grade tumors in the irradiated cohort of patients.[7] In a series from M.D. Anderson Cancer Center, ninety-two patients were treated with surgery for cerebral benign meningioma. Forty-eight, twelve, and thirty-two patients had gross total resection (GTR), subtotal resection (STR) with adjuvant radiation therapy, and STR alone, respectively. Twelve patients received radiation therapy as adjuvant treatment and 28 underwent radiation therapy as salvage treatment. Megavoltage machines were used. The median radiation dose was 54 Gy, mostly in conventional fractionation. With a median follow-up of 7.7 years, the 5-year PFS rates in patients treated with GTR and STR with or without radiation therapy were 77 and 52%, respectively ($p = 0.02$).[18] Among the patients who had STR, postoperative radiation therapy was associated with significantly better PFS (91%) at 5 years than with STR alone (38%).[18] However, the

overall survival did not differ among patients who had GTR, those who had STR and adjuvant radiation therapy, and those who underwent STR only. The authors concluded that postoperative radiation therapy was effective in the prevention of progression in patients with STR, but the optimal timing of radiation therapy could not be determined. A randomized trial comparing immediate and delayed radiation therapy was suggested by the authors.

Postoperative radiation therapy is therefore indicated in cases of subtotal resection and is associated with PFS and local control rates comparable to those in patients who had complete resection and superior to those in patients who had subtotal resection alone. Table 26-1 summarizes the results of selected studies comparing postoperative radiation therapy and surgery alone (complete or subtotal resection).

Radiation Therapy for Unresectable Meningiomas

Radiation therapy is often offered to patients who have meningiomas that are deemed unresectable because of technical difficulty or the patient's poor general medical condition. Data in the literature have demonstrated benefits in terms of improvement and stabilization of neurologic status. Radiation therapy is also associated with durable PFS in a significant proportion of patients. Several institutions have reported their treatment outcomes for this patient group.

Glaholm et al. reported the outcomes of 32 patients treated for unresectable meningiomas at Royal Marsden Hospital. Improvement in neurologic performance status occurred in 38% of the patients.[9] The reported 5-, 10-, and 15-year DFS rates were 53, 47, and 47%, respectively.[9] (The radiation therapy parameters were mentioned in the previous section.) The Joint Center for Radiation Therapy reported the treatment results of 19 patients with meningiomas who were treated with megavoltage radiation therapy after biopsy or without exploration. The mean radiation dose was 52.8 Gy utilizing conventional fractionation. With a median follow-up time of 45 months,

TABLE 26-2. Selected Studies of Patients with Unresectable Meningiomas Treated with Radiation Therapy.

Ref. no.	No. of patients	Endpoint	Local control
14	32	5-/10-/15-yr DFS	53%/47%/47%
18	7	Crude tumor control	86%
24	44	Crude tumor control	93%
25	11	Crude rate of neurologic improvement	82%
26	19	4-yr PFS	64%
32	9	5-yr PFS	80%

Abbreviations: PFS, progression-free survival; DFS, disease-free survival.

TABLE 26-3. Selected Studies Comparing Radiation Therapy and Surgery Alone for Recurrent Meningioma.

Ref.	No. of patients		Endpoint	Local control	
	Surgery	RT		Surgery	RT
21	15	10	10-yr LC	30%	89%
22	18	16	8-yr PFS	11%	78%
32	0	14	5-yr PFS	N/A	73%
33	27	16	Crude tumor control	37%	50%
34	0	10	5-yr PFS	N/A	41%

Abbreviations: RT, radiation therapy; PFS, progression-free survival; LC, local control.

the reported 4-year PFS was 64%.[12] Maire et al. described the results of 91 patients with meningiomas (44 with unresectable disease) treated with megavoltage radiation therapy to a median dose of 52 Gy at conventional fractionation. A 1.0- to 1.5-cm margin was placed around the gross tumor volume. The median follow-up for the 91 patients was 40 months. Out of the 44 patients with unresectable disease treated with primary radiation therapy, at least 41 (93%) were progression-free.[10]

In the University of Florida series, out of 7 patients with unresectable meningioma treated with radiation therapy of 50–55 Gy, tumor control was obtained in 6 (86%).[3] In an older series, Carella et al. reported a crude survival rate of 100% in 11 patients with nonhistologically confirmed meningiomas treated with megavoltage radiation therapy of 55–60 Gy over 6–6.5 weeks. With follow-up times ranging from 3 to 6 years, of the 11 patients treated, 9 (82%) had improvement of neurologic status and 2 (18%) had stable symptoms.[11] Pourel et al. reported outcomes of 9 patients treated with fractionated radiation therapy for unresected meningiomas. With a median follow-up of 45 months, the 5-year PFS was 80%.[19]

Primary radiation therapy appears to be effective in the treatment of unresectable meningioma in terms of tumor control and symptomatic improvement. Those series with shorter follow-up periods tend to show higher PFS compared to those with longer follow-up. Table 26-2 summarizes the results of selected studies of patients with unresectable meningiomas treated with radiation therapy.

Radiation Therapy for Recurrent Meningiomas

Salvage radiation therapy is often offered to patients with unirradiated recurrent meningiomas, either alone for unresectable cases or after repeat resection, and it appears to be superior to surgery alone for salvage.

In the study from UCSF, 16 patients with recurrent meningiomas were treated with radiation therapy over a period of 30 years. Orthovoltage machines were used to deliver radiation therapy in the earlier years, and megavoltage radiation therapy was given after 1950. The radiation dose was 30–40 Gy in the orthovoltage era and 45–55 Gy in the megavoltage era.[20] Out of the 16 patients treated, 8 (50%) had successful salvage. Compared to surgery alone for salvage, radiation therapy with or without resection was associated with better tumor control. In an early series from the University of Florida, Taylor and colleagues reported the treatment outcomes of 10 patients with recurrent meningiomas treated with conventionally fractionated megavoltage radiation therapy with a dose of 50–63 Gy.[6] A margin of 2–4 cm was placed around the gross tumor. The 10-year local control rate was 89% compared to 30% in patients who were managed with surgery alone for salvage.[6] The local control associated with salvage radiation therapy was similar to patients who underwent immediate postoperative radiation therapy. The Kyoto University series included 20 patients treated with megavoltage radiation therapy for recurrent meningioma. A margin of 1–2 cm was used. Radiation dose ranged from 50 to 61.2 Gy. Ten tumors were benign, and the remaining tumors were either atypical or anaplastic. The corresponding 5-year PFS rates were 41 and 30%, respectively.[21] Pourel et al. reported a 5-year PFS rate of 73% after a median follow-up time of 35 months in 14 patients with recurrent meningioma treated with conventional radiation therapy.[19] Miralbell et al. reported an 8-year PFS rate of 78% in the 16 patients treated with radiation therapy (photons with or without protons) for recurrent meningiomas, and it was significantly better than patients treated with surgery alone as salvage therapy.[7]

Overall, the literature supports the use of radiation therapy for the treatment of previously unirradiated recurrent meningioma, and the treatment outcomes are better than those with salvage surgery alone. Table 26-3 summarizes the results of selected studies comparing surgery and radiation therapy in patients with recurrent meningiomas. There is some suggestion that patients treated with immediate or delayed postoperative radiation therapy for meningioma have similar tumor control.[6,18] The question arises as to whether radiation therapy can be delayed in patients with subtotally resected meningiomas. This would be best answered through a randomized trial.

Radiation Therapy for Optic Nerve Sheath Meningiomas

The overall goal of treatment of optic nerve sheath meningioma is to preserve or improve visual function and to prevent intracranial extension. Because pial blood vessels of the intraorbital and intracanalicular portions of the optic nerve are incorporated in the growth of optic nerve sheath meningiomas, it is not always possible to achieve complete resection of these tumors without causing optic nerve infarction.[22] As a result, surgery is associated with a high rate of blindness and is not routinely recommended. Data in the literature have demonstrated that fractionated radiation therapy can stabilize vision in patients with optic nerve sheath meningioma.

Smith et al. reported their early experience with five patients treated with fractionated radiation therapy for optic nerve sheath meningiomas. Out of the five patients treated, four (80%) experienced improvement of tumor-related symptoms 2–10 months after treatment.[23] There was no evidence of tumor progression in all the five patients treated after a follow-up interval of 3–48 months.[23] Kennerdell et al. reported the results of fractionated radiation therapy for optic nerve sheath meningiomas in six patients. The radiation dose given was 55 Gy using conventional fractionation. All of the six patients treated had visual deterioration caused by tumor before radiation therapy, and all of them experienced improvement in their visual symptoms after treatment after 30–84 months.[24] None of the patients had tumor shrinkage or progression after treatment. These results were better than those of patients in the same series managed by observation or surgical resection alone. In a later series that included the six patients in the above study, Turbin et al. reported the treatment outcomes of 59 patients with optic nerve sheath meningiomas whose vision was better than no light perception. These patients were managed with either observation ($n = 13$), surgery ($n = 12$), surgery with radiation ($n = 18$), or radiation alone ($n = 16$).[25] The mean follow-up time was 150 months (range: 51–516 months). Patients treated with radiation therapy received 40–55 Gy in conventional fractionation. Visual acuity deteriorated significantly for the patients who underwent observation only, who underwent surgery only, and who underwent surgery with radiation. Patients who had radiation therapy alone showed an insignificant decrease in visual acuity. The complication rate was 33.3% in patients who underwent radiation therapy alone, 66.7% in patients who underwent surgery alone, and 62.5% in patients underwent surgery and radiation therapy.[25] The radiographic progression rate was 11% for patients who underwent radiation therapy alone compared to 31%, 58, and 50% for patients who underwent observation, surgery alone, and surgery and radiation therapy. The authors concluded that fractionated radiation therapy should be the initial treatment in optic nerve sheath meningioma patients when preservation of visual function would be a therapeutic goal.

The series mentioned above are older studies where patients were treated using older techniques. Narayan et al. from the University of Michigan reported the visual outcomes of 14 patients with optic nerve sheath meningioma who were treated with three-dimensional conformal radiation therapy (3DCRT) to doses ranging from 50.4 to 56 Gy (median: 54 Gy). The planning treatment volume was a 1-cm expansion around the gross tumor volume (defined as contrast-enhancing tumor on MRI). With a median follow-up of 51.3 months, five patients (36%) had a clinically significant improvement in visual acuity. Seven patients (50%) had stable visual acuity and only two (14%) had worsened visual acuity.[26] Clinically significant visual field improvement occurred in nine patients (64%). None of the patients developed radiographic progression. In terms of complications, one patient developed early radiation retinopathy, one experienced orbital pain, one developed dry eye, and two developed iritis.

Primary radiation therapy appears to yield the best therapeutic ratio in the management of optic nerve sheath meningioma compared to observation or surgery with or without radiation therapy. Because of its proximity to the eye, optic nerve and eye adnexae, more advanced radiation therapy techniques may decrease the complication rate. This is discussed in the preceding chapter.

Radiation Therapy for Atypical and Anaplastic Meningiomas

Surgery is the mainstay treatment for atypical and anaplastic meningiomas. However, because of the aggressive nature of these tumor types, postoperative radiation therapy is often given after surgical resection to reduce the risk of tumor recurrence. Because of the small number of patients and the variation in pathologic classification, the data in the literature on atypical and anaplastic meningiomas are difficult to interpret. The variation in the extent of resection in different studies further hinders data interpretation.

In the University of California, San Francisco, series, out of the 140 patients with meningiomas who underwent subtotal resections followed by fractionated radiation therapy, 23 had either atypical or anaplastic meningiomas. The reported 5-year survival rate and PFS rates for this subgroup were 58 and 48%, respectively.[17] The authors concluded that patients should receive at least 53 Gy to yield better outcomes and should receive radiation therapy immediately after surgery. In the Princess Margaret Hospital series, the authors reported the outcomes of 59 patients with atypical and anaplastic lesions who were treated with fractionated radiation therapy. Immediate fractionated radiation therapy was associated with improved PFS, DFS, and overall survival.[27] The minimum radiation dose used was 50 Gy. A 3- to 4-cm margin around the tumor was used. Dziuk et al. reviewed the results of 38 patients with malignant meningiomas treated at Baylor College of Medicine. With follow-up times ranging from 3 to 144 months, the 5-year DFS was 39% after total resection compared to 0% after subtotal resection ($p = 0.001$). For patients who had complete tumor resection, the 5-year DFS increased from 28% for surgery alone to 57% with postoperative radiation therapy.[28] Postoperative radiation therapy increased the 5-year DFS from 15 to 80% ($p = 0.002$). Postoperative radiotherapy improved the 2-year DFS from 50 to 89% ($p = 0.015$), but had no impact on 5-year DFS for recurrent malignant meningiomas. On multivariate analysis, the extent of resection, postoperative radiation therapy, and recurrence status were identified to be independent prognostic factors.[28] In a French series, Pourel et al. reported a 100% recurrence rate in seven patients with atypical or malignant meningiomas within 24 months after radiation therapy.[19] The authors recommended immediate postoperative radiation therapy for patients with atypical and anaplastic meningiomas because of their poor prognosis. Goyal et al. reviewed the outcomes of the 22 patients with atypical meningiomas treated at Cleveland Clinic Foundation. With a median follow-up of 5.5 years, eight of the 22 patients developed local recurrence. Patients undergoing gross total resection had a higher 10-year local control rate than those who had either a subtotal resection or a resection of unknown extent (87% vs. 17%; $p = 0.02$).[29] On univariate analysis, postoperative radiation therapy was not a factor that impacted local control.

Data in the literature support the use of immediate postoperative radiation therapy for patients with anaplastic or malignant meningiomas regardless of the extent of resection. The role of radiation therapy for atypical meningiomas is less clear. It is reasonable to take several factors into consideration when deciding whether to offer postoperative radiation therapy; these factors include the extent of resection, the presence of brain invasion, MIB-1 index (<4.2% vs. ≥4.2%), and the number of mitosis per 10 high power field (closer to 4 vs. closer to 20).[30] The presence of any adverse factors in atypical meningioma is an indication for postoperative radiation therapy.

Radiation Therapy Techniques and Doses

Modern conventional radiation therapy entails three-dimensional treatment planning, which allows conformal radiation dose distribution easily (Fig. 26-1). To achieve this, the planner should avoid putting beams at the exit paths of other beams. More advanced radiation delivery was discussed in the preceding chapter. The gross tumor volume (GTV) is typically defined by the intense contrast enhancement on computed tomography (CT) or magnetic resonance imaging (MRI). In general, MRI is superior to CT for GTV delineation, but the latter may be used for target delineation for patients not suitable for MRI. MRI-defined GTV is usually larger than CT-defined GTV but may not be completely inclusive of the latter. If there is MRI-CT fusion capability, the composite GTV may be used.

Margins varying from 1 to 4 cm around the gross tumor volume have been used in various studies.[3,9,16,17] In the modern three-dimensional conformal radiation therapy era, with the availability of high-resolution MRI and image fusion capabilities, it is possible to decrease the treatment margins because WHO grade 1 or benign meningiomas have sharp margins of demarcation between the tumor and the normal brain parenchyma. A clinical target volume (CTV) expansion to account for microscopic disease is usually not needed for WHO grade 1 tumors. It is reasonable to put a 0.5-cm margin around the

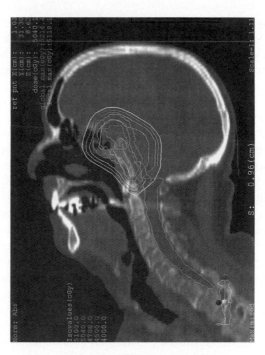

FIG. 26-1. Three-dimensional conformal radiation therapy plan for a skull base meningioma treated to a dose of 50.4 Gy in 28 fractions

GTV (tumor) to construct a planning treatment volume (PTV). A margin to account for the penumbra of the radiation beam is placed around the PTV. For WHO grade 2 (atypical) and grade 3 (anaplastic or malignant) tumors, a CTV expansion around the GTV (tumor) is needed to account for any possible microscopic disease, especially when there is brain invasion. If a WHO grade 2 or 3 tumor is completely resected, the surgical cavity or tumor bed becomes the CTV.

The recommended radiation doses for WHO grade 1 tumors and grade 2 and 3 tumors are 50.4–54 and 59.4 Gy, respectively. These recommendations are mainly based on the experience with these dose levels. A definite radiation dose response has not been demonstrated in meningioma. A recent dose escalation trial from Harvard University failed to show any difference in overall survival and local control between radiation doses of 55.8 cobalt gray equivalent (CGE) and 63 CGE.[31]

Radiation-Induced Toxicity

The acute toxicities associated with radiation therapy for intracranial meningiomas are usually well tolerated. Depending on the location of the tumor, those acute toxicities include fatigue, skin erythema, localized epilation, otitis externa, serous otitis media, and symptoms associated with raised intracranial pressure. Exacerbation of neurologic symptoms caused by the tumor is also possible. This can usually be ameliorated with the use of dexamethasone.

The late effects associated with radiation therapy depend on the location, the radiation dose delivered, and the radiation therapy technique used. Radiation-induced retinopathy and optic neuropathy could occur after radiation therapy for optic nerve sheath meningioma. If the ear is irradiated, hearing impairment and chronic otitis could occur. Other complications include hypopituitarism, radiation necrosis, memory deficit, and cognitive deficits. In the two largest meningioma series, the crude late complication rates were 2 and 3.6%, respectively.[9,17] Other series showed crude complication rates ranging from 0 to 16.7%.[6,7,12,18] Despite the fact that most of the patients treated in these series were treated prior to the 3DCRT era, the late complication rates were relatively low. With the advent of the current technology, the risk of complications should be further reduced. Advanced techniques are discussed in the preceding chapter.

Because of the close proximity of optic nerve sheath meningioma to the globe, optic nerve and the adnexae of the eye, the complication rates associated with conventional radiation therapy are typically higher than their counterparts in other locations. In the series by Turbin et al., 33% of the patients treated with radiation therapy alone developed major or permanent late complications.[25] Narayan et al. reported in their University of Michigan 3DCRT experience a complication rate of 36 % and all of them were eye (including eye adnexae) complications.[26] The eye complications could potentially be reduced utilizing advanced radiation techniques, which are discussed in the previous chapter.

Future Directions

Radiation therapy with or without surgery is an effective treatment for meningioma, especially for WHO grade 1 meningioma. However, the benefits of treatment have to be balanced against the potential resultant complications, which may affect patients' quality of life. With sophisticated treatment techniques such as intensity-modulated radiation therapy and fractionated stereotactic radiotherapy and new treatment modalities such as proton beam radiotherapy, the risk of treatment-related complications could potentially be decreased. These are covered in the previous chapter. Although postoperative radiation therapy typically improves PFS in patients with subtotally resected meningiomas, it does not impact overall survival. There are no randomized data comparing immediate and delayed radiation therapy for patients with subtotally resected meningiomas. To determine the optimal timing of postoperative radiation therapy, the European Organisation for Research and Treatment of Cancer (EORTC) is currently conducting a trial randomizing patients with subtotally resected or biopsied WHO grade 1 cerebral (excluding orbital) meningiomas to observation or postoperative radiation therapy or stereotactic radiosurgery (EORTC26021-22021). The primary endpoint of this study is the PFS. The secondary endpoints include quality of life, overall survival, the need for second surgery, acute neurotoxicity, and long-term neurotoxicity. Hopefully, this trial will provide us with more information on the optimal management of meningiomas.

References

1. Jaaskelainen J. Seemingly complete removal of histologically benign intracranial meningioma: late recurrence rate and factors predicting recurrence in 657 patients. A multivariate analysis. Surg Neurol 1986;26(5):461–9.
2. Mirimanoff RO, Dosoretz DE, Linggood RM, et al. Meningioma: analysis of recurrence and progression following neurosurgical resection. J Neurosurg 1985;62(1):18–24.
3. Condra KS, Buatti JM, Mendenhall WM, et al. Benign meningiomas: primary treatment selection affects survival. Int J Radiat Oncol Biol Phys 1997;39(2):427–36.
4. Levine ZT, Buchanan RI, Sekhar LN, Rosen CL, Wright DC. Proposed grading system to predict the extent of resection and outcomes for cranial base meningiomas. Neurosurgery 1999;45(2):221–30.
5. Barbaro NM, Gutin PH, Wilson CB, et al. Radiation therapy in the treatment of partially resected meningiomas. Neurosurgery 1987;20(4):525–8.
6. Taylor BW, Jr., Marcus RB, Jr., Friedman WA, et al. The meningioma controversy: postoperative radiation therapy. Int J Radiat Oncol Biol Phys 1988;15(2):299–304.
7. Miralbell R, Linggood RM, de la Monte S, et al. The role of radiotherapy in the treatment of subtotally resected benign meningiomas. J Neurooncol 1992;13(2):157–64.
8. Stafford SL, Perry A, Suman VJ, et al. Primarily resected meningiomas: outcome and prognostic factors in 581 Mayo Clinic patients, 1978 through 1988. Mayo Clin Proc 1998;73(10):936–42.
9. Glaholm J, Bloom HJ, Crow JH. The role of radiotherapy in the management of intracranial meningiomas: the Royal Marsden Hospital experience with 186 patients. Int J Radiat Oncol Biol Phys 1990;18(4):755–61.
10. Maire JP, Caudry M, Guerin J, et al. Fractionated radiation therapy in the treatment of intracranial meningiomas: local control, functional efficacy, and tolerance in 91 patients. Int J Radiat Oncol Biol Phys 1995;33(2):315–21.
11. Carella RJ, Ransohoff J, Newall J. Role of radiation therapy in the management of meningioma. Neurosurgery 1982;10(3):332–9.
12. Forbes AR, Goldberg ID. Radiation therapy in the treatment of meningioma: the Joint Center for Radiation Therapy experience 1970 to 1982. J Clin Oncol 1984;2(10):1139–43.
13. Melian E, Jay WM. Primary radiotherapy for optic nerve sheath meningioma. Semin Ophthalmol 2004;19(3–4):130–40.
14. Maier H, Ofner D, Hittmair A, et al. Classic, atypical, and anaplastic meningioma: three histopathological subtypes of clinical relevance. J Neurosurg 1992;77(4):616–23.
15. Jaaskelainen J, Haltia M, Servo A. Atypical and anaplastic meningiomas: radiology, surgery, radiotherapy, and outcome. Surg Neurol 1986;25(3):233–42.
16. Nutting C, Brada M, Brazil L, et al. Radiotherapy in the treatment of benign meningioma of the skull base. J Neurosurg 1999;90(5):823–7.
17. Goldsmith BJ, Wara WM, Wilson CB, et al. Postoperative irradiation for subtotally resected meningiomas. A retrospective analysis of 140 patients treated from 1967 to 1990. J Neurosurg 1994;80(2):195–201.
18. Soyuer S, Chang EL, Selek U, et al. Radiotherapy after surgery for benign cerebral meningioma. Radiother Oncol 2004;71(1):85–90.

19. Pourel N, Auque J, Bracard S, et al. Efficacy of external fractionated radiation therapy in the treatment of meningiomas: a 20-year experience. Radiother Oncol 2001;61(1):65–70.

20. Wara WM, Sheline GE, Newman H, et al. Radiation therapy of meningiomas. Am J Roentgenol Radium Ther Nucl Med 1975;123(3):453–8.

21. Kokubo M, Shibamoto Y, Takahashi JA, et al. Efficacy of conventional radiotherapy for recurrent meningioma. J Neurooncol 2000;48(1):51–5.

22. Dutton JJ. Optic nerve sheath meningiomas. Surv Ophthalmol 1992;37(3):167–83.

23. Smith JL, Vuksanovic MM, Yates BM, et al. Radiation therapy for primary optic nerve meningiomas. J Clin Neuroophthalmol 1981;1(2):85–99.

24. Kennerdell JS, Maroon JC, Malton M, et al. The management of optic nerve sheath meningiomas. Am J Ophthalmol 1988;106(4):450–7.

25. Turbin RE, Thompson CR, Kennerdell JS, et al. A long-term visual outcome comparison in patients with optic nerve sheath meningioma managed with observation, surgery, radiotherapy, or surgery and radiotherapy. Ophthalmology 2002;109(5):890–9; discussion 899–900.

26. Narayan S, Cornblath WT, Sandler HM, et al. Preliminary visual outcomes after three-dimensional conformal radiation therapy for optic nerve sheath meningioma. Int J Radiat Oncol Biol Phys 2003;56(2):537–43.

27. Milosevic MF, Frost PJ, Laperriere NJ, et al. Radiotherapy for atypical or malignant intracranial meningioma. Int J Radiat Oncol Biol Phys 1996;34(4):817–22.

28. Dziuk TW, Woo S, Butler EB, et al. Malignant meningioma: an indication for initial aggressive surgery and adjuvant radiotherapy. J Neurooncol 1998;37(2):177–88.

29. Goyal LK, Suh JH, Mohan DS, et al. Local control and overall survival in atypical meningioma: a retrospective study. Int J Radiat Oncol Biol Phys 2000;46(1):57–61.

30. Modha A, Gutin PH. Diagnosis and treatment of atypical and anaplastic meningiomas: a review. Neurosurgery 2005;57(3): 538–50.

31. Lopes VV, Chan A, Loeffler J, et al. A randomized radiation dose escalation trial in patients with recurrent or incompletely resected benign meningiomas treated with proton-photon irradiation. Int J Radiat Oncol Biol Phys 2003;57(suppl): S323–324.

27
Gamma Knife Surgery for Meningiomas

Jason Sheehan, Nader Pouratian, Charles A. Sansur, and Ladislau Steiner

Introduction

The Gamma Knife was developed and first built in the late 1960s as an alternative to open stereotactic lesioning for functional disorders. It has since become an indispensable neurosurgical tool used for the primary or adjuvant treatment of various intracranial pathologies. The Gamma Knife delivers a high dose of radiation in a single session to a stereotactically defined target by converging multiple beams of ionizing radiation. By creating a steep radiation dose fall-off around the target, radiation can be targeted to the lesion itself and damage to surrounding structures can be minimized. In part because of the limited scope of the pathology its treats (i.e., intracranial only), the Gamma Knife has become an extension of the neurosurgeon's therapeutic armamentarium.

For the treatment of meningiomas, there is no substitute at this time for extirpation. Indeed, numerous reports have confirmed that recurrence rates are directly related to the extent of resection. Gamma Knife surgery (GKS), and radiosurgery in general, therefore does not supplant open neurosurgical procedures. Rather, it allows safer treatment of meningiomas for which surgical resection is associated with exceedingly high rates of morbidity and mortality. The selection criteria for various treatments are not always clear and must be tailored to a patient's individual circumstances and expectations.

Pathophysiology of Gamma Knife Surgery

The Gamma Knife takes advantage of the natural difference in susceptibility of pathologic and normal tissue. The relative radioresistance of normal brain tissue relates to its low mitotic activity. The Gamma Knife further curtails injury to normal brain tissue by producing a rapid radiation fall-off and minimizing radiation to adjacent normal structures. The rate at which a total dose is applied is also important. A higher dose rate (same total dose applied over a shorter period of time or a larger dose in an equivalent amount of time) increases the lethality of a dose due to greater interference with intrinsic cellular repair mechanisms during irradiation. The significance of this effect is seen most clearly at a threshold dose rate of 1 Gy/min [1]. The normal tissue surrounding a target not only receives a markedly lower dose, but receives a lower dose rate as well.

In order to understand the radiobiology of a single high dose of radiation on normal brain, the effect of GKS on the normal parietal lobe of rats was studied. A dose of 50 Gy caused astrocytic swelling and fibrin deposition in capillary walls without changes in neuronal morphology or breakdown of the blood-brain barrier (BBB) at 12 months. At 75 Gy, more vigorous morphologic changes were seen in astrocytes within 4 months. In addition, necrosis, breakdown of the BBB, and hemispheric swelling were noted. At 120 Gy, astrocytic swelling occurred within 1 week of irradiation and necrosis was seen at 4 weeks, but it was not associated with hemispheric swelling [2].

By delivering the radiation dose in a single session, the Gamma Knife improves the effectiveness of the target dose by 2.5–3 times that of the same dose delivered in a fractionated manner. Although it is generally accepted that an increased effective radiation dose results in a greater rate of tumor control, little is really known about the pathophysiologic mechanisms of tumor control for Gamma Knife at the cellular level. Gamma Knife–mediated tumor control is due, at least in part, to radiation-induced DNA damage. Pathohistologic and imaging studies also suggest that GKS alters the microvascular supply of tumors. For example, reduced blood flow has been seen over time in meningiomas after GKS [3]. Early-responding tumors demonstrate the greatest reduction in blood flow. Other authors have proposed that the Gamma Knife may confer its effect by inducing apoptosis in proliferating cells [4,5]. It is noteworthy that the pathophysiologic effect of GKS does not seem to be tumor necrosis. For necrosis, higher doses than typically employed would be required.

Although an even dose distribution is an essential and basic concept in radiotherapy, there is some evidence that "hot spots" may be of benefit in GKS. When more than one isocenter is used to cover a target, the radiation dose distribution can become inhomogeneous. The resulting areas of local maxima are called "hot spots." Hot spots create islands of lethally injured cells that may enhance the cell kill in sublethal injury zones. Cells that are sublethally injured and are in the vicinity of lethally injured cells are more likely to undergo apoptosis than sublethally injured cells that are in the vicinity of other sublethally injured cells. Radiation geometry usually results in hot spots being located in the deep portions of the target. In tumors, this localization of hot spots may be particularly beneficial because this often corresponds to areas that receive the poorest blood supply and are therefore relatively hypoxic and less susceptible to radiation effects [6].

Although postulations regarding the pathophysiologic mechanisms of Gamma Knife may be speculative and premature, they may point the direction to future research.

Indications for Radiosurgery

Surgical resection of meningiomas has been the mainstay of treatment. Several compelling arguments favor surgery, including (1) seemingly difficult tumors can sometimes be removed safely; (2) surgery secures a tissue diagnosis; occasionally a tumor thought to be a meningioma on imaging is determined to be a different lesion; and (3) most meningiomas are benign tumors, and a "cure" can be achieved by complete resection. Advanced microsurgical and skull base surgical techniques have led to reduced morbidity and more thorough resections of meningiomas. Preoperative embolization has also led to decreased morbidity in select patients in whom the tumor blood supply may be difficult to access at the time of surgery [7]. Despite these advances, gross total resections, especially in the case of skull based meningiomas, tumors involving venous sinuses, and tumors with entwined cranial nerves, cannot always be accomplished without placing the patient at significant risk of morbidity and mortality. The goal of surgery should always be to preserve the quality of the patient's life, even if it means leaving residual tumor. Radiosurgery may therefore be utilized for patients with recurrent or residual meningiomas or as a primary treatment in patients with surgically inaccessible lesions that possess the typical imaging characteristics of meningiomas. Patients with atypical findings on magnetic resonance imaging (MRI) or computed tomography (CT) should undergo surgery to obtain a histologic diagnosis. This is critical because when GKS is used to treat tumors on imaging characteristics alone, the risk of an incorrect diagnosis may be as high as 2% [8].

Location plays a pivotal role in the selection of the appropriate treatment modality. Convexity meningiomas are usually treated with open surgery since they are amenable to complete resection. Skull base (including, for example, cavernous sinus and petroclival) and parasagittal meningiomas, on the other hand, are ideal lesions for radiosurgery due to their anatomy and associated surgical morbidity and mortality.

Skull base lesions are difficult to excise in their entirety without significant morbidity and mortality, especially cranial neuropathies and possible vascular injury. Many therefore opt to manage these tumors with subtotal resection followed by radiosurgery or radiosurgery alone. Subtotal resection may help to decompress important brain structures and yield a histologic diagnosis. Tumors within the parasellar compartment can be particularly difficult to remove with microsurgery without significant morbidity [9,10]. Residual tumor attached to still patent vascular or neural structures can be targeted with GKS, allowing less radical microsurgical resection and a lower incidence of morbidity. For GKS, a distance of at least 5 mm between the tumor and the optic apparatus is ideal. With a thin-cut stereotactic planning MRI and plugging (described in Methods section), GKS can be used to treat lesions within 2 mm of the optic apparatus. We tend to favor early treatment of skull base meningiomas rather than a "watch-and-wait" approach because of the favorable benefit to risk profile of radiosurgery.

Parasagittal meningiomas are challenging due to their association with the sagittal sinus and other major draining veins. If the sagittal sinus is occluded by the tumor, the tumor and the extent of the sinus involved can be completely resected. For those tumors with patent but partially invaded venous channels, especially in the middle or posterior third of the superior sagittal sinus, some tumor tissue must be left behind to avoid a venous infarction. Curative resection is rarely possible. While these residual tumors may be observed and repeat surgery performed once growth has occurred, the operative risk associated with repeat surgery is frequently higher than for the initial surgery. In patients with parasagittal meningiomas less than 3 cm in maximal diameter (<15 cc) and no progressive neurologic sequelae, radiosurgery is a reasonable first choice. For patients with larger lesions or those with progressive neurologic symptoms, resection followed by radiosurgery can be performed. Careful study of preoperative imaging helps determine if a staged approach (i.e., extirpation followed by radiosurgery) is necessary.

Methods

Perioperative Management

Although we have never had a patient have a seizure during therapy, the small but serious risk of a generalized seizure while the patient is secure within the Gamma Knife unit makes prophylaxis reasonable. We therefore place patients on a brief course of antiseizure medications prior to therapy. Patients are also empirically started on systemic steroids at the start of their therapy, and this is continued until the morning of postoperative day one. Although we have used steroids throughout our experience with GKS, their original purpose—to minimize vasogenic edema at the time of therapy—has never been documented as a problem. On the other hand, systemic steroids have proven indispensable in the event of the rare complication of edema after radiosurgical treatment of meningiomas.

Frame Placement and Imaging

The placement of the head frame is done in the operating room with monitered anesthesia. The patient is given intravenous sedation, usually short-acting narcotics (e.g., fentanyl) and propofol, until they are no longer responsive to verbal or moderate physical stimuli. Patients treated both before and since we have placed frames in the operating room have confirmed the preference for frame placement under anesthesia compared to the previous practice of frame placement using only local anesthetic. A simple strap with Velcro ends that is placed across the patient's head and fastened above the frame after it has been positioned appropriately obviates the needs for earplugs in the auditory canal, which can be painful. Care is taken to skew the placement of the frame in the direction of the pathology if it is far off the center of the brain. Care is also taken to not compress the ear against the frame for comfort.

After frame placement, a stereotactic contrast-enhanced MRI or CT is obtained since meningiomas are well visualized with contrast enhancement. For larger meningiomas, we also obtain a stereotactic angiogram, MR angiogram, or CT angiogram. This allows treatment to include the vascular supply when ideal treatment is not possible because of radiation dose constraints imposed by the treatment volume. The Heidelberg group proved that radiation occluded small nutrient vessels of meningiomas, providing the rationale for the treatment we have used since 1976.

Dose Planning and Selection

Dose planning is critical, especially in the case of skull base meningiomas in which the surgeon wants to avoid irradiating critical brain stem structures [11]. The dose must be planned so that the steepest isodose gradient of the dose distribution (usually between the 50 and 70% isodose lines) coincides with the periphery of the tumor. This may require several overlapping fields of radiation, each using a different collimator size and a separate stereotactic focal point. Changing the relative time of radiation at each target may also change the isodose distribution. Finally, the radiation field may be altered by blocking some of the radiation sources, also known as plugging. Plugging can be particularly useful in the treatment of skull base or parasellar meningiomas by creating an extremely steep dose gradient and thereby avoiding unnecessary radiation to the brain stem or cranial nerves. For larger tumors, staged treatment can also be considered.

Most groups, including our practice, use a prescription dose of 15–20 Gy [12,13]. In determining dose, one must consider not only tumor dose but also the radiation tolerance of adjacent structures, including cranial nerves and vasculature (discussed in Complications section). Lower doses of 13 or 14 Gy are therefore often used for treating cavernous sinus meningiomas due to the adjacency of critical structures, such as the optic apparatus. Some even argue that lower margin doses of 12 Gy afford the same degree of tumor control with a reduced risk of complications [14]. Unacceptably high rates of failure to control tumor growth have been reported with margin doses of 10 Gy or less [15].

Gamma Knife and Treatment

The Gamma Knife is comprised of a body that contains the radiation sources and a treatment couch that delivers the patient into the unit. Within the body are 201 Co^{60} source capsules, which are aligned with two internal collimators that direct the gamma radiation toward the center of the unit. A third external collimator helmet attaches to the treatment couch and the patient. The external collimator helmet is composed of 201 individual collimators that direct the gamma radiation to a common point of intersection, the isocenter. Each helmet is composed of fixed diameter apertures that create an isocenter of 4, 8, 14, or 18 mm diameter. The frame on the patient's head is fixed to the collimator helmet so that the area to be treated is at the isocenter.

The patient is positioned on the Gamma Knife couch, and the y and z coordinates for the first exposure are set on the head frame. The patient and the head frame are then secured within the collimator helmet and the x coordinate is set. At least two individuals, the operator and the person that sets the coordinates, confirm all settings. After confirming the exposure time, the entire couch is mechanically pulled into the body of the unit and the external collimator helmet locks into place with the internal collimators to commence treatment. After each exposure, the patient is withdrawn from the unit. The process is repeated for each isocenter.

At the end of the treatment, in the treatment suite, the frame is removed from the head by at least two people to prevent injury from the pins. Patients often report a sensation of tightening and discomfort during removal. Venous bleeding can usually be controlled with handheld pressure. Arterial bleeds can often be secured with an absorbable suture. The skin edges are opposed using steristrips for optimal cosmesis, and a modest head wrap is applied.

Results

In an initial report of GKS for meningiomas, the senior author had very limited enthusiasm for radiosurgical treatment of meningiomas [16]. However, over the years we have become more enthusiastic about GKS for meningiomas. Based upon experience, we no longer believe that "[m]icrosurgery should precede radiosurgery, and only in exceptional cases, such as old age or illness precluding surgery, should radiosurgery be a primary treatment of meningiomas" [16]. The indications for GKS of meningiomas have increased dramatically. This change in attitude is based upon the generally safe and effective application of radiosurgery for the treatment of meningiomas.

We have treated 329 meningiomas at the University of Virginia since 1989. The most recent evaluation of our material included 206 patients with meningiomas treated with GKS with a follow-up of 1–6 years. This included 142 patients treated for residual disease and 64 patients treated with GKS primarily. Tumor volume ranged from 1 to 32 cm³. These patients received an average of 38 Gy maximum dose (range 20–60 Gy) and an average margin dose of 14 Gy (range 10–20 Gy). Radiographic follow-up was available for 151 patients. Of the evaluated patients, 94 patients (63%) showed a volume decrease of at least 15% and 40 patients (26%) showed no change in size, corresponding to an 89% tumor control rate. Tumor growth was noted in 17 patients (11%). We now have long-term follow-up of 10–21 years in 31 meningiomas treated with GKS. Two thirds of these tumors have either shrunk significantly or remained stable. Among these were cases where only the vascular supply for the tumor (i.e., the nutritive vessel) was targeted. This has resulted in significant tumor shrinkage and lasting effect even in the long term.

The results of other centers are similar [8,16–21] (see Table 27-1). The University of Pittsburgh group recently reported long-term results in 85 patients whose meningiomas were treated with GKS. With a median follow-up of 10 years, they reported 53% of the tumors decreased in size and 40% were stable in size, corresponding to a 93% tumor control rate [22]. Kreil and colleagues similarly reported on 200 patients treated with GKS for meningiomas with a median follow-up of 7.9 years, finding that 56.5% of meningiomas demonstrated a decreased volume and 42.5% showed stable tumor volumes on follow-up [14]. Pollock and colleagues compared the efficacy of GKS with that of microsurgery for the treatment of meningiomas with an average diameter less than 35 mm. They concluded that progression-free survival after radiosurgery is equivalent to that after resection of a Simpson grade 1 tumor

and was superior to that after Simpson grade 2, 3, or 4 resections, confirming the efficacy of GKS, especially in tumors in which gross total resection is difficult to achieve due to anatomic constraints [23].

Skull Base Meningiomas

Outcomes for Gamma Knife treatment of skull base meningiomas have been reported extensively. At the Karolinska Hospital between 1987 and 1993, 40 patients with skull base meningiomas were treated with GKS with a median prescription dose of 16 Gy. Outcomes were assessed in these patients after a median follow-up of 9 years, revealing that tumor control was achieved in 87% of cases, including reductions in tumor volume in 33% of cases. Neurologic complications were observed in 11% of patients and tended to occur in those patients who received more than 20 Gy to the optic apparatus. Fewer complications were noted when more modern threshold doses for sensitive structures were administered. These tumor control rates are consistent with those published by other groups treating skull base meningiomas using GKS. Most reports have a median follow-up of approximately 3 years and report tumor control rates between 91 and 100%, with tumor shrinkage reported in 23–73% of treated skull base meningiomas [18,24–26].

Outcomes with respect to specific types of skull base meningiomas have also been reported (Figs. 27-1 and 27-2). The efficacy of GKS for treatment of petroclival meningiomas is similar to outcomes in other meningiomas. Subach and colleagues followed 62 patients who had petroclival meningiomas treated with GKS for a median of 37 months: 23% of the tumors decreased in volume, 68% demonstrated stable tumor volumes, and 8% grew [26]. Five patients (8%) experienced new cranial nerve palsies within 24 months of treatment, two of which resolved within 6 months. Roche and colleagues also specifically reported outcomes in petroclival meningiomas and

TABLE 27-1. Outcome of Radiosurgery for Meningiomas.

Author (year)	N	Follow-up (months)	Size Decrease (%)	Stable (%)	Increase (%)	Complications (%)	Improved (%)
Kondziolka (1991)[21]	50	12–36	54	38	2	6	—
Pendl (1997)[25]	97	48	39	56	5	5	—
Liscak (1999)[20]	67	2–60	52	48	0	4	36
Roche (2000)[19]	80	12–79	31	64	5	4	26
Lee (2002)[27]	159	2–145	34	60	6	7	29
Nicolato (2002)[17]	122	>12	61	36	3	3	—
Roche (2003)[18]	32	28–188	12	88	—	6	41
Kondziolka (2003)[22]	85	120	53	40	7	6	—
Flickinger (2003)[8]	219	2–164	—	—	3	5	—
Liscak (2004)[24]	176	36	73	25	2	15.5	63
Kreil (2005)[14]	200	60–144	57	42	2	3	42
Malik (2005)[30]	277	39	—	—	12	3–7	—
Pollock (2005)[13]	49	58	59	41	—	24	53
Steiner*	151	6–252	63	26	11	0	8

*Represents the series reported in this chapter.

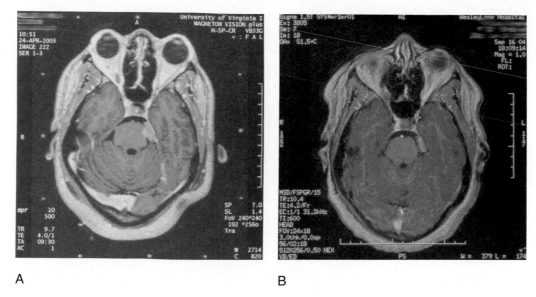

A   B

FIG. 27-1. (A) The patient is a 30-year-old woman with numbness in the left side of her face. An MRI revealed a left superior petrous meningioma with a volume of 2.7 cc. (B) Eighteen months post-GKS, the patient's tumor had markedly decreased in volume to only 0.5 cc

found that in 32 patients followed from 24 to 118 months, tumor control was achieved in 100% of patients but clinical status declined in 1 patient (4%) due to pontine infarction [18]. In the case of petroclival meningiomas, patients with large meningiomas with significant ventral brain stem compression are more susceptible to complications of treatment.

The efficacy of GKS for the treatment of cavernous sinus meningiomas has also been studied and characterized extensively (Fig. 27-3). Our series of 206 patients with follow-up included 112 patients with meningiomas involving the cavernous sinus. In 68% the tumor either disappeared or decreased

in volume, in 30% the tumors were unchanged on imaging, and in 2% they enlarged. Petroclival meningiomas involving the cavernous sinus were not included in this series and are to be evaluated in the future. Many groups have consistently reported excellent control rates of cavernous sinus meningiomas. Pollock and Stafford reported a 100% control rate in 49 patients with cavernous sinus meningiomas with a median follow-up of 58 months after GKS [13]. Similarly, Liscak and colleagues, who followed 67 patients between 2 and 60 months, reported a 100% tumor control rate (52% decrease in volume and 48% unchanged) [20]. Nicolato and colleagues

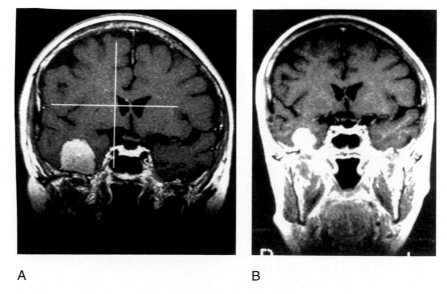

A   B

FIG. 27-2. (A) The patient is a 71-year-old woman who presented with headaches. Her preoperative MRI revealed a 9.6 cc right middle cranial fossa meningioma. (B) Five years following gamma knife surgery, the tumor had decreased in volume to 5.5 cc

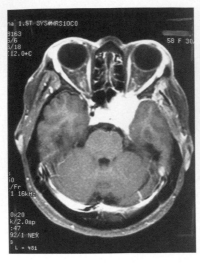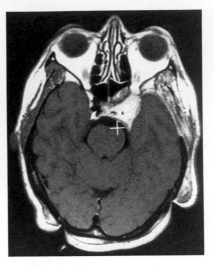

A   B

FIG. 27-3. (A) The patient presented with a history of progressive visual impairment in the left eye. An MRI obtained prior to GKS reveals a left cavernous sinus meningioma. The patient was status-post a microsurgical resection. The tumor volume was 11.3 cc. (B) An MRI obtained 5 years post-GKS reveals a marked reduction in the size of the tumor. At the time of this film, the tumor volume measured 7.8 cc

reported 98% tumor growth control in 156 patients they treated with GKS for cavernous sinus meningiomas with a median follow-up 49 months [17]. Additionally, they reported that clinical conditions were improved or stable in 97% of the 156 patients. Roche followed 92 patients who were treated with GKS for cavernous sinus meningiomas with a median follow-up of 30.5 months and found a 95% control rate [19]. The University of Pittsburgh group has similarly reported a 94% long-term tumor control rate [27].

Parasagittal Meningiomas Outcomes

Parasagittal meningiomas typically enjoy a similar response rate to GKS as other meningiomas in other locations. In a multicenter study of 203 patients with parasagittal meningiomas, the 5-year actuarial tumor control rate was 93% ± 4% for those who had radiosurgery as a primary therapy and 60% ± 10% for those who had upfront surgery [28]. The overall radiosurgical tumor control rate was 85% [28].

Atypical and Malignant Meningioma Outcomes

Atypical and malignant meningiomas usually demonstrate recurrence and aggressive growth regardless of the treatment modality (i.e., extirpation, radiosurgery, or radiation therapy). While GKS appears to work very well for benign meningiomas, the results for atypical and malignant meningiomas are less favorable. In a study from the University of Pittsburgh, Harris and colleagues reported 5-year progression-free survival rates of 83 and 72% for atypical and malignant meningiomas, respectively [29]. Kreil and colleagues reported less favorable results, reporting 5-year actuarial control rate of 49% in atypical meningiomas and 0% in malignant meningiomas

[30]. Ojemann and colleagues' results were similar to that of Kreil's report; they reported a 5-year progression-free survival of 26% in patients with malignant meningiomas treated with GKS, although outcomes were better in smaller sized tumors and in young patients [31]. Survival rates, as opposed to control rates, have also been reported for patients after GKS of atypical and malignant meningiomas. Five-year overall survival rates vary between 59 and 76% in patients with atypical meningiomas and 0 and 59% in patients with malignant meningiomas [29,31,32].

Radiation-Induced Meningioma Outcomes

It is well known that fractionated radiation therapy can induce meningiomas. The incidence of radiation-induced tumors following fractionated radiation therapy is 1.9% in 20 years. Some centers, including our own, have had limited yet favorable early experience with radiosurgical treatment of radiation-induced tumors. For example, the Mayo Clinic group recently reported a 100% 5-year local tumor control rate for 16 patients with radiation-induced tumors [33]. The median follow-up from the Mayo Clinic report was only 40.2 months. Although it is too early to know if such an approach is prudent, the concept of treating radiation-induced meningiomas with radiosurgery may have some interesting implications regarding the pathogenesis of intracranial tumors.

Clinical Outcomes

Many patients who present for management of meningiomas, especially skull base lesions, present with neurologic deficits, such as cranial nerve dysfunction. It is therefore important to evaluate outcomes with respect not only to tumor control but also to clinical outcomes. Gamma Knife surgery is regularly reported to be associated with improved cranial nerve function after treatment of skull base meningiomas. Pollock and colleagues, for example, reported that 12 out of 38 patients who presented with cranial neuropathies associated with cavernous sinus meningiomas had improvement in cranial nerve function on follow-up [13]. Roche and colleagues also reported on clinical outcomes in patients with cavernous sinus meningiomas treated with Gamma Knife. They reported that 23 of 54 patients with oculomotor palsies either improved or completely recovered, and 7 of 13 patients with trigeminal neuralgia improved or completely recovered [19]. Roche and colleagues reported similar success in Gamma Knife–treated petroclival meningiomas: 13 out of 32 patients treated with GKS for petroclival meningiomas had clinical improvement in cranial nerve dysfunction [18]. Kreil and colleagues reported that 96% of patients with skull base meningiomas treated with Gamma Knife had improved or stable neurologic status, with improvement noted in a broad range of areas, including vision and other cranial nerve functions, hemiparesis, ataxia, vertigo, seizures, and exophthalmus [14].

Factors Predicting Favorable Tumor Response

In addition to tumor grade, several other factors have also been implicated in improved outcomes. DiBiase and colleagues reported on imaging follow-up in 121 patients with a median follow-up of 4.5 years, reporting a 91.7% control rate and growth in 8.3% of tumors. They found that more effective treatment (i.e., greater disease-free survival and overall survival) was associated with tumor volumes less than 10.0 cc, female gender, a high conformality index, and dural tail inclusion in the treatment plan [34]. Kondziolka additionally notes that local tumor progression after radiosurgery was related to a history of prior resection and a history of multiple meningiomas [12]. Unlike the former study, they did not find a significant effect of patient age, margin dose, isodose, or tumor volume on tumor response.

Complications

All neurosurgical procedures, including GKS, have associated complications. The overall rate of complications with GKS of meningiomas is low (5–10%) and includes cranial neuropathies (accounting for the majority of the morbidity), vascular injuries (including, for example, carotid artery stenosis), posttreatment edema, cyst formation, and induction of new tumors [12,34,35]. Cranial neuropathies, accounting for approximately 75% of the overall 8.4% rate of complications reported by Pollock and colleagues, include, in order of decreasing frequency, trigeminal, abducens, optic, oculomotor,

facial, and vestibulocochlear palsies [35]. In long-term follow-up of 200 patients, Kreil and colleagues reported only one case of visual deterioration, one case of transient oculomotor palsy, and two cases of transient trigeminal neuralgia [14]. Malik and colleagues reported a similar rate of cranial neuropathies (7%), including involvement of the oculomotor, trigeminal, and facial nerves [30]. In our experience, we have had no long-term morbidity associated with GKS of meningiomas. However, a tumor without histologic diagnosis and with equivocal imaging characteristics in the pineal region was treated as a presumed meningioma, and bilateral edema of the basal ganglia occurred. This resulted in cognitive disturbances with incomplete recovery.

Cranial Neuropathies

Cranial nerve radiation tolerance is dependent upon the particular nerve and individual nerve involvement by the pathologic process requiring treatment. Of all the cranial nerves, the optic and acoustic nerves are the most sensitive to radiation. Their vulnerability is likely attributable to being central nervous system tracts, containing oligodendrocytes, carrying complex information, and their inability to regenerate after injury. Recommendations for upper limits of radiation to the optic apparatus range from 8 to 14.1 Gy [36–40], although optic neuropathy has been reported following a single 8 Gy dose [41]. Lee and colleagues found ~2% rate of visual deterioration after GKS of cavernous sinus meningiomas. After observing these complications, they recalculated optic nerve doses and found that the average dose to the nerve was 12 Gy [27]. In our practice, we make every effort to limit the dose to 8 Gy. Small volumes of the optic apparatus exposed to doses of 10 Gy or less may be acceptable in some cases [42,43]. Patient-to-patient variability likely depends on the extent of damage to the optic apparatus by tumor compression, ischemic changes, type and timing of previous interventions (e.g., fractionated radiation therapy and surgery), the patient's age, and the presence or absence of other co-morbidities (e.g., diabetes) [42,44].

The trigeminal and facial nerves, on the other hand, are more resilient. Accordingly, Kreil and colleagues reported two cases of GKS-induced trigeminal neuralgia (TN), but both were transient in nature [14]. The radiation tolerance of these nerves is best understood by comparing the incidence of neuropathies after GKS for trigeminal neuralgia (in which a small part of the nerve is treated with a high dose) with that seen after GKS for vestibular schwanommas (in which a longer length of the nerve is treated with a relatively low dose). In the treatment of TN, only one case of mild facial hypoesthesia was reported after treating 50–100 mm^3 of the trigeminal root entry zone treated with 60–80 Gy [45]. We have observed nine mild to profound hypoesthesias in trigeminal neuralgia patients treated with Gamma Knife doses of 50–90 Gy. In a larger group of small vestibular schwanommas treated with Gamma Knife with periphery doses of

10–25 Gy, the incidence of facial hypoesthesia was 19%. In the same 254 patients the incidence of facial paresis was 17%, although this was transient in all instances. The increased risk of neuropathy after treatment for vestibular schwanommas suggests that the length of nerve exposed to radiation might be the critical determinant for whether or not a cranial neuropathy develops.

The cranial nerves in the cavernous sinus are relatively robust and less susceptible to adverse radiation effects [14,37,43,46,47]. Neuropathies have not been seen with doses up to 40 Gy [37]. Pollock and Stafford reported 49 patients treated with GKS for cavernous sinus meningiomas and reported that 5 patients had new or worsened trigeminal dysfunction and one patient had new oculomotor palsy; it is unclear whether this is due to radiation effects or tumor progression [13]. On the other hand, 12 of 38 patients reported improvements in cranial nerve function. In our series of over 350 pituitary adenomas treated with GKS, 8 cases of cranial nerve palsies have been identified. The incidence of new cranial nerve palsies after GKS of sellar and parasellar lesions is concerning and warrants further investigation into the radiation tolerance of the contents of the cavernous sinus. We have not observed any neuropathies of CN IX–XII following GKS.

Vascular Injury and Carotid Artery Stenosis

Pollock and Stafford have documented ICA stenosis or occlusion in four patients after GKS (two with meningiomas and two with pituitary adenomas) [13]. Five other cases of carotid artery stenosis have been reported after Gamma Knife treatment of meningiomas. Patients were symptomatic in only two of these cases [19,48–50]. In our treatment of skull base meningiomas and pituitary adenomas with cavernous sinus extension, we have not observed any incidences of vascular stenosis or occlusion. This absence of stenosis is noted even though the internal carotid artery or portions of the circle of Willis, or its proximal branches, are often included in the treatment field. It is possible that the incidence of occlusion of smaller vessels is more common than recognized as the occlusion would occur slowly and compensatory changes could take place, preventing clinical syndromes from occurring. Regardless, the clinical impact is minimal.

Although Gamma Knife–related injury to the carotid and other arteries is rare, many have recommended limiting the dose to the carotid artery when possible. Pollock and colleagues have recommended that the prescription dose should be limited to less than 50% of the intracavernous carotid artery vessel diameter [49]. Shin and colleagues recommended restricting the dose to the internal carotid artery to less than 30 Gy [51].

Edema

Symptomatic perilesional edema after GKS has been reported in as few as 1% of patients [14] and as many as 25%

of patients [52]. In general, when it occurs, patients complain of severe headache and can be managed effectively with oral corticosteroids. Symptoms generally occur 1–6 months after treatment. The mechanism of edema formation is unclear, but studies consistently conclude that edema formation is far less likely in posterior fossa lesions [24]. On the contrary, edema is much more likely to occur in the setting of a parasagittal or superficially located meningioma [53,54]. Kondziolka and colleagues, in a multicenter study of parasagittal meningiomas, found a 3- and 5-year actuarial risk of developing symptomatic cerebral edema of 16% [28]. Another study reported that perilesional edema has been identified in up to 48% of patients who had superficially located meningiomas [55]. The anatomic distribution of post–Gamma Knife edema has led many to conclude that edema formation may be dependent on vascular anatomy and induction of vascular disturbances by the Gamma Knife. Patients with a history of pretreatment perilesional edema are at increased risk of developing symptomatic edema after treatment [54,56]. While it is difficult to predict who will develop such perilesional edema, many studies indicate that limiting the margin dose to 14 or 18 Gy may reduce the risk of edema.

Cyst Formation

Symptomatic cyst formation has also been reported after Gamma Knife of meningiomas in approximately 1–3 % of cases [32,57]. Shuto and colleagues, reporting on a series of 160 patients with 184 tumors whom they followed for 2 years, found new cyst formation in 5 tumors (one sphenoid ridge tumor, two petroclival tumors, one tentorial tumor, and one parasagittal meningioma) [57]. All affected patients had undergone prior surgery. Two patients had preoperative cysts that were exacerbated by GKS, and three had de novo cyst formation. Three of these patients required surgery secondary to symptomatic cyst formation [57]. The pathogenesis of post-irradiation cysts is not well understood but is assumed to be multifactorial and has been attributed to degenerative and secretory changes, radiation-induced ischemic necrosis, and intratumoral hemorrhage [57].

New Tumors

Radiation-induced tumors are a known complication of both fractionated radiotherapy and radiosurgery, although greater with the former. Two cases of glioblastoma multiforme have been reported after GKS for meningiomas [58,59]. Given the total number of meningiomas treated with GKS, this is an extremely rare event and should not necessarily temper the use of GKS in cases which GKS is indicated. We have observed two cases of radiation-induced meningiomas after Gamma Knife surgery of arteriovenous malformations in a total of 288 arteriovenous malformation patients with more than 10 years of neuroimaging follow-up.

Conclusions

The advantage of histologic diagnosis, debulking, and a chance of cure secures surgical extirpation as the procedure of choice for meningiomas. The ability of GKS to effectively treat small tumors with low morbidity argues strongly for minimizing morbidity during open procedures. This is especially true in locations where complete meningeal resection is impossible and thus the chance of recurrence is high. The option to treat residual tumor in critical or hard to reach locations should temper the ambition of total surgical removal. The tumors most amenable to GKS are less than 10–15 cm^3 in volume. The effectiveness of the therapy is most dependent upon the ability to define and treat the entire lesion. However, the desired result can also be obtained at times by treating the nutritive or feeding vessels of tumors (e.g., meningiomas).

References

1. Hall EJ, Marchese M, Hei TK, Zaider M. Radiation response characteristics of human cells in vitro. Radiat Res 1988;114:415–24.
2. Kamiryo T, Kassell NF, Thai QA, et al. Histological changes in the normal rat brain after gamma irradiation. Acta Neurochir (Wien) 1996;138:451–9.
3. Hawighorst H, Engenhart R, Knopp MV, et al. Intracranial meningeomas: time- and dose-dependent effects of irradiation on tumor microcirculation monitored by dynamic mr imaging. Magn Reson Imaging 1997;15:423–32.
4. Tsuzuki T, Tsunoda S, Sakaki T, et al. Tumor cell proliferation and apoptosis associated with the gamma knife effect. Stereotact Funct Neurosurg 1996;66(Suppl 1):39–48.
5. Marekova M, Cap J, Vokurkova D, et al. Effect of therapeutic doses of ionising radiation on the somatomammotroph pituitary cell line, gh3. Endocr J 2003;50:621–8.
6. Hopewell JW, Wright EA. The nature of latent cerebral irradiation damage and its modification by hypertension. Br J Radiol 1970;43:161–7.
7. Engelhard HH. Progress in the diagnosis and treatment of patients with meningiomas. Part I: Diagnostic imaging, preoperative embolization. Surg Neurol 2001;55:89–101.
8. Flickinger JC, Kondziolka D, Maitz AH, Lunsford LD. Gamma knife radiosurgery of imaging-diagnosed intracranial meningioma. Int J Radiat Oncol Biol Phys 2003;56:801–6.
9. Parkinson D. Lateral sellar compartment o.T. (cavernous sinus): history, anatomy, terminology. Anat Rec 1998;251:486–90.
10. Parkinson D. Extradural neural axis compartment. J Neurosurg 2000;92:585–8.
11. Rowe JG, Walton L, Vaughan P, et al. Radiosurgical planning of meningiomas: compromises with conformity. Stereotact Funct Neurosurg 2004;82:169–74.
12. Kondziolka D, Levy EI, Niranjan A, et al. Long-term outcomes after meningioma radiosurgery: physician and patient perspectives. J Neurosurg 1999;91:44–50.
13. Pollock BE, Stafford SL. Results of stereotactic radiosurgery for patients with imaging defined cavernous sinus meningiomas. Int J Radiat Oncol Biol Phys 2005;62:1427–31.
14. Kreil W, Luggin J, Fuchs I, et al. Long term experience of gamma knife radiosurgery for benign skull base meningiomas. J Neurol Neurosurg Psychiatry 2005;76:1425–30.
15. Ganz JC, Backlund EO, Thorsen FA. The results of gamma knife surgery of meningiomas, related to size of tumor and dose. Stereotact Funct Neurosurg 1993;61(Suppl 1):23–9.
16. Steiner L, Lindquist C, Steiner M. Meningiomas and gamma knife surgery. In: Al-Mefty O, ed., Meningiomas. New York: Raven Press, 1991:263–72.
17. Nicolato A, Foroni R, Alessandrini F, et al. Radiosurgical treatment of cavernous sinus meningiomas: experience with 122 treated patients. Neurosurgery 2002;51:1153–9; discussion 1159–61.
18. Roche PH, Pellet W, Fuentes S, et al. Gamma knife radiosurgical management of petroclival meningiomas results and indications. Acta Neurochir (Wien) 2003;145:883–8; discussion 888.
19. Roche PH, Regis J, Dufour H, et al. Gamma knife radiosurgery in the management of cavernous sinus meningiomas. J Neurosurg 2000;93(Suppl 3):68–73.
20. Liscak R, Simonova G, Vymazal J, et al. Gamma knife radiosurgery of meningiomas in the cavernous sinus region. Acta Neurochir (Wien) 1999;141:473–80.
21. Kondziolka D, Lunsford LD, Coffey RJ, Flickinger JC. Stereotactic radiosurgery of meningiomas. J Neurosurg 1991;74:552–9.
22. Kondziolka D, Nathoo N, Flickinger JC, et al. Long-term results after radiosurgery for benign intracranial tumors. Neurosurgery 2003;53:815–21; discussion 821–2.
23. Pollock BE, Stafford SL, Utter A, et al. Stereotactic radiosurgery provides equivalent tumor control to simpson grade 1 resection for patients with small- to medium-size meningiomas. Int J Radiat Oncol Biol Phys 2003;55:1000–5.
24. Liscak R, Kollova A, Vladyka V, et al. Gamma knife radiosurgery of skull base meningiomas. Acta Neurochir Suppl 2004;91:65–74.
25. Pendl G, Schrottner O, Eustacchio S, et al. Stereotactic radiosurgery of skull base meningiomas. Minim Invasive Neurosurg 1997;40:87–90.
26. Subach BR, Lunsford LD, Kondziolka D, et al. Management of petroclival meningiomas by stereotactic radiosurgery. Neurosurgery 1998;42:437–43; discussion 443–5.
27. Lee JY, Niranjan A, McInerney J, et al. Stereotactic radiosurgery providing long-term tumor control of cavernous sinus meningiomas. J Neurosurg 2002;97:65–72.
28. Kondziolka D, Flickinger JC, Perez B. Judicious resection and/or radiosurgery for parasagittal meningiomas: Outcomes from a multicenter review. Gamma knife meningioma study group. Neurosurgery 1998;43:405–13; discussion 413–4.
29. Harris AE, Lee JY, Omalu B, et al. The effect of radiosurgery during management of aggressive meningiomas. Surg Neurol 2003;60:298–305.
30. Malik I, Rowe JG, Walton L, et al. The use of stereotactic radiosurgery in the management of meningiomas. Br J Neurosurg 2005;19:13–20.
31. Ojemann SG, Sneed PK, Larson DA, et al. Radiosurgery for malignant meningioma: results in 22 patients. J Neurosurg 2000;93(Suppl 3):62–7.
32. Stafford SL, Pollock BE, Foote RL, et al. Meningioma radiosurgery: tumor control, outcomes, and complications among 190 consecutive patients. Neurosurgery 2001;49:1029–37; discussion 1037–8.

33. Jensen AW, Brown PD, Pollock BE, et al. Gamma knife radio-surgery of radiation-induced intracranial tumors: local control, outcomes, and complications. Int J Radiat Oncol Biol Phys 2005;62:32–7.

34. DiBiase SJ, Kwok Y, Yovino S, et al. Factors predicting local tumor control after gamma knife stereotactic radiosurgery for benign intracranial meningiomas. Int J Radiat Oncol Biol Phys 2004;60:1515–9.

35. Pollock BE. Stereotactic radiosurgery for intracranial meningiomas: indications and results. Neurosurg Focus 2003;14:e4.

36. Ove R, Kelman S, Amin PP, Chin LS. Preservation of visual fields after peri-sellar gamma-knife radiosurgery. Int J Cancer 2000;90:343–50.

37. Tishler RB, Loeffler JS, Lunsford LD, et al. Tolerance of cranial nerves of the cavernous sinus to radiosurgery. Int J Radiat Oncol Biol Phys 1993;27:215–21.

38. Girkin CA, CH C, Lunsford LD, et al. Radiation optic neuropathy after stereotactic radiosurgery. Ophthalmology 1997;104: 1634–43.

39. Stafford SL, Pollock BE, Leavitt JA, et al. A study on the radiation tolerance of the optic nerves and chiasm after stereotactic radiosurgery. Int J Radiat Oncol Biol Phys 2003;55:1177–81.

40. Chen JC, Giannotta SL, Yu C, et al. Radiosurgical management of benign cavernous sinus tumors: Dose profiles and acute complications. Neurosurgery 2001;48:1022–30; discussion 1030–2.

41. Tishler RB, Loeffler JS, Lunsford LD, et al. Tolerance of cranial nerves of the cavernous sinus to radiosurgery. Int J Radiat Oncol Biol Phys 1993;27:215–21.

42. Lundstrom M, Frisen L. Atrophy of optic nerve fibres in compression of the chiasm. Degree and distribution of ophthalmoscopic changes. Acta Ophthalmol (Copenh) 1976;54:623–40.

43. Leber KA, Bergloff J, Pendl G. Dose-response tolerance of the visual pathways and cranial nerves of the cavernous sinus to stereotactic radiosurgery. J Neurosurg 1998;88:43–50.

44. Rodriguez O, Mateos B, de la Pedraja R, et al. Postoperative follow-up of pituitary adenomas after trans-sphenoidal resection: MRI and clinical correlation. Neuroradiology 1996;38:747–54.

45. Noren G, Greitz D, Hirsch A, Lax I. Gamma knife surgery in acoustic tumours. Acta Neurochir Suppl (Wien) 1993;58:104–7.

46. Duma CM, Lunsford LD, Kondziolka D, et al. Stereotactic radiosurgery of cavernous sinus meningiomas as an addition or alternative to microsurgery. Neurosurgery 1993;32:699–704; discussion 704–5.

47. Jackson IM, Noren G. Role of gamma knife radiosurgery in acromegaly. Pituitary 1999;2:71–7.

48. Muramatsu J, Yoshida M, Shioura H, et al. [Clinical results of linac-based stereotactic radiosurgery for pituitary adenoma]. Nippon Igaku Hoshasen Gakkai Zasshi 2003;63:225–30.

49. Pollock BE, Nippoldt TB, Stafford SL, et al. Results of stereotactic radiosurgery in patients with hormone-producing pituitary adenomas: Factors associated with endocrine normalization. J Neurosurg 2002;97:525–30.

50. Lim YL, Leem W, Kim TS, et al. Four years' experiences in the treatment of pituitary adenomas with gamma knife radiosurgery. Stereotact Funct Neurosurg 1998;70(Suppl 1):95–109.

51. Shin M, Kurita H, Sasaki T, et al. Stereotactic radiosurgery for pituitary adenoma invading the cavernous sinus. J Neurosurg 2000;93(Suppl 3):2–5.

52. Singh VP, Kansai S, Vaishya S, et al. Early complications following gamma knife radiosurgery for intracranial meningiomas. J Neurosurg 2000;93(Suppl 3):57–61.

53. Chang JH, Chang JW, Choi JY, et al. Complications after gamma knife radiosurgery for benign meningiomas. J Neurol Neurosurg Psychiatry 2003;74:226–30.

54. Ganz JC, Schrottner O, Pendl G. Radiation-induced edema after gamma knife treatment for meningiomas. Stereotact Funct Neurosurg 1996;66(Suppl 1):129–33.

55. Kim DG, Kim Ch H, Chung HT, et al. Gamma knife surgery of superficially located meningioma. J Neurosurg 2005;102(Suppl): 255–8.

56. Kalapurakal JA, Silverman CL, Akhtar N, et al. Intracranial meningiomas: factors that influence the development of cerebral edema after stereotactic radiosurgery and radiation therapy. Radiology 1997;204:461–5.

57. Shuto T, Inomori S, Fujino H, et al. Cyst formation following gamma knife surgery for intracranial meningioma. J Neurosurg 2005;102(Suppl):134–9.

58. Loeffler JS, Niemierko A, Chapman PH. Second tumors after radiosurgery: Tip of the iceberg or a bump in the road? Neurosurgery 2003;52:1436–40; discussion 1440–2.

59. Yu JS, Yong WH, Wilson D, Black KL. Glioblastoma induction after radiosurgery for meningioma. Lancet 2000;356:1576–7.

28
Linear Accelerator Radiosurgery for Meningiomas

William A. Friedman

Introduction

Meningiomas are the most common benign primary brain tumor, with an incidence of approximately 7/100,000 in the general population. Surgery has long been thought to be the treatment of choice for symptomatic lesions and is often curative. Many meningiomas, however, occur in locations where attempted surgical cure may be associated with morbidity or mortality, such as the cavernous sinus or petroclival region (1–3). In addition, many of these tumors occur in the elderly, where the risks of general anesthesia and surgery are known to be increased. Hence there is interest in alternative treatments, including radiation therapy and radiosurgery, either as a primary or adjuvant approach.

This chapter will review all published experience on linear accelerator radiosurgery for meningiomas, with a detailed review of the methods and results obtained at the University of Florida.

Methods

Linear accelerator (LINAC) radiosurgery was first described in 1984 by Betti et al.(4). Colombo et al. described such a system in 1985 (5), and LINACs have subsequently been modified in various ways to achieve the precision and accuracy required for radiosurgical applications (6,7). In 1986, a team composed of neurosurgeons, radiation physicists, and computer programmers began development of the University of Florida LINAC-based radiosurgery system. This system has been used to treat over 2500 patients at the University of Florida since May 1988 and is in use at multiple sites worldwide.

Most LINAC radiosurgical systems rely on the same basic paradigm: A collimated x-ray beam is focused on a stereotactically identified intracranial target. The gantry of the LINAC rotates around the patient, producing an arc of radiation focused on the target (Fig. 28-1). The patient couch is then rotated in the horizontal plane and another arc performed. In this manner, multiple noncoplanar arcs of radiation intersect

at the target volume and produce a high target dose, with minimal radiation to surrounding brain. This dose concentration method is exactly analogous to the multiple intersecting beams of cobalt radiation in the Gamma Knife.

The target dose distribution can be tailored by varying collimator sizes, eliminating undesirable arcs, manipulating arc angles, using multiple isocenters, and differentially weighting the isocenters (8). More recently, some LINAC systems have also started to employ advanced beam shaping techniques, using multileaf collimators and intensity modulation. Achievable dose distributions are similar for LINAC-based and Gamma Knife systems. With both systems, it is possible to achieve dose distributions that conform closely to the shape of the intracranial target, thus sparing the maximum amount of normal brain. Recent advances in stereotactic imaging and computer technology for dose planning, as well as refinements in radiation delivery systems have led to improved efficacy, fewer complications, and a remarkable amount of interest in the various applications of Stereotactic radiosurgery (SRS). Perhaps of equal importance is the fact that increasing amounts of scientific evidence have persuaded the majority of the international neurosurgical community that radiosurgery is a viable treatment option for selected patients suffering from a variety of challenging neurosurgical disorders.

Treatment Technique

Although the details of radiosurgical treatment techniques differ somewhat from system to system, the basic paradigm is quite similar everywhere. Below is a detailed description of a typical radiosurgical treatment at the University of Florida.

Almost all radiosurgical procedures in adults are performed on an outpatient basis. The patient reports to the neurosurgical clinic the day before treatment for a detailed history and physical, as well as an in-depth review of the treatment options. The fundamental elements of any successful radiosurgical treatment include the following: head ring application, stereotactic image acquisition, treatment planning, dose selection, radiation delivery, and follow-up. All of these elements are

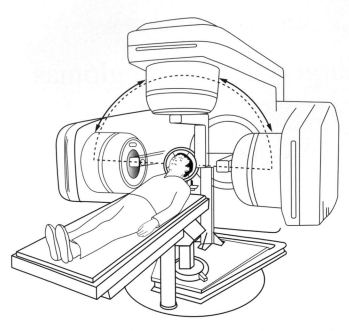

FIG. 28-1. The head of the linear accelerator rotates around the patient. The highly collimated x-ray beam is always focused on the stereotactic target, which has been moved to the center of the arc. A removable floorstand has been added to this system (University of Florida) to improve the accuracy of beam delivery

critical, and poor performance of any step will result in suboptimal results.

Head Ring Application

In general, patients 13 years of age and older are able to tolerate head ring application under local anesthesia. We usually premedicate with oral Valium. Those younger are treated under general anesthesia. The head ring must be applied such that the metal ring falls below the plane of the target. In general, if the top of the head ring is below the external auditory canal, the entire head can be imaged. Most stereotactic frames are anchored to the skull with metal-tipped pins. It is important that these pins have tips that will not produce artifact on computed tomography (CT) scan (aluminum or ceramic versus steel). Obviously, caution must be utilized to avoid placing one of the pins over a previous craniotomy, burr hole, or shunt. In general, head ring application takes about 5 minutes.

Stereotactic Image Acquisition

Patients undergo a volumetric magnetic resonance imaging (MRI) scan the day prior to treatment. The next morning, the patient arrives at 7:00 a.m. After head ring application, stereotactic CT scanning is performed. One-millimeter slices are obtained throughout the entire head. The stereotactic CT scan is transferred via Ethernet to the treatment-planning computer. Image fusion technology is used to fuse the patient's stereotactic CT to the previously acquired MRI images.

Treatment Planning

The primary goal of radiosurgery treatment planning is to develop a plan with a target volume that conforms closely to the surface of the target lesion, while maintaining a steep *dose gradient* (the rate of change in dose relative to position) away from the target surface in order to minimize the radiation dose to surrounding brain. A typical radiosurgical dose gradient will reduce the treatment dose to one-half the treatment dose over a 3-mm space. A number of treatment planning tools can be used to tailor the shape of the target volume to fit even highly irregular shapes (Fig. 28-2). Regardless of its shape, the entire lesion must lie within the target volume (the "prescription isodose shell"), with as little normal brain included as possible.

The volumetric MRI obtained the day before treatment is used to generate a "preplan." This plan can be generated manually or via a completely automated program (9) that will place multiple isocenters in such a way as to generate an optimally conformal prescription isodose line. The "preplan" is carefully examined and, if necessary, adjusted to generate the actual treatment plan. The technical methods of radiosurgery have been described at length in other publications (8).

A detailed discussion of dose planning is beyond the scope of this chapter. Suffice it to say that the radiosurgical team must develop considerable expertise using the available tools (multiple isocenters, beam weighting, intensity modulation, etc.) to be able to efficiently develop highly conformal radiosurgical plans.

Dose Selection

A peripheral dose of 12.5–15 Gy is appropriate for most meningiomas. The lower dose is used for larger tumors or those closer to critical brain structures. This dose range has proven effective at long-term tumor control and is also very unlikely to produce radiation-induced complications.

Radiation Delivery

The process of radiation delivery is the same for any radiosurgical target—careful attention to detail and the execution of various safety checks and redundancies are necessary to ensure that the prescribed treatment plan is accurately and safely delivered. When radiation delivery has been completed, the head ring is removed and the patient is observed for approximately 30 minutes and then discharged to resume her or his normal activities.

Follow-up

Standard follow-up after meningioma radiosurgery calls for an annual MRI scan for 5 years. At that point scan frequency is reduced to every 3 years.

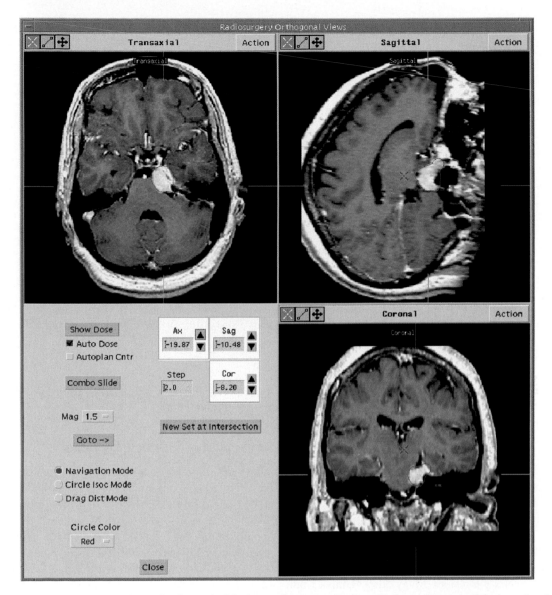

FIG. 28-2. Axial, sagittal, and coronal views of radiosurgical dosimetry for a petroclival meningioma. Because of the irregular shape, multiple isocenters are required to generate a conformal prescription isodose line

Results

Surgery remains the mainstay of treatment for many meningiomas. Simpson, in a classic paper, described the relationship between completeness of surgical resection and tumor recurrence (10). A Grade I resection, complete tumor removal with excision of the tumor's dural attachment and involved bone, has a 10% recurrence rate. A Grade II resection, complete resection of the tumor and coagulation of its dural attachment, has up to a 20% recurrence rate. Grade III resection is complete tumor removal without dural resection or coagulation. Grade IV resection is subtotal, and Grade V resection is simple decompression. Recurrence rates in the Grade IV and V groups basically reflect the natural history of the tumor, with high rates of recurrence over time. Unfortunately, some common meningioma locations, such

as the cavernous sinus or petroclival region, are not readily amenable to a complete dural resection or coagulation strategy because of location and the proximity of vital neural and vascular structures (Fig. 28-3). In addition, relatively high complication rates have been described for meningioma surgery in some locations and in the elderly.

Pollock and colleagues recently analyzed 198 patients with meningiomas less than 35 mm in diameter, treated with either surgical resection or Gamma Knife radiosurgery (11). Tumor recurrence was more frequent in the surgical resection group (12% vs. 2%). No statistically significant difference was detected in the 3- and 7-year actuarial progression-free survival rates between patients with Simpson Grade 1 resections and those who underwent radiosurgery. Progression free survival rates with radiosurgery were superior to Simpson Grade 2, 3, and 4 resections. Complications were lower in the radiosurgery group.

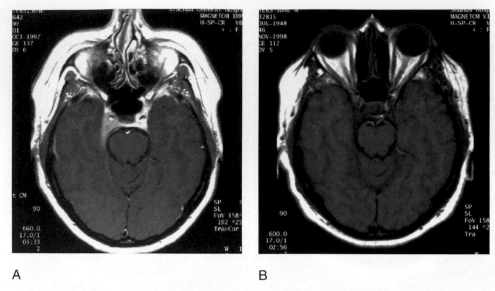

A   B

FIG. 28-3. (A) The enhanced MRI shows a right cavernous sinus lesion consistent with meningioma. It was treated with 12.5 Gy to the 70% isodose line, using 8 isocenters. (B) Enhanced MRI shows the same lesions 3 years later. The enhancement is gone and the lesion is barely visible

Flickinger evaluated tumor control and outcome in 219 meningiomas diagnosed by imaging criteria alone (12). The actuarial tumor control rate was 93% at 5 and 10 years. The actuarial rate of identifying a tumor other than meningioma was 2.3% at 10 years. The rate of radiation-induced complications was 5.3% in tumors treated after 1991 when MRI targeting and lower treatment doses were adopted.

Kondziolka reported on 99 consecutive patients who underwent meningioma radiosurgery (13). Ninety-three percent of these patients required no further surgery. Five to 10 years later, 96% of the patients believed that radiosurgery provided a satisfactory outcome. Radiation induced morbidity was seen in 5% and was generally transient. Many other Gamma Knife radiosurgery series (of up to 190 patients) document similar rates of tumor control and treatment morbidiy (13–26).

Multiple linear accelerator radiosurgical series have also been published (27–30). Hakim and colleagues described the largest such series, and the only one to report actuarial statistics (31). One hundred and twenty-seven patients with 155 meningiomas were treated. Actuarial tumor control for patients with benign tumors was 89.3% at 5 years. Six

patients (4.7%) had permanent radiation-induced complications (Table 28-1).

University of Florida Experience

Our early experience with 70 meningiomas was published in 1998 (32). Recently, a review of 210 patients was published (33). A retrospective analysis of all patients treated with linear accelerator (LINAC)–based radiosurgery for meningiomas between May 1989 and December 2001 was performed. All patients had follow-up for a minimum of 2 years, and no patients were excluded. A total of 210 patients were treated during the study interval. Actuarial local control for benign tumors was 100% at 1 and 2 years and 96% at 5 years. Actuarial local control for atypical tumors was 100% at 1 year, 92% at 2 years, and 77% at 5 years. Actuarial control for malignant tumors was 100% at 1 and 2 years, but only 19% at 5 years. Out of the 210 subjects, 13 (6.2%) experienced temporary radiation induced complications. Out of the 210 subjects, only 5 (2.3%) experienced permanent complications. All patients with permanent complications

TABLE 28-1. LINAC Radiosurgery for Meningiomas.

	Valentino (29) Rome, Italy (1993)	Chang (34) Stanford (1997)	Colombo (35) Vicenza, Italy (1998)	Hakim (31) Harvard (1998)	U. of Florida (32) (1998)
Number of patients	72	55	74	127	70
Mean marginal dose (Gy)	37 (1–4 fractions)	18.3 (12–25)	22.3 (18–26)	15 (9–20)	12.7 (10–20)
Tumor control	94%	98% (2 yr)	75% (8 yr)	89% (5 yr, benign)	100%
Complications					
Transient	3 (4%)	10 (18%)			2 (3%)
Permanent	0	4 (7%)	2 (3%)	4 (3%)	0

had malignant histology. This is the largest published linear accelerator meningioma experience.

References

1. Sekhar LN, Altschuler EM. Meningiomas of the cavernous sinus. In: Al-Mefty O, ed. Meningiomas. New York: Raven Press, 1991:445–60.
2. Sekhar LN, Jannetta PJ, Burkhart LE, Janosky JE. Meningiomas involving the clivus: a six-year experience with 41 patients. Neurosurgery 1990;27:764–81.
3. Sekhar LN, Swamy KS, Jaiswal V. Surgical excision of meningiomas involving the clivus: preoperative and intraoperative features as predictors of postoperative functional deterioration. J Neurosurg 1994;81:860.
4. Betti OO, Derechinsky VE. Hyperselective encephalic irradiation with a linear accelerator. Acta Neurochir Suppl 1984;33:385–90.
5. Colombo F. Linear accelerator radiosurgery. A clinical experience. J Neurosurg Sci 1989;33:123–5.
6. Friedman WA, Bova FJ. The University of Florida radiosurgery system. Surg Neurol 1989;32:334–42.
7. Lutz W, Winston KR, Maleki N. A system for stereotactic radiosurgery with a linear accelerator. Int J Radiation Oncol Biol Phys 1988;14:373–81.
8. Friedman WA, Buatti JM, Bova FJ, Mendenhall WM. LINAC Radiosurgery—A Practical Guide. Berlin: Springer-Verlag, 1998.
9. Wagner T. Optimal Delivery Techniques for Intracranial Stereotactic Radiosurgery Using Circular and Multileaf Collimators. Gainesville, FL: University of Florida, 2000.
10. Simpson D. The recurrence of intracranial meningiomas after surgical treatment. J Neurol Neurosurg Psychiatry 1957;20:22–39.
11. Pollock BE, Stafford SL, Utter A, et al. Stereotactic radiosurgery provides equivalent tumor control to Simpson Grade 1 resection for patients with small- to medium-size meningiomas. Int J Radiat Oncol Biol Phys 2003;55(4):1000–5.
12. Flickinger JC, Kondziolka D, Maitz AH, Lunsford LD. Gamma knife radiosurgery of imaging-diagnosed intracranial meningiomas. Int J Radiat Oncol Biol Phys 2003;56:801–6.
13. Kondziolka D, Levy EI, Niranjan A, et al. Long-term outcomes after meningioma radiosurgery: physician and patient perspectives. J Neurosurg 1999;91(1):44–50.
14. Kondziolka D, Lunsford LD, Coffey RJ, Flickinger JC. Stereotactic radiosurgery of meningiomas. J Neurosurg 1991;74:552–9.
15. Kondziolka D, Nathoo N, Flickinger JC, et al. Long-term results after radiosurgery for benign intracranial tumors. Neurosurgery 2003;53(4):815–21; discussion 821–2.
16. Kondziolka D, Niranjan A, Lunsford LD, Flickinger JC. Stereotactic radiosurgery for meningiomas. Neurosurg Clin North Am 1999;10:317–25.
17. Lee JY, Niranjan A, McInerney J, et al. Stereotactic radiosurgery providing long-term tumor control of cavernous sinus meningiomas. J Neurosurg 2002;97(1):65–72.
18. Stafford SL, Pollock BE, Foote RL, et al. Meningioma radiosurgery: tumor control, outcomes, and complications among 190 consecutive patients. Neurosurgery 2001;49(5):1029–37; discussion 1037–8.
19. Kobayashi T, Kida Y, Mori Y. Long-term results of stereotactic gamma radiosurgery of meningiomas. Surg Neurol 2001;55(6):325–31.
20. Pendl G, Eustacchio S, Unger F. Radiosurgery as alternative treatment for skull base meningiomas. J Clin Neurosci 2001;8(Suppl 1):12–4.
21. Pendl G, Schrottner O, Friehs GM, Feichtinger H. Stereotactic radiosurgery of skull base meningiomas. Stereotact Funct Neurosurg 1995;64:11–8.
22. Nicolato A, Ferraresi P, Foroni R, et al. Gamma knife radiosurgery in skull base meningiomas. Stereotact Funct Neurosurg 1996;66:112–20.
23. Nicolato A, Foroni R, Alessandrini F, et al. Radiosurgical treatment of cavernous sinus meningiomas: experience with 122 treated patients. Neurosurgery 2002;51(5):1153–9; discussion 1159–61.
24. Nicolato A, Foroni R, Alessandrini F, et al. The role of Gamma Knife radiosurgery in the management of cavernous sinus meningiomas. Int J Radiat Oncol Biol Phys 2002;53(4):992–1000.
25. Nicolato A, Foroni R, Pellegrino M, et al. Gamma knife radiosurgery in meningiomas of the posterior fossa. Experience with 62 treated lesions. Minim Invasive Neurosurg 2001;44(4):211–7.
26. Roche PH, Regis J, Dufour H, et al. Gamma knife radiosurgery in the management of cavernous sinus meningiomas. J Neurosurg 2000;93(Suppl 3):68–73.
27. Engenhart R, Kimmig BN, Hover KH, et al. Stereotactic single high dose radiation therapy of benign intracranial meningiomas. Int J Radiation Oncol Biol Phys 1990;19:1021–6.
28. Spiegelmann R, Nissim O, Menhel J, et al. Linear accelerator radiosurgery for meningiomas in and around the cavernous sinus. Neurosurgery 2002;51(6):1373–79; discussion 1379–80.
29. Valentino V, Schinaia G, Raimondi AJ. The results of radiosurgical management of 72 middle fossa meningiomas. Acta Neurochir 1993;122:60–70.
30. Villavicencio AT, Black PM, Shrieve DC, et al. Linac radiosurgery for skull base meningiomas. Acta Neurochir (Wien) 2001;143(11):1141–52.
31. Hakim R, Alexander III E, Loeffler JS, et al. Results of linear accelerator-based radiosurgery for inracranial meningiomas. Neurosurgery 1998;42:446–54.
32. Shafron DH, Friedman WA, Buatti JM, et al. LINAC radiosurgery for benign meningiomas. Int J Radiation Oncol Biol Phys 1999;43(2):321–7.
33. Friedman WA, Murad G, Bradshaw P, et al. Linear accelerator radiosurgery for meningiomas. J Neurosurg 2005;103:206–9.
34. Chang SD, Adler JR. Treatment of cranial base meningiomas with linear accelerator radiosurgery. Neurosurgery 1997;41:1019–27.
35. Colombo F, Francescon P. Clinical linear accelerator radiosurgery. In: Gildenberg PL, Tasker RR, eds. Textbook of Stereotactic and Functional Neurosurgery. New York: McGraw-Hill, 1998:757–62.

29
Brachytherapy for Meningiomas

P. Pradeep Kumar and Burak Sade

Introduction

Brachytherapy is defined, literally, as providing treatment from a short distance. Becquerel[1] discovered radioactivity in 1898, and radium was isolated by Pierre and Marie Curie[2] in the same year. In Paris in 1901, 3 years after radium was isolated, Pierre and Marie Curie suggested that a small radium tube may be inserted into a tumor for treatment, thus heralding the birth of brachytherapy (BT), more precisely, brachy radiation therapy (BRT). In 1895, Roentgen[3] discovered x-rays, and by 1897, Professor Freund demonstrated the disappearance of a hairy mole following treatment with x-rays, heralding the birth of external radiation therapy (EXRT).

Soon thereafter, both BRT and EXRT were used to treat neoplasms. Immediately, the users realized that when EXRT was used therapeutically, the radiation had to be fractionated into small doses and given over a long period of time to minimize the radiation damage to normal tissues surrounding the neoplasm and at the site of entry into the body, unlike BRT, which is delivered continuously from within the tumor. Thus, the time dose fractionation (TDF) formula for clinical use of EXRT was developed.[4–9] Even though multiple beam EXRT techniques, such as intensity modulated radiation therapy (IMRT) and Gamma Knife, minimize the reaction at the site of entry, still normal tissues immediately adjacent to the tumor target receive considerable radiation, which can be minimized in BRT where radiation is delivered from within the tumor.[10–15] In reality, no matter how EXRT is delivered, as far as the tumor dose delivery is concerned, it is suboptimal when compared to BRT (Fig. 29-1)

As newer sealed radioactive isotopes, such as Cs-137), Ir-192, I-125, and Pd-103), became available, removable and permanent BRT has been used either alone or in combination with EXRT to treat many neoplasms very successfully over the years.[16–23]

Advantages of Brachytherapy

Brachytherapy with I-125 has several important advantages in treating well-circumscribed slow-growing tumors, such as meningiomas, for the following reasons.[24,25]

Cytotoxic Effects of Iradiation

Cytotoxic effects of irradiation depend on the mitotic activity of the tumor cells. If the doubling time is long, such as in benign meningiomas, the mitotic phase of the tumor cells occurs at long intervals allowing the fractionated irradiation given for a few minutes per day to miss its cytotoxic action on the tumor[26–35] (Fig. 29-2A). .On the other hand, if the irradiation is continuous as with I-125 BRT over 24 hours a day for 80 days (effective life of I-125), the chances of catching the tumor cells during their mitotic activity at long intervals is much higher, making the treatment modality very effective[36–48] (Fig. 29-2B).

Tumor-Confined Dose Distribution

Even though EXRT with Gamma Knife and Linac can be shaped to confine to the tumor from outside, the conformity is better accomplished with I-125 brachytherapy from inside the tumor (Fig. 29-3).This type of tumor-confined dose distribution with I-125 brachytherapy from within the tumor also makes it much safer in treating recurrent skull base meningiomas following surgery or EXRT where the tissues surrounding the recurrent tumor are already damaged from previous treatment (Fig. 29-4). Continuous low-dose irradiation is also better tolerated.[49–56]

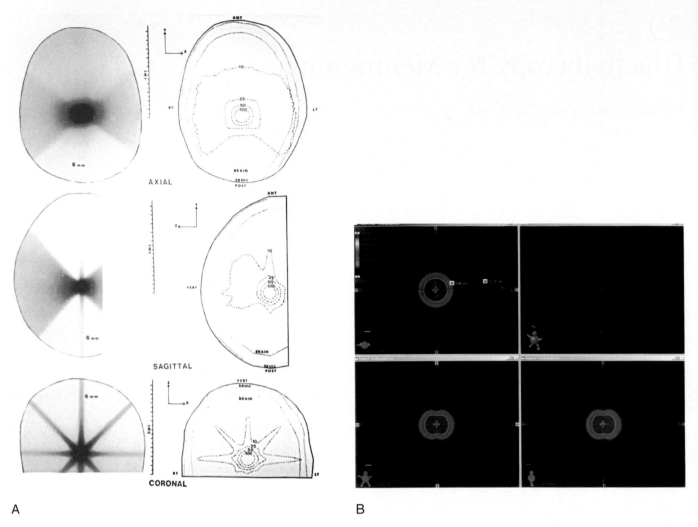

FIG. 29-1. (A) Dose distribution along *x, y, z* axes from linac external beam stereotactic radiation. (B) Dose distribution along *x, y, z* axes from brachytherapy using I-125 seed

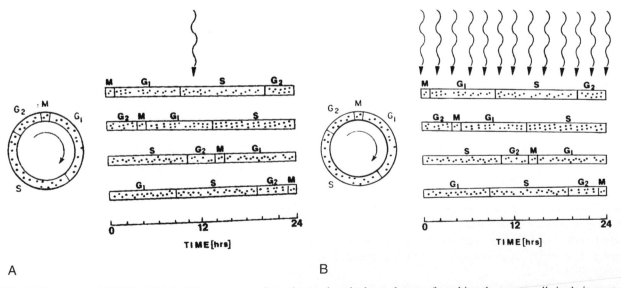

FIG. 29-2. (A) Fractionated EXRT, which is delivered over a few minutes, has the least chance of catching the tumor cells in their most radiosensitive mitotic (M) phase of their cell cycle. (B) Continuous irradiation with brachytherapy has a high probability of catching the tumor cells during the short-lived radiosensitive mitotic (M) phase of their cell cycle

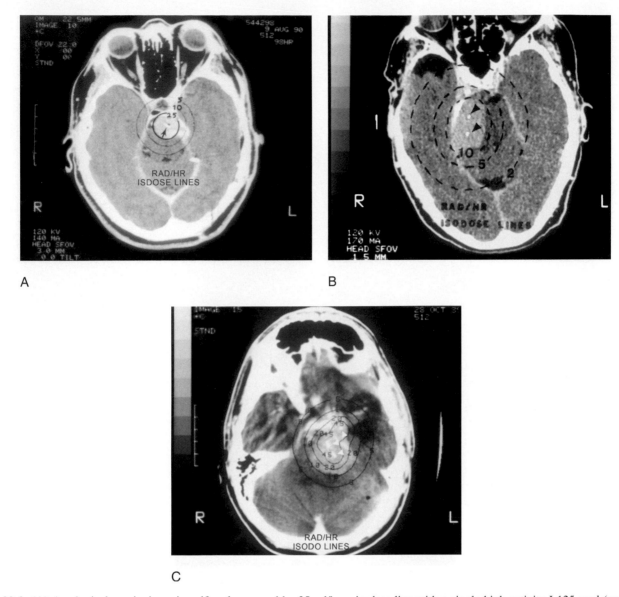

Fig. 29-3. (A) A spherical meningioma is uniformly covered by 25 rad/hour isodose line with a single high-activity I-125 seed (arrow) in the center of the tumor. (B) An oval meningioma is uniformly covered by 10 rad/hour isodose line with two high-activity I-125 seeds (arrow heads) implanted into the tumor at predetermined points.(C) An irregular meningioma is uniformly covered by 10 rad/hr isodose line with three high-activity I-125 seeds (arrow heads) implanted into the tumor at predetermined points

Local Anesthesia

I-125 brachytherapy is performed under local anesthesia, making it very safe for the elderly, especially those with comorbidities (Fig. 29-5). The real-time CT imaging of the entire implant procedure makes it a very accurate way of delivering radiation to the tumor[57] (Fig. 29-6).

One-Time Procedure

Since EXRT needs to be fractionated to minimize damage to the normal tissue, it involves multiple sittings for tumor localization and treatment.[31] In contrast, implantation of I-125 seed is a one-time procedure requiring no hospitalization, which is extremely convenient to the patient as well as being cost-effective.[58]

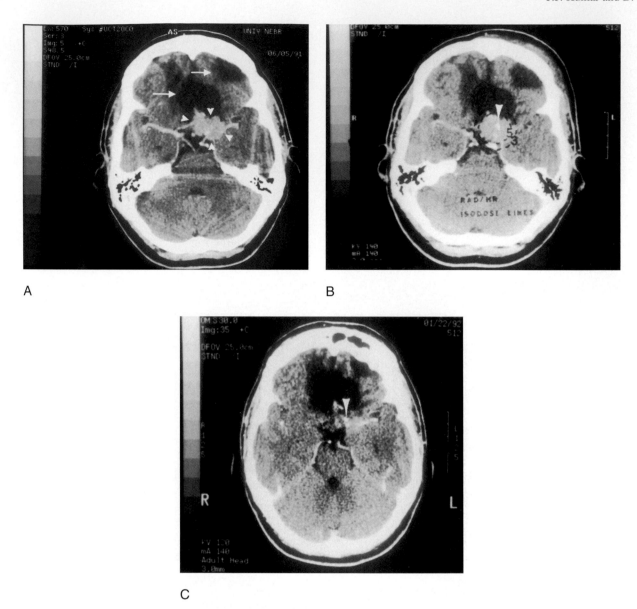

A

B

C

FIG. 29-4. (A) Head CT with contrast of a patient 7 years after surgery for a central skull base meningioma shows recurrent tumor (arrow heads) and large infarcts in both frontal lobes (arrows). (B) Head CT with contrast axial view, post I-125 seed implant, shows the seed in the center of the tumor shown in A (arrow head). The tumor is uniformly covered by 5 rad/hour isodose line. (C) CT head with contrast 6 months after the I-125 brachytherapy shows complete response of the recurrent meningioma with no additional infarcts in the brain. Arrowhead shows the decayed I-125 seed

FIG. 29-5. A very elderly female patient awake in prone position with the implant needle in position (arrow) through the stereotactic head frame. The whole procedure is done under local anesthesia and the patient is discharged home the same day

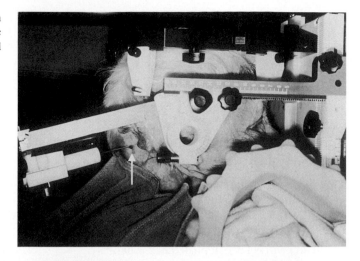

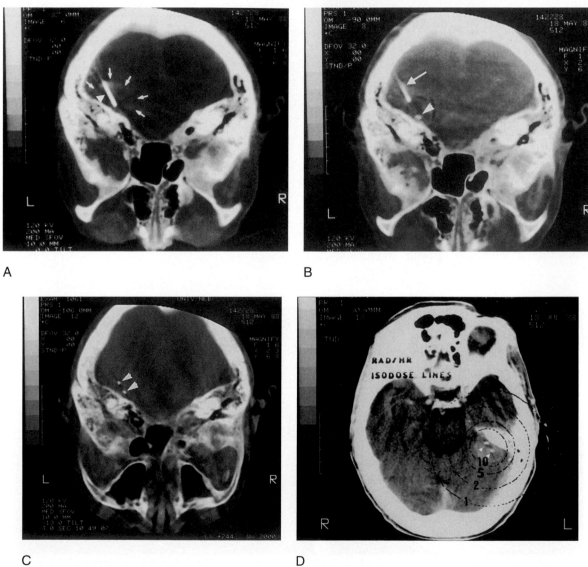

A

B

C

D

FIG. 29-6. (A) Real-time CT head in prone showing the implant needle tip (arrow head) inside the left CP angle meningioma (arrows). (B) Real-time CT head in prone showing the first I-125 seed (arrow head) in place and the implant needle tip (arrow) withdrawn, one centimeter from the seed. (C) Real-time CT head in prone showing two I-125 seeds (arrow heads) implanted into the left CP angle meningioma. The needle is removed. (D) Postimplant CT head with contrast axial view delineates the contrast enhanced left CP angle meningioma with two high-activity I-125 seeds (arrow heads). The tumor is uniformly covered by 10 rad/hour isodose line

Contraindications to Brachytherapy

Good Surgical Risk Patients

Since any kind of irradiation has late sequela resulting from its effects on normal tissues within and surrounding the tumor, surgery should always be the first choice in good surgical risk patients.[59–61]

Patients Requiring Immediate Decompression for Relief of Symptoms

Regression of meningiomas following irradiation is slow with a median time of 4 months (Fig. 29-7). If the patient needs immediate relief from pain or neurovascular deficits from nerve or vessel involvement, slow tumor regression following irradiation will not accomplish quick relief.[62]

Encased Functional Nerves and Vessels in the Tumor

Following irradiation, the meningioma becomes fibrotic and/or calcified, strangulating the encased nerves and vessels (Fig. 29-8). If they are still functional, strangulation will make them completely nonfunctional, resulting in serious neurologic and vascular deficits. However, the slow growth of benign meningiomas enables the development of collateral circulation as well as neurologic compensation in most patients. A good pretreatment clinical and imaging evaluation is essential to avoid these problems.[63,64]

Excessive Preexisting Calcification

Many benign meningiomas contain some amount of calcification because of their slow growth. Regression of a

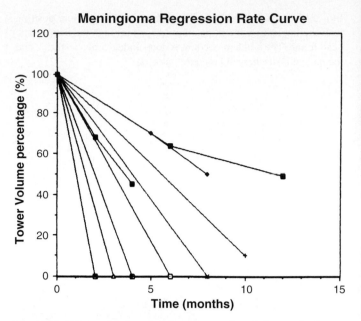

FIG. 29-7. Time-volume regression curves plotted for meningiomas treated with I-125 brachytherapy showed complete response from 2 to 8 months after implant (mean 4 months)

meningioma following irradiation will be limited to the noncalcified part of the tumor. If there is excessive pre-irradiation calcification, there will be minimal regression resulting in limited relief of symptoms caused by the tumor (Fig. 29-9). In this kind of situation, pre-irradiation surgical debulking will be a reasonable option, if it is not contraindicated.

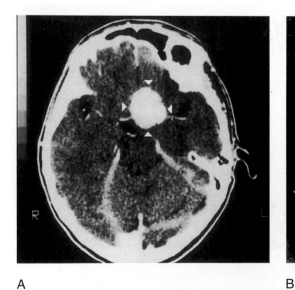

A

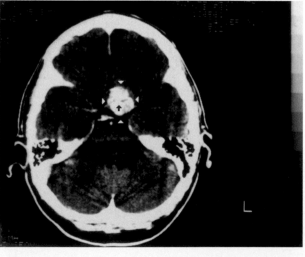

B

FIG. 29-8. (A) CT head with contrast axial view shows a clinoidal meningioma encasing both right and left middle cerebral arteries. (B) CT head with contrast axial view of the same patient in A 10 months after I-125 brachytherapy (arrow) showing marked regression of the tumor. However, the shrinkage of the tumor strangulates the encased vessels

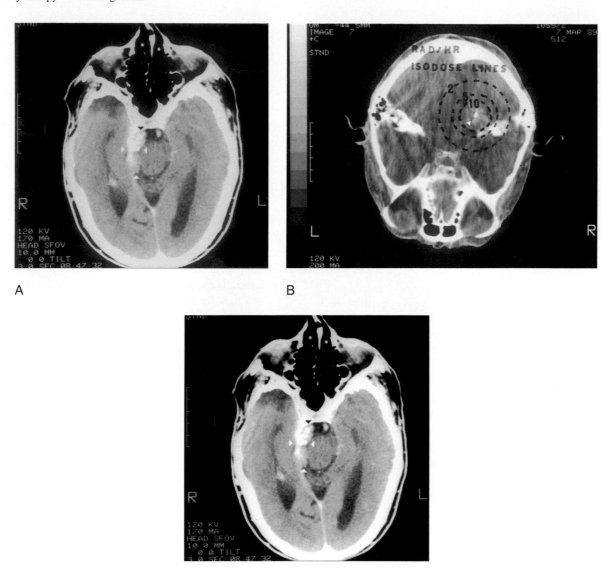

FIG. 29-9. (A) CT head without contrast axial view shows a right CP angle meningioma (arrow heads) with considerable calcification. (B) Postimplant CT scan of the patient in A showing the I-125 seed (arrow head). The tumor is covered by 10 rad/hour isodose line. (C) CT scan without contrast axial view of the same patient in A and B 13 months after the implant shows complete calcification of the entire tumor with very little reduction in the tumor size (arrowheads)

Definition of Response

If all the tumor cells are killed following irradiation, the entire tumor will be replaced by scar tissue and/or calcification. The scar tissue will shrink over a period of time and attain a nadir volume along with calcification, and remain stable thereafter. This is a complete response (CR). However, CR does not mean complete disappearance of the tumor, which will never happen in any tumor following irradiation (Fig. 29-10). On the other hand, if the tumor continues to regress during the follow-up period without reaching a nadir volume, it can be interpreted as partial response (PR). If there is no change in the dimensions of the meningioma beyond the median regression period, it can be interpreted as no response (NR).

Results and Complications

The literature is scant with respect to the reported results of meningiomas treated with brachytherapy. Even in the published series, the sizes of the study populations are limited.

According to the definition of various types of responses discussed above, the CR rate is 73% and the PR rate is 27% in the experience of the senior author.[62] This series consists of 15 meningiomas, in 13 of which the I-125 seeds were placed stereotactically and in 2 through craniotomy. The minimum tumor dose ranged from 100 to 500 Gy at a dose rate of 0.05–0.25 Gy/hour. In 2 patients with PR there was extensive calcification prior to implantation. If these patients were to be left out of the series, the CR then becomes 84%. The time period for the CR to take place

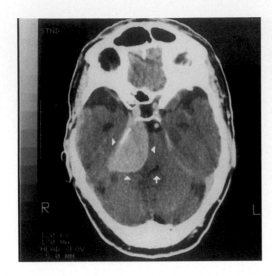

FIG. 29-10. CT scan with contrast axial view shows a large right CP angle meningioma (arrow heads) compressing the fourth ventricle (arrow). Multiple post I-125 brachytherapy follow up CT scans with contrast of the same patient repeatedly showed the same residual mass (scar tissue)

ranged from 2 to 8 months. In a series of 11 patients with primary or recurrent meningiomas, Obasi and colleagues reported that all patients had a decrease or stabilization in the size of the tumor at the last follow-up (median of 25 months).[65] In this study, the seeds were implanted stereotactically, and a total dose of 7000–10,000 cGY was applied with a dose rate of 5–10 cGy/hour. At the last follow-up, 45% of the patients still continued to experience reduction of their tumor size. Interestingly, this study has documented that all 3 of the patients who received a dose larger than 10,000 cGy developed radiation necrosis and vasogenic edema, as compared to 20% of patients with a dose less than or equal to 10,000 cGy, resulting in the overall incidence of 45% for development of radiation necrosis and/ or vasogenic edema..

In a relatively larger series consisting of 44 patients from Finland, Vuorinen and colleagues reported their results of 25 parasellar or clival meningiomas and 19 meningiomas of various locations in elderly patients. All had the Iodine-125 seeds placed stereotactically.[66] The total delivered dose was 100–150 Gy. The patients with parasellar or clival meningiomas had a median follow-up of 19 months and various degrees of shrinking was detected in 17 (68%) of the patients. In this series, 17 patients presented initially with deficits of cranial nerves III, IV, and VI, 8 (47%) of which improved following BRT. Interestingly, there was either new onset or worsening of facial numbness in 36% of the patients. Also, one patient experienced injury to the third cranial nerve during the implantation process. In their overall population, the incidence of seed misplacement was 4.5%.

In a group of 15 recurrent high-grade meningiomas with close follow-up, Ware and colleagues reported the median freedom from progression following I-125 BRT as 10 months and median survival as 2.4 years.[67] In this study, the seeds were placed in the surgical cavity following total or subtotal resection of the tumor. All of the patients had prior external beam radiation treatment. The mean follow-up following BRT was 3 years. Only 20% of patients had no recurrence at their last follow-up. There was no difference in the freedom from progression in patients who received high-dose versus low-dose treatment. In this series, the incidences of radiation necrosis and wound breakdown were reported as 27% each. The average time to occurrence was 11 months for necrosis and 8 months for wound breakdown.

Conclusion

Surgery should be the choice of treatment if the benefits outweigh the risks since radiation to any functioning structures, such as nerves and vessels, within or in the vicinity of tumoricidal radiation dose will result in delayed sequelae.

Irradiation is the treatment of choice when the risks of surgery outweigh its benefits. When irradiation is selected as the treatment choice, a meticulous pre-irradiation evaluation of neurovascular structures within and in the vicinity of the meningioma is essential for proper dosimetric and technical selection to avoid additional damage to these structures within the tumoricidal dose.

Brachytherapy appears to be a good therapeutic option due to its accuracy, simplicity, and biological superiority in treating slow-growing tumors, such as meningiomas, in very critical locations. However, because of its invasive nature, its use may be warranted in selected cases, which are not eligible for external radiation therapy.

Acknowledgment. Sincere appreciation to Sharron Phillips for her assistance in the preparation of this manuscript.

References

1. Becquerel H. Sur les radiations emises par phosphorescence. Compt Rend 1896;122:420.
2. Hall EJ. Radiobiology for the Radiologist, 3rd ed. Philadelphia: J. B. Lippincott Company, 1988:1–16.
3. Rontgen W. Über eine neue Art von Strahlen (vorläufige Mitteilung). Sitzungs-Berichte der Physikalisch-medicinischen Gesellschaft zu Wurzburg 1895;9:132.
4. Douglas BG, Fowler JF. The effect of multiple small doses of x rays on skin reactions in the mouse and a basic interpretation. Radiat Res 1976;66:401–426.
5. Ellis F. Dose time and fractionation: a clinical hypothesis. Clin Radiol 1969;20:1–7.
6. Fowler JF. 40 years of radiobiology: its impact on radiotherapy. Phys Med Biol 1984;29:97–113.
7. Parsons JT, Bova FJ, Million RR. A reevaluation of split-course technique for squamous cell carcinoma of the head and neck. Int J Radiat Oncol Biol Phys 1980;6:1645–1652.
8. Peters LJ, Withers HR, Thames HD. Radiobiological bases for multiple daily fractionation. In: Kaercher KH, Kogelnik HD, Reinartz G, eds. Progress in Radio-Oncology II. New York: Raven Press, 1982:317–23.

9. Withers HR. Cell cycle redistribution as a factor in multifraction irradiation. Radiology 1975;114:199–202.
10. Soyuer S, Chang EL, Selek U, et al. Radiotherapy after surgery for benign cerebral meningioma. Radiother Oncol 2004;71(1): 85–90.
11. Mendenhall WM, Morris CG, Amdur RJ, et al. Radiotherapy alone or after subtotal resection for benign skull base meningiomas. Cancer 2003;98(7):1473–82.
12. Mathiesen T, Kihlstrom L, Karlsson B, et al. Potential complications following radiotherapy for meningiomas. Surg Neurol 2003;60(3):193–8.
13. Bauman GS, Wong E. Re: new radiotherapy technologies for meningiomas: 3D conformal radiotherapy? Radiosurgery? Sterotactic radiotherapy? Intensity modulated radiotherapy? Proton beam radiotherapy? Spot scanning proton radiation therapy? Or nothing at all? Radiother Oncol 2004;73(2):251–2.
14. Deinsberger R, Tidstrand J, Sabitzer H, et al. LINAC radiosurgery in skull base meningiomas. Minim Invasive Neurosurg 2004;47(6):333–8.
15. Chuang CC, Chang CN, Tsang NM, et al. Linear accelerator-based radiosurgery in the management of skull base meningiomas. J Neurooncol 2004;66(1–2):241–9.
16. Schwaz G. An evaluation of the Manchester system of treatment of carcinoma of the cervix. Am J Roentgenol 1969;105:579.
17. Heyman J, Reuterwall O, Benner S. The radiumhemmet experience with radiotherapy in cancer of the corpus of the uterus. Acta Radiol 1941;22:11.
18. Henschke UK, Hilaris BS, Mahan GD. Afterloading in interstitial and intracavitary radiation therapy. Am J Roentgenol 1963;90:386.
19. Heyman J. The technique in the treatment of cancer uteri at radium-hemmet. Acta Radiol 1929;10:49.
20. Joslin CAF, Smith CW. The use of high activity ^{60}Co sources for intracavitary and surface mould therapy. Proc R Soc Med 1970;63:1029.
21. Meisberger LL, Keller R, Shalek RJ. The effective attenuation in water of the gamma rays of gold-198, iridium-192, cesium-137, radium-226 and cobalt-60. Radiology 1968;90:953.
22. Schulz RJ, Chandra P, Nath R. Determination of the exposure rate constant for ^{125}I using a scintillation detector. Med Phys 1980;7:355.
23. Krishnaswamy V. Dose distribution around an ^{125}I seed source in tissue. Radiology 1978;126:489.
24. Kumar PP. Cancer and state of the art in radiationoncology. Cancer J 1989;2(12): 461–470.
25. Kumar PP, Good RR, Skultety MF, et al. Absence of deleterious effects of 20,000- to 100,000-cGy iodine I-125 endocurietherapy on cerebral arteries. Endocurietherapy/Hyperthermia Oncology 1986;2:137–146.
26. Dizdaroglu M. Measurement of radiation-induced damage in DNA at the molecular level. Int J Radiat Biol 1992;61:175–9.
27. Ward JF. DNA damage produced by ionizing radiation in mammalian cells; identities, mechanisms of formation and reparability. Prog Nucleic Acids Mol Biol 1988;35:95–8.
28. Phillips MH, Griffin TW. Physics of high-linear energy transfer (LET) particles and protons. In: Perez CA, Brady LW, ed. Principles and Practice of Radiation Oncology. Philadelphia: Lippincott-Raven Publishers, 1997.
29. Griffin TW, Wambersie A, Laramore G, Castro J. International clinical trials in radiation oncology, high LET: heavy particle trials. Int J Radiat Oncol Biol Phys 1988;14:83–8.
30. Laramore GE, Griffin TW, Maor MH. Mixed beam radiation therapy for carcinoma of the prostate: results of a randomized RTOG trial. Int J Radiat Oncol Biol Phys 1985;11:1621–5.
31. Hellman S, Weichselbaum RR. Radiation oncology and the new biology. Cancer J Sci Am 1995;1:174–9.
32. Cox JD, Kline RW. Prostate biopsies after irradiation for adenocarcinoma. Int J Radiat Oncol Biol Phys 1983;9:229–32.
33. Barranco SC, Rmsdahl NM, Humphrey RM. The radiation response of human malignant melanoma cells grown in vitro. Cancer Res 1971;31:830–3.
34. Weichselbaum RR, Beckett MA. The maximum recovery potential of human tumor cells may predict clinical outcome in radiotherapy. Int J Radiat Oncol Biol Phys 1987;13:709–11.
35. Withers HR. In: Perez Ca, Brady LW, editors. Principles and Practice of Radiation Oncology. Philadelphia: JB Lippincott, 1987:67–98.
36. Mauceri HJ, Hanna NN, Wayne JD, et al. Tumor necrosis factor alpha (TNF-alpha) gene therapy targeted by ionizing radiation selectively damages tumor vasculature. Cancer Res 1996;56:4311–4.
37. Elkind MM. The initial part of the survival curve. Does it predict outcome of fractionated radiotherapy? Radiat Res 1988;114:425–8.
38. Elkind MM, Witmore GF. Radiobiology of Cultured Mammalian Cells. New York: Gordon and Breach, 1967.
39. Elkind MM. Fractionated dose radiotherapy and its relationship to survival curve shapes. Cancer Treat Rev 1976;3:2–6.
40. Elkind MM, Sutton H. Radiation response of mammalian cells grown in culture I. Repair of x-ray damage in surviving Chinese hamster cells. Radiat Res 1960;13:556–60.
41. Elkind MM, Sutton-Gilbert H, Moses WB, et al. Radiation response in cells in culture V. Temperature dependence of the repair of x-ray damage in surviving cells (aerobic and hypoxic). Radiat Res 1965;25:359–63.
42. Elkind MM. Sutton HG. X-ray damage and recovery in mammalian cells in culture. Nature 1959;184:1293–7.
43. Boothman DA, Bouvard I, Hughes EN. Identification and characterization of x-ray induced proteins in human cells. Cancer Res 1989;49:2871–4.
44. Carney DN, Mitchell JB, Kinsella T. In vitro radiation and chemotherapeutic sensitivity of established cell lines in human small cell lung cancer and large cell morphology variants. Cancer Res 1983;43:2806–9.
45. Kelland LR, Bingle L, Edwards S, et al. High intrinsic radiosensitivity of a newly established and characterized human embryonal rhabdomyosarcoma cell line. Br J Cancer 1989;59:160–3.
46. Peckman MJ. In: Steele GG, Adams GE, eds. The Biological Basis of Radiotherapy. New York: Elsevier; 1983:1–15.
47. Weichselbaum RR, Beckett MA, Vijayakumar S, et al. Radiobiological characterization of head and neck and sarcoma cell lines derived from patients prior to radiotherapy. Int J Radiat Oncol Biol Phys 1990;19:313–7.
48. Weichselbaum RR, Rotmensch J, Ahmed-Swan S, et al. Radiobiological characterization of 53 human tumor cell lines. Int J Radiat Oncol Biol Phys 1989;16:553–7.
49. Schell MC, Bova FJ, Larson V, et al. AAPM Report 54: Stereotactic radiosurgery. Am Assoc Physicists Med 1995.
50. Leksell LT. The stereotactic method and radiosurgery of the brain. Acta Chir Scand 1951;102:316–9.

51. Gill SS, Thomas DGT, Warrington AP, et al. Relocatable frame for stereotactic external beam radiotherapy. Int J Radiat Oncol Biol Phys 1991;20:599–603.

52. Sturm V, Kober B, Hover KH, et al. Stereotactic percutaneous single dose irradiation of brain metastases with a linear accelerator. Int J Radiat Oncol Biol Phys 1987;13:279–82.

53. Loeffler JS, Alexander E, Siddon RL, et al. Stereotactic radiosurgery for intracranial arteriovenous malformations using a standard linear accelerator. Int J Radiat Oncol Biol Phys 1989;17:673–7.

54. Mitsumori M, Shrieve DC, Alexander E, et al. Initial clinical results of LINAC-based stereotactic radiosurgery and stereotactic radiotherapy for pituitary adenomas. Int J Radiat Oncol Biol Phys 1998;42:573–80.

55. Kamerer D, Lunsford LD, Miller M. Gamma knife: an alternative treatment for acoustic neuromas. Ann Otol Rhinol Laryngol 1988;97:631–5.

56. Corn BW, Curran WJ, Shrieve DC, et al. Stereotactic radiosurgery and radiotherapy: new developments and new directions. Semin Oncol l998;24:707–14.

57. Patil AA, Kumar P, Leibrock LG. Response of extra-axial tumors to stereotactically implanted high-activity ^{125}I seeds. Stereotact Funct Neurosurg 1995;64:139–152.

58. Mathiesen T, Kihlstrom L, Karlsson B, et al. Potential complications following radiotherapy for meningiomas. Surg Neurol 2003;60(3):193–8; discussion 199–200.

59. McMullen KP, Stieber VW. Meningioma: current treatment options and future directions. Curr Treat Options Oncol 2004;5(6):499–509.

60. D'Ambrosio AL, Bruce JN. Treatment of meniongioma: an update. Curr Neurol Neurosci Rep 2003;3(3):206–14.

61. Curry WT, McDermott MW, Carter BS, et al. Craniotomy for meningioma in the United States between 1988 and 2000: decreasing rate of mortality and the effect of provider caseload. J Neurosurg 2005;102(6):977–86.

62. Kumar PP, Patil AA, Syh HW, et al. Role of brachytherapy in the management of the skull base meningioma, Cancer 1993;71:3726–3731.

63. Kumar PP, Good RR. Reversal of sixth nerve palsy in recurrent nasopharyngeal cancer with high-activity iodine-124 endocurietherapy. Endocurietherapy/ Hyperthermia Oncology 1987;3:91–95.

64. Kumar PP, Good RR, Cox Ta, et al. Reversal of visual impairment after interstitial irradiation of pituitary tumor. Neurosurgery 1986;18:82–84.

65. Obasi PC, Barnett GH, Suh JH. Brachytherapy for intracranial meningioma using a permanently implanted iodine-125 seed. Stereotact Funct Neurosurg 2002;79:33–43.

66. Vuorinen V, Heikkonen J, Brander A, et al. Interstitial radiotherapy of 25 parasellar/clival meningiomas and 19 meningiomas in the elderly. Analysis of short-term tolerance and responses. Acta Neurochir (Wien) 1996;138:495–508.

67. Ware ML, Larson DA, Sneed PK, et al. Surgical resection and permenant brachtherapy for recurrent atypical and malignant meningioma. Neurosurgery 2004;54:55–64.

30
Medical Therapy for Meningiomas

Glen H.J. Stevens and David M. Peereboom

If medals were given for effectiveness of treatment for progressive meningiomas from a historical perspective, medical management would collect the bronze behind radiotherapy and surgery. That placement has really not changed much today, but medical treatments do exist when surgery is not an option and patients have exhausted radiation. This chapter will highlight the historical use of hormonal/chemotherapy treatments that have most often been based on the molecular/immunologic rationale. What will be found, however, is a lack of phase III randomized trials with an abundance of small cohort and anecdotal trials that often mix benign and malignant meningiomas.

Hormonal Influences

Role of Endogenous Sex Steroids

Inference about meningiomas being under hormonal influence is based on several observations. It is well known that there is a preponderance of meningiomas in females versus males (2:1),[1] and meningiomas may increase in size during pregnancy and the luteal phase of the menstrual cycle[2] when progestin levels are high. The fluctuation in tumor size has been postulated to be secondary to direct trophic affects of gonadal hormones on meningioma cells, increased vascular engorgement, or steroid-induced fluid retention in the tumor.[3] It has also been suggested that some of the changes (growth) noted during pregnancy could be reversed postpartum.[4,5] There is also a well-known association of meningiomas with breast cancer,[6,7] and it is important to remind meningioma patients about self-breast exams and mammograms. Finally, meningiomas are rarely diagnosed during childhood before puberty, corresponding to the time of insignificant gonadal activity.[8] It is interesting, however that higher-grade meningiomas are seen more predominately in men[9] and that proliferation indices also tend to be higher in males.[10] If estrogen or progesterone can influence meningiomas, it would seem likely that receptors for these hormones could be found in association with meningiomas.

Meningioma Receptors

Estrogen Receptors

Estrogen receptors (ER) were first reported in association with meningiomas in 1979.[11] While ER have been found in association with meningiomas, the concentration of progesterone receptors (PR) is much greater, questioning the significance of ER.[12] Halper et al. studied ER and PR in meningiomas removed from 52 patients and found that the majority of the meningiomas expressed high-affinity PR using three different assay techniques, while ER were present in only a few meningiomas.[13] It is not surprising then that the use of antiestrogen drugs, such as tamoxifen, have yielded limited results.[14] In the Goodwin trial, 21 meningioma patients were treated with tamoxifen. Three patients had partial or minor responses of short duration, 6 remained stable for a median duration of 31+ months, and 10 (53%) demonstrated progression. Twenty-two percent reported subjective improvement. Another trial of this agent in six patients yielded one with a minor response.[15] Hence when ER are present, the question arises as to their exact role and significance. There was also one study that showed some response to the antiestrogen drug mepitiostane in meningioma patients.[16] In that case report, a 68-year-old woman with a history of gastric cancer was given mepitiostane for 2 years with a 73% regression of a suspected meningioma. Smith and Cahill suggest that although estrogen binding may be 30% in meningiomas it is primarily at low-affinity nonspecific receptors.[17] While it appears that ER can be found on meningiomas, their targeting for treatment purposes at this point seems limited.

Progesterone Receptors

Progesterone receptors (PR) are also found on meningiomas and are more prevalent than ER. They are again female predominant.[18] Progesterone receptors are seen more commonly in benign meningiomas and define a lower likelihood of tumor recurrence.[19,20] PR-negative meningiomas have been associated with a higher incidence of invasiveness, mitotic activity, and necrosis, as well as shorter disease-free intervals.[21,22] Conversly, the presence of PR can be considered a favorable prognostic factor for meningiomas. Mifepristone, also known as RU486, is an antiprogesterone and is a derivative of the progestine norethindrone.[23] Olsen et al. first reported on the effects of RU486 in meningioma tissue culture in 1986.[24] They found that RU486 inhibited growth (ranging from 18 to 36%) in three human meningioma cell lines that expressed ER and PR. These findings were then confirmed in in vivo and in vitro experiments.[25] Initial clinical trials by Grunberg and Lamberts suggested a mild benefit of RU486 in patients with meningiomas.[26,27] In the Grunberg trial, 12 patients were given RU486 at 200 mg/day, with 5 of those patients having at least a 10% decrease in tumor volume after a minimum of 6 months of treatment.[26] Two of the five responders later experienced progression of their meningioma. At least one patient withdrew from the trial secondary to side effects that were frequent and included fatigue (11/14) and gynecomastia in males (3/6). In the Lamberts trial, 10 patients with meningioma were also treated with 200 mg/day of RU486 and followed for 1 year.[27] Three patients had stable disease, four had progressive disease, and temporary regression was seen in three patients. Lamberts reported significant problems with nausea, fatigue, and anorexia in four patients that improved with prednisone replacement.[27] RU486 has known antiglucocorticoid activity, which complicates its prolonged use. A phase III double-blind randomized placebo-controlled trial of mifepristone conducted by the Eastern Cooperative Oncology Group (ECOG) in 193 meningioma patients showed no benefit.[28] Antiprogesterone drugs have a limited role in the treatment of recurrent meningioma.

Androgen Receptors

The role of androgen receptors (AR) in meningiomas is unknown. Androgen receptors have been found on meningiomas, and it has been suggested that AR rather than ER may regulate PR in meningiomas.[29] Carroll et al. found that more women (69%) than men with meningiomas express androgen receptor mRNA.[29] Testosterone has been shown to stimulate in vitro growth of meningioma cells.[30] There are currently no clinical trials investigating anti-androgen therapies.

Other Hormones

Somatostatin Receptors

Somatostatin receptors are found on meningiomas but vary in receptor density.[31] Why they are present and their exact role and function remain uncertain. The addition of octreotide (somatostatin agonist) in vitro can inhibit meningioma growth.[32] Garcia-Luna et al. gave octreotide subcutaneously to three patients with unresectable meningiomas at titrated doses of 1000, 900, and 1500 μg/24 hours for 16, 6, and 7 weeks,

respectively.[33] Computed axial tomography scans showed no change in tumor size, but all three patients noted some clinical improvement. Octreotide SPECT has been used clinically in the diagnosis of meningiomas from other intracranial tumors, taking advantage of the somatostatin receptors present in meningiomas.[34,35] There are currently no ongoing clinical trials investigating somatostatin agonists.

Prolactin Receptors

Muccioli et al. found prolactin receptors (PRL-R) in 62% of 60 resected meningiomas.[36] The PRL-R were unrelated to gender or histology. No PRL-R binding was noted from normal arachnoid cells. They also demonstrated that prolactin added to cell culture caused meningioma cells to grow. Conversely, dopamine inhibits in vitro growth of meningioma cells.[37] There are currently no clinical trials manipulating this relationship.

Chemotherapy

Chemotherapeutic drugs are usually cytotoxic or cytostatic in effect. World Health Organization (WHO) grade I meningiomas, which grow at a slow rate, may require a treatment strategy that is employed over many months or years and hence respond better to cytostatic therapies, while WHO III meningiomas (malignant) may respond better to cytotoxic drugs. Early clinical trials of adjuvant chemotherapy focused mostly on malignant meningiomas. Chamberlain treated malignant meningioma patients with cyclophosphamide/doxorubicin (Adriamycin™)/vincristine (CAV).[38] Fourteen patients with malignant meningioma received CAV 2–4 weeks after surgery and radiotherapy. There were three partial responders and 11 with stable disease with a median time to progression of 4.6 years (range 2.2–7.1 years). The median survival was 5.3 years with a range of 2.6–7.6 years. Four patients required CAV dose reductions, and three patients received fewer than the planned number of cycles due to myelosuppression. It is unknown, however, if the same results without the toxicity would have been achieved with surgery and radiotherapy alone without the addition of chemotherapy. This section will focus on the various chemotherapies employed in the treatment of meningiomas.

Hydroxyurea

Hydroxyurea is a ribonucleotide reductase inhibitor that has been used to treat various hematologic malignancies.[39] Hydroxyurea is used for long-term treatment of chronic myelogenous leukemia and sickle cell anemia.[40,41] Since hydroxyurea can be used in patients for long periods of time, it may be an ideal drug for WHO I and II meningiomas, which have a slow proliferation rate where prolonged exposure may be beneficial.[42] Hydroxyurea inhibits DNA synthesis by blocking the conversion of ribonucleotides to deoxyribonucleotides without affecting RNA or protein synthesis. Hydroxyurea is an antimetabolite that is orally absorbed, which allows ease of administration. Its effects appear to be specific to the S phase of the cell cycle. The molecular target is likely DNA synthesis mechanisms, and the drug causes surviving cells to be synchronized.[43] Hydroxyurea's mechanism of action hence makes it a good drug for use with other chemotherapeutic agents or in combination with radiation therapy.[44] Hydroxyurea inhibits human meningioma cell growth in culture and in xenograft transplantation models.[45] Scherll et al. were the first to report on the clinical responsiveness of human meningiomas treated with hydroxyurea.[46] In their study, four selected patients (three WHO I with progression and one malignant meningioma) received hydroxyurea at 20 mg/kg/day. The three patients with WHO I lesions decreased in size by 60, 74, and 15% during 5–10 months of treatment. The patient with WHO III meningioma had no recurrence for 24 months. None of the patients had significant bone marrow suppression. The authors hypothesized that treatment affect was secondary to induction of apoptosis. Based on these initial reports, Mason et al. treated 20 patients with progressive meningiomas (16 benign, 3 atypical, and 1 malignant) with hydroxyurea in a multicenter trial.[47] The mean patient age was 59 years with a Karnofsky Performance Score (KPS) of 80. Patients received a single dose of hydroxyurea of 20–30 mg/kg/day and were followed to progression or 2 years. Twelve patients with WHO I meningioma had stable disease for a median of 122 weeks, and two of those patients had clinical improvement with one partial response on imaging. Three WHO I meningioma patients had progression at 41, 55, and 66 weeks. For the three patients with WHO II tumors, progressive disease (PD) was noted at 12, 19, and 45 weeks and the WHO III patient had PD at 24 weeks. No patient had National Cancer Institute (NCI) grade 4 toxicity. For the 16 WHO I meningiomas the 1- and 2-year freedom from progression rates were 0.93 (SE 0.07) and 0.77 (SE 0.12), respectively, which were encouraging. Newton et al. reported on 21 meningioma patients treated with hydroxyurea.[48] Patients received hydroxyurea 20 mg/kg/day. Eighteen of 20 evaluable patients responded with stable disease ranging from 20 to 328+ weeks with a median time to progression of 176 weeks. Five of the stable patients progressed after 20, 56, 36, 216, and 56 weeks, respectively. Two patients had progressive disease after 10 weeks. They did report six patients with NCI grade 3 or 4 toxicity (four leukopenia and two anemia), although no patient who required filgrastim had an infectious complication. Eleven patients required dose reductions. They concluded that hydroxyurea had modest effects against residual meningiomas. Loven et al. examined hydroxyurea at 20 mg/kg/day in 12 patients (7 females, 5 males) with what they deemed slow-growing nonresectable meningiomas.[49] Six patients had received prior irradiation, and 10 had more than one prior surgery. Patients were followed with CT and by 201-Thalium single photoemission computed tomography every 3 months. During the study period, nine patients had progressive disease (10% increase in one diameter) with a median time to

progression of 13 months (range 4–24 months). Two patients were removed from the study within the first 3 months for early hematologic toxicity (one grade 3 anemia and one grade 4 thrombocytopenia) and one patient had a minimal response with tumor stabilization. Two other patients had grade 3–4 hematologic toxicity that was controlled by dose adjustments. There were no severe cases of nonhematologic toxicity, although there was one patient who had a nonhealing wound during his first 12 months of treatment. The Newton and Mason studies were published after the start of the Loven trial that was also stimulated by the Scherll data.[47–49] Loven et al. did not feel that hydroxyurea was an effective treatment for their population of nonresectable meningioma patients.[49] Rosenthal et al. reported on 15 progressive meningioma patients treated with hydroxyurea at 20 mg/kg/day as a single dose.[39] Patients were treated until progression or development of unmanageable toxicity. Two patients stopped treatment secondary to skin rashes that abated after stopping treatment. The rashes were NCI grade II and III. There were no treatment-related hospitalizations. There was one grade III hematologic toxicity and two additional patients who required dose reductions. Thirteen patients were evaluable for response to treatment. No complete or partial responses were noted. Eleven patients had stable disease for a median of 11 months, and two patients had progressive disease. Of the eleven stable disease patients, eight had progressive disease prior to starting hydroxyurea. Hahn et al. reported on 21 progressive or recurrent meningiomas (13 benign, 4 atypical and malignant, and 4 unproven histology).[50] They all had treatment with 3D-conformal radiation (55.8–59.4 Gy) and concurrent hydroxyurea for a minimum of 3 months at 20 mg/kg/day. Progression-free survival rates at 1 and 2 years were 84 and 77%, respectively. At the time of analysis, six patients had progressive disease at a median time to progression of 59 weeks. There were no documented cases of complete or partial response. Only one patient stopped hydroxyurea treatment due to gastrointestinal symptoms. Early clinical trials have supported the radiation sensitizing effects of hydroxyurea.[44] Levin reviewed early studies of hydroxyurea as a radiosensitzer in glioma patients.[51] The degree of benefit achieved with the addition of hydroxyurea to the radiation in the Hahn trial is unknown. A Southwest Oncology Group protocol (SWOG-S9811) completed accrual as of 06/01/05 using hydroxyurea alone in meningioma patients, and the results are pending.[52] It appears that hydroxyurea may have some utility in meningioma management as a single agent treatment or combined with radiation, but its exact role should be better defined once the SWOG data has been analyzed.

Temozolomide

Chamberlain et al. completed a prospective phase II study of temozolomide (TMZ) in 16 patients (11 female, 5 male) with refractory WHO I meningioma.[53] All patients had previously received surgery and involved-field radiotherapy and had progressive disease. None of the patients had received prior chemotherapy. Temozolomide was administered orally for 42 consecutive days every 10 weeks. The prolonged TMZ dosing was used to give maximal tumor exposure to drug and gave a 2.5-fold higher TMZ dose intensity as compared to the standard 5-day schedule given every 28 days.[54] Grade 3 or greater toxicity included anemia (25%), fatigue (18.7%), neutropenia (37.5%), seizures (6.3%), and thrombocytopenia (18.7%). No patient demonstrated a neuroradiographic complete or partial response. Three patients progressed after the first cycle, and all patients went off study secondary to disease progression. Time to tumor progression ranged from 2.5 to 5.0 months (median 5.0 months), and survival ranged from 4 to 9 months (median 7.5 months). They concluded that TMZ was not an active agent for the treatment of recurrent meningiomas.

Interferon-α2b

Interferons (IFN) are naturally occurring proteins that belong to a large class of glycoproteins called cytokines. They are produced by the immune system in response to various perturbations on the system including tumors.[55] Interferon-α has been reported to affect meningiomas in vivo and in vitro.[56,57] Interferons are thought to exert at least part of their antitumor effects on meningiomas through inhibition of angiogenesis.[58] Kaba et al. reported on the efficacy of IFN-α2b in the treatment of recurrent unresectable and malignant meningiomas.[56] Six patients (two WHO I, one WHO II, and three WHO III) received IFN-α subcutaneously at $4\,mU/M^2/day$, 5 days per week. Five patients had stabilization of their tumor, and one had slight progression with responses lasting 6–14 months (stable at time of publication). The toxicity was also reported as mild and tolerable, consisting mostly of flu-like symptoms and pain at the injection site. Two patients had mild leukopenia requiring dose reductions. While the data on IFN is limited in meningiomas, it appears to warrant additional consideration. Of interest, however, Drevelegas et al. reported on a multiple sclerosis patient with a documented intraventricular meningioma that grew while on interferon-β for 2 years.[60] They felt the growth was related to IFN stimulating platelet-derived growth factor receptors and/or downregulating transforming growth receptors that were both noted on the tumors. The investigators felt further studies were warranted.

Molecular Marker: Cyclooxygenase-2 (COX-2)

Another potentially interesting target for meningioma treatment is COX-2. Cyclooxygenase is the rate-limiting enzyme in the synthesis of prostaglandins from arachidonic acid.[61] COX-2 overexpression has been linked to tumorigenesis of colon, lung, and breast cancer.[62] COX-2 inhibitors have anti-inflammatory properties based on decreased prostaglandin production. Prostaglandins are thought to be involved in angiogenesis, increased cell proliferation, and suppression of apoptosis.[63] Celecoxib (Celebrex™) is a COX-2 inhibitor that produces a slow, time-dependent irreversible inhibition

of COX-2.[63] Ragel et al. examined the effect of COX-2 on meningiomas in vitro.[64] They measured COX-2 levels from surgically resected meningiomas and graded them from 0 to 4 using immunohistochemistry techniques. Western blot was also used to calculate human meningioma cell growth after treatment with celecoxib. They found high immunoreactivity (grade 4 staining) in 111/128 benign meningiomas and 6/7 atypical meningiomas. Western blot analysis of four surgical specimens that stained for COX-2 all displayed inhibited cell growth in a dose-dependent fashion and induced apoptosis by day 2 after exposure to celecoxib. Lin et al. found a relationship between meningioma grade and COX-2 expression.[65] Eighty-three surgical specimens from patients were evaluated. Tumor grade was determined using the 1993 and 2000 WHO criteria for meningioma grading. Using the WHO-93 grade, tumors with more aggressive pathology (benign, atypical, and malignant) had higher levels of COX-2. Using the WHO-2000 classification, however, the association between tumor grade and COX-2 expression was not significant ($p = 0.17$). This association provides a potential strategy for treatment although a planned Radiation Therapy Oncology Group (RTOG 0512) meningioma trial has been canceled secondary to the potential cardiac risk associated with COX-2 inhibitor use (See chapter 15).[66]

Emerging Therapies

Platelet-derived growth factor (PDGF) is overexpressed in meningiomas, which may in turn contribute to cell growth.[67] Imatinib (Gleevec™) is an inhibitor of specific protein tyrosine kinases targeted to PDGF.[68] Imatinib is currently being evaluated in clinical trials with meningiomas by several groups including the North American Brain Tumor Consortium (NABTC).[69,70]

Epidermal growth factor receptor (EGFR) overexpression has been well described in certain cancers, including glioblastoma multiforme.[71] Weisman et al. in 1987 helped to characterize EGFR status in meningiomas and suggested that it could be related to proliferation and or differentiation of meningioma cells.[72] Further work by Carroll et al. in 1997 in 27 meningioma surgical specimens also found EGFR expression and that activated EGFR could stimulate the Ras pathway through endogenous ligands.[73] The North American Brain Tumor Consortium has recently completed a phase I/II trial using the EGFR antagonist erlotinib (Tarceva™) in meningioma patients.[69] The final results of that trial are pending.

Since meningiomas are vascular tumors, there has also been an interest in exploring the use of antiangiogenesis agents other than IFN.[74] Cilengitide (EMD 121974) is thought to inhibit angiogenesis by blocking integrin function.[75] A phase I study of cilengitide (EMD 121974) in children with refractory primary brain tumors (including meningiomas) has been completed through the Pediatric Brain Tumor Consortium (PBTC-012), and the results are pending.[76]

Conclusion

There has been a concerted effort over the last 25 years to define targets for hormonal or chemotherapy-related management. While many different receptors have been identified on meningiomas and small cohort and phase II trials have initially appeared encouraging, no phase III trials have yet shown a response to pharmaceutical manipulation. The results of several phase II and III trials are currently pending. At present, trials using hydroxyurea have provided the best data for systemic treatment for recurrent meningiomas, but even these data are inconsistent. Newer receptor targets are being defined with the goal of providing targeted medical therapy.

References

1. Black PM. Hormones, radiosurgery and virtual reality: new aspects of meningioma management. Can J Neurol Sci 1997;24:302–306.
2. Bickerstaff ER, Small JM, Guest IA. The relapsing course of certain meningiomas in relation to pregnancy and menstruation. J Neurol Neurosurg Psychiatry 1958;21:89–91.
3. Chaudhuri P, Wallenburg HCS. Brain tumors and pregnancy. Europ J Obstet Gynec Reprod Biol 1980;11:109–114.
4. Roelvink NC, Kamphorst W, van Alphen HA, et al. Pregnancy-related primary brain and spinal tumors. Arch Neurol 1987;44:209–215.
5. Smith JS, Hinojosa AQ, Smith MH, et al. Sex steroid and growth factor profile of a meningioma associated with pregnancy. Can J Neurol Sci 2005;32:122–127.
6. Schoenberg BS, Christine BW, Whisnant JP. Nervous system neoplasms and primary malignancies of other sites. The unique association between meningiomas and breast cancer. Neurology 1975:25;705–712.
7. Markopoulos C, Sampalis F, Givalos N, et al. Association of breast cancer with meningioma. Eur J Surg Oncol 1998;24:332–334.
8. Poisson M. Sex steroid receptors in human meningiomas. Clin Neuropharmacol 1984;7:320–324.
9. Jaaskelainen J, Haltia M, Servo A. Atypical and anaplastic meningiomas: radiology, surgery, radiotherapy, and outcome. Surg Neurol 1986;25:233–242.
10. Matsuno A, Fujimaki T, Sasaki T, et al. Clinical and histopathological analysis of proliferative potentials of recurrent and nonrecurrent meningioma. Acta Neuropathol 1986;91:504–510.
11. Donnell M, Meyer G, Donegan W. Estrogen-receptor protein in intracranial meningiomas. J Neurosurg 1979;50:499–502.
12. Blankenstein MA, van der Meulin-Dijk C, Thijssen JHH. Assay of oestrogen and progestrin receptors in human meningioma cytosols using immunological methods. Clin Chim Acta 1987;165:189–195.
13. Halper J, Colvard DS, Scheithauer BW, et al. Estrogen and progesterone receptors in meningiomas: comparison of nuclear binding, dextra-coated charchol, and immunoperoxide staining assays. Neurosurgery 1989;25:546–553.
14. Goodwin JW, Crowley J, Eyre HJ, et al. A phase II evaluation of tamoxifen in unresectable or refractory meningiomas: a Southwest Oncology Group study. J Neurooncol 1993;15:75–77.
15. Markwalder TM, Seiler RW, Zava DT. Antiestrogenic therapy of meingiomas- a pilot study. Surg Neurol 1985;24:245–249.
16. Oura S, Sakurai T, Yoshimura G, et al. Regression of a presumed meningioma with the antiestrogen agent mepitiostane. Case report. J Neurosurg 2000;93:132–135.
17. Smith DA, Cahill DW. The biology of meningiomas. Neurosurg Clin North Am 1994;5:201–215.
18. Carroll R, Glowacka D, Dashner K, et al. Progesterone receptor expression in meningiomas. Cancer Res 1993;53:1312–1316.
19. Perry A, Cai D, Scheithauer B, et al. Merlin DAL-1, and progesterone receptor expression in clinicopathologic subsets of meningioma: a correlative immunohistochemical study of 175 cases. J Neuropathol Exp Neurol 2000;59:872–879.
20. Fewings P, Battersby R, Timperley W. Long-term follow up of progesterone receptor status in benign meningiomas: a prognostic indicator of recurrence? J Neurosurg 2000;92:401–405.
21. Hilbig A, Barbosa-Coutinho LM. Meningioma and hormone receptors: immunohistochemical study in typical and non-typical tumors. Arquiv Neuro Psiquiatria 1998;56:193–199.
22. Hsu DW, Efird JT, Hedley-Whyte ET. Progesterone and estrogen receptors in meningiomas: prognostic considerations. J Neurosurg 1997;86:113–120.
23. Spitz IM, Bardin CW. Mifepristone (RU 486)- A modulator of progestin and glucocorticoid action. NEJM 1993;329:404–412.
24. Olsen JJ, Beck DW, Schechte J, et al. Hormonal manipulation of meningioma in vitro. J Neurosurg 1986;65:99–107.
25. Matsuda Y, Kawamoto K, Kiya K, et al. Antitumor effects of antiprogesterones on human meningioma cells in vitro and in vivo. J Neurosurg 1994;80:527–534.
26. Grunberg SM, Weiss MH, Spitz IM, et al. Treatment of unresectable meningiomas with the anitiprogesterone agent mifepristone. J Neurosurg 1991;74:861–866.
27. Lamberts S, Tanghe H, Avezaat C, et al. Mifepristone (RU 486) treatment of meningiomas. J Neurol Neurosurg Psychiatry 1992;55:486–490.
28. Grunberg SM, Rankin C, Townsend J, et al. Phase III double-blind randomized placebo-controlled study of mifepristone (RU) for the treatment of unresectable meningioma. Proceedings of the American Society of Clinical Oncology Annual Meeting, Abstract No. 222, 2001, 20–56a.
29. Carroll RS, Zhang J, Dasher K, et al. Androgen receptor expression in meningiomas. J Neurosurg 1995;82:453–460.
30. Zava D, Markwalder T, Markwalder R. Biological expression of steroid hormone receptors in primary meningioma cells in monolayer culture. Clin Neuropharmacol 1984;7:382–388.
31. Reubi JC, Maurer R, Klijn JG, et al. High incidence of somatostatin receptors in human meningiomas:biochemical characterization. J Clin Endocrin Metabolism 1986;63-433–438.
32. Schulz S, Pauli SU, Schulz S, et al. Immunohistochemical determination of five somatostatin receptors in meningioma reveals frequent overexpression of somatostatin subtype sst2A. Clin Cancer Res 2000;6:1865–1874.
33. Garcia-Luna PP, Relimpio F, Pumar A, et al. Clinical use of octreotide in unresectable meningiomas: a report of three cases. J Neurosurg Sci 1993;37:237–241.
34. Schmidt M, Scheidhauer K, Luyken C, et al. Somatostatin receptor imaging in intracranial tumors. Eur J Nucl Med 1998;25:675–686.
35. Henze M, Strauss AD, Zabel SM, et al. Characterization of ^{68}Ga-DOTA-D-Phe^1-Tyr^3- octreotide kinetics in patients with meningiomas. J Nuc Med 2005;46:763–769.

36. Mucciolo G, Ghe C, Faccani G, et al. Prolactin receptors in human meningioma: characterization and biological role. J Endocrin 1997;153:365–371.

37. Schrell U, Fahlbusch R, Adams, E, et al. Growth of cultured human cerebral meningiomas is inhibited by dopaminergic agents. Presence of high affinity dopamine D1 receptors. J Clin Endorinol Metab 1990;71:1669–1671.

38. Chamberlain MC. Adjuvant combined modality therapy for malignant meningiomas. J Neurosug 1996;84:733–736.

39. Rosenthal MA, Ashley DL, Cher L. Treatment of high risk or recurrent meningioma with hydroxyurea. J Clin Neurosci 2002;9:156–158.

40. Kennedy BJ. Hydroxyurea therapy in chronic myelogenous leukemia. Cancer 1972;29:1052–1056.

41. Goldberg MA, Bougnara C, Dover GI, et al. Hydroxyurea and erythropoieten therapy in sickle cell anemia. Sem Oncol 1992;19(Suppl 9):74–81.

42. Hoshino T, Nagashima T, Murovic JA, et al. Proliferation potential of human meningiomas of the brain. A cell kinetics study with bromodeoxyuridine. Cancer 1986;58:1466–1472.

43. Yarbro JW. Mechanism of action of hydroxyurea. Semin Oncol 1992;19:1–10.

44. Sinclair WK. Hydroxyurea revisited: a decade of clinical effects studies. Int J Radiat Oncol Biol Phys 1981;7:631–637.

45. Schrell UM, Rittig MG, Anders M, et al. Hydroxyurea for treatment of unresectable and recurrent meningiomas I. Inhibition of primary human meningioma cells in culture and in meningioma transplants by induction of the apoptotic pathway. J Neurosurg 1997;86:845–852.

46. Scherll UM, Rittig MG, Anders M, et al. Hydroxyurea for treatment of unresectable and recurrent meningiomas. II. Decrease in the size of meningiomas in patients treated with hydroxyurea. J Neurosurg 1997;86:840–844.

47. Mason WP, Gentili F, MacDonald DR, et al. Stabilization of disease progression by hydroxyurea in patients with recurrent or unresectable meningioma. J Neurosurg 2002;97:341–346.

48. Newton HB, Scott SR, Volpi C. Hydroxyurea chemotherapy for meningiomas: enlarged cohort with extended follow-up. Br J Neurosurg 2004;18:495–499.

49. Loven D, Hardoff R, Sever ZB, et al. Non-resectable slow-growing meningiomas treated by hydroxyurea. J Neurooncol 2004, 67:221–226.

50. Hahn BM, Schrell UM, Sauer R, et al. Prolonged oral hydroxyurea and concurrent 3d-conformal radiation in patients with progressive or recurrent meningioma: results of a pilot study. J Neurooncol 2005;74:157–165.

51. Levin VA. The place of hydroxyurea in the treatment of primary brain tumors. Sem Oncol 1992:19(Suppl 9):34–39.

52. Southwest Oncology Group (SWOG): Swinnen LJ: Phase II study of hydroxyurea for unresectable meningioma: www.swog.org

53. Chamberlain MC, Denice D. Tsao-Wei, MS, et al. Temozolomide for treatment-resistant recurrent meningioma. Neurology 2004;62:1210–1212.

54. Khan RB, Raizer JJ, Malkin MG, et al. A phase II study of extended low-dose temozolamide in recurrent malignant glioma. Neurooncology 2002;4:39–43.

55. Muhr C, Gudjonsson O, Lilja A, et al. Meningioma treated with interferon-alpha, evaluated with ^{11}C–L-methionine positron emission tomography. Clin Cancer Res 2001;7:2269–2276.

56. Kaba SE, DeMonte F, Bruner JM, et al. The treatment of recurrent unresectable and malignant meningiomas with interferon alpha-2B. Neurosurgery 1997;40:271–275.

57. Zang ZJ, Muhr C, Wang JL. Interferon alpha inhibits the DNA synthesis induced by PDGF and EGF in cultured meningioma cells. Anticancer Res 1996;16:717–723.

58. Folkman J, Ingber D. Inhibition of angiogenesis. Semin Cancer Biol 1992;3:89–96.

59. Kirkwood JM, Strawderman MH, Ernstoff MS, et al. Interferon alpha-2B adjuvant therapy of high-risk resected cutaneous melanoma: The Eastern Cooperative Oncology Group Trial EST 1684. Clin Oncol 1996;14:7–17.

60. Drevelegas A, Xinou E, Karacostas D, et al. Meningioma growth and interferon beta-1b treated multiple sclerosis: coincidence or relationship? Neuroradiol 2005;47:516–519.

61. Pairet M, Engelhardt G. Distinct isoforms (COX-1 and COX-2) of cyclooxygenase: possible physiological and therapeutic implications. Fundam Clin Pharmacol 1998;10:1–17.

62. Umar A, Viner JL, Anderson WF, et al. Development of COX inhibitors in cancer prevention and therapy. Am J Clin Oncol 2003;26:S48–57.

63. Hines B, Brune K. Cyclooxygenase-2 10 years later. J Pharmacol Exp Ther 2002;300:367–375.

64. Ragel BT, Jensen RL, Gillespie DL, et al. Ubiquitous expression of cyclooxygenase-2 in meningiomas and decrease in cell growth following in vitro treatment with the inhibitor celecoxib: potential therapeutic applications. J Neurosurg 2005;103:508–517.

65. Lin CC, Kenyon L, Hyslop T, et al. Cyclooxygenase-2 (COX-2) expression in human meningioma as a function of tumor grade. Am J Clin Oncol 2003;26:S98–102.

66. Radiation Therapy Oncology Group (RTOG): www.rtog.org

67. Johnson MD, Okediji E, Woodard A, et al. Evidence for phosphatidylinositol 3-kinase-Akt-p70^{S6K} pathway activation and transduction of mitogenic signals by platelet-derived growth factor in meningioma cells. J. Neurosurg 2002;97:668–675.

68. Savage DG, Antman KH. Imatinib mesylate—a new oral targeted therapy. NEJM 2002;346:683–693.

69. North American Brain Tumor Consortium. Erlotinib in treating patients with recurrent malignant glioma or recurrent or progressive meningioma. http://clinicaltrials.com

70. National Cancer Institute trial: phase II trial of STI1571 (NSC716051) in patients with recurrent meningiomas; start date Sept 25 2003: http://www.ctf.org/clinical_trials/STI571meningioma.htm

71. Fleming TP, Saxena A, Clark WC, et al. Amplification and/or overexpression of platelet-derived growth factor receptors and epidermal growth factor receptors in human glial tumors. Cancer Res 1992;52:4550–4553.

72. Weisman AS, Raguet SS, Kelly PA. Characterization of epidermal growth factor receptor in human meningioma. Cancer Res 1987;47:2172–2176.

73. Carroll RS, Black PM, Zang J, et al. Expression and activation of epidermal growth factor receptors in meningiomas. J Neurosurg 1997;87:315–323.

74. Tatagiba M, Mirzai S, Samii M. Peritumoral blood flow in intracranial meningioma. Neurosurgery 1991;28:400–404

75. Burke PA, et al. Cilengitide targeting of alpha (v) beta (3) integrin receptor synergizes with radioimmunotherapy to increase efficacy and apoptosis in breast cancer xenografts. Cancer Res 2002;62:4263–4272.

76. Pediatric Brain Tumor Consortium: Phase I study of Cilengitide (EMD 121974) in children with refractory primary brain tumors (PBTC-012). www.clinicaltrials.gov

VI
Meningiomas by Location: Special Considerations, Surgical Technique, Outcome, Complication Avoidance

31
Convexity Meningiomas

Noojan J. Kazemi and Andrew H. Kaye

Convexity meningiomas, as their name implies, are tumors that arise from the convexity of the skull vault and have dural attachments that do not involve any of the dural venous sinuses and are not related to the falx or substantially to the skull base. Convexity meningiomas have the greatest potential for cure as they ideally lend themselves to total removal, including the involved dura.

Approximately 90% of all meningiomas are supratentorial, with around 15–19% being located in the region of the convexity (1,2). These meningiomas occur almost two to three times more frequently in females (3), with the uncommon malignant meningioma being more frequent in males (4).

Meningiomas arise from meningothelial or arachnoid cap cells present in the arachnoid (Pacchionian) granulations along the dura and in the arachnoid layers of the meninges; however, their etiology is not fully understood. As with all other meningiomas, increased incidence of convexity meningiomas is associated with radiotherapy (4–6). Convexity meningiomas are also associated with chromosomal abnormalities such as DNA loss in chromosome 22, a genetic abnormality found in NF-2 (7,8). Along with other tumors, there is an increased incidence of meningiomas in NF-2 (3).

Classification

Convexity meningiomas have traditionally been classified into several subtypes based on anatomic division: precoronal, coronal, postcoronal, paracentral, parietal, temporal, and occipital (4). The majority of convexity lesions are located with a component of the tumor anterior to the central sulcus as there is increased density of arachnoid granulations anterior and adjacent to the coronal suture.

Special Considerations

Operative Aims

The majority of convexity lesions can be removed totally, including involved dura, as well as any associated involved soft tissue and bone with a wide margin of dural resection. Even in instances of transdural bone and soft tissue invasion, a complete resection is still possible (9). Dural replacement with pericranium, fascia lata, or other form of dural substitute is always required (10). All the involved bone should be removed, and occasionally this involves discarding the bone flap and subsequent cranioplasty, but usually a radical drilling of the involved bone suffices.

Symptoms

The majority of patients will present with signs and symptoms of raised intracranial pressure, focal neurologic deficit, or seizures.

Convexity lesions around the precentral cortical area may result in contralateral weakness and focal motor seizures, while tumors of the postcentral area may result in sensory deficits. Speech disturbance may result from involvement of the Broca's and Wernicke's area of the dominant hemisphere. Visual deficits may arise from lesions overlying the temporal or occipital lobes.

Up to 40% of patients with convexity meningiomas experience seizures preoperatively (11).

Cerebral edema may be a feature of these lesions and may be associated with cortical invasion of the tumor. Pial vessel involvement may be implied by the presence of a large amount of cerebral edema.

Preoperative Investigations

In most cases of convexity meningioma, computed tomography (CT) will diagnose the lesion and may demonstrate calcification within it (Fig. 31-1). Magnetic resonance imaging (MRI) is the diagnostic test of choice, usually showing bright, uniform enhancement with gadolinium (Fig. 31-2). Often, a dural tail demonstrating enhancement of surrounding meninges is demonstrated—a characteristic sign of a meningioma (Fig. 31-3). Around 6% of all meningiomas can appear cystic on MRI and may be confused with metastasis (12). Contribution of major feeding vessels from the internal carotid artery

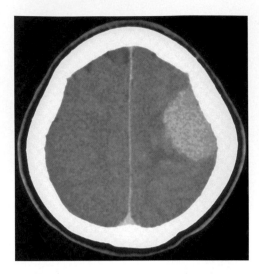

FIG. 31-1. Contrast-enhanced CT scan of a convexity meningioma

Growth Considerations

As meningiomas are not infrequently incidental findings, it is commonly thought that these tumors display a very low growth rate through life. Absolute growth rates of meningiomas vary between 0.03 and 2.62 cm³/year, with relative growth rates ranging between 0.48% and 72.2% (13). It has been suggested that surgical resection of meningiomas should be performed when the tumor growth rate is greater than 1 cm³/year (13,14). In the case of multiple convexity meningiomas, symptomatic lesions or those that display growth should be resected.

In the case of elderly patients, meningiomas often demonstrate a slower growth pattern (4,14). This fact, together with the increased incidence of morbidity and mortality from operative interventions in the elderly, may necessitate a more conservative approach to lesions in this group. Surgical treatment in this group is based on the neurologic condition and general health of the patient (15). Conservative treatment in the form of focused radiotherapy may be used, but as resection of convexity tumors is straightforward, surgery is usually the preferred treatment option. Thus the primary goal of convexity meningiomas, over and above lesions arising in other locations, is total tumor removal.

Particular care must be taken with convexity meningiomas that overlie the Sylvian fissure as the middle cerebral artery branches may adhere to the tumor capsule and are thus prone to injury during resection. This will be discussed later.

and venous drainage can be demonstrated on MR angiography and venography. Significant peri-tumoral edema is also shown (Fig. 31-4).

Digital subtraction angiography (DSA) is effective in demonstrating the vascularity of meningiomas, as well as its arterial feeders and venous drainage. In addition, angiography is useful for embolization of appropriate meningiomas. However, in the case of convexity meningiomas, much of the arterial supply is known to arise from the external carotid artery via branches of the middle meningeal artery and, in addition, embolization is usually not needed as feeding meningeal arteries can be occluded early in the operation. Where a meningioma has parasitized pial vessels, DSA may demonstrate these. There is a lower chance of an extrapial dissection being possible if pial vessels are visualized. The DSA will also demonstrate any additional internal carotid supply to a convexity lesion (Fig. 31-5).

Anesthetic Considerations

Steroid medication should commence immediately if there is evidence of cerebral edema and then tapered accordingly in the postoperative period.

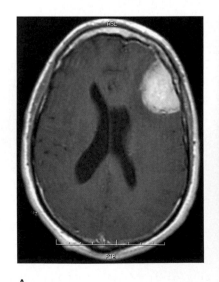

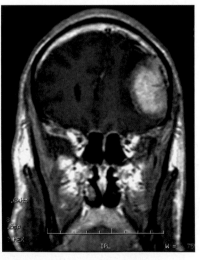

A   B

FIG. 31-2. Postgadolinium enhanced T1- weighted (A) axial and (B) coronal MRI of a convexity lesion

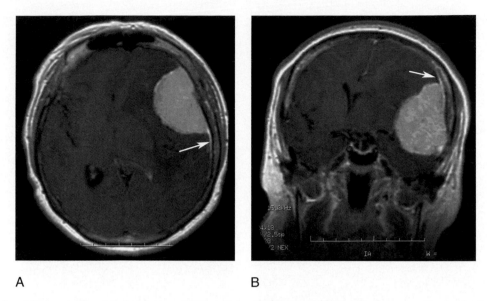

A B

FIG. 31-3. (A) Axial and (B) coronal gadolinium-enhanced T1-weighted MRI demonstrating the presence of a dural tail (white arrows) with some extension of the tumor mass into the Sylvian fissure

Anticonvulsants are commenced immediately upon diagnosis in the presence of any seizures, but also routinely continued for 3 months postoperatively in all patients, although there is some difference of opinion as to how long they should be continued. Preoperative optimization of cardiac and pulmonary function is necessary.

Significant blood loss may be encountered in cases of large or highly vascular tumors, and adequate preparation should be made in such situations. Other anesthetic management prior to surgery includes placement of an indwelling catheter and consideration for administering mannitol or furosemide for control of cerebral edema. Antibiotics are commenced at the induction of anesthesia and are continued for 24 hours after the operation.

Careful anesthetic application will minimize hemodynamic responses to intubation and surgery. It is important that there is no obstruction to the airway and cerebral venous drainage at any point. Care must be ensured that air embolism is detected at any stage, and where the head is elevated, a central venous catheter must be in position so as to aspirate air.

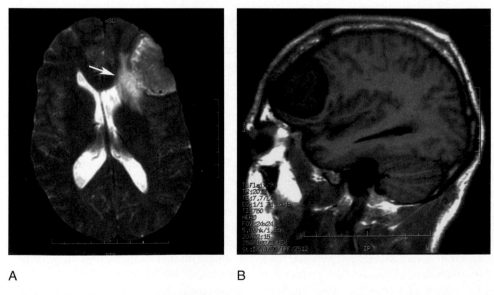

A B

FIG. 31-4. (A) T2-weighted axial MRI demonstrating peritumoral edema around the convexity lesion (white arrow). (B) T1-weighted sagittal image of the same lesion. The tumor demonstrates low signal before contrast

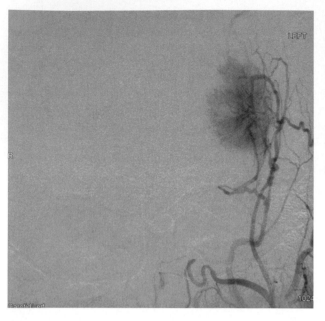
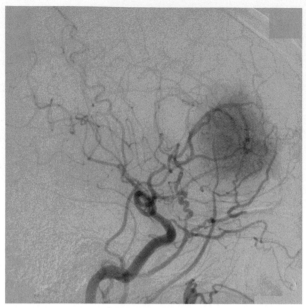

A   B

Fig. 31-5. (A) DSA image of external carotid run demonstrating external carotid supply to this convexity lesion. (B) DSA image of internal carotid artery run demonstrating significant internal carotid artery supply to the same lesion. Significant tumor blush is demonstrated on the DSA

Surgical Technique

Preoperative embolization is performed where appropriate (see Chapter 9), and frameless stereotactic navigation is utilized for all cases (see Chapter 21).

Patient Position

The patient is usually positioned such that the lesion is uppermost in the surgical field and the cranium is fixed in a three-point fixation headrest. If possible, the patient is positioned such that gravity is utilized and thus brain retraction minimized.

Adequate care is made to ensure that all pressure areas are padded, with special attention paid to the eyes, brachial plexus, and peripheral nerves. An adequate shave i s performed. Extreme care must be made to avoid any scrub solution running into the eyes with adequate cover of the eyes. The lesion is marked with the aid of neuro-navigation, and landmarks such as the superior sagittal sinus are also marked out.

Exposure

The skin flap is fashioned to ensure an adequate vascular base, and a semi-curved or bicoronal incision is often preferred as these provide good exposure and preserve scalp vascularity. This will also allow access to fascia if needed for dural repair. The use of frameless neuro-navigation software will ensure that the bone flap lifted is just beyond the margins of the tumor and the involved dura. The skin flap should extend at least 1–2 cm beyond the craniotomy so that it is entirely covered by the flap.

A free bone flap is preferred to an osteoplastic flap as this is less cumbersome to retract and eliminates excessive blood supply from branches of the external carotid artery. The bone flap must allow access to all the tumor margins and ideally expose an extra 1–2 cm beyond to allow adequate resection of involved dura, as well as for minor errors in the navigation system. The flap should be large enough to give access to safe exposure of associated vessels for vascular control as well as to be able to manage a change in operative approach.

Burr holes are placed, depending on the size of the tumor, circumferentially around a convexity meningioma tumor margin, and then a right-angled blunt dissector is utilized to separate the dura from bone in the directions of the adjacent burr holes. A high-speed craniotome is utilized to connect burr holes and cut the bone flap while securing hemostasis with bone wax to the bony edges. Hitching sutures between the dura and adjacent bone will control extradural bleeding beneath the bone margins, and this can be reinforced using oxidized cellulose (Surgicel) or absorbable gelatin sponge (Gelfoam). Arterial bleeders are controlled with diathermy. At this stage, if hyperostosis or tumor invasion of the bone has occurred, then the involved bone is drilled away. Rarely, if involvement is extensive, the bone flap is left out and a cranioplasty is later performed.

Operative Considerations

Particular attention should be paid to controlling involved vessels during dural opening as this will significantly reduce tumor vascularity. The major consideration with dural opening is to be aware of a tense dura indicating brain swelling. If this is not recognized at the outset, herniation of the cortex and subsequent brain infarction may occur. Cerebral swelling can be managed with elevation of the head, steroids, or use of diuretics such as mannitol or furosemide.

During dural opening, great care must be made to avoid damaging important draining veins that surround the tumor as these may be draining eloquent cortex. The dura is normally opened just beyond the margins of the lesion, and a circumferential dural flap is cut out, exposing minimal brain. An adequate margin of dura is created to ensure that the entire tumor is removed. With careful dissection, the arachnoid at the tumor–brain interface is divided and then a plane is developed between the brain and the tumor. This plane should be preserved as its maintenance minimizes injury to important vessels and cortex. The combined use of bipolar diathermy, microscissors, and sharp dissection is necessary to ensure an extrapial dissection. Recurrent and malignant convexity meningiomas may invade the brain, and hence control of the feeding vessels from the internal carotid artery may be required. Sharp dissection using magnification is routinely required. Often extensive central debulking is required to allow the tumor to collapse inward to allow better mobilization and removal of the lesion. This can be done with the aid of an ultrasonic aspirator. At all stages retraction of the brain must be minimized.

An important consideration for convexity meningiomas is where the lesion overlies the Sylvian fissure. Here, important branches of the middle cerebral artery may be adherent to the tumor capsule and must be carefully dissected free from the lesion to avoid neurologic injury. In this instance, dissection should commence in uninvolved areas of the capsule and proceed carefully by dissecting major vessels away, including large draining Rolandic veins in the eloquent cortex.

The other major consideration for convexity meningiomas involves where the dural attachment may extend over the floor of the anterior fossa, sphenoid wing, and the floor and anterior wall of the middle fossa. All of the involved dura should be removed if possible. The dural defect can usually be repaired by sewing a graft directly to the edge of the remaining dura. Particular attention is paid to securing hemostasis once the tumor mass is removed, and the dura is not closed until meticulous hemostasis is achieved. Bleeding is usually from the tumor, and if the plane of dissection between the tumor capsule and the brain is preserved, bleeding from the adjacent white matter is usually minimal.

Highly vascular lesions require vigilant hemostasis during the procedure, including the use of Avitene (microfibrillar collagen) and Surgicel. However, once dural feeding vessels are secured, vascularity can be easily controlled with diathermy and light pressure applied to a hemostatic agent. Preoperative embolization will minimize blood loss due to external carotid supply in highly vascular lesions.

A watertight dural closure should be achieved with convexity meningiomas minimizing postoperative cerebrospinal fluid leakage, infection, cortical scarring, and brain herniation. We prefer to utilize pericranium as a graft, but artificial dural substitutes or harvested fascia lata may also be utilized. The bone flap is replaced with small titanium plates after drilling out involved bone. Rarely, if tumor invasion is too extensive, the bone flap is discarded and a cranioplasty is later inserted. We secure the bone flap with titanium mini-plates, and the galea and skin are closed in layers.

Fluctuations in both arterial and central venous pressures should be strictly avoided postoperatively in order to minimize the risk of intracranial bleeding and cerebral edema.

Other Considerations with Convexity Meningiomas

Atypical and Malignant Meningiomas

Around 7% of meningiomas have atypical histology (WHO II) that correlates with more rapid growth and a worse clinical outcome (16). These atypical meningiomas often show an increase in cellularity, frequent mitoses, high nucleus-to-cytoplasm ratios, and prominent nucleoli (17). These lesions can be aggressive and have an increased likelihood for recurrence (18). Approximately 2% of meningiomas are malignant, and these show a high mitotic index with obvious necrosis (19). Clinically, malignant meningiomas may show frank brain invasion or metastatic spread. A significant determinant of outcome in atypical and malignant meningiomas is the extent of surgical resection (20).

Loss of alkaline phosphatase expression is an important prognostic factor in tumor recurrence (21,22) and is associated with deletion of the short arm of chromosome 1. Lesions with 1 q deletion recur in 60% of cases (23). Convexity meningiomas are unique as they are associated with an increased incidence of chromosome 22 q abnormalities. Chromosome 22 q changes are also found more in the transitional and fibrous subtypes of meningiomas, which occur more frequently in the convexity than other subtypes (24). As mentioned above, recurrence of convexity meningiomas is more frequent with tumors displaying atypical or malignant histologic features. Recurrent tumors also have an increased incidence of histologic atypia compared with the primary tumor (10). With recurrent lesions, microscopic clusters of meningioma cells or small nodules may be present in the dura adjacent to the tumor attachment. Further necessary resection poses greater risk of neurologic injury due to local scarring, with a higher incidence of postoperative complications.

En-Plaque Dural Spread

Preoperative imaging of convexity meningiomas will often show an extensive dural tail, but it is uncertain whether this represents direct dural invasion of meningioma cells or en-plaque dural extension of the tumor (10). Although the aim of convexity surgery is total resection, it may not be possible to excise the entire en-plaque component. However, it is important to perform as wide a margin of dural excision as feasible. Careful follow-up of these patients is essential, and if there is recurrent growth, further resection or radiation may be required.

Complications

The major operative complications concern immediate general and long-term neurologic outcomes.

Neurologic

Postoperative neurologic deficits may arise from cerebral edema or vascular injury. If venous drainage has been compromised or important cortical venous draining veins are taken, significant cerebral edema can arise. Hence the necessity of preserving cortical draining veins is emphasized.

Postoperative epilepsy and status epilepticus are potential complications, but their incidence is reduced with preservation of the cortical draining veins (25).

General

Meningiomas are associated with increased risk of thromboembolism in general, and particular attention needs to be paid to the risk of deep venous thrombosis or pulmonary embolism developing in elderly patients (26,27).

Myocardial infarction, anemia, or fluid balance irregularities are occasionally immediate postoperative complications of meningioma surgery.

Nuances and Lessons Learned

The major advances in meningioma surgery have involved improved diagnosis and better localization of the lesion. The introduction and development of frameless stereotaxy has meant that the tumor margins can be mapped out in a highly accurate fashion and its relationship to important adjacent vessels including the venous sinuses established. This has resulted in precise planning and placement of the skin and bone flaps to minimize exposure of normal adjacent brain. Most recurrent typical convexity lesions can be treated with repeat surgery, and radiotherapy is rarely used.

Other advances include better understanding of meningioma management in the setting of NF-2 patients. Such patients develop multiple and recurrent tumors, including meningiomas, and require careful planning of the timing and order of lesion resection.

Important operative nuances include:

1. Division of the arachnoid at the brain–tumor interface and then careful dissection between the tumor and the adjacent brain to develop a plane
2. Initial debulking of the lesion so as to allow the tumor capsule to be drawn in and then aid in furthering the tumor plane
3. Careful identification of feeding vessels as opposed to en-passent vessels. It is critical that such other vessels, including adjacent veins on the brain surface, not be taken so as to prevent venous infarction and cerebral edema
4. Exposure and preservation of MCA vessels in convexity lesions involving the Sylvian region

Prognosis

The prognosis for convexity meningiomas is very good as its accessible location allows for total resection (20). Simpson's classic landmark paper in 1957 (28) (Table 31-1) remains the benchmark for its demonstration of risk of recurrence being associated with completeness of tumor resection. This has since been confirmed by other authors (29,30).Complete resection, even if there is en-plaque growth, almost always excludes recurrence, although some believe complete resection now also refers to involved thickened arachnoid planes surrounding the tumor as well (9).

As mentioned above, recurrence is more frequent with atypical or malignant meningiomas, and follow-up is essential. The earlier a recurrence is detected, the smaller the tumor size and the better the chance that subsequent treatment will succeed. This is the case even with benign convexity lesions for which repeat surgery is the treatment of choice (4).

Radiotherapy may be indicated as an adjuvant therapy following removal of recurrent atypical or malignant convexity lesions, but complete macroscopic resection is still regarded as ideal treatment (31). Stereotactic radiosurgery with use of a LINAC or Gamma Knife system can also be utilized with lesions

TABLE 31-1. Simpson Grading for Resection of Intracranial Meningiomas.

Grade	Extent of resection	Recurrence rate (%)
I	Gross total resection of tumor including involved dura and bone	9
II	Gross total resection of tumor with coagulation of dural attachments	19
III	Gross total resection without resection or coagulation of dural attachments or of extradural extensions	29
IV	Partial resection of tumor	44
V	Simple decompression (biopsy)	N/A

Source: Ref. 28.

3 cm or smaller. Peritumorous changes and malignant transformation still form a hypothetical risk with radiosurgery, but this treatment may be appropriate for elderly patients or when the risks of anesthesia may be too high (32). Surgery remains the treatment of choice unless contraindicated by medical reasons.

Radiotherapy/radiosurgery holds some appeal for recurrent tumors with atypical or malignant features that are not accessible to surgery due to age or general patient condition. Chemotherapy with hydroxyurea has demonstrated positive results in control of tumor growth in a select group of patients (20–30%) (33). However, the role of chemotherapy appears to be limited in patients with convexity tumors.

References

1. Maxwell R, Chou S. Convexity meningiomas and general principles of meningioma surgery. In: Schmidek H, Sweet W, eds. Operative Neurosurgical Techniques, Indications and Methods. New York: Grune & Stratton, 1982:491–501.
2. Giombini S, Solero CL, Morello G. Late outcome of operations for supratentorial convexity meningiomas. Report on 207 cases. Surg Neurol 1984;22(6):588–94.
3. Al-Mefty O. Meningiomas. New York: Raven Press, 1991.
4. Hofmann B, Fahlbusch R. Surgical Management of convexity, parasagittal, and falx meningiomas. In: Schmidek H, Roberts D, eds. Operative Neurosurgical Techniques : Indications, Methods, and Results. Philadelphia: Elsevier Inc., 2006:721–38.
5. Harrison MJ, Wolfe DE, Lau TS, et al. Radiation-induced meningiomas: experience at the Mount Sinai Hospital and review of the literature. J Neurosurg 1991;75(4):564–74.
6. Mack EE, Wilson CB. Meningiomas induced by high-dose cranial irradiation. J Neurosurg 1993;79(1):28–31.
7. Rouleau GA, Wertelecki W, Haines JL, et al. Genetic linkage of bilateral acoustic neurofibromatosis to a DNA marker on chromosome 22. Nature 1987;329(6136):246–8.
8. Seizinger BR, Belamonte S, Atkins L. Molecular genetic approach to human meningioma:loss of genes on chromosome 22. Proc Natl Acad Sci USA 1987;84:5419–23.
9. Kinjo T, al-Mefty O, Kanaan I. Grade zero removal of supratentorial convexity meningiomas. Neurosurgery 1993;33(3):394–9; discussion 399.
10. Besser M. Convexity meningiomas. In: Kaye A, Laws Jr E, eds. Operative Neurosurgery. Churchill Livingstone, 2000:495–503.
11. Lieu AS, Howng SL. Intracranial meningiomas and epilepsy: incidence, prognosis and influencing factors. Epilepsy Res 2000;38(1):45–52.
12. Weber J, Gassel A, Hoch A, et al. Intraoperative management of cystic meningiomas. Neurosurg Rev 2003;26:62–6.
13. Nakamura M, Roser F, Michel J, et al. The natural history of incidental meningiomas. Neurosurgery 2003;53(1):62–70; discussion 71.
14. Yoneoka Y, Fujii Y, Tanaka R. Growth of incidental meningiomas. Acta Neurochir 2000;142(5):507–11.
15. Lieu AS, Howng SL. Surgical treatment of intracranial meningiomas in geriatric patients. Kaohsiung J Med Sci 1998;14(8):498–503.
16. Rohringer M, Sutherland G, Louw D, et al. Incidence and clinico-pathological features of meningioma. J Neurosurg 1984;71:665–72.
17. Delamone S, Flickinger J, Linggood R. Histopathologic features predicting recurrence of meningiomas foloowing subtotal resection. Am J Surg Pathol 1986;10:836–43.
18. Jaaskelainen J, Haltia M, Servo A. Atypical and anaplastic meningiomas: radiology, surgery, radiotherapy and outcome. Surg Neurol 1986;25:233–42.
19. Kleihues P, Cavenee W. Pathology and Genetics of Tumors of the Nervous System. Oxford: Oxford University Press, 2000.
20. Mirimanoff R, Donsoretz D, Linggood R, et al. Meningioma: analysis of recurrence and progression following neurosurgical resection. J Neurosurg 1985;62:18–24.
21. Muller P, Henn W, Niedermayer I, et al. Deletion of chromosome 1 p and loss of alkaline phosphatase indicate progression of meningiomas. Clin Cancer Res 1999;5:3569–77.
22. Ketter R, Henn W, Niedermayer I, et al. Predictive value of progression-associated chromosomal aberrations for the prognosis of meningiomas: a retrospective study of 198 cases. J Neurosurg 2001;95:601–7.
23. Steudel W, Feld R, Henn W, et al. Correlation between cytogenetic and clinical findings in 215 human meningiomas. Acta Neurochir Suppl (Wien) 1996;65:73–6.
24. Kros J, de Greve K, van Tilborg A, et al. NF2 status of meningiomas is associated with tumor localization and histology. J Pathol 2001;194:367–72.
25. Chan R, Thompson G. Morbidity, mortality, and quality of life following surgery for intracranial meningiomas. A retrospective study in 257 cases. J Neurosurg 1984;60:52–60.
26. Kallio M, Sankila R, Hakulinen T, et al. Factors affecting operative and excess long-term mortality in 935 patients with intracranial meningioma. Neurosurgery 1992;31:427–35.
27. Powers S, Edwards M. Prevention and treatment of thrombo-embolic complications in a neurosurgical patient. In: Wilkins R, Rengachary S, eds. Neurosurgery. New York: McGraw-Hill, 1985:406–10.
28. Simpson D. The recurrence of intracranial meningiomas after surgical treatment. J Neurol Neuropsychiatry 1957;20:22–39.
29. Melamed S, Sahar A, Beller A. The recurrence of intracranial meninigiomas. Neurochirurgia 1979;22:47–51.
30. Adegbite A, Khan M, Paine K, et al. The recurrence of intracranial meninigiomas after surgical treatment. J Neurosurg 1983;58:51–6.
31. Salazar O. Ensuring local control in meningiomas. Int J Radiat Oncol Biol Phys 1988;15:501–4.
32. Chang J, Chang J, Choi J, et al. Complications after gamma knife radiosurgery for benign meningiomas,. J Neurol Neurosurg Psychiatry 2003;74:226–30.
33. Schrell U, Rittig M, Anders M, et al. Hydroxyurea for treatment of unresectable and recurrent meningiomas. II: Decrease in the size of meningiomas in patients treated with hydroxyurea. J Neurosurg 1997;86:840–4.

32
Parasagittal Meningiomas

Jorge E. Alvernia and Marc P. Sindou

Introduction

Cushing and Eisenhardt (1) reported the parasagittal location as the most common in their series of 295 meningiomas (65/295 = 22%). The percentage of parasagittal meningiomas in the literature ranges from 16.8 to 25.6% (2). Whereas the initial classification within the group of parasagittal meningiomas was based on morphologic criteria (the global, nonhyperostosing type and the hyperostosing type), the most recent classifications are based on their location along the superior sagittal sinus.

The term parasagittal meningioma applies to those tumors involving the sagittal sinus and the adjacent convexity dura and falx. Although some meningiomas arising from the falx may occasionally involve sagittal sinus, most do not. Therefore, they have different clinical and surgical considerations. Different considerations also apply to the ones rising from the adjacent convexity and merely reaching the sagittal sinus without actually involving it. The attempt to subdivide meningiomas into groups was first made by Harvey Cushing in 1922 (1). He considered parasagittal meningiomas to be the most challenging at the time.

Cushing and Olivecrona (3) classified these tumors into three groups based on their relationship to the sagittal sinus: anterior (from crista galli to the coronal suture), middle (from the coronal to lamboid sutures), or posterior third (from the lamboid suture to the torcular). Classical teaching in neurosurgery has been that the anterior third of the sinus can usually be resected without morbidity, but acutely ligating the middle or posterior third of the sinus carries significant risk of venous infarction (4–8).

Surgery of meningiomas involving the sagittal sinus challenges the surgeon with a dilemma: leave the invasive fragment and have a higher rate of recurrence or attempt a total removal and have the venous circulation at risk. Current tendency is resection of the tumor mass outside the sinus wall(s) with coagulation of the remnant, followed if needed by an "en bloc" removal of the residual tumor when complete sinus occlusion occurs (9–11).

In the event of partial sinus invasion with a patent still-circulating sinus, resection of the invaded wall(s) requires patching of the defect to ensure the patency of the sinus. In cases where the sinus is totally occluded, the question whether to restore the venous circulation by performing a bypass following resection of a totally occluded sinus versus simple removal of its invaded portion without venous reconstruction is disputable (9,12–17). The development of collateral venous pathways in patients with totally occluded sagittal sinus, many argue, allows for complete removal of the invaded sinus with little risk for postoperative venous infarct, obviating the need for venous flow restoration. This may not, however, always be true. When surgery directly involving the sagittal sinus is considered, the benefits of surgery must far outweigh the risks (18,19).

Surgical risks of a radical removal have to be balanced with the therapeutic efficiency and limits of radiation therapy (20–28). Despite radiation's reported success, recurrence rate has been reported at 18–22% for tumor remnants attached to the dural sinuses. Presently, the refined stereotactic radiosurgical techniques play an increasing role in the treatment of meningiomas in "risky" locations, but long term effects and outcomes are still to be evaluated (29–34).

Special Considerations

The sagittal sinus is triangular in shape in cross section and increases gradually in size as it extends posteriorly (6). The superior sagittal sinus communicates with irregular venous cavities, i.e., the lateral venous lacunae, which lie in the dura mater on either side of it. In certain areas, the arachnoid projects into the venous sinuses to form the arachnoid illi. These are mushroom-shaped outpouchings of the subarachnoid space (SAS) that invaginate into them. They act like one-way valves to allow the cerebral spinal fluid (CSF) to flow into the veins and sinuses. Sometimes the arachnoid granulations may appear on magnetic resonance imaging (MRI) as a filling defect or a mass within a large dural sinus.

Each cerebral hemisphere has 8–12 external medial veins as well as a comparable number of internal medial cortical veins, all entering into the SAS. Apuzzo et al. (35), on a review of

100 angiograms, demonstrated that 70% of parasagittal venous drainage was evident within the sector 2 cm posterior to the coronal suture, whereas 30% was located in the anterior 2-cm region. Yamamoto et al. (36), also on a review of 100 angiograms, showed that 53% of the venous tributaries to the sagittal sinus entered the sinus within 2 cm anterior or posterior to the coronal suture (of these, 76% were located posterior to the coronal suture). These angiographic findings support the notion that sacrifice of the middle third of the sagittal sinus and their central tributary veins is risky. The sacrifice of the other groups of veins in the anterior or posterior thirds, unless they are of large caliber, does not appear so hazardous (2,6,37,38).

The anterior third extends from the crista galli to the coronal suture, the middle third from the coronal to the lamboid sutures, and the posterior third runs between the lamboid suture and the torcular herophili. Olivecrona was the first to introduce this distribution (37, 52, and 11%, respectively). Then Cushing and Eisenhardt (1) reported similar findings in their series (34, 57, and 9%, respectively). Collectively, the results of several reports show a preference of parasagittal meningiomas to grow in the middle third (39–41). Not only are there differences in the clinical presentation, but specific anatomic considerations make this topographical distribution important. The sagittal sinus is narrower in its anterior half and that the parasinoidal lacunae pachionian bodies and the veins entering the sinus are fewer in number and smaller than those behind the coronal suture, making the surgical approach easier in the anterior half. The growth of tumors of the middle third of the parasagittal sinus against the paracentral lobule and the precentral/postcentral gyri around the central sulcus makes them clinically evident early, explaining why they do not have the time to expand in size as do the tumors in the other two thirds.

The clinical characteristics are largely a matter of the tumor's proximity to the Rolandic fissure. Usually these patients present with motor or sensory seizures involving the contralateral lower extremity, as exemplified by Cushing's famous case of General Leonard Wood (1,2). Weakness of one side appears to be frequent, being the second most common presenting symptom following the seizures. Uniltral pyramidal signs are the principal physical findings, followed by sensory signs, papilledema, and dementia. In contrast to arising from the middle third, the ones from the anterior or posterior third have the chance to become quite large before detection. A long headache history and in some cases a frontal lobe syndrome in the anterior third and homonymous hemianopsia in the posterior third might be present. Midline calvarial bossing is considered by some authors to be the most valuable evidence of a large parasagittal meningioma. In reviewing 154 parasagittal meningiomas, Gauthier-Smith (42) found that anterior tumors most often present with headaches (36%) or mental status changes (36%), whereas tumors of the posterior third present with headaches (36%), visual symptoms (21%), focal seizures (21%), or mental status abnormalities (21%).

Different classifications of sinus invasion have been proposed by different authors (43). We have developed a single

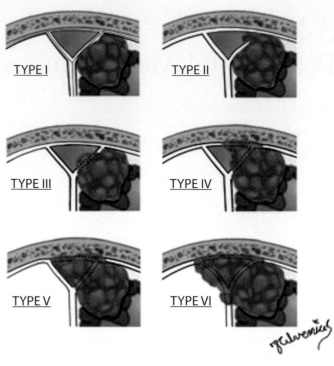

FIG. 32-1. Illustration showing personal classification. Type I: Meningioma attached to the outer surface of the sinus wall; Type II: lateral recess invaded; Type III: lateral wall invaded; Type IV: entire lateral wall and roof of the sinus both invaded; Type V: sinus totally invaded with one wall being free; Type VI: sinus totally invaded without any wall being free

classification scheme useful for surgical consideratioins (4–6,8,9). This classification developed for the parasagittal meningiomas may also be applied to those involving the torcular or the transverse sinus:

Type I:	Attachment to outer surface of the sinus wall
Type II:	Fragment inside the lateral recess
Type III:	Invasion of the ipsilateral wall
Type IV:	Invasion of the lateral wall and roof
Types V and VI:	Complete sinus occlusion, with or without one wall free, respectively (Fig 32-1)

Surgical Technique

Resection and venous repair are greatly facilitated by placing the patient in the semi-sitting position; this position allows a good venous return without significant risk of air embolism, likely because the relatively high level of intracranial venous pressure in these patients. Skin flap and craniotomy extend across the midline to permit visualization of both sides of the sinus, and approximately 3 cm proximal and distal margins from the occluded sinus is exposed. Care has to be taken to preserve the venous anastomotic pathways developed throughout the scalp, the pericranium, and the diploic venous channels. All of these have to be meticulously identi-

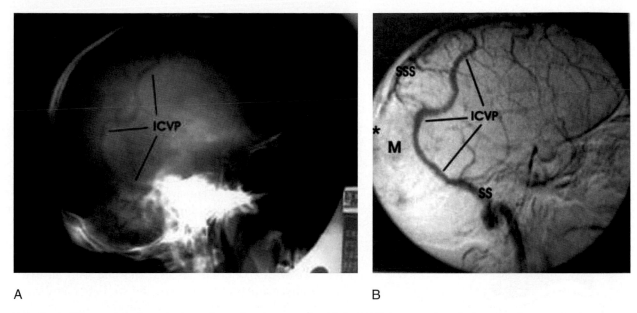

A   B

FIG. 32-2. Grade VI parasagittal meningioma located at the posterior third. (A) Plain x-ray; lateral view showing a major intraosseous collateral venous pathway (ICVP). (B) DSA, venous phase; lateral view showing the venous collateral from mid-third of superior sagittal sinus (SSS) to sigmoid sinus (SS). (Note complete occlusion of the posterior third SSS (*)

fied preoperatively on the venous phase of the DSA and also on plain x- ray of the skull (Fig 32-2). Because of frequent discrepancies between perspective images and intraoperative findings concerning intrasinusal fragments, the sinus should be explored through a short incision on the sinus wall.

Temporary control of venous bleeding from the sinus as well as from the afferent veins is usually achieved by packing small pledgets of hemostatic material (Surgicel, Johnson Medical; Viroflay, France) inserted within the lumen and inside the ostia of affluents, if necessary (Fig 32-3) (4–8,44–

46). We do not recommend inflated balloons because they do not easily pass through the sinus lumen (due to septation especially in the mid-third), and balloons may injure the sinus endothelium. Vascular clamps and aneurysm clips should be avoided due to their propensity to crush the sinus walls and to disrupt the afferent cortical veins. Bridging veins, especially in the Rolandic area, should be dissected free from the adjacent brain, dura, and tumor.

Venous reconstruction may be performed using patches (Fig. 32-3) or bypasses (Fig. 32-4) (38,47–63). We rec-

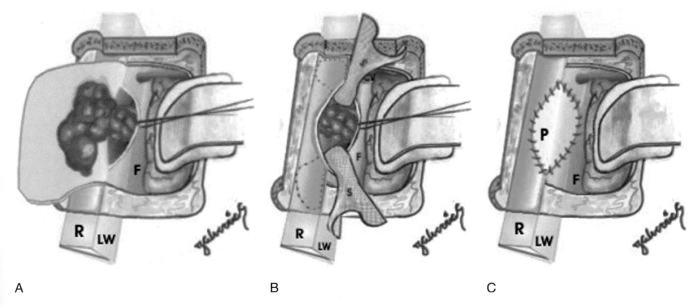

A   B   C

FIG. 32-3. Grade IV parasagittal meningioma—patching technique. (A) Exploration of the sinus lumen through a 3-cm opening, which allows identification of the intrasinusal tumoral fragment. (B) Control of the venous bleeding performed using pledgets of Surgicel(s). Vascular clamps and aneurysm clips are not used because they might injure sinus walls and avulse afferent bridging veins. (C) Venous reconstruction with patch performed using an autologous patch (fascia temporalis in this case). R, roof of SSS; LW, lateral wall of SSS; F, falx cerebri; S, Surgicel

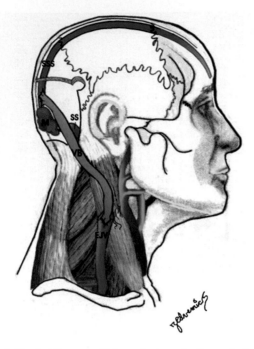

FIG. 32-4. Grade VI parasagittal meningioma in the posterior third—bypass technique. The bypass is performed with an autologous external jugular. This bypass is of the latero (in the SSS)–terminal (at the graft) type. The next step (not shown) will be resection of the totally occluded portion of the sinus

ommend for these purposes the use of two hemi-running sutures (prolene 8.0, laboratoire ETHNOR, Neuilly/Seine, France). Although autologous vein would appear to be the most appropiate material for use as a patch, vein harvesting seemed to us excessive for patching only. Locally situated dura mater or pericranium, or fascia lata, or, even better, the neighboring fascia temporalis are very good alternatives. Long autologous venous grafts harvested from the internal saphenous (more than 6 cm), or shorter ones from the external jugular vein may be used to bypass a totally occluded portions of the sinus.

To decrease the risk of bypass thrombosis after surgery, blood pressure, volume, and viscosity should be carefully monitored. Anticoagulation with heparin (two times control) administered as soon as the day after surgery and for 3 weeks, and then coumadin for 3 months, usually prevents clotting into the reconstructed sinus until reendothelization of the sinus is completed.

Regarding the tumor portion not attached to the sinus that must be removed before approaching the sinus, the steps can be succinctly described as follows: (1) intradural internal volume reduction (either by piecemeal removal with bipolar microcoagulation, microscissors, and microsuction or by means of an ultrasonic aspirator) and (2) sharp dissection of the tumor from the underlying cerebral cortex under high magnification.

Outcome/Complications

Local and General Morbidity

Despite the much discussed risk of air embolism in the semi-sitting position, we use this surgical position on a regular basis for all cases. In fact, in our personal series of 100 cases recently analyzed, just one air embolism case was diagnosed (1%). In this case the clinical course was uneventful.

Three patients developed a postoperative hematoma (3%): one a subacute subdural and two extradural hematomas. They all were evacuated without any permanent neurologic sequelae. It should be noted that none of these postoperative hematomas occurred in patients receiving postoperative anticoagulation. A postoperative infection rate in our series was 6%: three with a bone flap infection, two with a cerebral abscess, and one with an extradural empyema. All of these cases did well after antibiotic therapy and surgery. Hoessly and Olivecrona (3), in a series of 280 cases, reported systemic and local complications in 19 cases, postoperative hematoma in 1, exanguinations in 6, carotid thromboses in 2, cardiac insufficiency in 1, embolism in 2, "infections" in 3, and pneumonia in 4. Dimeco et al. (64), in a cooperative series of 108 cases, reported 5 patients with wound infections and 2 with a postoperative hematoma, one of whom had a fatal outcome and the other a poor clinical result after surgical evacuation. Unfortunately most of the other series (10,39,43) did not include outcome data in their reports.

Neurologic Morbidity and Mortality of Venous Origin

All authors dealing with parasagittal meningiomas agree on the importance of preserving the afferent (bridging) veins to the sinus (9,13,37,38,48,51,65), especially the ones of the central group in regard to the middle third sagittal sinus (as well as those located at the transversus sinus and the cerebral veins of Labbé) (5,6,40,41).

Avoidance of interrupting a partially occluded sagittal sinus is also a matter of general consensus. Conversely, aggressively resecting a totally occluded portion of a sinus, although traditionally accepted as safe, remains disputable; brain swelling, venous infarction, and subcutaneous CSF collection may occur when venous collateral circulation is impaired. In Olivecrona's series (3), which included 196 parasagittal meningiomas, all treated without venous reconstruction, morbidity amounted to 12.3%, half of which is attributed to venous damages. The 10% mortality rate resulted from 14 of the 109 tumors located at the middle (12.8%), 3 of the 31 at the posterior (9%), and 3 of the 56 at the anterior (5.3%) third. In Bonnal and Brotchi's series of 21 cases, one patient (4.7%) died after an en-bloc tumor resection without venous restoration (39). In another recent report consisting of 108 cases, brain swelling occurred in nine (8.9%) patients, three of whom had en bloc resection without venous reconstruction. Persistent subgaleal fluid collection occurred in 11 (10%), likely corresponding to a default in CSF reabsortion and/or persistent high intracranial pressure from venous origin (64). In our series, morbidity and mortality related to venous damage and/or absence of venous flow reconstruction were estimated at 8 and 3%, respectively. Perhaps these patients would have had a better outcome if they had undergone venous repair. But it might be that shaving of the tumor outside the sinus with secondary stereotactic radiation would have been less harmful. We really do not know.

The postoperative mortality after attempted total removal has clearly improved since the initial attempts of complete en-bloc resections performed decades ago by authors Hoessly and Oivecrona, who reported a 10.2% mortality rate for a series of 196 cases. Most likely, the improvement in microsurgical techniques and the repair of the venous system when a total surgical removal is attempted have dramatically changed the outcome in these patients. In our series of 100 cases, three patients (3%) died primarily from brain swelling, likely related to the surgical procedure. All of these patients had resection of the entire invaded portion of the sinus (type VI) without surgical venous flow restoration.

Complication Avoidance/Lessons Learned

Dural Sinus Reconstruction

Reconstructions in the venous system are not new; different techniques of dural sinus repair have been reported in the past few decades, as have encouraging results of anastomosing cortical veins to the sinus venous graft (53). Bonnal and Brotchi (39,40), Hakuba et al. (51), Bederson et al. (52), Sekhar et al. (61,62), Steiger et al. (63), and Schmid-Elsaesser et al. (60) have also reported satisfactory experience of patching with pieces of dura or autologous venous graft. In our series, 13 (86.6%) of the 15 repairs with dura or fascia were angiographically confirmed to be patent. Harvesting autologous veins, theoretically the best material for patching the venous system, seemed to us excessive for venous repairs. According to our experience, the best material is the thin and glossy fascia temporalis. When a synthetic graft (Goretex tube) was used, none remained patent in spite of anticoagulation therapy instituted. Therefore, we do not recommend synthetic grafts for repair of the venous system. When temporary occlusion of the sinus is required, the use of small pledgets of Surgicel within the lumen and at the ostia of the tributary afferents makes it simple. This technique was found to be much preferable to using aneurysm clips or balloons. As a matter of fact, clips or even temporary clamps were found to be damaging to the sinus walls. Balloons or silicone tubes (used as shunts) do not pass through the sinus lumen well due to the presence of septa, especially in the middle third of the sagittal sinus. Moreover, passing balloons or silicone tubes may avulse or traumatize the venous

endothelium, which increases the likelihood of intraluminal thromboses formation.

Whether a bypass is justified every time a total resection is attempted, or only in selected cases with proven high venous pressure, remains in debate. We are rather prone to consider doing it routinely, as performing a bypass in the extradural space presents little additional risk. However, another option is for the decision to be made after an intraoperative measurement of the intrasinusal pressure with an occlusion test.

Recurrence rate following aggressive gross total removal including the invaded sinus is relatively low compared to the rates from the literature reports for the same meningiomas but without the similar aggressive approach (Table 32-1). This favors tumor resection, not only of its outer portion but also of the fragment(s) invading the adjacent dural sinus. The lower recurrence rate following attempts of gross total resection (4% vs. 11–24%) supports our aggressive approach for these difficult tumors, rather than conservative removal of only the tumors outside of the sagittal sinus.

Achieving radical removal requires opening of the sinus, exploring its lumen and interrupting transiently its circulation, easily performed by occluding the proximal and distal sinus lumens of the opening with pledgets of Surgicel. Reconstruction is mandatory in the cases of incomplete occlusion and is considered optimal but highly useful in the cases with complete obliteration (Fig. 32-5.)

Outcome

Outcome was frequently problematic in cases with total occlusion of the dural sinuses that had resection without

TABLE 32-1. Historical Review of Surgical Series on Parasagittal Meningiomas.

paper (surgical series)	No. of cases	Year	Recurrence rate (%)	Median follow-up (yr)	Overall mortality (%)
Hoessly and Olivecrona[3]	196	1955	6	5	12.3
Simpson[10]	107	1957	19	5	?
Logue[13]	91	1975	11	?	4.4
Bonnal and[39] Brotchi	21	1978	14	?	4.7
Yashamita[34]	80	1980	14.6	5	?
Chan and Thompson[21]	16	1984	13	?	?
Mirimanoff[16]	38	1985	24	10	?
Jaaskelanen	136	1986	8	?	?
Philippon[32]	153	1986	14.4	10	?
Dimeco et al.[64]	108	2004	13.9	13	2
*Sindou and Alvernia	100	2008	4	8	3

* The current series presented in this chapter.

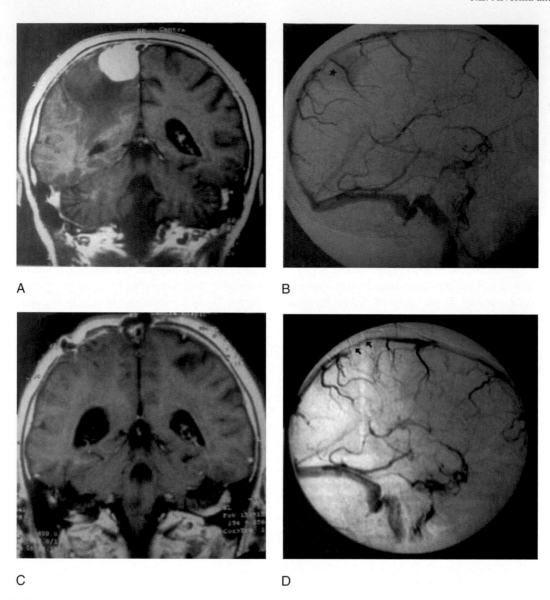

A   B

C   D

F ig. 32-5. Grade II parasagittal meningioma. (A) Preoperative T1-weighted MRI with gadolinium (coronal section) showing a right mid-third parasagittal meningioma from the lateral wall of the sagittal sinus. (B) Preoperative angiogram (lateral view, venous phase) showing sinus patency and tumor blush (*). (C) Postoperative T1-weighted MRI with gadolinium (coronal section) showing postoperative changes without evidence of tumoral remnant. The sinus was opened and the tumor into the lateral recess removed. (D) Postoperative angiogram (lateral view, venous phase) clearly showing sagittal sinus patency (black arrows)

venous reconstruction, as shown in the literature and in our series as well. The three deaths in our series corresponded to such circumstances; they were likely due to impairment of the naturally developed collateral channels caused during surgery. This poor outcome encountered earlier in our experience led us to be in favor of venous flow restoration. Because all bypasses with synthetic prosthesis (i.e., Goretex) occluded, even under the administration of anticoagulants, we believe that only autologous grafts should be utilized: external jugular vein for short graft, internal saphenous vein for longer ones. The higher morbidity rate in terms of neurologic complication

after surgical repair was encountered in the mid-third of the sagittal sinus, so working in this area mandates one to be particularly prudent when performing surgery in this region.

It should be pointed out that reconstruction of the sagittal sinus, either by patching or bypassing, did not increase the morbidity rate in our series, and the use of postoperative anticoagulation did not increase the rate of hemorrhagic complications.

We truly believe that attempts at total removal with venous repair should be considered favorably when dealing with meningiomas invading the dural sinuses.

Tumor Recurrence

In our personal series presented in this chapter, tumor recurrence rate was 4%, with a follow-up ranging from 3 to 23 years (mean 8 years). This percentage correlates well with Simpson's recurrence rate following a grade 1 resection, i.e., removal of the tumor and the surrounding dura and bone where involved (10). This relatively low rate seems to be due not only to the small number (only three) of atypical meningiomas that were encountered, but also to our policy of attempting in most cases radical resection including intrasinusal portion. To be noted, all four tumors with recurrence were located in the mid-third of the sagittal sinus, known to receive numerous and important afferent veins of the central group, making radical surgery more difficult to be accomplished. In the literature, recurrence rate varied from 6% as in Olivecrona's series (3), in which a majority of the patients had an "en bloc resection," to 24% in the Mirimanoff's series (16), with intermediate percentages in the other reported series (Table 32-1). Discrepancies in recurrence rates among different series are likely due to differences in the extent of resection, rather than histologic tumor types, although this cannot be established with certainty as only few series contained such information. Histologic characteristics in our series were not felt to have played a role in the propensity for recurrence, with the exception of the atypical meningiomas.

The recently refined radiosurgical techniques present therapeutic alternatives to radical surgery: either simple mass reduction with adjuvant radiosurgery or radiosurgery alone under certain conditions (4,12,23,25–28,30,31,66–69). Few publications contain results regarding specifically meningiomas of the parasagittal location (12). Several retrospective studies have suggested that radiotherapy is able to decrease the rate of local failure or progression after subtotal surgery of meningiomas to less than 20% at 5 years (25,26,29,30). Unfortunately, there has yet to be any randomized trials comparing radiosurgery and surgery for the treatment of these tumors (27).

Summary

Gross total removal of these tumors can be achieved without high morbidity or mortality. Our current management policy is the following: peeling of the external layer of the dural sinus wall should be performed in the cases with just an external layer invasion (Type I). In cases when only the lateral recess is invaded (Type II), removal of the intraluminal fragments through the recess followed by resuturing the recess or patching is adequate. In cases with partial occlusion of the sinus with one or two walls being invaded (Type III and IV), a patch is deemed sufficient. Conversely, when a complete occlusion of the sinus is demonstrated, as in the Type V (two walls invaded) or VI (three walls invaded), a bypass with external jugular or saphenous vein should be considered.

References

1. Cushing H, Eissendhardt L. Meningiomas: Their Classification, Regional Behavior, Life History, and Surgical End Results. Springfield, IL: Charles C Thomas,1938.
2. Wilkins R. Parasagittal meningiomas. In: Al-Mefty O, ed. Meningiomas. New York: Raven Press, 1991:329–343.
3. Hoessly GF, Olivecrona H. Report on 280 cases of verified parasagittal meningioma. J Neurosurg 1955;12:614–625.
4. Sindou M. Meningiomas invading the sagittal or transverse sinuses, resection with venous reconstruction. J Clin Neurosci 2001;8 (Suppl 1):8–11.
5. Sindou M, Alaywan F, Hallacq P. Chirurgie des grands sinus veineux duraux intracrâniens. In: Auque J (ed). Le sacrifice venue en neurochirurgie. Masson Paris. Neurochirurgie 1996;Suppl 1: 45–87.
6. Sindou M, Auque J. The intracranial venous system as a neurosurgeon's perspective. Adv Tech Stand Neurosurg 2000;26:131–216.
7. Sindou M, Hallacq P. Microsurgery of the venous system in meningiomas invading the major dural sinuses. In: Hakuba A, ed. Surgery of the Intracranial Venous System. New York: Springer, 1996:226–236.
8. Sindou M, Hallacq P: Venous reconstruction in surgery of meningiomas invading invading the sagittal and transverse sinuses. Skull Base Surg 1998;8: 57–64.
9. Sindou M, Hallacq P, Ojemann RG, Laws ER. Aggresive (Sindou, Hallacq) vs conservative (Ojemann, Laws) treatment of parasagittal meningiomas involving the superior sagittal sinus. Controversies in neurosurgery. In: Al Mefty O, Origitano TC, Harkey HL, eds. New York: Thieme, 1996:80–89.
10. Simpson D. The recurrence of intracranial meningiomas after surgical treatment. J Neurol Neurosurg Psychiatry 1957;20:22–39.
11. Black PM. Meningiomas. Neurosurgery 1933;32:643–657.
12. Kondziolka D, Flickinger JC, Perez B. Judicious resection and/ or radiosurgery for parasagittal meningiomas: outcomes from a multicenter review. Gamma Knife Meningioma Study Group. Neurosurgery 1998;43:405–413.
13. Logue V. Parasagittal meningiomas. Advances and technical standards in neurosurgery. In: Krayenbühl, ed. New York: Springer, 1975;2:171–198.
14. Kang JK, Jun SS, Sung WH, et al. Surgical management of meningioma involving the superior sagittal sinus. Surgery of the intracranial venous system. In: Hakuba A, ed. New York: Springer, 1996:252–259.
15. Levoshko LI, Voinov VI, Korotin VS. [Experience with surgery of parasagittal meningioma]. Vopr Onkol 1999;45:520–522.
16. Mirimanoff RO, Dosoretz DE, Ling good RM, et al. Meningioma: analysis of recurrence and progression following neurosurgical resection. J Neurosurg 1985;62:18–24.
17. Merrem G. [Parasaggital meningiomas. Fedor Krause memorial lecture]. Acta Neurochir (Wien)1970;23(2):203–216.
18. Oka K, Go Y, Kimura H, Tomonaga M. Obstruction of the superior sagittal sinus caused by parasagittal meningiomas: the role of collateral venous pathways. J Neurosurg 1994;81:520–524.
19. Waga S, Handa H. Scalp veins as collateral pathway with parasagitta. In: Torres RC, Frighetto L, De Salles AA, et al. Radiosurgery and stereotactic radiotherapy for intracranial meningiomas. Neurosurg Focus 14:e5, 2003l meningiomas occluding the superior sagittal sinus. Neuroradiology 1976;11:199–204.
20. Bauman GS, Wong E. Re: new radiotherapy technologies for meningiomas: 3D conformal radiotherapy? Radiosurgery?

Sterotactic radiotherapy? Intensity modulated radiotherapy? Proton beam radiotherapy? Spot scanning proton radiation therapy? Or nothing at all? [Radiother Oncol 2004;71(3):247–249]. Oncology 2004;73:251–252.

21. Chan RC, Thompson GB. Morbidity, mortality and quality of life following surgery for intracranial meningiomas: a retrospective study in 257 cases J Neurosurgery 1984;60:52–60.

22. Chang JH, Chang JW, Choi JY, et al. Complications after gamma knife radiosurgery for benign meningiomas. J Neurol Neurosurg Psychiatry 2003;74:226–230.

23. Chin LS, Szerlip NJ, Regine WF. Stereotactic radiosurgery for meningiomas. Neurosurg Focus 2003;14:e6.

24. Gagibov GA, Karaseva TA, Kuklina AS, et al. [Disorders of motor functions after removal of parasagittal meningiomas]. Zh Vopr Neirokhir Im N N Burdenko1985;24–30.

25. Kondziolka D, Nathoo N, Flickinger JC, et al. Long-term results after radiosurgery for benign intracranial tumors. Neurosurgery 2003;53:815–821.

26. Lundsford LD. Contemporary management of meningiomas: Radiation therapy as an adjuvant and radiosurgery as an alternative to surgical removal? J Neurosurg 1994;80:187–190.

27. Mirimanoff RO. New radiotherapy technologies for meningiomas: 3D conformal radiotherapy? Radiosurgery? Stereotactic radiotherapy? Intensity-modulated radiotherapy? Proton beam radiotherapy? Spot scanning proton radiation therapy… or nothing at all? Radiother Oncol 2004;71:247–249.

28. Linskey ME, Davis SA, Ratanatharathorn V. Relative roles of microsurgery and stereotactic radiosurgery for the treatment of patients with cranial meningiomas: a single-surgeon 4-year integrated experience with both modalities. J Neurosurg 2005;102 (Suppl):59–70.

29. Pollock BE, Stafford SL, Utter A, et al. Stereotactic radiosurgery provides equivalent tumor control to Simpson Grade 1 resection for patients with small- to medium-size meningiomas. Int J Radiat Oncol Biol Phys 2003;55:1000–1005.

30. Pollock BE. Stereotactic radiosurgery for intracranial meningiomas: indications and results. Neurosurg Focus 2003;14:e4.

31. Rogers L, Jensen R, Perry A. Chasing your dural tail: Factors predicting local tumor control after gamma knife stereotactic radiosurgery for benign intracranial meningiomas: In regard to DiBiase et al. (Int J Radiat Oncol Biol Phys 2004;60:1515–1519). Int J Radiat Oncol Biol Phys 2005;62:616–618.

32. Philippon J, Bataini JP, Cornu P, et al. Les méningiomas récidivants. Neurochirurgie 1986;(Suppl)1: 1–84.

33. Torres RC, Frighetto L, De Salles AA, et al. Radiosurgery and stereotactic radiotherapy for intracranial meningiomas. Neurosurg Focus 2003;14:e5.

34. Yashamita J Handa H, Iwaki K. Recurrence of intracranial meningiomas with special reference to radiotherapy. Surg Neurol 1980;14:33–40.

35. Apuzzo MLJ, Chikovani OK, Gott PS, et al. Transcallosal, interfornicial approaches for lesions affecting the third ventricle. Surgical considerations and consequences. Neurosurgery 1982;10:547–554.

36. Yamamoto I, Rhoton Jr AL, Sato O. Operative approaches to the third ventricle. Surgical anatomy for micronerosurgery (in Japanese). 1988;181–197.

37. Hakuba A: Surgery of the Intracranial Venous System. New York: Springer, 1996:619.

38. Hakuba A, Tsurund T, Ohata K, et al. Microsurgical reconstruction of the intracranial venous system. In: Hakuba A, ed. Surgery of the Intracranial Venous System. New York: Springer, 1996:220–225.

39. Bonnal J, Brotchi J. Surgery of the superior sagittal sinus in parasagittal meningiomas. J Neurosurg 1978;48:935–945.

40. Bonnal J, Brotchi J, Stevenaert A, et al. Excision of the intra-sinusal portion of rolandic parasaggital meningiomas, followed by plastic surgery of the superior of the superior longitudinal sinus. Neurochirurgie 1971;17: 341–354.

41. Bonnal J, Buduba C. Surgery of the central third of the superior sagittal sinus. Experimental study. Acta Neurochir (Wien) 1974;30:207–215.

42. Gauthier-Smith PC. Parasagittal and Falx Meningiomas. London: Butterworths,. 1970

43. Bonnal J.La chirurgie conservatrice et réparatrice du sinus longitudinal supérieure. Neurochirurgie 2001;28:147–172.

44. Sindou M, Mazoyer JF, Fischer G, et al. Experimental bypass for sagittal sinus repair. Preliminary report. J Neurosurg 1976;44:325–330.

45. Sindou M, Mazoyer JF, Pialat J, et al. [Experimental intracranial venous microsurgery. Bypass of the sagittal sinus for arterial or venous repair and preoperative measurement of the cerebral impedance in the dog]. Neurochirurgie 1975;21:177–189.

46. Sindou M, Mercier P, Bokor J, Brunon J. Bilateral thrombosis of the transverse sinuses: microsurgical revascularization with venous bypass. Surg Neurol 1980;13:215–220.

47. Donaghy RMP, Wallman LJ, Flanagan MJ, Numoto M. Sagittal sinus repair. Technical note. J Neurosurg 1973;38:244–248.

48. Hakuba A. Reconstruction of dural sinus involved in meningiomas. In: Al Mefty O, ed. Meningiomas. New York: Raven Press, 1991:371–382.

49. Kapp JP, Gielchinsky I, Petty C, Mc Clure C. An internal shunt for use in the reconstruction of dural venous sinuses.Technical note. J Neurosurg 1971;35:351–354.

51. Hakuba A, Huh CW, Tsujikawa S, Nishimura S. Total removal of a parasagittal meningioma of the posterior third of the sagittal sinus and its repair by autogenous vein graft. Case report. J Neurosurg 1979;51:379–382.

52. Bederson JB, Eisenberg MB. Resection and replacement of the superior sagittal sinus for treatment of a parasagittal meningioma: technical case report. Neurosurgery 1995;37:1015–1018.

55. Masuzawa H. [Superior sagittal sinus plasty using flax flap in parasagittal meningioma (author's transl)]. No Shinkei Geka 1977;5:707–713.

56. Meirowsky AM. Wounds of the dural sinuses. J Neurosurg 1953;10:496–514.

57. Menousky T, De Vries J. Cortical vein end-to-end anastomosis after removal of a parasagittal meningioma. Microsurgery 2002;22:27–29.

58. Sakaki T, Morimoto T, Takemurak, et al. Reconstruction of cerebral cortical veins using silicone tubing. J Neurosurg 1987;66:471–473.

59. Sakaki T, Morimoto T, Nakase H, et al. Revascularization of the dural sinus occluded by a meningioma using the saphenous vein graft. In: Hakuba A, ed. Surgery of the Intracranial Venous System. New York: Springer,1996:237–243.

60. Schmid-Elsaesser R, Steiger HJ, Yousry T, et al. Radical resection of meningiomas and arteriovenous fistulas involving critical dural sinus segments: experience with intraoperative sinus pressure

monitoring and elective sinus reconstruction in 10 patients. Neurosurgery 1997;41:1005–1018.

61. Sekhar LN, Tzortzidis FN, Bejjani GK, Schessel DA. Saphenous vein graft bypass of the sigmoid sinus and jugular bulb during the removal of glomus jugular tumors. Report of two cases. J Neurosurg 1997;86:1036–1041.

62. Sekhar LN: The exposure, preservation and reconstruction of cerebral arteries and veins during the resection of cranial base tumors. In: Sekhar LN, Schmamm Jr VL, eds. Tumors of the Cranial Base: Diagnosis and Treatment. Mount Kisko, NY: Futura, 1987:213–226.

63. Steiger HJ, Reulen HJ, Huber P, Boll J. Radical resection of superior sagittal sinus meningioma with venous interposition graft and reimplantation of the rolandic veins. Acta Neurochir (Wien) 1989;100:108–111.

64. Di Meco F, Li KW, Casali C, et al. Meningiomas invading the superior sagittal sinus: Surgical experience in 108 cases. Neurosurgery 2004;55(6):1263–1274.

65. Auque J. Le sacrifice veineux en neurochirurgie. Evaluation et gestion du risque. Neurochirurgie 1996;42(Suppl 1).

66. Black PM, Villavicencio AT, Rhouddou C, et al. Aggressive surgery and focal radiation in the management of meningiomas of the skull base: preservation of function with maintenance of local control. Acta Neurochir (Wien) 2001;143: 555–562.

67. Flickinger JC, Kondziolka D, Maitz AH, et al. Gamma knife radiosurgery of imaging-diagnosed intracranial meningioma. Int J Radiat Oncol Biol Phys 2003;56:801–806.

68. Singh VP, Kansai S, Vaishya S, et al. Early complications following gamma knife radiosurgery for intracranial meningiomas. J Neurosurg 2000;93(Suppl 3):57–61.

69. Stafford SL, Pollock BE, Foote RL, et al. Meningioma radiosurgery: tumor control, outcomes, and complications among 190 consecutive patients. Neurosurgery 2001;49:1029–1037.

33
Falcine Meningiomas

Chae-Yong Kim and Hee Won Jung

Introduction

Falcine meningioma originates from the falx cerebri and is defined by Cushing as a meningioma arising from the falx that is concealed completely by the overlying cortex and typically does not involve the superior sagittal sinus (1). However, in practice many falcine meningiomas involve the sagittal sinus. These meningiomas account for 9% of the 795 meningiomas that the authors have treated between 1990 and 2005.

Falcine meningiomas frequently have a dumbbell shape and invaginate into the medial aspects of both the left and right hemispheres. These tumors can be divided into the anterior, middle, and posterior types, depending on their origin in the falx (2). The anterior type arises from the falx located between the crista galli and the coronal suture, the middle type between the coronal suture and the lambdoid suture, and the posterior type between the lambdoid suture and the torcular Herophili. Yasargil classified falcine meningiomas as outer and inner types (3). The outer falcine meningiomas arise from the main body of the falx in the frontal (anterior or posterior), central parietal, or occipital regions. Inner falcine meningiomas arise in conjunction with the inferior sagittal sinus.

Special Considerations

Clinical Manifestations

The clinical signs and symptoms of these tumors are similar to those of parasagittal meningiomas. The clinical presentation is influenced by the location in the anterior, middle, or posterior third of the falx. Rarely, patients may have bilateral symptoms from a dumbbell-shaped tumor or spastic paraparesis from a large paracentral lesion. Visual hallucinations may occur in patients with the posterior type of lesion. Homonymous hemianopsia with macular sparing is also characteristic of posterior tumors.

Neuroradiologic Characteristics

Multiplanar magnetic resonance (MR) imaging is the current standard for preoperative evaluation of patients with falcine meningiomas. Coronal, sagittal, and axial T1-weighted gadolinium-enhanced sequences help define the anatomic location, size, and medial hemisphere involvement of these tumors. MR venography with a vertex view is important for demonstrating the nearby parasagittal draining veins that must be preserved during surgery.

Cerebral angiography is often helpful. In patients with these meningiomas, the pericallosal artery is often displaced, and the tumor may actually engulf it. The arterial phase of the angiogram or MR angiogram should be studied to determine the tumor's relationship to the anterior cerebral artery. A blood supply from the branches of the middle cerebral artery or the external carotid artery is more consistent with parasagittal meningiomas. Anterior falcine meningiomas are usually supplied by the anterior cerebral artery (ACA) or a tentorial branch of the ophthalmic artery. In large tumors, the exact origin of either parasagittal or falcine meningiomas may be difficult to determine. Parasagittal meningiomas are much more common than falcine meningiomas and are more likely to involve the bone; bone involvement appears as hyperostosis.

The venous phase of the angiogram is important because it provides significant information about whether the mass has invaded the sagittal sinus. It also provides information about the courses of many large draining veins around the mass, which must be clearly defineated preoperatives and preserved during surgery to prevent postoperative venous infarction.

Pathologic Characteristics

Any type of meningiomas can arise from falx. In our clinical experience, the transitional and meningothelial subtypes are most frequent, accounting for 68% (42 of 62 patients) of falcine meningiomas.

Special Considerations

Falcine and parasagittal meningiomas share the characteristics of sagittal sinus involvement, although much less commonly so with falcine tumors. Meningiomas in this area are defined in relation to the segment of the sinus they involve: anterior, middle, or posterior. The middle sinus is most frequently involved, and bilateral growth is common. The most important information about the tumor relates to the patency of the sinus, the type of sinus involvement, and the pattern of drainage from the cortical veins and their collateral vessels. Angiography is needed in some patients to prove the patency of the sinus, the anatomic location of the major cortical draining veins, and the pattern of flow. The sinus may be occluded, but the collateral cortical veins might give the impression that the sinus is still open or might show a newly developed diploid sinus. MR venography may be adequate to confirm occlusion of the sinus and show the major surrounding cortical veins. Signs of sinus occlusion include the disappearance of a segment of the superior sagittal sinus, a delay of venous drainage in the area of the obstruction, failure of the cortical vein to reach the sinus, and the clear reversal of normal venous flow.

Choosing the appropriate method of handling the involved sinus is the most important decision when treating falcine meningiomas. Decisions regarding the sinus management should be individualized for each patient according to several factors: the patient's age and symptoms, the patency of the sinus, the location of the tumor, and the cortical venous collaterals. A truly occluded sinus can be excised totally at any point. Preserving collateral venous channels becomes a vital part of the operation. The anterior third of the sinus can be excised with or without a graft or replacement. Tumor infiltration of one wall can be repaired primarily after the tumor is removed from the sinus. Recurrence is a problem and occasionally takes an aggressive course, which can extend along the entire dural sinus system, and makes curative removal during a subsequent operation impossible.

The second important factor to consider preoperatively is the involvement of the ACA by the tumor. Tumor engulfment of the ACA prevents safe total removal of the tumor. An intentional subtotal removal may be needed, and the surgeon should consider secondary treatment such as Gamma Knife radiosurgery or conventional radiation therapy.

Surgical Technique

The operative technique used for falcine meningiomas differs according to the tumor's location and the degree of sagittal sinus involvement. Cushing and Eisenhardt used a transcortical incision to expose most falcine meningiomas (1). However, with current microsurgical techniques and methods for improving intracranial compliance, including cerebrospinal fluid drainage, mannitol, and hyperventilation, a transcortical approach is rarely required.

An interhemispheric approach through a midline-crossing craniotomy is best for these meningiomas (4,5). For falcine meningiomas, the patient's position, scalp incision, and craniotomy are similar to those used for parasagittal meningiomas. An anterior- or middle-third type of tumor with a dumbbell shape requires a bicoronal or linear incision. For posterior-third tumors, a U-shaped flap based inferiorly that is wide enough to allow for a biparietal occipital craniotomy should suffice. The bone flap should extend 2–2.5 cm from the midline on both sides. The dura should be opened on the side of the nondominant hemisphere or the side of the larger component of a dumbbell-shaped tumor. The dural incision should be continued to the lateral portion of the superior sagittal sinus and the bleeding controlled with hemostatic clips.

In some cases, a bridging vein can be freed from the cortex for a few millimeters to give the required exposure without sacrificing the vein. A self-retaining retractor is placed. In the anterior-third type of tumor, it is usually possible to take the draining veins and the sagittal sinus, if needed, to complete the resection. The medial surface of the hemisphere should be gently retracted to identify the anterior and posterior limits of the tumor. Before internally decompressing the tumor, the anterior and posterior margins of the falx should be divided from superior to inferior, preferably with a 1-cm or greater margin from the tumor edge, to interrupt blood supply from the falx arteries.

The key to the operation is to perform an extensive internal decompression of the tumor with an ultrasonic aspirator and gradually draw the capsule into the area of decompression (3–5). Sometimes the tumor is transected parallel to the falx to more easily mobilize the capsule. In some patients, a bilateral exposure is required. At some point in the operation, depending on the size and configuration of the tumor, the falx is divided well away from the tumor attachment. The inferior sagittal sinus can be occluded. Great care must be taken not to injure the pericallosal and callosomarginal arteries.

Illustrative Case 1

A 47-year-old woman presented with chief complaints of headache and nausea for 3 months. She had a history of right-hand tremor for 3 years, which had worsened just before the time of presentation. At the time of admission, neurologic examination revealed right-sided 4+/5 weakness. MR images showed a large mass with a wide base in the middle third of the falx, which grew bilaterally but was more prominent on the left side (Fig. 33-1).

Angiography and embolization of the vessels feeding the tumor were performed a day before the operation. The tumor was supplied by the left occipital artery and left middle meningeal artery. After the Wada test, embolization of the left occipital artery feeders was performed using 150–250 micro PVA particles (Fig. 33-2).The bilateral interhemispheric approach was used through a midline-crossing frontoparietal craniotomy which allowed gross total removal of the tumor.

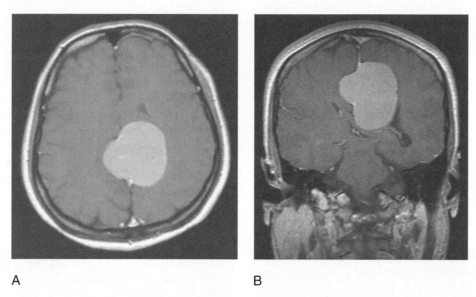

A   B

FIG. 33.1. Illustrative case 1. Magnetic resonance (MR) images show a 5.1 × 5.5 × 6.0 cm mass arising from the middle third of the falx cerebri and protruding bilaterally to both cerebral hemispheres, although predominantly to the left side. A, gadolinium-enhanced T1-weighted axial image; B, coronal image of same condition

With the patient in the prone position, the navigation system was used to design the craniotomy flap. The right side interhemispheric approach between the vein of Trolard and large draining veins of the parietal lobe was performed safely with minimal brain retraction. Sufficient internal debulking of the tumor and external dissection of the tumor margin while preserving the arachnoid plane was performed, and oxidized cellulose and cotton pledgets were used to prevent injury to the surrounding cerebral cortex and to protect the pericallosal arteries in the inferior margin of the dissection. The same technique was applied to the tumor on the left side of the falx. After removal of the tumor on both sides, the falx of tumor origin was excised. Gross total removal of the tumor and its origin was achieved with no intraoperative events.

The patient had transient right-sided weakness in the immediate postoperative period, which resolved fully 3 days after the operation. At the last clinical follow-up, her Karnofsky performance score (KPS) was 100 and there was no evidence of residual or recurrent tumor on MR images taken 22 months after the operation.

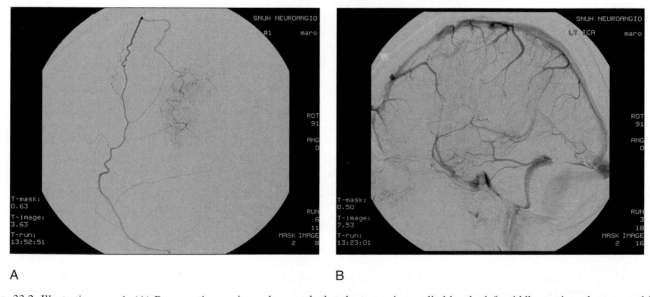

A   B

FIG. 33.2. Illustrative case 1. (A) Preoperative angiography reveals that the tumor is supplied by the left middle meningeal artery and left occipital artery. (B) It also shows downward depression of internal cerebral veins and the vein of Galen and patent superior sagittal sinus. The left occipital artery was superselected, and embolization was performed

Because this patient had no encased major arteries or sinus invasion and a good arachnoid plane, total removal of the mass was achieved successfully.

Illustrative Case 2

A 33-year-old woman presented with chief complaints of seizures, headache, and nausea for 9 months. At the time of admission, neurologic examination revealed no focal deficit. MR images showed a 35-mm mass with a wide base in the anterior third of the falx (Fig. 33-3). The tumor encased and compressed the ACA inferiorly and posteriorly (Fig. 33-3, white arrows in

A, black arrows in B, and arrowheads in C) and was accompanied by considerable peritumoral edema in both frontal lobes (Fig. 33-3A). It had a partly low signal intensity in T2-weighted image, suggesting a calcified consistency (Fig. 33-3A).

A bilateral interhemispheric approach was undertaken through a midline-crossing frontal craniotomy. The right side was approached first. The tumor had a hard and fibrotic consistency that prevented easy removal, and during internal debulking we found encased the ACA. It could not be separated from the surrounding mass and could not be dissected easily. The inferior part of the tumor encasing the ACA was left. Intraoperative Doppler analysis showed decreased ACA

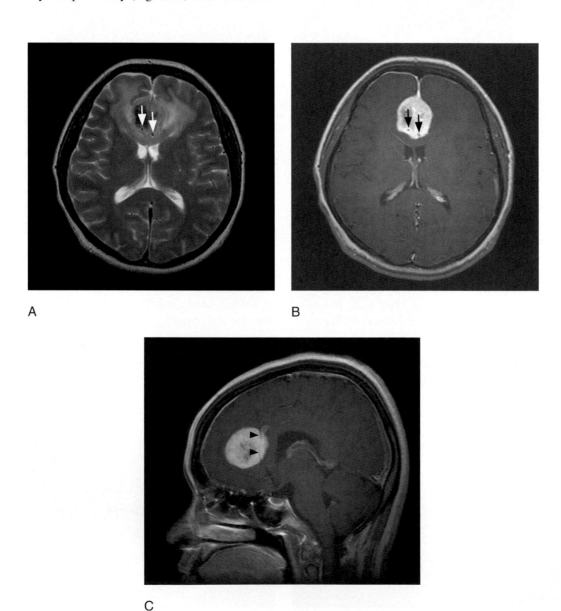

FIG. 33.3. Illustrative case 2. Magnetic resonance (MR) images show a 35-mm mass with a wide base at the anterior third of the falx cerebri. It encases and compresses the anterior cerebral artery (ACA) inferiorly and posteriorly (white arrows in A, black arrows in B, and arrowheads in C) and is associated with considerable peritumoral edema in both frontal lobes. The tumor has a partly low signal intensity in T2-weighted image, suggesting a fibrotic or hard consistency. A, T2-weighted axial image; B, gadolinium-enhanced T1-weighted axial image; C, sagittal image of the same condition

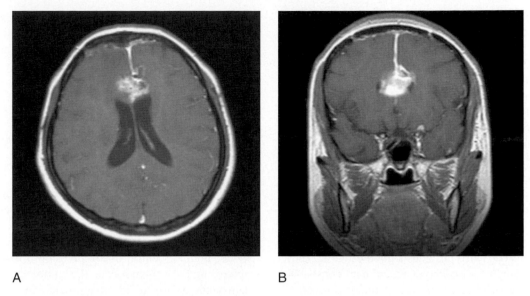

A   B

FIG. 33.4. Illustrative case 2. Magnetic resonance (MR) images taken 6 months after Gamma Knife radiosurgery. The images show the residual mass in the falx cerebri around anterior cerebral arteries. The mass is similar in size to that before radiosurgery. A, gadolinium-enhanced T1-weighted axial image; B, coronal image of the same condition

flow, and the patient was sent to the interventional neurovascular team immediately after wound closure for angiography and papaverine angioplasty. She recovered fully. For the residual mass stereotactic radiosurgery (Gamma Knife) was performed 6 months after the operation. At the last clinical follow-up, her KPS was 100 and there was no evidence of regrowth of the mass on MR images (Fig. 33-4).

The encasement of the major artery and the tumor's hard consistency make this type of operation difficult and increase the risk of postoperative morbidity.

Illustrative Case 3

A 49-year-old woman presented with chief complaints of headache and nausea for 6 months. At the time of admission, neurologic examination revealed right-sided (4+/5) weakness. No other neurologic deficit was observed. MR images showed large lobulated mass, which had a considerable peritumoral edema (Fig. 33-5) and low signal intensity in T2-weighted image, suggesting a hard consistency (Fig. 33-5A). The anterior cerebral arteries were encased, compressed, and deviated

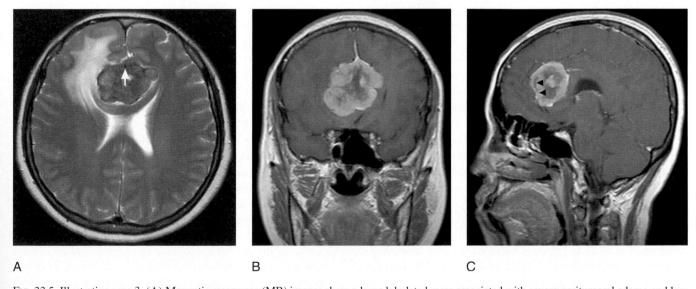

A   B   C

FIG. 33.5. Illustrative case 3. (A) Magnetic resonance (MR) images show a large lobulated mass associated with severe peritumoral edema and low signal intensity in T2-weighted image, suggesting a hard consistency. (B) The anterior cerebral arteries are encased, compressed, and deviated anteriorly by the tumor (white arrows in A and arrowheads in C). A, T2-weighted axial image; B, gadolinium-enhanced T1-weighted coronal image; C, sagittal image of the same condition

anteriorly by the tumor (Fig. 33.5, white arrows in A and arrowheads in C).

A bilateral interhemispheric approach was undertaken through a midline-crossing frontal craniotomy. The right side was approached first. The tumor had a very hard consistency and the ACA was noted to be encased, which was not dissected easily. Sufficient internal debulking of the tumor was not performed. The left-sided approach was performed under the same condition, and the ACA was torn. Primary arterial repair was performed in situ, and intraoperative Doppler analysis confirmed intact flow. Partial removal of the tumor and decompressive craniectomy were performed. The patient had transient right-sided weakness in the postoperative period. At the last clinical follow-up, her KPS was 80 and there was no evidence of regrowth of the mass on MR images. This case also provides a good example, showing that encasement of a major vessel and hard consistency of the tumor make the safe removal of tumor difficult. In selected patients with severe bilateral peritumoral edema, the surgeon should exercise the option of leaving the bone flap off after tumor resection.

Outcomes and Complications

At our institution, patients with falcine meningioma accounted for 68 of 795 meningiomas from 1990 to 2005. Forty-six patients were female and 22 male; their ages ranged from 14 to 77 years. The anterior third was the most frequently involved site (32 of 68 patients; 47%). The transitional and meningothelial types occurred in 44 (65%) of patients and a high grade (atypical and anaplastic) in three patients.

The tumor was totally removed in 58 patients. Seven had subtotal removal because of tumor involvement (or obliteration) of a major venous sinus (five involving the superior sagittal sinus and two invading the straight sinus). In two patients, subtotal resection was achieved because of ACA encasement by the tumor. In one additional patient, hard tumor consistency at the site of origin prevented total removal. We performed further surgery for recurrence in 10 patients over 16 years. No evidence of regrowth was evident in the remaining 58 patients, including those with subtotal removal. Stereotactic radiosurgery (Gamma Knife) for residual mass was performed in six patients. Postoperative adjuvant radiation therapy was done for high-grade meningiomas. The treatment policy for these high-grade meningiomas is discussed in another chapter of this book.

Complications in our series of 68 patients with falcine meningiomas included postoperative weakness, hemorrhagic infarction, cerebrospinal fluid leakage, and drug-induced toxic hepatitis. Fourteen patients had significant temporary deterioration of their neurologic status but recovered within weeks to months. Of the 68 patients, 63 had good outcome (no neurologic deficit or complications), three were better but had residual preoperative deficits, and two had a new postoperative deficit. One expired due to severe postoperative brain swelling and its complication despite aggressive management.

Complication Avoidance and Lessons Learned

Most falcine meningiomas can be removed through a unilateral exposure, which prevents traction and decreases the potential risk to the bridging veins bilaterally.

Early devascularization along the falx is preferred, and, for larger tumors, central decompression allows subsequent microsurgical separation of the tumor capsule from the surrounding arachnoid attachment. Sufficient internal debulking of the tumor and external dissection of the tumor margin off of the arachnoid plane using oxidized cellulose and cottonoid help prevent injury to the surrounding cerebral cortex and protect the pericallosal arteries in the inferior margin of the dissection. The pia should be preserved to maintain the integrity of the cerebral cortex.

Small vessels in the tumor wall should not be coagulated under the assumption that they are tumor feeders. Each should be dissected first to identify its complete course.

Preserving the cortical veins is crucial for preventing brain edema and postoperative complications. A preoperative venous-phase angiogram should be performed for this reason.

A critical area is the junction of the bridging veins traveling into the sinus. Frequently, these veins enter the two leaves of the dura before emptying into the sinus. These veins are vulnerable to injury when the bone flap is elevated, the dura is opened, or the tumor is resected.

The falx that is the origin of tumor should be widely excised beyond the area involved.

In the case of major artery encasement and hard tumor consistency, we recommend that the surgeon develop a plan to intentionally perform a subtotal removal of the tumor followed by radiosurgery or radiation therapy for the residual mass. It is also important to prepare for intraoperative vascular injury.

In the case of severe bilateral peritumoral edema and larger size mass, we recommend having a plan to leave out the bone flap after tumor resection.

Radiosurgery for intracranial meningiomas seems to be safe and effective. However, there are several reports that meningiomas of the convexity, parasagittal region, or falx cerebri have a higher incidence of peritumoral edema after radiosurgery than those of the skull base locations. Therefore, radiosurgery must be considered cautiously for treating falcine meningiomas.

References

1. Cushing H, Eisenhardt L. Meningiomas: Their Classification, Regional Behavior, Life History, and Surgical End Results. Springfield, IL: Charles C Thomas, 1938.
2. Lanman TH, Becker DP. Falcine meningiomas. In Al-Mefty O, ed. Meningiomas. New York: Raven Press, 1991:345–356.
3. Yasargil MG. Microneurosurgery of CNS tumors, IV-B. Stuttgart: Georg Thiem Verlag, 1996:134–165.
4. Al-Mefty O. Operative Atlas of Meningiomas. Philadelphia: Lippincott-Raven Press, 1998:383–450.
5. Tew JM, Van Loveren HR, Keller JT. Atlas of Operative Microneurosurgery, Vol. 2. Brain Tumors. Philadelphia: W.B.Saunders Company, 2001:8–26.

34
Olfactory Groove/Planum Sphenoidale Meningiomas

Douglas Fox, Vini G. Khurana, and Robert F. Spetzler

Introduction

Olfactory groove and planum sphenoidale meningiomas occur along the anterior cranial base overlying the area of the cribriform plate of the ethmoid bone, frontosphenoid suture, and planum sphenoidale. They compose as many as 10% of intracranial meningiomas.[1] The tumors are usually bilateral based on their midline origin, although they can also be unilateral.

Like most meningiomas, meningiomas of the anterior cranial base are typically benign and potentially curable. Thus, the extent of surgical resection is the most important predictor of recurrence.[2] Despite the benign pathology of meningiomas of the olfactory groove, their recurrence rates 10 years after surgical resection have ranged from 10 to 41%.[3,4] These high rates have been attributed to the difficulty in removing the tumor cells that invade the base of skull and paranasal sinuses.

In his 1957 grading system on meningiomas, Simpson thought that grade I resection was impossible given the risk of entry into the sinuses.[2] Ojemann[5] recommended removing the tumor and hyperostic bone but did not advise entry into the ethmoid sinuses unless tumor invasion was clearly defined. These tumors often extend caudally, compromising the bone of the skull base and the paranasal sinuses and complicating their removal. Tumor invades the orbits and nasal cavity in as many as 15% of cases.[1,6] Many authors have shown that the cranial base is the most common site of tumor recurrence, and failure to achieve radical resection of dural, bony, and paranasal sinus involvement leads to recurrence.[7–9] Cerebrospinal fluid (CSF) leakage is a significant complication after the radical resection of olfactory groove meningiomas, and appropriate reconstruction of the skull base is essential to minimize morbidity in these patients.

Olfactory groove and planum sphenoidale meningiomas are closely related to tumors of the tuberculum sellae, but their clinical presentations and surgical outcomes are very different. Given their proximity to the optic chiasm, tuberculum sellae tumors manifest early. Visual deficits are present even when the lesions are small. Given the paucity of symptoms associated with small tumors, early diagnosis of olfactory groove and planum sphenoidale meningiomas continues to be a problem. However, since the advent of cranial imaging with computed tomography (CT) and magnetic resonance imaging (MRI), these lesions are being identified earlier and at smaller sizes.

Anatomy of Olfactory Groove and Planum Sphenoidale

Olfactory groove meningiomas arise in the midline of the anterior cranial fossa over the cribriform plate and frontosphenoid suture. They often involve the area from the crista galli to the posterior planum sphenoidale.[5] The olfactory bulb and tract rest in the olfactory groove, which is formed by the cribriform plate and continues posteriorly beyond the ethmoidal spine (Fig. 34-1). Meningiomas that occur in the region of the olfactory groove are often symmetric and midline, but they can also be located eccentric to one side. The tumors can be associated with hyperostosis in the skull base. They can also thin or destroy the bone, leading to tumor invasion of the sinuses and, rarely, the orbits. With small tumors, the olfactory nerves can be preserved on one side as they lie on the lateral aspect of the tumor. With larger tumors, however, the nerves are thinned to such a degree that their preservation is almost impossible.[5]

The primary blood supply to these tumors is from the anterior and posterior ethmoid arteries. However, these tumors are also supplied by the meningeal branches from the ophthalmic artery, anterior cerebral arteries, anterior communicating artery, pial collaterals, and external carotid circulation (i.e., anterior branches of the middle meningeal artery). The anterior and posterior ethmoid arteries branch from the ophthalmic arteries and often collateralize with the meningeal arteries of the internal carotid arteries. These anastomoses place the ophthalmic artery and therefore vision at risk if embolization is pursued. Frontopolar arteries and other small

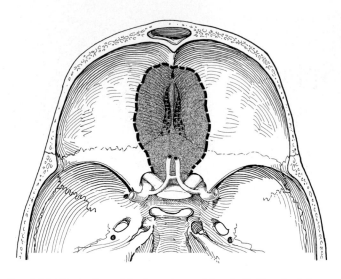

FIG. 34-1. Illustration of the bony base of the skull. The shaded area is the common site of tumors arising from the region of the olfactory groove. Note the relation of the optic chiasm and the anterior cerebral arteries. (With permission from Barrow Neurological Institute.)

branches of the anterior cerebral arteries may be sacrificed without consequence if they adhere to the posterior tumor capsule.[10]

Clinical Presentations

Given their location and slow growth, olfactory groove and planum sphenoidale meningiomas often obtain a significant size before they become symptomatic. Most patients with anterior cranial base meningiomas are women in the fifth and sixth decades of life. In series reported by Hentschel and DeMonte[1] and by Turazzi et al.,[11] more than 50% of patients had tumors larger than 6 cm. Most patients develop one or a combination of the following symptoms: subtle mental changes in cognition and personality, headaches, visual decline, and/or seizures. The onset of these symptoms is usually gradual and most often appreciated first by close family members.

Visual loss is usually limited to changes in acuity and restriction of the inferior fields. The visual symptoms associated with a planum sphenoidale meningioma often appear earlier than those associated with an olfactory groove meningioma because the former is closer to the optic apparatus than the latter. The visual loss is often more severe in one eye, but both are commonly involved. In contrast, inferior compression of the optic nerves and chiasm by tuberculum sellae meningiomas leads to unilateral or bilateral decreased acuity and often to incongruous visual field defects that resemble bitemporal hemianopsia.[12]

In Bakay's and Cares' series of olfactory groove meningiomas, visual symptoms and dementia were prominent at presentation.[7] In Ojemann's series, patients with olfactory groove meningiomas primarily had subtle mental deficits and headache, with relatively few visual findings.[5] Symon[10] believed that the most common symptom was visual loss, with the earliest finding being blurred vision in one eye related to central scotoma. He recommended close assessment of the central field with formal mapping.[10] Foster-Kennedy syndrome, classically described as pallor of the ipsilateral optic disc associated with papilledema of the contralateral optic disc, is very rare.[13] Symon[10] reported only one such case in his 40 patients.

Anosmia is not a typical presenting symptom, but it is often present on examination. In Bakay's and Cares' series of 36 patients, all had anosmia at presentation when examined.[7] Turazzi et al. noted that 27 of their 37 patients had anosmia when evaluated.[11]

Radiology

The radiographic appearance of meningiomas in the anterior cranial base is similar to the appearance of meningiomas in other locations. CT without contrast often shows a slightly hyperdense mass that enhances significantly after the administration of a contrast agent. CT is important for evaluation of the bony floor of the cranial base, allowing identification of hyperostosis and erosion that may assist in surgical planning. Coronal CT scans provide information about the entry of the tumor into the paranasal sinuses, although this information is also readily apparent on MRIs (Fig. 34-2).

The MRI appearance of meningiomas is isointense to brain on T1-weighted imaging and iso- to hyperintense on T2-weighted imaging. After the administration of gadolinium, the lesion should enhance significantly. At their periphery, meningiomas often have a tapered appearance called a dural tail.

MRI provides significant detail about the relation of the optic nerves and chiasm to the tumor. The anterior cerebral arteries and anterior communicating artery also can be identified on MRI (Fig. 34-3).

MR angiography allows further analysis of the vasculature involved or related to the tumor. Since the advent of MRI, catheter angiography is considered unnecessary.[5] Embolization is rarely necessary, given the significant risks of visual loss if embolization of the ethmoidal arteries is attempted given their relation to the ophthalmic artery.[14]

Rosen et al.[14] found no difference in the amount of surgical blood loss between tumors treated with and without preoperative embolization. However, other studies have found that preoperative embolization decreases blood loss.[15] Rosen et al.[14] reported that the rate of permanent neurologic deficits was less than 10%. However, they had two cases of monocular blindness, and the risk of a visual deficit associated with superselective angiography was 1.8%.

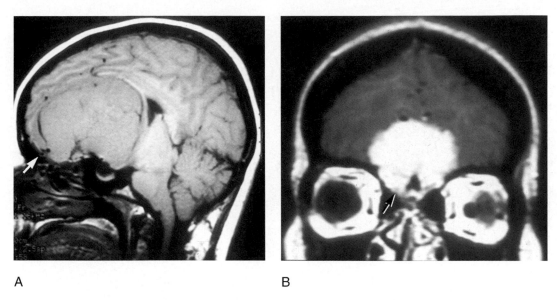

A   B

FIG. 34-2. (A) Sagittal and (B) coronal MRIs show extension of a meningioma into the paranasal sinuses (arrows). This tumor must be removed from the sinuses to minimize the risk of a recurrence

Nonsurgical Options

Because olfactory groove and planum sphenoidale meningiomas tend to be large at presentation, surgery is often the only option. Small tumors found incidentally in asymptomatic patients may be followed. Radiation, fractionated or stereotactic, is a treatment option, but it is usually reserved for residual tumor after surgical resection or for a recurrence. Patients with MRI findings consistent with meningioma who cannot tolerate surgery may be candidates for radiation without a pathologic diagnosis.

Surgical Techniques

Olfactory groove meningiomas are typically resected through a bifrontal craniotomy and subfrontal approach, which is the method that we prefer for large lesions (Fig. 34-4A).[1,11,16–19] Although there are various refinements to the technique, the subfrontal approach provides a wide exposure, minimizing the need to retract the frontal lobes. It also allows access to both sides of the posterior surface of the tumor. Planum sphenoidale tumors are more difficult to access because they involve the chiasmal apparatus due to their slightly more posterior position.

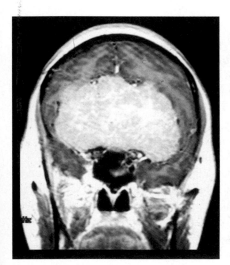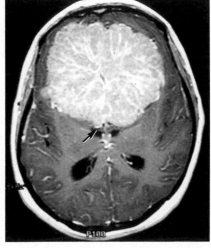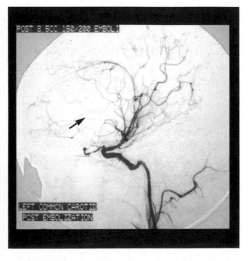

A   B   C

FIG. 34-3. Typical appearance of an olfactory groove meningioma on (A) coronal and (B) axial MRIs with contrast, which show that the large tumor has pushed the anterior cerebral arteries posteriorly (arrow). The displacement is better appreciated on (C) angiography, which is not routinely performed because these lesions are rarely embolized (arrow points to the center of the lesion)

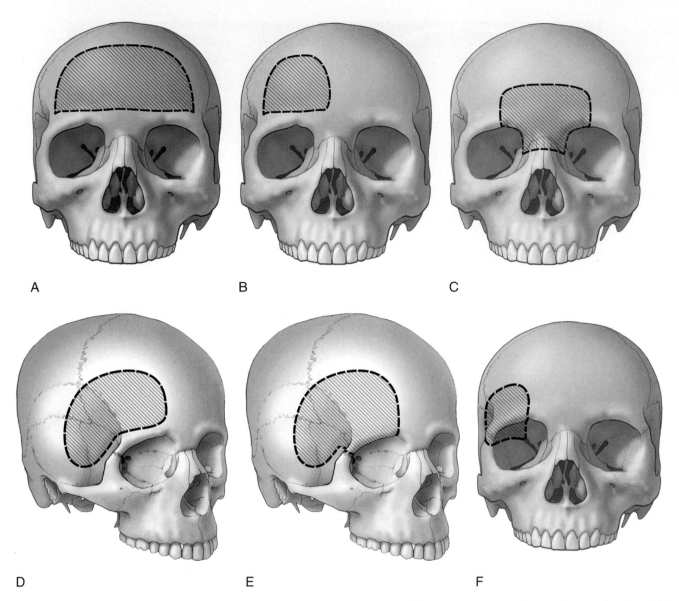

FIG. 34-4. Illustrations showing approaches for olfactory groove meningiomas: (A) bifrontal, (B) unifrontal, (C) bifrontal with the orbital bars, (D) pterional, (E) modified orbitozygomatic, and (F) an orbital osteotomy are all options for approaching this tumor. (With permission from Barrow Neurological Institute.)

The patient is positioned supine. The cranium is fixed in Mayfield-Kees three-pin fixation system with the head elevated and slightly extended. The craniotomy is performed with burr holes placed on each side of the sagittal sinus posteriorly and at the level of the MacCarty keyhole. The craniotomy is performed with a high-speed drill. About 1 cm of bone is left anteriorly along the orbital rim. The bone along the anteromedial aspect of the craniotomy is often irregular. Consequently, the outer table may need to be cut with a high-speed drill followed by fracture of the inner table. Dural tack-up sutures are used to control epidural bleeding.

The frontal sinus is almost routinely encountered and requires attention early. The mucosa should be removed from the free flap, and cauterization is used to remove the accessible

mucosa within the sinus. The sinuses are packed with bacitracin-soaked gel foam, and the pericranium is sewn in position over the open frontal sinuses as described by Ojemann.[5]

The dura is opened in a linear fashion on both sides over the medial inferior frontal lobe. Doing so allows the sagittal sinus to be divided at its anterior third after it has been tied with silk sutures. Next, the falx is cut to expose the tumor. Gentle retraction of the frontal lobes laterally and superiorly provides access to the tumor.

A unilateral approach can be used for smaller lesions (Fig. 34.4B). In the past some surgeons have recommended resection of a portion of the frontal lobe to improve access to the tumor.[10] Unilateral or bilateral orbital osteotomies offer a lower angle of approach and may minimize or obviate the need to retract the frontal lobe (Fig. 34-4C, F).[20] Thus, in our opinion, frontal lobe tissue should never be resected.

The tumor is readily identifiable and often has a thick capsule. It is important to dissect within the arachnoid plane surrounding the tumor to avoid damage to the surrounding brain and neurovascular structures. The capsule of the tumor is coagulated to shrink the lesion, and the process of devascularizing the tumor begins.

The blood supply typically enters from below the tumor. Thus, initial debulking of large tumors is necessary to expose the base of skull to interrupt the blood supply. Extensive internal decompression allows the surrounding structures to be identified and separated from the tumor capsule.

Next, attention is turned to the posterior aspect of the tumor. The surgeon must be vigilant to identify the anterior cerebral arteries and their respective branches. Several authors have noted that the frontopolar artery often adheres to the tumor. It may be released with microdissection but also can be sacrificed without consequence.[5,11]

The capsule is followed posteriorly to expose the sphenoid wing. The edge of the sphenoid wing can be traced medially to the anterior clinoid process and optic apparatus. The posterior arachnoid plane is often preserved, allowing complete removal of the tumor after internal debulking. If this plane has been violated by the tumor, caution is needed because important perforators from the anterior cerebral arteries must be preserved. Some authors recommend leaving tumor if the surgeon is unsure whether the small vessels encountered are feeding vessels or from the anterior cerebral arteries.[1]

After the bulk of the tumor has been removed, its dural attachment must be incised. Simple cauterization of the attachment is insufficient and is thought to leave the patient at high risk for a recurrence. Involved dura must be resected as completely as possible. Hyperostotic bone must be drilled until normal bone is identified because hyperostosis may be related to tumor invasion rather than to a reactive response.[21] If tumor enters the paranasal sinuses, it must be removed aggressively.[3] Given the historically low rate of tumor recurrence, many surgeons once thought that tumor invading the paranasal sinuses was not worth resecting. However, it is now known that the rate of recurrence correlates with bony and paranasal involvement.[3,22]

Historical Approaches

Symon[10] thought that a bifrontal craniotomy was needed only for large tumors and that a unilateral craniotomy was sufficient for smaller lesions. Removal of the right frontal lobe was advocated for exposure. A unilateral craniotomy often extends across the midline to include the sinus so that the falx and superior sagittal sinus can be divided. Olfaction is rarely preserved after resection, and Symon[10] did not believe that removing hyperostosis of the skull base was warranted given that the risk of recurrence was thought to be low.[11] Seeger[23] combined a bifrontal craniotomy with a unilateral subfrontal approach. Doing so

reduced retraction and potentially prevents venous compression because there is no need to elevate the frontal lobe.

Hassler and Zentner advocate a unilateral pterional approach with splitting of the lateral fissure (Fig. 34-4D).[24] The frontal sinus is avoided. The internal, middle, and anterior cerebral arteries and optic nerve are exposed and decompressed, initially by removal of the posterior aspect of the tumor. The hyperostotic area is then removed with a drill to devascularize the tumor. The falx is partially resected along with the crista galli, allowing the core of the contralateral tumor to be removed. The remaining tumor can be dissected freely from the brain.

Mayfrank and Gilsbach recommend an anterior interhemispheric approach.[25] The interhemispheric approach may have advantages over the subfrontal approach. First, it is easy to perform. Second, the relative risk of CSF leakage is reduced. Finally, the risk of infection is also lower because the frontal sinus is avoided. Mayfrank and Gilsbach thought that the subfrontal approach was limited because excessive retraction might be needed to expose the contralateral tumor. Furthermore, repair of skull base erosion or bony involvement can be difficult through a subfrontal approach.

A pterional craniotomy with an orbital osteotomy (Fig. 34-4E) has become a preferred option for anterior cranial base meningiomas and is our preferred approach for smaller tumors.[26] The pterional and modified orbitozygomatic approaches have several advantages. They provide a shorter distance to the tumor than the subfrontal exposure. The pterional and modified orbitozygomatic approaches also enable early detachment of the blood supply from the cranial base, thereby reducing blood loss. Removal of the orbital rim allows a lower angle of attack, potentially minimizing the need to elevate the frontal lobes. Early access to the tumor is obtained, and relieving CSF from the basal cisterns is facilitated. Identification of the vasculature at the onset of surgery, which allows identification and dissection of the arteries early in the surgery, is another advantage over the subfrontal approach. If involved, the anterior skull base can be drilled from this exposure, and the dura and anterior fossa floor can be reconstructed expeditiously. Complications can be associated with the modified orbitozygomatic approach, including CSF leakage, enophthalmos, and orbital entrapment. Removal of the orbital rim often results in violating the frontal sinus, but the increased risk of infection is minor.

Conclusion

Many different approaches are acceptable for the treatment of olfactory groove meningiomas. The choice is often based on the surgeon's experience and the size of the tumor. Typically, bilateral subfrontal approaches are used to access large lesions although the pterional or modified orbitozygomatic offer the advantage of identifying critical structures early in the surgery. Patients with visual loss or changes in mental status often improve after surgery. Given the low complication rates associated with contemporary neurosurgical techniques, patients can be optimistic about their outcomes. Preservation of contralateral olfactory function is also possible, especially with tumors less than 2 cm.[27] Because of the involvement of the skull base and the potential for entry into the paranasal sinuses, recurrence is a significant problem associated with olfactory groove meningiomas. These areas must be treated aggressively.[3] Once resection is complete, the surgeon must be facile with reconstruction of the skull base to prevent CSF leakage. These tumors are treatable and with aggressive removal may be associated with low recurrence rates.

Complication Avoidance/Lessons Learned

Surgical management of olfactory groove/planum sphenoidale meningiomas continues to be challenging. The advancement and wide use of cranial imaging has allowed for diagnosis to be made earlier and thus surgical removal is often easier and done prior to the patient experiencing neurologic deficits. The use of intraoperative navigation and microsurgical techniques has improved the surgeon's ability to deal with these difficult lesions. CSF leak and recurrence remain the most common postoperative problems, and thus aggressive removal and ability to reconstruct the floor of the anterior cranial fossa is a must for a surgeon dealing with these tumors. CSF diversion is important in the treatment of tumor that invades the floor of the anterior cranial fossa, allowing for reduced CSF pressure during healing. Avoidance of injury to the anterior cerebral arteries remains a top priority, and these vessels must be identified and preserved for optimal outcomes. Pterional or orbital approaches allow for quicker visualization of the vasculature and may be the preferred route if the tumor is of a smaller size.

References

1. Hentschel SJ, DeMonte F. Olfactory groove meningiomas. Neurosurg Focus 2003;15:E4.
2. Simpson D. The recurrence of intracranial meningiomas after surgical treatment. J Neurol Neurosurg Psychiatry 1957;20:22–39.
3. Obeid F, Al Mefty O. Recurrence of olfactory groove meningiomas. Neurosurgery 2003;53:534–42.
4. Mirimanoff RO, Dosoretz DE, Linggood RM, et al. Meningioma: analysis of recurrence and progression following neurosurgical resection. J Neurosurg 1985;62:18–24.
5. Ojemann RG. Olfactory grove meningiomas. In: Al Mefty O. Meningiomas. New York: Raven Press, 1991:383–94.
6. Derome PJ, Guiot G. Bone problems in meningiomas invading the base of the skull. Clin Neurosurg 1978;25:435–51.
7. Bakay L, Cares HL. Olfactory meningiomas. Report on a series of twenty-five cases. Acta Neurochir (Wien) 1972;26:1–12.
8. Mathiesen T, Lindquist C, Kihlstrom L, et al. Recurrence of cranial base meningiomas. Neurosurgery 1996;39:2–7.
9. Snyder WE, Shah MV, Weisberger EC, et al. Presentations and patterns of late recurrence of olfactory groove meningiomas. Skull Base Surgery 2000;10:131–9.
10. Symon L. Olfactory groove and surasellar meningiomas. In: Kayenbuhl H, ed. Advances and Technical Standards in Neurosurgery. New York: Springer-Verlag, 1977:69–71.
11. Turazzi S, Cristofori L, Gambin R, et al. The pterional approach for the microsurgical removal of olfactory groove meningiomas. Neurosurgery 1999;45:821–5.
12. Grisoli F, Diaz-Vasquez P, Riss M, et al. Microsurgical management of tuberculum sellae meningiomas. Results in 28 consecutive cases. Surg Neurol 1986;26:37–44.
13. Fukuyama J, Hayasaka S, Setogawa T, et al. Foster Kennedy syndrome and optociliary shunt vessels in a patient with an olfactory groove meningioma. Ophthalmologica 1991;202:125–31.
14. Rosen CL, Ammerman JM, Sekhar LN, et al. Outcome analysis of preoperative embolization in cranial base surgery. Acta Neurochir (Wien) 2002;144:1157–64.
15. Macpherson P. The value of pre-operative embolisation of meningioma estimated subjectively and objectively. Neuroradiology 1991;33:334–7.
16. Spektor S, Valarezo J, Fliss DM, et al. Olfactory groove meningiomas from neurosurgical and ear, nose, and throat perspectives: approaches, techniques, and outcomes. Neurosurgery 2005;57:268–80.
17. McDermott MW, Rootman J, Durity FA. Subperiosteal, subperiorbital dissection and division of the anterior and posterior ethmoid arteries for meningiomas of the cribriform plate and planum sphenoidale: technical note. Neurosurgery 1995;36:1215–8.
18. DeMonte F. Surgical treatment of anterior basal meningiomas. J Neurooncol 1996;29:239–48.
19. El Gindi S. Olfactory groove meningioma: surgical techniques and pitfalls. Surg Neurol 2000;54:415–7.
20. Tamaki N, Yin D. Giant olfactory groove meningiomas: advantages of the bilateral fronto-orbitonasal approach. J Clin Neurosci 1999;6:302–5.
21. Pieper DR, Al Mefty O, Hanada Y, et al. Hyperostosis associated with meningioma of the cranial base: secondary changes or tumor invasion. Neurosurgery 1999;44:742–6.
22. Christensen D, Laursen H, Klinken L. Prediction of recurrence in meningiomas after surgical treatment. A quantitative approach. Acta Neuropathol (Berl) 1983;61:130–4.
23. Seeger W. Microsurgery of the Cranial Base. New York: Springer-Verlag, 1983.
24. Hassler W, Zentner J. Pterional approach for surgical treatment of olfactory groove meningiomas. Neurosurgery 1989;25:942–5.
25. Mayfrank L, Gilsbach JM. Interhemispheric approach for microsurgical removal of olfactory groove meningiomas. Br J Neurosurg 1996;10:541–5.
26. Sekhar LN, Nanda A, Sen CN, et al. The extended frontal approach to tumors of the anterior, middle, and posterior skull base. J Neurosurg 1992;76:198–206.
27. Welge-Luessen A, Temmel A, Quint C, et al. Olfactory function in patients with olfactory groove meningioma. J Neurol Neurosurg Psychiatry 2001;70:218–21.

35
Tuberculum Sellae Meningiomas

Chang Jin Kim and Seok Ho Hong

Introduction

Tuberculum sellae (TS) meningiomas arise from the dura of the TS, chiasmatic sulcus, limbus sphenoidale, and diaphragma sellae. As they grow in the subchiasmal area compressing the optic nerves, TS meningiomas produce quite distinctive clinical, radiologic, and microsurgical features (Fig. 35-1) [1, 2]. The first report of a TS meningioma, in 1897, was as an incidental finding at an autopsy [3], and the first successful removal of this tumor was reported by Cushing in 1916 [4].

The clinical feature typical of TS meningiomas, primary optic atrophy with bitemporal hemianopsia in an adult with normal sella turcica on plain radiograph, has been recognized as a "suprasellar chiasmal syndrome" [1,4,5]. In most patients, however, visual loss appears to be asymmetric, in that the vision of one eye deteriorates earlier while that of the other eye stays relatively intact until the later stage [6–15]. The asymmetric nature of TS meningiomas has also been observed in preoperative magnetic resonance (MR) images, which show that the epicenter of the tumor is often slightly off the midline, although the main location is grossly on the central structures (Fig. 35-1). The laterality of the tumor epicenter has been reported to correspond to the side on which vision is more compromised [12]. Anterior-posterior views of cerebral angiograms show that dural feeders of the tumor, which appear to be stained in a "sunburst" fashion, are mostly off the midline, suggesting that the tumor does not originate in the exact midline microanatomically (Fig. 35-2).

The TS is a narrow bony ridge between the chiasmatic sulcus and the hypophyseal fossa (Fig. 35-3). The lateral end of the TS is just inferomedial to the intracranial orifice of the optic canal, through which the optic nerve travels to join the contralateral optic nerve at the chiasm [16,17]. During surgery, we have found that the majority of TS meningiomas arise from the dura of a relatively small area around the lateral end of the TS, just below the optic nerve. As the tumor grows, it compresses the ipsilateral optic nerve superiorly or superolaterally and causes it to deviate against the sharp edge of the falciform ligament (Fig. 35-3). Because of the anatomic proximity of

the lateral end of the TS to the optic canal, the tumor tends to extend into the optic canal underneath the nerve. Optic canal extension has been reported in 32–69.8% of patients with TS meningioma [18,19]. We similarly observed intracanalicular extension of the tumor in 24 of 41 (58.5%) patients with TS meningiomas. When the tumor continues to enlarge, the chiasm is compressed posteriorly or superiorly and the contralateral optic nerve is compressed laterally, resulting in visual compromise of the opposite eye in larger tumors. Although tumors arising from the exact midline may grow symmetrically and accordingly produce bilateral visual loss simultaneously, this is not observed frequently in clinical practice.

Recent progress in microsurgery has improved the surgical outcomes of skull base lesions, including TS meningiomas. Using advanced modern microsurgical techniques, the primary aim of surgery for TS meningioma is its complete resection, along with improvement or preservation of neurologic status.

Special Considerations

Clinical Presentation

TS meningiomas account for about 4–10% of all intracranial meningiomas [1,2,20–24]. These tumors mostly affect women [6–8,12,14,25,26], and the mean age at diagnosis is between 40 and 60 years [6–9,12,14,27]. The most common symptom at presentation is progressive asymmetric visual loss. The term "chiasmal syndrome," coined by Holmes and Sargeant in 1927, refers to a primary optic atrophy accompanying a bitemporal field defect in a patient with tumors in the TS [5]. To differentiate TS meningiomas from other suprasellar lesions, such as pituitary adenomas and chordomas, Cushing and Eisenhardt described TS meningioma as a "suprasellar meningioma" causing chiasmal syndrome [4]. The visual symptoms caused by these tumors, including loss of acuity slowly progressing to blindness in one eye followed by decreasing vision, usually in the temporal field of the other eye, were described by Grant and Hedges as "monotonously uniform" [28]. These findings have also been described elsewhere [6–8,11,12,14,21,29,30].

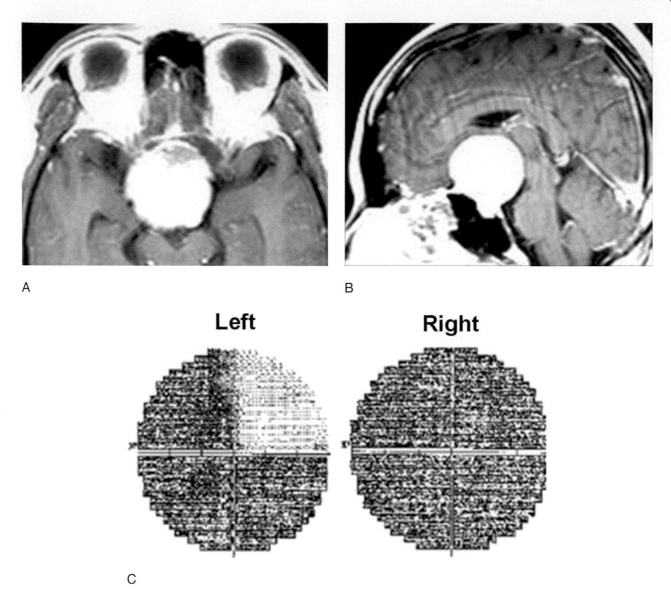

A   B

Left   Right

C

FIG. 35-1. Brain MR images of a 33-year-old female patient with visual failure. (A, B) A large suprasellar mass with strong homogeneous enhancement can be observed attached to the dura of the planum sphenoidale, chiasmatic sulcus, and TS area. (C) Perimetric examination showing that the right eye is totally blind; in the left eye, only the superior nasal quadrant remains, with a visual acuity of 0.2

In most patients with TS meningioma, visual loss starts insidiously and progresses slowly, except for rare cases of sudden onset or fluctuating courses. When we evaluated the preoperative perimetric findings in 41 patients managed between 1994 and 2003, we found that 36 of these patients showed asymmetric visual field defects (Fig. 35-4). Fundoscopic examination of 83 patients with TS meningiomas showed that only seven had normal optic discs, including one with equivocal findings [8]. Of the remaining 76 patients with abnormalities in the optic discs, 69 had optic disc pallor, 6 had Foster-Kennedy syndrome, and 1 had papilledema.

Headache is the second most common symptom in patient with TS meningioma, occurring in 21–54% of patients [6–9,14,26]. Although preoperative endocrinological disturbance is thought to be rare in these patients, if it

occurs, it is thought to occur later in the clinical course, with the most common endocrinopathy being hyperprolactinemia due to stalk compression [7,21,25,31,32]. Anosmia is also rare as are other neurologic problems, including mental status change, seizure, dizziness, and motor paralysis [8,9,14,29].

Radiologic Findings

Magnetic resonance (MR) imaging is the imaging modality of choice and is essential for diagnosis of TS meningiomas [33,34]. MR findings that differentiate these tumors from pituitary macroadenomas include (1) strong homogenous enhancement with gadolinium contrast; (2) suprasellar location of the tumor

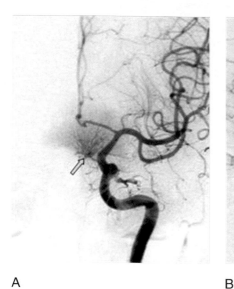
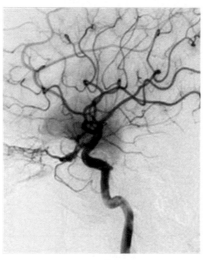

A   B

FIG. 35-2. Left internal carotid angiogram of a patient with TS meningioma. (A) Anterior-posterior view showing a typical "sunburst" tumor staining, where the point of convergence of tumor feeders is slightly off the midline. (B). Lateral projection showing that the feeders appear to be from the posterior ethmoidal artery, a branch of the ophthalmic artery, and showing that the internal carotid and anterior cerebral arteries are displaced by the tumor

epicenter; and (3) tapered extension of the enhanced mass into the surrounding dural base [35,36]. Thin-sectioned images with and without contrast enhancement in multiple planes, especially in coronal and sagittal sections, provide exquisite anatomic details showing the relationship of the tumor to neighboring structures. Careful review of MR images can determine whether the carotid arteries or the anterior cerebral arteries are encased by the tumor, information critical for surgery (Fig. 35-5).

Computed tomography (CT) scanning is also important in diagnosing TS meningiomas and planning for surgery. Thin-sliced CT images in the bone window setting provide important information on the bone anatomy of the TS area. Hyperostosis involving the TS and chiasmatic sulcus has been reported

[37]. Although cerebral angiography may not be always necessary, it can be useful because of its ability to delineate feeding vessels and to provide direct information regarding the surrounding vascular structures, such as displacement and narrowing of the vessels (Fig. 35-2). Recently, the authors have employed MR- or CT-based reconstructed angiograms in place of conventional angiograms, which are shown to be equally informative for these purposes (Fig. 35-6).

All of these radiologic findings should enable the surgeon to completely understand the three-dimensional topography of the tumor and its surrounding structures. This information will allow the surgeon to plan an optimal surgical strategy as well as perform proper microsurgical procedures according to individualized anatomic variations.

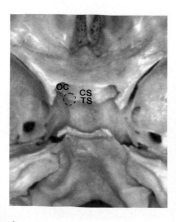
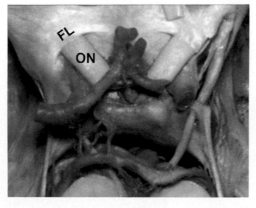
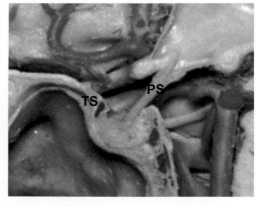

A   B   C

FIG. 35-3. Anatomic relationship of the tuberculum sella, optic nerve, internal carotid artery, anterior cerebral arteries, and pituitary stalk. (A) The lateral end of the TS (dashed circle), from which most TS meningiomas arise, is inferomedial and in close proximity to the optic canal. (B) The optic nerve is observed coming out of the optic canal under the falciform ligament. (C) Mid-sagittal section showing that the optic nerve is superior to the TS, and the pituitary stalk is posterior to the TS. Abbreviations: CS, chiasmatic sulcus; FL, falciform ligament; OC, optic canal; ON, optic nerve; PS, pituitary stalk

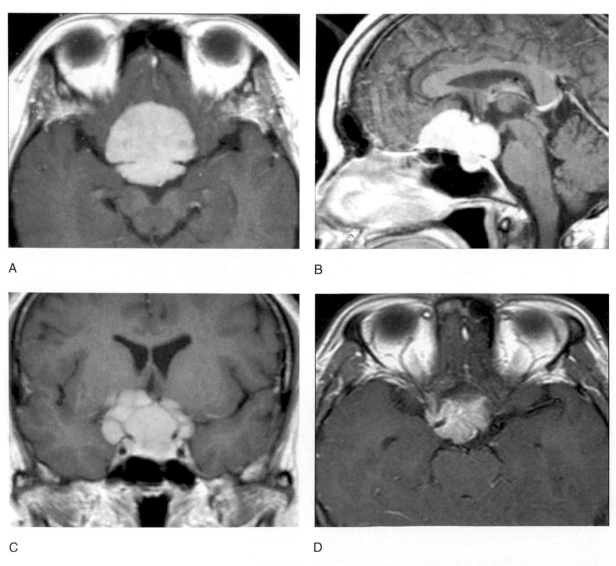

FIG. 35-4. The pattern of preoperative visual field defects in the 41 patients in the authors' series

FIG. 35-5. Brain MR images of a patient with TS meningioma. (A) Gadolinium-enhanced T1 axial section showing a homogeneously enhanced round suprasellar mass encasing both the internal carotid and middle cerebral arteries. (B) Gadolinium-enhanced T1 sagittal section showing that this mass has a broad dural base on the planum sphenoidale, chiasmatic sulcus, and TS, but the sella turcica is not enlarged. (C) Gadolinium-enhanced T1 coronal section showing the relationship of the internal carotid arteries, middle cerebral arteries, and anterior cerebral arteries on both sides of the mass. (D) Contrast-enhanced axial section brain MR image of a different patient showing tumor extension into the right optic canal

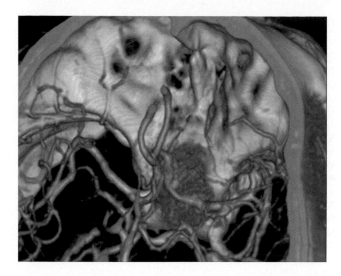

FIG. 35-6. Computerized tomography (CT) angiogram. A three-dimensional reconstructed image showing the relationship of the cerebral arteries to the tumor. The right anterior cerebral artery drapes the superior surface of the tumor as it branches from the right internal carotid artery, which is encased by the tumor

Treatment

The goals of surgery for TS meningiomas are (1) complete excision of the tumor with involved dural attachment and (2) preservation of the surrounding neurovascular structures, especially the optic nerves and cerebral arteries. Surgical outcomes have improved considerably in the last few decades, mainly due to advances in neuroradiologic and microsurgical techniques, in addition to increased understanding of microsurgical anatomy. Total removal of TS meningioma with acceptable morbidity and mortality rates has been achieved by current neurosurgical practice [6,7,9, 12,14,15,18,21,27]. Although radical excision is vital for lowering the rate of tumor recurrence [38], improvement or preservation of neurologic status should always be regarded as the ultimate, nonnegotiable goal of surgery.

Preoperative embolization of tumor feeders is usually not feasible since tumors are mostly fed from the posterior ethmoidal artery, a branch of the ophthalmic artery [39]. Radiation therapy, either external beam radiation or radiosurgery, is not considered as an initial therapeutic option for TS meningiomas. In contrast, radiotherapy may be used as an adjunctive treatment modality in patients with residual or recurrent tumors after primary surgery (see Chapters 25 and 26).

Surgical Techniques

Surgical approaches for TS meningiomas include the bifrontal approach, the unilateral subfrontal approach, the frontotemporal pterional approach, the orbitocranial or orbitozygomatic approach, the combined extradural and intradural approach, and the transsphenoidal approach

[19,25,40–46]. Among these, the bifrontal approach provides the widest surgical view and is regarded as the most suitable for very large tumors. The orbitocranial approach, in which the supraorbital bar is removed either in one piece together with the frontotemporal bone flap or in two separate pieces, shortens the working distance and provides additional basal exposure for surgery. It is advantageous because a surgeon can "look up" to visualize the superior pole of the tumor with minimal brain retraction [25,47]. Although the orbitozygomatic approach provides an excellent means to access lesions in the skull base, it is seldom necessary to use this approach in patients with TS meningiomas.

The combined extradural and intradural approach for TS meningiomas has been described [46] (see Chapter 36). Briefly, following frontotemporal craniotomy, the sphenoid wing, the orbital roof, and the anterior clinoid process are resected and the optic canal is opened extradurally, before removal of the intradural portion of the tumor. This approach has yielded excellent results [46]. In a similar approach, superior orbitotomy with the supraorbital ridge removal is performed in a single bone piece and extradural anterior clinoidectomy is performed after frontotemporal craniotomy, followed by the resection of the sphenoid wing [41]. In the transcranial-transsphenoidal approach for TS meningiomas, the anterior skull base is drilled out to expose the basal part of the tumor, and the optic canal and sphenoid sinus are opened before removal of the tumor [40].

The frontotemporal, the pterional, and the unilateral subfrontal approaches are thought to provide a sufficient surgical view in patients with TS meningiomas, with comparable outcomes and rates of complications as extensive skull base approaches [6,7,12,14,15,18,19,27,48]. Surgery for TS meningiomas consists primarily of "look-down" procedures. Thus, the superior orbital rim or orbital bar does not hinder surgical views if the craniotomy per se is low enough, to the level of the orbital roof (Fig. 35-7). In recent years, we

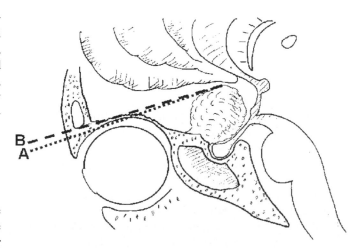

FIG. 35-7. Comparison of the inferior-superior viewing trajectory using the orbitocranial and basal fronto-temporal approaches

have preferred the basal frontotemporal approach over the orbitocranial approach, which we used more frequently in the earlier periods.

The transsphenoidal approach through the endonasal or transseptal route was recently introduced for TS meningiomas [42,44,49]. Because the lateral exposure is limited, this approach is thought to be applicable only in patients with small tumors (<2–3 cm in diameter) located in the midline. In addition, dissecting encased vessels or removing the mass extending into the optic canal is extremely difficult, and the dural opening cannot be closed by primary means, increasing the likelihood of cerebrospinal fluid (CSF) leakage and the risk of meningitis. Neurosurgeons require special training to work through a narrow and long operative route with or without a surgical endoscope. Only experts in transsphenoidal surgery or in endoscopic surgery with very high levels of related techniques and experiences should try this approach for TS meningiomas. The endoscopic for removal of meningiomas approach is described in Chapter 21.

Evolution of Surgical Approach from the Fronto-temporo-orbital to the Basal fronto-temporal Approach

In an earlier series of patients with TS meningiomas, we employed the fronto-temporo-orbital approach because it provided wider exposure and a wider angle of trajectory with a shorter working distance, and provided excellent inferior-superior viewing trajectories with minimal brain retraction. As our clinical experience increased, however, we found that the removal of the superior orbital rim did not offer an additional advantage if the frontal craniotomy was as low as the level of the anterior cranial base or of the orbital roof with only the thin orbital bony shell left over the periorbita by drilling away the sphenoid ridge and the orbital protuberances. The orbital roof is convex toward the frontal base and acts as an impediment to access the suprasellar area even after the orbital bar is removed (Fig. 35-7), and herniated orbital fat protruded through periorbital tearing after orbitotomy sometimes contributes to partial obstruction of the surgical view when the orbitocranial approach is performed, which seldom occurs in the frontotemporal approach.

When comparing the surgical results from skull base approaches [25,41,46] and those from pterional approaches using modern microsurgical techniques [7,12,48,50], there are no significant differences in the extent of resection, rate of visual improvement, and rate of mortality. Skull base approaches have yielded total resection rates of 67–100%, visual improvement rates of 25–77%, and mortality rates of 0–8.6%, whereas pterional approaches have yielded total resection rates of 80–100%, visual improvement rates of 40–80%, and mortality rates of 0–8.7% (Table 35-1).

TABLE 35-1. Reported Surgical Results.

Author, year	No. of cases	Total removal (%)	Visual improvement (%)	Mortality (%)
Cushing, 1938[a] [1]	24	54	53	21
Grant, 1956[a] [28]	30	12	50	20
Finn, 1974[a] [8]	83	67	60	13
Symon, 1984[a] [15]	68	76	63	7.4
Andrews, 1988 [6]	38	58	42	3
Almefty, 1985[b] [25]	35	91	25	9
Yasargil, 1996 [19]	112	100	40	0.9
Raco, 1999 [14]	69	91	51	7
Arai, 2000[b] [40]	21	100[c]	52	0
Zevgaridis, 2001 [51]	24	96	67	0
Fahlbusch, 2002 [7]	47	98	80	0
Jallo, 2002 [12]	23	87	55	9
Goel, 2002 [27]	70	84	70	3
Dolenc, 2003[b] [46]	35	100	77	—
Schick, 2005 [18]	53	91	38	4
Pamir, 2005 [48]	42	81	58	2
Authors' series[d]	41	95	70	0

[a]Macroscopic series.
[b]Skull base approaches.
[c]Including the cases of "almost total removal."
[d]Unpublished data.

Surgical Procedures

Corticosteroids, anticonvulsants, and antibiotics are administered preoperatively to all patients. The surgical approach is through the side with worse vision, which usually corresponds to the side of larger tumor extension, since optic canal unroofing and management of the tumor lateral to the optic nerve and the internal carotid artery are easier when performed from the ipsilateral side of the larger tumor extension. For tumors located exactly in the midline with no laterality of visual symptoms, the right side approach is preferred.

The patient is placed in the supine position with the head turned to the opposite side and extended slightly, thus allowing the frontal lobe to spontaneously fall downward due to gravity during surgery. Three-point skull fixation is applied.

Extradural Procedures

The skin incision starts from the point just anterior to the tragus and posterior to the superficial temporal artery, so that the artery is included in the flap. The excision extends further up behind the hairline and up to the midline in a curvilinear fashion. The temporalis fascia is incised along the skin incision and the temporalis muscle is split along the fascial incision using monopolar cautery. A combined skin and muscle flap is elevated and reflected anteriorly to expose the lateral part of the superior orbital rim and the base of the zygomatic process of the frontal bone. Three burr holes are made (Fig. 35-8 A). The key hole is made just behind the junction of the root of

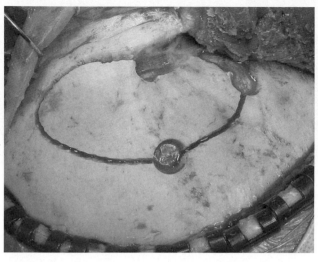
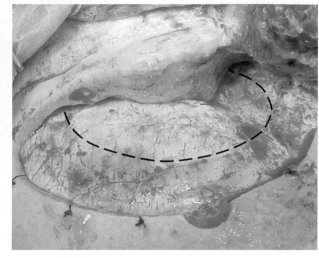

A   B

FIG. 35-8. Right basal frontotemporal craniotomy. (A) Position of the three burr holes and the low frontal cut. (B) The sphenoid ridge is generously drilled away, along with the orbital protuberances, and the frontal sinus is opened. The dural incision is indicated by a dashed line (B)

the zygomatic process of the frontal bone and the beginning
of the superior temporal line, thus exposing the dura of the lateral frontal base. A second burr hole is placed in the temporal
bone behind the sphenoid ridge, and a third burr hole is placed
on the superior temporal line about 4 cm posterior to the key
hole. The key hole and the temporal burr hole are connected
as low as possible using a high-speed drill and a rongeur. The
frontal cut is made from the key hole, extending medially just
above the superior orbital rim to reach the coronal plane of the
lateral two thirds of the superior orbital rim. The cut is then
turned up to the third burr hole in a curvilinear fashion. The
level of the frontal basal bone cut should be the same as that of
the frontal base. Finally, the temporal burr hole and the third
hole are connected and a bone flap is elevated. Before cutting
the bone with a high-speed drill, the dura must be separated
gently from the overlying bone to prevent dural tearing. After
multiple dural tack-up sutures, the sphenoid ridge lateral to
the superior orbital fissure is drilled away generously, leaving
only a thin layer of cortical bone over the orbit. The bony
protrusions on the rough frontal surface of the orbital roof are
also drilled away to make the frontal base flat. Extradural anterior clinoidectomy or optic canal unroofing is not routinely
performed. All of these procedures provide a similar range
of exposure as the orbitocranial approach if the orbital roof,
which is convex on the frontal base, is flattened sufficiently
by drilling.

A curvilinear dural incision is made around the sylvian
fissure from the temporal to the medial frontal base (Fig. 35-8B).
The inferiorly based dural flap is reflected and draped on the
bony orbit, with its edge sutured and pulled to secure an effective surgical view over the orbital ridge. The dural flap is kept
moist by applying wet cottonoid patties during intradural procedures. The lateral part of the inferior aspect of the frontal

lobe, the lateral portion of the sylvian fissure, and the anterior
pole of the temporal lobe are exposed.

Intradural Procedures

Under surgical microscope, the sylvian fissure is dissected and
opened widely from the distal to the proximal direction, exposing the middle cerebral artery. As the release of CSF during
sylvian dissection renders the brain slackened, the frontal lobe
starts to fall downward by gravity. Further medial arachnoid
dissection from the proximal sylvian fissure exposes the tumor.
Additional brain retraction using retractor blades is not usually
necessary. With the exposed temporal lobe covered with cottonoids, only the ipsilateral frontal lobe is retracted spontaneously. Elevating the arachnoid between the inferior surface of
the frontal lobe and the anterosuperior aspect of the tumor provides initial recognition of the tumor. The ipsilateral optic nerve
is usually found to be compressed superiorly or superolaterally,
flattened, and angulated against the falciform ligament as it
comes out of the optic foramen (Fig. 35-9; see also Fig. 35-12).
The internal carotid artery is found lateral to the optic nerve in
the line connecting the proximal middle cerebral artery and the
medial sphenoid ridge. When the optic nerve and the internal
carotid artery are completely covered by the tumor (Fig. 35-10),
which occurs occasionally, dissection should first be carefully
performed to identify the optic nerve and the carotid artery, but
only after thorough inspection to determine the relationship of
those vital structures to the underlying sphenoid.

Devascularization of the tumor is then performed to make
a red, hypervascular, and firm tumor into a white, hypovascular, and relatively soft tumor. This enables easier debulking
and further dissection of the tumor without bleeding (Fig. 35-11).
Devascularization starts from the most anterior part of the

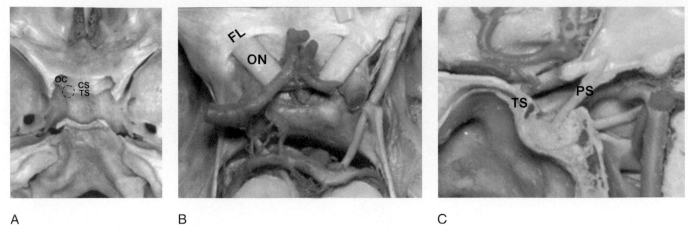

FIG. 35-9. Coronal MR of a relatively small-sized TS meningioma on the right side (A), operative view showing compression of the right optic nerve (B), and causing early visual disturbance ipsilaterally. Abbreviations: ICA, internal carotid artery; ON, optic nerve; T, TS meningioma

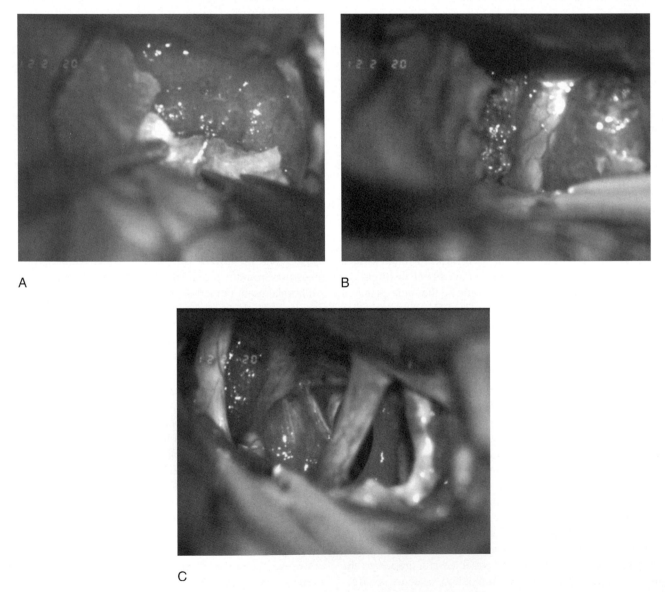

FIG. 35-10. Intraoperative photographs of a large TS meningioma (Multiplanar MR images presented in Fig. 35-5). (A) Initial exposure of the tumor, showing apparent encasement of the optic nerve and arteries. (B) Identification of the right optic nerve after careful dissection and removal of the anterior part of the tumor. (C) Identification of the pituitary stalk after complete removal of the tumor

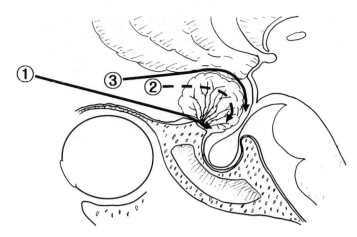

FIG. 35-11. Three base steps in microsurgery. Devascularization by coagulating the dural feeders and detachment from the dura ①, central debulking ②, and dissection from the surrounding tissue ③

tumor, medial to the optic nerves, applying bipolar coagulation between the tumor and the underlying dura. Devascularization then proceeds posteriorly, with each devascularized part of the tumor detached and removed piece by piece. This provides more working space, until most of the major feeding arteries from the dura around the lateral end of the TS inferomedial to the ipsilateral optic canal are coagulated and cut. Great care should be taken not to damage the ipsilateral optic nerve during devascularization of the feeders. The optic nerve is protected with cottonoids, and the exposed tip of the insulated bipolar forceps should be always kept away from the optic nerve. Sufficient and frequent saline irrigation is recommended for cooling and cleaning during coagulation.

The tumor is then debulked using an ultrasonic surgical aspirator or a pair of scissors (Fig. 35-11). As the remaining mass becomes smaller and there is more working space, dissection becomes easier. The tumor capsule is meticulously dissected from the surrounding structures while trying to keep the arachnoid layers unscathed. Initially, no attempt is made to remove the tumor from underneath the ipsilateral optic nerve. The optic nerve is under significant tension, until enough decompression has been accomplished. The tumor in the superior pole is dissected from the anterior cerebral arteries, with special attention paid not to injure the Heubner's artery or other perforating arteries. If these arteries are unintentionally injured, leading to vascular rupture, they should be repaired immediately by applying low-current bipolar cautery, by suturing the vessel wall, or by using microvascular surgical clips.

The medial aspect of the tumor is dissected from the contralateral optic nerve and the carotid artery by piecemeal removal. The contralateral optic nerve is usually displaced laterally by the tumor. The dissection proceeds posteromedially to the optic chiasm. The posteriorly displaced pituitary stalk is identified and the posterior portion of tumor is dissected from the interpeduncular fossa. The membrane of Liliequist provides an excellent dissection plane between the tumor and the surrounding structures. The tumor is removed from

the ipsilateral carotid artery and its perforators with great care, tracing the arachnoid plane. Finally, when sufficient decompression has been attained, the tumor is dissected from underneath the ipsilateral optic nerve, while taking extreme care not to apply tension to the optic nerve. It is recommended that great care be taken not to injure the optic nerve, since vision can recover even in eyes found preoperatively to be blind. Since it is often necessary to open the optic canal to mobilize the optic nerve, allowing the tumor to be resected from underneath the optic nerve, fine feeding arteries to the nerve should be preserved. Extreme adhesion between the tumor and the inferior surface of the optic nerve may make it infeasible to dissect the tumor without damaging the optic nerve. In these patients, it is better to leave a very thin layer of the tumor on the undersurface of the optic nerve. In our series of patients, this was one of the main reasons for incomplete resection of the tumor. When the tumor is observed to grow into the optic canal under the optic nerve, the canal is unroofed using a high-speed diamond drill after the dura around the optic canal is peeled off. To avoid a potentially disastrous accident, during which the rotating high-speed drill catches the cottonoids covering the brain and injures the adjacent vital structures, we have used an aluminum foil plate tailored to fit the working space for drilling. To protect the optic nerve from heat injury, continuous saline irrigation is used during drilling. The dura covering the optic nerve is excised, the optic nerve is gently mobilized, and the tumor extending into the canal is removed in a piecemeal fashion.

After complete resection of the tumor, the involved dura around the TS from which the tumor originated is excised and the involved hyperostotic bone is also drilled away, taking care not to enter the sphenoid or ethoid sinuses. CT images in bone window setting may give valuable information on bony structures, including the thickness of the involved bone. For elderly patients, the dura may be coagulated after tumor excision, depending on the case. The temporalis fascial flap, which had been harvested from the area posterior to the skin incision is fixed using fibrin glue on the area of dural defect or on the unintended opening into the sphenoid sinus (Fig. 35-12). Lumbar CSF drainage is not usually necessary.

Closure

After complete hemostasis, the dura is closed in a watertight fashion. Complete sealing of the dural closure without leakage is routinely checked by intradural saline filling with positive pressure through the last few stitches at the end of the closure. The bone flap is repositioned exactly into its original place and secured with miniplates and screws, which had been adjusted and attached during craniotomy, or with other rigid fixation devices. When the frontal air sinus is opened during craniotomy, the sinus mucosa is kept intact without resection. It is not necessary to obliterate or cranialize the opened frontal air sinus if watertight dural closure is achieved. To date, we have not experienced

342   C.J. Kim and S.H. Hong

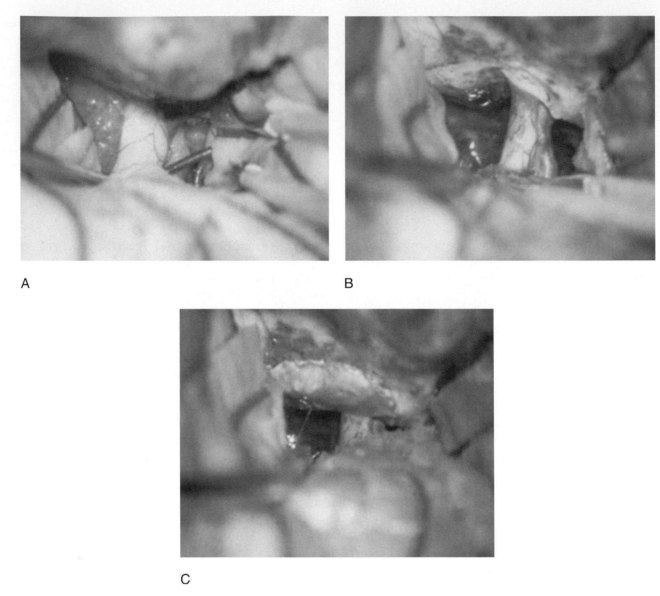

FIG. 35-12. Operative photograph of a medium-sized TS meningioma. (A) Tumor compression of the right optic nerve. (B) Complete removal of the tumor, along with its dural attachment and intracanalicular extension, after unroofing the optic canal. (C) Covering of the resected area with a temporalis fascia fixed with sutures and fibrin glue

complications such as CSF rhinorrhea, infection, or pneumocephalus with this maneuver. Drains are placed, one under the bone flap and another under the combined skin and muscle flap. We recommend that suction drains with negative pressure not be used. The combined skin and muscle flap is sutured back in layers.

Surgical Outcome

Advances in neuroimaging and microsurgical techniques along with better understanding of microsurgical anatomy have resulted in remarkable improvements in surgical outcomes in patients with TS meningioma (Table 35-1). Prior to the era of

microsurgery, mortality rates were mostly between 7 and 28% (Table 35-1), but ranged as high as 67% [31]. Following the introduction of operating microscope and microsurgical instruments, however, mortality rates have fallen to less than 10%. Mortality in the earlier series was often directly related to the surgical maneuvers utilized, which resulted in hemorrhage, hypothalamic failure from vascular injury, vasospasm, and brain swelling after surgery. In contrast, mortality in patients treated with microsurgical procedures is usually related to nonsurgical problems, such as pulmonary embolism, pneumonia, and sepsis [12,18,25,27,48]. During the first decade after the introduction of microsurgery in a series, however, mortality rate was reported to be still high, which was attributed to a lack of microsurgical expertise [14].

Among the prognostic factors that may influence surgical outcomes is the tumor size. Patients with tumors larger than 3 cm in diameter had mortality rates of 7.1–42%, whereas patients with tumors smaller than 3 cm in diameter had mortality rates of 0–4.4% [15,21,47]. Comparisons of mortality rates in patients with tumors larger and smaller than 4 cm in diameter showed that these rates were 5.7–32.1% for larger tumors and 1.4–14.8% for smaller tumors [14,24].

As mortality rates have become lower, the extent of resection for TS meningiomas has also been significantly improved (Table 35-1). Prior to the advent of microsurgery, the total resection rates were 12–76%, whereas after the introduction of microsurgery, these rates increased to 58–100% [19,40,46]. In some reports, total resections were reported in all patients [19,40,46].

While the rate of visual improvement after surgery was found to vary from 25 to 80% (Table 35-1), the employment of microsurgical techniques may also have affected visual outcome. Prior to the introduction of microsurgery, the visual improvement rate was reported to be 49–63%. Following the introduction of microsurgical techniques, the visual improvement rates have been generally higher, ranging as high as 80% [7]. Another factor that can influence visual outcome is patient age, with better vision after surgery more likely in patients younger than 40 or 60 years of age [7,18,30,48,51]. In contrast, gender has been found to have no effect on visual results [48,51].

The duration and severity of preoperative visual symptoms have been found to be prognostic of visual improvement after surgery [6,7,18,27,30,45,48,51]. Better results are obtained in patients with less than 6 months to 2 years of visual symptoms [6,7,18,30,45,48,51], although one study found that duration was not an absolute criterion for postoperative visual outcome [52]. Preoperative vision has also been shown to correlate well with visual outcome after surgery. Optic disc pallor on preoperative fundoscopic examination [7,18,27,30,48,51] and binocular involvement [7,48] have been reported to be associated with poor prognosis.

Tumor size has also been reported to be a prognostic factor for visual improvement. Patients with tumors larger than 3 cm in diameter have been reported to be more likely to have poor visual outcome after surgery [21,30,40,45], although this correlation was not observed in other reports [7,48,51]. Tumor extension into the optic canal [6,7,18], and significant peritumoral edema and increased vertical diameter of the tumor [48] have been found to be prognostic of poor postoperative vision. Some studies have reported a correlation between complete tumor resection and better visual outcomes [7,48], although other studies have not observed this correlation [45,51]. In addition, the presence of a clear arachnoid plane between the tumor and the surrounding nervous structures has been found to be a favorable prognostic factor for visual outcome [48,51].

We have performed surgery on a series of 41 patients between 1994 and 2003. We used the cranioorbital approach in the first 24 patients (58.5%), followed by the basal frontotemporal approach in 16 patients (39.0%) and the basal interhemispheric approach in one patient. Total resection was achieved in 39 patients (95.1%), Simpson grade I resection in 13 (31.7%), and grade II in 25 (61.0%). Subtotal resection was achieved in two patients (4.9%). The mortality rate was zero. Of the 30 patients for whom we had both pre- and postoperative visual assessments, 21 (70.0%) showed improvement in vision, 7 (23.3%) showed no change, and 2 (6.7%) showed deterioration.

Complications

Visual Complications

Visual function has been reported to worsen after surgery in 8.4–29% of patients with TS meningiomas [6,9,12,14,15,21,48,51,52]. Causes of visual deterioration may include direct mechanical damage from surgical manipulation, heat injury from electrical coagulation or drilling, prolonged compression by hematoma or surgical materials, ischemia induced by microvascular interruption of the optic nerve, migration of optic chiasm, and arachnoiditis [25].

Nonvisual Complications

Nonvisual complications may be caused by neurosurgical procedures or by perioperative medical problems. The rate of overall morbidity after surgery for TS meningioma has been reported to range from 15 to 38% [6,7,48]. Reported complications include hemorrhage or infarction from vascular injury, brain swelling related to brain retraction, anosmia, oculomotor palsy, diabetes insipidus, hypopituitarism, CSF leakage, meningitis, abscess, hydrocephalus, subdural hematoma, epidural hematoma, wound infection, seizure, pneumonia, sepsis, pulmonary embolism, deep vein thrombosis, and gastrointestinal bleeding [6,7,9,12,14,15,18,21,48,52].

Complication Avoidance

To avoid the complications described above and to improve surgical outcome, it is essential to expose the tumor adequately with basal exposure and to remove the tumor using meticulous microsurgical dissection. To avoid major complications related to surgery, it is vital to optimally expose the tumor, thus providing adequate surgical views with minimal brain retraction. To obtain a suitable visual trajectory, it is usually helpful to remove the sphenoid ridge and flatten the orbital excrescence by drilling. Wide dissection of the sylvian fissure allows sufficient CSF release and may also facilitate brain retraction without injury. We have found that forced retraction of the frontal lobe is not necessary, because gravity causes this lobe to fall backward spontaneously, providing a generous surgical window. Avoidance of any kind of forced retraction leads to the elimination of retraction-related complications.

Once the tumor is exposed, it is important to clearly identify the vital structures, including the optic nerves, the internal carotid arteries, and the anterior cerebral arteries. The tumor is devascularized by coagulating the arterial feeders from the dural base and detaching them from the dura. The central portion of the tumor is debulked, and the remaining capsule is dissected from the surrounding structure, while keeping the arachnoid plane. If the optic nerve is under significant tension due to tumor compression, dissection should be performed after sufficient decompression. It is recommended that the optic canal be unroofed to mobilize the optic nerve for dissecting the tumor portion extending into the canal. A high-speed microdrill and a diamond burr with continuous saline irrigation are recommended for unroofing the optic canal. In contrast, a punch or rongeur should not be used due to the risks of unintended pinching or compression, which could result in visual loss.

To lower the rate of recurrence, the attached dura and hyperostotic bone are resected whenever possible, especially in younger patients. Care should be taken not to open the sphenoid sinus during this procedure. The dural defect is covered with the temporalis fascial flap and fixed with fibrin glue.

When severe adhesion of the tumor to the surrounding vital structures hinders the likelihood of complete resection without surgical injury, a thin layer of the tumor is left to prevent serious complications.

To reduce the risk of CSF leakage, the dura should be closed in a watertight fashion, but it is not necessary to obliterate the opened frontal air sinus.

Summary

The majority of TS meningiomas arise from the dura around one lateral end of the TS, just inferomedial to the optic canal. As the tumor grows, it compresses the ipsilateral optic nerve superiorly or superolaterally against the sharp edge of the falciform ligament, and it compresses the contralateral optic nerve laterally. This results in characteristic asymmetric visual failure. Radical resection of the tumor without significant complication can be achieved in most patients using basal surgical exposure and meticulous microsurgical techniques.

While various skull base approaches provide excellent surgical routes to the suprasellar area, our experience suggests that the basal frontotemporal approach is suitable for resection of most TS meningiomas with good overall outcome. During surgery, technical considerations for protecting the surrounding neurovascular structures cannot be overemphasized. This will allow radical excision without surgery-related complications or neurologic deterioration.

References

1. Cushing H, Eisenhardt L. Suprasellar meningiomas. In: Meningiomas: Their Classificaiton, Regional Behaviour, Life History, and Surgical End Results. Baltimore: Charles C Thomas; 1938:224–49.
2. Olivercrona H. The suprasellar meningiomas. In: Handbuch der Neoruchirurgie. Berlin: Springer-Verlag, 1967:167–72.
3. Stirling J, Edin M. Tumor of the meninges in the region of the pituitary body, pressing on the chiasma. Ann Ophthalmol 1897(6):15–6.
4. Cushing H, Esenhardt L. Meningiomas arising from the TS with the syndrome of primary optic atrophy and bitemporal field defects combined with a normal sellae turcica in a middle-aged person. Arch Ophthalmol 1929;1:1–41, 168–206.
5. Holmes G, Sargent P. Suprasellar endotheliomata. Brain 1927;50:518–37.
6. Andrews BT, Wilson CB. Suprasellar meningiomas: the effect of tumor location on postoperative visual outcome. J Neurosurg 1988;69(4):523–8.
7. Fahlbusch R, Schott W. Pterional surgery of meningiomas of the TS and planum sphenoidale: surgical results with special consideration of ophthalmological and endocrinological outcomes. J Neurosurg 2002;96(2):235–43.
8. Finn JE, Mount LA. Meningiomas of the TS and planum sphenoidale. A review of 83 cases. Arch Ophthalmol 1974;92(1):23–7.
9. Gokalp HZ, Arasil E, Kanpolat Y, et al. Meningiomas of the tuberculum sella. Neurosurg Rev 1993;16(2):111–4.
10. Grant FC. Meningioma of the tuberculin sellae. AMA Arch Neurol Psychiatry 1952;68(3):411–2.
11. Gregorius FK, Hepler RS, Stern WE. Loss and recovery of vision with suprasellar meningiomas. J Neurosurg 1975;42(1):69–75.
12. Jallo GI, Benjamin V. TS meningiomas: microsurgical anatomy and surgical technique. Neurosurgery 2002;51(6):1432–39; discussion 9–40.
13. Krenkel W, Frowein RA. Proceedings: suprasellar meningiomas. Acta Neurochir (Wien) 1975;31(3–4):280.
14. Raco A, Bristot R, Domenicucci M, et al. Meningiomas of the TS. Our experience in 69 cases surgically treated between 1973 and 1993. J Neurosurg Sci 1999;43(4):253–60; discussion 60–2.
15. Symon L, Rosenstein J. Surgical management of suprasellar meningioma. Part 1: The influence of tumor size, duration of symptoms, and microsurgery on surgical outcome in 101 consecutive cases. J Neurosurg 1984;61(4):633–41.
16. Rhoton AL, Jr. The sellar region. Neurosurgery 2002;51(4 Suppl):S335–74.
17. Williams P, Bannister L, Berry M, et al. Skeletal system. In: Soames R, ed. Gray's Anatomy. 38th ed. Edinburgh: Churchill Livingstone, 1999:547–612.
18. Schick U, Hassler W. Surgical management of TS meningiomas: involvement of the optic canal and visual outcome. J Neurol Neurosurg Psychiatry 2005;76(7):977–83.
19. Yasargil M. Meningiomas. In: Yasargil M, ed. Microneurosurgery. New York: George Thieme Verlag, 1996:134–65.
20. Chan RC, Thompson GB. Morbidity, mortality, and quality of life following surgery for intracranial meningiomas. A retrospective study in 257 cases. J Neurosurg 1984;60(1):52–60.
21. Kadis GN, Mount LA, Ganti SR. The importance of early diagnosis and treatment of the meningiomas of the planum sphenoidale and TS: a retrospective study of 105 cases. Surg Neurol 1979;12(5):367–71.

22. Kallio M, Sankila R, Hakulinen T, et al. Factors affecting operative and excess long-term mortality in 935 patients with intracranial meningioma. Neurosurgery 1992;31(1):2–12.

23. MacCarty CS, Taylor WF. Intracranial meningiomas: experiences at the Mayo Clinic. Neurol Med Chir (Tokyo) 1979;19(7):569–74.

24. Solero CL, Giombini S, Morello G. Suprasellar and olfactory meningiomas. Report on a series of 153 personal cases. Acta Neurochir (Wien) 1983;67(3–4):181–94.

25. Al-Mefty O, Holoubi A, Rifai A, et al. Microsurgical removal of suprasellar meningiomas. Neurosurgery 1985;16(3):364–72.

26. Symon L, Jakubowski J. Clinical features, technical problems, and results of treatment of anterior parasellar meningiomas. Acta Neurochir Suppl (Wien) 1979;28(2):367–70.

27. Goel A, Muzumdar D, Desai KI. TS meningioma: a report on management on the basis of a surgical experience with 70 patients. Neurosurgery 2002;51(6):1358–63; discussion 63–4.

28. Grant FC, Hedges TR, Jr. Ocular findings in meningiomas of the TS. AMA Arch Ophthalmol 1956;56(2):163–70.

29. Ehlers N, Malmros R. The suprasellar meningioma. A review of the literature and presentation of a series of 31 cases. Acta Ophthalmol Suppl 1973:1–74.

30. Rosenstein J, Symon L. Surgical management of suprasellar meningioma. Part 2: Prognosis for visual function following craniotomy. J Neurosurg 1984;61(4):642–8.

31. Kunicki A, Uhl A. The clinical picture and results of surgical treatment of meningioma of the TS. Cesk Neurol 1968;31(2):80–92.

32. Shah RP, Leavens ME, Samaan NA. Galactorrhea, amenorrhea, and hyperprolactinemia as manifestations of parasellar meningioma. Arch Intern Med 1980;140(12):1608–12.

33. Chakeres DW, Curtin A, Ford G. Magnetic resonance imaging of pituitary and parasellar abnormalities. Radiol Clin North Am 1989;27(2):265–81.

34. Zimmerman CF, Schatz NJ, Glaser JS. Magnetic resonance imaging of optic nerve meningiomas. Enhancement with gadolinium-DTPA. Ophthalmology 1990;97(5):585–91.

35. Goldsher D, Litt AW, Pinto RS, et al. Dural "tail" associated with meningiomas on Gd-DTPA-enhanced MR images: characteristics, differential diagnostic value, and possible implications for treatment. Radiology 1990;176(2):447–50.

36. Taylor SL, Barakos JA, Harsh GRt, et al. Magnetic resonance imaging of TS meningiomas: preventing preoperative misdiagnosis as pituitary macroadenoma. Neurosurgery 1992;31(4):621–7; discussion 7.

37. Lee KF. The diagnostic value of hyperostosis in midline subfrontal meningioma. Radiology 1976;119(1):121–30.

38. Simpson D. The recurrence of intracranial meningiomas after surgical treatment. J Neurol Neurosurg Psychiatry 1957;20(1):22–39.

39. Nelson PK, Setton A, Choi IS, et al. Current status of interventional neuroradiology in the management of meningiomas. Neurosurg Clin N Am 1994;5(2):235–59.

40. Arai H, Sato K, Okuda, et al. Transcranial transsphenoidal approach for TS meningiomas. Acta Neurochir (Wien) 2000;142(7):751–6; discussion 6–7.

41. Ciric I, Rosenblatt S. Suprasellar meningiomas. Neurosurgery 2001;49(6):1372–7.

42. Couldwell WT, Weiss MH, Rabb C, et al. Variations on the standard transsphenoidal approach to the sellar region, with emphasis on the extended approaches and parasellar approaches: surgical experience in 105 cases. Neurosurgery 2004;55(3):539–47; discussion 47–50.

43. DeMonte F. Surgical treatment of anterior basal meningiomas. J Neurooncol 1996;29(3):239–48.

44. Jho HD. Endoscopic endonasal approach to the optic nerve: a technical note. Minim Invasive Neurosurg 2001;44(4):190–3.

45. Ohta K, Yasuo K, Morikawa M, et al. Treatment of TS meningiomas: a long-term follow-up study. J Clin Neurosci 2001;8(Suppl 1):26–31.

46. Dolenc V. Tuberuculum sellae meningiomas. In: Dolenc V, ed. Microsurgical Anatomy and Surgery of the Central Skull Base. Vienna: Springer-Verlag, 2003: 193–205.

47. Jane JA, Park TS, Pobereskin LH, et al. The supraorbital approach: technical note. Neurosurgery 1982;11(4):537–42.

48. Pamir MN, Ozduman K, Belirgen M, et al. Outcome determinants of pterional surgery for TS meningiomas. Acta Neurochir (Wien) 2005;147(11):1121–30.

49. Cook SW, Smith Z, Kelly DF. Endonasal transsphenoidal removal of TS meningiomas: technical note. Neurosurgery 2004;55(1):239–44; discussion 44–6.

50. Yasargil M. Pterional approach. In: Yasargil M, ed. Microneurosurgery. New York: George Thieme Verlag, 1996:36–50.

51. Zevgaridis D, Medele RJ, Muller A, et al. Meningiomas of the sellar region presenting with visual impairment: impact of various prognostic factors on surgical outcome in 62 patients. Acta Neurochir (Wien) 2001;143(5):471–6.

52. Grisoli F, Diaz-Vasquez P, Riss M, et al. Microsurgical management of TS meningiomas. Results in 28 consecutive cases. Surg Neurol 1986;26(1):37–44.

36
Anterior Clinoidal Meningiomas

Joung H. Lee and Burak Sade

Introduction

Clinoidal meningiomas (CM) are benign tumors arising from the meningeal covering of the anterior clinoid process (ACP). These tumors have been referred to by various other terms, such as medial or inner sphenoid wing meningiomas. In the literature predating the wide use of magnetic resonance imaging (MRI), CM was often reported under the loose category of "suprasellar," "perisellar," "parasellar" or "anterior fossa floor" meningiomas together with meningiomas of the tuberculum sellae, middle or lateral sphenoid wing, cavernous sinus and even the anterior fossa.[1–6] In large meningiomas encompassing both the cavernous sinus (CS) and the clinoidal region, the exact site of origin, based on preoperative imaging studies, or at times even after an intraoperative inspection, is often difficult to determine. In these large tumors, the clinoidal origin is assumed in our practice if greater than two thirds of the tumor is extracavernous in location. Those tumors extending to the clinoidal region, but originating from the tuberculum sella, optic canal, orbital roof, planum sphenoidale, middle or lateral aspects of the sphenoid wing, are not considered as CM.

Because of the proximity of the optic nerve (ON) to the ACP, patients with CM most commonly present with monocular visual deterioration, which is often unrecognized by patients until visual loss is severe and the tumor has reached a significant size. These tumors are often formidable to resect completely and safely, especially when their size becomes large enough to encircle, compress, and/or displace the adjacent ON, the internal carotid artery (ICA), its branches, and the oculomotor nerve. In the past, common morbidity associated with CM surgery included injury to the optic and oculomotor nerves, the ICA, and its branches. Mortality rate was as high as 32% in earlier series mainly due to major vessel injuries.[7] Total resection was possible in only a minority of cases, leading to early tumor recurrence and further deterioration of the patient. Many neurosurgeons, even today, recognizing the relatively high incidence of poor postoperative outcome for patients with these tumors, recommend conservative subtotal resection with or without postoperative radiation therapy or even a more conservative approach, using radiation as the sole treatment.[8] Additionally, most asymptomatic patients with CM are often observed with serial MRI scans.

During the past few decades, the primary goal of surgical management for patients with CM focused on maximizing the extent of resection and reducing the operative morbidity/mortality without any particular attention paid to enhancing visual outcome. In fact, reporting has been very limited regarding the patients' visual status. Moreover, the past views regarding postoperative visual recovery in patients with CM have been quite pessimistic. Poor visual outcome was previously attributed to an ischemic mechanism of preoperative visual loss, and visual deficits were considered mostly irreversible. At best, only a fraction of the patients with preoperative visual deterioration experienced visual improvement after removal of their CM (up to 30–40%), and many even noted visual worsening.[9,10] There is a clear need for further efforts directed at improving the overall outcome and, particularly, the visual outcome in patients with CM. Today, with advances in neuroimaging, which allows the detection of small tumors at the onset of symptoms, in addition to improved microsurgical techniques, skull base exposures, and neuroanesthesia, CM surgery can be far less risky. We propose that utilizing the surgical technique delineated in this paper, it is possible to attain gross total removal with minimal morbidity, and more importantly, to achieve postoperative visual improvement in the majority of patients with CM.

In 1983, Dolenc introduced an extradural technique of complete removal of the ACP.[11] This technique, described as a component of a more extensive approach, was originally advocated as a critical step necessary to gain safe entry into the CS for direct surgical management of intracavernous vascular lesions. Later, the "Dolenc approach" was utilized for CS tumors, clinoidal segment internal ICA and upper basilar aneurysms, and giant pituitary adenomas. Subsequently, a few others presented their experience with this technique, with some modifications, applied to surgery of a small number of parasellar/periclinoid region tumors such as craniopharyngiomas and suprasellar meningiomas.[12]

In this chapter we describe a skull base technique (SBT), modified from the original "Dolenc approach," consisting of extradural clinoidectomy coupled with optic canal unroofing and optic nerve sheath (ONS) opening. We also outline several key advantages provided by the SBT, and our current indications for its use. The advantages provided by the SBT include: (1) early localization and exposure of the ON and the adjacent ICA; (2) complete decompression and mobilization of the ON; (3) expansion of various operative windows; (4) facilitation of access to difficult locations; and (5) facilitation of aggressive removal of tumor, as well as the involved bone and dura.

Basic Principles of Meningioma Surgery

The same basic principles of meningioma surgery apply to CM removal as well, with minor modifications dictated primarily by the unique anatomic considerations inherent to the clinoidal region. These basic surgical principles, applicable to CM, may be summarized as follows: (1) optimal patient positioning, incision, bone removal; (2) when possible, tumor devascularization; (3) early localization, exposure, and decompression of the ON and ICA; (4) following the ON and ICA into the tumor; (5) internal tumor debulking; (6) extracapsular devascularization and dissection; (7) preservation of the adherent/surrounding neurovasculature; (8) removal of the involved bone and dura; and (9) dural reconstruction and closure.

Indications for the Skull Base Technique

Indications for the use of the SBT for CM (and other tumors in the periclinoid region) in our practice include those lesions: (1) causing ON or chiasmatic compression based on preoperative ophthalmologic evaluations; (2) encircling or covering the ON and ICA on preoperative MRI studies; (3) extending into the optic canal, subchiasmatic/infraoptic regions or the CS; (4) in patients with limited operative windows (e.g., patients with prefixed chiasm); and (5) causing extensive involvement of the surrounding bone and dura. When tumors are relatively small (2.5 cm or less) and not causing any significant preoperative visual deficits, surgical resection can be done utilizing standard pterional craniotomy without the added skull base exposure.

For relatively young patients—those with at least 15 years remaining in their life expectancy—we recommend surgery at the time of tumor detection regardless of the size, even in incidental tumors. This immediate intervention is a conscious attempt to provide these patients with total resection and the best possible outcome before these tumors become larger and pose increased surgical risks.

Surgical Technique

The surgical steps involved in the SBT utilized in removal of CM can be summarized as follow: (1) frontotemporal craniotomy; (2) sphenoid ridge drilling; (3) limited posterior orbitotomy; (4) posterolateral orbital wall removal (to completely decompress the superior orbital fissure); (5) optic canal unroofing; (6) complete extradural anterior clinoidectomy; and (7) dural opening, with dural incision extending into the falciform ligament and the ONS.

Positioning

After induction of general anesthesia, the patient is placed in the supine position, with the head fixed in a Mayfield 3-pin head-holder. The head is then rotated 30 degrees to the side contralateral to the tumor (Fig. 36-1). The head of the bed is elevated approximately 20 degrees.

Incision

A standard curvilinear frontotemporal incision is made starting just above the palpated zygoma, 1 cm anterior to the tragus, extending superiorly, then curving anteriorly from the superior temporal line to the midline, just to the limit of the hairline. The skin flap and the underlying temporalis fascia/muscle are elevated, and reflected anteriorly as separate layers.

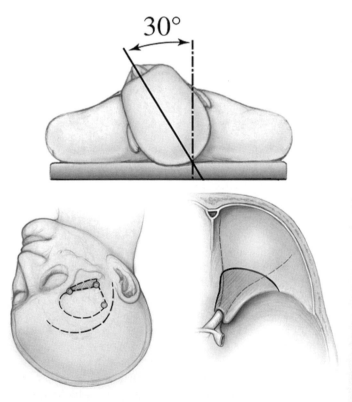

FIG. 36-1. The head of the bed is raised 15–20 degrees and the patient's head is rotated 30 degrees away from the side of surgery. A standard curvilinear incision is made behind the hairline. A frontotemporal craniotomy is turned following placement of three burr holes. The craniotomy flap is depicted by the broken line in the lower left picture, and the shaded area represents the bone drilled from the lateral sphenoid wing after performing the craniotomy. The shaded area in the lower right picture depicts the bone removed, including the lateral sphenoid wing, postero-lateral orbital wall, optic canal roof, and ACP

Craniotomy

A standard frontotemporal craniotomy is performed. The craniotomy is extended into the anterior frontal region by 1.5–2 cm from the "key hole," made parallel to the superior orbital rim to allow for subsequent extradural exposure of the orbital roof and optic canal. The size and shape of the frontal sinus is carefully appreciated from the preoperative MRI, so that if possible, entry into the lateral margin of the frontal sinus is avoided during the frontal extension of the craniotomy. If the frontal sinus is entered, it is repaired with a temporalis muscle graft followed by reinforcement with a pericranial flap.

Skull Base Technique

The lateral sphenoid ridge is drilled, followed by performing a limited posterior orbitotomy (Fig. 36-1). The sphenoid bone drilling is carried out by using a 6-mm round cutting burr. Orbitotomy and subsequent skull base drilling is then performed using a 4-mm coarse diamond burr. The posterolateral orbital wall is then removed to completely decompress the superior orbital fissure. The roof of the optic canal is then drilled with a diamond burr. During this stage, copious irrigation is critical in order to prevent potential ON damage by the heat generated from drilling. The bone overlying the optic canal is made "paper-thin" with the drill, following which the remaining bone is easily removed using a microdissector or a microcurette. While the medial aspect of the optic canal roof is being drilled, entry into the ethmoid or sphenoid sinus must be avoided. If an entry is made, a small temporalis muscle graft is used to cover the opening at the time of closure, further reinforced using a piece of blood-soaked gelfoam. This extradural dissection and exposure require some degree of frontal lobe retraction. Rather than using a fixed retraction system, we prefer "dynamic" retraction utilizing the suction tip held in one hand of the surgeon to gently retract the brain. Although many neurosurgeons advocate using lumbar cerebrospinal fluid (CSF) drainage, in our practice the lumbar drain is not used. We believe that the CSF in the subarachnoid space (including within the ONS) protects the brain and ON from intraoperative injury.

After exposure of the ON within the optic canal is completed, the dura is then circumferentially dissected off the ACP. The ACP is now ready to be removed. In situations of significant hypertrophy of the ACP, the center of ACP and hypertrophied optic strut is drilled, followed by removal of the remaining ACP by using a small straight-tipped Lempert rongeur. With nonhypertrophic ACP, removal can be done by gently manipulating the ACP to fracture the optic strut. During this maneuver, one must be careful to not cause any damage to the adjacent ON, ophthalmic artery, or the anterior loop of the ICA. If the "fracture technique" cannot be performed using minimal force, then the remainder of ACP can be drilled intradurally under direct visualization. Often, brisk venous bleeding is encountered from the triangular space occupied

by the removed ACP. This can be readily controlled by gently packing the extradural triangular space with a small piece of gelfoam. Aggressive packing should be avoided to minimize compressive injury to the ON or the oculomotor nerve. A brief summary of these extradural steps is as follows: (1) a standard fronto-temporal craniotomy; (2) lateral sphenoid wing removal; (3) posterior orbitotomy; (4) complete bone removal surrounding the superior orbital fissure; (5) optic canal unroofing; and (6) anterior clinoidectomy (Fig. 36-2).

Dural Opening

The dura is opened in two steps. First, a frontotemporal curvilinear opening is made centered over the sylvian fissure, followed by a second incision bisecting the dural flap directed toward the falciform ligament (Fig. 36-3). An operating microscope is brought in at this point, and the dural incision is continued from the falciform ligament along the length of the exposed ONS within the optic canal, extending to the annulus of Zinn. Cutting of the falciform ligament, and subsequently the ONS, is best performed by using a right-angle arachnoid knife or a "beaver blade." This completes the full exposure and decompression of the extradural ON, which can then be followed easily toward the tumor with exact knowledge of the ON's location (Fig. 36-3). The intradural ICA, located immediately lateral to the prechiasmatic ON, is easily identified by dissecting and removing tumor around the already exposed ON. In comparison, the lower picture in Fig. 36-3 depicts the conventional intradural exposure, not utilizing the SBT and opening of the ONS, in which the tumor is noted to be covering all the critical neurovascular structures.

Tumor Removal

Although the tumor may completely cover, circumscribe, and/or displace the intradural ON and the ICA, with the ON now exposed and decompressed, and with the intradural ICA localized, subsequent tumor removal can progress with ease. Moreover, as the ON is no longer compressed by the falciform

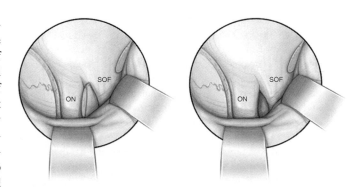

FIG. 36-2. Extradural view of the exposed intracanalicular optic nerve and the opened superior orbital fissure before and after complete removal of the ACP

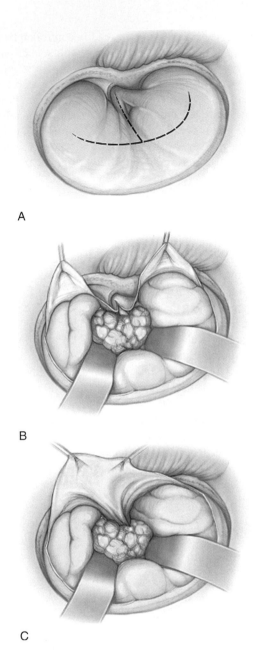

A

B

C

FIG. 36-3. The dural incision is made in two steps (A) First, a fronto-temporal curvilinear opening is centered on the sylvian fissure, followed by bisection of the dural flap extending across the falciform ligament and to the annulus of Zinn. View of a clinoidal meningioma following completion of the SBT and extending the dural incision into the optic sheath (B) The optic nerve is identified in the exposed optic canal and completely decompressed at the onset of tumor removal. Tumor resection progresses by following the optic nerve proximally. View of a clinoidal meningioma after the initial dural opening, utilizing conventional pterional craniotomy only (C) Upon exposure, the tumor is covering the critical neurovascular structures. The exact locations of the optic nerve and ICA are unknown to the surgeon, and the optic nerve remains in a compressed state. Tumor resection progresses slowly until the optic nerve and ICA are identified

ligament following complete opening of the ONS, the ON can now be safely manipulated and gently retracted to enlarge the interoptic and opticocarotid spaces during subsequent tumor

removal. The undersurface of the ON and chiasm is also readily and safely explored. In most cases, as the arachnoid plane around the ON and ICA is maintained, careful dissection of the tumor off of these critical neurovascular structures is possible. Tumor extension into the optic canal is also removed, with care exercised to prevent any damage to the ophthalmic artery. The tumor is removed, in large part, using suction and bipolar coagulation. In firm tumors, an ultrasonic aspirator or careful use of microscissors facilitates piecemeal removal. Central tumor debulking facilitates dissection of the tumor off of the surrounding critical neurovascular structures.

After initial debulking of the anterior aspect of the tumor, having established the exact intradural locations of the ON and ICA, attention may be directed at exposure and removal of the remainder of the tumor. The sylvian fissure is opened, and both the frontal and temporal lobes gently retracted. Particular attention is paid to preserve branches of the ICA and MCA. In large tumors, several arterial branches are often seen coursing into the tumor or around the capsule. Until their final course can be determined, confirming that these are indeed arterial branches feeding the tumor, the vessels should not be sacrificed. When dissecting the tumor off of the ON or the chiasm, fine vessels coursing on the undersurface (which provide the main blood supply) of the optic apparatus must be preserved. In dissecting the tumor extending into the suprasellar region, the pituitary stalk, which is usually displaced posteriorly and medially, must be recognized and preserved. Other neurovascular structures of critical importance include the oculomotor nerve, posterior communicating artery, anterior choroidal artery and their branches, which are encountered during dissection of the inferior pole, and the A1 and M1 main trunks and their branches, which are encountered during dissection/removal of the posterior segment.

When dealing with a large tumor (>5 or 6 cm), the senior author (JHL) prefers to approach the tumor by subdividing the tumor into several segments or poles: (1) the anterior segment—located directly above the anterior prechiasmatic ON and the proximal ICA (proximal to the posterior communicating artery). This is the anterior pole of the tumor, first encountered by following the intracanalicular ON proximally; (2) the lateral segment—located lateral to the ICA main trunk, dorsal to the ICA branches (posterior communicating and anterior choroidal arteries) and the oculomotor nerve, and includes the portion of the tumor extending into the middle fossa floor; (3) the medial segment—located medial to the ICA main trunk, surrounding or displacing the posterior prechiasmatic ON and optic chiasm; (4) the posterior segment—located posterior to the ICA bifurcation, sometimes circumscribing the MCA, ACA, and their branches; and (5) the inferior segment—located inferior to the optic chiasm and the ICA trunk and its branches, at times extending ventral to the oculomotor nerve. In this manner, the surgeon is, in his mind, removing five small manageable tumors, rather than one large formidable tumor.

Not infrequently, CM extends into CS by following the oculomotor nerve through the porous oculomotoris or via transdural penetration. The dural fold forming the porous oculomotoris is opened completely to allow decompression of the oculomotor nerve, and the CS may be explored if the tumor is soft and amenable to further removal. If the CS involvement is extensive and the tumor is fibrous, surgery is stopped after confirmation of the following: (1) gross-total resection of the intradural extracavernous portion of the tumor and removal of any accessible tumor-involved dura and bone; (2) decompression of the ON; and (3) decompression of the oculomotor nerve. Any involved dura not possible for removal is aggressively coagulated. Occasionally, the distal carotid dural ring may be involved by the tumor, which should also be removed down to the base. Any further bony hyperostosis is drilled using a 2- or 4-mm diamond burr, with care taken to not enter into the surrounding sphenoid or ethmoid sinuses.

Closure

The dura is reapproximated with multiple interrupted sutures. The dural defect along the skull base is covered with commercially available collagen dural substitute. No attempt is made for a watertight closure as this is neither necessary nor possible following extensive resection of the dura involved by tumor at the base of skull. The bone flap is replaced and secured with titanium mini-plates and screws. Closure of the temporalis muscle/facia and the scalp is then carried out in a routine fashion.

Outcome and Complications

The personal series of the senior author consisted of 46 patients with clinoidal meningiomas. Of these, 37 were female and 9 were male. Patient age ranged from 16 to 75 years, with an average age of 56. The tumor size varied between 10 and 80mm, with a mean of 36mm.

Extent of Resection

In 3 patients with relatively small tumors, a standard pterional approach was utilized, whereas in the remaining 43, SBT described in the preceding section of this chapter was added to the standard pterional craniotomy. Total resection (Simpson Grade I or II) was achieved in 33 patients (72%). The reason for subtotal resection was the involvement of CS in 8, distal carotid dural ring in 2 patients; adhesion to MCA in 2 and to ON in 1 patient. Intraoperatively, ACP hypertrophy was detected in 20 patients (43.5%) and tumor extension into the optic canal in 16 (34.8%).

Histology

Of the 46 meningiomas, 42 had Grade I histology, with the vast majority being meningothelial (37 patients). Four patients had transitional, and 1 had fibrous subtypes. Four patients had Grade II histology: 3 chordoid and 1 atypical subtypes.

Visual Outcome

Among these patients, 22 presented with visual deterioration. In 19 of them there was a combination of visual acuity loss and a field defect, whereas 3 of them presented with only a visual field defect. The roles of tumor size, ACP hypertrophy, and optic canal involvement by the tumor on preoperative visual status are summarized in Tables 36-1 through 36-3, respectively.

Nineteen of the 22 patients had postoperative neuro-opthalmological evaluation, and 16 of them had either normalization (5 patients) or improvement (11 patients) of their vision with an overall improvement rate of 73%, whereas 3 patients had no change. No patient in the entire series experienced visual deterioration following surgery (Fig. 36-4).

Neurologic Outcome and Complications

We evaluated the postoperative outcome by means of the Glasgow outcome scale (GOS); 42 patients had a GOS of 5 and 3 had a GOS of 4 at their first postoperative follow-up at 6 weeks. One patient died of pulmonary embolus during this period. Other complications seen in 7 patients (15%) were as follows (with 2 patients having multiple complications):

TABLE 36-1. Tumor Size and Preoperative Visual Status in 46 Patients with Clinoidal Meningiomas.

	Visual deficit	
Tumor size	Yes	No
≤20mm (n = 10)	4 (40%)	6 (60%)
21–40mm (n = 21)	11 (52.4%)	10 (47.6%)
≥41mm (n = 15)	7 (46.7%)	8 (53.2%)

TABLE 36-2. Anterior Clinoidal Process (ACP) Hypertrophy and Pre-Operative Visual Status in 46 Patients with Clinoidal Meningiomas.

	Visual deficit	
ACP hypertrophy	Yes	No
Yes (n = 20)[a]	13 (65%)	7 (35%)
No (n = 26)[b]	9 (34.6%)	17 (65.4%)

[a] Mean tumor size 38mm.
[b] Mean tumor size 34mm.

TABLE 36-3. Involvement of the Optic Canal (OC) by the Tumor and Pre-Operative Visual Status in 46 Patients with Clinoidal Meningiomas.

	Visual deficit	
OC involvement	Yes	No
Yes (n = 16)[a]	12 (75%)	4 (25%)
No (n = 30)[b]	10 (33.3%)	20 (66.7%)

[a] Mean tumor size 39mm.
[b] Mean tumor size 34mm.

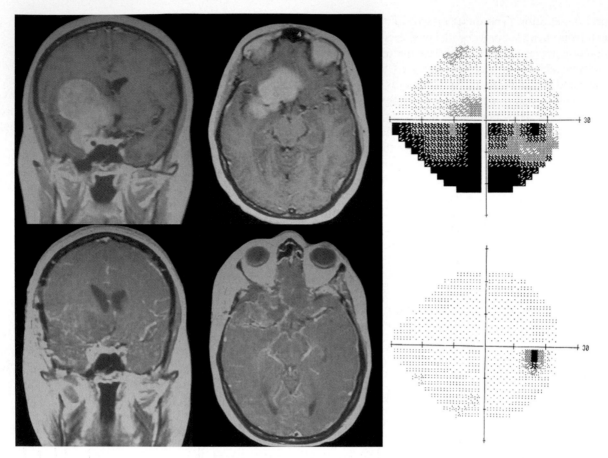

FIG. 36-4. (Upper row) Preoperative contrast-enhanced coronal and axial T1-weighted MR images of a patient who presented with a visual acuity of 20/80 and an inferior hemianopsia on the right. (Lower row) Postoperative contrast-enhanced coronal and axial T1-weighted MR images confirming aggressive subtotal resection and normalization of the visual acuity (20/20) and field defect

hydrocephalus necessitating a ventriculo-peritoneal shunt, new onset focal seizure, vasospasm, transient motor aphasia, venous hemorrhagic infarct of the frontal lobe, transient oculomotor and trochlear nerve palsies, meningitis, deep venous thrombosis, and gastrointestinal bleeding. With an average follow-up of 51 months, no recurrence was detected including the 4 patients with Grade II histology.

Literature specifically focusing on the outcome of CM is scant. Al-Mefty and Ayoubi have reported their results with 28 CM; they were able to achieve total resection in 83% patients.[9] Of these, 71% had a good or fair outcome. Ojemann described a more conservative surgical strategy, where he performed subtotal resection in all of his 17 patients, and 94% of these patients did well postoperatively.[8] Samii and Ammirati, in their analysis of 27 patients, achieved total resection in two thirds, with a good or fair outcome in 77%.[13] Risi et al,[10] and Puzilli et al,[14] have reported relatively lower total resection rates (58 and 63%, respectively), with slightly less favorable outcome rate in the 63–64% range.

A significant proportion of the patients with CM present with visual disturbances, and the literature focusing on the visual outcome of patients with these tumors is even more scarce. Six of the 20 patients (30%) in the series of Risi et al. had improvement of their vision following surgery, whereas another 6 had postoperative worsening.[10] Al-Mefty and Ayoubi have reported improvement in 6 out of 24 patients (25%), with preoperative visual disturbance and deterioration of vision in one patient.[9] Even in the hands of experienced surgeons with large series, the incidence of postoperative visual deterioration can be close to 20%.[15]

Advantages of the Skull Base Technique

The SBT provides significant advantages over the standard pterional technique in the management of CM. First of all, removal of the ACP provides improved exposure of the ON and the ICA, enhancing access to the pathology around these structures as well as within the optic canal.[16]

Second, by opening the optic nerve sheath (ONS) as an extension of the dural incision following anterior clinoidectomy, the ON can be decompressed and visualized early, and mobilized safely during surgery, thereby reducing the risk of intraoperative neurovascular injury.[16–18] In cases of large tumors encasing the ON and the ICA, the traditionally recommended surgical technique for removal has been to first identify the distal middle cerebral artery (MCA) branches and follow these vessels proximally toward the ICA with further tumor removal and dissection.[8,13,17,20,21] However, until the ICA and eventually the intradural ON are located, surgery progresses very slowly. More importantly, the risk of intraoperative neurovascular injury persists during surgery as the exact location of the ON and ICA remains unknown to the surgeon, and the ON remains compressed. During this time, any minor surgical retraction, dissection, or tumor manipulation may add further compression to the ON, especially against the falciform ligament. To avoid these critical problems, the ON can be exposed and simultaneously decompressed early in the surgery by unroofing the optic canal, followed by anterior clinoidectomy and then opening the ONS. The location of the optic canal and, hence, the intracanalicular segment of ON is fairly constant; only the intradural cisternal segment of ON varies in location depending on how the tumor causes nerve displacement during its growth. The exposed ON then can be followed from the optic canal proximally, toward the tumor in the intradural location. As tumor resection progresses further, the ICA can be readily found adjacent to the exposed distal intradural segment of the ON. Complete ONS opening, along the length of the nerve within the optic canal to the annulus of Zinn, relieves any focal circumferential pressure on the ON contributed by the falciform ligament. ON decompression, thus achieved, leads to reduced intraoperative injury to the nerve because the force of retraction is then dispersed over a much larger surface area.[17] If the tumor recurs, as the ON is already decompressed from the surrounding falciform ligament and optic canal, the patient's impending visual deterioration may be delayed.

Third, application of this technique results in expansion of important operative windows such as the optico-carotid[16] and carotico-oculomotor triangles.[22,23] This is of particular significance especially when the infraoptic or subchiasmatic regions need to be reached in the presence of a prefixed chiasm.

Fourth, because of the improved exposure by the expansion of the operative windows, access to difficult locations such as the CS, optic canal, and sella as well as the infraoptic and subchiasmatic regions is facilitated. For example, in our series 16 patients had extension of the tumor into the optic canal. Of these, 12 (75%) presented with visual loss. In these patients, removal of this component can only be achieved by the use of the SBT. SBT also provides increased exposure of the distal dural ring, facilitating aggressive tumor removal when the tumor encircles the ICA and involves the dural ring.

And last, all of the above advantages facilitate aggressive removal of the tumor as well as the surrounding dura and, if necessary, the involved bone.

Summary

The surgical steps involved in the SBT utilized in removal of CM can be summarized as follows: (1) frontotemporal craniotomy; (2) sphenoid ridge drilling; (3) limited posterior orbitotomy; (4) posterolateral orbital wall removal (to decompress the superior orbital fissure); (5) optic canal unroofing; (6) complete extradural anterior clinoidectomy; and (7) dural opening, with dural incision extending into the falciform ligament and the ONS.

The described SBT provides several critical advantages, which result in improved extent of resection and outcome.[24,25] These include: (1) early localization and exposure of the ON and ICA; (2) complete mobilization and decompression of the ON and ICA, which prevent or minimize intraoperative neurovascular injury; (3) expansion of various operative windows, particularly the opticocarotid triangle; (4) facilitation of access to difficult locations, especially in dealing with tumor extension into the orbit, sella, optic canal, CS, orbital apex, or the infraoptic and subchiasmatic regions; and (5) facilitation of aggressive removal of tumor as well as the involved bone and dura. The main goals of surgery are to achieve aggressive tumor removal with avoidance of intraoperative morbidity and, ultimately for those with preoperative compromised vision, to provide improvement in their visual function following surgery (Fig. 36-4). Utilizing the technique and principles outlined in this chapter, the senior author has achieved total resection in 72% and postoperative visual improvement in 73% of the patients with CM.

References

1. Bonnal J, Thibaut A, Brotchi J, Born J. Invading meningiomas of the sphenoid ridge. J Neurosurg 1980;53:587–599.
2. Klink DF, Sampath P, Miller NR, Brem H, Long DM. Long-term visual outcome after nonradical microsurgery in patients with parasellar and cavernous sinus meningiomas. Neurosurgery 2000;47:24–32.
3. Sleep TJ, Hodgkins PR, Honeybul S, Neil-Dwyer G, Lang D, Evans B. Visual function following neurosurgical optic nerve decompression for compressive optic neuropathy. Eye 2003;17:571–8.
4. Stafford SL, Perry A, Leavitt JA, Garrity JA, Suman VJ, Scheithauer B, Lohse CM, Meyer F. Anterior visual pathways meningiomas primarily resected between 1978 and 1988: the Mayo Clinic Rochester experience. J Neuroophthalmol 1998;18:206–10.
5. Rubin G, Ben David U, Gornish M, Rappaport ZH. Meningiomas of the anterior cranial fossa floor. Acta Neurochir (Wien) 1994;129:26–30.
6. Zevgaridis D, Medele RJ, Hischa AC, Steiger HJ. Meningiomas of the sellar region presenting with visual impairment: Impact of various prognostic factors on surgical outcome in 62 patients. Acta Neurochir (Wien) 2001;143:471–6.
7. Uihlein A, Weyand RD. Meningiomas of the anterior clinoid process as a cause of unilateral loss of vision: surgical considerations. Arch Ophthalmol 1953;49:261–70.

8. Ojemann RG. Management of cranial and spinal meningiomas. In: Selman W, ed. Clinical Neurosurgery. Vol 40. Baltimore: Williams & Wilkins, 1993:321–83.

9. Al-Mefty O, Ayoubi S. Clinoidal meningiomas. Acta Neurochirur 1991;(Suppl 53):92–7.

10. Risi P, Uske A, de Tribolet N. Meningiomas involving the anterior clinoid process. Br J Neurosurg 1994;8:295–305.

11. Dolenc VV. Direct microsurgical repair of intracavernous vascular lesions. J Neurosurg 1983;58:824–31.

12. Yonekawa Y, Ogata N, Imhof HG, Olivecrona M, Strommer K, Kwak TE, Roth P, Groscurth P. Selective extradural anterior clinoidectomy for supra- and parasellar processes. J Neurosurg 1997;87:636–42.

13. Samii, Ammirati M. Medial sphenoidal wing meningiomas. In: Sami M, ed. Surgery of Skull Base Meningiomas. Berlin: Springer-Verlag. 1993:35–41.

14. Puzilli F, Ruggeri A, Mastronardi L, Agrillo A, Ferrante L. Anterior clinoidal meningiomas: report of a series of 33 patients operated on through the pterional approach. Neuro-Oncology 1999;1:188–95.

15. Nakamura M, Roser F, Jacobs C, Vorkapic P, Samii M. Medial sphenoid wing meningiomas: clinical outcome and recurrence rate. Neurosurgery 2006;58:626–39.

16. Evans JJ, Hwang YS, Lee JH. Pre- versus post-anterior clinoidectomy measurements of the optic nerve, internal carotid artery and opticocarotid triangle: a cadaveric morphometric study. Neurosurgery 2000;46:1018–23.

17. Akabane A, Saito K, Suzuki Y, Shibuya M, Sugita K. Monitoring visual evoked potentials during retraction of the canine optic nerve: protective effect of unroofing the optic canal. J Neurosurg 1995;82:284–7.

18. Dolenc VV. A combined epi- and subdural approach to carotid-ophthalmic artery aneurysms. J Neurosurg 1985;62:667–72.

19. Al-Mefty O. Clinoidal meningiomas. In: Al-Mefty O, ed. Meningiomas. New York: Raven Press, 1991:427–43.

20. De Monte F. Surgical management of anterior basal meningiomas. J Neurooncol 1996;29:239–48.

21. Fohanno D, Bitar A. Sphenoidal ridge meningiomas. In: Symon L, ed. Advances and Technical Standards in Neurosurgery. Vol. 14. New York: Springer-Verlag. 1986:137–74.

22. Sade B, Kweon CY, Evans JJ, Lee JH. Enhanced exposure of the carotico-oculomotor triangle following extradural anterior clinoidectomy: a comparative anatomical study. Skull Base 2005;15:157–62.

23. Youssef AS, Abdel Aziz KM, Kim EY, Keller JT, Zuccarello M, van Loveren HR. The carotid-oculomotor window in exposure of upper basilar artery aneurysms: a cadaveric morphometric study. Neurosurgery 2004;54:1181–9.

24. Lee JH, Jeun SS, Evans J, Kosmorsky G. Surgical management of clinoidal meningiomas. Neurosurgery 2001;48:1012–21.

25. Tobias S, Kim CH, Kosmorsky G, Lee JH. Management of surgical clinoidal meningiomas. Neurosurg Focus 2003;14: Article 5.

37
Optic Nerve Sheath Meningiomas I: Aggressive Surgical Management

Werner Hassler and Uta Schick

Introduction

Optic nerve sheath meningiomas (ONSMs) represent 1–2% of all meningiomas, 1.7% of all orbital tumors, and about 35% of all intrinsic tumors of the optic nerve[1-3]. Thus ONSM represent a rare but nevertheless important entity due to their natural course of slowly progressive and unremitting loss of vision. Classical primary ONSM arise from the meningothelial cap cells of the arachnoid membrane surrounding the intraorbital optic nerve and may extend along the optic canal intracranially. Secondary ONSM extends from the planum sphenoidale, tuberculum sellae or anterior clinical process, into the subdural or subarachnoid spaces surrounding the nerve within the optic canal and, ultimately, within the orbit.[3-8] Most ONSMs are unilateral with 5% manifested bilaterally [2]. ONSM occurs predominantly in middle-aged women or in children.

The treatment of ONSM remains controversial, but includes surgery, radiotherapy, and plain observation. Complete surgical excision is thought to result in blindness in almost all cases.[9] When intracranial extension that threatens the optic chiasm or contralateral optic nerve is present, complete excision of the intracranial part via craniotomy has been described.[2,8,19] Complete neurectomy and tumor resection are also performed in cases of severe unilateral loss of vision accompanied by disfiguring proptosis. As surgical reports revealed a high morbidity in terms of visual loss and recurrences due to incomplete removal, other treatment options were debated.[2,11-14]

In adults with good vision, observation was often chosen as first method because of the slow growing nature of these tumors. Egan and Lessell[15] reported the natural history of 16 untreated patients, 11 of whom developed visual loss over a mean of 10.2 years.

Over the past years treatment plans for ONSM changed with intervention of precise fractionated and stereotactic radiotherapy. The role of radiation became more and more important since several authors have reported stabilization or even improvement of vision.[5,9,12,16-29] Radiation therapy is increasingly being offered to adults as primary therapy once mild to moderate vision loss develops.

We introduced a new classification system[30] in order to clarify the possible manifestations, and to guide optimal treatment modalities where surgical intervention and radiotherapy play a supplementary role. We present a single center series of 86 ONSMs treated over a 14-year period ($n = 63$ surgery only, $n = 7$ radiation only, $n = 16$ surgery and postoperative radiation).

Special Considerations

Clinical Features

Slowly progressive, painless loss of vision and proptosis are the cardinal features of ONSMs[4]. Other commonly reported clinical findings include afferent pupillary defect, color vision disturbance, visual field defect, optic disc edema, optic atrophy, and motility disturbance.[14]

Ophthalmoscopic examination may reveal optic nerve head swelling, contiguous macular edema, nerve pallor, or choroidal folds[29]. Optociliary shunt vessels may develop from compression of the central retinal vein in about one third of patients[2,9]. Mild to moderate proptosis (2–5 mm) is commonly present and may be the presenting sign.[22] Chemosis, lid edema, and limitation of motility may also be found.

Radiologic Findings

High field T1-weighted images with fat suppression and gadolinium contrast remain the procedure of choice for diagnosis of ONSM. The tumor is typically isointense to slightly hypointense to brain and optic nerve on T1-weighted images, and hyper- or hypointense on T2-weighted images.[29]

On thin computed tomography (CT) images there is hyperdense enhancement of the meninges surrounding a hypodense optic nerve ("tram track sign"). On noncontrast CT images linear or diffuse calcifications may be present.

Neuroimaging characteristics may also show tubular, globular, or even fusiform enlargement of the optic nerve.[31]

C-scan ultrasound imaging, a noninvasive, quantitative, and inexpensive method, provided optic nerve sheath diameters similar to those obtained by CT of the orbits.[32] This ultrasound showed the optic nerve up to 15 mm behind the globe.

Pathology and Pathogenesis

Primary ONSMs arise from the arachnoid cap cells surrounding the intracanalicular or intraorbital portion of the nerve and are almost always intimately associated with the nerve, giving rise to its tendency to surround the nerve.[5] This results in a concentric thickening of the optic nerve diameter. ONSMs extend posteriorly into the annulus of Zinn. Therefore, ONSMs cannot be resected completely without compromising the integrity of the optic nerve.[33]

Aggressive ONSMs are known with infiltration of the globe or optic nerve. Thus, deterioration of visual acuity may also result from direct tumor invasion into the intracranial optic nerve ($n = 4$). Infiltration of the globe occurred in 2 patients and infiltration of the cavernous sinus in 4 patients. Irregular margins in the orbit implied local invasion.[34]

Location

Tumor location seems to have an important impact on the evolution of visual function. Onset of visual loss in ONSM at or near the orbital apex is thought to be followed by rapid and progressive further loss[1,11] and a higher risk of intracranial extension. We were also able to identify intracanalicular location as a negative factor for visual acuity. Saeed et al. demonstrated that tumors with posterior components in the orbit had more frequent intracranial involvement. Intracranial extension was more frequent and had a greater growth rate in younger patients.[34] In cases in which ONSM involves the intracanalicular portion of the nerve, up to 38% incidence of contralateral nerve involvement was reported.[2]

Classification

A new classification system based on the tumor location and extent is provided to clarify the possible manifestations of ONSM (Fig. 37-1). Treatment modalities are derived according to the different types and subtypes.

Type I is located purely intraorbital ($n = 11$). Type Ia is restricted to a flat extension around the optic nerve ($n = 2$). Type Ib is manifested as a large bulbiform mass ($n = 6$), growing concentrically around the optic nerve with marked proptosis. Type Ic shows exophytic tumor growth upon the optic nerve ($n = 3$).

Type II is located intraorbitally with extension through the optic canal or superior orbital fissure ($n = 39$) (Fig. 37-1). Type IIa is manifested as intraorbital tumor with tumor growth through the optic canal ($n = 35$) (Fig. 37-2A). Type IIb involves the orbital apex ($n = 4$) and the superior orbital fissure, and sometimes even infiltrates the cavernous sinus.

Type III is located intraorbitally with large intracranial tumor extension (more than 1 cm) ($n = 36$). Type IIIa

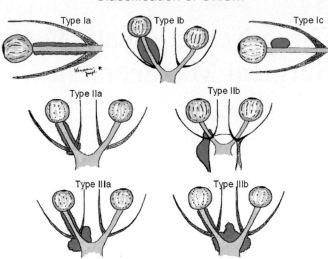

Classification of ONSM

Type Ia Type Ib Type Ic

Type IIa Type IIb

Type IIIa Type IIIb

FIG. 37-1. Schematic drawing of different types and subtypes of ONSM according to their location. Type I—purely intraorbital: (Ia) flat tumor extension around the optic nerve, (Ib) large extension around the optic nerve, (Ic) exophytic tumor upon the optic nerve. Type II—intraorbital with extension through the optic canal or superior orbital fissure: (IIa) intraorbital tumor with tumor growth through the optic canal, (IIb) tumor of the apex, superior orbital fissure, cavernous sinus. Type III—intraorbital and large intracranial tumor extension: (IIIa) intraorbital and intracranial extension to the chiasm, (IIIb) intraorbital and large intracranial extension to the chiasm, contralateral optic nerve, and planum sphenoidale. (From Ref. 30.)

extends to the chiasm ($n = 28$). Type IIIb involves the chiasm up to the contralateral optic nerve and planum sphenoidale ($n = 8$).

Intracranial extension could be diffuse grass-like (65%) or nodular (35%).

Treatment Recommendations

After review of the latest articles[16,20–29] we would like to recommend radiotherapy without biopsy as the treatment of choice in flat purely intraorbital ONSM (type Ia) (Fig. 37-1) once mild vision loss develops or tumor enlargement is determined by serial imaging. Otherwise these tumors should only be observed. Purely intraorbital tumors manifesting as a large mass (type Ib) around the optic nerve should only be operated on to treat painfully uncomfortable eyes without useful vision. Otherwise these tumors can be observed and radiated once visual decline begins to occur. Type Ic tumors with large exophytic parts should be operated on.

Tumors with involvement of the optic canal (type IIa) and questionable intracranial extension with visual decline should be explored with intradural or extradural bony decompression of the optic canal. Then, the intracranial tumor is removed with preservation of the feeding vessels. The intraorbital part involving the distal optic nerve still facilitating

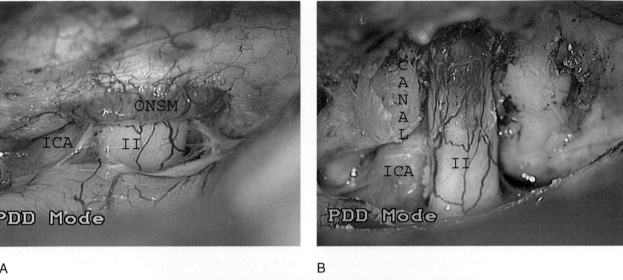

A   B

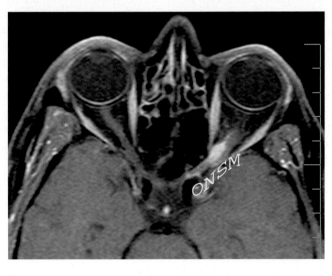

C

Fig. 37-2. Intraoperative photographs of ONSM and radiographic findings. (A) Intraoperative photograph of meningioma Type IIa coming out of the optic canal, surrounding the optic nerve, and preserved arachnoid (ONSM optic nerve sheath meningioma, II optic nerve, ICA internal carotid artery). (B) Intraoperative photograph following decompression of the optic canal and tumor removal around the optic nerve (II optic nerve, ICA internal carotid artery, canal: bony decompression of the optic canal). (C) Preoperative T1-weighted enhanced MRI with fat suppression showing the ONSM extension from the apex through the optic canal into the intracranial space (ONSM optic nerve sheath meningioma)

useful vision should not be removed. Radiation should be the next treatment option for these subtotally resected tumors.

Type IIb tumors of the apex should be biopsied to verify histology. An extradural decompression of the optic canal and superior orbital fissure is recommended. The intracavernous part should be radiated.

Specific indications for surgery are intracranial extension (type III) to prevent involvement of the contralateral optic nerve and resect the intracranial tumor mass. These patients should first undergo intracranial resection with intra- or extradural decompression of the optic canal. IIIa subtype already extends to the chiasm, and the tumor around the optic nerve

is resected. IIIb subtype reaches the contralateral optic nerve, and the tumor is removed from the planum sphenoidale, chiasm, and optic nerves. The intraorbital part should be radiated once visual decline has occurred.

Surgical Technique

Almost all operations are performed via a unilateral frontotemporal approach. This pterional approach is well described in the literature.[35–37] Craniotomy is extended to the middle of the orbital rim and 1 cm above the margin. For intradural procedures, the sylvian fissure is routinely opened. Drainage of cerebrospinal fluid (CSF) is performed by opening the basal cisterns and by lumbar drainage. The ipsilateral optic nerve and carotid artery are identified and the intracranial tumor is first coagulated and resected along the dura around the optic canal. Preservation of the small feeding vessels between the carotid artery and the optic nerve is important and can be achieved by removing the tumor within the arachnoidal plane. At this step mainly irrigation instead of coagulation should be used. The ipsilateral optic canal should always be exposed. We favor early lateral opening of the falciform ligament to relieve the compression of the optic nerve caused by the ligament. The dura is resected around the optic canal and the bony optic canal is decompressed. The drilling should begin laterally until the floor of the optic canal is reached to prevent any contact to the nerve. Finally, the optic canal is unroofed. In case of opening the medially located sphenoid sinus or ethmoidal cells, subcutaneous tissue with fibrine glue is applied. The optic nerve sheath is opened until the annulus of Zinn is reached (beyond this area the tumor removal is not safe). The tumor around the optic nerve and the involved dura are carefully removed. In tumors infiltrating the nerve, resection is limited to the exophytic part. In blind patients with disfiguring painful proptosis, the optic nerve is transsected and the intraorbital part aggressively removed.

In tumors without intracranial extension, an extradural approach is favored with sphenoid ridge drilling, posterior orbitotomy, and decompression of the superior orbital fissure and unroofing of the optic canal.

Tumors with exophytic intraorbital mass are amenable to excision via a lateral orbitotomy.

During the last year we changed our technique of decompression and performed an extradural decompression of the optic canal in five patients. This extradural drilling is much easier, more extensive, and safer for the optic nerve, avoiding any damage. The final step of intradural tumor removal remains unchanged.

Orbitozygomatic resection is used by some authors to treat orbital or sphenocavernous meningiomas.[38–40] However, in ONSMs we do not attempt a complete excision of the tumor. In our opinion, the orbitozygomatic approach is too extended to perform subtotal resections in infiltrative ONSMs.

Surgical Data

The standard approach utlized was the intradural pterional approach in 55 patients with decompression of the optic canal and no resection of the intraorbital flat tumor around the optic nerve. In 12 patients a combined intra- and extradural approach with intradural inspection of the optic nerve was performed. Extradural approach with posterior orbitotomy was restricted to 10 patients with purely intraorbital meningiomas. Two patients were operated on via a lateral orbitotomy. Totally, 7 patients underwent open diagnostic biopsy. Nine patients with amaurosis and prechiasmal involvement of the optic nerve underwent transsection of the optic nerve. Orbital

invasion by the tumor extended beyond the optic nerve into the globe in 2 patients, and enucleation of the eye was carried out by an ophthalmologist.

Outcome/Complications

Outcome and Surgery

The natural history of ONSM is a progressive loss of vision,[2,3,10,15,16,20,25,30] but left untreated, ONSMs may extend intracranially to the contralateral side, resulting in bilateral blindness. However, these tumors are not associated with mortality or significant neurologic morbidity except visual deterioration [5].

Only rare cases of visual improvement after microsurgical resection of ONSMs have been reported, but these cases represent a subset that are located far anteriorly, just posterior to the globe.[10,12,20] Other surgical series reported a high rate of visual complications (30–40%), such as central retinal artery occlusion, motility disturbances, visual field defects, and a high rate of recurrence (65%).[1,2,10] Therefore, surgical excision has been used to treat blind, uncomfortable, or unsightly eyes, to reduce the risk of intracranial extension or contralateral extension, and to treat young patients, in whom a higher biological activity is presumed.[1,2,8,10,14] In patients with tumors confined to the optic canal, decompression of the canal may be associated with vision stabilization for years. Optic sheath opening along the length of the nerve within the optic canal to the annulus of Zinn relieves any focal circumferential pressure on the optic nerve.[33] Conversely, Saeed et al.[34] could not detect preservation of vision by optic sheath decompression. If there is evidence of tumor spread across the planum sphenoidale and useful vision is still present, only the intracranial part of the tumor with preservation of the optic nerve can be removed to prevent spread to the contralateral optic nerve.[8]

In larger surgical series,[41,42] only 2 of 21 patients with anteriorly located tumors showed improved vision. In Kennerdell's series,[10] 7 patients with functional visual acuity remained stable for 2–10 years following subtotal resection. However, his group experienced loss of vision in the majority of cases. Delfini et al.[11] support surgery in patients with progressive symptoms, despite its resulting in more than 80% decline in vision. Verheggen et al.[43] demonstrated an improvement of visual acuity in intracanalicular and intraorbital meningiomas in 89% of the patients postoperatively. Rosenberg et al.[44] evaluated 20 surgically treated patients with 69% stable or improved vision postoperatively. In the series of Roser et al.[13] patients with sudden visual loss (less than 5 months prior to surgery) showed improvement following surgery, consisting of decompression of the optic nerve and subtotal resection of the tumor. These patients gained visual function for a mean time of 60 months with acceptable risk of morbidity and still having the feasibility of radiotherapy in the future.

Outcome (Personal Data)

In our series, visual deterioration was observed in 11 patients postoperatively and improvement in 6 patients (Table 37-1). Sixty-two patients maintained their vision. Thus, we were able to demonstrate that it is possible to perform surgery without it resulting in significant visual loss.

At discharge, the postoperative visual acuity did not significantly differ from the preoperative visual acuity. Patients remained stable within the three different visual categories (Table 37-1). Patients with good preoperative vision preserved this quality ($n = 32$), and only 6 patients' vision worsened (Table 37-1). Poor vision did only improve in 2 patients postoperatively and remained unchanged in 22 patients (Table 37-1). Only in the group with fair vision did 4 patients' vision improve and 5 worsen (Table 37-1). Sixty-two of 79 patients remained unchanged. Preoperative vision highly correlated with postoperative vision. Age did not correlate with the pre- or postoperative visual acuity. The type of tumor had no significant impact on the postoperative visual acuity.

Proptosis resolved completely in 4 patients, incompletely in 14 patients, and remained unchanged in 13 patients. Ocular motility recovered in 7 patients. However, postoperative new transient ptosis and/or oculomotor paresis were seen in 4 patients each.

Complications (Personal Data)

Two patients suffered from infarction (1 partial infarction of the contralateral MCA area with aphasia, 1 complete infarction of the ipsilateral MCA area with hemiparesis). Four patients had a temporary cerebrospinal fluid fistula and were sufficiently treated by lumbar drainage. Two epidural hematomas required reoperation, and 2 subdural hygromas were punctured. Two patients suffered from an epileptic seizure in the first postoperative week. One patient required antibiotic therapy for meningitis. The transient morbidity rate was 13.9%, and the permanent morbidity rate 2.5%.

Follow-up (Personal Data)

At follow-up, 3 patients showed a delayed improvement following surgery (Table 37-2). Visual outcome following surgery in ONSM usually is closely associated with time. In our

TABLE 37-1. Visual Outcome in 79 Patients Immediately Following Surgery[a].

Variable	Preop no. of patients	Postop no. of patients		
		Good	Fair	Poor
Visual acuity				
Good	38	32	2	4
Fair	17	4	8	5
Poor	24	2	0	22
Total	79	38	10	31

[a]Visual categories: Snellon notation ≥0.5 (=5/10) good vision, <0.5–>0.1 (=5/50) fair vision, ≤0.1–0 no useful or bad vision.

TABLE 37-2. Visual Outcome in 79 Patients at Follow-up[a].

Variable	Postop no. of patients	No. of patients at FU		
		Good	Fair	Poor
Visual acuity				
Good	38	30	2	6
Fair	10	1	5	4
Poor	31	1	1	29
Total	79	32	8	39

[a]Visual categories: ≥0.5 (=5/10) good vision, <0.5–>0.1 (=5/50) fair vision, ≤0.1–0 no useful or bad vision.

series, visual acuity became worse in those with long duration of preoperative symptoms prior to intervention.

Vision at delayed follow-up significantly differed from the immediate postoperative vision. However, most patients still remained stable within the three different groups. Patients with good postoperative vision preserved this vision ($n = 30$), but 8 patients' vision worsened (Table 37-2). Poor vision did not improve at follow-up ($n = 29$) except in 2 patients. In the group with fair vision, 1 patient's vision improved and 4 patient's vision worsened (Table 37-2). Sixty-four of 79 patients remained unchanged. The type of the tumor did not significantly influence the visual acuity at delayed follow-up. However, the worst vision was seen in type Ia and IIIb tumors.

Growth of Residual Tumor (Personal Data)

Growth of residual tumor was found in 13 cases (16.5%) 59.2 months (mean, range 14–98 months) postoperatively. Three of these tumors with good vision were further treated with radiotherapy. Eight meningiomas with intracranial extension were reoperated, and 2 clinically asymptomatic tumors were only observed. Two patients suffered from multiple intracranial meningiomas. The duration of follow-up positively correlated with the growth of residual tumor. Eight tumor progressions were seen more than 60 months postoperatively. Neither the extent of initial resection, nor the approach, nor the subtype, influenced the incidence of tumor progression.

Radiotherapy

The application of stereotactic radiosurgery or three-dimensional conformal beam fractionated radiotherapy provides increasing evidence for the benefit of radiotherapy in ONSM.[5,20,22,24,26]

Turbin et al.[9] provided substantial data indicating that conventional radiation therapy was associated with the best visual outcome during follow-up period. They recommended fractionated external beam radiation (5000–5500 cGy). Visual acuity fell significantly in the "observation-only" (13 patients), "surgery-only" (12 patients), and "surgery-with-radiation" groups (16 patients). Eighteen patients had received only radiation and did not show a significant decrease in visual acuity.

Liu et al.[20] presented a series of 5 patients undergoing stereotactic radiotherapy by use of 1.8 Gy fractions to a cumulative dose of 45–54 Gy with dramatic improvement in visual acuity, visual field, and color vision within 3 months after SRT in 4 patients. Moyer et al.[24] reported a patient recovering vision after three-dimensional conformal radiotherapy for ONSM.

Andrews et al.[16] reported a series of 30 patients with different locations of meningiomas (29% intraorbital, 36% optic canal, 3% chiasm, 18% chiasm and optic canal, 9% middle and posterior fossa) who underwent CF-SRT with a 6-MeV LINAC. Of 24 optic nerves with useful vision before CF-SRT, 22 demonstrated either stability (12 nerves) or improvement (10 nerves).

Pitz et al.[26] reported the results of 15 patients with ONSMs undergoing stereotactic fractionated conformal radiation with 54 Gy. Visual acuity improved in 1 patient and the visual field in 6 patients. Visual outcome in the other patients remained unchanged. This study is remarkable because of the visual improvement after radiation without side effects. Stereotactic three-dimensional conformal fractionated radiation seems to be superior to conventional fractionated radiation.

Narayan et al.[25] demonstrated the effectiveness of three-dimansional conformal radiation therapy ($n = 14$) in controlling tumor growth while improving ($n = 5$) or preserving ($n = 7$) vision in most patients.

Some patients with ONSM have a stable course for many years, and a few may even show slight improvement. The routine application of radiation therapy may unnecessarily expose some patients to complications and should be reserved for those patients whose visual function declines under observation.[15] Radiotherapy is still associated with relevant treatment-related morbidity up to 33% including retinopathy, persistent retinitis, dry eye, neuronal damage to the optic nerve resulting in visual loss, and late pituitary dysfunction.[9,25,29,45] Radiation-induced optic neuropathy may occur from months to years after treatment. Factors that contribute to optic neuropathy are an excess of 60 Gy and fraction doses greater than 1.9 Gy.[46] The mechanism of injury is unknown but has been postulated to be the damage to endothelial cells of blood vessels.[3]

As these effects can occur even very long time after treatment, the clinical data to definitively determine the long-term incidence of complications are still maturing.[21]

Radiotherapy does not lead to an acute decrease in tumor volume in all cases and therefore cannot be recommended in cases of rapid visual decline, where surgery is indicated to immediately alleviate pressure to visual structures. Postoperative tumor remnants provide smaller and safer targets for adjuvant radiotherapy.[13]

Radiotherapy (Personal Data)

In our study, 16 patients with ONSM underwent postoperative radiotherapy. Seven patients underwent radiotherapy without surgery.

Eighteen of the meningiomas received stereotactic fractionated conformal radiation (50–60 Gy). Four patients underwent conventional radiation (dose range 44–54 Gy) over 6 weeks. One recurrent tumor was treated with Gamma Knife (14 Gy). Vision improved in 3 patients, remained unchanged in 13 patients, and deteriorated in 7 patients.

Complication Avoidance/Lessons Learned

Our standard surgical procedure consists of decompression of the optic canal, intracranial tumor removal, and no resection of the intraorbital tumor. It should be the goal to resect as much tumor as possible, to open the bony canal to alleviate compressive ischemia without manipulation of the optic nerve to minimize visual loss.

There are different mechanisms for preoperative optic nerve injury: ischemia, compression, demyelization, and tumor invasion.[12,33] Compressive mechanical injury leads to small vessel compromise and demyelization, especially in patients with a long duration of visual loss before surgery. Assuming that there is no additional intraoperative trauma to the optic nerve, incomplete or no recovery of visual function after surgery may imply chronic severe preoperative ischemic or compressive damage and demyelization. In our study, preoperative disc pallor was a negative factor for visual improvement. The bony optic canal is not enlarged in ONSMs, and the tumor in the canal compresses the optic nerve. This compressive injury can at least be reversed by surgical bony decompression of the optic canal. This is the main argument in favor of surgery.

In the past, 10 intracranial extensions were detected intraoperatively and not suspected on preoperative magnetic resonace imaging (MRI) scans. On the other hand, intracranial extension could not be confirmed in 3 patients. Nowadays, fat-suppression techniques and high magnetic field MRI scans focused on the optic nerve usually answer the question of intracanalicular involvement. On very rare occasions, small tumors located within the optic canal remain impossible to detect using neuroimaging. Such lesions are discovered only during exploratory craniotomy.[22]

Resection of ONSM usually remains subtotal. As radiation has been proved to be effective, there is no need to attempt complete excision for the tumor in the apex, superior orbital fissure or cavernous sinus. Residual tumor can be irradiated. We also know that there may be direct tumor invasion into the optic nerve. In these cases resection should be limited to the exophytic part.

Seven of our cases had classic definitive MRI findings ("tram-tracking sign"), all of whom underwent radiotherapy without biopsy. In case of uncommon tumor progression or progressive clinical deterioration, histology should be confirmed. There may always be some cases of sarcoid or other uncommon lesions (e.g., lymphoma) mimicking OSMN. At least in our orbital series of more than 650 patients, there were 4 cases of suspected meningiomas that were histologically proven to be sarcoidosis, lymphoma, benign lymphatic hyperplasia, and aspergillosis. The fusiform variety may be confused with glioma. Therefore, radiation without tissue diagnosis should only be considered for patients with classic clinical and radiographic findings of ONSM.

New techniques, including stereotactic radiosurgery, conformal radiation, and intensity modulation have been developed to reduce the complications of radiotherapy. Radiotherapy has taken on a new role and is increasingly being offered to adults as primary therapy once mild to moderate vision loss develops. Thus we were compelled to rethink our surgical treatment and had to declare radiotherapy as the new standard of care except for those with a mass effect intracranially. Seven patients with intraorbital ONSM and visual decline were treated with radiation only. Sixteen patients with residual tumors underwent postoperative radiotherapy.

The tumor type had no significant prognostic relevance to the evolution of visual acuity. However, type Ia and IIIb tumors presented with a bad visual acuity at follow-up. Five of the IIIb tumors showed bilateral intraorbital tumor growth. In the future, it would be preferable to perform radiotherapy at an earlier point in time on these tumors.

The most common operative causes of morbidity include visual loss, CSF leak, and tumor recurrence. In the resection of these tumors, the most important complication is neural or vascular injury, and careful attention must be taken to preserve small feeding vessels and the ophthalmic artery. The optic nerve has to be treated gently not to produce vasospasm of the vasa vasorum of the optic nerve. Subcutaneous fat is placed around the optic nerve following decompression to avoid a CSF fistula.

Summary

Intraorbital ONSM does grow intracranially and may form a large intracranial mass. Our classification system differentiates among intraorbital, intracanalicular or intrafissural, and combined intraorbital and intracranial types of ONSMs.

Treatment options including radiotherapy, surgery, and observation may be recommended based on this classification. If visual function is good, observation alone can be employed in intraorbital ONSM until progression is noticed. The role of radiotherapy has to be reevaluated and offered to adults once mild vision loss develops in intraorbital ONSMs. Surgery with decompression of the optic canal and intracranial tumor resection is favored for tumors with intracanalicular and intracranial extension. In case of residual or recurrent tumor growth, surgery should be followed by radiotherapy.

References

1. Castel A, Boschi A, Renard L, et al. Optic nerve sheath meningiomas: clinical features, functional prognosis and controversial treatment. Bull Soc Belge Ophthalmol 2000; 275:73–8.
2. Dutton JJ. Optic nerve sheath meningiomas. Surv Ophthalmol 1992; 37:167–83.
3. Cantore WA. Neural orbital tumors. Curr Opin Ophthalmol 2000; 11:367–71.
4. Mafee MF, Goodwin J, Dorodi S. Optic nerve sheath meningiomas: role of MR imaging. Radiol Clin N Am 1999; 37:37–58.
5. Miller NR. Radiation for optic nerve meningiomas: Is this the answer? Ophthalmology 2002; 109:833–4.
6. Mourits MP, van der Sprenkel JW. Orbital meningiomas, the Utrecht experience. Orbit 2001; 20:25–33.
7. Shimano H, Nagasawa S, Kawabata S, et al. Surgical strategy for meningioma extension into the optic canal. Neurol Med Chir (Tokyo) 2000; 40:447–52.
8. Volpe NJ, Gausas RE. Optic nerve and orbital tumors. Neurosurg Clin N Am 1999; 10:699–715.
9. Turbin RE, Thompson CR, Kenderell JS, et al. A long-term visual outcome comparison in patients with optic nerve sheath meningioma managed with observation, surgery, radiotherapy, or surgery and radiotherapy. Ophthalmology 2002; 109:890–900.
10. Kennerdell JS, Maroon JC, Malton M, et al. The management of optic nerve sheath meningiomas. Am J Ophthalmol 1988; 106:450–7.
11. Delfini R, Missori P, Tarantino R. Primary benign tumors of the orbital cavity: Comparative data in a series of patients with optic nerve glioma, sheath meningioma or neurinoma. Surg Neurol 1996; 45:147–54.
12. Fineman MS, Augsburger JJ. A new approach to an old problem. Surv Ophthalmol 1999; 43:519–24.
13. Roser F, Nakamura M, Martini-Thomas R, et al. The role of surgery in meningiomas involving the optic nerve sheath. Clin Neurol Neurosurg 2006; 108:470–6. Epub 2005 Sep 6.
14. Wright JE, McNab AA, McDonald WI. Primary optic nerve sheath meningioma. Br J Ophthalmol 1989; 73:960–6.
15. Egan RA, Lessell S. A contribution to the natural history of optic nerve sheath meningiomas. Arch Ophthalmol 2002; 120: 1505–8.
16. Andrews DW, Faroozan R, Yang BP, et al. Fractionated stereotactic radiotherapy for the treatment of optic nerve sheath meningiomas: preliminary observations of 33 optic nerves in 30 patients with historical comparison to observation with or without surgery. Neurosurgery 2002; 51:890–904.
17. Baumert BG, Villa S, Studer G, et al.. Early improvement in vision after fractionated stereotactic radiotherapy for primary optic nerve sheath meningioma. Radiother Oncol 2004; 72:169–74.
18. Kwon Y, Bae JS, Lee do H, et al. Visual changes after gamma knife surgery for optic nerve tumours. Report of three cases. J Neurosurg 2005; 102(Suppl):143–6.
19. Landert M, Baumert BG, Bosch MM. The visual impact of fractionated stereotactic conformal radiotherapy on seven eyes with optic nerve sheath meningiomas. J Neuroophthalmol 2005; 24:86–91.
20. Liu JK, Forman S, Hershewe GL, et al. Optic nerve sheath meningiomas: visual improvement after stereotactic radiotherapy. Neurosurgery 2002; 50:950–7.
21. Melian E, Jay M. Primary radiotherapy for optic nerve sheath meningioma. Semin Ophthalmol 2004; 19:130–40.
22. Miller NR. Primary tumours of the optic nerve and its sheath. Eye 2004; 18:1026–37.
23. Moster ML. Detection and treatment of optic nerve sheath meningioma. Curr Neurol Neurosci Rep 2005; 5:367–75.
24. Moyer PD, Golnik KC, Breneman J. Treatment of optic nerve sheath meningioma with three-dimensional conformal radiation. Am J Ophthalmol 2000; 5:694–6.

25. Narayan S, Cornblath WT, Sandler HM, et al. Preliminary visual outcomes after three-dimensional conformal radiation therapy for optic nerve sheath meningioma. Int J Radiat Oncol Biol Phys 2003, 56:537–43.

26. Pitz S, Becker G, Schiefer U, et al. Stereotactic fractionated irradiation of optic nerve sheath meningioma: a new treatment alternative. Br J Ophthalmol 2002; 86:1265–8.

27. Radhakrishnan S, Lee MS. Optic nerve sheath meningiomas. Curr Treat Options Neurol 2005; 7:51–5.

28. Richards JC, Roden D, Harper CS. Management of sight-threatening optic nerve sheath meningioma with fractionated stereotactic radiotherapy. Clin Exp Ophthalmol 2005; 33:137–41.

29. Turbin RE, Pokorny K. Diagnosis and treatment of orbital optic nerve sheath meningioma. Cancer Control 2004; 11:334–41.

30. Schick U, Dott U, Hassler W. Surgical management of meningiomas involving the optic nerve sheath. J Neurosurg 2004; 101:951–9.

31. Carrasco JR, Penne RB. Optic nerve sheath meningiomas and advanced treatment options. Curr Opin Ophthalmol 2004; 15:406–10.

32. Garcia JP, Finger PT, Kurli M, et al. 3D ultrasound coronal C-scan imaging for optic nerve sheath meningioma. Br J Ophthalmol 2005; 89:244–5.

33. Lee JH, Jeun SS, Evans J, et al. Surgical management of clinoidal meningiomas. Neurosurgery 2001; 48:1012–7.

34. Saeed P, Rootman J, Nugent RA, et al. Optic nerve sheath meningiomas. Ophthalmology 2003; 110:2019–30.

35. Hassler WE, Eggert H. Extradural and intradural microsurgical approaches to lesions of the optic canal and the superior orbital fissure. Acta Neurochir (Vienna) 1985; 74:87–93.

36. Mauriello JA, Flanagan JC. Surgical approaches to the orbit. In: Mauriello JA, Flanagan JC, ed. Management of Orbital and Ocular Adnexal Tumors and Inflammations. New York: Springer-Verlag, 1990:149–69.

37. Rohde V, Schaller K, Hassler W. The combined pterional and orbitocygomatic approach to extensive tumors of the lateral and latero-basal orbit and orbital apex. Acta Neurochir (Vienna) 1995; 132:127–30.

38. Day JD. Cranial base surgical techniques for large sphenocavernous meningioma: technical note. Neurosurgery 2000; 46:754–60.

39. Ducic Y. Orbitozygomatic resction of meningiomas of the orbit. Laryngoscope 2004; 114:164–70.

40. McDermott MW, Durity FA, Rootman J, et al. Combined fronto-temporal-orbitozygomatic approach for tumors of the sphenoid and orbit. Neurosurgery 1990; 26:107–16.

41. Ito M, Ishizawa A, Miyaoka M, et al. Intraorbital meningiomas. Surgical management and role of radiation therapy. Surg Neurol 1988; 29:448–53.

42. Cristante L. Surgical treatment of meningiomas of the orbit and optic canal: a retrospective study with particular attention to the visual outcome. Acta Neurochir (Wien) 1994; 126:27–32.

43. Verheggen R, Markakis E, Muhlendyck H, et al. Symptomatology, surgical therapy and postoperative results of sphenoorbital, intraorbital-intracanalicular and optic sheath meningiomas. Acta Neurochir Suppl (Wien) 1996; 65:95–8.

44. Rosenberg LF, Miller NR. Visual results after microsurgical removal of meningiomas involving the anterior visual system. Arch Ophthalmol 1984; 102:1019–23.

45. Subramanian PS, Bressler NM, Miller NR. Radiation retinopathy after fractionated radiotherapy for optic nerve sheath meningioma. Ophthalmol 2004; 111:565–7.

46. Parson JT, Bova FJ, Fitzgerald CR. Radiation optic neuropathy after megavoltage external-beam irradiation: analysis of time-dose. Int J Radiat Oncol Biol Phys 1994; 30:753–63.

38

Optic Nerve Sheath Meningiomas II: Conservative Management with Fractionated Stereotactic Radiotherapy

David W. Andrews and James J. Evans

Background

Radiosurgery has become an important treatment alternative to surgery for a variety of intracranial lesions. As currently practiced, it has in fact replaced surgery as a standard of care in some instances, complements surgery as a postoperative adjunct in others, and most commonly represents an alternative to surgery or the only treatment option. Radiosurgery techniques have evolved quickly with the development of new technologies, enabling more complex yet more efficient treatment plans. As a consequence, these technologies have broadened radiosurgery applications and improved radiosurgery outcomes. Among these newer techniques, treatments involving fractionated stereotactic radiation, referred to as fractionated stereotactic radiotherapy (FSR), have emerged as a consequence of linear accelerators designed for and dedicated to stereotactic techniques. Without the logistical constraints of retrofitted general purpose linear accelerators used in radiation oncology, often available only once or twice a week, dedicated units have enabled the design of treatment paradigms that strive for an ideal treatment based on the radiobiology of the target and dose-limiting contiguous tissues. This chapter will summarize our 12-year experience with the Varian 600SR, initially with the Radionics software more recently modified to a Novalis shaped beam radiosurgery unit, and our practice of FSR for both primary and secondary optic nerve sheath meningiomas (ONSM)

ONSM represent one third of all optic nerve tumors, but are comparatively rare among meningiomas.[1] These tumors can arise intraorbitally from arachnoid cap cells within the fibrous dural capsule of the optic nerve. Alternatively, they may represent secondary extensions from an intracranial site. ONSM typically exhibit a meningotheliomatous or transitional histology and are classified as benign under the World Health Organization (Helsinki) grading system for meningiomas. As with intracranial meningiomas, middle-aged females are most often affected.[2,3] A salient symptom is early visual loss, presumably from a combination of compression and circulatory interference of the optic nerve as the tumor enlarges within the dural sheath.[4] Common signs include optic atrophy and optociliary shunt vessels.[5,6] It is postulated that chronic compression of the intraorbital portion of the optic nerve produces gradual obstruction of the central retinal vein, thus preventing the normal passage of venous blood from the retina through the central retinal vein to the cavernous sinus. Optociliary veins represent a collateral drainage route that bypasses the central retinal vein and exit from the orbit via the choroidal circulation and its anastomoses. While long-term survival is likely, the vast majority of untreated patients will progress to complete blindness in the affected eye.[7]

Patients with useful vision and no documented tumor growth have traditionally been observed while surgery has been reserved for patients with progressive symptoms or evidence of tumor growth.[5] Due to their intimate circumferential relationship to the optic nerve and central retinal artery and vein, ONSM have historically been extremely difficult to resect surgically even with modern microneurosurgical techniques.

Until the advent of FSR, the role of traditional radiation therapy in optic nerve sheath meningiomas had been controversial and largely unexplored with few published reports. Arguments against this modality include frequent lack of radiographic response to radiation and potential postradiation injury of the optic nerve and uninvolved optic apparatus.[8,9] However, recent reports in the literature including our own have demonstrated the potential efficacy of radiation therapy in preserving or improving vision.[7,10–13] Indeed, several other authors have since suggested radiation therapy as an adjuvant therapy for incompletely resected tumors or as the primary management of ONSM.

Diagnostic Imaging and Differential Diagnosis of Primary ONSM

Diagnosis of primary ONSM is readily made with fat-suppressed gadolinium-enhanced magnetic resonance imaging (MRI),[14] which reveals the classic "tram-track" appearance

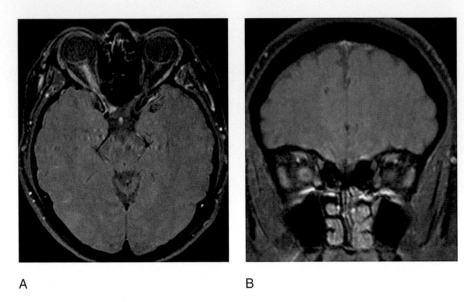

A   B

FIG. 38-1. (A) Fat-suppressed axial T1-weighted gadolinium-enhanced image of right primary ONSM in a patient with associated visual loss; (B) Fat-suppressed coronal T1-weighted gadolinium-enhanced view

of the tumor in axial view and "bulls-eye" appearance in the coronal view (Fig. 38-1).

Without fat supression, this tumor is obscured by periorbital fat and thus can easily be missed on MRI scans. Despite this characteristic appearance, a differential diagnosis should include neurosarcoid,[11,15] demyelinating optic neuritis,[16] and, least likely, optic nerve glioma.[17] We have noted that, in addition to an MR appearance like ONSM, neurosarcoid also avidly takes up the radionuclide octreotide, a radioisotope invariably taken up by meningiomas.[11]

Optical Coherence Tomography

We are routinely performing optical coherence tomography (OCT) which is a noninvasive, noncontact method yielding accurate cross-sectional in vivo imaging of retinal nerve fiber layer (RNFL) thickness.[18,19] OCT imaging can detect and measure changes in tissue thickness with micrometer-scale sensitivity and has proven to be quite sensitive and reliable in the detection of retinal fiber layer loss due to compressive optic neuropathies, often before clinical manifestations of visual loss. OCT is now widely used in serial assessments of patients with glaucoma, diabetic neuropathy, and macular holes, but no reports have yet emerged for serial assessments of ONSM. We are currently quantifying pre- and post-treatment RNFL in patients with primary and secondary ONSM, and these data may have prognostic significance as we advance in the FSR practice of ONSM. Particularly for patients with secondary ONSM, we have been recommending FSR if OCT

reflects unambiguous retinal nerve fiber layer loss, even in patients with intact vision. We have followed patients with normal OCT at 6-month intervals with MRI, visual fields, and OCT.

Review of Treatment Outcomes for ONSM

Table 38-1 summarizes the current experience with focused radiation techniques for treatment of ONSM.

Three publications have compared FSR outcomes to nonradiation management including either observation or surgery followed by observation[20,24,26] for primary and/or secondary ONSM. Two publications including our own are featured in Table 38-2. Neither surgery nor observation yields any likelihood of visual improvement, whereas FSR yields visual improvements ranging from 25 to 80% for visual fields and 8–86% for refracted visual acuity (Table 38-1). With FSR, the combined likelihood of improvement or stabilization climbs to a range of 92–100% for visual fields and 86–100% for visual acuity. In a more detailed follow-up ophthalmologic analysis of outcomes in a subset of these patients, we have noted improvements in not only visual fields (Fig. 38-2) but also refracted visual acuity and color perception.[27]

These rates compare favorably to considerably lower vision preservation rates after surgery or observation (Table 38-2). When compared to observation or surgery, visual outcomes were significantly better, and we concluded that patients with ONSM should be treated upfront solely on radiographic diagnostic criteria.

TABLE 38-1.

Author (Ref.), date	N^a	Isodose prescription	Visual outcome		
			Perimetry	Acuity	Color vision
Fractionated stereotactic radiotherapy					
Andrews (20), 2002	24	1.8 Gy/50. 4–54 Gy	▲42%	▲N/A	▲ N/A
			▸ 50%	▸ N/A	▸ N/A
			▾ 8%	▾ N/A	▾ N/A
Liu (21), 2002	5	1.8 Gy/45–54 Gy	▲ 80%	▲ 60%	▲ 40%
			▸ 20%	▸40%	▸ 60%
			▾ 0	▾ 0	▾ 0
Pitz (22), 2002	12	1.8 Gy/50.4 Gy + 2 × 3.6 Gy boost	▲ 42%	▲ 8%	▲ N/A
			▸ 58%	▸ 92%	▸ N/A
			▾ 0	▾ 0	▾ N/A
Becker (23), 2002	24	1.8 Gy/54 Gy	▲ 25%	▲27%	▲ N/A
			▸ 71%	▸ 73%	▸ N/A
			▾ 4%	▾ 0	▾ N/A
Landert (24), 2005	7	1.8 Gy/54 Gy	▲ 66%	▲ 86%	▲ N/A
			▸ 29%	▸ 0	▸ N/A
			▾ 5%	▾ 14%	▾ N/A
3-D conformal radiation					
Narayan (25), 2003	14	1.8–2 Gy/50. 4–56 Gy	▲ 100%^{b}	▲ 36%	▲ N/A
			▸ 0	▸ 50%	▸ N/A
			▾ 0	▾ 14%	▾ N/A

$^a N$ = eyes with measureable function before treatment.
^{b} Only 9/14 had baseline visual fields and 9/9 had improvement.
▲ = improvement in function; ▸= no change in function; ▾ = loss of function.

TABLE 38-2.

Author (Ref.), date	N	Visual field outcomes		
		FSR or RT alone (N)	Surgery alone (N)	Observation alone (N)^a
Andrews (20), 2002	50	▲ 42% (10)	▲ 0	▲ 0
		▸ 50% (12)	▸16% (5)	▸30% (3)
		▾ 8% (2)	▾ 67% (21)	▾70% (7)
Landert (24), 2005	13	▲ 66% (4)	▲ N/A	▲ 0
		▸ 29% (2)	▸ N/A	▸ 50% (3)
		▾ 5% (1)	▾ N/A	▾ 50% (3)

^{a} Only visual acuity data available.
▲ = improvement in function; ▸ = no change in function; ▾ = loss of function.

than light perception at diagnosis, 13 patients were observed only, 12 had surgery only, 18 received radiation alone, and 16 had surgery and radiation. Irradiated patients received between 40 and 55 Gy of conventional multiport or conformal external beam radiation. Ratio acuity scores revealed that visual acuity fell significantly for observed only, surgery only, and surgery with radiation groups, whereas the radiation only group manifested a decrease in visual acuity that was not significant.

These data are further supported by the analysis of Turbin et al.[26] These authors retrospectively compared the outcomes of 64 patients with diagnosed primary ONSM treated with either observation, surgery, radiotherapy, or a combination of surgery and radiotherapy. Of 59 patients with vision greater

Radiobiological Principles of FSR for ONSM

Fractionated radiotherapy has been used to treat patients with cranial base tumors over the last half-century. Stereotactic radiosurgery has made the treatment of cranial base tumors far more precise with modern imaging and versatile three-dimensional treatment planning software which, through dose volume histograms, maximizes dose to target with high conformality and minimizes dose to contiguous normal structures. Two exceptions are optic nerve sheath meningiomas and acoustic neuromas, where these cranial nerves are intrinsic to the target volume. As special sensory cranial nerves, injury to sensory function occurs much more frequently than either sensory or motor function in mixed cranial nerves, reflecting a lower threshold for injury. Low daily doses of radiation and a cumulative dose below a threshold value, however, have proven to be safe for the optic nerves and more recently for the cochlear nerve. We will advance arguments based on published data that tumors involving or near special sensory cranial nerves, when treatment is indicated, should be treated with FSR utilizing daily conventional fraction sizes.

Single doses of 15 or 54 Gy in 30 daily fractions both result in excellent control of meningiomas. The SRS dose of 15 Gy,

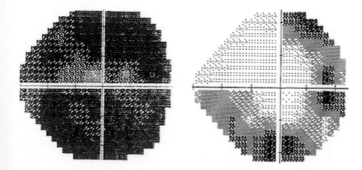

FIG. 38-2. Humphrey automated perimetry (24-2 central threshold) of left visual field in patient with left ONSM at pretreatment (left) and with documented improvement in central vision at 46 weeks after FSR (right)

however, exceeds the generally accepted single-dose tolerance of the optic nerves (8–10 Gy) for treatment of ONSM and may be associated with a risk of optic neuropathy approaching 78% at ≥15 Gy dose prescriptions. For fractionated radiotherapy, decades of experience have led to guidelines for normal tissue tolerance. For optic nerve and chiasm, guidelines have evolved that have proven to be extremely safe and are generally based on the recommendation initially made in 1992 by Goldsmith,[28] later corroborated by a large retrospective analysis by Parsons, who also established a daily dose of 1.9 Gy as safe.[29]

Based on the assumption that 15 Gy in a single fraction and 54 Gy in 30 fractions are biologically equivalent, the α/β ratio for meningiomas may be calculated based on the linear quadratic formula:

$$BED\ (Gy) = D(1 + d/\alpha/\beta)$$

where D is the total dose, d is the dose per fraction, and α/β is the characteristic constant associated with the particular tissue in question. Assuming $BED_1 = BED_2$ for tissue of an unknown α/β:

$$D_1(1+d_1/\alpha/\beta) = D_2 (1+d_2/\alpha/\beta) \text{ or } \alpha/\beta$$
$$= (D_1 \times d_1 - D_2 \times d_2)/D_2 - D_1$$

For meningiomas using the assumption of equivalent BED for 15 Gy in a single fraction ($d_1 = 15$ Gy) and 54 Gy in 30 fractions ($d_2 = 1.8$ Gy):

$$\alpha/\beta = (15 \times 15) - (54 \times 1.8)/(54 - 15) = 3.28 \text{ Gy}$$

and the corresponding BED is calculated as:

$$BED = 15(1+15/3.28) = 54(1+1.8/3.28) = 83.6 \text{ gy}$$

It has been clearly established that the radiation tolerance to the optic nerves and chiasm depends on the total dose of radiation and the dose per fraction. Goldsmith et al. proposed a model predicting the total dose associated with a low risk of optic neuropathy when various doses per fraction were prescribed:

$$\text{Optic ret dose} = \text{Dose (cGy)}/ N^{0.53}$$

Shrieve et al. applied these formulas to the treatment of parasellar meningiomas where the optic apparatus is a dose-limiting structure.[30] If the optic ret tolerance of 890 is observed and the α/β is assumed to be $3.28 \pm 10\%$, a range of doses from a minimum of 46 Gy in a minimum of 22 fractions to 54 Gy in 30 fractions is necessary to achieve tumor control and an acceptable rate of optic neuropathy.

An assumption in this analysis is that vision is intact at the inception of treatment. The natural history of primary optic nerve sheath meningiomas or meningiomas that encroach upon the optic apparatus reflects progressive visual loss to blindness in the affected eye. Assumptions regarding the morbidity of radiation treatment must in these cases be weighed against the morbidity associated with the natural history of the disease. If radiation optic neuropathy, for example, occurred at rates of 5–10% in a median range of 4–6 years,

and the natural history reflected rates of visual loss to blindness at 80–90% over a broader median range of 6–10 years, the therapeutic benefit would outweigh the treatment-related morbidity, even if as high as a 10% rate of optic neuropathy is assumed.

Technique

We commissioned the world's first installation of a linear accelerator designed for and dedicated to stereotactic radiosurgery and fractionated stereotactic radiotherapy in 1994.[31] Since then, we adopted a treatment technique which incorporates stereotactic technique with conventional daily doses of radiation. These dose-fraction protocols are designed to optimize therapeutic effect while minimizing treatment-related morbidities. Our rationale for a conventional fraction FSR paradigm stems from our belief that special sensory cranial nerves, notably the optic nerves and the cochlear nerves, are more sensitive to any therapeutic intervention including radiation therapy.[20,32] Drawing from previously reported observations documenting injury thresholds for the optic nerves after radiation for head and neck cancers, we have adopted a 1.8 Gy daily fraction schedule, and for both primary and secondary ONSM we have achieved both high tumor control rates and actuarial visual improvement after FSR (discussed below). Pretreatment patient preparation involves the customized design of a lightweight relocatable frame based on either an upper arch Reprosil dental mold (Gill-Thomas-Cosman frame) or a thermoplast mask of the face. Either template is adapted to the frame and yields a reproduceable and accurate frame relocation each time it is applied for treatment. On this day both magnetic resonance imaging (MRI) and computed tomography (CT) data are obtained, in the latter case with a fiducial cage attached. Due to the high spatial fidelity of CT data, the CT dataset is an obligatory imaging dataset for treatment planning. Both imaging datasets are electronically transferred to the treatment planning workstation, where they are fused into one composite image for treatment planning purposes. The patient is discharged home and returns for outpatient treatment inception usually a week to 10 days later.

The Novalis treatment-planning workstation provides a number of planning options ranging from dynamic arc treatment to conformal static arcs or stereotactic IMRT. At our institution, most treatment plans involve a single isocenter treatment with five noncoplanar arcs utilizing the dynamic arc method. With mini-multileaf collimation, this technique allows for both high target conformality and high dose homogeneity, variables commonly considered to yield the highest therapeutic index. More complex cranial base lesions are treated with either conformal arc or, if highly irregular concave surfaces are involved, stereotactic IMRT. Treatment planning is highly effective and efficient due to the software design which is capable of parallel treatment plans for comparison (Fig. 38-3).

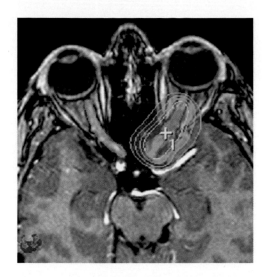

FIG. 38-3. Axial T-1 weighted image of left ONSM treated with dynamic arc FSR. Dose prescription was 1.8 Gy to the 91% isodose line in daily fractions over 5 weeks to a total dose of 52.2 Gy. Organs at risk (OARs) include optic nerves

Clinical Outcomes

We have treated 126 patients to date with either primary ($N = 32$) or secondary ($N = 94$) optic nerve sheath meningiomas. Patients with unambiguously documented pre-treatment visual status and follow-up visual data identified by chart review are designated in Table 38-3.

Nine patients are either at follow-up too early for assessment or their ophthalmologic data are incomplete or missing, and 29 patients have either normal vision, light perception only, or no light perception. We included 88 remaining patients with serviceable but compromised vision (down to finger count only) eligible for assessment of visual improvement after FSR treatment, including 18 primary ONSM and 71 patients with secondary ONSM.

After our preliminary observations,[20] we are now documenting greater rates of visual recovery at longer follow-up, particularly for secondary ONSM where the median time to visual improvement was over twice the median time for

improvement for primary ONSM (see below). It remains unclear why the response time is longer for secondary ONSM at this point, but prospective examination with data including OCT of both groups may provide clues.

The pathophysiology of visual loss from both primary and secondary ONSM clearly must involve a compressive component, since optociliary vessels reflect occlusion of the central retinal vein. Mechanical decompression leads to disappearance of this collateral circulation,[33] but FSR also achieves this finding without ostensible change in ONSM tumor volume,[34] suggesting a restitution of normal optic nerve vascular physiology independent of any change in tumor size.

Primary Optic Nerve Sheath Meningiomas

We initiated conventional fraction FSR in 1995 after we commissioned the first Varian 600SR, and taking advantage of our strong affiliation with Wills Eye Hospital, addressed a large population of patients with both primary and secondary ONSM. Based on the data published by Parsons et al., we initiated a dose fraction FSR program of 1.8 Gy daily fractions to a cumulative dose of 54 Gy (Table 38-1) and published our initial results involving 33 optic nerves in 30 patients in 2002. These data reflected a 90% actuarial visual preservation rate. One patient with primary ONSM lost vision after treatment, which was scored as treatment-related visual loss despite lack of adequate follow-up data to determine whether visual loss was actually related to treatment failure. This patient is lost to follow-up.

Our current results reflect durable improvement in vision at a median follow-up of 247 weeks (range 15–490 weeks) (Fig. 38-4a) with one reported case of radiation-induced optic neuropathy (Fig. 38-4b) in 18 patients with serviceable vision. Sixteen of 18 patients experienced visual improvement. The actuarial rate of visual improvement (13 with compromised fields, 4 with diminished acuity, and 1 with diplopia) was 96% (Fig. 38-3), and the median time to visual improvement was 21 weeks. Visual loss was noted in only one patient at 82 weeks, and this was ascribed to treatment.

Secondary Optic Nerve Sheath Meningiomas

Ultimately the management of patients with serviceable (central acuity preserved) or measureable (LPO) vision should be considered by a multidisciplinary team, which includes radiosurgeons and cranial base surgeons. Surgical series have described excellent treatment outcomes with visual recovery, particularly when the optic nerve is decompressed at the orbital apex. It is important to note that the surgical goal is early identification of the optic nerve, extradural bony decompression (anterior clinoidectomy and unroofing of the optic canal), and division of the falciform ligament and opening of the optic sheath (35). Treatment options for secondary ONSM include surgical removal and/or radiation. Based on our experience and

TABLE 38-3.

Visual status	Primary ONSM (N)	Secondary ONSM (N)
Normal vision	2	4
Field compromise	16	30
Acuity compromise	4	24
Acuity and field compromise	0	12
Diplopia	1	1
LPO	2	0
NLP	7	14
TOTAL	**32**	**85**

LPO Light perception only
NLP No Light perception

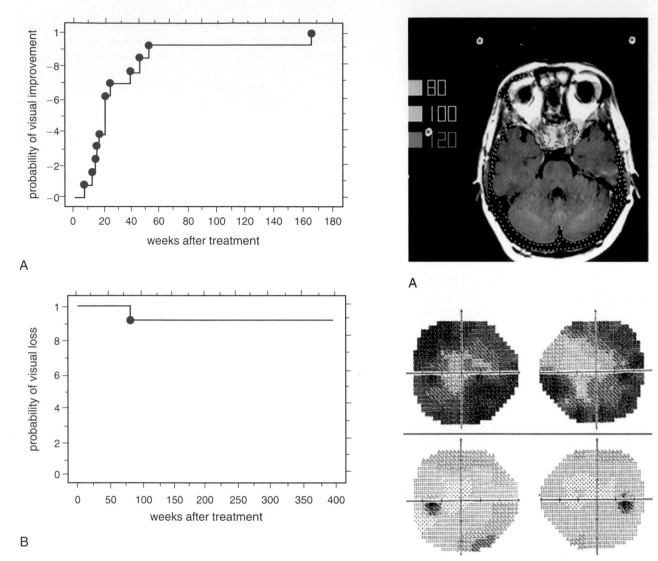

A

B

FIG. 38-4. (A) Kaplan Meyer curve of probability of visual improvement in patients with primary ONSM after FSR who presented with serviceable (central) vision but documented visual compromise; (B) Kaplan Meyer curve of probability of visual loss in patients with primary ONSM after FSR

FIG. 38-5. (A) Axial fused MR/CT with color wash of treatment plan for a planum sphenoidale meningioma with invasion of both orbital apices and bilateral visual loss. Dose was 1.8 Gy to the 70% isodose surface; (B) upper panel: Humphrey perimetry before treatment; lower panel: perimetry at 129 weeks follow-up revealing marked improvement in both fields

literature review, the only radiation technique which yields significant therapeutic benefit is FSR (Fig. 38-5).

We have treated 94 patients with secondary ONSM, 71 of whom had serviceable but compromised vision before FSR treatment. Forty-seven of these patients had evaluable follow-up visual data. Our current results reflect durable improvement in vision at a median follow-up of 286 weeks (range 54–576 weeks) (Fig. 38-6a), with three cases of radiation-induced optic neuropathy (Fig. 38-6b). Thirty-one of 47 patients experienced visual improvement for a raw visual improvement rate of 66%. As with primary ONSM, the actuarial rate of visual improvement was 96% (Fig. 38-6a), but the median time to visual improvement was more than twice as long at 52 weeks. Visual loss was noted in three patients at 6, 11, and 60 months.

In the lattermost case, this patient had undergone cranial irradiation as a child for lymphoma, and this patient was at an increased risk of visual loss after FSR treatment of a clinoidal meningioma.

Comments and Summary

FSR has proven to be a safe and effective means of managing both primary and secondary ONSM. Due to the compelling outcomes for primary ONSM in particular, FSR

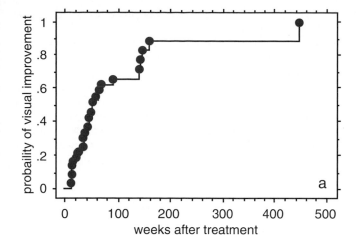

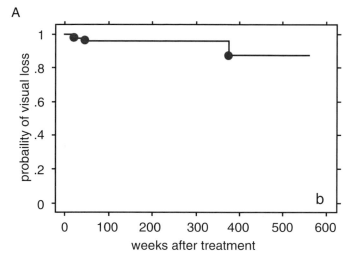

FIG. 38-6. (A) Kaplan Meyer curve of probability of visual improvement in patients with secondary ONSM after FSR who presented with serviceable (central) but compromised vision; (B) Kaplan Meyer curve of probability of visual loss in patients with secondary ONSM after FSR

should be considered a standard of care for the treatment of this disease. Compared to the natural history of visual loss, treatment with FSR should be recommended if any associated visual compromise is documented, including preclinical RNFL loss quantified by OCT. We have an even greater optimism of long-term excellent visual outcomes with the advent of dynamic collimation, which achieves much higher dose homogeneity along the axis of the optic nerve with the dynamic arc technique (Fig. 38-2).

The optimal treatment for secondary ONSM associated with visual loss remains unclear. Surgery still remains an important intervention for patients with visual loss and/or proptosis due to invasion of the orbit. We have demonstrated that FSR is an important treatment alternative with compelling outcomes reflecting visual improvement by a noninvasive means. Only prospective studies will determine if these outcomes are supe-

rior to surgery, particularly for patients with poor vision prior to intervention. We feel that optical coherence tomography will provide important data that may guide the treatment algorithm.

References

1. Leonard DW, Bolger WE. Minimally invasive approach for biopsy of an optic nerve sheath tumor. Otolaryngol Head Neck Surg 1999;120(5):776–9.
2. Alper MG. Management of primary optic nerve meningiomas. Current status—therapy in controversy. J Clin Neuroophthalmol 1981;1(2):101–17.
3. Wright JE, McNab AA, McDonald WI. Primary optic nerve sheath meningioma. Br J Ophthalmol 1989;73(12):960–6.
4. Wright JE, Call NB, Liaricos S. Primary optic nerve meningioma. Br J Ophthalmol 1980;64(8):553–8.
5. Muci-Mendoza R, Arevalo JF, Ramella M, et al. Optociliary veins in optic nerve sheath meningioma. Indocyanine green videoangiography findings. Ophthalmology 1999;106(2):311–8.
6. Sibony PA, Krauss HR, Kennerdell JS, et al. Optic nerve sheath meningiomas. Clinical manifestations. Ophthalmology 1984;91(11):1313–26.
7. Dutton JJ. Optic nerve gliomas and meningiomas. Neurol Clin 1991;9(1):163–77.
8. Wara WM, Sheline GE, Newman H, et al. Radiation therapy of meningiomas. Am J Roentgenol Radium Ther Nucl Med 1975;123(3):453–8.
9. Delfini R, Missori P, Tarantino R, et al. Primary benign tumors of the orbital cavity: comparative data in a series of patients with optic nerve glioma, sheath meningioma, or neurinoma. Surg Neurol 1996;45(2):147–53; discussion 53–4.
10. Dabbs CB, Kline LB. Big muscles and big nerves. Surv Ophthalmol 1997;42(3):247–54.
11. Fineman MS, Augsburger JJ. A new approach to an old problem. Surv Ophthalmol 1999;43(6):519–24.
12. Kennerdell JS, Maroon JC, Malton M, Warren FA. The management of optic nerve sheath meningiomas. Am J Ophthalmol 1988;106(4):450–7.
13. Sarkies NJ. Optic nerve sheath meningioma: diagnostic features and therapeutic alternatives. Eye 1987;1(Pt 5):597–602.
14. Mafee MF, Goodwin J, Dorodi S. Optic nerve sheath meningiomas. Role of MR imaging. Radiol Clin North Am 1999;37(1): 37–58, ix.
15. Ing EB, Garrity JA, Cross SA, Ebersold MJ. Sarcoid masquerading as optic nerve sheath meningioma. Mayo Clin Proc 1997;72(1):38–43.
16. Cornblath WT, Quint DJ. MRI of optic nerve enlargement in optic neuritis. Neurology 1997;48(4):821–5.
17. Liauw L, Vielvoye GJ, de Keizer RJ, van Duinen SG. Optic nerve glioma mimicking an optic nerve meningioma. Clin Neurol Neurosurg 1996;98(3):258–61.
18. Kanamori A, Nakamura M, Matsui N, et al. Optical coherence tomography detects characteristic retinal nerve fiber layer thickness corresponding to band atrophy of the optic discs. Ophthalmology 2004;111(12):2278–83.
19. Blumenthal EZ, Williams JM, Weinreb RN, et al. Reproducibility of nerve fiber layer thickness measurements by use of optical coherence tomography. Ophthalmology 2000; 107(12):2278–82.

20. Andrews DW, Faroozan R, Yang BP, et al. Fractionated stereotactic radiotherapy for the treatment of optic nerve sheath meningiomas: preliminary observations of 33 optic nerves in 30 patients with historical comparison to observation with or without prior surgery. Neurosurgery 2002;51(4):890–902; discussion 3–4.

21. Liu JK, Forman S, Hershewe GL, et al. Optic nerve sheath meningiomas: visual improvement after stereotactic radiotherapy. Neurosurgery 2002;50(5):950–5; discussion 5–7.

22. Pitz S, Becker G, Schiefer U, et al. Stereotactic fractionated irradiation of optic nerve sheath meningioma: a new treatment alternative. Br J Ophthalmol 2002;86(11):1265–8.

23. Becker G, Jeremic B, Pitz S, et al. Stereotactic fractionated radiotherapy in patients with optic nerve sheath meningioma. Int J Radiat Oncol Biol Phys 2002;54(5):1422–9.

24. Landert M, Baumert BG, Bosch MM, et al. The visual impact of fractionated stereotactic conformal radiotherapy on seven eyes with optic nerve sheath meningiomas. J Neuroophthalmol 2005;25(2):86–91.

25. Narayan S, Cornblath WT, Sandler HM, et al. Preliminary visual outcomes after three-dimensional conformal radiation therapy for optic nerve sheath meningioma. Int J Radiat Oncol Biol Phys 2003;56(2):537–43.

26. Turbin RE, Thompson CR, Kennerdell JS, et al. A long-term visual outcome comparison in patients with optic nerve sheath meningioma managed with observation, surgery, radiotherapy, or surgery and radiotherapy. Ophthalmology 2002;109(5):890–9; discussion 9–900.

27. Behbehani RS, McElveen T, Sergott RC, et al. Fractionated stereotactic radiotherapy for parasellar meningiomas: a preliminary report of visual outcomes. Br J Ophthalmol 2005;89(2):130–3.

28. Goldsmith BJ, Rosenthal SA, Wara WM, Larson DA. Optic neuropathy after irradiation of meningioma. Radiology 1992; 185(1):71–6.

29. Parsons JT, Bova FJ, Fitzgerald CR, et al. Radiation optic neuropathy after megavoltage external-beam irradiation: analysis of time-dose factors. Int J Radiat Oncol Biol Phys 1994;30(4):755–63.

30. Shrieve DC, Hazard L, Boucher K, Jensen RL. Dose fractionation in stereotactic radiotherapy for parasellar meningiomas: radiobiological considerations of efficacy and optic nerve tolerance. J Neurosurg 2004;101(Suppl 3):390–5.

31. Das IJ, Downes MB, Corn BW, et al. Characteristics of a dedicated linear accelerator-based stereotactic radiosurgery-radiotherapy unit. Radiother Oncol 1996;38(1):61–8.

32. Andrews DW, Suarez O, Goldman HW, et al. Stereotactic radiosurgery and fractionated stereotactic radiotherapy for the treatment of acoustic schwannomas: comparative observations of 125 patients treated at one institution. Int J Radiat Oncol Biol Phys 2001;50(5):1265–78.

33. Brazier DJ, Sanders MD. Disappearance of optociliary shunt vessels after optic nerve sheath decompression. Br J Ophthalmol 1996;80(2):186–7.

34. Mashayekhi A, Shields JA, Shields CL. Involution of retinochoroidal shunt vessel after radiotherapy for optic nerve sheath meningioma. Eur J Ophthalmol 2004;14(1):61–4.

35. Lee JH, Jeun SS, Evans J, Kosmorsky G. Surgical management of clinoidal meningiomas. Neurosurgery 2001;48(5):1012–9; discussion 9–21.

39
Lateral and Middle Sphenoid Wing Meningiomas

Benoit J.M. Pirotte and Jacques Brotchi

Introduction

Definition

Meningiomas account for approximately 13–19% of all intracranial tumors. Meningiomas of the skull base locations constitute 40% of all intracranial meningiomas. Of these, about one half occur in the sphenoid wing.[1-3] Sphenoid wing meningiomas then account for more or less 20% of intracranial meningiomas and represent a real surgical challenge due to their invasion of the bone and their proximity to main arteries and cranial nerves. Anatomically, the sphenoid wing extends from the anterior clinoid process to the pterion with the greater wing constituting the outer third and the lesser wing the inner two thirds. The greater wing and the lateral half of the lesser wing represent the lateral and middle portions of the sphenoid wing.[2-7]

Classification

The first description of sphenoid wing meningiomas, given in 1938 by Cushing and Eisenhardt,[8] classified them into three groups: (1) deep, inner or clinoidal; (2) middle or alar; and (3) outer or pterional. Lateral and middle sphenoid wing meningiomas represent the groups 2 and 3 in that classification.

Later on, Bonnal et al.[4,5] and Brotchi and Bonnal[6] divided sphenoid wing meningiomas into five groups that raised specific surgical problems: (A) deep or clinoidal or sphenocavernous; (B) invading en plaque of the sphenoid wings; (C) invading en masse of the sphenoid wings which combines the features of groups A and B; (D) middle ridge meningiomas; and (E) pterional or sylvian point meningiomas (Fig. 39-1). Al-Mefty[1,9] made a subdivision of clinoidal meningiomas into three groups. All these classifications are based on surgical considerations and related to operative strategy and challenge. Many of the surgical principles used in the treatment of meningiomas were described in the classic two-volume work published by Cushing and Eisenhardt.[8] The modern management of meningiomas has been summarized in two books,

Meningiomas, edited by Al-Mefty, and *Meningiomas and Their Surgical Management*, edited by Schmidek, published in 1991 and in related articles.[1-15]

Special Considerations

More accessible and resectable than clinoid meningiomas, lateral and middle sphenoid wing meningiomas are often included in the general chapter of sphenoid wing meningiomas and discussed together with the clinoidal meningiomas. The very challenging surgical considerations of clinoid meningiomas (also called medial sphenoid wing meningiomas) have been addressed and studied in specific chapters because of their relationship with the cavernous sinus, oculomotor and optic nerves, as well as the internal carotid artery and its branches.[2,9] The surgical management of lateral and middle sphenoid wing meningiomas has been rarely addressed specifically, probably because they are more accessible than the clinoidal type, but also because they often extend to the inner portion of the sphenoid wing. Although considered as the most resectable tumors, lateral and middle sphenoid wing meningiomas are neurosurgically challenging because of their high rates of recurrence, partly due to the frequent bone involvement.

Specific Clinico-Radiologic and Surgical Challenge

Lateral and middle sphenoid wing meningiomas may extend to the inner portion of the sphenoid wing and involve partially the clinoid process. Indeed, it is not uncommon that dissection has to deal with the internal carotid artery and the optic nerve. Additionally, hyperostotic reactions may cause infiltration and compression on the intraorbital structures, the sylvian veins, and the superior orbital fissure. Clinical features unique to this group of meningiomas include exophtalmus, transient diplopia due to oculomotor nerve dysfunction, peri-orbital pain or numbness in the territory of the V1 branch, progressive visual loss, and seizures. Compression

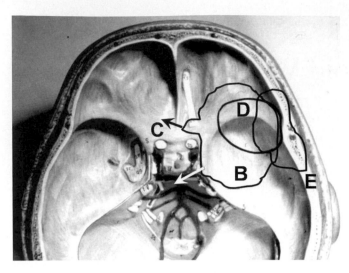

Fig. 39-1. Sphenoid wing meningiomas divided into five groups raising specific surgical difficulties: (A—not shown) deep or clinoidal or sphenocavernous; (B) invading en plaque of the sphenoid wings; (C) invading en masse of the sphenoid wings; (D) middle ridge (lesser wing) meningiomas; (E) pterional or lateral (greater wing and pterion) meningiomas (From Refs. 4, 5, and 7.)

of the sylvian veins may generate fronto-temporal brain edema at the time of the diagnosis.[2,4–6,11,16]

Specific Surgical Indications

Lateral and middle sphenoid wing meningiomas should be operated after diagnosis when they are symptomatic, even when symptoms are limited to an isolated exophthalmus, pterional pain, or diplopia. Al-Mefty mentioned that the indication should be individualized, taking into consideration the age, the neurologic status and symptoms, the arterial circulation, the extent of tumor involvement, and the tumor behavior.[1,9] In patients older than 70 or if the diagnosis is done by chance without any peritumoral brain edema, a progression in tumor size should be demonstrated on repeated magnetic resonance imaging (MRI) follow-up, before considering surgery. However, when the tumor is extended to the optic canal, surgery is always indicated to avoid extension towards the optic sheath and to the midline.

Specific Preoperative Workup

Decisions regarding the treatment of sphenoid wing meningiomas are often difficult. There are several specific questions and features that must be considered prior to deciding on surgery:[8]

Is it actually a meningioma? Special attention should be paid to bony structures on computed tomography (CT)/MR images. Particular attention should be given to the anterior clinoid process. When the anterior clinoid process is missing, an osteolytic malignant tumor mass such as a metastasis or a

chordoma might be suspected. A preoperative CT scan with bony windows is therefore useful to check whether the bone is hyperostotic or eroded.

Where does the tumor blood supply come from? The tumor may be vascularized by branches of the external carotid artery, by branches of the internal carotid artery, or even fed by both. A careful analysis of the MR angiography sequences is recommended to assess the degree and origin of the feeding meningeal arterial branches of these meningiomas, particularly the branches that could come from the internal carotid artery to feed the tumor. Although MR angiography is accurate for this purpose,[16,18] we still recommend performing a selective angiography in cases that show a rich or unusual tumor vascularization, and a tumor diameter exceeding 4 cm. Angiography might remain necessary to depict the tumor's vascularity and the blood supply and to determine the feasibility of preoperative embolization. [17–21]

What relationship does the meningioma have to the adjacent arteries and veins? Internal carotid artery and its branches may be displaced, stretched, or encased. Precise anatomy of arteries and veins (including the dominant and collateral veins) is important to know in order to reduce the risk of surgical vascular injury. Today, the best tools showing the vessels inside and around the meningioma are MRI and MR angiography, which provide great safety for surgical dissection. MR venography might also help to assess the number, the size, and the compression of sylvian veins in huge lateral sphenoid wing meningiomas.

What are the tumor boundaries and the limits of dural invasion? The dural invasion may be very extensive in "en plaque" meningiomas (our B and C groups) (Fig. 39-1). Gadolinium-enhanced T1-weighted MR sequences are very accurate to assess the tumor limits and invasion of the dura. However, dural enhancement doesn't necessarily mean that the dura is invaded but is highly suggestive. Nevertheless, the resection of the enhanced dura is mandatory to lessen the risk of recurrence.

What is the extent of invasion in the skull base and cranio-facial cavities? It is very important to know whether the tumor invades the pterygo-maxillary fossa, parapharyngeal space, and Eustachian tube. Indeed, the long-term prognosis of meningiomas in terms of recurrence is closely correlated to the degree of tumor removal. One should, therefore, aim to achieve gross total removal such as reflected by the Simpson grade I or II.[22] It is also important to assess the extent of bone invasion, since hyperostotic bone often means tumor invasion. Coronal sections (CT scan and MRI) are the best tools to study the extension of the meningioma into the skull base and cranio-facial cavities. Furthermore, one should pay attention to the risk of cerebrospinal fluid (CSF) leakage when ethmoid or sphenoid sinuses must be opened during surgery.

Are the optic nerves and tract involved? It is of great benefit to know before surgery the potential intimacy between the meningioma and the optic nerves in order to avoid postoperative visual deficit. A neuro-ophthalmological examination is mandatory before surgery when the meningioma extends towards the clinoid process. A tumoral extension to the optic canal may, however, exist without any clinical deficit. Coronal MRI views are very helpful for assessing that issue and for making appropriate intraoperative decisions.

Is the pituitary stalk of concern? The pituitary stalk may be intimately involved by juxta-sellar meningiomas. Therefore, an endocrinological workup is also mandatory. However, normal endocrine parameters do not exclude a surgical adherence of the pituitary stalk to the tumor.

Why is exophthalmus present? Exophthalmus may be due to bony hyperostosis, orbital invasion by the meningioma, or cavernous sinus involvement. It is very important to know if the cavernous sinus is involved and to remember that its tumoral invasion may be encountered without any cranial nerve deficit. One must understand before surgery the cause of the exophtalmus. Coronal MRI views are essential.

Why is diplopia present? The two major causes of diplopia are orbital and cavernous sinus invasion. Rarely, diplopia may be due to a herniated tumoral bud into the posterior fossa between the upper brain stem and the tentorial free edge. In such a situation, the third and the fourth cranial nerves may be adherent to the tumor. Sagittal, axial, and coronal MRI views are essential in the preoperative planning. Careful dissection must avoid nerve damage, which can occur if the tumor is aggressively mobilized.

Summarized Preoperative Workup

In all cases of lateral and middle sphenoid wing meningiomas, the preoperative planning requires a CT scan with bony windows, a three-dimensional multiplanar gadolinium-enhanced MRI, and MR sequences of MR angiography and venography. When lateral and middle sphenoid wing meningiomas extend to the clinoid process and the cavernous sinus, an internal/external carotid artery selective angiography workup is mandatory. In juxta-sellar extension, we like to perform a neuro-ophthalmological and endocrinological workup. The question of a preoperative embolization should be raised in all cases, and performed when branches feeding the tumor arise from the external carotid system only.

Surgical Technique

Surgical Considerations

Surgery is the gold standard treatment of sphenoid wing meningiomas. Since the chance of total removal during a second operation is much smaller than during the first one and the complication rate higher, the objective of the operation should be the total removal of the meningioma at first surgery in every procedure. However, one should keep in mind that complete removal implies total removal of the tumor, including the dural attachment and bone that is involved by the tumor. The completeness of the surgical removal is the single most important prognostic factor. From our experience, hyperostotic bone must be considered as a tumoral bone.

However, this goal must always be tempered by surgical judgment, recognizing that the first priority is to try to preserve or improve neurologic function. Neurologic deficits can occur, even in experienced hands, but everything should be done to avoid them. Bone removal is not easy to achieve when the tumor goes far inferiorly into the cranio-facial cavities, encases the internal carotid artery, and its branches or the cranial nerves.

Indications for Alternative Therapies

Quality of life must always be kept in view, which is why other alternative treatments have been considered, such as radiotherapy, radiosurgery, hormonal therapy, and chemotherapy.[23–27] For patients in whom total removal of the tumor carries significant risk of morbidity, it is better to leave some tumor and plan to observe the patient. In some patients the tumor may remain stable indefinitely. In others reoperation at a future date or radiosurgery is indicated. Radiosurgery has nowadays accumulated enough patients treated and length of follow-up. Radiosurgery, especially with the Leksell Gamma Knife device, can be considered as a safe and effective treatment for focal tumors left in place along the sphenoid wing that allows tumor shrinkage and clinical improvement in short-term and long-term observation.[24,26] The cavernous sinus is for us an important surgical boundary, beyond which surgery is rarely performed. We consider a new postoperative diplopia as a major deficit. This is the reason why we recommend limiting the surgical resection to the extracavernous portion of the meningioma when it is obviously impossible to achieve a total removal without injuring the internal carotid artery and/or cranial nerves. In that situation, we apply Leksell Gamma Knife radiosurgery on the small tumor remnant located in the cavernous sinus.

For indications for other alternative therapies, such as chemo- or hormonal therapy, there are no randomized prospective data.[1,23] It is too early to draw any conclusion or advice in this regard, but these options should be kept in mind for the future.

Indications for Specific Approaches

Neuronavigation is helpful in sphenoid wing meningioma surgery because of the fixed bony landmarks, which can help safely localize the carotid artery and its major branches during the microdissection, especially when they are encased by the tumor. Image guidance has become a new standard in skull base neurosurgery in our practice.

Anesthesia Technique

Patients are operated on under general anesthesia using intravenous Pentothal, sufentanyl, and cis-atracrium. After endotracheal intubation anesthesia is maintained with isoflurane. Venous and arterial blood pressures are monitored through central venous and radial arterial lines. Administration of an anticonvulsant medication (Diphenylhydantoin 1 g) and antibiotics (Cefazoline 2 g) is started with the general anesthesia. After induction of anesthesia and insertion of a catheter in the bladder, 10–20 mg of furosemide are given and 100 g of mannitol are administered intravenously during the exposure. Two doses of Sólumedrol 40 mg are administered further during surgery. Lumbar CSF drainage is no longer performed since microdissection allows one to open the basal cistern with sufficient brain relaxation.

Neurophysiologic Monitoring

Intraoperative neurophysiologic monitoring is not mandatory for surgery of sphenoid wing meningiomas. However, EMG monitoring with electrodes directly inserted into the lateral rectus, superior rectus, and superior oblique muscles may be helpful when the meningioma invades the orbit or has some intimate contacts with the third and fourth cranial nerves.

Surgical Procedure

The key considerations in tumor removal include: (1) careful positioning of the patient and a well planned incision to give adequate exposure; (2) early interruption of the blood supply to the tumor; (3) internal decompression of the tumor using the cavitron, cautery loops, and/or bipolar coagulation; (4) careful dissection of the tumor capsule, gradually displacing it into the area of decompression, dividing vascular and arachnoid attachments as they are encountered, and minimizing retraction on the surrounding brain tissue; (5) removal of involved dura and bone when possible; and (6) reconstruction of dural defects, when indicated, with a free graft of pericranial tissue or fascia.

Patient Positioning and Initial Exposure

The patient lies in a supine position with the head fixed in a Mayfield clamp to secure it from any movement. Except for groups D and E, which are close to convexity, we open widely the basal cisterns to help the brain relaxation. In groups B and C, the head is turned about 30 degrees to the opposite side (45 degrees in groups D and E), moderately hyperextended and elevated from heart level by giving a 20-degree angle to the table. When neuronavigation is used, reference points are registered and the microscope is calibrated at that stage.

The choice of the opening is chosen according to careful preoperative neuroradiological study. We prefer a simple large pterional flap for most of sphenoid wing meningiomas keeping the frontal sinus intact, allowing for easy entry into the orbit by removal of the lateral roof and wall, keeping the periorbita intact. When the tumor invades the orbit and the periorbita, we use a pteriono-orbital approach, which can be extended to the zygoma.

In the pterional approach, we deflect the skin, galea, pericranium, and muscle in one layer to avoid injury to the frontal branch of the facial nerve.[28] For the pteriono-orbital flap, great care is taken to preserve the supraorbital nerve. When the zygoma has to be sectioned, the superficial and deep layers of the fascia temporalis are incised along the zygomatic arch 10 mm posterior and parallel to the course of the frontal branches of the facial nerve. The arch is then dissected subperiostally, and cut. The muscle can be detached from the temporal fossa and retracted downward or kept on the bone flap when we want to keep them both together.

A technical detail concerning the key-hole is that the burr hole should ideally be placed to expose the orbit and the frontal fossa simultaneously. One must see through it the orbital roof separating the periorbita from the frontal dura.

Exposure of the Tumor and Resection

The dura is opened under the microscope in a semicircular fashion centered on the pterion.

Group B and C meningiomas. In groups B and C, the sylvian fissure is opened. Frontal and temporal lobes are separated and gently kept away with a self-retaining retractor. Great care is taken to protect the sylvian veins. We always search for the distal branches of middle cerebral artery first which we follow from the distal to medial direction. This is a safe maneuver to find the middle and anterior cerebral arteries and then the internal carotid artery itself. By going straight on the skull base, one can injure the carotid artery and the optic nerve. Neuronavigation will perhaps modify that concept, but in the meantime we find it safer to go distally first. The tumor is debulked either with the ultrasonic aspirator or with bipolar cutting or coagulation and scissors when the tumor consistency is hard. Great care must be taken with the adjacent arteries and nerves when using the ultrasonic aspirator. This instrument does not differentiate between the tumor and the surrounding critical neurovascular structures as can the surgeon! Every small artery must be preserved and dissected. Lenticulostriate arteries may be stretched or encased and are very fragile. By following the arteries, the brain is progressively separated from the meningioma, giving access to the optic nerves and tract, which are dissected. Similarly, the pituitary stalk displaced medially by the tumor is dissected and preserved. We never lose the arachnoidal membranes during dissection. They represent the best natural protection for arteries and cranial nerves and are very useful for separating the third cranial nerve, the posterior communicating artery, and anterior thalamic or lenticulostriate perforating arterial branches.

When the tumor mass has been removed, the invaded dura and bone are resected. We stop at the boundary of the cavernous sinus, whose lateral and superior walls are often superficially involved. It is possible to peel these walls to achieve aggressive tumor removal with cautious bipolar coagulation. The last problem concerns bone and orbital invasion. The whole hyperostotic bone should be removed from the pterion

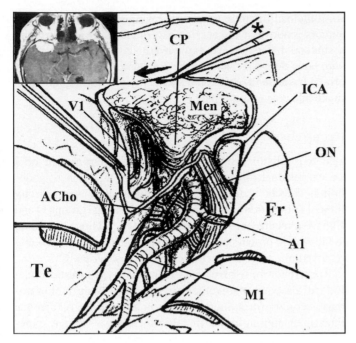

FIG. 39-2. Drawing showing a left-sided operative view after the resection of a middle sphenoid wing meningioma (Men) extending to the anterior clinoid process (CP) and just before the removal of the dura (*) covering the sphenoid wing. The temporal (Te) and frontal (Fr) brain retractors allow to see the internal carotid artery (ICA), the anterior cerebral artery (A1), the middle cerebral artery (M1), the optic and ophtalmic nerves (ON and V1 respectively), and the anterior choroidal artery (ACho)

to the sphenoid body by opening the foramen rotundum, the foramen ovale, and the superior orbital fissure whenever necessary. The use of high-speed drills with diamond burrs and irrigation is recommended. One should be very cautious with Zinn's common tendinous ring, whose removal compromises the ocular mobility and stability. The supraorbital rim and orbital roof may be removed and the optic canal opened. In group B and C (largely invading) meningiomas, the anterior clinoidal process must absolutely be removed since it is very often the starting point of recurrence. When the tumor spreads into the lower part of the orbit and the nasoethmoidal cells, a second operation through an anterior approach[11] is a possibility. An alternative is a combined fronto-temporal and lateral infratemporal fossa approach to the skull base[28] or a transmalar or transzygomatic approach through a subciliary incision (Figs. 39-3 and 39-4).[10]

Group D meningiomas. Group D meningiomas are easier to remove. The sylvian fissure is superficially opened. The only difficulty may come from the dural entry point of the sylvian veins into the sphenoparietal sinus. In the absence of preoperative MR venography revealing other collateral veins allowing division of the sylvian vein, it must absolutely be preserved with a piece of dura around it, sometimes with a small nub of tumor left in place.

Group E meningiomas. In group E, the operation will essentially concern bone, dura, and periorbita. A very wide opening of the roof and lateral wall of the orbit must be performed, taking care to keep the periorbita intact. After removal of as much hyperostotic bone as possible with the help of drills, one

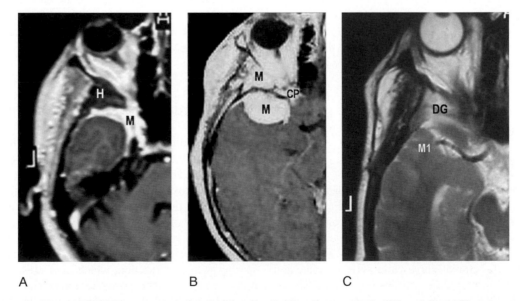

A   B   C

FIG. 39-3. Preoperative T1-weighted MR sequences after Gd injection (A, B) and postoperative T2-weighted MR sequences (C) of a middle sphenoid wing meningioma (M) with hyperostosis (H) extending to the left anterior clinoid process (CP). C shows the dural graft (DG) into the empty space left by drilling of the hyperostosis and the proximity of the M1 segment of the middle cerebral artery (M1)

is ready to open the periorbita. If done earlier, orbital fat will herniate and reduce the surgical space. When involved, the periorbita must be removed, but care should be taken not to injure extraocular muscles and Zinn's annulus. Finally, these tumors may sometimes invade maxillary and malar bones and require complex surgery.

Closure and Reconstruction

Closure must be planned before surgery. But before closing, one should have a very clean operative field, without any bleeding from the skull base. Hemostasis should be meticulous. The dura is sutured in a watertight manner either primarily or with pericranial or fascia lata graft. If the sinus cavities have been opened, they should be plugged with muscle or fat. If the opening is wide, and it is covered with a sutured dural graft. Any potential CSF leakage should be avoided. Bone flap is cosmetically replaced using either nonresorbable sutures or microplates whose location has been planned before opening the bone. When cut, the zygomatic arch is reattached with microplates. Orbital rim can nicely be reconstructed with either a rib or a piece of split bone flap of the convexity. The temporal muscle is sutured to the fascia at the orbital rim and along the temporal bone when separated from the skin. Otherwise, it is sutured at its posterior margin only and the skin closed in two layers.

Postoperative Care

These patients should be monitored in the intensive care unit for a minimum of 24 hours. During the first postoperative day, we usually perform a CT scan to assess for postoperative hematoma or pneumocephalus. When the main arteries have been dissected, ultrasonic Doppler is performed daily for one week for presence of vasospasm. Most patients are given steroids at least 48 hours before the operation and longer if there is significant brain edema. Postoperatively, the steroids are tapered off over 5 days or longer, depending on the degree of cerebral edema and the patient's condition.

Outcome/Complications

Complication Rate and Quality of Tumor Removal

The complication rate of lateral and middle sphenoid wing meningiomas is much lower than that of clinoid and medial sphenoid wing meningiomas. We reported no mortality in the series, including those which extended to the clinoid process (groups B and C). Groups D and E showed no morbidity, especially for the cranial nerves and sylvian veins, and the removal was total in all cases (Simpson grade I). Groups B and C showed 37% of patients with visual impairment and oculomotor palsy. The rate of total removal (Simpson grade I and II) was 50% in group B, while partial removal

was obtained in group C sphenoid wing meningiomas. Other authors report that in cases of cavernous sinus involvement, a subtotal but extensive extracavernous removal combined with bony decompression of the cranial nerves at the superior orbital fissure and optic canal frequently produced good functional and cosmetic results.[14]

Recurrence

One must distinguish true recurrence from regrowth of a known residual tumor. MR imaging with injection of gadolinium detects recurrence. Meningiomas that were strictly limited to the middle and lateral sphenoid wing (groups D and E) have a recurrence rate of less than 10%.[25] Those extending to the clinoid process or the cavernous sinus may be subtotally removed in a large number of cases in most series.[1,2,4–13]

Recurrence may also arise from the hyperostotic bone. Indeed, osseous involvement in sphenoid wing meningiomas accounts for subtotal resection and higher recurrence rates than meningiomas in other locations.[14] In our experience, we have observed that recurrence of lateral and middle sphenoid wing meningiomas extending medially usually starts from the anterior clinoid process. Therefore, resecting the anterior clinoid process might help to reduce the recurrence rate.[4,5]

Simpson et al. have observed a recurrence rate of 9% for patients with total removal of the tumor, including the site of attachment.[22] For patients with total removal of the tumor except for the site of dural attachment, which was simply cauterized, the recurrence rate was 19%. Interestingly, recurrence usually happens, on average, 5 years after surgery. Recurrence after 10–15 years is very unusual. Tumor recurrence in patients who had gross total removal of the intradural mass, but no resection or coagulation of the dural attachment site or involved bone, were noted in 29% of cases. Recurrence could also be due to regional multicentricity, which could explain some recurrences after initial removal which was thought to be "total."

Complication Avoidance/Lessons Learned

One of the main risks of this surgery is missing some important preoperative information regarding the tumor extension and the intimate relationship with cranial nerves and vessels. That can be avoided by a meticulous clinical and radiologic evaluation. If the surgical exposure is not adapted to the specific location of meningioma, removal will be hazardous or suboptimal.

Frontal branch of the facial nerve. Every detail is important, starting with skin incision, which must preserve the branches of the facial nerve. Bad cosmetic results may happen with bone removal without adequate reconstruction. However, it is mandatory to remove all the hyperostotic bone to protect against recurrence. Therefore, frontal, pterional, facial, and orbital repair is often necessary. We do not hesitate to do it in collaboration with surgeons specialized in cosmetic correction.

Watertight dural suture. CSF fistula may lead to meningitis and may compromise the results of superb tumor removal. A meticulous technique is necessary for sinus plugging and dural repair.

Brain retraction. Exposing the sphenoid wings requires some surgical room. We gain it by making a large enough basal bone opening, by putting the head in the correct position, and by CSF aspiration by opening the sylvian and opticochiasmatic fissures. The greatest enemy of the neurosurgeon is the brain retractor, which may cause extended neurologic deficits.

Oculomotor and optic nerves. A postoperative diplopia is a major handicap. To avoid it, great care must be taken with third and fourth cranial nerve dissection and the cavernous sinus exploration. A postoperative loss of vision is highly disabling. We never put any retractor on the optic nerve. We do it slightly on the carotid artery and pay attention when drilling the optic canal. We always provide copious irrigation to prevent thermal injury of the nerve.

Perforating arteries. Motor deficit may occur if anterior thalamic or lenticulostriate arteries are injured. One must be sure that the vessel is going to the meningioma only before coagulating and dividing it. This is not easy with stretched or encased vessels, but patience is our best ally.

Summary

Since the chance of total removal during a second operation is much smaller than during the first one and the complication rate higher, the most appropriate surgical treatment of lateral and middle sphenoid wing meningiomas, and the objective in every procedure, should be total removal of the meningioma at first surgery. One should keep in mind that complete removal implies total removal of the tumor, including the dural attachment and bone that is involved with the tumor. The completeness of surgical removal is the single most important prognostic factor. However, this goal must always be tempered by surgical judgment, recognizing that the first priority is to try to preserve or improve neurologic function. For this reason it is very important to adapt the strategy correctly with a complete and accurate preoperative workup.

References

1. Al-Mefty O, ed. Meningiomas. New York: Raven Press Ltd., 1991.
2. Ojemann RG. Meningiomas: clinical features and surgical management. In: Wilkins RH, Rengachary SS, eds. Neurosurgery. New York: McGraw-Hill, 1985:635–654.
3. Schmidek HH, ed. Meningiomas and Their Surgical Management. Philadelphia: W B Saunders Company, 1991.
4. Bonnal J, Brotchi J, Born J. Meningiomas of the sphenoid wings. In: Sekhar LN, Schramm VL Jr., eds. Tumors of the Cranial Base: Diagnosis and Treatment. Mount Kisco, NY: Futura Publishing, 1987:373–392.
5. Bonnal J, Thibaut A, Brotchi J, Born J. Invading meningiomas of the sphenoid ridge. J Neurosurg 1980;53:587–599.
6. Brotchi J, Bonnal J. Lateral and middle sphenoid wing meningiomas. In: Al-Mefty O, ed. Meningiomas. New York: Raven Press, 1991:413–425.
7. Brotchi J, Levivier M, Raftopoulos C, Noterman J. Invading meningiomas of sphenoid wings. What must we know before surgery? Acta Neurochir 1991;(Suppl. 53):98–100.
8. Cushing H, Eisenhardt L. Meningiomas: Their Classification, Regional Behaviour, Life History and Surgical Results. Springfield, IL: Charles C Thomas, 1938.
9. Al-Mefty O. Clinoidal meningiomas. J Neurosurg 1990;73: 840–849.
10. Basso AJ, Carrizo A. Sphenoid ridge meningiomas. In: Schmidek HH, ed. Meningiomas and Their Surgical Management. Philadelphia: W.B. Saunders Company, 1991:233–241.
11. Derome PJ, Guiot G. Bone problems in meningiomas invading the base of the skull. Clin Neurosurg 1978;25:435–451.
12. Ojemann RG. Surgical management of olfactory groove, suprasellar and medial sphenoid wing meningiomas. In: Schmidek HH, ed. Meningiomas and Their Surgical Management. Philadelphia: WB Saunders Company, 1991:242–259.
13. Philippon J, Bataini JP, Cornu P, et al. [Recurrent meningioma]. Neurochirurgie 1986;32 (Suppl 1):1–84.
14. Roser F, Nakamura M, Jacobs C, et al. Sphenoid wing meningiomas with osseous involvement. Surg Neurol 2005;64:37–43.
15. Shrivastava RK, Sen C, Costantino PD, Della Rocca R. Sphenoorbital meningiomas: surgical limitations and lessons learned in their long-term management. J Neurosurg 2005; 103:491–497.
16. Bozzao A, Finocchi V, Romano A, et al. Role of contrast-enhanced MR venography in the preoperative evaluation of parasagittal meningiomas. Eur Radiol 2005;15:1790–1796.
17. Neumaier Probst E, Grzyska U, Westphal M, Zeumer H. Preoperative Embolization of intracranial meningiomas with a fibrin glue preparation. AJNR Am J Neuroradiol 1999;20: 1695–1702.
18. Engelhard HH. Progress in the diagnosis and treatment of patients with meningiomas. Part I: Diagnostic imaging, preoperative embolization. Surg Neurol 2001;55:89–101.
19. Latchaw RE. Preoperative intracranial meningioma embolization: technical considerations affecting the risk-to-benefit ratio. AJNR Am J Neuroradiol 1993;14:583–586.
20. Richter H-P, Schachenmayr W. Preoperative embolization of intracranial meningiomas. Neurosurgery 1983;13:261–268.
21. Wakhloo AK, Jüngling FD, Velthoven van V, et al. Extended preoperative polyvinyl alcohol microembolization of intracranial meningiomas: assessment of two embolization techniques. AJNR Am J Neuroradiol 1993;14:571–582.
22. Simpson D: The recurrence of intracranial meningiomas after surgical treatment. J Neurol Neurosurg Psychiatry 1957;20:22–39.
23. Hahn BM, Schrell UM, Sauer R, et al. Prolonged oral hydroxyurea and concurrent 3d-conformal radiation in patients with progressive or recurrent meningioma: results of a pilot study. J Neurooncol 2005;74:157–165.
24. Metellus P, Regis J, Muracciole X, et al. Evaluation of fractionated radiotherapy and gamma knife radiosurgery in cavernous sinus meningiomas: treatment strategy. Neurosurgery 2005;57:873–886.

25. Morita A, Coffey RJ, Foote RL, et al. Risk of injury to cranial nerves after gamma knife radiosurgery for skull base meningiomas: experience in 88 patients. J Neurosurg 1999;90: 42–49.

26. Roche PH, Regis J, Dufour H, et al. Gamma knife radiosurgery in the management of cavernous sinus meningiomas. J Neurosurg 2000;93(Suppl 3):68–73.

27. Zachenhofer I, Wolfsberger S, Aichholzer M, et al. Gamma-knife radiosurgery for cranial base meningiomas: experience of tumor control, clinical course, and morbidity in a follow-up of more than 8 years. Neurosurgery 2006;58:28–36.

28. Mickey B, Close L, Schaefer S, Samson D. A combined fronto-temporal and lateral infratemporal fossa approach to the skull base. J Neurosurg 1988;68:678–684.

40
Orbitosphenoid Meningiomas

Eric H. Sincoff and Johnny B. Delashaw, Jr.

Introduction

Orbitosphenoid meningiomas present a challenge to the neurosurgeon in terms of surgical management and treatment options. To assist the neurosurgeon devise an optimal treatment plan for patients that present with an orbitosphenoid meningioma, collaboration with colleagues from otolaryngology, ophthalmology, plastic surgery, and radiation oncology is essential. Orbitosphenoid meningiomas were described by Cushing and Eisenhardt in 1938[1] as meningioma en plaque. Over the past several decades, as understanding of the associated anatomy and pathology of these lesions has developed,[2] overall knowledge of these lesions has also improved. In the last 20 years advancements in skull base approaches, such as neuronavigation and modern imaging techniques, have allowed surgeons to be more aggressive with regard to primary resection of these lesions.[3] While complete surgical excision of meningiomas with preservation of function continues to be the surgical goal, sphenoid wing meningiomas with orbital extension have historically exhibited high rates of recurrence, estimated at 35–50%.[4–6] Advances in stereotactic radiation techniques have allowed patients a longer recurrence and symptom-free interval, but these tumors present difficulty because of their proximity to the optic nerve.[7–9] This chapter will focus on the surgical and nonsurgical management of orbitosphenoid meningiomas, and a few case examples are presented.

Special Considerations

Description and Presentation

As with all meningiomas, orbitosphenoid meningiomas arise from arachnoid cap cells that are associated with the arachnoid granulations and follow neural structures through their foramina.[10] Orbitosphenoid meningiomas are usually secondary lesions of the orbit arising from the sphenoid. This is in comparison to the rarer primary meningiomas of the orbit that arise

from the optic nerve sheath and then spread to the sphenoid bone producing hyperostosis.[11] Orbitosphenoid meningiomas can be considered a subtype of the more general classification of sphenoid wing meningiomas and are essentially sphenoid wing meningiomas with orbital extension. A classification scheme for sphenoid wing meningiomas was first proposed by Cushing and Eisenhardt in 1938 and describes the inner or clinoidal, the middle or alar, and the outer or pterional meningiomas.[1,8] Since that time, several classification schemes for sphenoid wing meningiomas have been described. However, Cushing and Eisenhardt's original description provides a useful starting point with which to describe orbitosphenoid meningiomas. Orbitosphenoid meningiomas may originate from any and all of the subtypes described by Cushing, but usually are associated with the en plaque (or hyperostosing) meningiomas of the lateral sphenoid wing[12] that have extension into the orbit and often involve the cavernous sinus. These lesions can involve the orbital apex with associated hyperostosis compressing the contents of the orbit and the optic nerve.[2] Furthermore, these lesions can extend into the anterior, middle, infratemoporal/zygomatic fossae as well as the paranasal sinuses.

Orbitosphenoid meningiomas, as with most meningiomas, are more common in females.[2,3,12] The most common presenting complaint is proptosis and retroorbital pain.[3,4,8,13] Patients may also present with optic neuropathy, which is more common in recurrent cases, decreased facial sensation in the maxillary and ophthalmic divisions of the trigeminal nerve due to cavernous sinus involvement, and diplopia.[4] Visual field deficits tend to occur in cases with optic nerve compression and/or encasement.[14]

Relevant Anatomy

A discussion of the relevant anatomy pertaining to orbitosphenoid meningiomas is essential in presenting their surgical and nonsurgical management. The bony orbit is comprised of seven bones: ethmoid, frontal, lacrimal, maxilla, palatine, sphenoid, and zygomatic (Fig. 40-1A). The optic canal lies at the

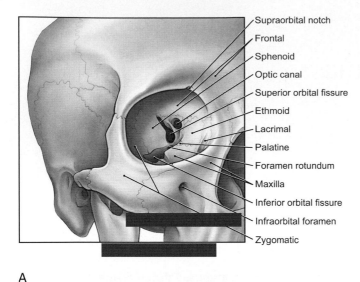

A

B

Fig. 40-1. (A) Diagramatic representation of the right orbit, from an anterior perspective. The seven bones that make up the orbit (ethmoid, frontal, lacrimal, maxilla, palatine, sphenoid, and zygomatic) are visible. The superior and inferior orbital fissures are also visible. (B) Diagrammatic representation of the orbital apex, from an anterior perspective, detailing CN III, IV, V1, V2, and VI. Additionally, the optic nerve can be seen passing through the annular tendon to which the extraocular muscles attach. The superior and inferior divisions of CN III, nasocilliary nerve, and CN VI also pass through the annular tendon

superomedial orbital apex and through it pass the optic nerve and ophthalmic artery. The superior orbital fissure is bounded by the greater and lesser wings of the sphenoid and medially by the sphenoid body. The optic strut separates the superior orbital fissure from the optic canal. Through the superior orbital fissure the III, IV, V1, VI cranial nerves and superior ophthalmic vein pass. The inferior orbital fissure, bounded by the greater wing of the sphenoid, body of sphenoid, maxilla, zygomatic, and palatine bones, does not communicate with the intracranial space. Through the inferior orbital fissure pass the zygomatic and infraorbital branches of the maxillary nerve and the inferior ophthalmic vein (Fig. 40-1B).

The dura of the middle fossa passes through the superior orbital fissure to become the periorbita of the orbit. This periorbita encases the orbital contents and is contiguous with the periosteum of the skull. The annular tendon surrounds

the optic foramen at the orbital apex and is adjacent to the superior orbital fissure. All of the extraocular muscles except the inferior oblique have their insertion on the annular tendon. Through the annular tendon pass cranial nerves II, the inferior and superior divisions of III, VI, and the nasociliary nerve. The lacrimal and frontal branches of V1 and cranial nerve IV do not pass through the annular tendon (Fig. 40-1B).

Most approaches for orbitosphenoid meningiomas involve a supralateral approach with resection of the lateral and superior orbital walls and involve opening the bony superior orbital fissure. Opening of the superior orbital fissure is a natural extension of sphenoid wing resection. This resection can, if necessary, be carried medially if resection of the clinoid is required or if opening the optic canal is required. Tumors invading the periorbita that actually extend into the orbital contents necessitating surgical exploration of the orbit require familiarity with the detailed anatomy of the orbit. The relevant surgical anatomy of the orbit is through a superior and lateral perspective. Approaching the orbit superiorly via resection of the orbital roof, the first structure encountered overlying the levator palpebrae is the frontal nerve. More laterally overlying the lateral rectus lies the lacrimal nerve. The abducens nerve enters the lateral rectus via its medial surface, and lying medial to the abducens nerve is the inferior division of the oculomotor nerve located deep to the superior rectus and supplying the inferior and medial rectus muscles. Overlying the superior oblique is the trochlear nerve, and deep to the superior oblique, lies the anterior extension of the nasociliary nerve with its medial branches, and anterior and posterior ethmoidal nerves (Fig. 40-2). Since the density of critical neural structures is greater laterally than medially, approaches

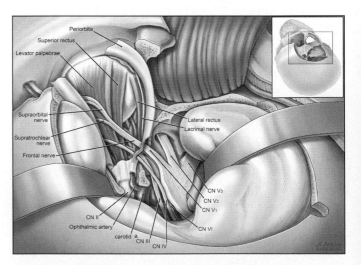

Fig. 40-2. Diagramatic representation of the orbit from a superolateral surgical perspective as would be observed in a modified orbitozygomatic craniotomy after resection of the orbital roof and anterior clinoid. The levator palpebrae muscle is visible with the overlying frontal nerve. The lateral rectus and superior rectus muscles are also visible. The exposure extends to the cavernous sinus where CN III, IV, V1, V2, and VI are visible. The cavernous carotid is seen passing within the cavernous sinus beneath the clinoid

to the orbital contents should proceed medially, although this is not always possible.

The superior orbital fissure lies at the anterior extent of the cavernous sinus through which cranial nerves III, IV, V1, and VI pass. Except for cranial nerve VI, the cranial nerves lie in the lateral wall of the cavernous sinus between the dura propria and the cerebral dura. These two layers of the dura can be separated and present a cleavage plane extending from the superior orbital fissure anteriorly to the foramen ovale posteriorly, allowing meningiomas that have not penetrated the cavernous sinus and the associated cranial nerve sheaths of the lateral cavernous sinus wall to be resected (Fig. 40-2). The dura of the superior wall of the cavernous sinus extends anteriorly over the optic canal as the falciform ligament and posteriorly as the anterior and posterior petroclinoid folds that blend into the tentorium (Fig. 40-3). Within the cavernous sinus lies the cavernous carotid artery and cranial nerve VI. The cavernous sinus can be entered via the Parkinson's triangle between cranial nerves IV and V1. However, we do not advocate this unless the patient has nonfunctional vision of the associated eye. Also relevant is the anterolateral triangle bounded by cranial nerves V1 (medial border) and V2 (lateral bordes). The middle fossa bone forming the floor of the anteromedial triangle is the lateral wall of the sphenoid sinus (Fig. 40-4).

Imaging

Imaging of orbitosphenoid meningiomas typically involve magnetic resonance (MR) imaging to define the extent of the lesion and the lesion's relationship to the surrounding structures.[15] Computed tomography (CT) imaging can play a special role in defining the degree of hyperostosis of the sphenoid bone and orbit but cannot be relied upon to exclude residual or recurrent meningioma.[4] Orbitosphenoid meningiomas can present on CT scans and MR images with hyperostosis alone with absent dural

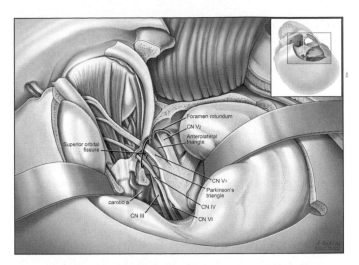

Fig. 40-4. The cavernous sinus showing Parkinson's triangle between IV and V1 through which the cavernous sinus may be entered. Also visible is the anterolateral triangle bounded by V1 and V2 through which the sphenoid sinus can be entered

enhancement. The imaging characteristics can on occasion be mistaken for fibrous dysplasia. These patients can also present similarly with proptosis and diplopia.

Assessment of the size of the paranasal sinuses surrounding the superiomedial and medial orbit as well as the sphenoid sinus may also alert the clinician to a meningioma involving the orbit or sphenoid. These paranasal sinuses can enlarge as a reaction to the meningioma in a condition called pneumosinus dilitans and may alert the clinician to perform further imaging, especially in patients presenting with visual symptoms and optic neuropathy.[16,17] Angiography can play a role if embolization or carotid sacrifice is being contemplated.[18]

Pathology

Orbitosphenoid meningiomas have similar predisposing characteristics to other meningiomas including prevalence in females, ionizing radiation, and type 2 neurofibromatosis.[18] These lesions can have extensive interosseous involvement without dural involvement resulting in proptosis and optic nerve compression.[19] Changes can occur in the optic disc and the surrounding fundus, and optic disc edema and optociliary veins in the setting of progressive visual loss may be observed.[20]

Surgical Technique

Several surgical approaches to orbitosphenoid meningiomas have been described.[4,12,21–26] The extent of the involvement of the orbit, cavernous sinus and paranasal sinus, in addition to possible requirement for optic nerve decompression at the optic canal, dictate what type of approach is required. Smaller lesions can be addressed with a pterional craniotomy followed by opening the superior orbital fissure and optic canal as necessary. Lesions

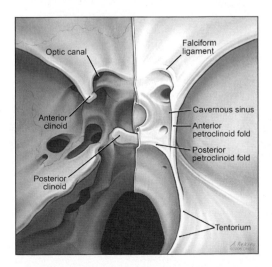

Fig. 40-3. A superior view of the optic canal, clinoid processes, cavernous sinus, and anterior and posterior petroclinoid folds as they blend into the tentorium

with a larger degree of orbital involvement may require an orbital osteotomy with exposure of the superior and lateral orbit. Lesions with paranasal sinus involvement may require a craniofacial approach and opening of the maxillary, sphenoid, and ethmoidal sinuses. Young patients presenting with nonfunctional vision due to large tumor burden within the orbit may undergo orbital exenteration to achieve curative resection.

We prefer the modified one-piece orbitozygomatic approach in which the orbital roof is fractured and an osteotomy of the frontal process of the zygomatic bone is performed. The remaining orbital roof is resected posteriorly as far as necessary to decompress the optic nerve and resect the tumor. We have not found an osteotomy of the zygomatic arch to improve exposure in most cases unless the tumor extends into the infratemporal fossa. Depending on the extent of the lesion, an osteoplastic technique can be utilized. An extradural clinoidectomy is preferred to an intradural clinoidectomy as it provides some protection to the optic nerve and can be performed with an extradural opening of the optic canal.[27–30]

Preoperative Evaluation

Patients with orbitosphenoid meningiomas require the usual preoperative clearance as for any craniotomy. To obtain an accurate preoperative assessment of patients' preoperative visual function, patients should have a preoperative neuro-ophthalmic assessment, including dilated fundus exam and

Goldmann peripheral field testing. Otolaryngologic evaluation should include CT of the sinuses if paranasal sinus involvement is an issue.

Surgical Technique

At induction we administer a 10-mg dose of dexamethasone. A first-generation cephalosporin is used for prophylaxis, in most cases. If a large paranasal sinus component is present and a craniofacial resection is required, we prefer to use an ampicllin-sulbactam or similar antibiotic regimen with continued use for 3 days postoperatively. To decrease the degree of brain retraction necessary, a lumbar drain is used in most cases.[31] The lumbar drain remains in place postoperatively in cases with sinus involvement requiring a craniofacial approach. As a caution, lumbar drains do have potential serious morbidity, especially when drainage is continued postoperatively.[32] Therefore, prolonged use of a lumbar drain postoperatively, must be weighed against the potential morbidity.

The surgical technique for a modified orbitozygomatic approach involves positioning the patient supine in a Mayfield headholder with the head slightly rotated contralateral to the side of surgery and with the neck extended. Craniofacial resection and requirements for free flap harvest, if necessary, must also be considered when positioning and draping. A minimal hair shave is performed just along the incision line. A bicoronal incision is planned from just anterior to the tragus extending to

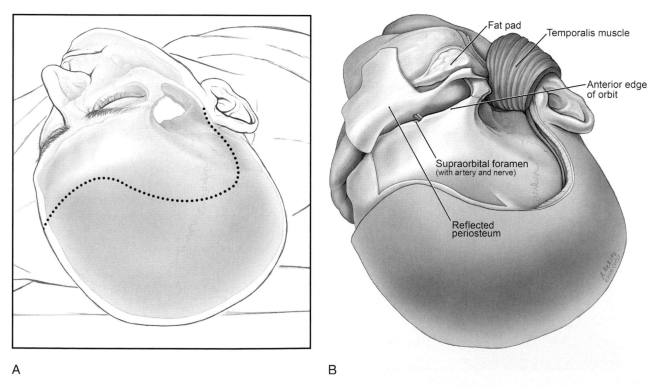

A   B

FIG. 40-5. (A) Diagramatic representation of patient positioning and the bicoronal skin incision. (B) Bicoronal skin incision and interfascial dissection have been performed and the temporalis muscle has been reflected inferiorly. The anterior edge of the orbit, the supraorbital nerve and the foramen are identified

the contralateral superior temporal line (Fig. 40-5A). We have observed and others have reported no increase in wound infections with a minimal hair shave.[33–35] The bicoronal incision is taken down through the galea but not the periosteum. The scalp flap is elevated utilizing an interfascial technique to protect the frontalis nerve.[36,37] Although others advocate a subfascial or submuscular technique,[38] we find the interfascial technique provides an easier plane to dissect over the zygoma. The periosteum is reflected as a separate layer and protected with moist 4 × 4 s. Towel clamps are used to secure the anteriorly reflected skin flap and are secured to a stockinette with rubber bands and Allis clamps attached to the operating table. The temporalis fascia and muscle are then incised and elevated in an inferior to superior manner to protect the deep temporalis neurovascular supply,[39,40] and retracted with a towel clamp (Fig. 40-5B). The periorbita is dissected off of the orbit superiorly and laterally, and the supraorbital nerve is dissected from its notch or fractured at its foramen. By using a cottonoid with an elevator between the inner bony surface of the orbit and the periorbita, it is often possible to prevent tearing of the periorbita.

Once the soft tissue dissection is completed, the craniotomy flap can be undertaken. Burr holes are drilled at the keyhole, the temporal squama, and just superior to the superior temporal line. Optionally, the keyhole burr hole can be drilled simultaneously into the orbit and the anterior fossa. The dura is then stripped from the undersurface of the flap. The initial cut is made with a craniotome with footplate and extends from the temporal squama burr hole superiorly to the burr hole just above the superior temporal line and anteriorly to the orbit just lateral to the supraorbital notch. The next cut extends from the temporal squama burr hole, parallel to the zygomatic arch and as low as possible on the temporal squama, anteriorly, and then turns superiorly towards the sphenoid ridge until stopped by the bony ridge. A cut then proceeds from the keyhole to the sphenoid ridge. The craniotome without the footplate attachment is then used to make the final cuts. A cut is made that extends across the orbital ridge and roof connecting to the initial cut made with the footplate attachment. Then a cut is made extending across the lateral orbital and frontal process of the zygoma ending at the keyhole. The final cut is across the sphenoid ridge so that it fractures when the flap is elevated (Fig. 40-6A). Osteotomes are then used at the orbital roof and the lateral orbital wall so that the orbital roof fractures easily when the flap is elevated and is fractured (Fig. 40-6B,C). Optionally, if the keyhole extends into the orbit, an inferiorly directed cut can be made along the lateral orbit ending at the

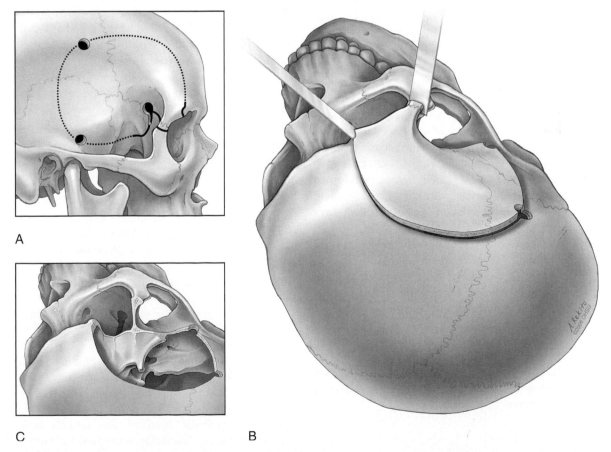

A

C   B

FIG. 40-6. (A) Modified one-piece orbito-zygomatic craniotomy burr hole placement: (------) drill with footplate, (——) drill without footplate. (B) Modified one-piece orbito-zygomatic craniotomy after the soft tissue work has been completed showing the bone cuts and fracturing technique for elevating the bone flap. (C) Schematic view of the skull with initial bone flap removed and partial resection of orbital roof

inferior orbital fissure and then extended anteriorly across the frontal process of the zygoma. Using this optional technique slightly more orbital exposure can be obtained.

In cases of nonfunctional vision in which there is widespread infiltration of the orbit, orbital exenteration may be undertaken.[41] Orbital exenteration proceeds first by extradurally identifying the optic nerve and ophthalmic artery. The optic nerve is then transected and the artery ligated and cut. Orbital exenteration can be undertaken intracranially or extracranially; we prefer the intracranial technique as it is a natural extension of the modified orbito-zygomatic craniotomy.[42] The orbital contents can then be resected by dissecting about the periorbita and removing the globe and surrounding orbital contents. In an attempt to improve cosmesis, resection of the eyelid is not routinely performed. Consideration of a forearm, abdominal rectus, or lattisimus dorsi free flap should be made when orbital exenteration is undertaken, especially in cases with paranasal sinus involvement.[43,44] In some cases the temporalis muscle and fascia can be used as a flap to seal off the orbit and sinuses, avoiding the need for microvascular anstomosis.[45]

If there is cavernous sinus involvement and the eye is nonfunctional, cavernous sinus exenteration may also be undertaken. We do not advocate exploration of the cavernous sinus in cases of functional vision and refer such patients for postoperative radiosurgery.[4] In cases where cavernous sinus exenteration is being contemplated, balloon test occlusion should be undertaken, and if indicated plans for extracranial to intracranial bypass made.[46]

Reconstruction of patients with large orbitosphenoid meningiomas with paranasal sinus involvement and/or orbital exenteration can represent a formidable challenge. Of primary concern is a watertight dural closure, supplemented if needed with a dural graft. Additionally, fibrin glue or one of the other dural sealant products presently available can be used to further seal the dural suture line. The temporalis muscle or a free flap can be used to seal the paranasal sinuses and orbit from the intranranial space in cases with large communications to the intracranial space. In cases without tumor involvement of the sinuses, but with entry into the frontal sinus, the vascularized pericranium can be used to seal off the frontal sinus by sandwiching it between the open sinus and the bone flap. The pericranium can also be used to seal off the ethmoidal air cells from the intracranial space if they are entered during resection. Any portion of the bone flap with hyperostosis or gross tumor involvement must be resected. The bone flap is then replaced and split calvarial bone graft, titanium mesh, and hydroxyapatite bone cement can be used to reconstruct the greater sphenoid wing and orbit as necessary.[2,3,42,47,48] In cases of complete involvement of the bone flap where it must be discarded, reconstruction can be undertaken at a later time with a computer generated flap.

Radiosurgery

Radiosurgery and conventional radiation can play a very important role in the management of patients with orbito-

sphenoid meningiomas.[4,6,8,9,46,49] Radiotherapy allows control of cavernous sinus and orbital disease in patients with functional vision. New techniques such as Cyberknife or a linear accelerator (LINAC) allow radiosurgery to be undertaken in a fractionated manner for orbital lesions.[50,51] Other radiosurgical techniques such as proton beam therapy can also be used.[7]

The role of chemotherapy for orbitosphenoid meningiomas and meningiomas in general remains to be defined. Hydroxyurea has been reported by some to control meningioma growth in cases of unresectability or recurrence.[52]

Case Examples

Case One

In this case example, we describe a 68-year-old female who presented with a 6-month history of right eye pain and headaches. On physical exam extraocular movements were intact and visual fields were full. The patient demonstrated no cranial nerve abnormalities with the exception of a slightly decreased sensation in the right V2 distribution. Remaining neurologic and physical exams were unremarkable.

MR imaging demonstrated a right-sided sphenoid wing meningioma with orbital involvement and associated hyperostosis (Fig. 40-7A, B). A right-sided pterional craniotomy was undertaken with resection of any hyperostotic bone. All dural tail attachments were canterized. Reconstruction was performed with titanium mesh and hydroxyapatite bone cement. Six-month follow-up MR images showed no evidence of tumor and the patient reported some headache relief (Fig. 40-7C, D).

Case Two

In this case example, we describe a 40-year-old female with a history of intermittent right eye ptosis and associated eye pain. On physical exam there was evidence of some mild right eye ptosis. Extraocular movements were full, and the patient demonstrated no visual field abnormalities. Remaining neurologic and physical exams were unremarkable.

MR imaging revealed a sphenoid wing meningioma with involvement of the anterior temporal dura (Fig. 40-8A, B). Additionally, there was hyperostosis of the sphenoid wing, orbital roof, and lateral orbital wall resulting in compression of the superior orbital fissure contents. It was felt that this compression was causing the oculomotor nerve dysfunction resulting in mild intermittent ptosis of the right eye. A modified orbito-zygomatic approach was initially contemplated, but concerns about fracturing a thickened orbital roof led to a decision to perform a pterional approach and drill off the orbital roof. The bone encountered was quite thickened and of abnormal texture. A large amount of bone was resected

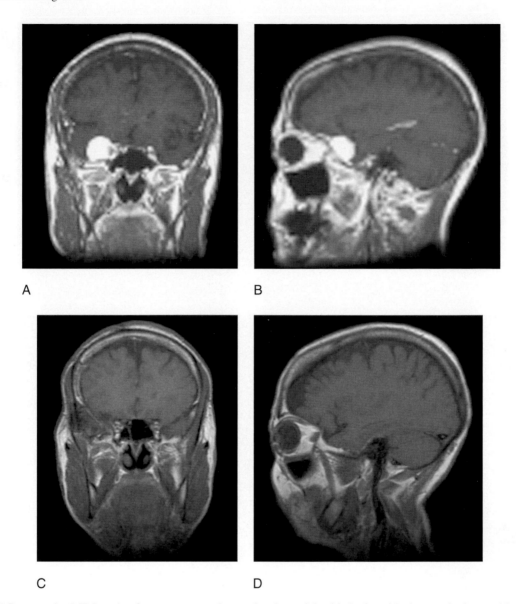

FIG. 40-7. (A, B) Preoperative MR imaging from case example one showing a right sided sphenoid wing meningioma with orbital extension. (C, D) Six-month follow-up MR imaging from case example one showing no evidence of recurrence

from the orbital roof, and the entire bony superior orbital fissure was opened. Additionally, some of the anterior clinoid was resected, but the optic canal was not opened as it was not compromised by hyperostotic bone. Once the extradural bone resection was completed, the anterior temporal dura was resected as it was involved with tumor. A dural graft was placed and the bone flap replaced after resecting from it the hyperostotic bone. Reconstruction was undertaken with titanium mesh and hydroxyapatite bone cement. Postoperative CT scan demonstrated good resection of hyperostotic bone (Fig. 40-8C, D).

Summary and Lessons Learned

Orbitosphenoid meningiomas are lesions that for the most part are sphenoid wing meningiomas with some degree of orbital involvement. Key elements that must be considered in the operative and nonoperative treatment of patients harboring such lesions include: preoperative visual function, degree of hyperostosis, optic canal involvement, cavernous sinus involvement, and paranasal sinus involvement. The experience of the senior author has changed the management of such lesions at our institution over the years.

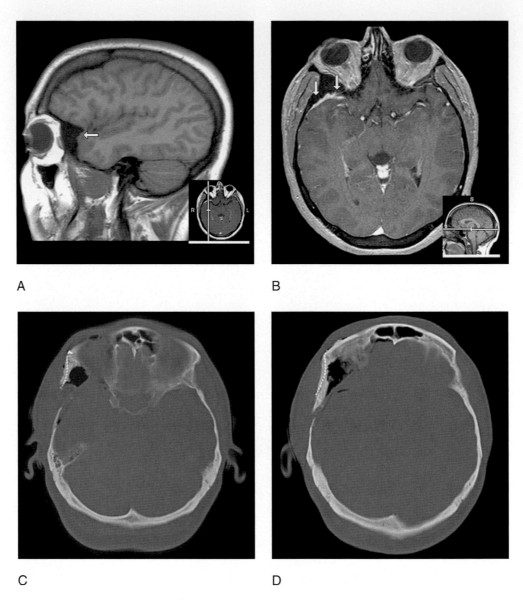

FIG. 40-8. (A, B) Preoperative MR imaging from case example two showing a right-sided sphenoid wing meningioma with associated hyperostosis and involvement of the superior orbital fissure and anterior temporal dura. (C, D) Postoperative CT from case example two showing good resection of hyperostotic bone

One of the lessons learned is that cavernous sinus exploration in a patient with functional vision is not worth the resulting ophthalmoplegia. Therefore, we do not enter the cavernous sinus unless the patient presents with nonfunctional vision. Instead, we resect the tumor not involved with the cavernous sinus and refer such patients for radiosurgery of the cavernous tumor. Another lesson learned is that in cases of extensive hyperostosis involving the orbital roof, a two-piece orbito-zygomatic craniotomy or a pterional craniotomy with extensive drilling of the orbital roof may be safer than our standard one-piece modified orbito-zygomatic craniotomy. The concern is that if the flap should fracture too posteriorly on the orbital roof, the optic nerve and carotid artery may be placed at risk. Furthermore, we do not advocate drilling the optic canal unless there is compromise of the canal by tumor or hyperostosis. Such drilling only places the uninvolved optic nerve at risk. In cases of optic canal and/or clinoidal involvement, we advocate an extradural approach to optic canal opening and clinoidectomy. We believe that an extradural approach affords some protection of the optic nerve and carotid during drilling.

The senior author's experience has also taught us not to underestimate the importance of cosmesis and appropriate reconstruction. We use titanium mesh and bone cement to reconstruct the resected sphenoid wing and use care in handling the temporalis muscle to avoid an unsightly temporal hollow. We have also noted that extensive orbital roof reconstruction is not necessary and that orbital pulsations resolve over time.

Orbitosphenoid meningiomas can represent difficult lesions for surgical and nonsurgical management. However, with knowledge of the associated anatomy and the collaboration of associated specialties, these lesions can be treated with good outcome.

References

1. Cushing H, Eisenhard L. Meningiomas: Their Classification, Regional Behavior, Life History, and Surgical End Results. Springfield, IL: Charles C Thomas, 1938.
2. Shrivastava RK, Sen C, Costantino PD, et al. Sphenoorbital meningiomas: surgical limitations and lessons learned in their long-term management. J Neurosurg 2005; 103(3):491–7.
3. Sandalcioglu IE, Gasser T, Mohr C, et al. Spheno-orbital meningiomas: interdisciplinary surgical approach, resectability and long-term results. J Craniomaxillofac Surg 2005; 33(4):260–6.
4. Maroon JC, Kennerdell JS, Vidovich DV, et al. Recurrent sphenoorbital meningioma. J Neurosurg 1994; 80(2):202–8.
5. Adegbite AB, Khan MI, Paine KW, et al. The recurrence of intracranial meningiomas after surgical treatment. J Neurosurg 1983; 58(1):51–6.
6. Mirimanoff RO, Dosoretz DE, Linggood RM, et al. Meningioma: analysis of recurrence and progression following neurosurgical resection. J Neurosurg 1985; 62(1):18–24.
7. Miralbell R, Cella L, Weber D, et al. Optimizing radiotherapy of orbital and paraorbital tumors: intensity-modulated X-ray beams vs. intensity-modulated proton beams. Int J Radiat Oncol Biol Phys 2000; 47(4):1111–9.
8. Abdel-Aziz KM, Froelich SC, Dagnew E, et al. Large sphenoid wing meningiomas involving the cavernous sinus: conservative surgical strategies for better functional outcomes. Neurosurgery 2004; 54(6):1375–83; discussion 83–4.
9. Bauman GS, Wong E. Re: new radiotherapy technologies for meningiomas: 3D conformal radiotherapy? Radiosurgery? Stereotactic radiotherapy? Intensity modulated radiotherapy? Proton beam radiotherapy? Spot scanning proton radiation therapy? Or nothing at all? [Radiother Oncol 2004;71(3):247–249]. Radiother Oncol 2004; 73(2):251–2.
10. Roser F, Nakamura M, Jacobs C, et al. Sphenoid wing meningiomas with osseous involvement. Surg Neurol 2005; 64(1):37–43.
11. Boulos P, Dumont AS, Mandell JW, Jane JA. Meningiomas of the orbit: contemporary considerations. Neurosurg Focus 2001;10(5).
12. Carrizo A, Basso A. Current surgical treatment for sphenoorbital meningiomas. Surg Neurol 1998; 50(6):574–8.
13. Honeybul S, Neil-Dwyer G, Lang DA, et al. Sphenoid wing meningioma en plaque: a clinical review. Acta Neurochir (Wien) 2001; 143(8):749–57; discussion 58.
14. Wilson WB. Meningiomas of the anterior visual system. Surv Ophthalmol 1981; 26(3):109–27.
15. Charbel FT, Hyun H, Misra M, et al. Juxtaorbital en plaque meningiomas. Report of four cases and review of literature. Radiol Clin North Am 1999; 37(1):89–100, x.
16. Miller NR, Golnik KC, Zeidman SM, et al. Pneumosinus dilatans: a sign of intracranial meningioma. Surg Neurol 1996; 46(5):471–4.
17. Lloyd GA. Orbital pneumosinus dilatans. Clin Radiol 1985; 36(4):381–6.
18. Black PM. Meningiomas. Neurosurgery 1993; 32(4):643–57.
19. Henchoz L, Borruat FX. Intraosseous meningioma: a rare cause of chronic optic neuropathy and exophthalmos. Klin Monatsbl Augenheilkd 2004; 221(5):414–7.
20. Ellenberger C. Perioptic meningiomas. Syndrome of long-standing visual loss, pale disk edema, and optociliary veins. Arch Neurol 1976; 33(10):671–4.
21. Columella F, Testa C, Andreoli A. Radical resection and reconstruction in spheno-ethmoidal-orbital tumors. Report of 3 cases. J Neurosurg Sci 1974; 18(3):198–205.
22. Day JD. Cranial base surgical techniques for large sphenocavernous meningiomas: technical note. Neurosurgery 2000; 46(3):754–9; discussion 9–60.
23. Honeybul S, Neil-Dwyer G, Lang DA, et al. The transzygomatic approach: a long-term clinical review. Acta Neurochir (Wien) 1995; 136(3–4):111–6.
24. Lauritzen C, Vallfors B, Lilja J. Facial disassembly for tumor resection. Scand J Plast Reconstr Surg 1986; 20(2):201–6.
25. Schepers S, Ioannides C, Fossion E. Surgical treatment of exophthalmos and exorbitism: a modified technique. J Craniomaxillofac Surg 1992; 20(7):313–6.
26. Seifert V, Dietz H. Combined orbito-frontal, sub- and infratemporal fossa approach to skull base neoplasms. Surgical technique and clinical application. Acta Neurochir (Wien) 1992; 114 (3–4):139–44.
27. Delashaw JB, Jr., Tedeschi H, Rhoton AL. Modified supraorbital craniotomy: technical note. Neurosurgery 1992; 30(6):954–6.
28. Delashaw JB, Jr., Jane JA, Kassell NF, et al. Supraorbital craniotomy by fracture of the anterior orbital roof. Technical note. J Neurosurg 1993; 79(4):615–8.
29. Schwartz MS, Anderson GJ, Horgan MA, et al. Quantification of increased exposure resulting from orbital rim and orbitozygomatic osteotomy via the frontotemporal transsylvian approach. J Neurosurg 1999; 91(6):1020–6.
30. Balasingam V, Noguchi A, McMenomey SO, et al. Modified osteoplastic orbitozygomatic craniotomy. Technical note. J Neurosurg 2005; 102(5):940–4.
31. Telischi FF, Landy H, Balkany TJ. Reducing temporal lobe retraction with the middle fossa approach using a lumbar drain. Laryngoscope 1995; 105(2):219–20.
32. Samadani U, Huang JH, Baranov D, et al. Intracranial hypotension after intraoperative lumbar cerebrospinal fluid drainage. Neurosurgery 2003; 52(1):148–51; discussion 51–2.
33. Dvilevicius AE, Machado S, do Rego JI, et al. [Craniotomy without trichotomy: analysis of 640 cases]. Arq Neuropsiquiatr 2004; 62(1):103–7.
34. Bekar A, Korfali E, Dogan S, et al. The effect of hair on infection after cranial surgery. Acta Neurochir (Wien) 2001; 143(6):533–6; discussion 7.
35. Siddique MS, Matai V, Sutcliffe JC. The preoperative skin shave in neurosurgery: is it justified? Br J Neurosurg 1998; 12(2):131–5.
36. Yasargil MG, Reichman MV, Kubik S. Preservation of the frontotemporal branch of the facial nerve using the interfascial temporalis flap for pterional craniotomy. Technical article. J Neurosurg 1987; 67(3):463–6.
37. Pekar L, Blaha M, Schwab J, et al. [Craniotomy and the temporal branch of the facial nerve]. Rozhl Chir 2004; 83(5):205–8.
38. Coscarella E, Vishteh AG, Spetzler RF, et al. Subfascial and submuscular methods of temporal muscle dissection and their relationship to the frontal branch of the facial nerve. Technical note. J Neurosurg 2000; 92(5):877–80.

39. Oikawa S, Mizuno M, Muraoka S, et al. Retrograde dissection of the temporalis muscle preventing muscle atrophy for pterional craniotomy. Technical note. J Neurosurg 1996; 84(2):297–9.
40. Kadri PA, Al-Mefty O. The anatomical basis for surgical preservation of temporal muscle. J Neurosurg 2004; 100(3):517–22.
41. Lin HF, Lui CC, Hsu HC, et al. Orbital exenteration for secondary orbital tumors: a series of seven cases. Chang Gung Med J 2002; 25(9):599–605.
42. McDermott MW, Durity FA, Rootman J, et al. Combined fronto-temporal-orbitozygomatic approach for tumors of the sphenoid wing and orbit. Neurosurgery 1990; 26(1):107–16.
43. Gok A, Erkutlu I, Alptekin M, et al. Three-layer reconstruction with fascia lata and vascularized pericranium for anterior skull base defects. Acta Neurochir (Wien) 2004; 146(1):53–6; discussion 6–7.
44. Izquierdo R, Origitano TC, al-Mefty O, et al. Use of vascularized fat from the rectus abdominis myocutaneous free flap territory to seal the dura of basicranial tumor resections. Neurosurgery 1993; 32(2):192–6; discussion 7.
45. Kiyokawa K, Tai Y, Inoue Y, et al. Efficacy of temporal musculopericranial flap for reconstruction of the anterior base of the skull. Scand J Plast Reconstr Surg Hand Surg 2000; 34(1):43–53.
46. George B, Ferrario CA, Blanquet A, et al. Cavernous sinus exenteration for invasive cranial base tumors. Neurosurgery 2003; 52(4):772–80; discussion 80–2.
47. Papay FA, Zins JE, Hahn JF. Split calvarial bone graft in cranio-orbital sphenoid wing reconstruction. J Craniofac Surg 1996; 7(2):133–9.
48. Leake D, Gunnlaugsson C, Urban J, et al. Reconstruction after resection of sphenoid wing meningiomas. Arch Facial Plast Surg 2005; 7(2):99–103.
49. Maguire PD, Clough R, Friedman AH, et al. Fractionated external-beam radiation therapy for meningiomas of the cavernous sinus. Int J Radiat Oncol Biol Phys 1999; 44(1):75–9.
50. Bhatnagar AK, Gerszten PC, Ozhasaglu C, et al. CyberKnife Frameless Radiosurgery for the treatment of extracranial benign tumors. Technol Cancer Res Treat 2005; 4(5):571–6.
51. Andrews DW, Faroozan R, Yang BP, et al. Fractionated stereotactic radiotherapy for the treatment of optic nerve sheath meningiomas: preliminary observations of 33 optic nerves in 30 patients with historical comparison to observation with or without prior surgery. Neurosurgery 2002; 51(4):890–902; discussion 3–4.
52. Schrell UM, Rittig MG, Anders M, et al. Hydroxyurea for treatment of unresectable and recurrent meningiomas. II. Decrease in the size of meningiomas in patients treated with hydroxyurea. J Neurosurg 1997; 86(5):840–4.

41
Cavernous Sinus Meningiomas: Conservative Surgical Management

Burak Sade and Joung H. Lee

Introduction

The idea that cavernous sinus meningiomas (CSM) might be operable lesions was revolutionized by the work of Dolenc in the 1980s.[1] Following his pioneering dissection techniques, the concept of aggressive resection of CSM gained popularity among many surgeons in late 1980s and early 1990s with the additional advances made in skull base surgery techniques.

Early Experience with Cavernous Sinus Meningiomas

O'Sullivan and colleagues reported total tumor resection in 8 of 39 patients.[2] These authors stated that the most important factor dictating the possibility of total resection was the involvement of the internal carotid artery (ICA). In their series, gross total removal could rarely be achieved due to the holocavernous extension of the tumor in most instances. Approximately 20% of their patients experienced new onset of cranial nerve deficits related to extraocular motility (EOM). In the subgroup of patients with more extensive involvement, and, therefore, in whom only subtotal resection was possible, new-onset oculomotor and trigeminal nerve deficits were seen in up to one third of the patients. Interestingly, with a mean follow-up of 2 years, tumor recurrence was seen in 25% of patients who had complete resection and in only 6% who had subtotal resection.

In the series of 38 patients with CSM, De Monte and colleagues achieved total resection in 76% of the patients.[3] From their raw data, the incidence of new-onset oculomotor and trigeminal nerve deficits were 13 and 19%, respectively. In the same series, one third of the patients with preoperative abducens nerve deficit improved. In 12 patients with more than 10 years of follow-up, both patients with subtotal resection showed regrowth, whereas the recurrence was seen in 10% of totally resected tumors.

De Jesus and colleagues reported on their experience with 119 patients, 61% of whom had total resection.[4] The cranial nerve outcome was not detailed in this study. However, the recurrence and regrowth rates were similar for the totally and subtotally resected meningiomas, respectively. With a mean follow-up of 34 months, recurrence was seen in 10% of patients who had total resection, whereas regrowth rate was 15% in those who underwent subtotal resection. The recurrence-free survival was 94% at 3 years and 81% at 5 years in the total resection group, whereas the rates were 87 and 62%, respectively, for the latter group.

The focus of the study by Knosp and colleagues, which consisted of 59 CSM, was on the cranial nerve outcome.[5] In their study, the extent of resection and the recurrence/regrowth data was not assessed. Their results showed that improvement of existing deficit was seen in 43% of oculomotor and 50% of abducens nerve palsies, whereas the deficit worsened in 58% of trochlear and 21% of the ophthalmic division of the trigeminal nerve. The improvement of the oculomotor nerve was only observed in partially impaired nerves, suggesting that decompression of the nerve should be addressed in a timely manner.

Changes in the Management Paradigm to a More Conservative Approach

More recently, a more conservative treatment management strategy has evolved for CSM. Couldwell and colleagues recommend subtotal resection and decompression of the cavernous sinus with the goal of improving the cranial nerve outcome, and minimizing the size of the tumor for subsequent radiosurgical treatment.[6] With the introduction of more conformal techniques, intensity-modulated radiation treatment and stereotactic radiosurgery have become important options for these lesions. Subtotal resection of the extra- and/or intracavernous component of the tumor, along with radiation therapy, have shown similar tumor control rates as earlier series with more extensive surgery, while exhibiting more favorable cranial nerve outcomes. Pamir and colleagues compared the outcome of patients who had undergone radical resection or subtotal resection with radiosurgery and those who were treated with radiosurgery alone.[7] They found that extracavernous resection followed by radiosurgery was as affective as radical surgery, and in terms of cranial nerve morbidity and third-year tumor volume control, conservative approach yielded better results.

In the series of Nicolato and colleagues in their experience with 122 patients who were treated with Gamma Knife radiosurgery either as the only treatment or as an adjunct to surgery, 5-year actuarial progression-free survival was 96.5% with a median follow-up of 4 years.[8] The median dose to the tumor margin was 14.6 Gy. Their results showed that the number of patients with shrinkage of the tumor following treatment showed an increase with a longer follow-up. In the series of Lee and colleagues on 159 patients, 5- and 10-year actuarial tumor control rates were reported as 93%.[9] The median dose to the tumor margin was 13 Gy. Neurological status improved 29% and worsened in 9% of the patients in this series. Maruyama and colleagues reported a 5–year actuarial tumor control rate of 94% with a median dose of 16 Gy.[10] The improvement of cranial nerve function was significantly better in the radiosurgery-alone group.

As an alternative to Gamma Knife, linear accelerator radiosurgery has also been reported as an effective treatment option. Spiegelmann and colleagues reported a 97% tumor control rate with a median follow-up of 36 months and mean radiation dose of 14 Gy to the tumor margin in 42 patients.[11] In this series, 4% of the patients had new-onset trigeminal neuropathy and 3% had new visual field defect. In the group with existing deficits, 29% of the patients with trigeminal neuropathy and 22% with oculomotor nerve palsy improved.

Brell and colleagues reported on their results of 30 patients who were treated with fractionated stereotactic radiotherapy.[12] The median radiation dose was 52 Gy, with a daily fraction

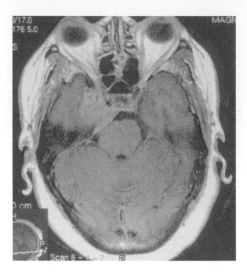

FIG. 41-1. Postcontrast T1-weighted axial image of a patient who presented with intermittent diplopia and visual blurring. The patient had a history of pulmonary sarcoidosis. In this case, the decision was to proceed with surgery with the goals of (1) definitive tissue diagnosis, (2) debulking of the mass for the improvement of future radiation treatment planning, and (3) decompression of cranial nerve's II and III.

of 2 Gy, and the median follow-up was 50 months. The 4-year actuarial local progression-free survival was 93%. Half of the patients had improvement of their symptoms, whereas 7% deteriorated. In the study of Metellus and colleagues, the results of fractionated radiotherapy were compared with those of Gamma Knife radiosurgery.[13] Both groups included primary and postsurgical cases, but the tumor size was larger in the radiotherapy group. Median follow-up was 88 months for

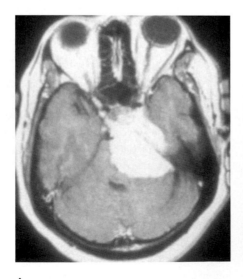

A

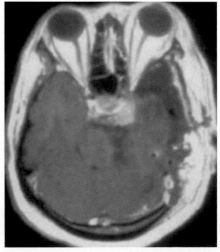

B

FIG. 41-2. (A) Postcontrast T1-weighted axial image of a patient with a left petroclival meningioma with cavernous sinus invasion. (B) Subtotal resection was achieved in two stages to provide sufficient tumor debulking for subsequent radiosurgery treatment

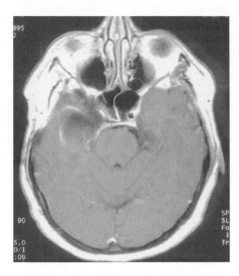

FIG. 41-3. Postcontrast T1-weighted axial image of a patient following exenteration of the right cavernous sinus with its recurrent meningioma including the cavernous segment of the internal carotid artery

the radiotherapy and 63 months for the radiosurgery group, and the actuarial progression-free survival was 94% for both groups. Clinical improvement was seen in a higher number of patients in the radiotherapy group, but transient and permanent morbidity was higher in this group also.

Over the years, our practice has also evolved toward a more conservative management strategy. In our practice, we consider the inclusion of surgery in the management of CSM under the following conditions:

1. Decompression of cranial nerves—mainly the optic or the oculomotor nerves—to improve functional outcome
2. Confirmation of tissue diagnosis when the neuroimaging studies, or the patient's history not classic for a meningioma (Fig. 41-1)
3. Debulking of the tumor when there is a significant extracavernous portion to prepare the patient for Gamma Knife (Fig. 41-2)
4. Exenteration of the cavernous sinus including the internal carotid artery (following a balloon occlusion test) in patients who no longer have serviceable vision or oculomotor function and in whom previous surgery or radiation treatment has failed (Fig. 41-3)

Surgical Strategy

In approaching the cavernous sinus, we use a standard frontotemporal craniotomy followed by sphenoid ridge drilling, limited posterior orbitotomy, and posterolateral orbital wall removal to completely decompress the superior orbital fissure. In our experience, the addition of the zygomatic osteotomy has not been necessary. Following these steps, we then proceed with the unroofing of the optic canal and then removal

of the anterior clinoid process extradurally. Finally, dura is opened with dural incision extending into the falciform ligament and the optic nerve sheath. The details of the extradural skull base technique used in approaching the CSM is similar to the technique used in the surgical management of anterior clinoidal meningiomas and is detailed in the relevant chapter and literature.[14]

During the extradural dissection, prior to the removal of the anterior clinoidal process, the sphenotemporal dural fold is dissected by peeling the medial temporal dura off of the lateral cavernous sinus wall, thereby providing complete extradural exposure of the cavernous sinus, as well as the second and third divisions of the trigeminal nerve. Tissue sampling or removal of the tumor can be performed through the various operative triangles of the cavernous sinus, depending on the goal of the surgery.

Utilization of this technique provides many advantages, such as early localization and exposure, as well as mobilization and decompression of the optic nerve and ICA. The operative goal is achieved at this point if decompression of the optic nerve is the primary goal of the surgery. In selected cases, decompression of the oculomotor nerve may be warranted. In those cases, the dural fold forming the porous oculomotoris is opened completely to allow decompression of the oculomotor nerve, and the cavernous sinus may be explored through its superior wall if the tumor is soft and amenable to further removal. Fibrous texture of the tumor is a limiting factor in many cases. The skull base technique summarized above enlarges the carotico-oculomotor triangle[15] and therefore enhances the exposure at this stage.

It has been shown by anatomic studies that microscopic infiltration of the ICA by the tumor can be seen in as much as 42% of the patients with CSM.[16] Invasion of the ICA can be present even in the absence of narrowing in the preoperative angiographic studies.[17] A more substantial removal of tumor lateral to and not encompassing the ICA can be possible as compared to tumors that involve the ICA and/or extend medial to it. Abdel-Aziz and colleagues have reported a 92% total resection rate for the former group of tumors, as compared to none in the latter group[18] It is also important to remember that the trigeminal nerve and the Gasserian ganglion also seem to be prone to invasion despite the lack of any neurologic deficits, and the pituitary gland can be involved as well through the thin dural barrier.[17]

Summary

With the advances of more conformal radiation treatment options, subtotal resection combined with radiation treatment, or radiation treatment alone, has replaced the concept of radical surgery as the primary treatment option for CSM. With the increasing concerns for the quality of life, this new management strategy offers comparable disease control, with much less cranial nerve morbidity.

References

1. Dolenc V. Direct microsurgical repair of intracavernous vascular lesions. J Neurosurg 1983;58:824–31.
2. O'Sullivan MG, van Loveren HR, Tew JM Jr. The surgical respectability of meningiomas of the cavernous sinus. Neurosurgery 1997;40:238–47.
3. De Monte F, Smith HK, al-Mefty O. Outcome of aggressive removal of avernous sinus meningiomas. J Neurosurg 1994;81:245–51.
4. De Jesus O, Sekhar LN, Parikh HK, Wright DC, Wagner DP. Long-term follow-up of patients with meningiomas involving the cavernous sinus: recurrence, progression, and quality of life. Neurosurgery 1996;39:915–20.
5. Knosp E, Perneczky A, Koos WT, Fries G, Matula C. Meningiomas of the space of the cavernous sinus. Neurosurgery 1996;38:434–44.
6. Couldwell WT, Kan P, Liu JK, Apfelbaum RI. Decompression of cavernous sinus meningioma for preservation and improvement of cranial nerve function. J Neurosurg 2006;105:148–52.
7. Pamir MN, Kilic T, Bayrakli F, Peker S. Changing strategy of cavernous sinus meningiomas: experience of a single institution. Surg Neurol 2005;64(Suppl 2):S58–66.
8. Nicolato A, Foroni R, Alessandrini F, Bricolo A, Gerosa M. Radiosurgical treatment of cavernous sinus meningiomas: experience with 122 treated patients. Neurosurgery 2002;51:1153–9.
9. Lee JY, Niranjan A, McInerney J, Kondziolka D, Flickinger JC, Lunsford LD. Stereotactic radiosurgery providing lon-term tumor control of cavernous sinus meningiomas. J Neurosurg 2002;97:65–72.
10. Maruyama K, Shin M, Kurita H, Hawahara N, Morita A, Kirino T. Proposed treatment strategy for cavernous sinus meningiomas: prospective study. Neurosurgery 2004;55:1068–75.
11. Spiegelmann R, NIssim O, Menhel J, Alezra D, Pfeffer MR. Linear accelerator radiosurgery for meningiomas in and around the cavernous sinus. Neurosurgery 2002;51:1373–80.
12. Brell M, Villa S, Teixidor P, Lucas A, Ferran E, Marin S, Acebes JJ. Fractionated stereotactic radiotherapy in the treatment of exclusive cavernous sinus meningioma: functional outcome, local control, and tolerance. Surg Neurol 2006;65:28–34.
13. Metellus P, Regis J, Muracciole X, Fuentes S, Dufour H, Nanni I, Chinot O, Marin PM, Grisoli F. Evaluation of fractionated radiotherapy and gamma knife radiosurgery in cavernous sinus meningiomas: treatment strategy. Neurosurgery 2005;57:873–86.
14. Lee JH, Sade B, Park JH. A surgical technique for removal of clinoidal meningiomas. Neurosurgery 2006;59(Suppl 1):ONS 108–14.
15. Sade B, Kwon JT, Evans JJ, Lee JH. Enhanced exposure of the carotico-oculomotor triangle following extradural anterior cliniodectomy: a comparative anatomical study. Skull Base 2005;15:157–62.
16. Kotapka MJ, Kalia KK, Martinez AJ, Sekhar LN. Infiltration of the carotid artery by cavernous sinus meningioma. J Neurosurg 1994;81:252–5.
17. Sen C, Hague K. Meningiomas involving the cavernous sinus: histological factors affecting the degree of resection. J Neurosurg 1997;87:535–43.
18. Abdel-Aziz KM, Froelich S, Dagnew E, Jean W, Breneman JC, Zuccarello M, van Loveren HR, Tew JM Jr. Large sphenoid wing meningiomas involving the cavernous sinus: conservative surgical strategies for better functional outcomes. Neurosurgery 2004;54:1375–84.

42
Temporal Bone Meningiomas

Mario Sanna, Maurizio Falcioni, Abdelkader Taibah, and Sean Flanagan

Introduction

Temporal bone (TB) meningiomas are rare lesions that may be classified into two distinct groups: lesions originating in the TB and lesions originating outside the TB and invading the bone during their growth.[1]

Primary meningiomas of the TB have been rarely reported, and from a histopathologic point of view this term should be reserved to lesions truly originating from the TB. However, the real existence of this entity is presently questioned after a literature review by Chang et al.,[1] who found that no "primary meningioma" reported in the literature had been evaluated with magnetic resonance imaging (MRI); this makes it impossible to completely exclude the possibility of a far more frequent intracranial meningioma with secondary temporal bone invasion.

In our opinion the only lesions that should be considered primary TB meningiomas are the rare geniculate ganglion (GG) meningiomas;[2] these tumors originate from meningeal cells that can be found in the GG, a completely extradural site.

Meningiomas of the internal auditory canal (IAC)[3] are another entity included in the TB meningiomas; this classification is appropriate from a pure anatomic point of view, because the IAC is a component of the TB, even if, from a clinical point of view, they may be better considered posterior fossa meningiomas.

Secondary invasion of the TB may occur in meningiomas originating from different locations, mainly the middle cranial fossa (MCF), the posterior cranial fossa and the jugular foramen.[4] The tendency to infiltrate bone has been documented exclusively in en plaque meningiomas, while the globular types tend to remain confined in the intradural space.[1,5] The different origin, pattern of growth, and spread of these lesions make particularly difficult any attempt of classification and treatment standardization.

Spread Through the Temporal Bone

GG Meningiomas

GG meningiomas originate from arachnoid cell rests displaced during embryogenesis and lying within the sheath of the facial nerve (FN).[6] They tend to have a globular shape and grow into the middle ear cleft, following the path of least resistence. Real GG meningiomas are clearly separated by the MCF dura and do not infiltrate the bone, even though they erode the bone during their growth (Fig. 42-1).

IAC Meningiomas

IAC meningiomas originate from the arachnoid granulations situated along the dural lining of the canal walls.[7] During their growth, they tend to engulf the contents of the IAC. Displacement of such contents may be found in any direction, depending on the site of dural origin of the tumor. Extension usually occur into the cerebellopontine angle (CPA), with invasion of the inner ear rarely reported (Fig. 42-2).[7–9]

Secondary Meningiomas of the Temporal Bone

Invasion of the TB from its external surfaces occurs slowly, usually in the form of finger-like projections invading preformed routes such as pneumatized cells and vascular channels.[6] Involvement of the pneumatic system, tympanic cavity, and Eustachian tube seems to happen Predominantly along the submucosal plane. While involvement of the TB is accompanied by a bony resorption, the endosteal layer of the inner ear capsule is usually resistant to invasion, sparing the membranous labyrinth in the majority of the cases (Fig. 42-3).[6]

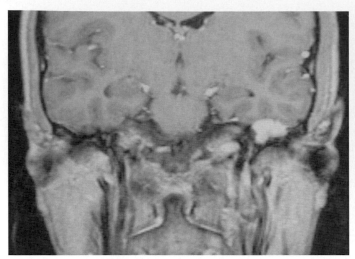

Fig. 42-1. Coronal MRI of a geniculate ganglion meningioma, protruding inferiorly into the middle ear cleft

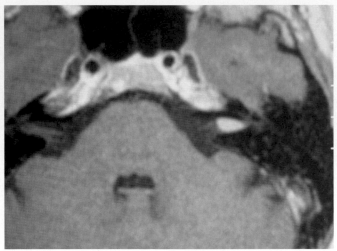

Fig. 42-2. Axial MRI of an internal auditory canal meningioma. The lesion appears indistinguishable from a vestibular schwannoma

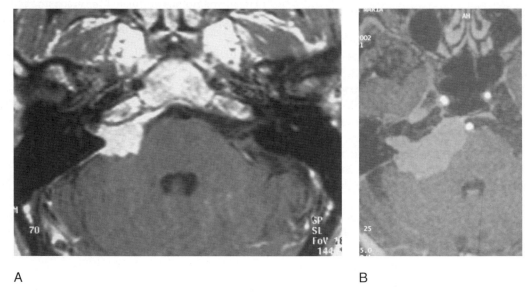

A   B

Fig. 42-3. (A) Axial MRI of a CPA meningioma with invasion of the internal auditory canal. Note the characteristic dural tail on both the anterior and posterior borders of the lesion and the broad attachment to the posterior surface of the temporal bone. (B) Axial MRI of another CPA meningioma. Also in this case a broad attachment to the posterior surface of the temporal bone is clearly visible, as well as the eccentric tumor location with respect to the internal auditory canal

Diagnosis

GG Meningiomas

GG meningiomas may produce the symptoms of a middle ear mass, mainly conductive hearing loss, frequently associated with facial weakness. When reaching the middle ear cleft, the mass may become visible on otomicroscopy as a retrotympanic lesion, usually appearing reddish. There are no specific signs that can direct the diagnosis, and the diagnostic doubt

must prompt the clinician to ask for radiologic investigation. A sensorineural component of the hearing loss due to erosion of the otic capsule is rarely encountered.

IAC Meningiomas

Meningiomas can produce the symptoms of any lesion located into the IAC, mainly tinnitus, sensorineural hearing loss, and unsteadiness. While true vertigo spells, facial weakness, or hemifacial spasm are found more frequently than in vestibular

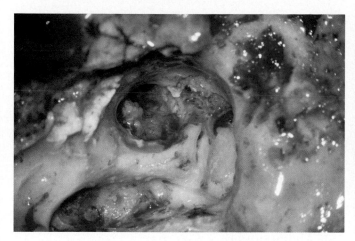
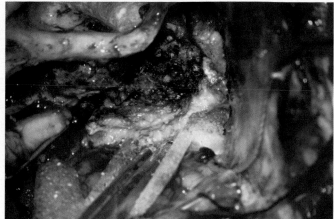

A   B

FIG. 42-4. (A) Intraoperative view of a left-sided meningioma operated on through the transotic approach. Note the presence of the lesion at the level of the hypotympanum. (B) Similar case as in Fig. 42-3, but this example on the left side. Once the posterior fossa dura has been opened, the component of the meningioma into the cerebellopontine angle and the internal auditory canal comes clearly into view

schwannoma (VS), they remain rare.[3] The presence of these symptoms should alert the clinician on the possibility of a tumor different from VS.

While CPA meningiomas are frequently asymptomatic until they reach considerable size, due to their capability to encircle nerves and vessels, IAC meningiomas tend to be symptomatic early, probably because of the limited space available within the IAC to accommodate their growth.

Tumors with Secondary Involvement of the Temporal Bone

Due to the different possibilities of origin of meningiomas infiltrating the TB, the presentation of these lesions may be extremely variable. However, because of the tendency of all en plaque meningiomas to produce cranial nerve deficits only late during their course, the first symptoms of their presence are often related to the TB invasion. The most frequent presentation is represented by a conductive hearing loss due to invasion of the middle ear. This can occur in two different ways: direct involvement of the ossicular chain or, more frequently, occlusion of the Eustachian tube with consequent secondary secretory otitis media.[5] In the first case, it may be possible to detect on otoscopy a retrotympanic mass[10] or a polipoid lesion in the external auditory canal. This situation usually prompts the clinician to further investigations.

The presence of a secretory otitis represents a more insidious presentation, and very often the patient is treated with common medications and/or ventilation tube insertion for a long time before reaching the correct diagnosis.[5] However, the signs that should alert the clinician are the persistence of the conductive

hearing loss despite any treatment and the constant appearance of othorrea following the ventilation tube insertion.

Another less frequent possibility is the development of a cholesteatoma secondary to the presence of the meningioma. This can happen through different ways: erosion of the walls of the external auditory canal by the meningioma and subsequent skin invagination, or presence of the meningiomas into the external auditory canal with medial skin entrapment. However, also in these situations, the clinician is prompted to ask for additional investigations. Naturally the simultaneous presence of cranial nerve deficits related to the intracranial extension makes it mandatory to investigate the patient with an MRI.

Radiologic Examination

GG Meningiomas

On bone algorithm computed tomography (CT), GG meningiomas appear like a mass eroding the TB and in continuity with the GG area. The lesion has the same CT characteristics as the more common petrous bone cholesteatoma and FN schwannoma, even if the borders of the bony erosion are usually not clearly defined.

On MRI, the same lesion appears hypointense on T1 and hyperintense on T2, with enhancement after gadolinium infusion.[2] Enhancement may be heterogeneous, sometimes resembling hemangiomas.[11] The differentiation from FN schwannomas or hemangiomas, on MRI, is difficult because they also have a favorite site of occurrence at the level of the GG.[11] In contrast, petrous bone cholesteatomas do not enhance after gadolinium infusion.

IAC Meningiomas

IAC meningiomas are not visible on bone algorithm CT and show the same features of VS on MRI (hypointensity on T1, hyperintensity on T2, and enhancement after gadolinium infusion). The characteristics that usually differentiate meningiomas from VS (asymmetric relationship with the IAC, broad attachment to the posterior surface of the TB, and the presence of a dural tail)[4] are clearly visible only after extension into the CPA.

The presence of an enhancement of the IAC dura described by Asoaka[12] has not been confirmed by other reports.

Tumors with Secondary Involvement of the Temporal Bone

Radiologic investigation of en plaque meningiomas with invasion of the TB may present some difficulties. In fact, when an MRI is done as an initial radiographic examination because the patient is affected by neurologic symptoms, the bone infiltration may not be particularly evident, with the possibility resulting in an incorrect surgical planning through approaches that do not allow a complete control of the bone (as in the retrosigmoid approach). For this reason, in presence of an en plaque meningioma the radiologic workup should always be completed with a CT scan with bone algorithm in order to better visualize the possible bony involvement.

On the contrary, patients complaining of symptoms referrable to the middle ear are usually investigated with a CT with bone algorithm, with the consequent possibility of missing signs of presence of the disease outside the temporal bone. These signs are represented mainly by diffuse hyperostosis with hairy borders.[13] The presence of this aspect on the CT scans makes it mandatory to further investigate the patient with an MRI to detect the intracranial component of the en plaque meningioma.

While posterior fossa and MCF meningiomas invading the TB usually show unmistakable features, jugular foramen meningiomas may be sometimes confused with paragangliomas and lower cranial nerve schwannomas. Conventional angiography is of invaluable help in differentiating doubtful cases and is mandatory because the surgical planning may change completely in relation with the tumor nature.

Treatment Modalities

GG Meningiomas

The extreme rarity of these tumors frequently leads to the misdiagnosis of FN schwannomas or hemangiomas. However, the issue is of secondary significance because their treatment follows the same concepts of other FN tumors. The most important element is represented by the preoperative FN status. Patients with normal FN function are monitored radiologically, while patients with FN palsy are surgically treated.

There is not unanimous agreement on the best treatment for patients showing a grade II or III weakness, because there are pros and cons for conservative and aggressive therapy. Conservative treatment allows the patient to still maintain satisfactory FN function for an unpredictable period of time, while surgery leads to nerve interruption and grafting in almost all of the cases, with consequent complete palsy and no possibility to recover a function better than grade III.[14] On the contrary, results of grafting are directly related to the duration of the preoperative deficits, with the best results obtained in patients in whom the FN deficit lasted for a short preoperative time prior to detection.[14]

IAC Meningioma

Preoperative treatment planning is often based on the incorrect diagnosis of VS. The available management options include surgical removal through one of the three most adopted approaches (translabyrinthine, retrosigmoid, and middle cranial fossa), radiologic monitoring, and stereotactic radiosurgery. Even if, due to the rarity of the lesion, there are no reported series on observation of intracanalicular meningiomas, stereotactic radiosurgery does not seem a valuable treatment modality in pure intracanalicular lesion without any sign of growth.

When tailoring the best treatment for any single case it should be taken into account that, even if the general principles are the same as when dealing with VS, meningiomas need special consideration:[1] they may be a little more difficult to remove without any FN insult because the position of the nerve is less predictable;[2] hearing preservation has been less frequently reported; and[3] a radical removal has to include the involved dura.

Tumors with Secondary Involvement of the Temporal Bone

Any attempt to classify the possible treatment modalities when dealing with meningiomas with infiltration of the temporal bone is a difficult task, in particular because of the multitude of different intracranial extension that may accompany the bone invasion. In fact, even if the TB component is often responsible for the symptomatology, the overall judgment on the benefit to surgically treat the lesion is mainly based on size and extension of the intracranial component. The slow growth that often characterizes these lesions means that it is common to diagnose huge en plaque tumors which remained completely asymptomatic but for the component into the TB. Consideration should be made of the following factors:[1] patient's age and general conditions;[2] probable postsurgical neurological deficits; and[3] possibility of radical removal. Alternative options are radiologic monitoring, conventional stereotactic radiosurgery, and partial removal alone or associated with radiotherapy of the tumor remnant.

All different options have pros and cons; however, due to the high rate of postoperative neurologic deficits usually associated with aggressive removal of huge lesions and the high rate of recurrence, presently it seems appropriate to reserve radical surgical procedure only for young patients and in the presence of a reasonable possibility of radical removal. While these kinds of meningiomas may be theoretically managed conservatively for a long time, sometimes the TB infiltration creates situations like secondary cholesteatoma or chronic otitis, requiring some sort of surgical treatment at least at the level of the TB. Stereotactic radiosurgery is usually not adopted as the first choice of treatment, but reserved for lesions showing clear growth.

Surgical Approaches

GG Meningiomas

There can be different possibilities ranging from small lesions centered on the GG to larger lesions with massive involvement of the middle ear cleft. In the first instance it is usually possible to remove the lesion through a MCF approach. This approach, in presence of a limited extension of the tumor, allows the surgeon to preserve the hearing and perform the graft to reconstruct the FN.[15] However, the MCF approach does not permit any control of the majority of the tympanic segment of the FN due to the presence of the lateral semicircular canal; therefore, for larger tumors with extension into the middle ear, it may be necessary to combine the MCF with a transmastoid approach in order to better control the tumor extension into the middle ear cleft.[16] If required, the incus may also be removed and repositioned (in the same or a second stage surgery).

A larger lesion, occupying the entire middle ear, in which there is no possibility to reconstruct the ossicular chain, is better approached through a subtotal petrosectomy in order to obtain complete control of the lesion. In the presence of protrusion of the lesion into the MCF, the approach is enlarged through a craniotomy to permit superior dural retraction. In the rare instance of erosion of the cochlea, a transcochlear (TC)[17,18] approach allows the largest available approach without additional deficits.

The tumors are usually well dissected from the MCF dura because of the absence of any infiltration, and this situation leads to the possibility of establishing a clear cleavage plane. Anatomic preservation of the FN is only occasionally achieved, and the majority of surgeries must be completed with a nerve reconstruction procedure.

IAC Meningiomas

The three classic approaches available for treatment of IAC lesions may be adopted in cases of meningiomas.[3] However, in the rare cases in which the diagnosis is suspected preoperatorely, it should be noted that a removal of the dural attachment of the lesion is usually required, and this is often located at the

level of the fundus of the IAC. This makes the RS approach less well suited for meningiomas, because of the impossibility to directly control the fundus. Another specific consideration is that the contents of the IAC may be engulfed or displaced without any typical pattern, depending exclusively on the site of origin of the meningioma. Due to additional manipulation of the FN required during tumor removal, when hearing is not an issue, the translabyrinthine is by far the most appropriate approach for IAC meningiomas.

Tumors with Secondary Involvement of the Temporal Bone

Due to the variability of size, locations, and symptoms of meningiomas invading the TB, there are many different surgical treatments available. These may be subdivided in those intended to solve the symptoms produced by the TB infiltration and those targeted to remove of the meningioma. Among the first group, the simplest surgical treatment, which is ventilation tube insertion to resolve a secondary secretory otitis, has shown no effectiveness due to persisting discharge and conductive hearing loss,[5] and this should be disregarded as a treatment modality.

In the presence of a secondary otitis media or cholesteatoma, when it is not indicated to remove the meningioma, the target of the surgery is simply to eradicate the middle ear infection. The safest solution is represented by a subtotal petrosectomy accompanied by blind sac closure of the external auditory canal and middle ear obliteration. Even if this inevitably results in a conductive hearing loss of 50–60 dB, every other attempt to preserve the middle ear will end up in a failure with recurrence due to the presence of the meningiomatous infiltration of the bone.

When the aim of surgery is total or subtotal removal of the meningioma, the approach should be selected carefully in order to be able to reach every intended extension of the lesion: intracranially, into the TB, and extracranially. Presently there is a large variety of skull base approaches available for the surgeons; however, the selected approach in the specific case must absolutely include complete exposure of the TB. Therefore, the classic retrosigmoid approach that allows only a very limited control of the posterior surface of the TB is excluded from consideration.

In the presence of meningiomas growing into the MCF with infiltration of the tegmen, a subtotal petrosectomy may be extended superiorly with a large craniotomy. In huge lesions, a further extension of the approach may be obtained with temporary displacement of the zygomatic arch.

Posterior cranial fossa lesions with infiltration of the TB are best approached through a translabyrinthine or a transotic route, depending on the amount of temporal bone invasion. For huge tumors extending anteriorly into the prepontine cistern, a TC approach may be indicated, especially if FN weakness is already present preoperatively. All these lateral routes in fact allow a complete control of progressively larger areas of the TB, so that the surgeon theoretically has the possibility to completely eradicate the lesion, including the involved dura and bone.

Jugular foramen lesions with extension to the TB need to be approached through a route that allows control of the jugular foramen. A petro-occipital transsigmoid approach[19] very often perfectly suits this kind of lesion, permitting control of the intra- and extradural components of the tumors without any unnecessary sacrifice of the hearing and/or FN. Unfortunately, the possibility of sparing hearing and FN is mainly dependent on the extent of the meningioma into the temporal bone; however, when required the petro-occipital transsigmoid approach may be easily combined with a translabyrinthine or a transotic approach, allowing control of any possible tumoral extension at the level of the middle ear and/or otic capsule. Adopting an infratemporal type A approach to anteriorly displace the FN in order to better control any involvement of the carotid artery is rarely required.

Follow-Up

As in the majority of skull base lesions, meningiomas of the TB need prolonged follow-up. This should be tailored to the type of tumor and the specific patient. IAC and GG meningiomas usually may be considered cured after 5–7 years from the surgery; aggressive lesions, however, especially if only partially removed, require prolonged follow-up and often adjunctive treatments.

References

1. Chang CYJ, Cheung SW, Jackler RK. Meningiomas presenting in the temporal bone: the pathways of spread from an intracranial site of origin. Otolaryngol Head Neck Surg 1998;119:658–64.
2. Falcioni M, Piccirillo E, Taibah A, et al. Meningiomas intrinsic to the geniculate ganglion. Skull Base Surg 2001;11:297–32.
3. Bacciu A, Piazza P, Di Lella F, Sanna M. Intracanalicular meningioma: clinical features, radiologic findings and surgical management. Otol Neurotol (in print)
4. Irving RM. Meningiomas of the internal auditory canal and cerebellopontine angle. In: Tumors of the Temporal Bone. Jackler RK, Driscoll CLW, ed. Philadelphia: Lippincott Williams & Wilkins, 2000:219–35.
5. Ayache D, Trabalzini F, Bordure P, et al. Serous otitis media reveling temporal en plaque meningioma. Otol Neurotol 2006;27:992–8.
6. Nager GT. Meningiomas involving the temporal bone. In: Pathology of the Ear and the Temporal Bone. Baltimore: Williams & Wilkins 1993:623–4.
7. Nager GT, Masica DN. Meningiomas of the cerebello-pontine angleand their relation to the temporal bone. Laryngoscope 1970;80:863–95.
8. Brookler KH, Hoffmann RA, Camins M, et al. Trilobed meningioma: ampulla of posterior semicircular canal, internal auditory canal and cerebellopontine angle. Am J Otol 1980;1:171–3.
9. Ishikawa N, Komatsuzaki A, Tokano H. Meningioma of the internal auditory canal with extension into the vestibule. J Laryngol Otol 1999;113:1101–3.
10. Sanna M, Russo A, De Donato G, et al. Color Atlas of Otoscopy: From Diagnosis to Surgery. 2nd ed. Stuttgart/New York: Georg Thieme Verlag, 2002:150–8.
11. Falcioni M, Russo A, Taibah A, et al. Facial nerve tumors. Otol Neurotol 2003;24:942–7.
12. Asaoka K, Barrs DM, Sampson JH, et al. Intracanalicular meningioma mimicking vestibular Schwannoma. AJNR 2002;23:1493–6.
13. Vrionis FD, Roberton JH, Gardner G, Heilman C. Temporal bone meningiomas. Skull Base Surg 1999;9:127–39.
14. Falcioni M, Taibah A, Russo A, et al. Facial nerve grafting. Otol Neurotol 2003;24:486–9.
15. Sanna M, Khrais T, Mancini F, et al. The Facial Nerve in Temporal Bone and Lateral Skull Base Microsurgery. Stuttgart/New York: Georg Thieme Verlag, 2006:86–148.
16. Gersdorff M, Brucher JM, Vilain J. Primary meningioma of the geniculate ganglion: apropos of a case. Rev Laryngol Otol Rhinol 1992;113:51–4.
17. Sanna M, Mazzoni A, Gamoletti R. The system of the modified transcochlear approaches to the petroclival area and the prepontine cistern. Skull Base Surg 1996;6:221–5.
18. Sanna M, Saleh E, Russo A, et al. Atlas of Temporal Bone and Skull Base Surgery. Stuttgart/New York: Georg Thieme Verlag, 1995:52–61.
19. Mazzoni A, Sanna M. A posterolateral approach to the skull base: the petro-occipital transsigmoid approach. Skull Base Surg 1995;5:157–67.

43
Posterior Clinoidal Meningiomas

Takeo Goto and Kenji Ohata

Introduction

Posterior clinoidal (PC) meningioma is a very rare and challenging skull base tumor to neurosurgeons. There have been scant reports regarding surgical strategy for this tumor (1,2). Samii et al. reported a case of PC meningioma successfully resected in staged operations combining lateral suboccipital approach and pterional approach (2). Dolenc emphasized rarity of the tumor. In his series of meningiomas of the central skull base treated in the last 20 years, he had only six cases, representing 0.7% of central skull base meningiomas (1,2). He indicated that the tumors may be reached via transcavernous-transsellar approach and be removed totally without additional deficits except transient oculomotor nerve palsy (1). In this chapter we describe our experience with five cases of PC meningiomas encountered in the last 20 years, resected via the presigmoidal transpetrosal approach (3–5).

Special Considerations

The posterior clinoid process (PCP) is located postero-laterally to the pituitary stalk, postero-medially to the entrance to cavernous sinus of the oculomotor nerve and just behind the C1-2 segment of the internal carotid artery (ICA). Meningioma arising from the PCP would compress the pituitary stalk anteriorly, the oculomotor nerve laterally or infero-laterally, and the C1-2 segment of the ICA and its branches superiorly or anteriorly as the tumor enlarges. If the tumor expands far anteriorly, the optic nerve and optic chiasm will be shifted superiorly or antero-superiorly. Therefore, diplopia and visual disturbance may be common presenting symptom(s). Some large PC tumors may also cause hydrocephalus by compressing the third ventricle.

In radiologic evaluations, attachment of the tumor at the PCP is very small and dural tail sign is not usually detected. Some PC meningiomas are preoperatively misinterpreted as other parasellar tumors (6). Some neurosurgeons may also confuse PC meningioma with anterior clinoidal (AC) meningioma. The direction of the ICA compression may help in differentiating PC meningioma from AC meningioma. The ICA is often shifted posteriorly in the case of AC meningioma but anteriorly in the case of PC meningioma.

Surgical Technique

Selection of the Surgical Approach

Surgery for PC meningioma requires the following five steps: (1) devascularization of the tumor at the PCP; (2) exposure of the oculomotor nerve; (3) dissection of the tumor from the ICA and its branches, such as the anterior choroidal artery; (4) dissection from the pituitary stalk and the hypothalamus; and (5) dissection from the optic chiasm and nerve.

Samii et al. suggested that the first and second steps could be performed with a standard lateral suboccipital approach, followed by the final three steps being carried out with a pterional approach (2). Combination of these two approaches should be suitable for relatively small and soft PC meningiomas.

Another approach to the lesion is a transcavernous-transsellar approach (1,7). This approach can accomplish all five steps in one stage. However, it has several disadvantages. In the transcavernous-transsellar approach, as the ICA and its branches are shifted anteriorly, the direct exposure of the tumor may be hindered. There are inherent surgical risks in removing the tumor through the narrow spaces between perforators of ICA, especially in the hands of inexperienced surgeons. Moreover, peeling off the outer layer of cavernous sinus lateral wall, which is required in this approach, sometimes obstructs venous return from the sphenoparietal sinus to the sphenobasal vein, which could be the main drainage of cerebral venous flow as PC meningioma usually obstructs the inferior petrosal sinus. Additionally, early detection of the oculomotor nerve is difficult in this approach.

The presigmoid transpetrosal approach (3,4) circumvents the disadvantages of the previous two approaches. In the last

T. Goto and K. Ohata

20 years, five PC meningiomas have been removed by this approach at our institute.

Position and Skin Incision

The patient is placed in a lateral park-bench position. A curvilinear pterional skin incision begins anterior to the tragus, 5 mm behind the superior temporal artery, and stops approximately 4 cm before reaching the midline anteriorly. An additional postero-temporal extension of incision is made beginning at the previous incision 1.5 cm above the uppermost part of the ear cartilage down to 2 cm medial to the tip of the mastoid process (Fig. 43-1A). The temporal muscle is separated subperiosteally from temporal squama, zygomatic arch, and mastoid process. The suboccipital muscles and upper part of the insertion of the sternocleidomastoid muscle are also elevated subperiosteally (Fig. 43-1B).

Craniotomy

Following the standard temporo-occipito-suboccipital craniotomy, the outer table of the mastoid process is split to prevent the postoperative cosmetic deformity. This maneuver is easily accomplished with a reciprocating saw. The sigmoid sinus is carefully exposed down to its short horizontal segment. The zygomatic arch is cut with a sagittal saw. If the superior border of the tumor is very high, the superior wall of the mandibular joint and middle cranial base 1 cm lateral to the foramen spinosum should be cut and reflected downward (oticocondylar osteotomy) (8) (Fig. 43-1C).

Extent of Petrosectomy

A retractor is used to protect the sigmoid sinus, and petrosectomy is then performed. The posterior and anterior semicircular canals are partially drilled to preserve hearing.

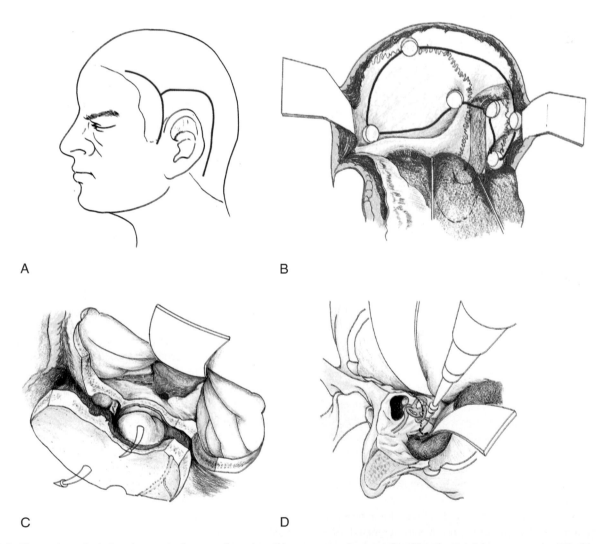

A   B

C   D

FIG. 43-1. Illustrations depicting the surgical steps of presigmoid transpetrosal approach with oticocondylar osteotomy: (A) skin incision; (B) location of burr holes and the extent of the craniotomy; (C) oticocondylar osteotomy; (D) petrosectomy with partial labyrinthectomy. (From Ohata K, Baba M. Surgical Anatomy of the Skull Base. Tokyo: Miawa Shoten, 1996)[4]

The petrosal ridge is removed up to the level of the internal auditory meatus. The medial petrous ridge is resected over the internal auditory meatus (Fig. 43-1D). If the tumor extends tentorial infratentorially, anterior petrosectomy is required. During epidural procedure, significant attention is given to the extent of dural elevation from the middle cranial base. Where venous return is limited to the sphenobasal veins and venous plexus around the foramen ovale, dural elevation from the middle cranial base should be restricted to preserve those venous returns.

Dural and Tentorial Incisions

The petrosal dura is opened, leaving a 5-mm dural fringe on the anterior margin of the sigmoid sinus and on the inferior margin of the superior petrosal sinus. The subtemporal dural incision is extended as far anteriorly as possible. Its medial extent is directed along the posterior margin of the gasserian ganglion (Fig. 43-2A). The superior petrosal sinus is transected immediately posterior to the trigeminal nerve. The tentrium is divided from the point of the transaction of the superior petrosal sinus to its hiatus just behind the dural entrance of the trochlear nerve (Fig. 43-2B).

Tumor Removal

Gentle elevation of the temporal lobe gives wide exposure of the tumor above and below the trochlear nerve (Fig. 43-2C). At the early stage of the operation, it is possible to coagulate the feeding arteries from the posterior clinoid process. After internal decompression of the tumor, proximal oculomotor nerve can be usually found in the interpeduncular cistern. Tracing the oculomotor nerve from the normal proximal side

to the involved distal side is the important surgical strategy to prevent unexpected injury of the nerve. Involved ICA and its branches, which are commonly displaced antero-superiorly, then can be safely dissected under direct vision from the postero-lateral side through this approach. This approach can also provide direct exposure to the inferior surface of the optic chiasm, pituitary stalk, and hypothalamus.

If the tumor extends anteriorly under the optic nerve, it will not be reached safely through this approach. Orbitozygomatic approach should be added for removal of far anterior extension of PC meningiomas (9).

Closure

After tumor removal, the dural defect is closed watertight, and abdominal fat tissue soaked with fibrin glue is inserted into the epidural space. The temporo-occipito-suboccipital bone flap, outer table of the mastoid process are replaced and fixed with titanium miniplates.

Outcome and Complications

PC meningioma is very rare, and to our knowledge there has not been any reported series detailing surgical outcome except a case report (2). We present surgical results of our five cases here.

The patients included two males and three females, who ranged in age from 45 to 58 years (mean 51.6 years). One patient (Case 1) had a small tumor, the maximum diameter of which was 2 cm, and the other four patients (Cases 2–5) had a large tumor more than 4 cm in diameter. One small tumor (Case 1) and two large tumors (Cases 2, 5) were totally

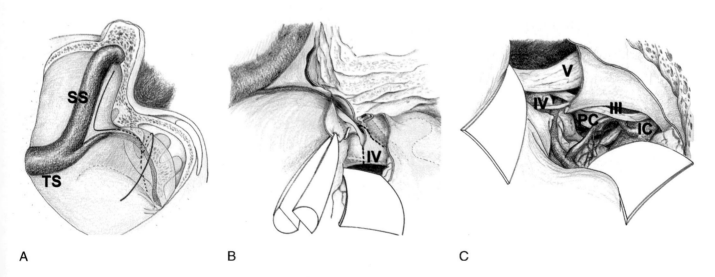

A   B   C

FIG. 43-2. Diagrams illustrating the surgical steps after petrosectomy: (A) dural incision (solid line shows the extent of dural incision); (B) tentorial incision; (C) operative view around the posterior clinoid process through the presigmoid transpetrosal approach. TS, transverse sinus; SS, sigmoid sinus; PC, posterior clinoid process; IC, internal carotid artery; III, oculomotor nerve; IV, trochlear nerve; V, trigeminal nerve. (From Ohata K, Baba M. Surgical Anatomy of the Skull Base. Tokyo: Miawa Shoten, 1996.)[4]

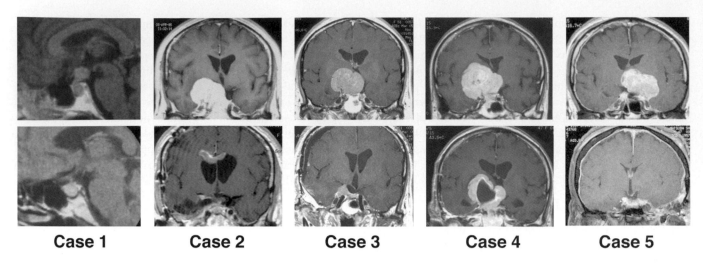

Case 1   **Case 2**   **Case 3**   **Case 4**   **Case 5**

FIG. 43-3. Pre- and postoperative MR images of the presented five cases. The upper row shows preoperative images and the lower row shows postoperative images, respectively

removed by presigmoidal transpetrosal approach in one stage. One large tumor (Case 3), which had extreme anterior expansion, was near totally resected with a combination of transpetrosal approach and orbitozygomatic approach. One huge fibrous tumor (Case 4) was partially removed to avoid surgical complications (Fig. 43-3). Postoperative oculomotor nerve palsy, visual disturbance, and cerebral infarction from the injury of perforators have not occurred in our five cases.

Summary

Posterior clinoidal meningioma is a challenging skull base tumor to neurosurgeons. Small or soft PC meningioma may be treated with standard approaches such as combined lateral suboccipital and pterional approaches or a transcavernous-transsellar approach. In some large PC meningiomas it is very difficult to safely dissect the tumor from the surrounding neurovascular structures, even if the tumor seems soft on the preoperative radiologic studies. In our limited experience with five cases of PC meningiomas over the last 20 years, the presigmoid transpetrosal approach has served us well, resulting in excellent patient outcome.

References

1. Dolenc VV. Microsurgical Anatomy and Surgery of the Central Skull Base. New York: Springer, 2003:212–216.
2. Nakamura M, Samii M. Surgical management of a meningioma in the retrosellar region. Acta Neurochir (Wein) 2003;145:215–220.
3. Hakuba A, Nishimura S, Jang B. A combined retroauricular and preauricular transpetrosal approach to clivus meningioma. Surg Neurol 1988;30:108–116.
4. Ohata K, Baba M. Presigmoidal transpetrosal approach. In: Hakuba A, ed. Surgical Anatomy of the Skull Base. Tokyo: Miwa Shoten, 1996:109–139.
5. Ohata K, Tamami T, Goto T, et al. Surgical removal of retrochismatic craniopharyngiomas with transpetrosal approach. Oper Techn Neurosurg 2003;6(4):200–204.
6. Abe T, Matsumoto K, Homma H, et al. Dorsum sellar meningioma mimicking pituitary macroadenoma: case report. Surg Neurol 1999;51:543–547.
7. Dolenc VV, Sklap M, Sustersic J, et al. A transcavernous-transsellar approach to the basilar tip aneurysms. Br J Neurosurg 1987;1:251–259.
8. Ohata K, Baba M. Otico-condylar approach. In: Hakuba A, ed. Surgical Anatomy of the Skull Base. Tokyo: Miwa Shoten, 1996:37–65.
9. Hakuba A, Liu S, Nishimura S. The orbitozygomatic infratemporal approach: a new surgical technique. Surg Neurol 1986;26:271–276.

44
Petroclival and Upper Clival Meningiomas I: An Overview of Surgical Approaches

Marcus L. Ware, Svetlana Pravdenkova, Kadir Erkmen, and Ossama Al-Mefty

Classification and Incidence

Petroclival meningiomas, by definition, are tumors that originate in the upper two thirds of the clivus at the petroclival junction medial to the fifth cranial nerve.[1,2] These tumors often displace the brain stem and the basilar artery to the opposite side. Petroclival meningiomas may be in the posterior fossa alone, or may span the middle and posterior cranial fossae. These tumors may also involve the posterior cavernous sinus through the Meckel's cave. Sphenopetroclival lesions are the most extensive of these lesions. They invade the posterior cavernous sinus and grow into the middle and posterior fossae. The bony clivus and the petrous apex are involved and the sphenoid sinus is invaded. Clival meningiomas originate from the midline clivus. They displace the basilar artery and brainstem posteriorly. Meningiomas arising from the lower third of the clivus are defined as foramen magnum lesions. Posterior fossa meningiomas arising lateral to the trigeminal nerve are termed petrosal meningiomas and are divided into anterior and posterior petrosal meningiomas.

The incidence of meningiomas in the general population varies between 2 and 15 per 100,000 people and increases with age.[3] Meningiomas account for 20% of all primary intracranial neoplasms and 25% of all intraspinal tumors.[3] Most meningiomas are benign and grow slowly.[4] Of intracranial meningiomas, 10–15% are located in the posterior fossa and only 3–10% of posterior fossa meningiomas are petroclival meningiomas.[5]

Clinical Presentation

The mean age at presentation in these patients is the mid-40s with a very wide range.[5] The typical presentation of the petroclival meningioma is that of an insidious onset. The clinical presentation can be divided into four groups based upon involvement of cranial nerves, mass effect on the cerebellum, brain stem compression, and increased intracranial pressure, either from the tumor mass or obstructive hydrocephalus.[6,7]

Cranial neuropathies are commonly associated with petroclival meningiomas, with the fifth and eighth cranial nerves being the most frequently involved.[5,8] Facial nerve involvement occurs in nearly half of these patients (2,7,9). In addition, several cases have been reported of trigeminal neuralgia associated with contralateral posterior fossa tumors.[10–13] The lower cranial nerves are involved in nearly one third of these cases.[2,7] Cranial nerves III, IV, and VI, despite their proximity and ultimate involvement of tumor, are symptomatic in less than half of the cases.[2,14] Cerebellar signs, which occur in nearly 70% of cases, are the most frequently identified clinical findings in these patients.[5,8,9,15] Headache is the most frequent complaint.[5] Long tract signs and somatosensory deficits, consistent with brain stem compression, are quite variable. Spastic paresis is reported in 15–57% of patients and somatosensory deficit has been reported in 15–20% of patients.[5]

Management of Patients with Petroclival Meningiomas

Because meningiomas are usually benign and slow growing, patients may harbor these tumors for years without ill effects. Not every patient with a meningioma requires immediate treatment. Smaller tumors in asymptomatic patients may be followed with serial magnetic resonance imaging (MRI) scans without significant morbidity.[16] We recommend treatment of meningiomas that are larger, those that show evidence of growth or aggressive features, or if the patient becomes symptomatic. Meningiomas can be treated with surgical resection, radiosurgery, or conventional fractionated radiation therapy. Surgical treatment of meningiomas is still the gold standard of treatment for tumors at first presentation. Complete resection of benign meningiomas is associated with high cure rates.[17,18] The use of radiosurgery in the treatment of petroclival meningiomas has grown greatly over the past decade, both as initial therapy and as an adjuvant to surgical resection.[19–24] However, only relatively smaller tumors can be treated with radiosurgery. Conformal fractionated radiation therapy may be used to treat tumors of all sizes and sites.[25,26] In cases of patients who cannot tolerate surgery and harbor tumors that require treatment, we recommend treatment with either radiosurgery or with conformal fractionated radiation therapy. Because radiosurgery and conformal radiation may be associated with secondary malignancies[27–34] and may not reduce the mass effect of larger tumors,[35–37] we recommend surgical resection in cases of younger patients with larger or growing tumors. In cases where a subtotal resection was achieved surgically, we follow benign meningiomas for evidence of progression prior to treatment with radiosurgery or conformal radiation therapy. Patients with higher grade meningiomas are treated with adjuvant radiation therapy after tumor resection and pathologic analysis.

Preoperative Evaluation

In addition to a complete history and physical examination, patients with petroclival meningiomas require extensive imaging to define their lesions as part of their preoperative evaluation. The size of the tumor, its location, and extent of middle fossa and posterior fossa involvement should be defined by MRI and/or computed tomography (CT) imaging. Knowledge of the arterial anatomy would allow the surgeon to remove the blood supply to the tumor while leaving en passé arteries intact. A detailed knowledge of the venous anatomy is important in deciding on tumor approach as some approaches are more challenging with specific venous drainage patterns. We therefore recommend that each patient has MR angiography (MRA) and MR venography (MRV) prior to surgery. We reserve angiogram for cases where there is abnormal arterial or venous anatomy seen on MRA and MRV that would influence our choice of surgical approach.

Zygomatic Anterior Petrosal Approach

Description of Approach

The patient is placed supine on the operative table with the trunk flexed to allow elevation of the patient's trunk and head, and the ipsilateral shoulder is elevated using a shoulder roll. The head is rotated towards the contralateral side and the vertex is lowered to place the neck in extension. A curvilinear incision is made from anterior to the tragus at the level of the zygomatic arch and is continued behind the hair to the midline. The flap is rotated anteriorly. The superficial and deep layers of the temporalis fascia are elevated with the skin flap to protect the frontal branch of the facial nerve. The zygomatic arch is cut anteriorly and posteriorly, and the temporalis muscle is elevated and retracted inferiorly. A craniotomy is made along the floor of the middle fossa and crossing the sphenoid wing. The dura mater is elevated from the floor of the middle fossa until the middle meningeal artery is encountered. This vessel

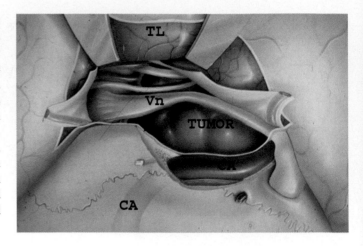

Fig. 44-1. Illustration of the exposure provided by the anterior petrosal approach. The petrous apex has been resected, the middle fossa dura mater has been opened, and the tentorium has been cut after coagulation of the superior petrosal sinus. TL, temporal lobe; Vn, trigeminal nerve; CA, carotid artery

is then coagulated and cut. This dissection is continued and the foramen ovale and the third division of the trigeminal nerve are identified. The greater superficial petrosal nerve is identified and dissected to prevent traction injury. The dura mater is dissected from the lateral wall of the cavernous sinus along the third and second divisions of the trigeminal nerve until the gasserian ganglion is exposed and the trigeminal impression is encountered (Fig. 44-1). The petrous apex is then drilled medial to the carotid artery, extending from the trigeminal impression to the internal auditory meatus (IAM), exposing the posterior fossa dura. The dura is then opened along the base of the temporal lobe. The superior petrosal sinus is coagulated and cut to allow opening of the tentorium to the incisura, thus allowing exposure to the posterior cranial fossa.

History of Approach

The anterior petrosal approach was first described by Bochenek and Kukwa.[38] This approach consisted of drilling of the petrous apex through the middle fossa to expose the cerebellopontine angle and cutting the tentorium to better visualize the brain stem and basilar artery. Kawase and colleagues modified this approach in order to expose the lower basilar artery and then petroclival and sphenopetroclival tumors.[39–41]

Benefits of Approach

The anterior petrosal approach is best suited for smaller petroclival meningiomas that do not extend below the IAM (Fig. 44-2). Tumors that extend farther into the posterior fossa and lateral to the IAM require the posterior petrosal approach. The anterior petrosal approach has the added benefit of allowing improved visualization of the clivus across the midline. If a

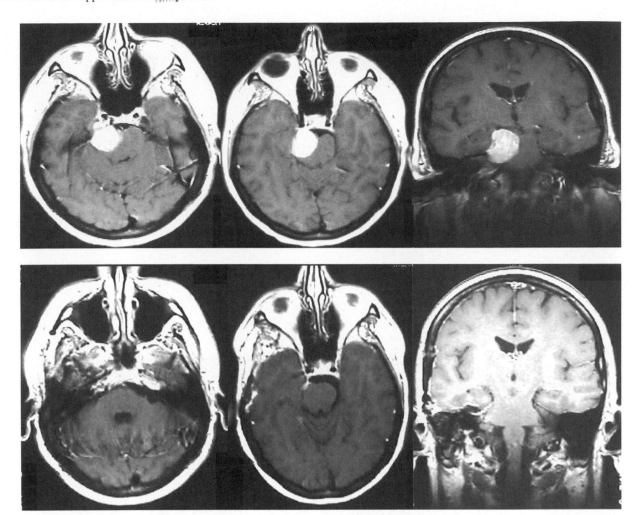

FIG. 44-2. Preoperative (upper row) and postoperative (lower row) T_1-weighted MR images of a patient who underwent resection of a petroclival meningioma via a zygomatic anterior petrosal approach

tumor extends more medially or across midline, the posterior approach may yield limited exposure. An anterior middle fossa approach should be used alone or as an addition to a posterior petrosal approach to provide exposure of the tumor across the midline. In addition, this approach provides excellent exposure of the tumors that invade the posterior cavernous sinus.

Limitations of Approach

The anterior petrosal approach is limited in its ability to expose tumors deeper in the posterior fossa and requires more manipulation of the trigeminal nerve. The trigeminal nerve is the center of exposure of the anterior petrosal approach, and tumor resection occurs in the spaces above and below the nerve. Manipulation of the trigeminal nerve introduces the possible complication of deafferentation pain within the trigeminal distribution that is often difficult to manage.

Posterior Petrosal Approach

Description of Approach

The patient is positioned supine with the head turned to the opposite side and the ipsilateral shoulder raised slightly. The skin incision is made extending from the zygoma anterior to the tragus and extending in a curvilinear fashion behind the ear to below the mastoid process. The skin flap is rotated anteriorly and inferiorly, and the temporal fascia is incised and reflected inferiorly in continuity with the sternocleido-mastoid muscle. The temporalis muscle is cut along the superior edge of the incision and retracted inferiorly and anteriorly. Four burr holes are placed straddling the transverse sinus: two in the posterior fossa and two supratentorially. A single bone flap is created covering the middle and posterior fossae (Fig. 44-3). The transverse-sigmoid sinus junction is exposed with the craniotomy. The mastoid cortex

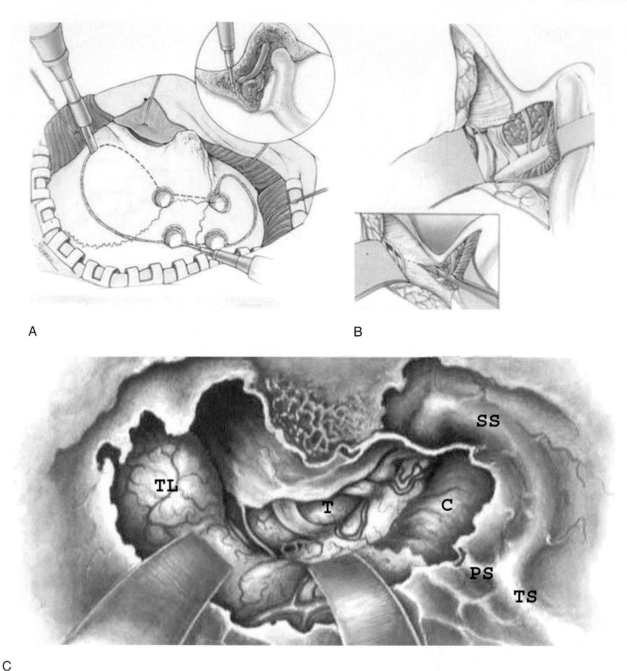

FIG. 44-3. Illustration of the exposure provided by the posterior petrosal approach. (A) Approach after the temporalis and sternocleidomastoid muscle have been cut and retracted. (B) Exposure prior to opening the dura of the middle fossa and splitting the tentorium. (C) Full exposure provided by this approach. TL, temporal lobe; T, tumor, C, cerebellum; SS, sigmoid sinus; TS, transverse sinus; PS, superior petrosal sinus

is cored and cut, and a mastoidectomy is performed, exposing the presigmoid dura mater and keeping the bony labyrinth intact. The sigmoid sinus is skeletonized to the jugular bulb. The dura is opened along the floor of the temporal fossa and in the presigmoid region. Care is taken to locate and protect the vein of Labbé at its insertion into the transverse sinus. The superior petrosal sinus is coagulated or occluded with a clip, and then it is cut to connect the dural openings. The tentorium is sectioned in a parallel plane to the petrous ridge and across the incisura after the surgeon locates and preserves the fourth cranial nerve insertion. The posterior temporal lobe is elevated and the sigmoid sinus is retracted posteriorly, allowing access to the supra- and infratentorial spaces.

History of Approach

The more extensive, hearing-sacrificing translabyrinthine approach was originally pioneered by Morrison and King[42] and exposed the cerebellopontine angle through drilling of the mastoid and labyrinth and cutting of the tentorium. This approach was modified by Hakuba et al.,[43] with the addition of posterior fossa craniotomy to the labyrinthectomy. The transcochlear approach was described by House et al.[44] to allow more complete exposure of the cerebellopontine angle. In this approach, the facial nerve is mobilized in the temporal bone from the stylomastoid foramen to its entrance into the internal auditory canal. This allows for additional bone resection and greater exposure. However, this exposure involves direct manipulation of the facial nerve and increases the risk of facial nerve injury. Al-Mefty et al.[2] described the retrolabyrinthine approach, which had the goal of maintaining exposure without sacrificing the hearing or facial nerve function. Other groups have used the retrolabyrinthine approach with good success of tumor resection and hearing preservation.[45–47] The posterior petrosal approach has also been used in the treatment of vascular lesions in the posterior fossa.

Benefits of Approach

The posterior petrosal approach may be used to provide exposure of tumors deeper within the posterior fossa, lateral to the IAM (Fig. 44-4). The petrous resection is retrolabyrinthine, allowing for preservation of hearing. Of patients who underwent a posterior petrosal or combined petrosal approach in a recent series, the hearing preservation rate was 92%.[48] In addition, this approach allows for exposure with minimal temporal lobe retraction and reduces the operating distance to the petroclival junction. This is the approach of choice for larger petroclival tumors and for those that extend below the IAM. Resection of the petrous temporal bone increases surgical exposure of the petroclival region by allowing a more lateral view of the brain stem and petroclival groove.

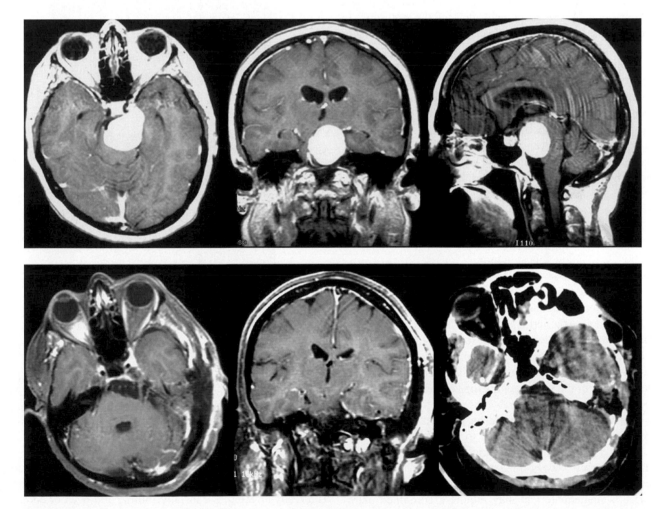

FIG. 44-4. Preoperative (upper row) and postoperative (lower row) T_1-weighted MR images of a patient who underwent resection of a petroclival meningioma via posterior petrosal approach. This tumor was a large petroclival meningioma extending below the IAM in a patient with intact hearing

The retrolabyrinthine posterior petrosal approach requires mobilization of the sigmoid sinus.[1] This requires skeletonization and exposure from the transverse sinus to the jugular bulb to provide enough length to be able to retract the sinus. In addition, a posterior fossa craniotomy is required to allow room for displacement of the sinus. Finally, the sigmoid sinus cannot be mobilized until the tentorium is cut to untether the sinus. Once these steps are performed, the sinus can be mobilized posteriorly, allowing adequate exposure.

Limitations of Approach

Many of the complications of this approach are encountered when retracting the mobilized sigmoid sinus or in cutting the tentorium. Although some surgeons advocate transection of the sigmoid sinus to allow better access,[49–53] we feel that this is not necessary for sufficient exposure and carries a risk of insufficient venous outflow. Any injury to the sinus requires meticulous repair. The posterior petrosal approach may present a higher risk in patients who have a dominant or single sigmoid sinus on the side of the tumor, in patients with a transverse sinus that do not connect to the torcular herophili, and in patients with the venous drainage through the tentorium. In patients with a dominant or single sigmoid sinus ipsilateral to the tumor, retraction of the sinus may lead to venous congestion during the operation and injury to the sinus could lead to more serious complications (Fig. 44-5). In patients whose transverse sinuses do not connect at the torcular herophili, the venous drainage may be completely split with one hemisphere draining through the superior sagittal sinus and the other through the deep venous system. Thus, retraction of the dominant or single sinus could also lead to venous congestion of the hemisphere that is drained by this structure. In patients with sinus drainage through the tentorium, care must be taken not to transect the tentorium in a way that disrupts this drainage. In these cases, the tentorium should be cut medially and laterally to the tentorial sinus and tumor resection may proceed above and below this structure.

The anatomy of the vein of Labbé is also critical in this approach.[54] In cases where the vein of Labbé inserts into the superior petrosal sinus in the tentorium before the transverse-sigmoid sinus junction, care must be taken to keep this drainage from being severed. In these cases, the insertion of the vein should be inspected closely during dural opening to ensure that the incision through the tentorium is made anterior to the insertion of the vein, keeping the venous drainage to the temporal lobe in continuity.

In a number of cases, the posterior petrosal approach may provide inadequate tumor exposure to allow complete resection. In cases of patients with a high jugular bulb, the presigmoid approach may be inadequate to allow exposure. In patients with tumors that cross the midline of the clivus, this exposure is inadequate and may require a combined petrosal approach. In addition, in cases with tumor in the anterior corner of the petroclival groove and the posterior cavernous

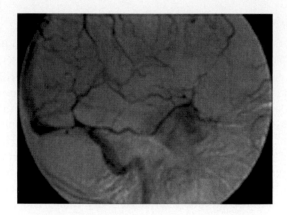

A

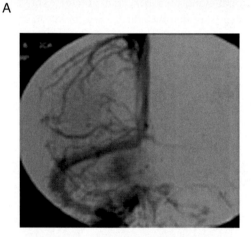

B

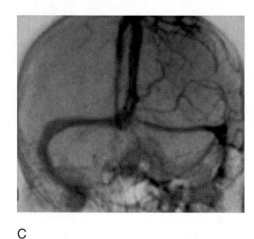

C

FIG. 44-5. Venous phase angiogram demonstrating venous anatomy reviewed prior to petrosal approaches. (A) Case in which the vein of Labbé empties into the tentorium. (B) Case in which the dominant sigmoid sinus is ipsilateral to the tumor. (C) Case in which the transverse sinuses are not connected at the torcular

sinus, the labyrinth may obstruct the surgeon's view, making complete tumor removal impossible. In cases where hearing is already affected, a translabyrinthine approach or complete petrosectomy should be considered. In cases where hearing is intact a combined petrosal approach should be considered.

Combined Petrosal Approach

Description of Approach

The skin incision is similar to that described for the posterior petrosal approach. The anterior limb of the incision can be carried up to the midline to allow the skin flap to be reflected anteriorly. The superficial temporal artery is preserved on the muscle layer. The skin is reflected anteriorly along with the temporal fascia to preserve the frontal branch of the facial nerve. The zygomatic arch is cut anteriorly and posteriorly, and the temporalis muscle is reflected inferiorly. The bone flap is similar to the posterior petrosal flap, although it is extended farther anteriorly along the floor of the middle fossa and crosses the sphenoid wing. The mastoid cortex is cored and removed. The mastoid is drilled to skeletonize the labyrinth and the petrous apex is also drilled. The dura mater is opened in a similar fashion to the description of the posterior petrosal approach, but the incision is extended farther anteriorly along the floor of the middle fossa (Fig. 44-6). The dura mater along the floor of the temporal fossa can be connected with a dural incision along the sphenoid wing to expose the sylvian fissure as well. The tentorium is incised anteriorly to the incisura posterior to the trochlear nerve insertion and is connected with a tentorial cut paralleling the superior petrosal sinus from the posterior direction. With this exposure, the tumor can be approached through the petrous bone anterior and posterior to the labyrinth and middle ear apparatus.

History of Approach

The combination of the anterior and posterior approaches can further extend the exposure, taking advantage of the benefits of each individual approach. This approach was first described by Hakuba et al.,[43] who combined the preauricular and post-

auricular transpetrous approaches, including resection of the labyrinth and endolymphatic sac. The cochlea and ossicles of the ear were left intact with an attempt to preserve hearing. Among the eight patients treated using this approach, seven had hearing loss. Partial resection of the labyrinth has been described by Sekhar et al.[55] as a technique that has the potential to preserve hearing while extending the temporal exposure. This approach was used in a series of 36 patients, with 80% preservation of hearing. The technique was slightly modified by another group[56,57] with similar hearing preservation rates. Anatomic studies have demonstrated an increase in horizontal exposure with labyrinth resection,[58,59] although other groups have found that partial labyrinth resection does not supplement the critical exposure required for resection of tumors in the petroclival region.[60] Moreover, Sekhar advocates that the extra exposure gained with the partial labyrinthectomy and petrous apicectomy is secondary to the resection of the petrous apex.[55] Thus, the combined petrosal approach as described takes advantage of the ability to resect the petrous apex from the middle fossa exposure as opposed to increasing the risk of hearing loss with a partial labyrinthectomy.

Benefits of Approach

The combined petrosal approach is optimal for patients with large petroclival tumors who have serviceable hearing.[61] This exposure takes advantage of the benefits of both anterior and posterior petrosal approaches, while saving hearing and facial nerve function. Specifically, one can resect large tumors in the posterior fossa below the IAM through the posterior petrosal exposure while using the anterior petrosal exposure to visualize the midline clivus, ventral brain stem, the contralateral side, and the anterior cavernous sinus (Fig. 44-7). In addition, this approach allows exposure of the petrous apex and

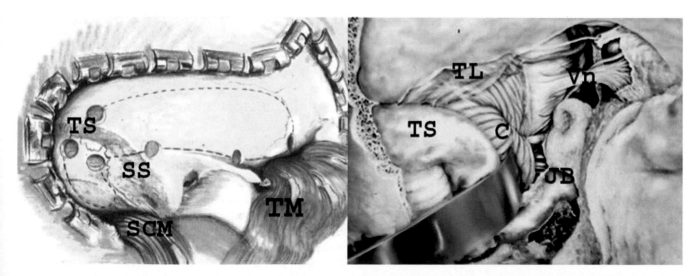

FIG. 44-6. Illustration of exposure provided by the combined petrosal approach. The panel on the left shows the approach after the temporalis and sternocleidomastoid muscle have been cut and retracted. The panel on the right shows the full exposure provided by this approach. TM, temporalis muscle; SCM, sternocleidomastoid muscle; TL, temporal lobe; T, tumor, C, cerebellum; SS, sigmoid sinus; TS, transverse sinus; Vn, trigeminal nerve; JB, jugular bulb

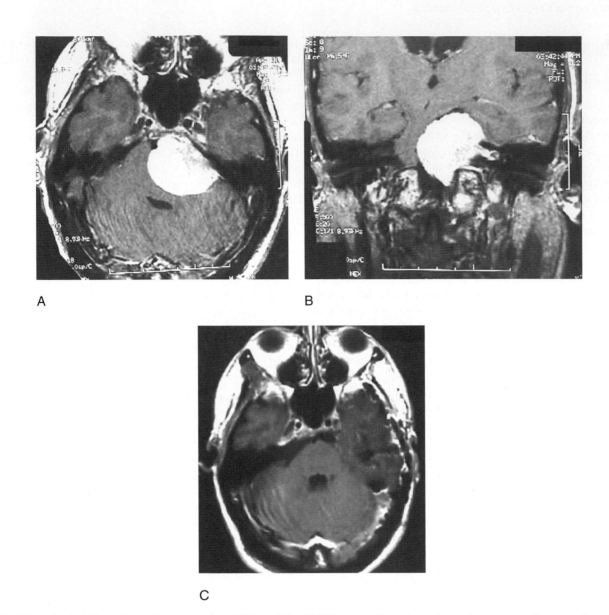

FIG. 44-7. Preoperative (A and B) and postoperative (C) T_1-weighted MR images of a patient who underwent complete resection of a large petroclival meningioma via the combined petrosal approach

the Meckel's cave. The ability to expose the ventral brainstem allows visualization of the basilar artery and perforating vessels, providing a safer approach to resection.

Limitations of Approach

Just as this approach combines the benefits of the anterior and posterior petrosal approaches, the risks of the combined petrosal approach is the sum of the risks of each of these individual approaches. While performing the anterior petrosal portion of this approach, there is a similar risk to the trigeminal nerve and internal carotid artery. While performing the posterior portion of this approach, there is a risk to the sigmoid sinus being retracted. However, in cases of large tumors that extend across the midline of the clivus with a significant amount of tumor in the posterior fossa, the risks are well worth the benefits of increased exposure.

Complete Petrosectomy

Description of Approach

The skin incision is similar to the combined petrosal approach. As the skin is reflected anteriorly, the external auditory canal is sectioned and closed in a blind sac. The mastoidectomy is performed, followed by a labyrinthectomy. The facial nerve is then skeletonized along its course through the temporal bone and is left within a thin bone canal for protection. The tympanic membrane and inner ear ossicles are resected. The petrous apex and cochlea are then drilled to complete the petrosectomy. This approach allows unobstructed lateral visualization of the petroclival, clival, and cavernous sinus regions (Fig. 44-8)

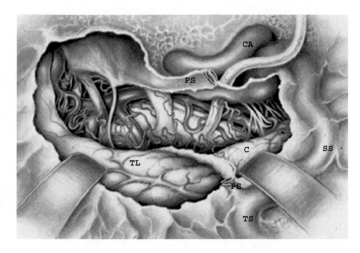

FIG. 44-8. Illustration of the exposure provided by the total or complete petrosectomy approach. TL, temporal lobe; C, cerebellum; SS, sigmoid sinus; TS, transverse sinus; PS, superior petrosal sinus

History of Approach

In 1976, House and Hitselberger first described the transcochlear approach (44). This approach was a forward extension of the translabyrinthine approach, where the facial nerve is mobilized and the cochlea removed. This approach was modified by Jenkins and Fisch, who achieved a more anterior exposure by removing the external auditory canal and the tympanic membrane (62). The final modification of this technique to allow wider resection of petroclival meningiomas was the addition of tentorial section to allow better supratentorial access (63).

Benefits of Approach

In patients with large tumors and loss of hearing, the complete petrosectomy allows the most extensive surgical exposure. Removal of the inner ear apparatus connects the posterior and anterior exposures, allowing a true anterior, lateral, and posterior approach to the petroclival region, and to all areas into which these tumors extend (Fig. 44-9).

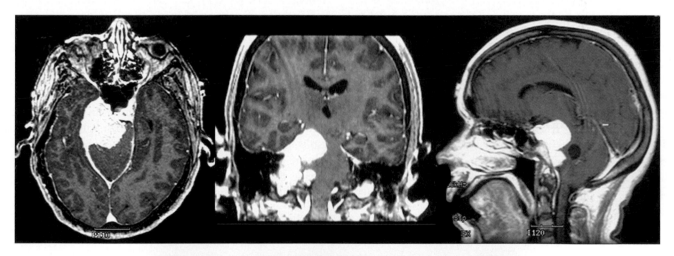

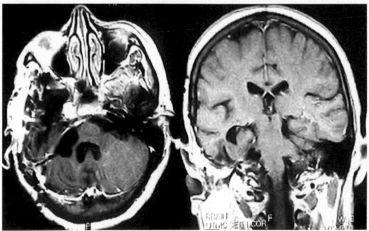

FIG. 44-9. Preoperative (upper row) and postoperative (lower row) T$_1$-weighted MR images of a patient who underwent resection of a petroclival meningioma after complete petrosectomy. This tumor was a large petroclival meningioma extending below the IAM in a patient without serviceable hearing in the right ear

Limitations of Approach

The limitation of this approach is the longer preparation time required to drill the entire petrous bone. Often we will stage these procedures, performing the exposure on one day and following with tumor resection on the following day. Additionally, there is risk of injury to the facial nerve because the exposure requires skeletonizing the nerve along its course through the temporal bone. Leaving a thin shell of bone surrounding it during exposure can decrease the risk of facial nerve injury. In this series, new facial weakness developed in two patients, and two experienced worsening of preoperative facial weakness. It is difficult to assess whether this symptom is secondary to the surgical exposure or to dissection of the tumor, because patients who undergo complete petrosectomy often have tumors that involve the facial nerve.

Choice of Surgical Approach

The choice of surgical approach should be dictated by a number of factors. The size and location of the tumor, the extent of bone infiltration by the tumor, and the patient's arterial and venous anatomy are among the most critical factors determining the choice of approach. We have already described the approaches that we commonly use to surgically remove petroclival meningiomas. We will briefly review the criteria that we use in choosing the surgical approach for resection of petroclival meningiomas (Fig. 44-10). Prior to surgery, each patient receives an MRI, MRV, CT, and hearing test. Patients with small tumors that are superior to the IAM are operated using the anterior petrosal approach. Patients with larger tumors that do not cross the midline of the clivus are operated using the posterior petrosal approach if their hearing is intact,

while those whose hearing is impaired are operated using the total petrosectomy. The combined petrosal approach is used for those patients who have large tumors extending across the clivus and for those patients who have large tumors that involve the anterior cavernous sinus.

Complications of Approaches to Petroclival Tumors

One of the major concerns of treating patients with petroclival meningiomas with surgical resection is the risk of complications. However, advances in microsurgical techniques have greatly reduced the risks associated with these surgeries.[7,15,42,61,64,65] In a previous publication, the senior author (OA) reported results for 97 patients who were treated with petroclival and sphenopetroclival meningiomas between 1995 and 2005[48] At the time of that publication 28 patients were operated using the zygomatic anterior petrosal approach, 27 underwent a posterior petrosal approach, 34 underwent the combined petrosal approach, and 8 underwent a complete petrosectomy. Exposure-related complications occurred in 8 patients. There were no cases of trigeminal neuralgia after the zygomatic anterior petrosal approach. Only 5 (8%) of the patients who were operated using the posterior petrosal and combined petrosal approaches experienced hearing loss. Ten patients (10%) in this series had cerebral spinal leakage. Only 3 patients (3%) required surgical repair of this leakage, and 2 patients (2%) developed postoperative meningitis. Given these results, we concluded that the surgical approaches described here are safe when used under the correct circumstances and provide the surgeon with the exposure to carefully remove these challenging tumors.

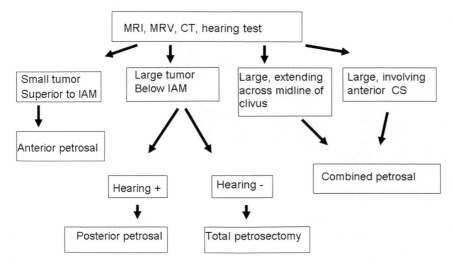

Fig. 44-10. Algorithm for surgical approach. This diagram illustrates our algorithm for choosing the surgical approach for patients with petroclival meningiomas. IAM, internal auditory meatus; CS, cavernous sinus

References

1. Al-Mefty O: Operative Atlas of Meningiomas. Philadephia, Lippincott-Raven, 1988.
2. Al-Mefty O, Fox JL, Smith RR: Petrosal approach for petroclival meningiomas. Neurosurgery 1988;22:510–517.
3. Rachlin J, Rosenblum M: Etiology and biology of meningiomas, in Al-Mefty O (ed): Meningiomas. New York, Raven, 1991, pp 22–37.
4. Wilson CB: Meningiomas: genetics, malignancy, and the role of radiation in induction and treatment. The Richard C. Schneider Lecture. J Neurosurg 1994;81:666–675.
5. Pieper D, Al-Mefty O: Petroclival/sphenopetroclival meningiomas, in Robertson JT, Coakham HB, Robertson JH (eds): Cranial Base Surgery. London, Churchill Livingstone, 2000, pp 449–472.
6. Cherington M, Schneck SA: Clivus meningiomas. Neurology 1966;16:86–92.
7. Hakuba A, Nishimura S, Tanaka K, Kishi H, Nakamura T: Clivus meningioma: six cases of total removal. Neurol Med Chir (Tokyo) 1977;17:63–77.
8. Voss NF, Vrionis FD, Heilman CB, Robertson JH: Meningiomas of the cerebellopontine angle. Surg Neurol 2000;53:439–446; discussion 446–437.
9. Mayberg MR, Symon L: Meningiomas of the clivus and apical petrous bone. Report of 35 cases. J Neurosurg 1986;65:160–167.
10. Cappabianca P, Mariniello G, Alfieri A, de Divitiis E: Trigeminal neuralgia and contralateral mass. J Neurosurg 1997;86:171–172.
11. Grigoryan YA, Onopchenko CV: Persistent trigeminal neuralgia after removal of contralateral posterior cranial fossa tumor. Report of two cases. Surg Neurol 1999;52:56–60; discussion 60–51.
12. Haddad FS, Taha JM: An unusual cause for trigeminal neuralgia: contralateral meningioma of the posterior fossa. Neurosurgery 1990;26:1033–1038.
13. Mase G, Zorzon M, Capus L, et al.: Trigeminal neuralgia due to contralateral meningioma of the posterior cranial fossa. J Neurol Neurosurg Psychiatry 1994;57:1010.
14. Hakuba A, Nishimura S: Total removal of clivus meningiomas and the operative results. Neurol Med Chir (Tokyo) 1981;21:59–73.
15. Bricolo AP, Turazzi S, Talacchi A, Cristofori L: Microsurgical removal of petroclival meningiomas: a report of 33 patients. Neurosurgery 1992;l31:813–828; discussion 828.
16. Yano S, Kuratsu J: Indications for surgery in patients with asymptomatic meningiomas based on an extensive experience. J Neurosurg 2006;105:538–543.
17. Miller DC: Predicting recurrence of intracranial meningiomas. A multivariate clinicopathologic model—interim report of the New York University Medical Center Meningioma Project. Neurosurg Clin N Am 1994;5:193–200.
18. Simpson D: The recurrence of intracranial meningiomas after surgical treatment. J Neurol Neurosurg Psychiatry 1957;20:22–39.
19. Iwai Y, Yamanaka K, Yasui T, et al.: Gamma knife surgery for skull base meningiomas. The effectiveness of low-dose treatment. Surg Neurol 1999;52:40–44; discussion 44–45.
20. Linskey ME, Davis SA, Ratanatharathorn V: Relative roles of microsurgery and stereotactic radiosurgery for the treatment of patients with cranial meningiomas: a single-surgeon 4-year integrated experience with both modalities. J Neurosurg 2005;102 (Suppl):59–70.
21. Roche PH, Pellet W, Fuentes S, et al.: Gamma knife radiosurgical management of petroclival meningiomas results and indications. Acta Neurochir (Wien) 2003;145:883–888; discussion 888.
22. Stafford SL, Pollock BE, Foote RL, et al.: Meningioma radiosurgery: tumor control, outcomes, and complications among 190 consecutive patients. Neurosurgery 2001;49:1029–1037; discussion 1037–1028.
23. Subach BR, Lunsford LD, Kondziolka D, et al.: Management of petroclival meningiomas by stereotactic radiosurgery. Neurosurgery 1998;42:437–443; discussion 443–435.
24. Zachenhofer I, Wolfsberger S, Aichholzer M, et al.: Gamma-knife radiosurgery for cranial base meningiomas: experience of tumor control, clinical course, and morbidity in a follow-up of more than 8 years. Neurosurgery 2006;58:28–36; discussion 28–36
25. Goldsmith B, McDermott MW: Meningioma. Neurosurg Clin N Am 2006;17:111–120, vi.
26. Noel G, Bollet MA, Calugaru V, et al.: Functional outcome of patients with benign meningioma treated by 3D conformal irradiation with a combination of photons and protons. Int J Radiat Oncol Biol Phys 2005;62:1412–1422.
27. Kaido T, Hoshida T, Uranishi R, et al.: Radiosurgery-induced brain tumor. Case report. J Neurosurg 2001;95:710–713.
28. Kleinschmidt-Demasters BK, Kang JS, Lillehei KO: The burden of radiation-induced central nervous system tumors: a single institution s experience. J Neuropathol Exp Neurol 2006;65:204–216.
29. Kranzinger M, Jones N, Rittinger O, et al.: Malignant glioma as a secondary malignant neoplasm after radiation therapy for craniopharyngioma: report of a case and review of reported cases. Onkologie 2001;24:66–72.
30. Salvati M, Frati A, Russo N, et al.: Radiation-induced gliomas: report of 10 cases and review of the literature. Surg Neurol 2003;60:60–67; discussion 67.
31. Shamisa A, Bance M, Nag S, et al.: Glioblastoma multiforme occurring in a patient treated with gamma knife surgery. Case report and review of the literature. J Neurosurg 2001;94:816–821.
32. Sheehan J, Yen CP, Steiner L: Gamma knife surgery-induced meningioma. Report of two cases and review of the literature. J Neurosurg 2006;105:325–329.
33. Shin M, Ueki K, Kurita H, Kirino T: Malignant transformation of a vestibular schwannoma after gamma knife radiosurgery. Lancet 2002;360:309–310.
34. Yu JS, Yong WH, Wilson D, Black KL: Glioblastoma induction after radiosurgery for meningioma. Lancet 2000;356:1576–1577.
35. Couldwell WT, Cole CD, Al-Mefty O: Patterns of skull base meningioma progression after failed radiosurgery. J Neurosurg 2007;106:30–35.
36. Liscak R, Kollova A, Vladyka V, et al.: Gamma knife radiosurgery of skull base meningiomas. Acta Neurochir Suppl 2004;91:65–74.
37. Milker-Zabel S, Zabel-du Bois A, Huber P, et al.: Fractionated stereotactic radiation therapy in the management of benign cavernous sinus meningiomas : long-term experience and review of the literature. Strahlenther Onkol 2006;182:635–640.
38. Bochenek J, Kukwa A: An extended approach through the middle cranial fossa to the internal auditory meatus and the cerebellopontine angle. Acta Otolaryngol 1975;410–414.
39. Kawase T, Shiobara R, Toya S: Anterior transpetrosal-transtentorial approach for sphenopetroclival meningiomas: surgical method and results in 10 patients. Neurosurgery 1991;28:869–875; discussion 875–866.

40. Kawase T, Shiobara R, Toya S: Middle fossa transpetrosal-transtentorial approaches for petroclival meningiomas. Selective pyramid resection and radicality. Acta Neurochir (Wien) 1994;129:113–120.

41. Kawase T, Toya S, Shiobara R, Mine T: Transpetrosal approach for aneurysms of the lower basilar artery. J Neurosurg 1985;63:857–861.

42. Morrison AW, King TT: Experiences with a translabyrinthine-transtentorial approach to the cerebellopontine angle. Technical note. J Neurosurg 1973;38:382–390.

43. Hakuba A, Nishimura S, Jang BJ: A combined retroauricular and preauricular transpetrosal-transtentorial approach to clivus meningiomas. Surg Neurol 1988;30:108–116.

44. House WF, Hitselberger WE: The transcochlear approach to the skull base. Arch Otolaryngol 1976;102:334–342.

45. Canalis RF, Black K, Martin N, Becker D: Extended retrolabyrinthine transtentorial approach to petroclival lesions. Laryngoscope 1991;101:6–13.

46. Couldwell WT, Fukushima T, Giannotta SL, Weiss MH: Petroclival meningiomas: surgical experience in 109 cases. J Neurosurg 1996;84:20–28.

47. Daspit CP, Spetzler RF, Pappas CT: Combined approach for lesions involving the cerebellopontine angle and skull base: experience with 20 cases–preliminary report. Otolaryngol Head Neck Surg 1991;105:788–796.

48. Erkmen K, Pravdenkova S, Al-Mefty O: Surgical management of petroclival meningiomas: factors determining the choice of approach. Neurosurg Focus 2005;19:E7.

49. Cantore G, Delfini R, Ciappetta P: Surgical treatment of petroclival meningiomas: experience with 16 cases. Surg Neurol 1994;42:105–111.

50. Hwang SK, Gwak HS, Paek SH, et al.: The experience of ligation of transverse or sigmoid sinus in surgery of large petroclival meningiomas. J Korean Med Sci 2002;17:544–548.

51. Malis LI: The petrosal approach. Clin Neurosurg 1991;37:528–540.

52. Megerian CA, Chiocca EA, McKenna MJ, et al.: The subtemporal-transpetrous approach for excision of petroclival tumors. Am J Otol 1996;17:773–779.

53. Spetzler RF, Daspit CP, Pappas CT: The combined supra- and infratentorial approach for lesions of the petrous and clival

54. Sakata K, Al-Mefty O, Yamamoto I: Venous consideration in petrosal approach: microsurgical anatomy of the temporal bridging vein. Neurosurgery 2000;47:153–160; discussion 160–151.

55. Sekhar LN, Schessel DA, Bucur SD, Raso JL, Wright DC: Partial labyrinthectomy petrous apicectomy approach to neoplastic and vascular lesions of the petroclival area. Neurosurgery 1999;44:537–550; discussion 550–532.

56. Horgan MA, Delashaw JB, Schwartz MS, et al.: Transcrusal approach to the petroclival region with hearing preservation. Technical note and illustrative cases. J Neurosurg 2001;94:660–666.

57. Kaylie DM, Horgan MA, Delashaw JB, McMenomey SO: Hearing preservation with the transcrusal approach to the petroclival region. Otol Neurotol 2004;25:594–598; discussion 598.

58. Chanda A, Nanda A: Partial labyrinthectomy petrous apicectomy approach to the petroclival region: an anatomic and technical study. Neurosurgery 2002;51:147–159; discussion 159–160.

59. Horgan MA, Anderson GJ, Kellogg JX, et al.: Classification and quantification of the petrosal approach to the petroclival region. J Neurosurg 2000;93:108–112.

60. Miller CG, van Loveren HR, Keller JT, et al.: Transpetrosal approach: surgical anatomy and technique. Neurosurgery 1993;33:461–469; discussion 469.

61. Cho CW, Al-Mefty O: Combined petrosal approach to petroclival meningiomas. Neurosurgery 2002;51:708–716; discussion 716–708.

62. Jenkins HA, Fisch U: The transotic approach to resection of difficult acoustic tumors of the cerebellopontine angle. Am J Otol 1980;2:70–76.

63. Thedinger BA, Glasscock ME, 3rd, Cueva RA: Transcochlear transtentorial approach for removal of large cerebellopontine angle meningiomas. Am J Otol 1992;13:408–415.

64. Al-Mefty O, Ayoubi S, Smith RR: The petrosal approach: indications, technique, and results. Acta Neurochir Suppl (Wien) 1991;53:166–170.

65. Angeli SI, De la Cruz A, Hitselberger W: The transcochlear approach revisited. Otol Neurotol 2001;22:690–695.

regions: experience with 46 cases. J Neurosurg 1992;76:588–599.

45

Petroclival and Upper Clival Meningiomas II: Anterior Transpetrosal Approach

Takeshi Kawase, Kazunari Yoshida, and Koichi Uchida

Introduction

Skull base meningiomas can be removed through a narrow surgical corridor, provided that the attachment and the feeders are included in the surgical exposure. The anterior transpetrosal approach[1,2] is a kind of "key hole skull base surgery" with the above concept for removal of petroclival tumors. The surgical steps are:[1] epidural exposure of the dura overlying the tumor;[2] coagulation of the feeders;[3] decompression of the internal content;[4] retraction of the tumor margin toward the attachment;[5] dissection of the slackened nerves and vessels around the tumor; and[6] removal of the tumor margin with the dural attachment. The indications, limitations, the surgical technique, and our surgical results are presented in this chapter.

Advantages and Disadvantages of the Anterior Transpetrosal Approach

The advantages of the approach are as follows, compared to the suboccipital approach:[1] one stage surgery is possible even if the tumor extends into the middle fossa or the Meckel's cave;[2] tumor bleeding can completely be controlled by coagulation of feeders (the tentorial artery and the middle meningeal artery) before internal decompression;[3] low manipulation injury to the cranial nerves VII–X, accessed anterior to the facial nerve;[4] no retraction damage to the cerebellum and brain stem; and[5] higher radicality by removal of the tentorial or the petrous dural attachment.

The advantages compared to the presigmoid approach[3,4] are low risk of venous complication, without the need for exposing the sigmoid sinus and the vein of Labbé, and shorter operation time for the bony pyramid removal. The disadvantages are its contraindications for broad-based tumors and the necessity for technical training.

Classification of Petroclival Meningioma and Indication of Anterior Transpetrosal Approach

Meningiomas of the petroclival region are classified into the following five types, according to the tumor extension on magnetic resonance imaging (MRI) (Table 45-1). Cerebellopontine angle meningiomas (i.e., ventral petrous) or lower clival meningiomas are excluded from the series.

Upper Clival

The tumors originate around the orifice of the Meckel's cave, and the attachment is limited to the upper half of the clivus or the tentorium, medial to the internal auditory meatus (IAM). Invasion into the Meckel's cave is common (Fig. 45-1a).

Sphenoclival

These tumors extend into the middle fossa or the cavernous sinus from the clivus (Fig. 45-1b).

Petroclival

These tumors have a wide attachment extending posterior or inferior to the IAM (Fig. 45-1c).

Mid-Clival

This rare group of tumors have a main origin from and dural attachment on the central clivus.

Central Skull Base

These rare tumors show bilateral extension in the central skull base (i.e., suprasellar, parasellar, and clivus).

TABLE 45-1. Clinical Features of 94 Operated Meningiomas Extending into Petroclival Area.

Type of tumor	No. of Patients	%	
Upper clival	55	(58.5%)	70 cases operated by APA
Sphenoclival	15	(16.0%)	
Petroclival	13	(13.8%)	
Mid-clival	4	(4.3%)	
Central skull base	7	(7.4%)	
Total	94	(100%)	

The anterior transpetrosal approach (APA) is indicated for upper clival (UC) and sphenoclival (SC) types. The indication is limited not by the tumor size, but by the size of the tumor attachment. The lower limit of the surgical exposure by APA is the line between the mid-clivus and IAM, and the radical tumor resection could be expected if the attachment is limited within this space (Fig. 45-2). For petroclival (PC)-type tumors, the posterior transpetrosal or suboccipital approach is added (5). For other tumors, various approaches are utilized with the goal of maximal tumor removal. In this chapter, the surgical technique of APA and the surgical results for 70 patients with the UC or Sphenoclival (SC) types are presented. The surgical technique for typical PC type tumor, discussed in other chapters, was excluded from this series.

Preoperative Preparations

MRI T1 with contrast and T2 images and temporal bone targeted computed tomography (CT) images are prepared before surgery. Angiography is necessary for large tumors, but MR angiography has replaced conventional angiography for small sized tumors. Preoperative embolization is necessary only in patients with tumor feeders from the ascending pharyngeal or the middle meningeal artery. The following surgical tools are prepared: a surgical drill, ultrasonic aspirator (Sonopet M&M Co., Ltd, Tokyo, Japan), neuroendoscope attached to the microscope (OME-8000, Olympus Co., Ltd, Tokyo, Japan), and the "Skull Base Instrument Set," which contains the following microsurgical tools: Sugita's hooked retractors, tumor retractors, and variable dissectors (Mizuho-ika Co., Ltd, Tokyo, Japan). Facial nerve monitoring is optionally used.

Spinal drainage may be employed preoperatively to reduce compression of the temporal lobe. In the case of large tumors, the trigone of the lateral ventricle can be punctured for continuous cerebrospinal fluid (CSF) drainage. The patient is placed in supine position with a pillow inserted under the shoulders, and the upper body is elevated 20 degrees. The patient's head is rotated laterally with the head flexed downward. The correct lateral head position is important to facilitate the exposure and identification of the inner structures of the temporal bone as the surgery progresses.

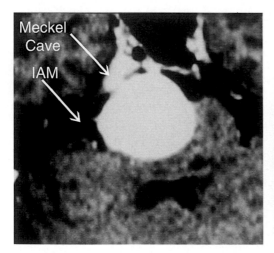

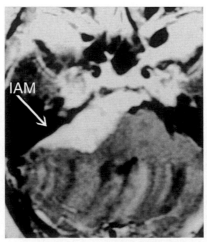

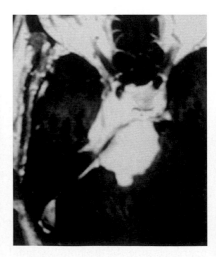

A   B   C

FIG. 45-1. Classification of petroclival meningiomas. (A) Upper clival type (UC), limited laterally by the internal auditory meatus (IAM), commonly involving Meckel's cave. (B) Sphenoclival type (SC), extending into the middle fossa or cavernous sinus. (C) Petroclival type (PC), with broad attachment extending posterior to the IAM. The anterior petrosal approach is indicated for UC and SC subtypes

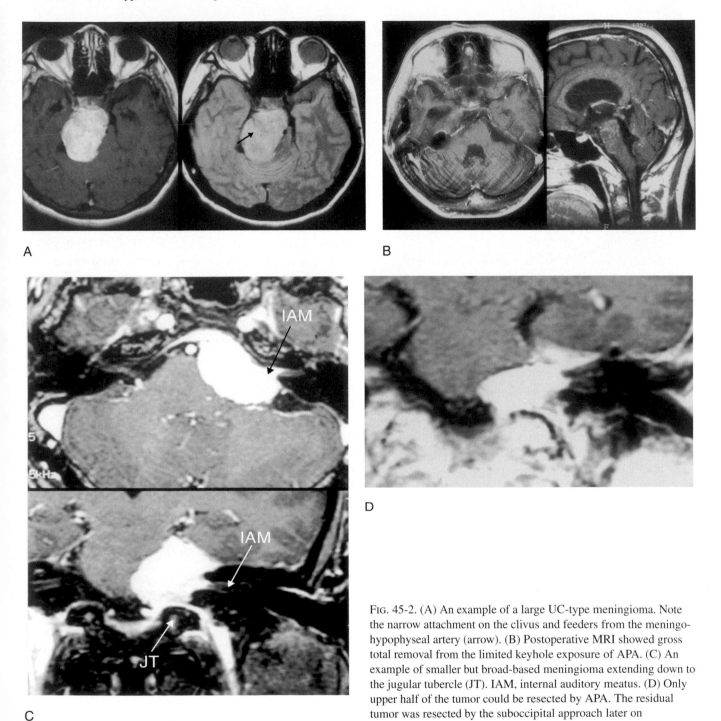

Fig. 45-2. (A) An example of a large UC-type meningioma. Note the narrow attachment on the clivus and feeders from the meningo-hypophyseal artery (arrow). (B) Postoperative MRI showed gross total removal from the limited keyhole exposure of APA. (C) An example of smaller but broad-based meningioma extending down to the jugular tubercle (JT). IAM, internal auditory meatus. (D) Only upper half of the tumor could be resected by APA. The residual tumor was resected by the suboccipital approach later on

Surgical Technique

Skin Incision and Craniotomy

A U-shaped scalp incision is made above the ear (Fig. 45-3) and the anterior limb of the incision is made straight to avoid injuring the upper facial nerve. The base of the "U" incision is made along the superior temporal line, and a fascial flap of sufficient size is created for use during closure.

In patients with SC-type tumors showing higher tumor extension above the posterior cliniod process, the zygomatic arch is removed (zygomatic petrosal approach)[7] to reduce the retraction damage on the temporal lobe. A question mark skin incision is made along the auricle. For subgaleal dissection close to the orbital rim, the subgaleal fat pad must be left attached to the galeal side to avoid the upper facial nerve injury. After exposing the zygomatic arch, it is cut by a surgical saw in two points. The temporal muscle is freed

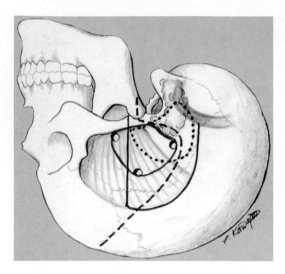

FIG. 45-3. Skin incision and the craniotomy site for APA (solid line) and zygomatic petrosal approach (broken line). The dotted line is a craniotomy for posterior petrosal approach

from the skull and tacked interiorly to allow the "look-up" surgical view for the superior part of the tumor in the parasellar region.

The bone spur of the zygomatic arch, the external auditory meatus, and the squamous suture are the pertinent landmarks for craniotomy. The craniotomy is centered low above the mandibular joint and the external auditory meatus. It is created along the outer margin of the squamous suture, and it is not necessary to expose the sigmoid sinus. An additional bone drilling under the roof of the zygoma is important to expose the foramen spinosum (Fig. 45-4).

Exposure and Resection of the Pyramid

The petrous pyramid is exposed epidurally until the petrous rim is identified. CSF drainage is helpful for the exposure. The foramen spinosum, which is located in the floor of the middle fossa, is identified, and the middle meningeal artery (MMA) is coagulated and divided. Venous bleeding around the foramen ovale must be controlled with oxycellulose cotton. Greater and lesser superficial petrosal nerves can be confirmed by their dural adhesion at the pyramid at a point posterior to the foramen ovale, coursing along in parallel in bony grooves. They are dissected carefully with the attached periosteal dural layer. This interdural dissection is extended anteriorly to the mandibular nerve, reducing tension of the dura. The trigeminal impression is exposed on the pyramidal apex (Fig. 45-5). Location of the semicircular canal can be identified from the arcuate eminence, an important posterior landmark on the pyramid. In some cases it is not prominent, and the semicircular canal must be confirmed from the target bone CT.

The internal auditory canal (IAC) is slightly anterior to the eminentia arcuata, at a depth of 7 mm from the bone surface. The geniculate ganglion is located on the proximal extension line of the greater superficial petrosal nerve (GSPN), at the intersection of the line between the external and internal auditory meatuses. The cochlea is located deep in the bone in the angle of the two lines formed by the GSPN and the IAC. From the surgeon's viewpoint, the carotid artery and Eustachian tube are lateral to the GSPN. A line of maximal bone resection with preservation of the auditory structure is shown in Fig. 45-5. It is medial to the GSPN, anterior to the eminentia arcuata, and superior to the internal auditory canal. Depth of

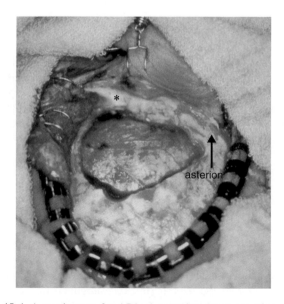

FIG. 45-4. A craniotomy for APA. A complete bone resection under the root of zygoma (*) is most important. (From Neurol Surg 1998; 26:304–313, with author's permission.)

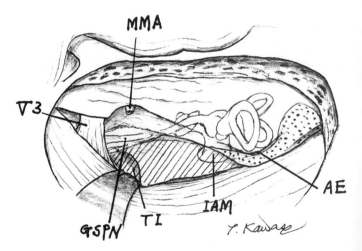

FIG. 45-5. Epidural exposure of the pyramid. The interdural layer is dissected to preserve the greater superficial petrosal nerve (GSPN), and the dissection line is extended on the mandibular nerve (V3) to reduce the tension of the dura. The superior semicircular canal is under the arcuate eminence (AE). The shaded is the area of bone resection. For large tumors extending along the tentorium, the bone resection is extended around the semicircular canal (dotted). TI, trigeminal impression; MMA, middle meningeal artery

the pyramidal apex is deeper in the anterior part, and the depth must be confirmed to follow the dural layer of the posterior fossa. Overdrilling toward the clivus may injure the abducens nerve as it enters the Dorello's canal, and the drilling must be finished at a point 5 mm medial to the trigeminal nerve. The diamond burr or Sonopet® (M&M Company, Tokyo, Japan) is recommended to preserve the dura mater for final bone resection. The bone resection must be carried out completely until none of the bone spur remains on the rim. The limited bone resection does not expose the petrous carotid artery.

Dural Incision

The basal dura of the middle fossa is incised 2 cm inward toward the superior petrosal sinus (SPS), and the incision is extended in a T-shape along the sinus. In a tumor showing middle fossa extension, it must be removed from the tentorium. Next an aperture in the posterior fossa dura is made under the SPS, and the petrosal vein and anterior inferior cerebellar artery are confirmed in the cerebellopontine angle cistern. In larger tumors, the cistern is packed with the tumor. The SPS is double-ligated at the point anterior to the junction of petrosal vein, so that the venous flow can be preserved (Fig. 45-6). This step is followed by a tentorial incision, and care must be taken not to injure the trochlear nerve around the tentorial notch. Both sides of the tentorial leaflet are tacked with sutures.

Opening Meckel's Cave and Detachment of Feeders

Location of the trigeminal nerve varies depending on the origin of tumors (8) (Fig. 45-7). The trigeminal nerve deviates laterally and compressed under the tentorium in

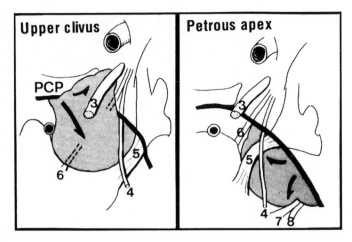

FIG. 45-7. Variation of the course of trigeminal nerve V depending to the site of the tumor attachment. (A) V nerve courses lateral to the tumor, which originates from clivus. (B) V nerve courses medial or inferior to the tumor, which originates from petrous apex or the tentorium

a tumor originating from the clivus, whereas it is deviated medially or inferiorly in a tumor originating from the petrous apex or the tentorium, respectively. In either case, the trigeminal nerve can be confirmed at the portal of the Meckel's cave. A 1-cm dural incision along the Meckel's cave exposes the plexiform part of the trigeminal nerve as well as the invaded tumor in the cave (Fig. 45-8). This step increases mobilization of the trigeminal nerve and enlarges the space between the tentorium and the trigeminal nerve, where the tentorial artery originates. Removal of the tumor in the Meckel's cave is followed by coagulation of the feeding arteries from the tentorial artery at the tumor attachment (Fig. 45-9).

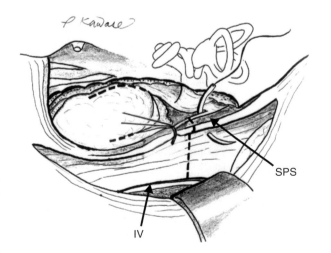

FIG. 45-6. Dural incision. The middle fossa dura has already been cut in a "T" shape, and the tentorium is exposed. Double ligations are made on the superior petrosal sinus (SPS), and the tentorium is incised with the SPS. Do not incise the tentorium anteriorly, so as not to injure the cranial nerves IV and V underneath. (Modified from Op Tech Neurosurg 1999; 10–17, with the author's permission.)

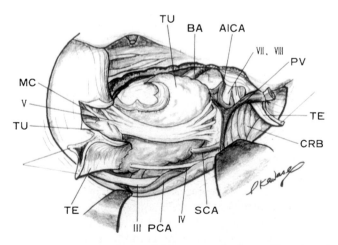

FIG. 45-8. Exposure of the clival type meningioma. The trigeminal nerve V is mobilized by opening the Meckel's cave (MC). TU, tumor; TE, tentorium; CRB, cerebellum; BA, basilar artery; AICA, anterior inferior cerebellar artery; SCA, superior cerebellar artery; PCA, posterior cerebral artery; PV, petrosal vein. (From Op Tech Neurosurg 1999; 10–17, with the author's permission.)

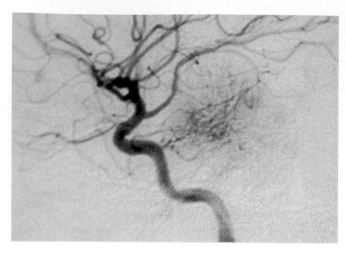

A

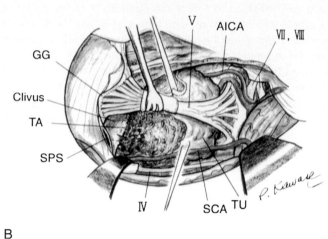

B

FIG. 45-9. (A) Tumor feeders from the tentorial artery in a petroclival meningioma. (B) Coagulation of the feeders between the IV and V cranial nerves after mobilization of those nerves. TA, tentorial artery; GG, Gasserian ganglion; SPS, superior petrosal sinus; TU, tumor. (From Op Tech Neurosurg 1999; 10–17, with the author's permission.)

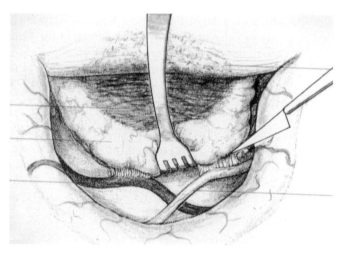

FIG. 45-10. Internal tumor decompression is followed by retraction of the tumor margin toward the tumor base by using a hooked tumor retractor. Enough surgical space is obtained for sharp dissection of the marginal structures, which are returning to their normal position

Removal of the Tumor

Complete hemostasis and softening of the tumor enables easy internal tumor decompression by ultrasonic aspirator. The superior cerebellar artery and the trochlear nerve have the highest incidence to be encased by the tumor, and they must carefully be dissected. Retraction of the tumor margin toward the tumor base with the tumor retractor slackens all the surrounding structures, returning them to their normal position, and giving enough space for sharp dissection in the key hole (Fig. 45-10). Flexible angle change of the microscope is necessary for optimal exposure of the tumor in its entirety.

During removal of the tumor margin, special care must be given to the abducens nerve running medial to the tumor, and VII, VIII cranial nerves and AICA located inferior to

the tumor. The arachnoid layer is commonly preserved separating the nerve complex from the tumor. Also, it is not uncommon that the tumor is covered by elongated and fanned trigeminal nerve complex in the clival type meningiomas (Fig. 45-8).

The most risky aspect of the surgery pertains to the tumor adhesion to the perforating arteries from basilar artery. If they are encased, a thin layer of the tumor must be left to prevent injury to the perforating arteries. After removal, III–VIII cranial nerves are inspected with a 70-degree angled neuroendoscope.

Closure

The drilled petrous apex and opened air cells on the rim of the craniotomy are covered with pieces of abdominal subcutaneous fat and fixed with fibrin glue. An additional reinforcement with temporal fascial flap is sutured with dura mater to prevent CSF rhinorrhea and accumulation under the scalp. The subdural air accumulation is replaced with artificial CSF. The cranial bone flap is fixed with titanium plates, and temporal muscle is reapproximated. The scalp is sutured in two layers in a routine fashion.

Surgical Results

Seventy patients with the UC- or SC-type meningiomas were operated utilizing the APA technique. The tumor size was large (≧40 mm) in 23 cases, medium (25–39 mm) in 26 cases, small (<25 mm) in 21 cases. The tumor invaded the Meckel's cave in 44 cases (62.8%) and cavernous sinus in 17 cases (24.3%). The cavernous sinus tumor had been removed until 1997, but these were left untouched thereafter to avoid ocular dysfunction (Fig. 45-11). Gross total tumor resection (no residual tumor on postoperative MRI) was achieved in 52 patients (74.3%), subtotal resection (more than 90%)

TABLE 45-2. Surgical Results of 70 Upper Clival or Sphenoclival Meningiomas Operated by the Anterior Transpetrosal Approach.

Extent of surgical resection	No of Patient	(%)
Gross total	52	(74.3%)
Subtotal (≧90%)	17	(24.3%)
Partial (<90%)	1	(1.4%)
Total	70	(100%)

in 17 (24.3%), and partial resection (<90%) in one patient (Table 45-2). Most of the residual tumor was in the cavernous sinus, or on the brain stem.

Postoperative Course and Surgical Complications

The postoperative course was uneventful in 48 (68.5%) patients. Their postoperative complications are catergorized as follows: vascular, cranial nerves, and others.

The major vascular complication was injury to the basilar perforating arteries adherent to the tumor, which occurred in 4 patients (5.7%; Fig. 45-12). Therefore, a thin layer of the tumor is no longer aggressively removed in cases of dense adhesion on the brain stem, especially in patients with perifocal edema in the brain stem, noted on preoperative T2-weighted MR images (2,9), or those with thick capsules. The residual tumor is controlled by Gamma Knife (Fig. 45-13).

The major cranial nerve complication was double vision, either by IV or VI cranial nerve injury, and it was permanent in 5 (7.1%) patients. Permanent abducens palsy forced the patient to cover the affected eye in their daily life, but this was not necessary for patients with trochlear nerve palsy. Permanent facial palsy occurred in 4 (5.7%) patients due to overstretching the GSPN or inappropriate resection of the pyramid, and 2 of these patients underwent hypoglossal-facial anastomosis. More than half of the patients in the series had facial hypesthesia of various degrees, which was well tolerated by the patients except for one patient who was bothered by significant paresthesia. Preoperative complaint of trigeminal neuralgia disappeared in all 5 patients. Preop-

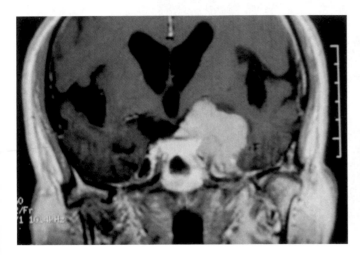

A

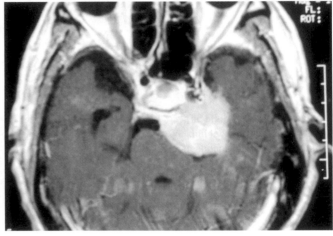

B

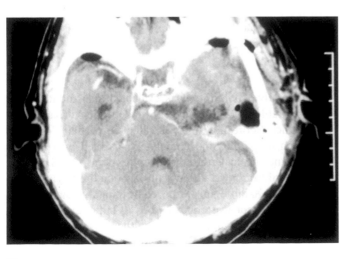

C

FIG. 45-11. (A) A case of SC-type meningioma, an coronal view. (B) An axial view showing extension into the cavernous sinus. (C) Postoperative contrast CT. Supra- and infratentorial meningioma was removed with the tentorium by the zygomatic petrosal approach. A small part of the cavernous sinus tumor was not removed

petrosectomy, etc.). The extent of what can be accomplished through each operative corridor may be influenced by tumor consistency, vascularity, and adherence to critical neurovascular structures. On a case-by-case basis, the surgical exposure afforded by each component of the approach will vary because of patient-specific anatomy and pathology (e.g., high jugular bulb, nonaerated mastoid, location of the brain stem, etc.) and should be factored into preoperative surgical plan.

Clival Zones

In an attempt to simplify the complex task of designing an appropriate surgical strategy for petroclival meningiomas, Aziz et al.[8] developed the concept of clival zones. *Zone I* (upper

zone) extends from the dorsum sellae to the upper border of the internal auditory canal. *Zone II* (middle zone) extends from the upper border of the internal auditory canal to the upper border of the jugular tubercle, and includes the central clival depression. *Zone III* (lower zone) extends from the upper border of the jugular tubercle to the lower edge of the clivus (Fig. 46-1).

Tumors with a dural base in Zone I are best addressed via a subtemporal, anterior petrosectomy approach. The boundaries

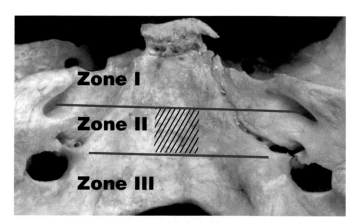

A

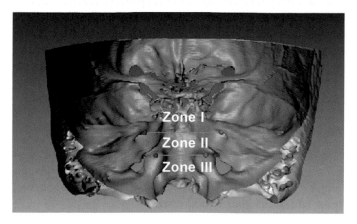

B

FIG. 46-1. The three clival zones. (A) Photograph of a dry human skull showing the three clival zones separated by solid lines. Zone I (upper zone) extends from the dorsum sellae to the upper border of the internal auditory canal. Zone II (middle zone) extends from the upper border of the internal auditory canal to the upper border of the jugular tubercle. The central clival depression is shown by the hatched area. Zone III (lower zone) extends from the upper border of the jugular tubercle to the lower edge of the clivus. (B) Three-dimensional reconstructed image of a human cadaver skull base demonstrating the three clival zones, which can be easily identified on reconstructed clinical data. (From Ref. 8.)

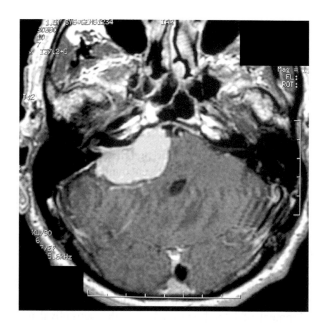

A

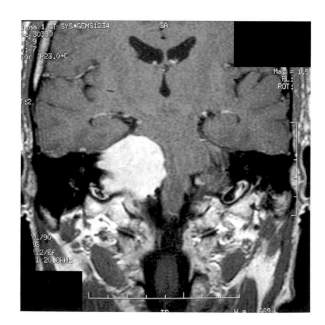

B

FIG. 46-2. T1-weighted, gadolinium-enhanced, axial (A) and coronal (B) magnetic resonance image (MRI) images of a Zone I + II petroclival meningioma

of the anterior petrosectomy exposure are the petrous segment of the internal carotid artery (lateral), the internal auditory canal (inferior), and the trigeminal root (anterior) with exposure extending from CN III down to the internal auditory canal. The anterior petrosectomy is also essential for lesions that cross the midline of the clivus.[9]

Zone II tumors are best approached via a posterior petrosectomy (retrolabyrinthine approach). The boundaries of a posterior petrosectomy are CN IV (superior), the jugular bulb (inferior), the sigmoid sinus (posterior), and the bony labyrinth (anterior). Of note, tumors with a dural attachment in the central clival depression are virtually impossible to completely resect via a standard, retrolabyrinthine posterior petrosectomy. Total resection often requires either a translabyrinthine or transcochlear approach with or without mobilization of the facial nerve. Figure 46-2 provides an example of a patient who underwent a combined approach during surgical resection of a petroclival meningioma that occupied Zones I and II.

Lesions extending below the jugular foramen into Zone III require a retrosigmoid dural opening. However, when portions of the medulla "cap" a meningioma in this location, we recommend the addition of a transcondylar component to the overall surgical approach strategy. This additional block provides the surgeon with a more lateral trajectory, thus avoiding unnecessary retraction of the medulla that might be necessary through a standard retrosigmoid approach. For lesions with suprasellar extension into the region above Zone I, a frontotemporal craniotomy with orbitozygomatic osteotomy (FTOZ) may be considered.

Armed with multiple surgical options, potential components of a complex approach can include the anterior petrosectomy, posterior petrosectomy, retrosigmoid/transcondylar approach, and FTOZ. Knowing the advantages and limitations of these various approaches, the surgical team can incorporate two or more of these components into a patient-tailored, combined approach.

Surgical Technique—Combined Approach

Our surgical approach to petroclival meningiomas uses a single-session, combined anterior and posterior petrosectomy. Additional components, which are described in previous chapters, can be added as needed.

Patient Position

The patient is positioned in the lateral oblique (park-bench) position with the neck in slight flexion to open the occipitocervical angle. The thorax is elevated with the patient's head tilted toward the floor until the zygoma becomes the apex of the surgical field. A lumbar drain is placed for cerebrospinal fluid (CSF) drainage during the procedure. Neurophysiologic monitors are placed and image guidance systems are registered.

FAQ: Do you routinely use a lumbar drain?

Yes. Controlled CSF drainage is useful for both the anterior and posterior portions of this approach. During anterior petrosectomy, brain relaxation through CSF release aids in extradural temporal lobe retraction. During the posterior petrosectomy when a retrosigmoid craniotomy is not added, the cisterna magna may be difficult to expose, thereby resulting in cerebellar protrusion through the dural opening. Postoperatively, use of a lumbar drain facilitates sealing of the fat graft and obliteration of the mastoid space.

Skin Incision

The skin incision consists of two limbs. The anterior limb begins just anterior to the tragus at the level of the zygomatic arch, continues anteriorly in a curvilinear fashion behind the hairline, and ends near the midline. For this portion of the incision, a hair-sparing technique can be used. The posterior limb begins 6 cm behind the ear, below the level of the mastoid tip, and continues in a curvilinear manner around the ear to end on the anterior limb of the incision 4 cm above the pinna. An interfascial technique is used to expose the zygoma while protecting the frontotemporal branch of the facial nerve.[10] The frontal scalp flap is reflected anteriorly. Care is taken to leave the attachment of the masseter muscle intact on the inferior aspect of the zygomatic arch. The zygomatic arch is downfractured. The temporal component of the scalp flap is then reflected inferiorly. The temporalis muscle is incised along the superior temporal line leaving a fascial cuff for later repair and reflected anteriorly and inferiorly (Fig. 46-3).

Craniotomy

The craniotomy is designed as a one-piece temporal-suboccipital craniotomy flap that exposes the temporal dura, transverse and sigmoid sinuses, and posterior fossa dura overlying the cerebellum. Critical to the safe creation of this flap is the correct placement of the four necessary burr holes and the proper sequencing of the bone cuts. Initially, two lateral burr holes are placed above and below the asterion, on either side of the transverse-sigmoid junction. Two medial burr holes are placed above and below the superior nuchal line, isolating the transverse sinus. The temporal portion of the bone flap is generated by connecting the lateral burr hole situated above the asterion to the medial burr hole situated above the transverse sinus using the craniotome. The suboccipital portion of the bone flap is generated by connecting the lateral burr hole (situated below the asterion) to the medial burr hole (situated below the transverse sinus). The remaining island of bone overlying the sinus can then be removed after careful epidural dissection using the craniotome for the medial cut overlying the transverse sinus; a combination of the drilling and dissection is used for the lateral cut overlying the transverse sigmoid junction (Fig. 46-4).

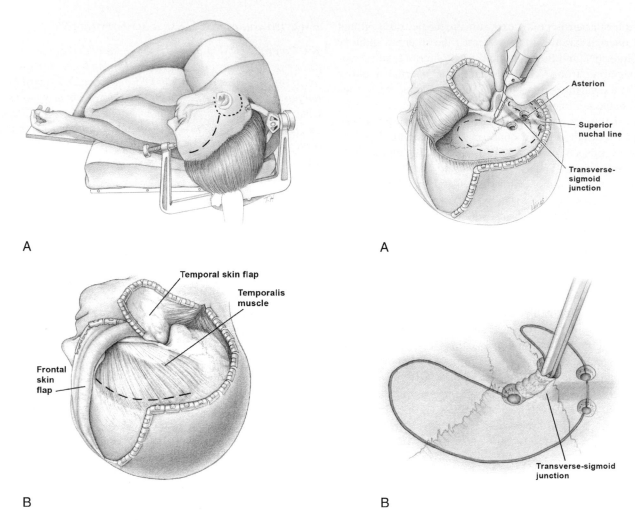

A

B

FIG. 46-3. Skin incision for the combined approach.(A) Extension of the neck brings the zygoma to the apex of the surgical field. The two components of the incision include one for the combined temporal-suboccipital craniotomy (dotted line) and the other for fronto-temporal extension of the craniotomy (dashed line). (B) Temporal skin flap is reflected inferiorly. Frontal skin flap is reflected anteriorly. Hemostatic clips are placed on the skin edges. Incision of the temporalis muscle cuff is shown. (From Ref. 7.)

A

B

FIG. 46-4. Bone cuts for the combined approach. (A) Temporalis muscle is reflected anteroinferiorly, leaving a superior fascial cuff. Entry burr boles are positioned at the most anterior mastoid point and below the asterion, which are above and below the transverse-sigmoid junction, respectively. A second set of burr holes placed above and below the superior nuchal line isolates the transverse sinus. Craniotome is used to connect the burr holes for the subtemporal craniotomy and retrosigmoid craniotomy first. (B) Transverse sinus, which can be dissected from the overlying bone, is crossed using the craniotome. Final cut across the transverse-sigmoid junction from the most anterior mastoid point to the asterion should be made carefully because the sinus rises dramatically into a groove in the bone. After the overlying bone is thinned with a cutting burr, the final bone cut is made with a punch and the bone flap is then elevated. (From Ref. 7.)

FAQ: Do you always use a large craniotomy?

No. If a smaller approach is considered acceptable, only a small temporal craniotomy is made to facilitate the anterior petrosectomy. The neuro-otologist then extends the mastoidectomy to remove the temporal plate, uncovers the sigmoid sinus, and removes 5–8 mm of retrosigmoid bone.

Posterior Petrosectomy

At this point, the neuro-otology service performs the posterior petrosectomy with the intention to open a working channel centered on the internal auditory canal. In a patient with normal hearing, drilling of the petrous bone is restricted to the retro-labyrinthine part; the posterior semicircular canal marks the anterior limit of the resection, thus becoming the major obstacle to an unobstructed view. Careful drilling of the bone surrounding the posterior semicircular canal, until it appears as a blue line, is mandatory to ensure that the maximal possible exposure is obtained before proceeding to the intradural stage. Access to the tumor in this exposure is purely through the presigmoid dura; this access can, once again, seem exceedingly narrow at first inspection.

The final working space is determined by two factors. The first factor is the degree of pneumatization of the mastoid.

The greater the extent of pneumatization of the mastoid, the further back the sigmoid sinus lays, and therefore the greater is the surface area of the presigmoid dura (also called Trautman's triangle). Nothing can be done to modify this aspect of the patient's anatomy. The second factor relies on the ability to mobilize the transverse-sigmoid junction posteromedially, thereby increasing the width of the presigmoid space. This key step during the posterior petrosectomy approach requires removal of bone posterior to the sigmoid sinus, either by drilling or turning a small retrosigmoid bone flap.

Anterior Petrosectomy

After completion of the posterior petrosectomy, the neurosurgical team resumes the case and performs the subtemporal exposure in preparation for the anterior petrosectomy. Exposure preparation for anterior petrosectomy starts with careful elevation of the temporal lobe dura from the middle fossa floor. Coagulation and cutting of the middle meningeal artery is necessary to allow retraction; this initially is an extradural exposure, and CSF drainage through a lumbar drain facilitates elevation of the temporal lobe.

Elevation of the dura from posterior to anterior direction permits identification and preservation of the greater superficial petrosal nerve (GSPN). Care is taken to properly distinguish the true ridge of the petrous bone from the indentation created by the superior petrosal sinus. Self-retaining retractors are placed behind the true ridge of the petrous pyramid to allow for appropriate exposure during drilling.

Exposure through an anterior petrosectomy is always surprisingly narrow, unless the tumor itself has expanded the petrous apex. Two steps are mandatory to unlock the approach and provide an adequate working space. The first step is to ascertain that maximal drilling of Kawase's triangle has been accomplished. In our opinion, the only reliable landmarks that

ensure the maximal available space is obtained (before the dura is opened) are the adequate exposure and visualization of the petrous ICA as the lateral limit and the IAC as the inferior limit. The second step is the section of the superior petrosal sinus and tentorium cerebelli when the procedure reaches the intradural stage. During this second step, care is taken not to injure the CN V, which is often compressed by the tumor against the tentorium and the superior petrosal sinus; this nerve is very vulnerable as it crosses the petrous apex, en route to the gasserian ganglion.

After opening the presigmoid dura parallel to the sigmoid sinus, the temporal dura is opened parallel to the middle fossa floor. Finally, a relaxing incision is made in the supratentorial dura along the line of the transverse sinus with great care not to injure the vein of Labbé. After these cuts are made, the superior petrosal sinus is clipped and cut, and the tentorium is incised all the way to the incisura. The tentorial cut is directed in a slightly anterior trajectory. A posterior trajectory will cause the surgeon to ride up along the tentorium, away from the incisura. With completion of these steps, gentle retraction of the transverse-sigmoid junction posteromedially can significantly increase the width of the presigmoid space (Fig. 46-5).

Closure

Closure begins with reapproximation of the dura using a combination of interrupted and running suture. A watertight dural closure is impossible because of dural resection at the petrous apex. Mastoid air cells are thoroughly waxed, and the mastoid antrum is plugged with a piece of temporalis muscle. Gaps in the dural closure are covered with dural substitute. A dural sealant is used to reinforce all interfaces and suture lines. A free fat graft is used to fill in the defect in the mastoid. The bone flap is rigidly fixed into position with titanium miniplates. The temporalis is split to cover the fat graft, and interrupted sutures are used to resuspend the temporalis muscle to the fascial cuff

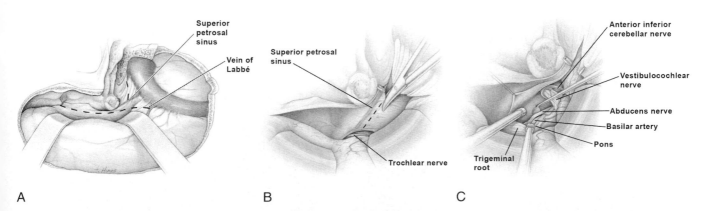

A   B   C

FIG. 46-5. Dural opening for the combined approach. (A) Dura between the sigmoid sinus and petrous apex is exposed. Surgeon makes a dural incision in the posterior fossa dura (anterior to the sigmoid sinus) and in the middle fossa dura (superior to the petrosal sinus). This incision continues posteriorly to the transverse sigmoid junction. Care is taken to avoid injuring the vein of Labbé. (B) Superior petrosal sinus and tentorium are incised ventrally toward the incisura in a course directed posterior to the entry of the trochlear nerve into the tentorial edge. (C) Gently applying 10-mm self-retaining retractors to the posterior temporal lobe, the surgeon exposes the medial temporal lobe, lateral pons, basilar artery, and cranial nerves V through VIII. (From Ref. 7.)

of the superior temporal line. A subgaleal drain is inserted and connected to continuous aspiration. After the galea is closed with interrupted suture, the skin is closed with staples.

Outcomes and Potential Complications

Although there are numerous published series on petroclival meningiomas,[3,11–14] few reports have outcome data specific for patients who underwent combined approaches. In a report of seven patients with petroclival meningiomas operated on via a combined approach, Cho and Al-Mefty[11] achieved gross total resection in five of these patients; there was no mortality and one patient lost hearing after surgery. In a series of 97 patients with petroclival meningiomas, Erkmen et al.[9] noted rates of 8% for hearing loss and 15% for CSF leak for the 34 patients who underwent a combined petrosal approach.

Complication Avoidance/Lessons Learned

A number of critical steps during a combined petrosal approach represent avoidable pitfalls. The first point in the operation when an easily avoidable problem arises is during bone removal over the transverse sinus. Careful identification of the bony landmarks, including the asterion, can help to avoid unintended sinus injury and serves during image guidance for planning the location of the burr holes. The combination of burrs and punches to make the lateral cut helps to avoid sinus injury.

During extradural dissection, risk of injury to the temporal lobe can be reduced by adequate brain relaxation via lumbar drainage. Dissection of the middle fossa floor, in a posterior-to-anterior direction, protects the GSPN from inadvertent avulsion. During the dural opening, careful identification of the vein of Labbé is essential to avoid injury. If the vein drains into the superior petrosal sinus rather than the transverse

sinus, additional effort may be required to identify the superior petrosal sinus anterior to the entry of the vein of Labbé so that the sinus may be sacrificed without venous compromise.

The fourth cranial nerve is at risk during division of the tentorium. Early identification of the nerve in the subarachnoid space before completion of the tentorial cut is essential to injury avoidance. The fifth cranial nerve is at risk during ligation and division of the superior petrosal sinus. Care must be taken during the placement of the clips to the sinus to avoid catching a portion of the nerve in the clip blades. Dorello's canal and cranial nerve VI can be avoided during the anterior petrosectomy by using the inferior petrosal sinus as a limit to drilling.

Once again, tumors with a dural attachment in the central clival depression are virtually impossible to completely resect via a standard retrolabyrinthine posterior petrosectomy. Complete resection requires more radical drilling, via either a translabyrinthine or transcochlear approach, with or without mobilization of the facial nerve. In light of the additional morbidity associated with these approach extensions, especially in patients with serviceable hearing, we favor leaving a small amount of residual tumor and reserving radiosurgery for tumor control in this location when appropriate (Fig. 46-6).

In some cases, there is significant T2 signal change within the brain stem, which indicates that the dissection plane will be poor. In these patients, we favor leaving a thin layer of tumor on the brain stem surface rather than risking injury with aggressive resection. However, resection of enough tumor is critical to untether the brain stem and allow for re-expansion (Fig. 46-7).

In situations when the surgical strategy requires a combination of anterior and posterior approaches, a staged procedure should be considered. In clinical practice, two major factors should be considered when contemplating staging versus a single operative session (Fig. 46-8). First, one should avoid compromising optimal surgical positioning to accommodate a single-stage combined approach. Second, the length of time required for each component of the procedure should be realistically assessed.

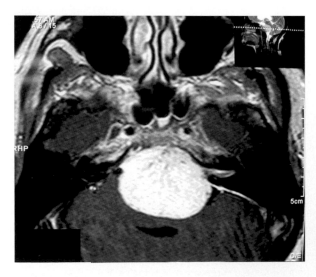
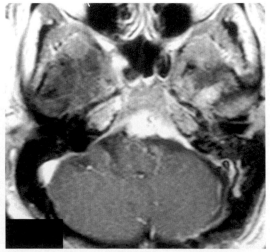

A   B

FIG. 46-6. MRI scans revealing a petroclival meningioma. (A) Preoperative scan shows tumor extending into Zones I–III. (B) Postoperative scan shows residual tumor in the central clival depression and around the basilar artery

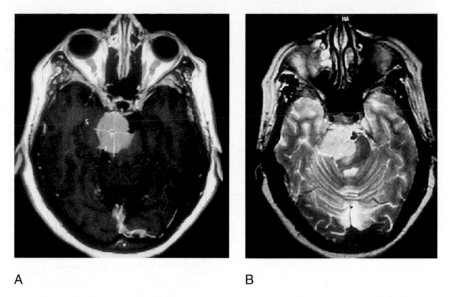

FIG. 46-7. MRI scan demonstrating a right-sided petroclival meningioma. (A) Preoperative T1-weighted, gadolinium-enhanced scan. (B) T2-weighted image demonstrates increased signal intensity in the brain stem representing pial invasion

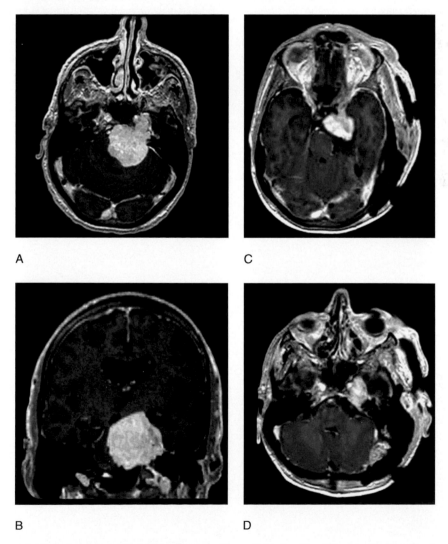

FIG. 46-8. Preoperative axial (A) and coronal (B) MRI scans revealing a Zone I + II + III petroclival meningioma with cavernous sinus involvement. The posterior petrosectomy approach was performed as the first portion of a staged procedure. (C) Postoperative axial MRI images demonstrating residual tumor in Zone I and the cavernous sinus after the posterior approach only. (D) Future extracavernous tumor removal via the anterior approach is planned as a staged procedure. Decompression of the brain stem is also noted

Summary

In dealing with these difficult petroclival and upper clival lesions, we design our approaches on a patient-by-patient basis by using a component-based strategy that is built on the unique anatomic features of both the tumor and its surrounding anatomy. By having options in the armamentarium, the skull base team can design an approach by adding appropriate components for optimal exposure and safe resection. A thorough understanding of the relationships these tumors can have with critical neurovascular structures can minimize morbidity and mortality and maximize patient benefit.

References

1. Campbell E, Whitfield RD. Posterior fossa meningiomas. J Neurosurg 1948;15:131–153.
2. Hakuba A, Nishimura S, Tanaka K, et al. Clivus meningioma: six cases of total removal. Neurol Med Chir (Tokyo) 1977;17:63–77.
3. Al-Mefty O, Fox JL, Smith RR. Petrosal approach for petroclival meningiomas. Neurosurgery 1988;22:510–517.
4. Kawase T, Shiobara R, Toya S. Middle fossa transpetrosal-transtentorial approaches for petroclival meningiomas. Selective pyramid resection and radicality. Acta Neurochir (Wien) 1994;129:113–120.
5. Miller CG, van Loveren HR, Keller JT, et al. Transpetrosal approach: surgical anatomy and technique. Neurosurgery 1993;33:461–469.
6. Oghalai JS, Jackler RK. Anatomy of the combined retro-labyrinthine-middle fossa craniotomy. Neurosurg Focus 2003;14:e8.
7. Tew JMJ, van Loveren HR, Keller JT. Atlas of Operative Microneurosurgery. Vol. 2. Philadelphia, W.B. Saunders Company, 2001.
8. Abdel Aziz KM, Sanan A, van Loveren HR, et al. Petroclival meningiomas: predictive parameters for transpetrosal approaches. Neurosurgery 2000;47:139–150.
9. Erkmen K, Pravdenkova S, Al-Mefty O. Surgical management of petroclival meningiomas: factors determining the choice of approach. Neurosurg Focus 2005;19:E7.
10. Yasargil MG, Reichman MV, Kubik S. Preservation of the frontotemporal branch of the facial nerve using the interfascial temporalis flap for pterional craniotomy. Technical article. J Neurosurg 1987;67:463–466.
11. Cho CW, Al-Mefty O. Combined petrosal approach to petroclival meningiomas. Neurosurgery 2002;51:708–716.
12. Couldwell WT, Fukushima T, Giannotta SL, Weiss MH. Petroclival meningiomas: surgical experience in 109 cases. J Neurosurg 1996;84:20–28.
13. Little KM, Friedman AH, Sampson JH, et al. Surgical management of petroclival meningiomas: defining resection goals based on risk of neurological morbidity and tumor recurrence rates in 137 patients. Neurosurgery 2005;56:546–559.
14. Sekhar LN, Swamy NK, Jaiswal V, et al. Surgical excision of meningiomas involving the clivus: preoperative and intraoperative features as predictors of postoperative functional deterioration. J Neurosurg 1994;81:860–868.

47
Petrous Meningiomas I: An Overview

H. Maximilian Mehdorn and Ralf M. Buhl

Introduction

Meningiomas of the cerebello-pontine angle (CPA) and the ventral petrous area account for approximately 8–23% of intracranial meningiomas or approximately 10–15% of the tumors in the CPA.[1–3] Nakamura et al.[1] presented a selected series of 421 CPA meningiomas, which seems to represent the largest series presented so far from a single institution. Clinical symptoms leading to diagnosis lasted from 1[4] to 4 years[5] and include the symptoms which are characteristic for lesions of the CPA: symptoms of the cranial nerves (CNs) V–VIII, in the order of the predominance (6), hearing loss (73%), cerebellar signs (32%), trigeminal neuropathy (16%), and facial nerve dysfunction (16%). In addition, depending on their size symptoms of compression of the pons such as gait disturbance and obstructive hydrocephalus in 10–20% of these patients were observed.[7,8] Rarely trigeminal neuralgia, even on the contralateral side, due to mass effect[9] or hemifacial spasm,[10–12] dizziness and vertigo, symptoms of the lower cranial nerves, have been reported. As with other CPA tumors, meningiomas can also be asymptomatic for a long period of time or be discovered during cranial imaging for other reasons.

Similar to vestibular schwannomas because of frequent involvement of the internal auditory meatus and early involvement of hearing, these tumors have been evaluated and managed both by neurosurgeons and otologic skull base surgeons. Both surgical disciplines should join efforts to optimize therapy for these tumors located in a challenging area, particularly also because symptoms may lead patients initially to otologists. In the following, however, a rather neurosurgical perspective is outlined to describe access to and treatment of these meningiomas, with a special reference given as to when otologic cooperation is particularly appreciated.

The region of concern can be divided into different smaller regions. Although one could differentiate these regions according to the anatomy of arachnoid cisterns as described by Yasargil,[17] this is, in meningiomas, only helpful to a limited degree. A more useful way is to divide the CPA using the cranial

nerves themselves as landmarks, particularly the internal auditory canal (IAC)[13–15] According to this system, the CPA region would then be divided into a region anterior and another one posterior to the virtual line of exit of the CNs. Furthermore, the anterior and the posterior regions could each be divided into an upper, middle and lower third, according to the CNs: the uppermost region would be between the tentorium and the CNs VII/VIII, the middle region between the CNs VII/VIII and the lower CNs, and the lowest region extending further down into the foramen magnum. Nakamura[16] divided the CPA meningiomas according to their position in relation to the internal acoustic canal (IAC).

From the surgical point of view, the most important differentiation is whether the origin of the tumor is located anterior or posterior to the foramina through which the cranial nerves leave the intradural space. Additionally, the location of tumor origin largely dictates the surgical limitations or risks of surgery, and ultimately the patient's outcome.

Special Considerations

Preoperative Imaging

A variety of approaches to the CPA has been suggested: In neurosurgical practice, the suboccipital-retrosigmoid or "lateral suboccipital"[17] is the favored approach, followed by temporo-occipital craniotomy and presigmoidal approach or a combination of those.[16,18,19] The preoperative imaging should help the surgeon to understand the surgical anatomy of the lesion and its important surrounding structures in order to select the best approach to the tumor to obtain the highest degree of surgical resectability with least morbidity.

Imaging of the petrous bone, its pneumatization and extension, and the surrounding venous sinus system is of primary importance. The bone data can be obtained using thin-slice computed tomography (CT) imaging, which can also be used as a basis for neuronavigation. High-resolution, thin-slice CT, with bone window setting may furthermore be useful to demonstrate focal or extended hyperostosis—spicula and other alterations—in the petrous bone indicative of the origin of the meningioma (which is not always correct) and to better differentiate between meningioma and acoustic neurinoma (Fig. 47-1).

Tumor imaging is best achieved using magnetic resonance imaging (MRI) with standard protocols including T1- and T2-weighted images without and with contrast. Since the knowledge of possible contact to nerve and vascular structures is very important prior to planning surgery, heavily T2-weighted MR imaging[20] and three-dimensional (3D) MP-RAGE and 3D CISS sequences[21] may be used. Imaging of the contact to the brain stem with edema formation is best visualized using T2 sequences. Furthermore, the access to large meningiomas of the CPA, particularly those arising in or reaching the rostral petrous bone, may require information concerning the venous

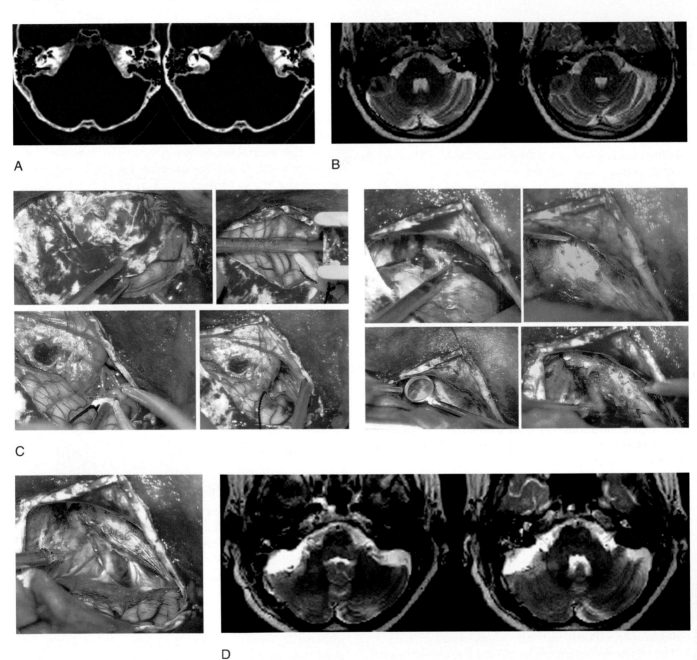

FIG. 47-1. A 74-year-old patient presenting with headaches, dizziness, and somewhat unstable gait. (A) CT scan of the petrous bone demonstrates hyperostosis at the origin of the meningioma. (B) MRI scan (axial T2 FSE) shows meningioma and surrounding structures. (C) Intraoperative view of meningioma at different stages of removal—note that (a) due to CSF drainage no retraction is required and the tumor is delivered easily after disrupting its origin; (b) complete removal with drilling of hyperostosis and coagulation of remnants on the dura. (D) Postoperative MRI scan showing complete tumor removal and re-expansion of the cerebellar hemisphere—CNs are well visualized

drainage in the area, in order to decide the direction—laterally—and thereby extension of the surgical access route. In order to have the liberty to intraoperatively occlude a sigmoid sinus, if needed, the patency, the size, or its "dominance" should be assessed, which can be done with good quality MR images. This attention should further be directed towards possible obstruction of the extracranial venous outflow at the level of the jugular bulb or the jugular veins, since anesthesiologic venous catheters and suboptimal positioning of the patient may additionally hinder the venous outflow, which could result in a difficult if not treacherous access route when approaching a deep-seated lesion in the presence of a swollen cerebellum.

While angiography may be helpful in huge tumors to determine the need for preoperative embolization, it has been replaced by MRA if only the vascular anatomy of the venous system needs to be determined. CT data can be fused with previous MRI data in order to save money and time but still allow for implementation of all relevant imaging data for surgical neuronavigation.

Differential Diagnosis

Differential diagnosis for CPA meningiomas (CPAM), on the basis of noncontrast and contrast MRI scan, include vestibular schwannoma (VS), metastatic intradural tumors, chordomas, and other tumors[15,22] and far less frequently giant aneurysms of the vertebral or the basilar artery. While the latter can usually be ruled out easily, the VS can be particularly difficult to differentiate (Fig. 47-2). On one hand, a meningioma may invade the IAC or originate from the dura of the canal both anterior and posterior to the nerves VII or VIII.[18,23] On the other hand, even in small (1.5 cm maximal length) VS, a contrast enhancement of the dura may extend in a tail-like fashion onto the intracranial dura representing the vascularity seen during surgery around the IAC. The same can hold true for purely intradural metastases, particularly in breast cancer and melanomas where the petrous bone is usually not invaded by the tumor.[24] The dural tail sign can be seen both on the dura of the petrous bone and the tentorium, making it very difficult, if not impossible, to differentiate the origin of the meningioma. Additionally, the origin of the meningioma may extend into both areas as well, crossing or invading the inner

wall of the venous sinuses. Furthermore, particularly in large meningiomas or meningiomas of the lower CPA region, special

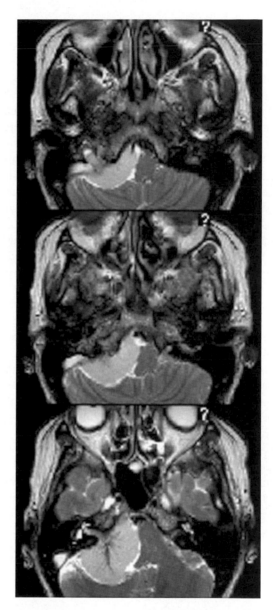

A

FIG. 47-2. A 50-year-old patient presenting with vertigo, severe gait ataxia, headaches, and hearing problems on her right ear. (A) MRI scan (T2-weighted CLE) showing large meningioma possibly arising below and around the IAC producing marked compression of the brain stem; note (top) the stroma delineation; (B) the surface against the cerebellar hemisphere with areas of captured CSF making dissection at least in this region easier; (bottom) invasion of the canal for CN VII/VIII and foramina of the lower CNs; the nerves themselves cannot be identified in this scans due to the size of the tumor. (B) Immediate postoperative MRI scans showing marked edema formation in the cerebellar hemisphere and persistent displacement of the brain stem. After a stormy course, good recovery with some swallowing difficulty and facial palsy followed

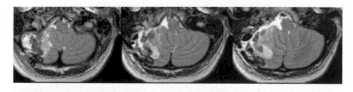

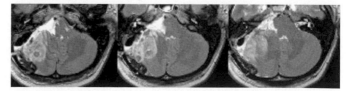

B

attention should be given to the extension of the meningioma into the foramina of the lower CNs.

Indication for Surgery

In this chapter, indications for surgery will be discussed while alternative treatment options such as Gamma Knife or radiation will be left to the appropriate chapters in this book. Since these tumors present mostly through signs of contact to the cranial nerves and only rarely through symptoms of intracranial pressure or compression of the pons and hydrocephalus, usually the indication for surgery is based on the assumption that symptoms do not disappear when nothing is done and that surgical removal of such a lesion is easier when smaller. On the other hand, special consideration must be given to the natural history of the tumor and to the probable results of surgical removal, particularly in elderly patients.[25,26]

Unfortunately, little or nothing is known about the natural history of the meningiomas of the CPA when they are small, since they are mostly operated upon, while those patients who present with large tumors and are not operated usually die from cardiopulmonary failure. To better explain the relative risks of surgery to the patient, it would be interesting to know more about the growth rate of a meningioma in a particular patient before he or she is recommended to undergo surgery. (See chapters 6 and 20). So far, radiographic examinations may not be particularly helpful in an individual patient to predict the growth with reasonable accuracy. Therefore, if justified on the clinical basis, a short period of a "wait-and-see attitude" may sometimes help to identify the growth rate for a specific meningioma and facilitate the decision for surgery once the tumor has grown on serial MRI scans.[27] Recommendation for surgery must be considered very carefully if the patient has only one remaining hearing ear ipsilaterally (28). One has to remind oneself in this scenario, however, that the diagnosis based on imaging alone remains unclear to a certain degree, and the patient should be advised accordingly. It has been reported that a suspected meningioma of the CPA was, upon growth on serial MRI scans, operated on and proved to be a melanoma.[29] Also, combinations of different tumors may occur in the same patient.[30,31]

Preoperative Evaluation

Once indication for surgery has been fully discussed with the patient, specific preoperative evaluation may include otologic examination, including auditory brain stem evoked potentials, neuro-ophthalmologic evaluation, gait analysis, somatosensory and motor-evoked potentials, and neuropsychological testing. The latter is becoming more and more important as not only survival but the quality of life in the pre- and postoperative phase becomes more and more important to the patients and families.[32]

While preoperative embolization of a meningioma may be helpful for some locations, in meningioma of the CPA, it is rarely indicated. The reason is the arterial supply to these tumors that usually comes through branches of the artery of Bernasconi-Cassinari, which does not lend itself for embolization except when particularly large. In the instances of large tumors, particular care should be taken to the possibility of intra- or immediate postembolization swelling of the meningioma. Ischemia of the CNs is always a risk of embolization in this region.

Surgical Access to Meningiomas of the CPA

In general, surgical access to a meningioma of the CPA is the same as for other tumors of this region. However, one has to try to define the area of tumor origin, which should (if possible) be attacked in the very early part of operation in order to devitalize the meningioma and thus reduce its volume. In the following, the most common neurosurgical access route to these tumors, i.e., the suboccipital retroauricular retrosigmoid approach,[17,19] will be presented in detail. This approach has also been advocated by some otologic surgeons[33] for patients with functional hearing, which should be preserved if possible. However, in the literature other approaches are well described, including those performed together with or by the otologic colleagues.[34] The translabyrithine[2] or retrolabyrinthine,[35] extended translabyrithine with transapical extension,[36] combined transpetrosal, combined transtemporal,[37] far lateral/transcondylar, middle cranial fossa, and extended middle cranial fossa[38] as well as some of these approaches combined with a transtentorial approach[39,40] may be considered depending on the tumor size and origin.

Positioning of the patient follows the general rules of access to the posterior fossa through the lateral suboccipital retromastoid approach. It is important to have the head sufficiently high in position above the heart in order to reduce intracranial pressure. About half of the neurosurgeons—including the authors—seem to prefer the park-bench position. Other authors[41,42] prefer the sitting or semisitting position in order to facilitate relaxation of the structures of the posterior fossa and cleansing of the surgical field by simple irrigation. The authors have never used this position for meningioma, so the problem of venous air embolism does not need to be considered for the positioning described here.

In the authors' institution, the head is fixed in the Mayfield headholder and the patient positioned in a modified park-bench position, slightly turned away from the side of the tumor, the shoulder supported in order to facilitate the access. One has to carefully plan the access route to the tumor particularly when performing a "keyhole" approach. The patient's shoulder should be kept in mind as a potential obstacle (which should not be for delicate surgery), particularly when the tumor is in the upper part of the CPA extending upwards along the lower surface of tentorium, and when the patient has a short or thick neck. The table is positioned in such a manner that the head is the highest part of the body. This requires some degree of inclined positioning and bending of the table in order to prevent the patient from slowly sliding downward. The patient is additionally secured by tape or a belt, so turning the table along the patient's axis into various positions is possible, suitable for different directions taken during various steps of the procedure. If neuronavigation is utilized in order to facilitate the angle and area of approach, the fiducials are now registered and the approach is calculated. The pins of the Mayfield headholder should be positioned in such a fashion as to allow for applying a Budde-Halo® or other ring system carrying the self-retaining brain retractors in such a fashion that the ring system does not hinder various access angles.

Additionally, intraoperative measurement of evoked potentials, especially the auditory evoked brain stem potentials, as well as facial (and other cranial) nerve monitoring should be used to alert the surgeon before irreversible damage occurs to the structures by retraction of nerves and/or vessels and/or local direct damage. Its value has repeatedly been stressed by many neurosurgeons.[42–47]

The skin is incised according to the approach required, its exact location and extent depending on the size of the tumor and the size and location of the transverse and sigmoid sinuses, while the degree of pneumatization of the petrous bone is no longer considered important as long as a careful closure of these structures is achieved at the end of surgery, using some muscle graft from the nuchal muscles or some abdominal fat secured to the bone with fibrin glue or similar suitable materials. The craniotomy is usually performed using a high-speed drill. We prefer to place a burr hole over the cerebellar hemisphere where the bone is thinnest, and the trephination is carried out as far laterally as possible, as required for good view to the medial aspect of the tumor while its medial border is determined by the size and attachment of the tumor to the petrous bone. Its upper border should be on or slightly above the transverse sinus, and its upper lateral angle should be close to 90° in order to allow for a dural opening as far laterally and upwards as possible. The center of the craniotomy in cranio-caudad direction is placed according to the height of the center of the tumor so that the upper and the lower margins of its extension can be reached. The dura is usually incised in a semicircular or L-shaped fashion, its base oriented toward the sigmoid sinus. If difficult lateral access to the tumor is suggested from the size of tumor and displacement of the cerebellar hemisphere, as a routine, the dural opening should be carried out caudad enough to facilitate opening of the cisterna magna and release of cerebrospinal fluid (CSF). This often facilitates the lateral approach even with or without as little retraction as possible of the cerebellar hemisphere, in the park-bench position. A preoperatively placed lumbar drainage may serve the same purpose but has never been used in the author's experience, for fear of downward herniation of the cerebellum into the foramen magnum prior to opening of the dura.

The arachnoid membranes of the lateral cisterns should be dissected carefully in order to ease access to the meningioma of the CPA. The intensity of contact between the arachnoid membranes and the dorsal aspect of the meningioma usually implies the degree of "surgical aggressiveness" of the meningioma, i.e., the degree of intimacy of contact between

the meningioma and the surrounding structures, particularly the cranial nerves and the vessels to and from the brain stem. This, in turn, foretells early during surgery the potential for intraoperative damage that could be inflicted to the patient, and extreme care should be exercised. When a meningioma respects the arachnoid membranes, dissection is easier and internal decompression by means of suction and/or ultrasound dissection can be achieved during the initial phase without too much fear of nerve and vessel injury. In the authors' impression, meningiomas which respect the arachnoid plane are usually also softer and better suctioned than meningiomas which do not respect the arachnoid membranes. Internal decompression then allows for rapid access to the origin of the meningioma in order to reduce its vascularization and further ease the tumor resection. Often bony spicula, hyperostosis, and /or the internal stroma structure visible in the MRI or CT scan, and even better seen during the initial phase of internal meningioma decompression, will point to the origin of the meningioma. In this case, after initial tumor decompression, rapid attention should be directed toward coagulating this area. It may become necessary to broadly coagulate the dura and thereby expose a feeding artery or several small arteries, which may bleed severely for a short time, during which they can be visualized and obliterated. If it cannot be coagulated using bipolar coagulation, it may be helpful to obliterate the artery within its bony canal by simply drilling the bony structures with a high-speed diamond drill without simultaneous water irrigation, thus causing heat sufficient for coagulating the artery and obliterating its canal with the bone powder.

When the meningioma is slowly removed, the surrounding structures reappear. Depending on the degree of aggressivity of meningioma attachement, it may be more or less difficult, or even impossible, to completely dissect the nerves and vessels free from the meningioma without damaging some fibers. This is true for all cranial nerves, to a lesser extent for the arteries and veins. In this situation, it may be safer to leave a small remnant of meningioma tissue than irreversibly damaging the nerve fibers.

Meningiomas extending into the canal or the foramina of the CN are particularly challenging with respect to the degree of surgical resection. Often, a major part of the dorsal bony aspect of the foramina needs to be drilled away in order to be able to look into the lateral part of the foramen.

In our experience as well as in others', the meningiomas of the CPA anterior to the internal acoustic canal are often softer and more easily removed with suction than meningiomas originating posterior to the IAC. This rule may compensate for the more difficult access and difficulties in dissecting the cranial nerves involved within the meningioma or displaced by the lesion. Meningiomas originating anterior to the CNs usually push the CNs posteriorly and widen the distance between them, allowing access to the origin of the tumor; however, in larger meningiomas it may become very difficult to distinguish the CNs during dissection and internal decompression. Then a very careful dissection is necessary, following the fibrous bands which may separate various compartments of the meningioma and may encase either nerve fibers or small arteries—mostly branches of the posterior inferior cerebellar artery. If anatomy allows, again in these cases it may be very helpful to start dissection of the meningioma at its origin.

Upon completion of the tumor removal and once excellent hemostasis has beeen achieved, special care should be given to the watertight dural closure. When bone drilling or craniotomy has opened pneumatic cells, they need to be sealed carefully using fibrin glue and muscle grafts locally prepared from the neck muscles or other material easily attaching to the remaining dura. Larger cavities in the bone should be filled with fat preferentially taken from the abdominal wall. The use of a lumbar drainage can be helpful to divert intracranial CSF flow and reduce intracranial pressure until the inner wound has sealed sufficiently. Use of steroids is mandatory in order to prevent perioperative brain swelling; perioperative use of antibiotics as single shot infusion is routinely used in our institution.

Particular Surgical Considerations

Brain Retraction

Retraction of the cerebellar hemsiphere should be kept as short as possible. If required, it should be used only intermittently in order to reduce contusional damage to the hemisphere. We usually cover the cerebellar hemisphere either with a piece of glove cut to the size of the approach or Surgicel® prior to the placement of cottonoid upon which the retractor blade is positioned. This allows for smooth and easily reversible retraction.

Superior Petrous Vein

This vein drains a major part of the cerebellar hemisphere and the brain stem, so it might be wise to preserve it as much as possible.[47] In this respect, dissection of the venous complex in its arachnoid sleeve may be helpful; however, if interrupting it becomes necessary, coagulation and cutting should be done before it tears off of the sinus. There seems to be no clear correlation between coagulation of this vein and brain stem damage, at least as evaluated by evoked potentials.[48]

Sinus Walls

Once a sinus wall has been injured inadvertently or the sinus has been opened deliberately, care must be taken to prevent air embolism, particularly in the sitting position, and the appropriate steps need to be taken, first preventing further connection between the sinus and the air by putting a patty on the hole and by raising the intravenous pressure by ventilation. Then, a gelfoam patty soaked with fibrin glue usually allows for sinus wall reconstruction when patiently applied with gentle pressure. If the hole in the sinus wall is too big to be occluded in this manner and when the sinus is required for cerebral drainage one should apply a larger piece of Tissudura ® or other available material in order to rensconstruct the wall. Gentle and patient pressure is mandatory while coagulation of the fibrin glue and sealing of the hole takes place.

High Jugular Bulb

In this context one should plan surgical access with the full set of anatomic data in mind. Also, the position of the jugular bulb can become important when drilling off the bony attachment of the meningioma since a high bulb[49] can pose a major risk of intraoperative bleeding.

Cranial Nerves

While the rule "the thinner the nerve, the higher the risk during manipulation" certainly holds true for CNs in the posterior fossa, dissection of the nerves III, V, VII, VIII and the lower cranial nerves IX–XII may be—due to their fiber structure—as difficult and time-consuming as that of the CNs IV and VI, the former being mostly covered by the arachnoid membranes and compressed againgst the tentorium, the latter often being pushed anteriorly out of the surgical access route. Most frequent damage to the VI nerve may occur at its point of entry into Dorello's canal.

Posterior Fosssa Circulation

When cerebellar veins such as the superior petrosal vein are compressed by the meningioma, they can be damaged during dissection. If the surgeon expects this to occur he or she should coagulate and cut the vein deliberately prior to damaging it to minimize intraoperative bleeding.

Cerebellar Arteries

Arterial supply to the tumor often comes also from cerebellar arteries, particularly in large meningiomas. In these instances, care must be taken to preserve these arteries and veins in the capsule whenever possible, mostly when the vessels are large and encased in the arachnoid membranes or the capsule itself, particularly when one works close to the brain stem since they are important for its supply.

Radical Removal

If one tries to preserve quality of life, it is usually impossible to perform a radical removal of a meningioma of the CPA in the sense of "Simpson Grad O" as defined by Al-Mefty et al. (50). Problems which may be relevant in this regard are the meningioma ingrowth into the internal acoustic canal, or the other foramina, or its origin in the dural lining of these structures. Also, it may be difficult to dissect the tumor from the nerves or their vasculature. A particular problem may be the fibers of the trigeminal nerve, which could be spread widely apart by the meningioma, thus causing dissection even more cumbersome.

Samii et al.[1] reported rates of total removal (Simpson I) of 86.1% in meningioma with dural involvement around the IAC, while Bassiouni et al.[51] reported only 27.5%[14/51] Simpson Grade I removal in meningiomas around the posterior petrous bone. However, one should try to perform a radical removal by any means possible, because the first operation is the operation that decides the future for the patient—whether he or she has to live with a reasonable fear of recurrent tumor or not.

Complete tumor removal should include the drilling of the spiculae and hyperostotic bone, not only, as mentioned before, to obtain good hemostasis on the origin of the meningioma, but also to remove tumor nodules extending into this bone.

"Dural Tail"

When a meningioma has been nearly completely removed, often strands of fibrous tissue suggestive of the "dural tail" seen on MRI with contrast may extend further along the borders. Since these strands indeed may harbor tumor cells, they should be removed carefully while paying attention not to damage the entry areas of the CNs, particularly the CN VI. Also, we have frequently observed that once the strands are removed, they may re-present or be so firmly attached to the inner layer of the dura that bleeding points from the preclival sinus system may be opended (partcularly in meningiomas of the anterior petrous area and their extension onto the clivus). Again, these bleeding points must be carefully sealed by bipolar coagulation.

Results

Complete tumor removal with high quality of life is the primary goal of surgery and can be achieved in approximately 50% (27–86%) of the patients. Clinical outcome after surgery is reported to be normal life in 86%,[51] performance status basically unchanged at a follow-up of 12 months[52] or normal or minimally disabled in 22/26.[53] Hearing could be preserved in 9/10 patients using the retrosigmoid approach[33] or in 82%[55] to 90%[1] of patients with preoperative functional hearing; normal facial function was preserved in 65%.[11/17] Anecdotal reports[56] or reports on a larger series[55] show improvement of hearing deficit following total removal of large meningiomas via the retrosigmoid approach.[57] As Schaller[58] and others pointed out, the results are better for the retromeatal tumors as compared to the premeatal tumors, although retromeatal tumors tend to be bigger than premeatal meningiomas.

Mortality rates are presented between 0%,[16,19,26,54] 2.5%,[5,52] and 4.8–5%.[6,8] Also, in our series of 44 patients with meningioma of the CPA, 0% mortality was achieved.

Major surgical compications in the largest published series presented in 1996 by Matthies[55] were CSF leakage in 8%, requiring revision in 2%, and hemorrhage in 3%, requiring

surgical intervention in 2%.[52] Facial nerve paresis or paralysis was encountered in 17%, and reconstruction was necessary in 7%. Other authors present less favorable results[6] with a facial palsy rate of 30%.

Since gross total resection (Simpson grade I) can only be achieved in a limited number of patients (e.g., 57% in 52), follow-up radiotherapy should be considered as deemed appropriate.

Summary

Meningiomas around the cerebellopontine angle, in particular those arising ventral to the IAC, still present a major surgical challenge. Depending on their origin and size, the standard neurosurgical approach via a lateral retromastoidal retrosigmoid craniotomy can be sufficient or may be extended in order to achieve a radical tumor resection while preserving cranial nerve and brain stem functions. Modern imaging techniques have helped to understand the microsurgical neuroanatomy and the postoperative results.

References

1. Nakamura M, Roser F, Dormiani M, et al. Intraoperative auditory brainstem responses in patients with cerebellopontine angle meningiomas involving the inner auditory canal: analysis of the predictive value of the responses. J Neurosurg 2005;102:637–42.

2. Cueva RA, Mastrodimos B. Approach design and closure techniques to minimize cerebrospinal fluid leak after cerebellopontine angle tumor surgery. Otol Neurotol 2005; 26:1176–81.

3. Magliulo G, Zardo F, Bertin S, et al. Meningiomas of the internal auditory canal: two case reports. Skull Base 2002; 12:19–26.

4. Garcia-Navarrete E, Sola RG. Aspectos clínicos y quirúrgicos de los meningiomas de la base del cráneo. III. Meningiomas de la fosa posterior. Rev Neurol 2002 ; 34:714–23.

5. Gerganov V, Bussarsky V, Romansky K, et al. Cerebellopontine angle meningiomas. Clinical features and surgical treatment. J Neurosurg Sci 2003; 47:129–35.

6. Voss NF, Vrionis FD, Heilman CB, Robertson JH. Meningiomas of the cerebellopontine angle. Surg Neurol 2000; 53:439–46

7. Pirouzmand F, Tator CH, Rutka J. Management of hydrocephalus associated with vestibular schwannoma and other cerebellopontine angle tumors. Neurosurgery 2001; 48:1246–53.

8. Mallucci CL, Ward V, Carney AS, et al. Clinical features and outcomes in patients with non-acoustic cerebellopontine angle tumours. J Neurol Neurosurg Psychiatry 1999; 66:768–71.

9. Sepehrnia A, Schulte T. Trigeminal neuralgia caused by contralateral cerebellopontine angle meningioma - case report. Zentralbl Neurochir 2001; 62:62–4.

10. Cancelli I, Cecotti L, Valentinis L, et al. Hemifacial spasm due to a tentorial paramedian meningioma: a case report. Neurol Sci 2005; 26:46–9.

11. Galvez-Jimenez N, Hanson MR, Desai M. Unusual causes of hemifacial spasm. Semin Neurol 2001; 21:75–83.

12. Iwai Y, Yamanaka K, Nakajima H. Hemifacial spasm due to cerebellopontine angle meningiomas–two case reports. Neurol Med Chir (Tokyo) 2001; 41:87–9.

13. Schaller B, Merlo A, Gratzl O, Probst R.Premeatal and retro-meatal cerebellopontine angle meningioma. Two distinct clinical entities. Acta Neurochir (Wien) 1999;141(5):465–71.

14. Yuguang L, Chengyuan W, Meng L, et al. Neuroendoscopic anatomy and surgery of the cerebellopontine angle. J Clin Neurosci 2005; 12:256–60.

15. Bonneville F, Sarrazin JL, Marsot-Dupuch K, et al.Unusual lesions of the cerebellopontine angle: a segmental approach. Radiographics 2001;21(2):419–38.

16. Nakamura M, Roser F, Mirzai S, et al. Meningiomas of the internal auditory canal. Neurosurgery 2004; 55:119–27.

17. Yasargil MG Microneurosurgery. Vols I, IVB. Stuttgart, Thieme, 1996.

18. Roser F, Nakamura M, Dormiani M, et al. Meningiomas of the cerebellopontine angle with extension into the internal auditory canal. J Neurosurg 2005; 102:17–23.

19. Jiang YG, Xiang J, Wen F, Zhang LY. Microsurgical excision of the large or giant cerebellopontine angle meningioma. Minim Invasive Neurosurg 2006; 49:43–8.

20. Kumon Y, Sakaki S, Ohue S, et al. Usefulness of heavily T2-weighted magnetic resonance imaging in patients with cerebellopontine angle tumors. Neurosurgery 1998; 43:1338–43.

21. Held P, Fellner C, Fellner F, et al. MRI of inner ear and facial nerve pathology using 3D MP-RAGE and 3D CISS sequences. Br J Radiol 1997; 70:558–66.

22. Ahlhelm F, Nabhan A, Naumann N, et al. Tumoren der Schädelbasis Radiologe 2005;45(9):807–15.

23. Langman AW, Jackler RK, Althaus SR. Meningioma of the internal auditory canal. Am J Otol 1990; 11:201–4.

24. Quint DJ, McGillicuddy JE. Meningeal metastasis of the cerebellopontine angle demonstrating "dural tail" sign. Can Assoc Radiol J 1994; 45:40–3.

25. Buhl R, Hasan A, Behnke A, Mehdorn HM. Results in the operative treatment of elderly patients with intracranial meningioma. Neurosurg Rev 2000; 23:25–9.

26. Nakamura M, Roser F, Dormiani M, et al. Surgical treatment of cerebellopontine angle meningiomas in elderly patients. Acta Neurochir (Wien) 2005;147(6):603–9.

27. Zeitouni AG, Zagzag D, Cohen NL. Meningioma of the internal auditory canal. Ann Otol Rhinol Laryngol 1997; 106:657–61.

28. Driscoll CL, Jackler RK, Pitts LH, Brackmann DE. Lesions of the internal auditory canal and cerebellopontine angle in an only hearing ear: is surgery ever advisable? Am J Otol 2000; 21:573–81.

29. Kan P, Shelton C, Townsend J, Jensen R. Primary malignant cerebellopontine angle melanoma presenting as a presumed meningioma: case report and review of the literature. Skull Base 2003; 13:159–166.

30. Tsukamoto H, Hikita T, Takaki T. Cerebellopontine angle meningioma associated with cranial accessory nerve neurinoma–case report. Neurol Med Chir (Tokyo) 1994; 34:225–9.

31. Wilms G, Plets C, Goossens L, et al. The radiological differentiation of acoustic neurinoma and meningioma occurring together in the cerebellopontine angle. Neurosurgery 1992; 30:443–5.

32. Buhl R, Huang H, Gottwald B, et al. Neuropsychological findings in patients with intraventricular tumors. Surg Neurol 2005; 64:500–3.

33. Batra PS, Dutra JC, Wiet RJ. Auditory and facial nerve function following surgery for cerebellopontine angle meningiomas. Arch Otolaryngol Head Neck Surg 2002; 128:369–374.

34. Saleh EA, Taibah AK, Achilli V, et al. Posterior fossa meningioma: surgical strategy. Skull Base Surg 1994; 4:202–12.

35. Alliez JR, Pellet W, Roche PH. Avantages de l'abord rétro-labyrinthique pour l'exérèse des méningiomes insérés au pourtour du coude du sinus latéral. Neurochirurgie 2006; 52:419–31.

36. Sanna M, Agarwal M, Jain Y, et al. Transapical extension in difficult cerebellopontine angle tumours: preliminary report. J Laryngol Otol 2003;117(10):788–92.

37. Leonetti JP, Anderson DE, Marzo SJ, et al. Combined transtemporal access for large (>3 cm) meningiomas of the cerebellopontine angle. Otolaryngol Head Neck Surg 2006; 134:949–52.

38. Danner C, Cueva RA. Extended middle fossa approach to the petroclival junction and anterior cerebellopontine angle. Otol Neurotol 2004; 25:762–8.

39. Le Garlantezec C, Vidal VF, Guerin J, et al. Approches thérapeutiques des méningiomes de l'angle ponto-cérébelleux et de la face postérieure du rocher. A propos de 44 cas Rev Laryngol Otol Rhinol (Bord) 2005; 126:81–9.

40. Thedinger BA, Glasscock ME 3rd, Cueva RA. Transcochlear transtentorial approach for removal of large cerebellopontine angle meningiomas. Am J Otol 1992;13(5):408–15.

41. Nakamura M, Roser F, Dormiani M, et al. Facial and cochlear nerve function after surgery of cerebellopontine angle meningiomas. Neurosurgery 2005; 57:77–90.

42. Nakamura M, Roser F, Dormiani M, et al. Intraoperative auditory brainstem responses in patients with cerebellopontine angle meningiomas involving the inner auditory canal: analysis of the predictive value of the responses. J Neurosurg 2005;102(4):637–42.

43. Nakamura M, Roser F, Dormiani M, et al. Facial and cochlear nerve function after surgery of cerebellopontine angle meningiomas. Neurosurgery 2005; 57:77–90.

44. Romstock J, Strauss C, Fahlbusch R. Continuous electromyography monitoring of motor cranial nerves during cerebellopontine angle surgery. J Neurosurg 2000; 93:586–93.

45. Kombos T, Suess O, Kern BC, et al. Can continuous intraoperative facial electromyography predict facial nerve function following cerebellopontine angle surgery? Neurol Med Chir (Tokyo) 2000; 40:501–5.

46. Wedekind C, Klug N. Recording nasal muscle F waves and electromyographic activity of the facial muscles: a comparison of two methods used for intraoperative monitoring of facial nerve function. J Neurosurg 2001;95:974–8.

47. Strauss C, Neu M, Bischoff B, Romstock J. Clinical and neurophysiological observations after superior petrosal vein obstruction during surgery of the cerebellopontine angle: case report. Neurosurgery 2001; 48:1157–9.

48. Gharabaghi A, Koerbel A, Lowenheim H, et al. The impact of petrosal vein preservation on postoperative auditory function in surgery of petrous apex meningiomas. Neurosurgery 2006; 59(1 Suppl 1):ONS68–74.

49. Akaishi K, Hongo K, Tanaka Y, Kobayashi S. Cerebellopontine angle meningioma with a high jugular bulb. J Clin Neurosci 2001; 8:452–4.

50. Kinjo T, al-Mefty O, Kanaan I. Grade zero removal of supratentorial convexity meningiomas. Neurosurgery1993; 33: 394–9.

51. Bassiouni H, Hunold A, Asgari S, Stolke D. Meningiomas of the posterior petrous bone: functional outcome after microsurgery. J Neurosurg 2004; 100:1014–24.

52. Roberti F, Sekhar LN, Kalavakonda C, Wright DC. Posterior fossa meningiomas: surgical experience in 161 cases. Surg Neurol 2001; 56:8–20.

53. Lange M, Duc LD, Horn P, et al. Cerebellopontine angle meningiomas (cpam)—clinical characteristics and surgical results. Neurol Neurochir Pol 2000;34(6 Suppl):107–13.

54. Pomeranz S, Umansky F, Elidan J, et al. Giant cranial base tumours. Acta Neurochir (Wien) 1994; 129:121–6.

55. Matthies C, Carvalho G, Tatagiba M, et al. Meningiomas of the cerebellopontine angle. Acta Neurochir Suppl 1996; 65:86–91.

56. Katsuta T, Inoue T, Uda K, Masuda A. Hearing restoration from deafness after resection of a large cerebellopontine angle meningioma–case report. Neurol Med Chir (Tokyo) 2001; 41:352–5.

57. Grey PL, Baguley DM, Moffat DA, et al. Audiovestibular results after surgery for cerebellopontine angle meningiomas. Am J Otol 1996; 17:634–8.

58. Schaller B, Heilbronner R, Pfaltz CR, et al. Preoperative and postoperative auditory and facial nerve function in cerebellopontine angle meningiomas. Otolaryngol Head Neck Surg 1995; 112:228–34.

48
Petrous Meningiomas II: Ventral, Posterior and Superior Subtypes

Burak Sade and Joung H. Lee

Introduction

Despite the relatively small size of the petrous bone, meningiomas arising from this region constitute a heterogeneous group of tumors in regards to surgical considerations, operative risks, outcome, and tumor histology.

In the literature, there is a lack of standardized terminology for meningiomas arising from the posterior surface of the petrous bone. For instance, some authors include all meningiomas arising from the posterior surface of the petrous bone in their definition of "posterior petrous meningiomas".[1,2] Others prefer the term "cerebellopontine angle meningioma" for the same group of tumors.[3–5] The term "Petrous pyramid" meningiomas has also been used. Sekhar has classified posterior fossa meningiomas into five groups, and according to this classification, some of Type II, III, and IV meningiomas can be referred to as petrous meningiomas.[6]

In this chapter we present our series of petrous meningiomas (PM), in which we aim to assess the operative outcome and tumor histology according to the site of tumor origin in reference to the internal auditory canal (IAC). A retrospective review of 58 patients operated by the senior author between June 1994 and June 2006 was performed. The site of tumor origin was assessed intraoperatively. Tumors were classified in reference to the IAC as posterior petrous meningiomas (PPM), superior petrous meningiomas (SPM), and ventral petrous meningiomas (VPM). Petroclival, clival, tentorial, and jugular foramen/tubercle meningiomas were strictly excluded from the analysis. All patients were operated via a simplified suboccipital retrosigmoid approach, which was described in detail previously.[7]

Review of Our Series

There were a total of 58 patients: 29 PPM (Fig. 48-1), 8 SPM (Fig. 48-2), and 19 VPM (Fig. 48-3). In two patients there were multiple tumors with different sites of origin along the petrous bone, and therefore, these were not included in the analysis.

Symptoms

Of the 56 patients, 25% presented with gait imbalance, 23% with hearing loss, 21% with headache attributable to the tumor, and 14% with either facial numbness or trigeminal neuralgia, whereas in 29% of the patients, the tumor was detected incidentally. The incidence of symptoms according to the site of origin is detailed in Table 48-1.

Tumor Size

The overall tumor size was 29.6 ± 12.9 mm (11–60 mm), which did not show any significant difference among the groups: 31.5 ± 15.1 mm (11–60 mm) in PPM, 23.9 ± 6 mm (15–23 mm) in SPM, and 29.6 ± 11.2 mm (15–52 mm) in VPM.

Extent of Tumor Resection

Gross-total tumor resection (Simpson Grade I–II) was achieved in 84% of the patients and was significantly higher in PPM and SPM (Table 48-2).

Complications

New-onset hearing loss was the most common operative complication (11%), followed by new-onset permenant deficits of cranial nerves 6, 7, 9, and 10 (21%), seen exclusively in the VPM group. Postoperative cerebrospinal fluid (CSF) rhinorrhea was seen in 7% and was again more frequent in VPM. Other complications consisted of cerebrospinal fluid (CSF) leak from the wound and cerebellar hematoma for PPM, and chemical meningitis in the VPM group. Details of operative complications according to the site of tumor origin are outlined in Table 48-3.

Involvement of the Internal Auditory Canal by the Tumor

Overall, tumor involvement of the IAC was detected in 23% of the patients, which did not show any significant difference among the groups: 21% in PPM, 25% in SPM, and 26% in VPM.

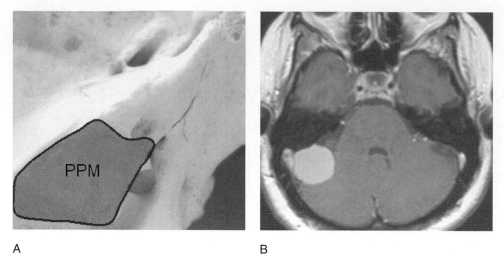

FIG. 48.1. (A) Site of origin in posterior petrous meningiomas (PPM). (B) Postcontrast T1-weighted MRI of a patient with PPM. Note the distance of the tumor from the internal auditory canal

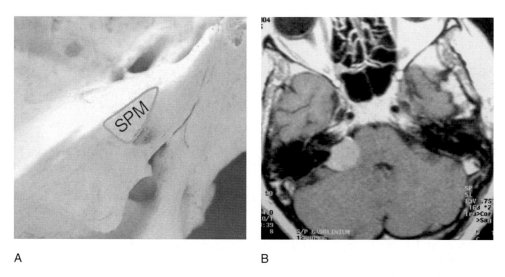

FIG. 48.2. (A) Site of origin in superior petrous meningiomas (SPM). (B) Postcontrast T1-weighted MRI of a patient with SPM showing the lower pole of the tumor at the level of the internal auditory canal

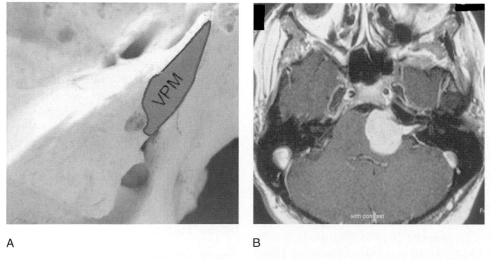

FIG. 48.3. (A) Site of origin in ventral petrous meningiomas (VPM). (B) Postcontrast T1-weighted MRI of a patient with VPM. Note the osseous hypertrophy ventral to the internal auditory canal at the site of tumor origin

TABLE 48.1. Incidence of Symptoms According to the Site of Origin of the Tumor.

Site of origin	Symptoms				
	Gait imb.	H/A	Hearing loss	Trigeminal	Incidental
PPM ($n = 29$)	10 (34%)	7 (24%)	6 (21%)	2 (7%)	7 (24%)
SPM ($n = 8$)	—	2 (25%)	3 (38%)	1 (13%)	3 (38%)
VPM ($n = 19$)	4 (21%)	3 (16%)	4 (21%)	5 (26%)	6 (32%)

H/A, headache.

TABLE 48.2. Extent of Tumor Resection According to the Site of Tumor Origin.

Site of origin	Extent of tumor resection	
	GTR (Simpson I–II)	STR
PPM ($n = 29$)	28 (97%)	1 (3%)
SPM ($n = 8$)	8 (100%)	—
VPM ($n = 19$)	11 (58%)	8 (42%)

GTR, gross-total resection; STR, subtotal resection.

TABLE 48.3. Operative Complications According to the Site of Tumor Origin.

Site of origin	Operative complications			
	Hearing loss	Other CN def.	Rhinorrhea	Miscellaneous
PPM ($n = 29$)	—	—	1 (3%)	2 (7%)
SPM ($n = 8$)	—	—	—	—
VPM ($n = 19$)	6 (32%)	4 (21%)	3 (16%)	1 (5%)

CN, cranial nerve.

TABLE 48.4. Role of Internal Auditory Canal Involvement.

IAC involvement	Preop HL	Postop HL (new onset)	GTR
Yes ($n = 13$)	10 (77%)	2 (15%)	10 (77%)
No ($n = 43$)	3 (7%)	4 (9%)	37 (86%)

IAC, internal auditory canal; HL, hearing loss; GTR, gross-total resection.

TABLE 48.5. Histologic Subtype According to the Site of Tumor Origin

Site of origin	Tumor histology		
	Meningothelial	Fibrous	Other
PPM ($n = 29$)	8 (27%)	20 (69%)	1 (3%)
SPM ($n = 8$)	2 (25%)	5 (62%)	1 (13%)
VPM ($n = 19$)	13 (68%)	2 (11%)	4 (21%)

Involvement of the IAC was associated with the presence of preoperative hearing loss, but did not affect the incidence of postoperative new-onset hearing loss or extent of resection (Table 48.4).

Tumor Histology

The most common histologic subtype found in the entire group of PM was fibrous (48%), followed by meningothelial (41%). However, meningothelial was the most common histology in the VPM subgroup (Table 48-5).

Discussion

As stated earlier, the lack of standardized terminology in meningiomas arising from the posterior surface of the petrous bone makes it difficult to compare the available data in the literature. In our series, we included the meningiomas exclusively arising from the petrous bone, lateral and posterior to the petro-occipital sulcus, and excluded meningiomas of the surrounding locations such as tentorium, petroclival/clival region or jugular foramen/tubercle. The rationale for doing so was[1] to clarify and accurately use the term "petrous meningioma" to refer specifically to the site of tumor origin

and[2] to acknowledge the variation of surgical challenges and nuances between VPM and meningiomas of the other sites mentioned above.

Surgical Approaches

Surgery of PM is fraught with difficulties because of the frequent involvement of the cranial nerves V–XI as well as the critical vascular structures of the cerebellopontine angle, which renders complete resection challenging and also increases the incidence of postoperative cranial nerve morbidities. In general, the most commonly used surgical techniques consist of suboccipital retrosigmoid or variants of transpetrosal approaches.

While the suboccipital retrosigmoid approach is preferred in the vast majority of tumors located posterior to the IAC, the use of both retrosigmoid and transpetrosal techniques have been advocated by various authors in the surgical management of meningiomas ventral to the IAC[3–5,8–13] with similar operative outcomes. The technical details, advantages, and disadvantages of each of these approaches have been well discussed in the literature and are not the main focus of this chapter.

Operative Outcome

Our results are in parallel with those published previously, in that meningiomas arising from posterior to the IAC have a more favorable outcome with much less cranial nerve morbidity as compared to tumors located ventrally.[1,2,12,14] In our series, new-onset hearing loss following surgery and other cranial nerve deficits exclusively occurred in the VPM group (32% of new-onset hearing loss and 21% other CN deficit in VPM as compared to none in PPM or SPM). The working area in the surgical management of VPM consists of operative windows between the tentorium and CN V, between CN V and CN VII/VIII complex, and between CN VII/VIII complex and CN IX/X, which increases the risk of operative injury to these structures, especially the cochlear nerve, which is known to be very sensitive even to minor traction. Postoperative new-onset permenant facial nerve palsy was seen in only one patient with VPM in our series. The results of Nakamura and colleagues also suggest a more favorable facial nerve outcome in CPA meningiomas when the site of tumor origin is superior or posterior to the IAC [14]. In our experience the incidence of postoperative CSF rhinorrhea was also higher in VPM. This may be the result of drilling of the site of tumor origin in our practice whenever feasible to ensure gross-total resection. In the case of VPM, when an air cell is violated, it might be less visible as compared to a site along the posterior petrous bone. In this context, it is important to emphasize the fact that gross-total resection has been less achievable (58%) in VPM, whereas almost all of PPM and SPM had Simpson Grade I or II resection.

Involvement of the Internal Auditory Canal

In our series the extension of the tumor into the IAC was associated with preoperative hearing loss, in that in patients with tumor inside the IAC, hearing loss was 10 times more frequent. However, involvement of the IAC did not affect the extent of resection or the incidence of new-onset postoperative hearing loss. Nakamura and colleagues also found a higher incidence of preoperative facial weakness and hearing loss and less favorable facial nerve and hearing outcomes in tumors involving the IAC.[14] In their series of 72 patients with CPA meningiomas involving the IAC, Roser and colleagues compared the group of tumors which had a site of origin outside the IAC and secondary involvement of the IAC with tumors in which the site of origin was inside the IAC. They found that drilling of the IAC did not influence the postoperative outcome in the former group, but the outcome was much less favorable regardless of the drilling status in the latter group.[15]

Tumor Histology

In our experience, the tumor histology showed significant difference in VPM as compared to PPM or SPM. In VPM, 68% of the tumors had meningothelial subtype, whereas 69% of PPM and 62% of SPM had fibrous histology. We have previously shown that meningiomas of the central skull base, which includes the ventral petrous region, are predominantly of the meningothelial subtype.[16] Numerous findings at the cellular and embryologic levels raise a possibility that these central skull base meningiomas may actually be unique

tumors among meningiomas.[16] This topic is discussed in detail elsewhere in this book. Of interest, fibrous histology was the predominant subtype in PPM and SPM, which was almost five times higher than the overall incidence of fibrous meningiomas in our overall series of intracranial meningiomas. Wu and colleagues also reported a higher incidence of fibrous histology in their type I tumors, which they define as tumors lateral to the IAC.[2]

Conclusion

VPM are different tumors in their histology (meningothelial) and operative outcome. The predominance of meningothelial histology may suggest a different tumorigenesis compared to PPM or SPM, where the fibrous subtype is much more prevalent.

VPM should be viewed as a distinct group of tumors in their surgical consideration, histology, and outcome. On the other hand, PPM and SPM have a similar outcome and tumor histology and, therefore, can be viewed as a single group.

References

1. Bassiouni H, Hunold A, Asgari S, Stolke D. Meningiomas of the posterior petrous bone: functional outcome after microsurgery. J Neurosurg 2004;100:1014–24.
2. Wu ZB, Yu CJ, Guan SS. Posterior petrous meningiomas: 82 cases. J Neurosurg 2005;102:284–9.
3. Matthies C, Carvalho G, Tatagiba M, Lima M, Samii M. Meningiomas of the cerebellopontine angle. Acta Neurochir 1996;(Suppl 65):86–91.
4. Thomas NWM, King TT. Meningiomas of the cerebellopontine angle. A report of 41 cases. Br J Neurosurg 1996;10:59–68.
5. Voss NF, Vrionis FD, Heilman CB, Robertson JH. Meningiomas of the cerebellopontine angle. Surg Neurol 2000;53:439–47.
6. Roberti F, Sekhar LN, Kalavakonda C, Wright DC. Posterior fossa meningiomas: surgical experience in 161 cases. Surg Neurol 2001;56:8–21.
7. Yamashima T, Lee JH, Tobias S, Kim CH, Chang JH, Kwon JT. Surgical procedure "Simplified retrosigmoid approach" for C-P angle lesions. J Vlin Neurosci 2004;11:168–71.
8. Abdel Aziz KM, Sanan A, van Loveren HR, Tew JM, Keller JT, Pensak ML. Petroclival meningiomas: predictive parameters for transpetrosal approaches. Neurosurgery 2000;47:139–52.
9. Bricolo AP, Turazzi S, Talacchi A, Cristofori L. Microsurgical removal of petroclival meningiomas: a report of 33 patients. Neurosurgery 1992;31:813–28
10. Couldwell WT, Fukushima T, Giannotta SL, Weiss MH. Petroclival meningiomas: surgical experience in 109 cases. J Neurosurg 1996;84:20–8.
11. Goel A, Muzumdar D. Conventional posterior fossa approach for surgery on petroclival meningiomas: a report on an experience with 28 cases. Surg Neurol 2004;62:3323–40.

12. Liu JK, Gottfried ON, Couldwell WT. Surgical management of posterior petrous meningiomas. Neurosurg Focus 2003;14(6): Article 7.
13. Samii M, Tatagiba M, Carvalho GA. Resection of large petroclival meningiomas by the simple retrosigmoid route. J Clin Neurosci 1999;6:27–30.
14. Nakamura M, Roser F, Dormiani M, Matthies C, Vorkapic P, Samii M. Facial and cochlear nerve function after surgery of cerebellopontine angle meningiomas. Neurosurgery 2005;57:77–90.
15. Roser F, Nakamura M, Dormiani M, Matthies C, Vorkapic P, Samii M. Meningiomas of the cerebellopontine angle with extension into the internal auditory canal. J Neurosurg 2005;102:17–23.
16. Lee JH, Sade B, Choi E, Golubic M, Prayson R. Meningothelioma as the predominant histological subtype of midline skull base and spinal meningiomas. J Neurosurg 2006;105:60–4.

49
Foramen Magnum Meningiomas

Luis A.B. Borba and Benedicto O. Colli

Introduction

Although meningiomas account for almost 20% of brain tumors, only 1.8–3.2% arises at the foramen magnum (FM).[1-3]

In their monograph on meningiomas, Cushing and Eisenhardt divided foramen magnum meningiomas into two groups: craniospinal and spinocranial tumors.[2] The craniospinal type arose above the foramen magnum ventral to the neuraxis and projected downward, displacing the medulla and cervical spinal cord. The spinocranial type was found dorsal or dorsolateral to the spinal cord and projected upward into the posterior fossa cisterns.

Recently, George et al. defined as foramen magnum meningiomas those arising anteriorly from the inferior third of the clivus to the superior edge of the C2 body, laterally from the jugular tubercle to the C2 laminae and posteriorly from the anterior border of the occipital squama to the spinal process of C2.[4,5] The dentate ligament divided the foramen into anterior and posterior compartments. The foramen magnum meningioma has the main dural attachment in the anterolateral face of the foramen in 70%, anterior in 15%, posterolateral in 10%, and posterior in 5% of the cases.[1,3,6]

Clinical Signs

As with all meningiomas, there is a female predominance for foramen magnum meningiomas. They become symptomatic in the fourth to sixth decades of life, and a few cases in the pediatric population have been reported.[7]

The clinical signs and symptoms are extremely variable and the wide variety is related to the great amount of neural structures in the area.[8] Headache, occipital radicular pain, cervical pain, long tract deficits, lower cranial nerve palsies, muscular atrophy of limbs, and cerebellar disturbance are the main signs and symptoms.

Diagnosis

Contrast computed tomography (CT) is diagnostic in 75% of patients with foramen magnum meningioma.[4] Magnetic resonance imaging (MRI) is the choice for the diagnosis of foramen magnum lesions. T1-weighted images demonstrate the tumor, its main dural attachment and extension to the clivus, spinal canal, and sometimes inside the skull base foramina.

Differential Diagnosis

The slow-growing pattern makes clinical diagnosis difficult, and very often the interval between the first symptoms and the diagnosis is great.[1] The insidious, often remitting, course may simulate cervical spondylosis, multiple sclerosis, syringomyelia, or chiari malformation.

Treatment

Despite the advance of alternative therapies, surgery remains the treatment of choice for the management of foramen magnum meningiomas.[8-12]

Preoperative Evaluation

The appropriate surgical plan is developed after a complete neurologic and radiologic examination. The status of the lower cranial nerve (LCN) is a crucial issue before proceeding with the surgical treatment. Preoperative impairment of LCN may indicate a tracheostomy before surgery. Sometimes, a long-term LCN deficit can be compensated by the contralateral side. A tracheotomy is mandatory in the presence of new postoperative lower cranial nerve deficit.

The radiologic evaluation must include a CT of the craniocervical junction to depict bone abnormalities and the normal anatomy of the area. The size of occipital condyle and lateral mass of C1, as well as the angle between these structures in the axial view, are important factors to consider in the surgical decision of large bony removal.[13–16] MRI studies of cervical spine are mandatory because an asymptomatic compression of spinal cord by degenerative discoarthrosis can cause a neurologic deterioration related to the patient positioning during surgery.[4]

Besides the improvements in diagnostic modalities, surgical techniques, and postoperative management, intraoperative neurophysiologic monitoring contributes to an improved outcome of skull base surgery. Electroencephalogram (EEG) monitoring and somatosensory evoked potentials (SSEPs) are routinely made in patients with skull base lesions. Monitoring of lower cranial nerves is a useful and safe procedure during surgery of FM meningiomas. Tumor adherence or close proximity to the nerves makes them vulnerable to injury. Spontaneous electromyography (EMG) activity alerts the surgeon to the possibility of damage to these structures.

Choice of Surgical Approach

A wide variety of surgical techniques has been described for removal of foramen magnum meningiomas,[1,5,6,9,10,12,13,17–20] and the choice of the surgical approach is the main point of controversy in its management.[9,10,12,13,15,17,18,20–23]

Transoral transclival removal of foramen magnum meningiomas was advocated by Miller and Crockard,[24] who described two cases of successful removal. However, the difficulty to repair the dura to avoid a cerebrospinal fluid (CSF) leak is the main concern with this approach. Endoscopic removal has been recently tried with similar problems. Goel et al.[18] reported a series of 17 cases operated by this approach, many of them located anteriorly or anterolaterally in the foramen magnum. Total removal was obtained in 82% of the patients. Despite excellent results, the author emphasizes that all tumors were considered to be giant in relation to the foramen magnum. It is well known that the larger the tumor, the easier its removal is utilizing the corridor and space created by the tumor.[9,13] The so-called conventional suboccipital approach described by Goel et al.[18] is actually a posterolateral approach with exposure of the foramen magnum without drilling the occipital condyle or transposing the vertebral artery. Samii et al[23] reported 38 patients with 40 meningiomas of the craniocervical junction. Fifteen were spinocranial and 25 craniocervical according to the dural attachment. Standard midline or lateral suboccipital approaches, with or without laminectomy, were sufficient for the great majority of cases.

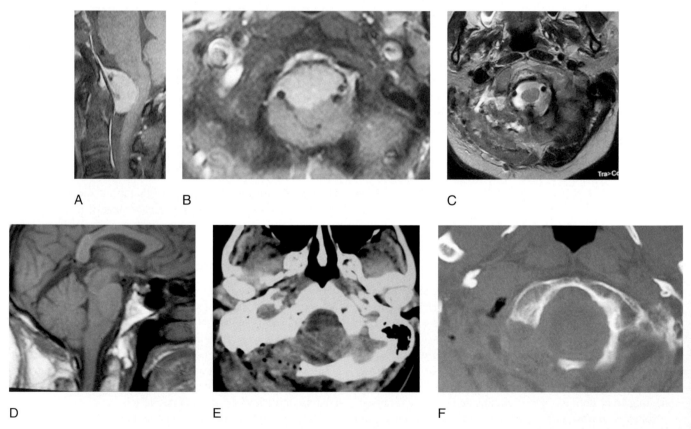

A   B   C

D   E   F

FIG. 49.1. A 45-year-old female with a history of progressive tetraparesis without lower cranial nerve deficits. (A, B) The T1-weighted MRI images with contrast depict a mass located anteriorly in the foramen magnum with a dural tail. (C–F) The postoperative MRI and CT scan show the absence of residual tumor and the extent of bone removal

In seven cases, a partial removal of the condyle was needed. Total removal was achieved in 12 of 15 spinocranial (80%) and 13 of 25 craniocervical (52%) tumors. Margalit et al.[22] reviewed 42 cases of foramen magnum tumors with an anterior or anterolateral location. A meningioma was diagnosed in 18 patients. Vertebral artery mobilization at the dural entry point was performed in all patients; however, partial condyle resection was made in 8 patients. A Simpson grade I resection was achieved in 55% of the patients. They concluded that condyle removal may be needed depending on the extent and location of foramen magnum tumors and their specific pathology. Arnautovic et al.[9] reported 18 cases of ventral foramen magnum meningiomas, all of them originating from the lower clivus with extension to the foramen magnum area. Radical removal was achieved in 75% of the patients. A high

incidence of LCN deficits illustrates the extreme complexity of such tumors (Fig. 49-1 and 49-2).

The topic to be addressed is what type of tumor we are dealing with. The craniospinal tumor of Cushing used to have a more anterior and wide dural attachment in the foramen magnum with superior extension to the clival area. Its surgical removal is more demanding, and currently a more lateral approach, afforded by the removal of the occipital condyle and sometimes the jugular tubercle, allows a better view, providing a wider field of vision to perform a radical removal. This type of tumor should be managed as a clival tumor. The spinocranial tumor of Cushing has a different type of dural attachment, either posterior or posterolateral in the foramen magnum. However, a clear arachnoid plan is found between the tumor and the surrounding neural and

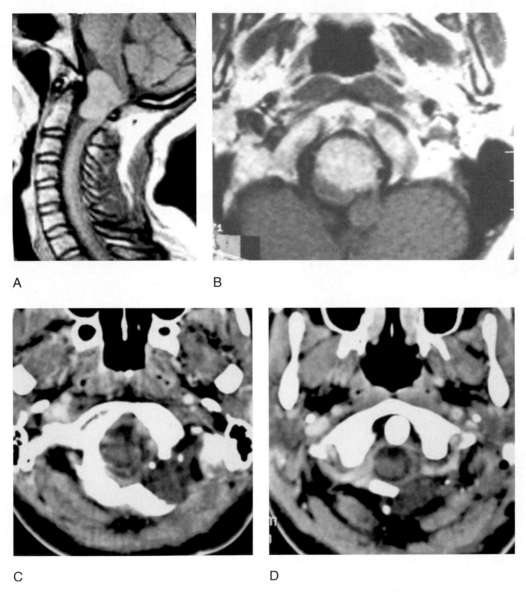

A

B

C

D

FIG. 49-2. A 48-year-old female with a short history of tetraparesis. (A, B) The T1-weighted MRI images with contrast show a tumor located anteriorly in the foramen magnum without a dural tail. (C, D) The postoperative CT scan depicts the bony removal with preservation of the occipital condyle

vascular structures, allowing a safe tumor resection without extensive bony removal.

Surgical Approach

The surgical approaches used by us to treat 12 patients with foramen magnum meningiomas during the last 6 years are described below (Fig. 49-3).

The patients are operated under general anesthesia. The endotracheal tube is placed using an endoscope to avoid neck manipulation. The patients are placed in the lateral position with the side of the tumor upward, the ipsilateral shoulder displaced anteriorly, and the head slightly rotated ipsilaterally to keep the parallel lateral view. A "C"-shape incision is made with the upper limb at the level of the external auditory meatus, the posterior limb in the midline, and

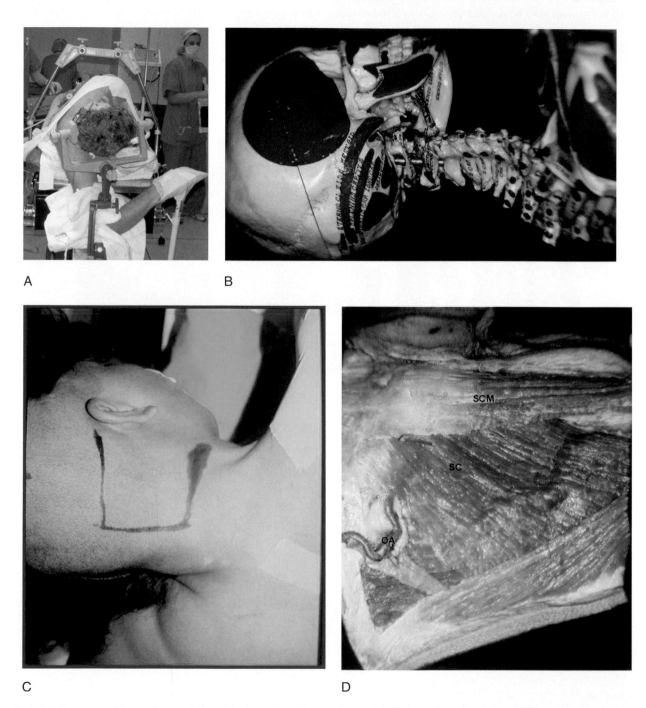

A

B

C

D

FIG. 49-3. (A) Lateral position with an anterior displacement of the shoulder and a slight ipsilateral rotation of the head to keep it parallel to the floor. (B) The bony anatomy can be seen in the lateral position, providing a straight access to the anterior foramen magnum. (C) A "C"-shape incision is used with its center in the mastoid tip.

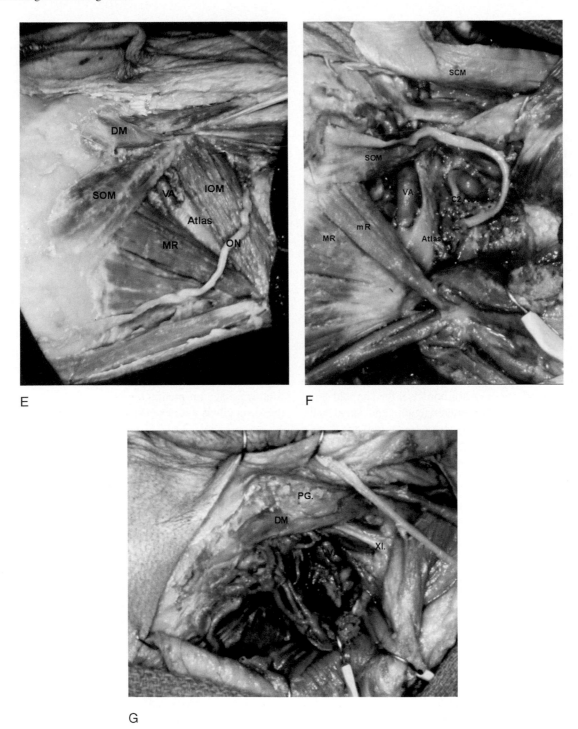

E

F

G

FIG. 49-3 (continued) (D, E) The SCM is displaced laterally exposing the splenius capitis, and the semispinalis and the longissimus capitis are mobilized medially, exposing the suboccipital triangle. (F, G) The superior and inferior oblique muscles and the major and minor rectus muscles are exposed. The V3 segment of the vertebral artery can be seen inside the triangle

the inferior incision at the level of the C_3–C_4 vertebrae. The skin flap is displaced laterally, and the posterior and superior limbs of the sternocleidomastoid muscle are detached from the mastoid process and displaced anteriorly, exposing the splenius capitis, the posterior limb of the digastric muscle, and the lavator scapulae muscle.[16] These muscles are detached from the mastoid process and displaced inferiorly and medially, providing exposure of the suboccipital triangle formed by the superior and inferior obliques and major and minor rectus muscles. Inside this triangle, the posterior arch of the atlas and the horizontal segment of the vertebral artery can be seen. Removal of these small muscles will expose the vertebral artery from the axis to the entry point in the foramen magnum. Generally the posterior branch of the C2 root can be followed laterally by crossing just superior to the vertebral artery in its segment from C2 to C1. The venous plexus surrounding the vertebral artery is kept in place to reduce bleeding.

Lateral craniectomy or craniotomy of the posterior fossa is performed, enlarging the foramen magnum to expose the sigmoid sinus, and the ipsilateral posterior arch of C1 is also removed. Sometimes hemilaminectomy of C2 is also necessary. The vertebral artery is totally exposed from the axis to the entry point into the dura of the foramen magnum. The decision to remove the occipital condyle and to mobilize the vertebral artery is made based on the tumor type. For tumors with anterior origin or arising from the inferior clivus, the vertebral artery is displaced after opening the foramen transversarium of C1, allowing resection of the posterior third of the occipital condyle. A good landmark to limit the bony removal is the identification of the condylar vein.[9,16] The hypoglossal canal is located at the junction of the posterior and middle thirds of the condyle.[16] The jugular tubercle is a small bony protuberance located superior to the condyle, and its removal provides better exposure of the LCN in the jugular foramen.[15] For tumors with anterolateral origin, the vertebral artery is kept in place and the condyle is not removed. The dura mater is opened parallel to the posterior border of the sigmoid sinus, extending inferiorly to the foramen magnum and spinal canal. This allows exposure of the posterior fossa and spinal canal and lateral displacement of the vertebral artery. The tumor is removed in a piecemeal fashion with a combination of coagulation and suction. An ultrasonic aspirator is helpful to decrease the size of large tumors. After tumor removal, the dura is closed watertight and the muscles are reinserted into their original place.

Our approach differs basically from that of Margalit et al.[22] and Arnautovic et al.[9] regarding surgical position, incision, and muscle dissection. We prefer the lateral view allowed by the lateral position independent of the extent of bone removal. The skin incision and the muscle dissection permit dislocation of soft tissue laterally and medially, respectively, making the surgical field shallow and wider. The proximal extracranial control of the vertebral artery is important for tumor dissection from the intradural segment of this vessel. Although some authors strongly believe that removal of the occipital condyle and mobilization of the vertebral artery are crucial for the surgical resection of anterior foramen magnum meningiomas,[9,12,20] it is our understanding that the surgical approach for the resection of these tumors should be tailored for each case. Tumors classified as craniospinal generally are more difficult to resect. A wide lateral craniectomy with a partial mastoidectomy and partial resection of the occipital condyle and mobilization of the vertebral artery give a more lateral and short access to the mass, facilitating its resection.[9,12,20]

Resection of the occipital condyle and mobilization of the vertebral artery are not necessary in spinocranial foramen magnum meningiomas because these tumors generally behave as spinal meningiomas with an arachnoid plane between the tumor and adjacent neurovascular structures and a narrow attachment to the dura. In this subtype of tumor the lateral position and muscle dissection are sufficient to provide an excellent view of the tumor.

Results

Miller and Crockard[24] described two cases of successful removal of FM meningiomas through transoral transclival approach, and total removal was obtained through endoscopic removal by Goel et al.[18] in 82% of 17 patients. However, the difficulty to repair the dura to avoid a CSF leak is the main concern with these approaches. Samii et al.[23] reported total removal in 12 of 15 spinocranial (80%) and 13 of 25 craniocervical (52%) meningiomas of the craniocervical junction using standard midline or lateral suboccipital approaches, with or without laminectomy and partial removal of the condyle. Margalit et al.[22] achieved Simpson grade I resection in 55% of 18 patients with meningiomas of the foramen magnum of the anterior or anterolateral location with partial condyle resection performed in 8 patients. Arnautovic et al.[9] reported radical removal in 75% of the 18 patients with ventral foramen magnum meningiomas, all of them originating from the lower clivus with extension to the foramen magnum area.

Mortality and Morbidity

Morbidity related to the resection of foramen magnum meningiomas is directly related to the location and extension of the tumor. Craniospinal tumors are closely related to the LCN, and dysfunction of these LCN is not uncommon in the postoperative period and should be treated aggressively to avoid severe pulmonary complications. Arnautovic et al.[9] reported a high incidence of LCN deficits after removal of ventral foramen magnum meningiomas, illustrating the extreme complexity of such tumors. The presence of preoperative LCN deficits is associated with a better prognosis due to previous adaptation to the dysfunction. De novo LCN deficits may be catastrophic if not addressed intensively. New permanent motor deficits are not common. However, temporary exacerbation of a previous deficit is frequent, but recovery is the rule.

Despite the recent advances in technology and modern microsurgery techniques, surgical resection of foramen magnum meningiomas remains a challenge for neurosurgeons. The origin and the pattern of growth are the main points predicting a safe resection of the mass. An extensive skull base approach may be helpful but is not essential in all patients with foramen magnum meningiomas. The management of these tumors should be tailored to each patient to adopt the best and safest way to remove the tumor avoiding surgical morbidity (Fig. 49-4).

Even the less invasive approaches can have serious morbidity. Miller and Crockard,[24] using transoral transclival approaches, and Goel et al.,[18] using endoscopic removal,

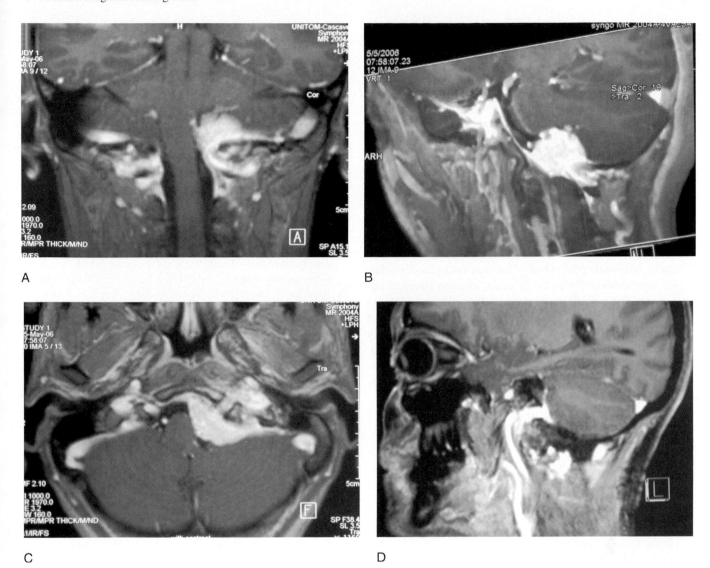

A

B

C

D

FIG. 49-4. A 45-year-old female with a history of neck pain, hemiparesis, and hemiatrophy of the tongue. (A, B) The T1-Weight MRI images with contrast depict a tumor with invasion of the hypoglossal canal and jugular foramen. A partial removal was planned to avoid additional cranial nerve deficit (C, D)

reported that the difficulty of repairing the dura to avoid a CSF leak is the main concern with these approaches.

Personal Results

Total removal of the tumor was achieved in 9 patients, subtotal in 2, and partial resection in 1 patient. The first patient with subtotal removal was a 53-year-old female with an en plaque meningioma which extended extradurally, invading the bone of the occipital condyle and expanding intradurally en plaque to the jugular foramen. Her only preoperative symptom was occipital neuralgia. Dural enhancement surrounding the occipital condyle was not removed to avoid severe instability in an oligosymptomatic patient. An MRI after a 3-year follow-up demonstrated a decrease of contrast enhancement and no

tumor regrowth. The second patient was a 47-year-old male with a diffuse meningioma attached anteriorly and extending posteriorly. The dura of the inferior clivus was not removed, and the tumor progressively regrew, invading the foramina of the cranial nerves and compressing the medulla. The patient died of respiratory complications 4 years later. The case of partial removal involved a patient with an invasion of the jugular foramen without any symptoms of cranial nerve deficits. In this case we preferred to leave some residual tumor to avoid LCN deficits. At a short follow-up of 8 months, it did not show any signs of regrowth.

The occipital condyle was partially removed in 7 patients. In these cases, the tumor growth occurred from the clivus to the spinal canal with its main attachment point located in the lower clivus and in the anterior border of the foramen magnum, and the tumors were classified as clivospinal tumors. In

5 patients, partial removal of the condyle was not necessary because the main point of attachment was located inferior to the anterior or anterolateral border of the foramen magnum. In this situation a clear plane between the tumor and the surrounding neurovascular structures provided by an arachnoid layer from the spinal canal to the clivus was found. These tumors were classified as spinoclival tumors.

Postoperative complications occurred in 2 patients. The first was a 42-year-old female with a large clivospinal tumor with invasion of the hypoglossal canal. During the preoperative period we decided to resect the tumor in the canal to assure a radical removal. During the postoperative period a transitory bilateral palsy of the IX, X, and XII cranial nerves were found. After intense therapy, the swallowing dysfunction improved dramatically and dysphonia improved after 3 months. The same patient had a CSF leak and hydrocephalus, which were managed with the insertion of a ventriculoperitoneal shunt. The second case was a 63-year-old male with an anterior spinocranial tumor with severe myelopathy who had a slight worsening of motor deficit at early follow-up, but with dramatic improvement after 6 months of follow-up. The preoperative deficits improved in all patients within a short follow-up period. The most dramatic recovery was from a motor weakness. There was no surgical mortality in this series.

References

1. Boulton MR, Cusimano, MD: Foramen magnum meningiomas: concepts, classifications, and nuances. Neurosurg Focus 2003;14(6):Article 10.
2. Cushing H Eisenhardt L: Meningiomas: Their Classification, Regional Behavior, Life History, and Surgical End Results. Springfield, IL: Charles C Thomas, 1938.
3. Yasargil MG, Mortara RW, Curcic M: Meningiomas of the basal posterior fossa. Adv Tech Stand Neurosurg 1980;7:1–115.
4. George B: Meningiomas of the foramen magnum. In: Schimidek III (ed): Meningiomas and their surgical management. Philadelphia: W.B. Saunders, 1991:459–70.
5. George B, Lot G, Boissonet H. Meningioma of the foramen magnum: A series of 40 cases. Surg Neurol 1997;47:371–79.
6. Meyer FB, Ebersold MJ, Reese DF: Benign tumors of the foramen magnum. J Neurosurg 1984;61(1):136–42.
7. Stein BM, Leeds NE, Taveras JM, Pool JL: Meningiomas of the foramen magnum. J Neurosurg 1963;20:740–51.
8. Sawaya RA: Foramen magnum meningioma presenting as amyotrophic lateral sclerosis. Neurosurg Rev 1998;21(4):277–80.
9. Arnautovic KI, Al-Mefty O, Husain M: Ventral foramen magnum J Neurosurg 2000;92(Suppl 1):71–80.
10. Bertalanffy H, Seeger W: The dorsolateral, suboccipital, transcondylar approach to the lower clivus and anterior portion of the craniocervical junction. Neurosurgery 1991;29(6):815–21.
11. Menezes AH, Traynelis VC, Fenoy AJ, et al.: Honored guest presentation: surgery at the crossroads: craniocervical neoplasms. Clin Neurosurg 2005;52:218–28.
12. Sekhar LN, Wrught DC, Richardson R, Monacci W: Petroclival and foramen magnum meningiomas: surgical approaches and pitfalls. J Neurooncol 1996;29:249–59.
13. Baldwin HZ, Miller CG, van Loveren HR, et al: The far lateral/combined supra- and infratentorial approach. A human cadaveric prosection model for routes of access to the petroclival region and ventral brain stem. J Neurosurg 1994;81(1):60–8.
14. Spektor S, Anderson GJ, McMenomey SO, et al: Quantitative description of the far-lateral transcondylar transtubercular approach to the foramen magnum and clivus. J Neurosurg 1963;20:740–51.
15. Suhardja A, Agur AM, Cusimano MD: Anatomical basis of approaches to foramen magnum and lower clival meningiomas: comparison of retrosigmoid and transcondylar approaches. Neurosurg Focus 2003;15;14(6):e9.
16. Wen HT, Rhoton AL Jr, Katsuta T, de Oliveira E: Microsurgical anatomy of the transcondylar, supracondylar and paracondylar extensions of the far lateral approach. J Neurosurg 1997;87:555–85.
17. Babu RP, Sekhar LN, Wright DC: Extreme lateral transcondylar approach: technical improvement and lessons learned. J Neurosurg 1994;81:49–59.
18. Goel A, Desai K, Mazumdar D. Surgery on anterior foramen magnum meningiomas using a conventional posterior suboccipital approach: a report on an experience with 17 cases. Neurosurgery 2001;49:102–7.
19. Kratimenos GP, Crockard HA: The far lateral approach for ventrally placed foramen magnum and upper cervical spine tumours Br J Neurosurg 1993;7(2):129–40.
20. Sen CN, Sekhar LN. An extreme lateral approach to intradural lesions of the cervical spine and foramen magnum. Neurosurgery 1990;27:197–207.
21. David CA, Spetzler RF: Foramen magnum meningiomas. Clin Neurosurg 1997;44:467–89.
22. Margalit NS, Lesser JB, Singer M, Sen C: Lateral approach to anterolateral tumors at the foramen magnum: Factors determining surgical procedure. Neurosurgery 2005;56(2):324–36.
23. Samii M, Klekamp J, Carvalho G: Surgical results for meningiomas of the craniovertebral junction. Neurosurgery 1996;39:1086–95.
24. Miller E, Crockard HA: Transoral transclival removal of anteriorly placed meningiomas at the foramen magnum. Neurosurgery 1987;20(6):966–8.

50
Cerebellar Convexity Meningiomas

Roberto Delfini, Antonio Santoro, and Angelo Pichierri

Introduction

Cerebellar convexity (CC) meningiomas are rare. A small number of series reported in the literature are often included in the wider coverage of posterior fossa meningiomas, and therefore, an accurate metanalysis is not possible. Nevertheless, it may be assumed that they account is not possible for 8.5–18% of the posterior fossa meningiomas and represent about 1.5% of all meningiomas.[1–22]

Classification

In 1938, Cushing and Eisenhard published their surgical series of meningiomas in which they describe the pathology in detail.[3] In this book they also proposed the first classification of posterior fossa (PF) meningiomas. They encountered only three cases of pure CC meningiomas (about 1% of their entire series). In 1953, Castellano and Ruggiero categorized PF tumors into five groups: cerebellar convexity, tentorium, posterior petrous, clivus, and foramen magnum.[3] Subsequently, different nomenclatures have been proposed by several authors,[13,20,23–27] particularly regarding lesions of clivus, medial tentorium, and petrous bone. The most important and recent work on cerebellar convexity meningiomas was carried out in 1991 by Kobayashi and Nakamura, who wrote a comprehensive chapter on the topic in the book *Meningiomas* by Al-Mefty.[9]

Traditionally, cerebellar convexity meningiomas have been categorized according to their location into three types: medial, lateral, and superior.[9] However, taking into consideration anatomic criteria, we prefer to classify these meningiomas into four groups.[7,19,22]

Group A: Pure convexity meningiomas arising from the dura over the posterior convexity of the cerebellum. As mentioned above, Cushing and Eisenhard encountered only three cases of meningioma without attachments to the tentorium or the sinuses (Figs. 50-1 to 50-3).

Group B: Inferior peritorcular meningiomas arising from or invading the inferior wall of the torcular Herophili or the medial transverse sinus (Fig. 50-4).

Group C: Parasinusal meningiomas arising in the angle beween the petrous and convexity dura. These tumors may include the wall of the sigmoid and lateral transverse sinuses. The major part of cerebellar convexity meningiomas belongs to this subgroup (Fig. 50-5).

Group D: Meningiomas with secondary invasion of cerebellar convexity/fossa. This is the case of the rare intraosseus meningiomas of the posterior fossa[22] and of other posterior fossa meningiomas with a consistent dural attachment in the cerebellar convexity (Fig. 50-6).

Clinical Features

There is no well-defined clinical pattern characterizing these lesions. Often the patient is asymptomatic until the tumor becomes large enough to cause signs and symptoms of increased intracranial pressure and hydrocephalus.[9,14] Sometimes the patient may present with headache or progressive cerebellar dysfunction ipsilateral to the tumor.[9,14]

An elevation of intracranial venous pressure may occur in case of dural sinus invasion, expecially in the peritorcular meningiomas. For this reason, a small tumor growing inwardly into a sinus can cause early florid clinical symptoms.[7]

The clinical picture can be devious and mistaken for one of the more familiar diseases, particularly when false localizing signs occur. In the latter case, diplopia, trigeminal neuralgia, facial nerve palsy, hearing disturbance, tinnitus on the contralateral side, lower cranial nerve signs, truncal ataxia, and even bulbar palsy have all been reported and were attributed to the brain stem compression or to the cranial nerves stretching at the edges of dural orifices of the posterior fossa.[9,28,29,30,31]

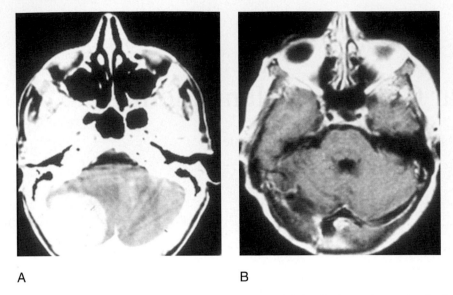

FIG. 50-1. A 72-year-old woman presenting with a long-standing occipital cephalgia, dizziness, dysmetria, dysdiadochokinesis, and dysgraphia. Two days before admission, two episodes of emesis occurred. (A) CT scan revealed a group A right cerebellar meningioma. The patient underwent a right suboccipital craniotomy. (B) One-month follow-up MRI showing the total extirpation of the lesion

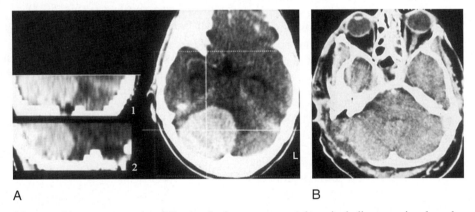

FIG. 50-2. A 70-year-old man with an acute and rapidly developing symptomatology including emesis, slurred speech, and progressive disturbances of consciousness leading to coma. (A) A preoperative CT scan with coronal (1) and sagittal (2) reconstructions showed a group A right cerebellar meningioma. The patient underwent an emergency surgery. (B) Postoperative CT scan showing the craniectomy and the total removal of the lesion

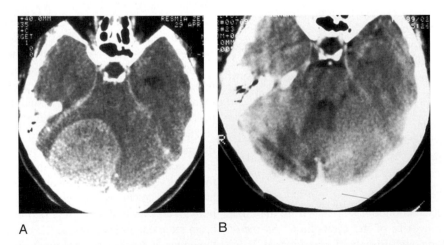

FIG. 50-3. A 43-year-old woman with a long-standing dizziness, subjective vertigo, nystagmus, and cerebellar ataxia. One month before presentation, progressive dysgraphia and slurred speech started. During the week before admission, she had five episodes of emesis. (A) Preoperative CT scan showing a group A right cerebellar meningioma. The patient underwent a right suboccipital craniotomy. (B) A postoperative CT scan shows the results of the operation

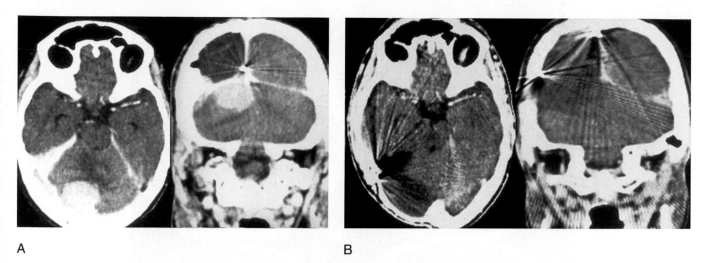

A   B

Fig. 50-4. A 58-year-old man previously operated on for a supratentorial meningioma presented to our department 19 years later with ceph-algia, cerebellar ataxia, dizziness, dysdiadochokinesis, and subjective vertigo. (A) CT scan with coronal reconstructions showing a group B cerebellar meningioma arising from the cerebellar convexity and involving the medial half of the transverse sinus until its confluence into the torcular Herophili. The patient underwent a right suboccipital craniotomy, and an intraoperative occlusion test of transverse sinus was performed. As the test was well tolerated, the sinus was closed and removed together with the meningioma. (B) Postoperative CT scan show-ing the results of the operation

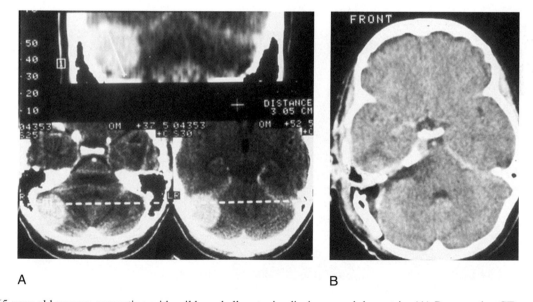

A   B

Fig. 50-5. A 65-year-old woman presenting with mild cerebellar ataxia, dizziness, and dysmetria. (A) Preoperative CT scan with coronal reconstructions shows a group C right cerebellar meningioma arising from the angle between the petrous bone and convexity dura. The patient underwent the extirpation of the lesion via a retrosigmoid approach. (B) Early postoperative CT scan showing the craniotomy and the results of the intervention

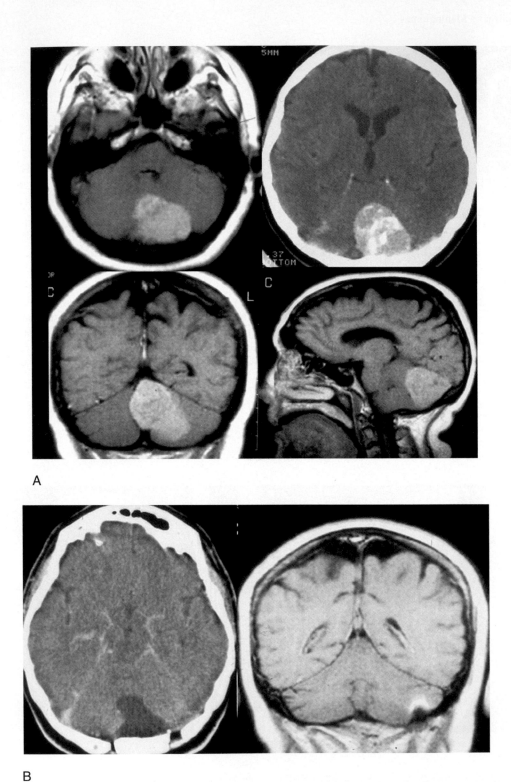

FIG. 50-6. A 77-year-old woman with cephalgia, cerebellar ataxia, dysmetria, and explosive voice. (A) Preoperative imaging (CT and MRI) showing a group D cerebellar meningioma. The dural attachment of the lesion was upon the cerebellar convexity and, with a minor component, on the inferior surface of the cerebellar tentorium. The lesion was removed via a midline suboccipital approach and peeling of the lesion from the torcular Herophili was performed. Afterwards, the dural base was coagulated. (B) Postoperative imaging (CT and MRI) showing the results of the intervention

Eventually, these meningiomas are often discovered incidentally on imaging study done for other reasons.

Imaging Characteristics

The neuroradiologic appearance of these lesions does not differ from other meningiomas. Magnetic resonance imaging (MRI) gives the most useful information, such as the location of the tumor and its possible attachment to the tentorium.[9,14,19]

Recently, in cases in which a study of venous sinus status is needed, the increased accuracy of combined contrast-enhanced and phase-contrast MR venography has reduced the diagnostic gap with the angiography.[32] However, angiography is still the gold standard procedure, which allows: (1) a precise examination of the sinuses; (2) an assessment of tolerance of sinus obliteration by means of a direct endovascular cannulation and subsequent balloon occlution test;[7] and (3) a therapeutic embolization of the major feeding vessels of the tumor.[20] In most cases, branches of external carotid artery or the posterior meningeal branch of the vertebral artery are seen to feed the tumor.[9,33] In the group A lesions, embolization may not be necessary as the blood supply comes straight through the convexity dura.[14]

Surgical Considerations

Surgery is indicated when the patient has neurologic symptoms.[19] An adequate head position is important to keep intracranial venous pressure relatively low (between 0 and 15mmHg).[9] The head is positioned higher than the heart, tilting the cranial half of the operating table about 30 to 45 degrees.[9]

Group A meningiomas can be approached with the patient in the prone position and with the head slightly flexed. A linear or a reverse U-shaped skin incision can be used.[9] The incision is carried through all layers of the scalp and pericranium, which are then elevated and held retracted over a rolled sponge.[7] The craniotomy can be uni- or bilateral according to the location of the tumor and of the invasion of the occipital sinus that can be sacrified. Removal is accomplished by a repetitive series of internal debulking and extracapsular microdissection. A careful dissection of the tumor from the surrounding cerebellar cortex and cortical vesels is needed to avoid damage of the vermian branch of the posterior inferior cerebellar artery and of cerebellar venous drainage, which can cause postoperative cerebellar strokes or edema.[9]

Group B meningiomas can be approached with the patient in prone position. In cases with secondary supratentorial invasion, the Concorde position may be useful for performing a combined suboccipital/transtentorial/occipital approach.[7,9] The skin incision varies according the number of peritorcular quadrants containing tumor. After suboccipital craniotomy, a piecemeal rongeuring of bone is the safest method of dural

exposure.[7] Infiltrated or hyperostotic bone should be removed and discarded. This pathologically modified bone greatly increases the risk of unroofing a venous sinus.[7]

Sindou proposed six types of invasion of intracranial venous sinus walls. We can use this classification for transverse sinus and torcular Herophili invasion distinguishing four situations:[34]

Type I: attachment to outer surface. Often the tumor merely abuts or is attached to the sinus by arachnoidal adhesions. In these cases a layer of dural attachment over the sinus can often be peeled off.[19]

Type II: lateral recess invaded. A resection of intraluminal fragment is possible. The defect is then repaired, resuturing the sinus wall (8.0 monofilament suture) or reconstructing it with dural clips. The sinus should be opened and closed sequentially and in small portions as the tumor is progressively removed.[7]

Type III: lateral wall invaded. If the surgeon decides for a gross total removal of the lesion, the consequent sinus defect should be repaired with an autologous or heterologous patch graft.

Type IV to VI: massive invasions with entire lateral wall and roof invaded. A reconstruction is possible either with patches or with a venous bypass. In our experience, these procedures are much more hazardous. In fact, the surgical procedure in itself becomes more complex for the patient positioning (the semi-sitting position has been advocated in these cases), due to consequent risks of air embolism, and to the more extensive operative exposure required (3cm all along the margins of the involved sinus). The results of an aggressive treatment of meningiomas invading torcular or transverse sinuses (reconstruction with bypass, wide sinus wall resections) shows a mortality of 3.6%.[34] On the other hand, even when these specific meningiomas are subtotally removed, a very low rate of recurrences is observed.[9,19,20] Therefore, we think that it is preferable to leave a small portion of the tumor behind and either treat the residue with radiosurgery or follow the tumor growth over time.[7,9,18,35]

The dural attachment to the sinus surface or the residual fragment should always be coagulated with bipolar cautery, regardless of the degree of sinus invasion described above.[7]

Group C meningiomas are usually separated from the cranial nerves by cerebellar tissue, but in very large tumors there may be only a thin layer of arachnoid.[9,19] In this type of tumor, the same approach can be used as described for cerebellopontine angle tumors with patient in 3/4 prone position with rotation of the head. An Italic S-shaped skin incision made in the retroauricular region allows a wide view of occipital bone and asterion. Subsequently, a suboccipital craniotomy or craniectomy can be used to access the retrosigmoid region. The lateral limit of bone aperture should be far enough to allow adequate tumor exposure.[9]

Sindou classification and the above-mentioned pitfalls may be used also in this group to manage the contingent sinus invasion. If the tumor invades a nondominant transverse (at preoperative radiologic imaging right sinuses are often dominant) or sigmoid sinus with a good tolerance to the occlusion tests or if, in the minority of cases, the sinus is almost completely occluded, it may be sacrificed.[9,19,27,36] On the contrary, a reconstruction is needed if the sinus cannot be resected. Interruption of a transverse sinus should be medial to the junction of the vein of Labbé and the transverse sinus.[7] Closure is begun only after the integrity of the sinuses is confirmed during a Valsalva maneuver.[7]

Group D meningiomas should be treated according to the prevalent site of origin of the meningioma.

The use of electroneurophysiology (somatosensory evoked potential, auditory brain stem response) are useful for monitoring brain stem function.[9] Dural reconstruction can be performed by using a heterologous dural patch graft (e.g., bovine pericardium). Relief of neurologic manifestations and the prevention of further tumor growth are the goals of surgical treatment.[7]

Results

With the advent of microsurgical techniques, the results have generally been good to excellent, with good outcome and no recurrence even in the cases of subtotal resection due to sinus invasion.[9,19,20] The eventuality of a catastrophic outcome is solely dependent on mismanagement of the dural sinuses. Failure to repair a sinus or closure of a previously patent sinus are often life-threatening and, in other cases, accompanied by severe neurologic deficits.[7]

Incomplete removal or recurrence can be treated by reoperation if tumor regrowth becomes symptomatic. In these cases, some authors have also proposed radiation as an efficent alternative treatment, but further studies are needed to set the role of stereotactic radiosurgery or fractionated radiation therapy (in cases of extensive dural spread). However, recent reports suggest that radiosurgery seems to be an effective adjuvant modality treatment for World Health Organization (WHO) grade I lesions with subtotal or partial removal. A combined radiosurgery treatment associated with fractionated irradiation for the far less common WHO grade II/grade III residual or recurrent tumors may also be considered.[18]

Our Experience

Between 1990 and 2005, we encountered 37 cases of cerebellar convexity meningiomas. The main data for these patients are summarized below:

Location	Cases	Excision	Outcome	Complications	Reccurrence
Group A	4	Total	Good	No	No
Group B	9	Total (7)	Good	No	1 case treated with radiosurgery
		Subtotal (2)			
Group C	16	Total (13)	Good	No	No
		Subtotal (3)			
Group D	8	Total (7)	Good	No	1 case reoperated after 8 years
		Subtotal (1)			

References

1. Campbell E, Whitfield RD. Posterior fossa meningiojmas. J Neurosurg 1948;5:131–53.
2. Castellano F, Ruggiero G. Meningiomas of the posterior fossa. ACTA Radiol (Suppl) 1953;104:1–117.
3. Cushing HW, Eisenhardt L. Meningiomas: their classification, regional behavior, life history and surgical results. Springfield, ILs: Charles C Thomas, 1938.
4. D'Errico A. Meningiomas of the cerebellar fossa. J Neurosurg 1950;7:227–32.
5. Grand W, Bakay L. Posterior fossa meningiomas. A report of 30 cases. ACTA Neurochir (Vienna) 1975;32:219–233.
6. Grigoryan YA, Onopchenko CV. Persistent trigeminal neuralgia after removal of controlateral posterior cranial fossa tumor. Report of two cases. Surg Neurol 1999;52:56–61.
7. Harsh IV GR. Torcular and peritorcular meningiomas. In Neurosurgical operative atlas. Setti S. Rengachary 2000;5(1):13–21.
8. Hubschmann OR, Krieger AJ. Posterior fossa meningiomas. NJ Med 1987;84:185–9.
9. Kobayashi S, Nakamura Y. Cerebellar convexity meningiomas. In Al-Mefty O, ed. Meningiomas. New York: Raven Press, 1991:495–501.
10. Landeiro. Posterior fossa craniotomy. Arq Neuropsiquiatr 2000;58(1):169–73.
11. MacCarty CS, Taylor WF. Intracranial meningiomas: experiences at Mayo Clinic. Neurol Med Chir (Tokyo) 1979;19:569–74.
12. Markham JW, Fager CA, Horrax G, Poppen JL. Meningioomas of the posterior fossa. Their diagnosis, clinical features and surgical treatment. AMA Arch Neurol Psychiatr 1955;74:163–170.
13. Martinez R, Vaquero J, Areitio E et al. Meningiomas of the posterior fossa. Surg Neurol 1983;19:237–43.
14. McDermott MW, Wulson CB. Meningiomas. In: Youmans JR, ed. Neurological Surgery, 4th ed. Philadelphia: WB Saunders, 1996:2782–825.
15. McKinney PA, Beale MD, Kellner CH. Electroconvulsive therapy in a patient with a cerebellar meningioma. J ECT 1998;14(1):49–52.
16. Mirimanoff RO, Dosoretz DE, Linggod RM, et al. Meningioma: analysis of recurrence and progression following neurosurgical resection. J Neurosurg 1985;62:18–24.
17. Nagano T, Saiki I, Kanaya H. Multiple meningiomas in the posterior fossa. Surg Neurol 1985;23:425–7.
18. Nicolato A, Foroni R, Pellegrino M, et al. Gamma Knife radiosurgery in meningiomas of the posterior fossa: experience with 62 treated lesions. Minim Invasive Neurosurg 2001;44:211–217.
19. Ojemann RG. Cerebellar convexity meningioma. Clin Neurosurg 1992;40(17):321–383.
20. Roberti F, Sekhar LN. Posterior fossa meningiomas: surgical experience in 161 cases. Surg Neurol 2001;56:8–21.
21. Russel JR, Bucy PC. Meningiomas of the posterior fossa. Surg Neurol 1953;23:183–92.
22. Yamazaki T, Tsukada A, Uemura K, et al. Intraosseous meningioma of the posterior fossa. Neurol Med Chir (Tokyo) 2001;41:149–153.
23. Cudlip SA, Wilkins PR, Johnston FG, et al. Posterior fossa meningiomas: surgical experience in 52 cases. Acta Neurochir (Wien) 1998;140:1007–1012.
24. Mayberg MR, Symon L. Meningiomas of the clivus and apical petrous bone. Report of 35 cases. J Neurosurg 1986;65: 136–42

25. Sekhar LN, Wright DC, Richardson R, Monacci W. Petroclival and foramen magnum meningiomas: Surgical approach and pitfalls. J Neuro Oncol 1996;29:249–59.

26. Spallone A, Makhmudov UB, Mukhamedjanov DJ, Tcherekajev VA. An attempt to define the role of skull base approaches in their surgical management. Surg Neurol 1999;51:412–20.

27. Yasargil MG, Mortora RW, Curcic M. Meningiomas of basal posterior cranial fossa. In: Krayenbuhl H et al., eds. Advances and Technical Standard in Neurosurgery. Vienna: Springer-Verlag, 1980:3–115.

28. Kumar A, Mafee M, Torok N. Anatomic specificity of central vestibular signs in posterior fossa lesions. Ann Otol Rhinol Laryngol 1982;91:510–5.

29. Nagahiro S, Matsukado Y, Uemura S. Posterior fossa meningioma with special reference to false localizing sign. Neurol Med Chir (Tokyo) 1998;22:421–8.

30. O'Connel JEA. Trigeminal false localizing signs and their causation. Brain 1978;101:119–142.

31. Shenoy SN, Raja A. Acute aspiration pneumonia due to bulbar palsy: an initial manifestation of posterior fossa convexity meningioma. J Neurol Neurosurg Psychiatry 2005;76:296–8.

32. Bozzao A, Finocchi V, Romano A, et al. Role of contrast-enhanced MR venography in the preoperative evaluation of parasagittal meningiomas. Eur Radiol 2005;15:1790–6.

33. Salamon GM, Combalbert A, Raybaud C, Gonzalez J. An angiographic study of meningiomas of the posterior fossa. J Neurosurg 1971;35:731–41.

34. Sindou M. Meningiomas invading the sagittal or transverse sinuses, resection with venous reconstruction. J Clin Neurosci 2001;8(Suppl 1):8–11.

35. Chang JH, Chang JW, Choi JY, et al. Complications after gamma knife radiosurgery for benign meningiomas. J Neurol Neurosurg Psychiatry 2003;74:226–30.

36. Scott M. The surgical management of meningiomas of the cerebellar fossa. Surg Gynecol Obstet 1972;135:545–50.

51
Tentorial Meningiomas

Khaled A. Aziz, Sebastien C. Froelich, Philip Theodosopoulos, and John M. Tew, Jr.

Introduction

Tentorial meningiomas account for 2–6% of all intracranial meningiomas.[1] Tentorial meningiomas can arise from the lateral and posterior portion of the tentorium near or adjacent to the major venous sinuses or from the medial portion (i.e., tentorial incisura) near or adjacent to critical neurovascular structures. Three-dimensional understanding of the radiographic pathoanatomy of tentorial meningiomas is required to design the appropriate surgical approaches. Anatomic and radiologic features important in classification and selection of the appropriate surgical approach for treatment are reviewed.

Anatomic Considerations

Dura

The dura is composed of a periosteal layer that faces the bone and a meningeal layer (dura propria) that faces the brain. The meningeal dura propria folds inward to form the falx cerebri, tentorium cerebelli, falx cerebelli, and diaphragm sellae. The tentorium is rigidly attached to the temporal and occipital bones. The lateral edge is attached to the petrous ridge, where it divides to form the superior petrosal sinus. The posterior edge is attached to the inner surface of the occipital bone; it divides along the internal occipital protuberance and the edges of the shallow osseous groove to form the torcular Herophili and transverse sinuses.

The tentorium cerebelli covers the cerebellum and forms a free dural edge around the brain stem called the tentorial incisura. The anterior end of each free edge is attached to the petrous apex and the anterior and posterior clinoid processes. The attachments to the petrous apex and clinoid processes form three dural folds: the anterior and posterior petroclinoid folds and the interclinoid fold. Between these folds is located the oculomotor trigone through which the oculomotor and trochlear nerves enter the cavernous sinus. The posterior petroclinoid fold extends from the petrous apex to the posterior clinoid process. The anterior petroclinoid fold extends from the petrous apex to the anterior clinoid process. The interclinoid fold covers the ligament extending from the anterior to the posterior clinoid process.

Tentorial Arterial Blood Supply

The falx cerebri, falx cerebelli, and tentorium are supplied by the basal and convexity branches of the meningeal arteries. By receiving contribution from branches of the cerebral arteries, the falx cerebri, falx cerebelli, and tentorium make an anastomotic pathway between the dural and parenchymal arteries. The tentorium receives supratentorial and infratentorial arterial contributions (Fig. 51-1). The supratentorial feeders are the medial and lateral tentorial branches of the cavernous segment of the internal carotid artery (ICA) medially, and branches of the middle meningeal artery anterolaterally, respectively. The infratentorial feeders are the most superior extensions of the jugular branch of the ascending pharyngeal artery; these feeders are occasionally the tentorial branch of the posterior cerebral artery medially, occipital artery laterally, and posterior meningeal artery posteriorly. The lateral two thirds of the tentorium and its edge along the transverse sinus are supplied primarily from the petrosal and occipital arcades. The petrosal (basal) arcade, which follows the superior petrosal sinus, is composed of the lateral tentorial artery, branches from the petrous and petrosquamosal trunk of the middle meningeal artery, and lateral branch of the dorsal meningeal artery. The occipital arcade is composed above the tentorium by the petrosquamosal trunk and occipital branches of the middle meningeal artery, and below the tentorium by the occipital and posterior meningeal arteries. The medial third of the tentorium is supplied by the medial (marginal) tentorial artery (i.e., artery of Bernasconi and Cassinari); this tentorial branch of the meningohypophyseal trunk also contributes to the supply of the dural segment of the oculomotor and trochlear nerves. This area may also infrequently receive a contribution from a dural branch of the posterior cerebral artery (i.e., artery of Schechter).[2]

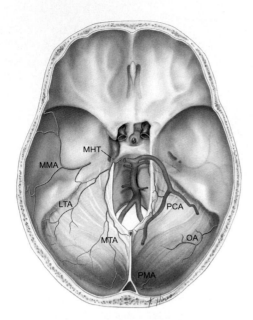

FIG. 51-1. Drawing of the arterial blood supply of the tentorium. Supratentorial feeders of the tentorium arise from the meningohypophyseal trunk (MHT), including the medial (Bernasconi and Cassinari) tentorial artery (MTA), lateral tentorial artery (LTA), branches of the middle meningeal artery (MMA), and branches of the posterior cerebral artery (PCA). Infratentorial feeders of the tentorium arise from branches of the ascending pharyngeal artery, branches of the occipital artery (OA), and posterior meningeal artery (PMA). (Courtesy of the Mayfield Clinic.)

The meningohypophyseal trunk gives rise to the medial and lateral tentorial arteries. The lateral tentorial artery, also known as the basal tentorial artery, commonly arises as a single trunk from the cavernous segment of the ICA. The lateral tentorial artery enters the tentorium along its attachment to the petrous ridge and supplies the tentorial area lateral to that supplied by the medial tentorial artery.[2]

Tentorial Venous Drainage

Understanding the venous anatomy of the tentorium is critical. Complications after the intraoperative sacrifice of veins in the posterior fossa have been reported. Cerebellar infarction or hemorrhage may result from division of the bridging veins between the superior surface of the cerebellum and the tentorium.[3,4] The terminal ends of numerous surface veins form these bridging veins. Therefore, sacrifice of those bridging veins is more hazardous than sacrifice of the veins on the surface of the cerebellum.

Hemispheric bridging veins more often occur in the medial (37.5%) or intermediate (37.5%) third of the cerebellar hemisphere than in the lateral third (25%).[5] Distance from the midline to the most medial hemispheric bridging vein averaged 22.1 mm. Distance between the two most medial (left and right) hemispheric bridging veins averaged 44.4 mm.[6] Although a single cerebellar bridging vein can be sacrificed because of its well-developed anastomoses, sacrifice of multiple bridging veins can lead to postoperative complications[3,4]

Four distinct complexes identified in the posterior temporal venous drainage include the lateral (Labbé) complex in 100%, anteroinferior complex in 70%, medial-inferior complex in 38%, and posteroinferior complex in 88%.[7] Veins enter the sinus as three basic geometric configurations: first, a candelabra of veins that unite to form one large draining vein; second, multiple independent draining veins; and third, venous lakes that run in the tentorium before entering the sinuses. A vein or veins that enter the tentorium cannot be assumed to be an insignificant temporal lobe vein because the vein(s) may be dominant, draining isolated portions of the temporal lobe. Sectioning the tentorium may result in sacrifice of the dependent venous drainage and may be, in part, responsible for observed cases of venous infarctions. Should a venous lake be identified, modification of the tentorial transsection to avoid sacrifice is recommended. The majority of draining venous complexes (90%) enters the tentorium 1.5–2.0 cm from the sigmoid-transverse-superior petrosal junction.[7]

Dural sinuses are formed between the outer wall periosteal dura and inner wall dura propria, except for the straight sinus that is only formed by the dura propria. The torcular Herophili (confluence of sinuses) is formed by the union of the superior sagittal sinus, straight sinus, and transverse sinuses. The

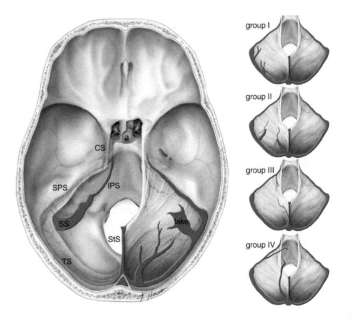

FIG. 51-2. Drawing of the venous sinuses of the tentorium shows classification into four groups according to their drainage pattern. Group I (69%): sinuses receive bridging veins from the cerebral hemispheres draining into the superior surface of the tentorium. Group II (89%): sinuses receive bridging veins from cerebellar hemispheric and vermian veins into the inferior surface of the tentorium. Group III (42%): many small veins form small sinuses. Group IV (8%): rare type formed by veins, which can be major venous drainage, running through the tentorial edge to form a tentorial sinus. CS, cavernous sinus; SPS, superior petrosal sinus; IPS, inferior petrosal sinus; SS, sigmoid sinus; TS, transverse sinus; StS, straight sinus. (Courtesy of the Mayfield Clinic.)

torcular is usually asymmetric and shows multiple variations in its tributaries[8]. This asymmetry is detectable in preoperative magnetic resonance venography (MRV) or venogram; detection of this feature is vital in tentorial meningiomas, especially with sinus invasion.

Tentorial venous (sinuses) lakes are venous channels formed between the leaflets of the tentorium more than 1 cm away from the entry into the transverse sinus where one or more veins from various venous complexes converge. Veins draining into the tentorium cannot be assumed to be insignificant because they may represent a dominant venous drainage.[5,7] Tentorial sinuses have been dissected and explored in cadavers.[5] These sinuses can be demonstrated in MRV with contrast and in the venous phase of cerebral angiography. Tentorial sinuses are classified into four groups according to their drainage pattern[5] (Fig. 51-2).

Nerovascular Relationships

The region of the medial tentorial free edge (incisura) has been classified as anterior, middle, and posterior spaces.[9] The anterior incisural space, which is located anterior to the midbrain and pons, extends above the optic chiasm to the lamina terminalis, and below the chiasm and third ventricular floor to the interpeduncular fossa. In addition to the optic tract, the anterior space contains the third and fourth cranial nerves that enter the roof of the cavernous sinus, crural cistern, medial temporal lobe and uncus, and lateral surface of the midbrain. The anterior incisural space contains the posterior communicating artery (PCoA), anterior choroidal artery, and basilar bifurcation. The medial posterior choroidal artery arises from the proximal part of the posterior cerebral artery (PCA) in the anterior incisural space; it courses parallel and medial to the PCA through the middle incisural space to reach the posterior incisural space. The PCA and superior cerebellar artery (SCA) arise in the anterior space and pass around the brain stem to reach the middle and posterior incisural spaces. The main vein of the anterior incisural space is the basal vein of Rosenthal. This vein originates below the anterior perforated substance, courses posterolaterally around the cerebral peduncle, and continues below the optic tract and medial to the uncus. The basal vein courses through the anterior, middle, and posterior incisural spaces and finally empties into the vein of Galen.

The middle incisural space is located superiorly between the temporal lobe (medial to the temporal horn) and midbrain, and is located inferiorly between the cerebellum and upper brain stem. It contains the trochlear and trigeminal cranial nerves, crural and ambient cisterns, anterior choroidal artery, PCA, and SCA. The anterior choroidal artery enters the middle incisural space below the optic tract and passes through the choroidal fissure near the inferior choroidal point to supply the chord plexus in the temporal horn. The PCA enters the middle incisural space between the cerebral peduncle and uncus to give off several cortical branches that cross the free edge to reach the inferior surface of the temporal and occipital lobes. These branches include the lateral posterior choroidal and thalamogeniculate arteries that course medial to the free edge. The lateral posterior choroidal arteries course superolaterally through the choroidal fissure and around the pulvinar to reach the choroid plexus in the temporal horn and atrium. The basal vein of Rosenthal courses along the upper part of the cerebral peduncle below the pulvinar to reach the posterior incisural space; this vein may rarely terminate in a tentorial sinus (lake) in the free edge at this level (Type IV).

The posterior incisural space is located between the posterior midbrain and tentorial edge. This space corresponds to the pineal region with the quadrigeminal plate at the center. The quadrigeminal cistern is situated posterior to the quadrigeminal plate. As the major cistern in the posterior incisural space, it communicates superiorly with the posterior pericallosal cistern, inferiorly with the cerebellomesencephalic fissure, and inferolaterally with the posterior part of the ambient cistern located between the midbrain and the parahippocampal gyrus. Occasionally, the quadrigeminal cistern communicates with the velum interpositum—a space that extends forward into the third ventricular roof between the splenium and pineal gland. The trunks and branches of the PCA and SCA course into the posterior incisural space. The PCA bifurcates into the calcarine and parieto-occipital arteries near where it crosses above the free edge. The medial posterior choroidal arteries enter the posterior incisural space and enter the velum interpositum to supply the choroid plexus in the third ventricular roof and lateral ventricular body. As the lateral posterior choroidal artery passes around the posteromedial surface of the pulvinar, it gives branches to the thalamus along the way and then passes through the choroidal fissure to supply the choroid plexus in the atrium. The posterior incisural space has the most complex venous structures in the human brain. The internal cerebral and basal veins with their tributaries converge on the vein of Galen, which passes below the splenium to enter the straight sinus at the tentorial apex.

Radiologic Considerations

Diagnostic studies are essential for selection of the surgical approach and are the most critical aspect of operative planning for tentorial meningiomas. A thorough interpretation of magnetic resonance imaging (MRI), MRV, angiography, and venography is critical. MRI provides anatomic localization of the tumor, including dural origin, extent of growth above and below the tentorium, and relationship to the surrounding neurovascular structures. MRI will also show any brain stem infiltration in cases of incisural types. T1- and T2-weighted signal changes are diagnostic for invasion of the brain stem pia matter.[10,11] Assessment of the extent of edema surrounding the tumor is important because it may indicate impairment of venous drainage or aggressive tumor pathology. An angiogram helps in identification of the tumor's blood supply and displacement of major arteries. Preoperative arterial embolization of the external carotid blood supply and tentorial branches of the cavernous segment of the ICA may be helpful in reducing intraoperative blood loss.[12] Venogram and/or MRV will allow the surgeon to assess dominance of venous sinuses, patency of the dural sinuses, identification of tentorial sinuses if possible, and evaluation of the posterior temporal lobe drainage.

Classification and Surgical Approach

Tentorial meningiomas are classified on the basis of the site of tentorial attachment.[13,14] Our classification, which is based on the surgical approach for each tentorial location, divides tentorial meningiomas into the anterior, middle, and posterior groups (Fig. 51-3 and Table 51-1).

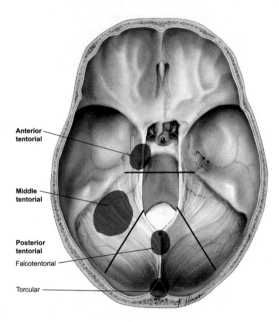

FIG. 51-3. Our classification of tentorial meningiomas is based on the surgical approach for each tentorial region. This classification divides tentorial meningiomas into the anterior, middle, and posterior groups. (Courtesy of the Mayfield Clinic.)

TABLE 51-1. Distribution of Lesions According to our Proposed Classification with the Surgical Approach Used.

Type	Subtype	Surgical approach
Anterior	Incisural	Pterional, frontotemporal orbitozygomatic
Middle	Supratentorial	Subtemporal
	Infratentorial	Lateral suboccipital
Posterior	Supratentorial	Occipital transtentorial
	Infratentorial	Supracerebellar infratentorial
	Torcular	Combined occipital transtentorial and supracerebellar infratentorial

Source: Courtesy of the Mayfield Clinic.

Anterior Tentorial Meningiomas

Anterior tentorial meningiomas (Yasargil T1) are approached using a frontotemporal craniotomy (pterional approach) (Fig. 51-4). The patient is placed in the supine position with the head rotated 30 degrees so that the zygoma is the highest point in the surgical field. Addition of an orbitozygomatic osteotomy minimizes brain retraction and facilitates the line of sight to the anterior incisural space. Anterior clinoidectomy and optic foraminotomy are performed based on the tumor extension. Extradural mobilization of the lateral wall of the cavernous sinus is added in cases where tumors extend into the cavernous sinus. The optic and carotid cisterns are opened, followed by opening of the sylvian fissure from the proximal to distal direction. The tumor is identified within the carotid-oculomotor window. The oculomotor and trochlear nerves are usually stretched in the superiolateral aspect of the tumor's capsule. The tumor is approached from the lateral to medial direction; the tentorium and tumor capsule are cauterized. Debulking starts within the carotid-oculomotor window between the oculomotor and trochlear nerves.[15] The trigeminal nerve might be displaced posteriorly. Bleeding from the posterior cavernous sinus is controlled with small pieces of Oxycel. Tumor extension into the cavernous sinus is not aggressively chased. Rather it is treated postoperatively with focused-beam radiation therapy.

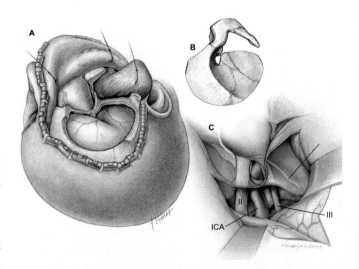

FIG. 51-4. Frontotemporal approach to an anterior incisural meningioma. (A, B) A one-piece frontotemporal orbitozygomatic craniotomy is performed. (C) After an anterior clinoidectomy and optic foraminotomy are performed, the optic and carotid cisterns are open followed by opening the sylvian fissure. The tumor is identified within the carotid-oculomotor window. This approach allows working channels in the carotid-oculomotor window and window between cranial nerves III through V. ICA, internal carotid artery; II, optic nerve; III, oculomotor nerve; IV, trochlear nerve. (From Ref. 16.)

Middle Tentorial Meningiomas

Middle tentorial meningiomas are divided into infratentorial and supratentorial tumors.[14] Supratentorial tumors are approached using a subtemporal craniotomy with zygomatic osteotomy (Fig. 51-5). The patient is placed in the lateral position with the superior sagittal sinus parallel to the floor; the head is tilted down 15 degrees to achieve gravity retraction. Anterior petrosectomy can be added for better control of the infratentorial portion of the tumor.[16] Devascularization of the tumor is achieved with extradural control of the middle meningeal artery and cautery of the middle fossa dura. The dura is opened parallel to the temporal lobe, which is then gently retracted. The tumor is approached from the lateral to medial direction. The trochlear and trigeminal cranial nerves are stretched on the superior aspect of the tumor capsule; the cranial nerves 7 and 8 will be displaced on the posterior aspect. The tumor is devascularized and debulked between the cranial nerve widows. The posterior cerebral and superior cerebellar arteries are displaced on the medial aspect of the tumor capsule. The medial portion of the tumor is dissected at the last stage of resection from the PCA, SCA, and brain stem. Resection of the medial portion is performed only when there is a well-preserved pia-arachnoid plane. Pial invasion by tumor precludes total resection. Great care must be exercised to avoid neurovascular injury.

The infratentorial middle tentorial tumors are approached with a lateral suboccipital craniotomy (SOC) (Fig. 51-6).[17] The patient is placed in the lateral oblique position; a standard SOC exposes the transverse sinus superiorly and sigmoid sinus laterally. Opening of the cisterna magna and the cerebellomedullary cistern to release the cerebrospinal fluid (CSF) is essential to relax the cerebellum before placement of any retraction system. The fifth, seventh, and eighth cranial nerve complex are located ventral to the tumor. Tumor vascularization is reduced by bipolar coagulation of the tentorial and posterior fossa dural attachment. After debulking of the tumor, its capsule can then be safely and meticulously dissected from the cerebellar surface, trying to keep the arachnoid plane intact between the tumor and cerebellar cortex. In the absence of any arachnoidal planes, the tumor can be dissected from the pia of the cerebellar cortex. While dissecting the anterior portion of the capsule, the surgeon can identify cranial nerves 5, 7, and 8. Use of electrophysiologic monitoring probes is essential at this stage of dissection. After review of the MRV and/or venogram to avoid jeopardizing the posterior temporal lobe venous drainage, as mentioned previously, resection of the tentorial origin is always recommended to achieve a tumor-free margin. Resection of the transverse sinus is only necessary if the sinus is fully infiltrated and occluded by the tumor.

Posterior Tentorial Meningiomas

Posterior tentorial meningiomas are approached using an occipital transtentorial approach for tumors in the supratentorial space

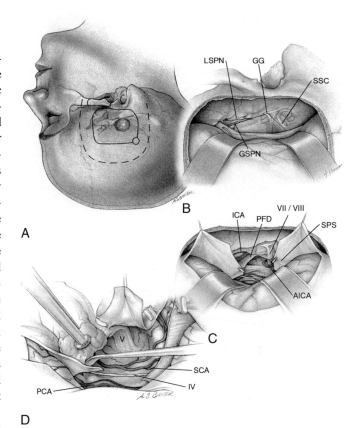

FIG. 51-5. Subtemporal approach with anterior petrosectomy to a supratentorial middle incisural meningioma. (A) Patient is placed in the lateral position with the superior sagittal sinus parallel to the floor. Skin incision (dashed line) for a subtemporal craniotomy with zygomatic osteotomy (solid line) and anterior petrosal approach. (B) Extradural exposure of the floor of the middle cranial fossa after subtemporal craniotomy. Glasscock's and Kawase's triangles are outlined on the middle fossa floor. The boundaries of Glasscock's triangle are laterally, a line from the foramen spinosum to the facial hiatus; medially, the greater superficial petrosal nerve (GSPN); and at the base, V3. Boundaries of Kawase's triangle are laterally, the GSPN; medially, the petrous ridge; and at the base, the arcuate eminence. The ICA is exposed in Glasscock's triangle. The posterior fossa dura is exposed down to the level of the inferior petrosal sinus by resection of the bone of Kawase's triangle. (C) Intradural exposure achieved with anterior petrosectomy when coupled with temporal craniotomy, section of inferior temporal lobe dura, elevation of temporal lobe, sacrifice of superior petrosal sinus (SPS) (shown with two titanium clips applied), section of tentorium cerebelli, and opening of posterior fossa dura. (D) Trochlear (IV) and trigeminal (V) cranial nerves are stretched on the superior aspect of the tumor's capsule, and cranial nerves VII and VIII will be displaced on the posterior aspect. Tumor is devascularized and debulked between the cranial nerves widows. Posterior cerebral and superior cerebellar arteries are displaced on the medial aspect of the tumor's capsule. Medial portion of the tumor is dissected at the last stage of resection from the posterior cerebral artery (PCA), superior cerebellar artery (SCA), and brain stem. AICA, anterior inferior cerebellar artery; LSPN, lesser superficial petrosal nerve; GG, geniculate ganglion; SSC, superior semicircular canal; PFD, posterior fossa dura. (From Ref. 16.)

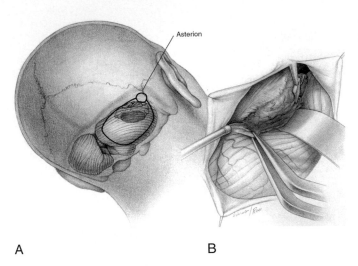

Asterion

A   B

Fig. 51-6. Lateral suboccipital approach to an infratentorial middle tentorial meningioma. (A) Key-hole burr hole is placed inferomedial to the asterion to avoid injury of the transverse-sigmoid junction in performing the lateral suboccipital craniotomy (line). (B) Dural opening and dural leaves are reflected along the sinus edges. Tumor vascularization is reduced by bipolar coagulation of the tentorial and posterior fossa dural attachments as well as the tumor capsule. (From Ref. 16.)

and using a suboccipital supracerebellar infratentorial approach for tumors with infratentorial extension.[18] This category also includes falcotentorial and torcular meningiomas.

The patient is positioned in the lateral oblique position for lesions with a supratentorial origin, with the tumor side down to facilitate gravity retraction (Fig. 51-7). The dura is opened in a cruciate manner to base the flaps on the superior sagittal and transverse sinuses. Depending on the depth along the straight sinus where the tumor is attached, dissection proceeds up to the falcotentorial junction. Devascularization of the tumor includes bipolar of the surrounding exposed dura, including bridging vessels between the tumor and dura and tumor capsule. For posteriorly located lesions, part of the dura can be excised, including the straight sinus if it is occluded by tumor. The straight sinus should not be occluded if patent. For falcotentorial lesions, interval debulking of the tumor mass is followed by incisions of the tentorium and falx leaves to create a tumor-free margin.

After control of the straight sinus is achieved with hemoclips, the sinus is incised posteriorly and then anteriorly, with care taken not to tear bridging veins between the anterior portion of the tumor capsule and confluence of veins. These bridging veins between the tumor capsule and the veins of Galen and Rosenthal are controlled with the bipolar coagulation. After the inferior surface of the tumor is retracted, arachnoid adhesions with the midbrain and the superior cerebellar surface are dissected.

Posterior tentorial meningiomas that have a primary infratentorial attachment are approached using the supracerebellar infratentorial approach (Fig. 51-8). The patient is placed in the lateral oblique position with the head flexed about 15 degrees, positioning the tentorium in a horizontal plane. A bilateral suboccipital craniotomy is performed. After opening the dura, the

occipital sinus is controlled with hemoclips and the falx cerebelli is reflected superiorly with the dural leaf based on the torcula. A safe working corridor, about 1.2 cm on either side of midline (total approximately 2.5 cm), will avoid disturbing cerebellar bridging veins.[6] This corridor brings the surgeon to the superior vermian and precentral cerebellar veins, which can be coagulated. Tumor devascularization, sectioning of the straight sinus, and tumor dissection are performed as discussed in the posterior tentorial supratentorial type.

Lesions that span the infra- and supratentorial space to a significant degree are approached by combining the approach to the supratentorial aspect of the tumor with the infratentorial approach. Examples of this are torcular meningiomas that are approached via a combined supracerebellar-infratentorial and occipital-transtentorial approach. Dissection is carried out as described in each section above, although it is tailored to the extent of the lesion. Radical subtotal resection with preservation of the confluent sinuses is indicated in patients with a patent torcular; resection with excision of the torcular is recommended for patients with an occluded torcular.

Outcomes and Complications

The primary goal of surgery for meningiomas is gross total resection that includes the involved dura. Sectioning of the transverse sinus during surgery for tentorial meningiomas to achieve total resection should be based on thorough evaluation of preoperative venogram or MRV and intrasinus pressures. The sectioning point should be medial to the venous point of the main posterior temporal lobe drainage to avoid postoperative temporal hemorrhagic infarction. For cases with partially occluded sinuses, the literature shows no major differences in recurrence rates between total (including infiltrated sinus) versus subtotal resections.[14] Complications from resection of tentorial meningiomas can be due to either surgical approach or surgical resection. The major complications during surgical approaches occur as the result of venous injuries either to the transverse or sigmoid sinuses, injury of the posterior temporal venous drainage (vein of Labbé), or sacrifice of critical bridging veins or venous lakes.[3–5,7] Complications from resection can vary according to the tumor location and the potential injuries of the cranial nerves, and blood vessels to the brain stem, brain, or cerebellum.

Clinical Series

In our series of 34 patients with tentorial meningiomas operated on in the last 6 years, 29 patients recovered back to their normal baseline activities and three patients had fair outcomes of moderate disability (disabled but independent). Two patients had poor outcomes of severe disability (conscious but disabled, dependent for daily life) due to vascular injuries of the brain stem and perforations to the PCA. Both patients had tumors of the tentorial incisura. There were no mortalities.

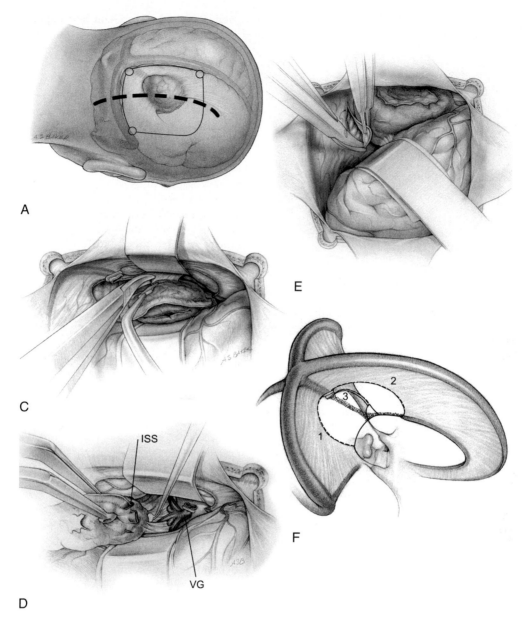

FIG. 51-7. Occipital transtentorial approach to a falcotentorial meningioma. (A) Patient is positioned in the lateral position, with the tumor side down for gravity retraction. A linear skin incision (dashed line) and craniotomy flap (solid line) edges just lateral to the superior sagittal sinus and superior to the transverse sinus. The falcotentorial junction containing the straight sinus (SS) is followed to reach the tumor capsule. (B) After extracavation and debulking of the tumor mass, incisions of the tentorium and falx leaves are made. (C) The straight sinus is controlled with hemoclips and incised posteriorly then anteriorly. (D) Bridging veins between the tumor capsule and the veins of Galen (VG) and Rosenthal are controlled with the bipolar, microscissors, and hemoclips. Inferior surface of the tumor is then retracted and arachnoid adhesions with the midbrain and the superior cerebellar surface are dissected with Rosen dissector. ISS, inferior sagittal sinus. (E) Dural sinuses, tentorium, and falx cerebri are seen. Notice the resected dura (dash line) and resected portion of the straight sinus. 1, tentorial; 2, falx cerebri; 3, straight sinus. (From Ref. 16.)

Goals for Safe Treatment of Tentorial Meningiomas

Safe surgical resection should be the principal goal in treating tentorial meningiomas. Safe resection is defined as either gross total resection with preservation of neurovascular structures or subtotal resection in which residual tumor remains attached to neurovascular structures for subsequent radiation therapy or observation.

Understanding the pathoanatomy of each tentorial meningioma subtype and demonstration of the arterial and venous anatomy of the tentorium and brain are essential in executing the safe resection of tentorial meningiomas. The first goal is to choose the optimal surgical corridor that exposes the dural base of the tumor

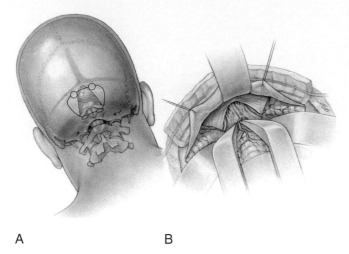

A   B

FIG. 51-8. Supracerebellar infratentorial approach to a falcotentorial meningioma. (A) Bilateral suboccipital craniotomy. (B) After opening the dura, the dural leaf is seen based on the torcular. A working corridor, about 1.2 cm on either side of midline, brings the surgeon to the superior vermian and the precentral cerebellar veins, which are controlled with the bipolar. (From Ref. 16.)

adequately and preserves venous drainage. The second goal is careful appreciation of the preoperative venous anatomy to determine the extent of tumor involvement and potential collateral damage. In general, a patent straight sinus is unsafe to sacrifice, while a patent transverse sinus may be sacrificed between the sinus confluence and transverse sigmoid junction medial to the venous point. Use of image guidance helps to plan a less invasive approach and to identify venous sinuses, tumor landmarks, location of critical structures (e.g., brain stem), and degree of subtotal resection. The third goal is early devascularization of the tumor from the underlying dura; following this tumor debulking should be performed, and finally the tumor capsule can then be circumferentially dissected from the important arterial and venous anatomy. Preservation of the arachnoidal plane is important. The fourth goal is resection of the tentorial origin as extensively as possible to create a tumor-free margin.

Summary

Tentorial meningiomas can be classified into subtypes according to their location and optimal surgical corridor. Precise preoperative planning can be designed after thorough evaluation of MRI, MRA, MRV, and/or angiogram and venogram to identify anatomic location, blood supply, and venous relationships. Safe surgical resection should be the principal goal in treating tentorial meningiomas; resection can include the addition of less invasive skull base techniques if needed to maximize exposure and minimize brain retraction. Subtotal resection is an important goal when critical neurovascular structures are

involved. Residual tumors can be followed radiologically or treated with focused-beam radiation therapy.

References

1. Castellano F, Ruggiero G. Meningiomas of the posterior fossa. Acta Radiol Suppl 1953; 104:1–177.
2. Martins C, Yasuda A, Campero A, et al. Microsurgical Anatomy of the Dural Arteries. Neurosurgery 2005; 56(Operative Neurosurgery Suppl 2):211–251.
3. Bruce JN, Stein BM. Complications of surgery for pineal region tumors. In: Post KD, Friedman ED, McCormick P, ed.Postoperative Complications in Intracranial Neurosurgery. New York: Thieme, 1993:74–86.
4. Page LK. The infratentorial-supracerebellar exposure of tumors in pineal area. Neurosurgery 1977; 1:36–40.
5. Matsushima T, Suzuki SO, Fukui M, et al. Microsurgical anatomy of the tentorial sinuses. J Neurosurg 1989; 71:923–928.
6. Ueyama T, Al-Mefty O, Tamaki N. Bridging veins on the tentorial surface of the cerebellum: a microsurgical anatomic study and operative considerations. Neurosurgery 1998; 43:1137–1145.
7. Guppy KH, Origitano TC, Reichman, OH, et al. Venous drainage of the inferolateral temporal lobe in relationship to transtemporal/transtentorial approaches to the cranial base. Neurosurgery 1997; 41:615–620.
8. Bisaria KK. Anatomic variations of the venous sinuses in the region of the torcular Herophili. J Neurosurg 1985; 62:90–95.
9. Rhoton AL. Tentorial incisura. Neurosurgery 2000; (The Posterior Cranial Fossa: Microsurgical Anatomy and Surgical Approaches Suppl) 47(3):S131–S153.
10. Kawase T, Shiobara R, Toya S. Anterior transpetrosal-transtentorial approach for sphenopetroclival meningiomas: surgical method and results in 10 patients. Neurosurgery 1991; 28:869–876.
11. Sekhar LN, Swamy NK, Jaiswal V, et al. Surgical excision of meningiomas involving the clivus: Preoperative and intraoperative features as predictors of postoperative functional deterioration. J Neurosurg 1994; 81:860–868.
12. Gökalp HZ, Arasil E, Erdogan A, et al. Tentorial meningiomas. Neurosurgery 1995; 36:46–51.
13. Hischam B, Anja H, Siamak A, et al. Tentorial Meningiomas: Clinical Results in 81 Patients Treated Microsurgically. Neurosurgery 2004; 55:108–118.
14. Yasargil MG, Mortara RW, Curcic M. Meningiomas of the basal posterior cranial fossa. Adv Tech Stand Neurosurg 1980; 7:3–115.
15. Samii M, Carvalho GA, Tatagiba M, et al. Meningiomas of the tentorial notch: Surgical anatomy and management. J Neurosurg 1996; 84:375–381.
16. Tew JM Jr, van Loveren HR, Keller JT. Atlas of Operative Microneurosurgery, Vol. 2: Brain Tumors. Philadelphia, W.B. Saunders, 2001.
17. Sekhar LN, Jannetta PJ, Maroon CJ. Tentorial meningiomas: surgical management and results. Neurosurgery 1984; 14:268–275.
18. Ammerman JM, Lonser RR, Oldfield EH. Posterior subtemporal transtentorial approach to intraparenchymal lesions of the anteromedial region of the superior cerebellum. J Neurosurg 2005; 103:783–788.
19. Muthukumar N, Konziolka D, Lunsford LD, et al. Stereotactic radiosurgery for tentorial meningiomas. Acta Neurochir (Wien) 1998; 140:315–321.

52
Torcular, Transverse, and Sigmoid Sinus Meningiomas

Jorge E. Alvernia and Marc P. Sindou

Introduction

Meningiomas located in the torcular, transverse, and sigmoid sinus (SS) regions are dangerous tumors to deal with. In the presence of a totally occluded sinus, the question whether to restore the venous circulation by performing a bypass when a completely occluded sinus is resected, rather than just remove the tumor and the obstructed segment of the sinus without venous reconstruction, is a matter of great debate. In the cases with partial sinus invasion by the tumor, and due to the presence of bilateral lateral sinus drainage, the sacrifice of one side could technically be performed without impunity in some cases. Unfortunately, and as shown in this chapter, the multiple anatomic variants compel the surgeon to be especially cautious in terms of resecting a tumor invading the dural sinuses without reconstructing them, even in cases when a collateral circulation is already developed (1,2).

The neurosurgeon dealing with these kinds of tumors should be familiarized not just with the anatomy of this region (3,4), but also with the different techniques of venous repair when needed (5–11). Although today radiosurgery provides an additional treatment option for these tumors (12), surgery provides in most cases the only definitive way to cure these patients, as shown in our personal series, especially in the atypical or malignant variants, in which no tumor recurrence was found after a follow-up ranging from 3 to 23 years (8 years on average).

Special Considerations

The average diameter of the transverse sinus (TS) is 8–10mm, but commonly the diameter differs in size between the left and right sides. One TS may drain symmetrically (20%) (Fig. 52-1A) or asymmetrically (55%) (Fig. 52-2A). In 25%, one TS alone drains the superior sagittal sinus (SSS) or the straight sinus, depending on the configuration of the torcular Herophili (Fig. 52-2B) (1). In fact, Bisaria found in a study of 110 cranial cavities that this sinus confluence varied from a common pool to merely a potential confluence, depending upon the presence of incomplete or complete partitions of dura mater. Rare variants were also shown in this study such as a SSS and a straight sinus seeming to fork, and the forks from both sinuses joining to form the TS. Other anatomic variants, such as double straight sinuses draining into one TS and a TS originating from a tentorial vein, were also described (13).

As to the tentorial sinuses cerebelli, Muthukumar, in a study of 80 fresh cadaveric cranial cavities, encountered them in 86%. The author classified these as medial, middle, and lateral. The medial ones (25% of the total) had a branching "staghorn" configuration and drained into the straight sinus, the torcular herophili, and the medial third of the TS (these being the most richly vascularized), whereas the ones located in the middle third (50% of the cases) did not present with this branching pattern, and size varied from small to medium. On the other hand, those located laterally (25%) were smaller than the other types and tended to drain into the junction of the TS and superior petrosal sinus (SPS) or into the lateral one third of the TS (14).

It is important to remember that the TS may be atresic in 17% of the cases, with the remaining SS draining the inferior cerebral veins (vein of Labbé) (Fig. 52-2C) (1).

The SS usually receives the superior and inferior petrosal sinuses and sometimes veins from the lateral pons and the medulla. It often anastomoses with scalp veins by way of the mastoid or hypoglossal canals via condyloid emissary veins. The SS may also be atresic, in which case the ipsilateral TS and its tributaries drain towards the opposite side. The superior petrosal sinus (SPS) drains the petrosal vein as well as some cerebellar and inferior cerebral veins and may anastomose with the sylvian veins. Sometimes the petrosal sinus and the vein of Labbé may have a common trunk (Fig. 52-1B).

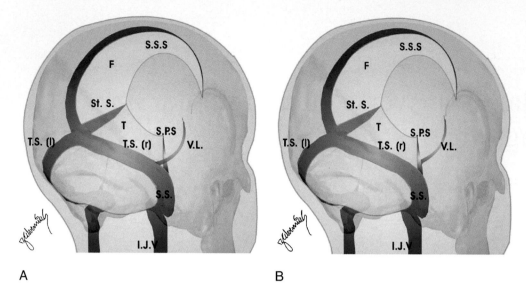

FIG. 52.1. (A) Balanced system: When both lateral sinuses are seen to be well developed on venous angiogram, the sacrifice of one does not entail surgical risk if the sacrifice is performed below of the vein of Labbé and the superior petrosal vein. (B) Venous anatomic variant showing, for instance, a common trunk for the vein of Labbé and the superior petrosal sinus at the sinodural angle. Particular care and attention must be paid to venous anatomic variants like this before any sacrifice is decided. S.S.S, superior sagittal sinus; F, falx; St. S., straight sinus; T, tentorium; T.S. (r), transverse sinus right side; T.S. (l), transverse sinus left side; S.P.S, superior petrous sinus; V.L, vein of Labbé; S.S, sigmoid sinus; I.J.V, internal jugular vein

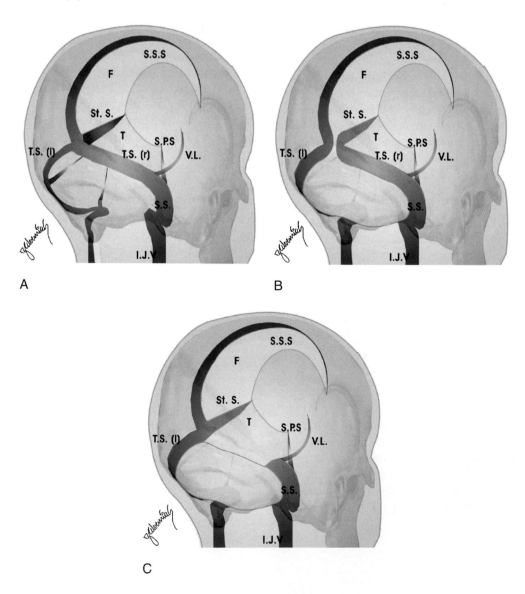

In the treatment of meningiomas involving the torcular, TS, and SS, it is important to consider the different variants and to establish before any surgical approach the presence or not of a "balanced" TS venous drainage, not only from magnetic resonance (MR) and MR venogram, but also from venous phase of digital subtraction angioplasty (DSA). Regarding the sinus classification of sinus invasion, the classification used for parasagittal meningioma is adequate—Type I: Attachment to outer surface of a sinus wall; Type II: Fragment inside a lateral recess; Type III: Invasion of one wall; Type IV: Invasion of two walls; Types V and VI: Complete sinus occlusion, with or without one wall free, respectively (1,5).

Due to the differences in presentation and surgical approaches, these meningiomas can be conveniently divided into three categories as follows: (1) those invading the torcular or adherent to it, (2) those invading the TS, arising either from the tentorium or the superior aspect of the cerebellum, and (3) those invading the SS that may come from the posterior part of the petrous bone or as an extension from the jugular foramen.

Torcular Meningiomas

In 1887, Birdsall and Weir reported the first effort at removal of a peritorcular meningioma; their case, only the fifth intracranial operation for a tumor ever reported, ended unfortunately in fatal postoperative hemorrhage. But it was not until later that Oppenheim and Krause reported the first successful removal of a parasagittal and peritorcular meningioma.

Rarely do the dural sinuses converge symmetrically at a central point beneath the internal occipital protuberance. Rather, torcular venous channels are usually asymmetric and septate. Cushing and Eisenhardt's torcular meningiomas constituted 16% of their 77 parasagittal tumors. In most of the other series, torcular tumors comprise about 1% of intracranial meningiomas. In fact, as stated by Malis, the one good thing about torcular meningiomas is their rarity (1,15,16).

In Cushing and Eisenhardt's series, the signs and symptoms reflected either compression of the occipital lobe or cerebellum or intracranial hypertension referable to obstruction of venous flow. Headache was global in half of the patients. The other half complained of occipital and suboccipital pain, probably resulting from distorsion of the surrounding dura. Neck pain and stiffness might have indicated incipient tonsillar herniation. All patients had papilledema. At least half also had homonymous field cuts suggestive of occipital compression and supratentorial presence.

Cerebellar signs, indicating infratentorial tumor extension, included ataxia, dysmetria, hypotonia, and nystagmus. Presumably, the slow growth of peritorcular meningiomas allows gradual development of sufficient collateral flow to preclude the presence of sudden thrombosis of a partially occluded dominant sinus.

Usually the middle meningeal and occipital branches from the external carotid artery, the meningeal branches of the vertebral artery, and the tentorial branches of the cavernous internal carotid artery are the feedings arteries.

Transverse Sinus Meningiomas

Usually the meningiomas that involve the transverse sinus come either from the cerebellar convexity or from the tentorium.

Cerebellar Convexity/Superior Type

The cerebellar convexity meningiomas classically are divided in three types: medial, lateral, or superior. Typically the superior ones are the most likely to invade the transverse sinus. Characteristic symptoms of this kind of meningioma are few. The patient may present with headache, progressive cerebellar signs, signs of increased intracranial pressure, and symptoms of hydrocephalus (17).

Tentorial Meningiomas

Several classifications of tentorial meningiomas have been proposed based on the sites of tumor origin as determined at surgery. Briefly the tentorial meningiomas may be classified simply as follows: (1) medial, subdivided into anterior, middle, and posterior, (2) lateral with anterior, middle, and posterior groups, and (3) falcotentorial (para-straight sinus) meningiomas.

However, with large tumors it may be difficult to determine the actual site of origin. In the majority of cases, the bulk of the tumor grows infratentorially and frequently provides characteristic clinical symptoms, such as headache and truncal ataxia. Commonly the meningiomas that invade the lateral sinus are posterolateral and falcotentorial in origin (18–24).

Sigmoid Sinus Meningiomas

Sigmoid sinus meningioma refers in most cases either to "meningioma of the posterior surface of the petrous pyramid" or to a meningioma arising from the jugular foramen. The term

FIG. 52.2. (A) Unbalanced system: A predominant unilateral drainage (as in most of the cases—usually to the right), the sacrifice of the nondominant side might be performed as long as it is done below of the vein of Labbé and superior petrosal vein. (the only unbalanced system when technically a venous sacrifice might be done) (B) Split system: Accounts for the cases when the posterior deep venous system is drained through one lateral sinus and the posterior superficial venous system is drained through the contralateral one (any sacrifice of this system will entail catastrophic consequences). (C) One transverse sinus is absent. Any sacrifice of this system will entail catastrophic consequences as well. S.S.S, superior sagittal sinus; F, falx; St. S., straight sinus; T, tentorium; T.S. (r), transverse sinus right side; T.S. (l), transverse sinus left side; S.P.S, superior petrous sinus; V.L, vein of Labbé; S.S, sigmoid sinus; I.J.V, internal jugular vein

introduced by Samii and Ammiratti, the "posterior petrous pyramid," is useful and denotes the site of dural attachment tending to exclude those meningiomas not originating from this region but growing in close relation to it. Actually, those located posterior to the internal auditory meatus (IAM) are more likely to invade the SS. Classically these tumors present with cerebellar symptoms whereas those anterior to it usually cause decreased hearing. Regarding the meningiomas arising from the jugular foramen, they usually present with lower cranial nerve deficit (25,26).

Surgical Technique

Resection and venous repair in most of these cases is performed by placing the patient either in the sitting position for torcular meningiomas (Fig. 52-3A) or in the park bench position for those involving the transverse or sigmoid sinus. Although the sitting position may entail some risk of venous embolism, it is strongly advised in torcular cases because of its convenience to have a straightforward venous bleeding control of the different torcular

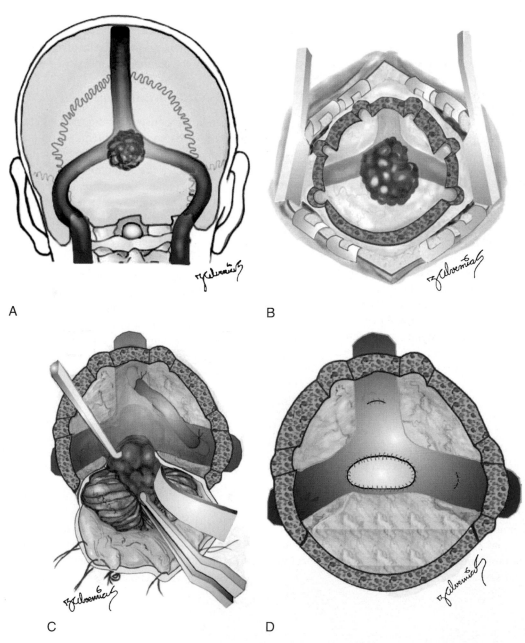

A   B

C   D

FIG. 52.3 (A) Torcular meninigoma. The sitting position in these cases allows a convenient exposure of all the corners around the tumor, decreases the amount of venous bleeding, and provides easier access to the neck when necessary for bypass. (B) Craniotomy for torcular meningiomas should display at least 2 cm of dura tumor-free around the meningioma, including 2–3 cm of SS and TS away from the tumor on both sides. (C) When removing the intrasinusal portion of torcular meningiomas, a temporary synthetic catheter from the sagittal sinus to the transverse sinus is an alternative to the use of pledgets of surgical for control bleeding. (D) Torcular patching with autologous graft (fascia lata) and removal of the temporary synthetic venous pontage

corners. Conversely, for those located on the TS and SS, the park bench usually provides an adequate exposure. An inverted U-shaped incision for the torcular and an inverted J-shaped incision for the sigmoid and transverse sinus meningiomas with an associated craniotomy extending across the midline above and below the sinus to permit patching or primary suture when needed, is strongly encouraged. It should be noted that a 2-cm dural free margin around the tumor is advisable to allow a complete resection and to have enough room for venous repair or bypass when needed. Special care has to be taken to preserve the venous anastomotic pathways developed throughout the scalp, the pericranial and the diploic venous channels, when craniotomy is performed. A meticulous preoperative evaluation identifying the venous

phase of the DSA and the intradiploic venous channels on plain x-ray of the skull is recommended (27–30). When in doubt about a residual intrasinusal fragment, a short wall incision should always be performed for inspection (1,2,5).

Temporary control of venous bleeding from the sinus, as well as from the afferent veins, may be achieved just by packing small pledgets of hemostatic material (Surgicel, Johnson Medical, Viroflay, France) within the sinus lumen. Venous reconstruction may be performed using patches (Figs. 52-3 and 52-4) or bypasses (Fig. 52-5). For these purposes two hemi-running sutures (prolene 8.0, laboratoire ETHNOR, Neuilly/Seine, France) are enough. Locally situated dura mater, pericranium, or fascia lata, or even better the neighboring fascia, are very good alternatives. Long autologous venous grafts harvested

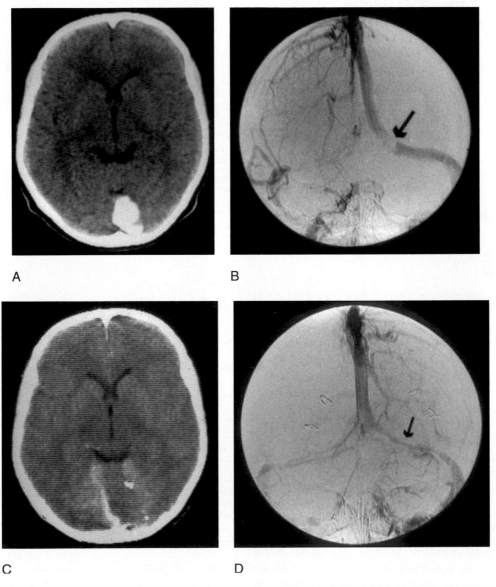

A

B

C

D

FIG. 52.4. Grade III torcular meningioma. (A) Preoperative head CT with contrast displaying a meningioma in relation to the inion. (B) Preoperative angiogram (venous phase) showing a torcular meningioma occluding completely the right transverse sinus and partially occluding the left one (arrows). (C) Postop CT showing complete removal of the meningioma. (D) Postop angiogram (venous phase) displaying patency of both lateral sinus

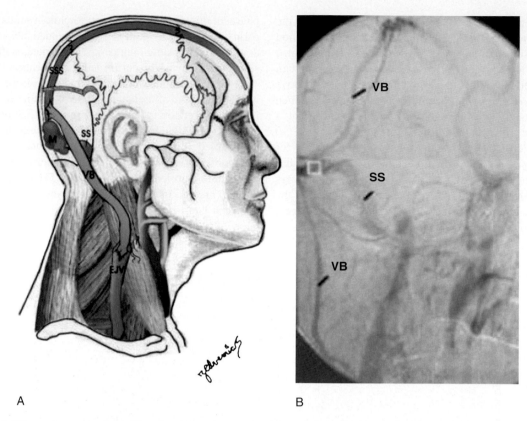

A   B

FIG. 52.5. Grade VI torcular meningioma. Drawing (A) and postoperative angiogram (B) showing the surgical bypass from SSS to EJV with an autologous saphenous vein (used because of the need for a long graft, i.e., more than 6 cm) in a case of complete occlusion of the torcular. SSS, superior sagittal sinus; SS, sigmoid sinus; VB, venous bypass (saphenous vein); M, meningioma; EJV, external jugular vein

from the internal saphenous vein (more than 6 cm) (Fig. 52-5) or shorter from the external jugular vein may also be used to bypass a totally occluded portions of the sinus. (Table 52-1)

To decrease risk of bypass thrombosis after surgery, anticoagulation with heparin (two times control PTT) for 3 weeks followed by Coumadin for 3 months is usually recommended in the reconstructed sinus until re-endothelization is achieved.

Regarding the part not attached to the sinus, the operative steps can be succinctly described as follows: (1) intradural volume reduction (either by piecemeal removal with bipolar microcoagulation, microscissors, and microsuction or by means of an ultrasonic aspirator) and (2) sharp dissection of the tumor from the underlying cerebral cortex under high magnification.

Torcular Meningioma

Temporizing surgical measures, such as optic nerve sheath fenestration to relieve visual deficits arising from elevated intracranial pressure or ventriculoperitoneal shunting of obstructive hydrocephalus, have been reported, especially in cases whereby the patient condition precludes any kind of

TABLE 52.1. Tumor Types and Surgical Techniques.

Location	Type	Surgical technique used
Torcular	Type V right TS/ Type IV left TS	Extraction of intratorcular fragment and patching
Torcular	Type IV rifght TS/ Type IV left TS	Extraction intratorcular fragment + patching (undertemporarily shunt)
Torcular	Total occlusion of posterior third of SSS and Torcular (Type VI)	Sino-extrajugular bypass with saphenous vein
Transverse	Type III	Removal of invaded wall and clippage of the lateral wall free tumor edges
Transverse	Type IV	Bypass to the internal jugular vein
Transverse	Type IV	Bypass to the external jugular vein
Transverse	Type VI	No venous reconstruction
Transverse	Type III	patching wall
Sigmoid	Type III	Extrasinusal removal, coagulation of wall invaded
Sigmoid	Type III	Extrasinusal removal, coagulation of wall invaded
Sigmoid	Type IV	Removal of two invaded walls and proximal and distal sinus packing

major surgical intervention. The choice of operative approach depends on the tumor size and location, the nature of sinus involvement, and the goals of surgery. Although a unilateral occipital craniotomy or a unilateral suboccipital craniectomy is considered in "unilateral cases" for some authors (24), our policy in these cases is to completely expose the torcular corners to get a complete control of the torcular.

The sitting position is strongly recommended. An inverted U-shaped incision with its apex at the lambda and its base between the mastoid processes usually provides an excellent exposure. Bone is usually removed through a free flap occipital craniotomy and/or suboccipital craniectomy. Some authors recommend piecemeal removal by rongeuring the bone over the venous sinuses. In the cases presented, bone was carefully removed using the free bone flap technique and was detached from the underlying tumor with a Penfield dissector.

When tumor invasion is limited to the outer layer of the sinus (Type I), just a simple peeling should be enough. If one corner (Type II) or wall (Type III) is invaded, the sinus wall should be opened and the tumor removed. The sinus is then reconstructed either with a direct running suture or an autologous patch respectively.

Some authors feel that sequentially opening and closing small segments of the sinus as the tumor is progressively removed from the sinus avoids venous bleeding and decreases the likelihood of venous infarct. The protocol for these presented cases involves temporarily introducing pledgets of Surgicel proximally and distally to the invaded segment to momentarily occlude the venous circulation.

Removal of a meningioma involving more than two sinus walls (Type IV–VI) definitely needs consideration for a temporary or definitive shunt depending whether a patch is performed or not. A shunt from the superior sagittal sinus to the transverse sinus during isolation and repair of a tumor-invaded torcular Herophili is recommended for these cases, as shown in the Fig. 52-3. In cases with complete venous wall involvement (Type VI of our classification) the recommendation certainly is a definitive venous bypass (Fig. 52-5).

Transverse Sinus Meningiomas

As a general rule, the approach to this kind of meningioma starts with the interception of skin and dural tumor feeders coming from the occipital artery and/or posterior auricular artery and middle and posterior meningeal branches, respectively, in the early phase of surgery, to facilitate total tumor removal with reduced blood loss. In these cases a combined supra- and infratentorial craniotomy is usually indicated, as shown in the Fig. 52-6A. The dura is to be opened in a circumferential fashion around the tumor and incised parallel to the venous sinuses in order to disconnect the dural middle meningeal feeders coming from above, dural tentorial feeders (Bernasconi-Cassinari artery branches) coming from anterior, and the dural meningeal posterior feeders coming from inferior location, as displayed in Fig. 52-6B.

With regard to approaches, the supratentorial is used for the portions of the tumor above the tentorium mainly for the removal of tentorial or falcotentorial meningiomas (Fig. 52-6C). The suboccipital approach is used to remove the inferior extension of the tentorial meningiomas or cerebellar meningiomas invading the transverse sinus. A combined (supra- and subtentorial) approach "as a glance"—if not at the beginning, at least at the end—should be done in order to verify complete tumor removal.

The major question as to whether the involved sinus should be resected with the tumor is addressed during surgery only after considering the major morbidity associated with sinus transection. If the sinus is completely occluded and there is a compensatory venous drainage as confirmed by angiography, the involved sinus can be resected with impunity.

If the collateral circulation is not well developed and radical removal subjects the patient at risk of neurologic deficit, a reoperation may be undertaken after collateral circulation has developed. Sekhar et al. (22) insist that a sinus invaded with tumor should be resected and reconstructed with dural leaves or with a saphenous vein graft in young patients where compensatory venous drainage has not developed yet.

Because of the early occlusion of synthetic bypasses, namely Goretex, experienced with parasagittal meningiomas, only autologous grafts are recommended—external jugular for short graft and internal saphenous vein for longer ones (1,2,5). The use of anticoagulants as shown in the parasagittal series did not increase the complication rate.

The absence of neurologic deterioration encountered after surgical repair in the lateral sinus prompted the attempt at total resection. Primary closure when just one lateral recess is invaded, and patching when at least one sinus wall is free of tumor ,should be attempted. In the case of complete sinus obstruction with partial or total involvement of the torcular by the tumor, accompanied by a nonfunctional contralateral lateral sinus, a temporary bypass (from proximal and distal to the tumor) plus patching (in Type V), if possible, or a definitive bypass with jugular or saphenous vein (in Type VI) is recommended.

Regarding tentorial meningiomas invading the transverse sinus a combined supra- and infratentorial approach is always recommended (32,33). Special care must be taken to avoid venous avulsion when doing either one of the approach (vein of Labbé and cerebellar veins, respectively).

When approaching a falcotentorial meningioma, the falx and tentorium may be sectioned, with subsequent retraction of the occipital pole which usually has a few, if any, bridging veins allowing a wide exposure of the tumor. For some authors the major benefit of this approach is the fact that the surgeon can frequently coagulate and section the feeding arteries of the tumor before dissecting the tumor mass. For these tumors other authors, such as Nagashima and Kobayashi, have reported the use of a radial graft interposition between the straight and right lateral sinuses to achieve a complete tumor removal of a torcular herophili hemangiopericytoma (34). The cases reported in our series use either external jugular or saphenous vein grafts (1,2,5).

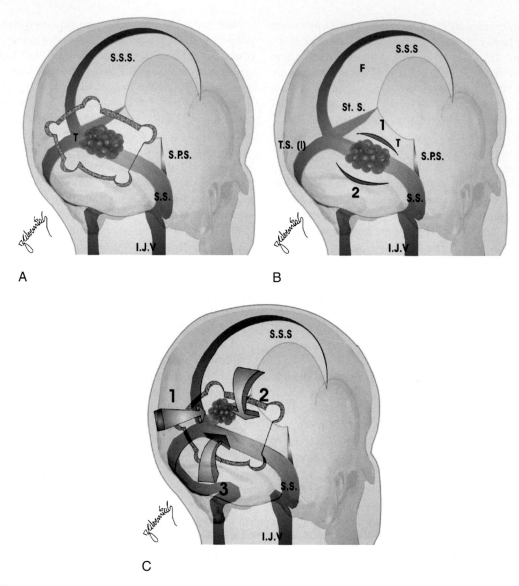

FIG. 52.6. (A) Classical craniotomy for TS meningiomas providing adequate dural exposure including the torcular and the inferior part of the superior sagittal sinus. (B) Dural incision disconnecting the meningeal feeders. 1. Dural tentorial feeders (Bernasconi-Cassinari artery branches). 2. Dural posterior meningeal artery feeders. (C) When approaching falcotentorial meningiomas, the same craniotomy described for transverse meningiomas allows mixed approaches: 1, interhemispheric; 2, supratentorial; 3, infratentorial. S.S.S, superior sagittal sinus; F, falx; St. S., straight sinus; T, torcular; T.S. (l), transverse sinus left side; S.P.S, superior petrous sinus; S.S, sigmoid sinus; I.J.V, internal jugular vein

In some selected cases, because of the particular disposition of the lateral sinus to be devoid of bridging veins draining directly into it an because of the presence of intraluminal septae, it is felt that aneurysm clips may be used, as shown in Fig. 52-7 (1).

Sigmoid Sinus

The so-called posterior pyramid tumors are usually approached mainly through a lateral suboccipital craniectomy or craniotomy with the patient in the semi-sitting or three-quarter prone position, with the head in a Mayfield frame flexed and turned 30 degrees toward the side of the lesion.

The bone over the sinus may be removed using a high-speed drill after careful dural separation. A few diploic or emissary veins draining into the sinus may be encountered. These are coagulated away from the sinus and sharply transected. If a hole or small tear is made in the sinus, it is usually packed with gelfoam and larger tears need to be sutured.

In these cases the foramen magnum is opened as much as possible, avoiding the vertebral artery, but removing as much of the medial aspect of the condyle as neccesary. The posterior arches of C1 and C2 are removed unilaterally. Opened mastoid air cells are sealed with fat and fascia lata. No foreign material as bone wax is necessary, because it does not provide good sealing and even favors late ear granuloma development. Hemostasis

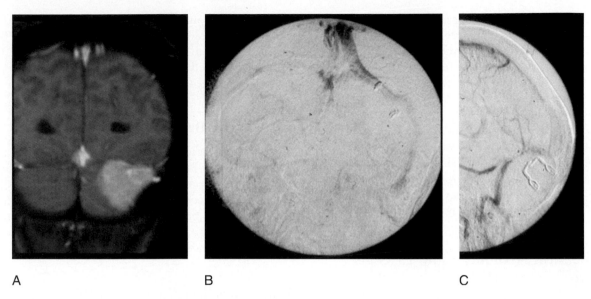

A   B   C

FIG. 52.7. (A) Preop brain MRI with contrast showing a posterior fossa convexity meningioma invading the left transverse sinus. (B, C) Postop angiogram: anteroposterior and lateral view respectively (venous phase) showing (unique) left transverse sinus, patent after tumor intrasinusal resection, and posteroinferior recess repair, using two angled clips (Sugita type)

is secured and double- checked with a Valsalva maneuver that will sometimes reveal venous bleeding not previously obvious. Ultimately, the dura is closed in a watertight fashion using an autologous tissue such as fascia lata. Again, it is not necessary to use heterologous or synthetic material for this procedure. The muscles and skin are closed with separate layers as usual, and a compressive dressing is then applied for about one week.

Outcome and Complications

In this current series of meningiomas involving the major sinuses, eight cases were presented in previous publications (5): three located in the torcular and five in the transverse sinus. For this chapter, three additional cases have been added, all of which were meningiomas invading the SS. No focal general morbidity was found in this overall series.

Neurologic Morbidity and Mortality

Overall, the protocol for all cases, except the SS ones, was to attempt total removal, avoiding any venous sacrifice and restoring the venous flow either with primary repair, patching, or venous bypass when an accessory venous drainage was not guaranteed (Table 52-2). In this series, there was morbidity or mortality in the removal of meningiomas using this protocol. Certainly the presence of bilateral drainage in some of these cases favored the outcome.

For the current series, performing patching or bypassing to restore the venous flow did not increase the morbidity rate, nor did the use of postoperative anticoagulation.

Although our series comprised just 11 cases, when taking into account the cases of meningiomas involving the superior

TABLE 52-2. Tumor Types and Surgical Results.

Location	Type	Simpson	POP patency	Outcome	Recurrence
Torcular	Type V right TS/I Type IV left TS	(+)	Favorable	(−)	
Torcular	Type IV rifght TS/Type IV left TS	I	(+)	Favorable	(−)
Torcular	Total occlusion of posterior third of SSS and Torcular (Type VI)	I	(+)	Favorable	(−)
Transverse	Type III	I	(+)	Favorable	(−)
Transverse	Type IV	I	?	Favorable	(−)
Transverse	Type IV	I	?	Favorable	(−)
Transverse	Type VI	I	NA	Favorable	(−)
Transverse	Type III	I	(+)	Favorable	(−)
Sigmoid	Type III	II	(+)	Favorable	(−)
Sigmoid	Type III	II	(+)	Favorable	(−)
Sigmoid	Type IV	I	NA	Favorable	(−)

NA: Nonapplicable.
(?): Patient did not consent the POP angiogram.
Favorable: Karnofsky 90–100.

sagittal sinus, it further supports that attempting total removal of the tumor with venous repair can be considered favorably when dealing with meningiomas invading the torcular or lateral dural sinuses.

Tumor Recurrence

In our personal series, tumor recurrence rate was 0%, with a follow-up ranging from 3 to 23 years (mean of 8 years). This percentage is expected from Simpson's general classification when resection of class I (complete removal with excision of dural attachment) or II (complete removal with coagulation of dural attachment) is carried out (Table 52-2). This relatively low rate seems due in part to the absence of atypical meningiomas encountered in this series and to the attempt at macroscopic total removal in these cases.

Due to the small number of cases in this series involving the SS where a Simpson II resection was performed, a definitive statement regarding recurrence cannot be drawn. However, it is felt that in this particular subgroup when a venous reconstruction cannot be done for whatever reason, a postoperative course of radiation should be always considered.

Complication Avoidance and Lessons Learned

Air Embolism

In this series, there was one case of an air embolism. This complication ocurred with one patient in the sitting position and was uneventful. It is clear that the surgical position and the amount of sinus wall or sinus exposure increases the risk of an air embolism, but it was felt that the likelihood of a life-threatening condition was low if adequate technique and abundant irrigation was used while the sinuses were opened. Recommendations for these cases include continuous irrigation with water over the surgical field and close end-tidal CO_2 monitoring with a central line in place in order to remove air when needed.

Blood Loss

Due to the common hypervascularization of these tumors, a painstaking analysis of the preoperative images has to be done. There is great value in obtaining preoperative four vessel DSA including venous phase for all cases. A preoperative embolization of the external carotid branches should be done if available.

When planning the skin and bone flap, a previous knowledge of the arterial and bone feeding channels is extremely important in order to design a tailored approach which allows both an adequate tumoral devascularization and a convenient surgical exposure without putting the skin at risk of postoperative infection or scalp necrosis from a decreased blood supply (35–37).

Bridging Vein Avulsion

Although the transverse and sigmoid sinuses have of a small number of bridging veins draining into them, particular attention has to be paid whenever the occipital lobe and cerebellum are retracted. In cases of supratentorial occipital approaches, especially when the transverse-sigmoid junction has to be displayed, great care is needed to avoid tearing the vein of Labbé or causing accidental avulsion of the brinding

veins. The same attention is needed when retracting down the cerebellum in order to avoid tearing the cerebellar bridging veins draining into the straight and tentorial sinuses. Again, a preoperative careful assessment of the DSA venous phase is always encouraged.

Brain Tumor Bed Injury Prevention

A preoperative assessment based on the "pial tumoral blush" and the amount of peritumoral edema gives some clues as to the extent of tumor's invasiveness. In fact, there is a direct correlation between the tumor size, the amount of edema and "tumoral blush" coming from the pial vascularization, and the absence of an adequate plane of cleavage between the tumor and the underlying brain cortex (35–37).

Dural Sinus Sacrifice

When both lateral sinuses are well developed (or approximately equal in size), interruption of one lateral sinus might theoretically be tolerated because of drainage of all tributary veins above the occluded area by the opposite side. Distally, the remaining part of the lateral sinus would continue to drain its tributaries into the internal jugular vein.

Occlusion of a lateral sinus that is totally draining the SSS is associated with a high risk of bilateral hemispheric brain swelling. Occlusion of a lateral sinus totally draining the straight sinus would also have dangerous consequences for brain deep-venous circulation. Occlusion of the SS on the side of an absent or atresic transverse sinus would lead to temporal lobe infarction due to the absence of drainage of the intracranial venous system. In the instance where the vein of Labbé drains into the superior petrosal sinus, division of the tentorium at the transverse-sigmoid junction must be avoided, as it might cause venous infarction of the temporal lobe (1,2).

Cerebrospinal Fluid Leakage

In order to avoid CSF leakage, all cases must undego a watertight closure of the dura mater with autologous fascia lata. In the case of mastoid cell opening, a plug and closure with fat and/or fascia lata is strongly recommended. Synthetic and heterologous material is not recommended.

Summary

When dealing with meningiomas invading the torcular, TS, or SS, a preoperative venous assessment by means of a DSA with venous phases is of paramount importance.

Achieving radical removal requires opening of the sinus, exploring its lumen, and interrupting transiently its circulation. The latter can easily be performed by occluding the proximal and distal luminal openings with pledgets of Surgicel. Reconstruction is mandatory in the event of incomplete occlusion and may be beneficial in cases with complete obliteration.

When the torcular is invaded by a meningioma, a bypass (either definitive or temporary) plus patching has to be considered. In cases of incomplete occlusion, the resected wall(s) should be repaired with patching. An autologous graft harvested from fascia lata or fascia temporalis appears to be adequate. Harvesting a venous graft for patching, although theoretically of superior quality, seemed to us rather excessive.

References

1. Sindou M, Auque J. The intracranial venous system as a neurosurgeon's perspective. In: Advances and Technical Standards in Neurosurgery. New York: Springer-Verlag, 2000: 26.
2. Sindou M, Auque J, Jouanneau E. Neurosurgery and the intracranial venous system. Acta Neurochir Suppl 2005; 94:167–175.
3. Ziyal IM, Ozgen T. Landmarks for the transverse sinus and torcular herophili. J Neurosurg 2001; 94(4):686–687.
4. Tubbs RS, Salter G, Oakes WJ. Superficial surgical landmarks for the transverse sinus and torcular herophili. J Neurosurg 2000; 93(2):279–281.
5. Sindou M. Meningiomas invading the sagittal or transverse sinuses, resection with venous reconstruction. J Clin Neurosci 2001; 8(Suppl 1):8–11.
6. Hakuba A. Surgery of the Intracranial Venous System. New York: Springer, 1996:619.
7. Hakuba A. Reconstruction of dural sinus involved in meningiomas. In: Al-Mefty O (ed). Meningiomas. New York: Raven Press, 1991:371–382.
8. Hakuba A, Tsurund T, Ohata K, et al. Microsurgical reconstruction of the intracranial venous system. In: Hakuba A (ed). Surgery of the Intracranial Venous System. New York: Springer, 1996:220–225.
9. Sindou M, Alaywan F, Hallacq P. Chirurgie des grands sinus veineux duraux intracrâniens. In: Auque J (ed). Le Sacrifice Venue en Neurochirurgie. Neurochirurgie 1996; (Suppl 1):45–87.
10. Sindou M, Hallacq P. Venous reconstruction in surgery of meningiomas invading the sagittal and transverse sinuses. Skull Base Surg 1998; 8:57–64.
11. Sindou M, Mazoyer JF, Fischer G, et al. Experimental bypass for sagittal sinus repair. Preliminary report. J Neurosurg 1976; 44:325–330.
12. Hodes JE, Sanders M, Patel P, Patchell RA. Radiosurgical management of meningiomas. Stereotact Funct Neurosurg 1996; 66(1–3):15–18.
13. Bisaria KK. Anatomic variations of venous sinuses in the region of the torcular Herophili. J Neurosurg 1985; 62(1):90–95.
14. Muthukumar N, Palaniappan P. Tentorial venous sinuses: an anatomic study. Neurosurgery 1998; 42(2):363–371.
15. Harsh IV G, Wilson C. Meningiomas of the peritorcular region. In: Al-Mefty O (ed). Meningiomas. New York: Raven Press, 1991:363–369.
16. Borges-Fortes A. Torcular meningioma; transtentorial tumor. Hospital (Rio J) 1952; 42(3):329–338.
17. Kobayashi S, Nakamura Y. Cerebellar convexity meningiomas. In: Al-Mefty O (ed). Meningiomas. New York: Raven Press, 1991:495–501.
18. Hostalot C, Carrasco A, Bilbao G, et al. Tentorial meningiomas. Report of our series. Neurocirurgia (Austr) 2004; 15(2):119–127.

19. Bret P, Guyotat J, Madarassy G, et al. Tentorial meningiomas. Report on twenty-seven cases. Acta Neurochir (Wien) 2000; 142(5):513–526.
20. Rostomily RC, Eskridge JM, Winn HR. Tentorial meningiomas. Neurosurg Clin N Am 1994; 5(2):331–348.
21. Gokalp HZ, Arasil E, Erdogan A, et al. Tentorial meningiomas. Neurosurgery 1995; 36(1):46–51.
22. Sekhar LN, Jannetta PJ, Maroon JC. Tentorial meningiomas: surgical management and results. Neurosurgery 1984; 14(3):268–275.
23. Bassiouni H, Hunold A, Asgari S, Stolke D. Tentorial meningiomas: clinical results in 81 patients treated microsurgically. Neurosurgery 2004; 55(1):108–116.
24. Sugita K, Yoshio S. Tentorial meningiomas. In: Al Mefty O (ed). Meningiomas. New York: Raven Press, 1991:357–361.
25. Samii M, Ammirati M. Cerebellopontine angle meningiomas. In: Al-Mefty O (ed). Meningiomas. New York: Raven Press, 1991:503–515.
26. Prabhu SS, DeMonte F. Complete resection of a complex glomus jugulare tumor with extensive venous involvement. Case report. Neurosurg Focus 2004; 17(2):E12.
27. Kuroiwa T, Ogawa D, Ukita T, et al. Hemodynamics of the transverse sinus using cine angiography. No Shinkei Geka 1995; 23(4):311–314.
28. Carriero A, Magarelli N, Samuele F, Palumbo L, Bocola V, Iezzi A. [The torcular Herophili: the diagnostic pitfalls in TOF 3D magnetic resonance angiography]. Radiol Med (Torino) 1994; 87(4):441–446.
29. Strasberg Z, Kirschberg G, Tuttle RJ, Holgate RC. Meningioma of torcular simulating dural arteriovenous malformation. Can Med Assoc J 1977; 117(6):582–583.
30. Convers P, Michel D, Brunon J, Sindou M. Dural arteriovenous fistulas of the posterior cerebral fossa and thrombosis of the lateral sinus. Discussion of their relations and treatment apropos of 2 cases. Neurochirurgie; 32(6):495–500.
31. Sindou M, Mercier P, Bokor J, Brunon J. Bilateral thrombosis of the transverse sinuses: microsurgical revascularization with venous bypass. Surg Neurol 1980;13:215–220
32. Uchiyama N, Hasegawa M, Kita D, Yamashita J. Paramedian supracerebellar transtentorial approach for a medial tentorial meningioma with supratentorial extension: technical case report. Neurosurgery 2001; 49(6):1470–1473.
33. Castro I, Christoph DH, Landeiro JA. Combined supra/infratentorial approach to tentorial meningiomas. Arq Neuropsiquiatr 2005; 63(1):50–54.
34. Nagashima H, Kobayashi S, Takemae T, Tanaka Y. Total resection of torcular herophili hemangiopericytoma with radial artery graft: case report. Neurosurgery 1995; 36(5):1024–1027.
35. Alvernia JE, Sindou MP. Preoperative neuroimaging findings as a predictor of the surgical plane of cleavage: prospective study of 100 consecutive cases of intracranial meningioma. J Neurosurg 2004; 100(3):422–430.
36. Sindou M, Alaywan M. Role of pia mater vascularization of the tumour in the surgical outcome of intracranial meningiomas. Acta Neurochir (Wien) 1994; 130(1–4):90–93.
37. Alaywan M, Sindou M. Prognostic factors in the surgery for intracranial meningioma. Role of the tumoral size and arterial vascularization originating from the pia mater. Study of 150 cases. Neurochirurgie 1993; 39(6):337–347.

53
Falcotentorial and Pineal Region Meningiomas

Ivan Radovanovic and Nicolas de Tribolet

Introduction

Meningiomas arising at the falcotentorial junction and in the pineal region are rare and account for about 1 % of all intracranial meningiomas. Moreover, few reports in the modern literature describe these lesions, and to-date less than 100 cases are documented.

Historically, meningiomas of the falcotentorial junction were described as a subtype of meningiomas of the posterior falx by Cushing and Eisenhardt in their seminal work on meningiomas in 1938 (1). However, previous surgical reports can be found in works by Olivecrona in 1934 (2) and Balado and Tiscornia in 1927 (3). There have also been controversies as to the exact definition of pineal region meningiomas since their first description by Sachs in 1962 (4) and then Piatt and Campbell in 1983(5). This initial series included meningiomas of the falcotentorial junction. In contrast, Stein stated that only meningiomas of the velum interpositum and freely lying in the pineal region should be considered as pineal region meningiomas (6). More recently, Konovalov considered all meningiomas in the vicinity of the pineal gland irrespective of their insertion on the falcotentorial dura as meningiomas of the pineal region (7). In contrast, Tung and Apuzzo distinguish pineal region meningioma arising from the falcotentorial junction and secondarily extending into the pineal region and the posterior third ventricle from meningiomas taking origin from the velum interpositum without dural attachment occupying the pineal region and the posterior third ventricle (8). We will describe the falcotentorial junction and pineal region meningiomas together and mention nuances in their respective management when necessary.

Special Considerations

Classification

Yasargil's classification of tentorial meningiomas is the most used and defines 10 types of tumors according to their location on the cerebellar tentorium. Falcotentorial meningiomas are referred as T3–T8 (8–10) (Fig. 53.1A). Falcotentorial meningiomas can be further divided according to their insertion and projection on sagittal magnetic resonance imaging (MRI) as anterior or posterior and superior or inferior, and on axial MRI as midline symmetrical and midline asymmetrical (11–13) (Fig. 53-1B). Pineal region meningiomas can be classified as free-lying masses in the pineal space without dural attachment, tumors attached to the tentorium and/or the falx without functional compromise of the venous system, or tumors with attachment but with occlusion of the galenic system (7).

In 1995, Asari et al. collected 38 surgical patients with falcotentorial meningiomas described in the literature (13). Since then another 53 falcotentorial and pineal region meningiomas were described in various series (7,9,14–16) for a total number of 91. The proportion of these tumors ranges from 0.3 to 1% of different meningioma series (7,14,15)

Clinical Presentation and Natural History

The most prominent and frequent presenting clinical symptoms or signs of falcotentorial and pineal region meningiomas are headaches, gait disturbances, mental changes, papilloedema, and, less frequently, hearing impairment, visual disturbances, pyramidal deficits, diplopia or other cranial nerve deficits, urinary incontinence, or Parinaud's sign. Obstructive hydrocephalus is present in the majority of the cases at the time of diagnosis as pineal region and falcotentorial meningiomas are often discovered when the tumors are already large due to the paucity and relative unspecific character of the symptoms. Several authors have noted the infrequency of Parinaud's sign compared with other pineal region tumors. In our experience of nine falcotentorial meningiomas, Parinaud's sign was never present preoperatively.

Diagnostic Studies

MRI is nowadays the gold standard diagnostic tool for meningiomas. Falcotentorial meningiomas appear as other

485

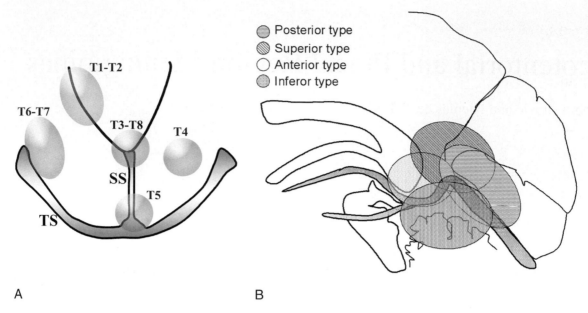

Fɪɢ. 53-1. (A) Classification of tentorial meningiomas according to their origin from the tentorium; falcotentorial meningioma are T3–T8. (B) Classification of falcotentorial meningiomas according to saggital imaging

intracranial meningiomas on MRI: they are iso- or hypointense on T1 and T2 sequences, and they enhance more or less homogeneously upon gadolinium injection on T1-gated sequences (Fig. 53-2A,C, and E). Asari et al. found a correlation between homogeneous enhancement and meningotheliomatous features at histology as well as between heterogeneous enhancement and transitional or malignant histology (12). MRI is also used to study the invasion of meningiomas into the falcotentorial dura, which often do but may not necessarily enhance. The role of angio-MRI to study the arterial supply and especially the patency of the venous system is not clear, but it still remains inferior to digital subtraction angiography (DSA).

DSA allows studying details of the vascular anatomy, which is highly complex in this region. The arterial supply of tumors attached to the falcotentorial dura comes mainly from the internal carotid artery (ICA) meningeal branches supplying the falx and the tentorium, especially the Bernasconi-Cassinari tentorial artery (Fig. 53-3A, B). In addition, vascularization from the following arteries is common: the posterior choroidal arteries, the superior cerebellar artery (SCA), the posterior cerebral artery (PCA), the pericallosal arteries, and the meningo-hypophyseal trunk branches. Feeding from branches of the external carotid artery (ECA), such as the occipital artery, is frequent as well. Meningiomas of the velum interpositum freely lying in the pineal region are frequently attached to the tela choroidea and are more often supplied by posterior choroidal arteries (7,8,12,13,15,17).

Asari et al. have carefully studied the displacement of the arterial and venous systems by falcotentorial meningiomas (13,18). The PCA is generally displaced in the quadrigeminal cistern and the posterior choroidal arteries are displaced anteroinferiorly. The vein of Galen and the internal cerebral veins are displaced anteriorly and inferiorly (Fig. 53-3C) by anterior and superior tumors, and superiorly by inferior falcotentorial meningiomas. Occlusion or stenosis of the straight sinus and the vein of Galen is common (Fig. 53-3C, D); however, compromise of the internal cerebral veins or the basal veins of Rosenthal is less frequent. Occasionally a blood flow inversion can be seen in these veins (Fig. 53-3D). It must, however, be kept in mind that not visualizing a venous sinus or a vein encased in a tumor on DSA does not mean that the structure is occluded and that it could be safely sacrificed without meticulous intraoperative examination. Collateral circulation often develops (Fig. 53-3C, D). Embolization of these tumors has been described as difficult and often not possible, and therefore, the usefulness of such a procedure remains unclear.

Surgical Technique

General Considerations

From a surgical point of view, falcotentorial and pineal region meningiomas represent challenging lesions that sum up the complexity of surgical approaches to the pineal region and of meningioma resection in deep locations.

Surgery of pineal region and falcotentorial meningiomas shares much with surgical techniques for other pineal and pineal region tumors, which can be accessed by the occipital transtentorial approach or the infratentorial supracerebellar approach. However, surgery is rendered more difficult by the specific features of meningiomas such as dural attachments, which in meningiomas are deeply located and difficult to approach, as well as venous sinus invasion, which compromise the deep venous flow draining vital cerebral structures.

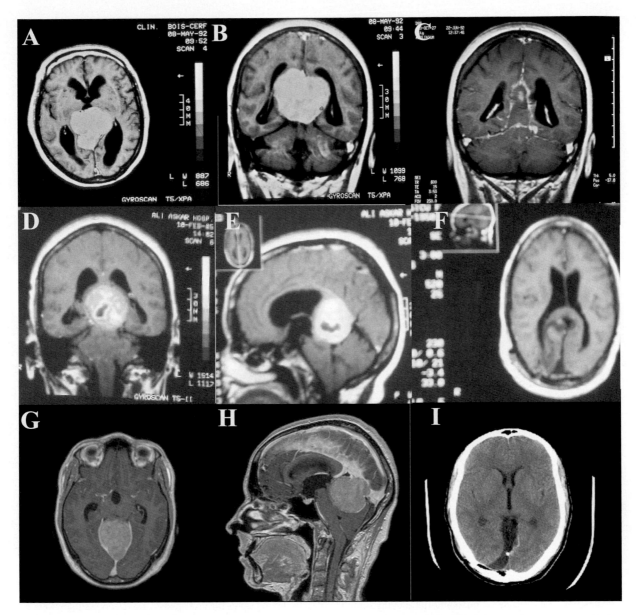

FIG. 53-2. Radiologic aspects of falcotentorial meningiomas. (A) Axial T1-weighted enhanced MRI picture showing the typical homogeneous aspect of a meningioma with anterior extension. This 60-year-old female presented with intracranial hypertension, short-term memory loss, gait ataxia, and urinary incontinence. (B) Coronal MRI section of the same case as A, showing the mainly supratentorial extension of the tumor. In this case no collateral venous channels could be demonstrated. (C) Postoperative T1-weighted gadolinium-enhanced MRI showing complete removal. The patient recovered completely except for left homonymous hemianopia, which disappeared 2 years later. (D, E) Coronal and sagittal T1-weighted enhanced MRI picture of another superior and anterior type falcotentorial meningioma. (F) Postoperative MRI shows total tumor revoval as well as right occipital lobe retraction-induced damage resulting in permanent hemianopia. (G, H) Axial and sagittal T1-weighted enhanced MRI pictures of a falcotentorial meningioma with mainly infratentorial extension (inferior type) in a 40-year-old female. (I) Postoperative CT scan showing total tumor removal without evidence of occipital lobe damage; the patient experienced transient metamorphopsia in the immediate postoperative period

Particular attention should be paid to the deep venous structures and the collateral channels, which have to be preserved at all cost. The straight sinus can be excised if it is occluded but must be preserved if it is patent, even at the cost of leaving a small piece of tumor, which can be treated by radiosurgery later.

History and Choice of Approach

Several surgical approaches to the pineal gland, including meningiomas of this region, have been described in the last century.

First, Dandy used a parietal parasagittal transcallosal approach, which occasionally also required an occipital lobectomy (19).

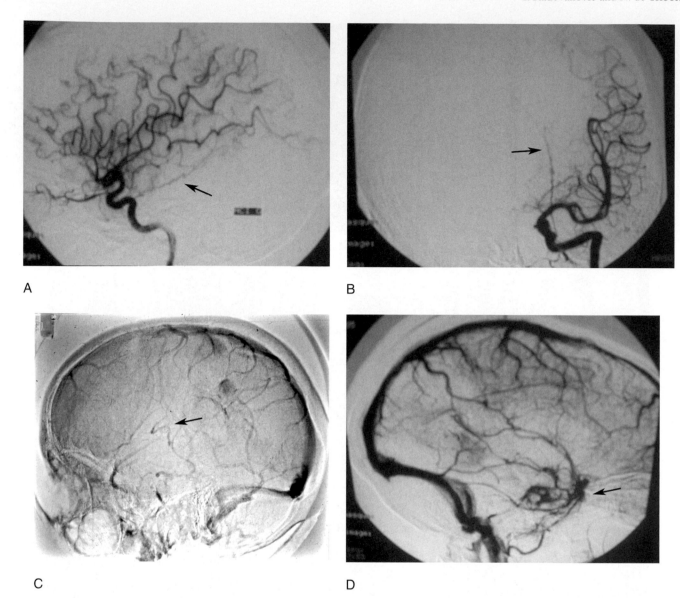

Fıg. 53-3. Angiographic aspects of falcotentorial meningioma. (A, B) DS angiography (arterial phase, right carotid injection) in antero-posterior and lateral views of the patient described in Fig. 53-2G and H showing vascularization of the tumor by a prominent Bernasconi-Cassinari tentorial artery (arrows). (C) Venous phase of the left carotid angiogram of the case described in Fig. 53-2A and B showing complete occlusion of the straight sinus and forward displacement of the internal cerebral veins (arrow). In this case no collateral venous channels could be demonstrated. (D) Venous phase of the case described in Fig. 53-2G and H showing straight sinus occlusion, no visualization of the basal veins of Rosenthal, but an inverted blood flow is seen in these veins on the vertebral angiograms (not shown) with drainage in the cavernous sinus (arrow)

This approach was subsequently favoured by several authors. Further, Van Wagenen described the transventricular approach (20). However, these approaches were plagued by high morbidity and mortality mainly because of lack of modern microsurgical techniques and anesthesia. These approaches to the pineal region are no longer used.

Krause was the first to describe and successfully use the infratentorial supracerebellar approach in three cases (21). In the microsurgical era, Stein further developed and popularized this approach during the 1970s (6,22,23).

Finally, the right suboccipital approach was performed by Poppen (24). This method required extensive lifting of the occipital

lobe after cerebrospinal fluid (CSF) drainage from a ventricular catheter. This technique was modified by Jamieson, who preferred mobilizing the occipital lobe laterally rather than superiorly (25).

The occipital transtentorial and the infratentorial supracerebellar approaches are nowadays accepted as the main standard techniques accessing the pineal region, including for meningiomas of this region.

Occipital Transtentorial Approach (24,26–29)

The occipital transtentorial approach can be performed with the patient in a prone, park-bench (semi-prone), or sitting position. In the park-bench position, which we currently favor, the head is flexed forward with the nose pointed down, allowing the occipital lobe to fall aside with the aid of gravity. At the beginning of our experience we used to favor the sitting position, as advocated by Lapras (27,30). In the sitting position the head is flexed anteriorly to prevent the occipital lobe dropping backward, thus allowing an easier gravity-supported retraction. The standard preventive measures against air embolism including a central venous line, esophageal Doppler, and end-tidal CO_2 monitoring are mandatory and should be installed by an experienced neuro-anesthesiologist team, although we have never experienced significant air embolism during the occipital approach.

The side of the approach is chosen considering the direction of tumor extension, the shape of the torcular, and the location of major occipital bridging veins, although in general, large cortical bridging veins are rarely present in the occipital area. All this taken into consideration, we usually prefer approaching from the right side whenever possible.

The skin incision is made in an inverted U-shape over the right occipital region starting 1.5 cm on the left of the occipital protuberance, extending upward parallel to the midline, next turning right, and finally downward to reach the right mastoid (Fig. 53-4A). This should allow exposing at least 2 cm of the sagittal suture superiorly and the occipital protuberance inferiorly. Two burr holes on the midline, one over the torcular and another 6 cm away and upward, allow detaching the dura from the superior sagittal sinus and the torcular Herophili. An occipital bone flap exposing 2 cm of the transverse sinus, the torcular, and 6 cm of the superior sagittal sinus is elevated. The medial cut should extend 1 cm beyond the sagittal sinus to the left (Fig. 53-4A). The dura is opened in an inverted C-shape and turned over the superior sagittal sinus, exposing

the occipital lobe. The incision does not run along and parallel to the transverse sinus but extends obliquely down to the torcular, leaving a sleeve of dura that will prevent the occipital pole bulging backwards. The dural flap is suspended toward the controlateral side with some traction on the sagittal sinus. The occipital horn of the ipsilateral ventricle is tapped to release CSF. The falx and tentorium are exposed and the tumor is visualized (Fig. 53-5A). As mentioned above, no large occipital bridging veins are usually present; however, when such veins are encountered, they could limit significantly the exposure. Nevertheless, they should be preserved as their sacrifice might cause a hemorrhagic infarction of the occipital lobe as we have encountered in one of our cases of pineal tumor.

The surgeon then proceeds in the unilateral interhemispheric space between the falx and the medial side of the occipital lobe. In the sitting position a retractor is necessary to lift the occipital lobe aside, but when the patient is in the park-bench position, most of the time the procedure can be done without placing any retractors on the occipital lobe, which falls down with gravity and is deflated by CSF drainage. The straight sinus is followed until the incisura of the tentorium is exposed. The tentorial incision is made postero-anteriorly and begins 2 cm anterior to the torcular and 0.5 cm lateral to the straight sinus and proceeds parallel to the sinus until the falcotentorial junction is reached (Fig. 53-5B). Great care should be taken not to injure the vein of Galen, which is sometimes adherent to or covered by the falcotentorial dura.

In the case of falcotentorial meningiomas, the tumor usually encases the straight sinus and the falcotentorial junction. The tentorial incision is then made laterally to the tumor and proceeds again postero-anteriorly to the free tentorial edge interrupting the vascular supply on the way (Fig. 53-5B). The venous channels and lakes of the tentorium can cause significant bleeding,

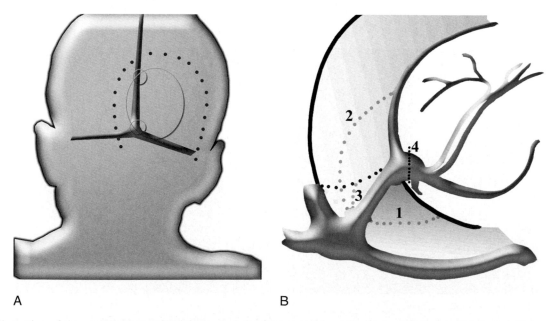

A   B

FIG. 53-4. Illustration of the occipital transtentorial approach for falcotentorial meningiomas. (A) Inverted U-shape incision over the right occipital region, burr holes over the torcular and superior sagittal sinus and craniotomy. (B) Order of incision—1: right tentorium; 2: falx along the superior border of the tumor; 3: left tentorium; 4: vein of Galen

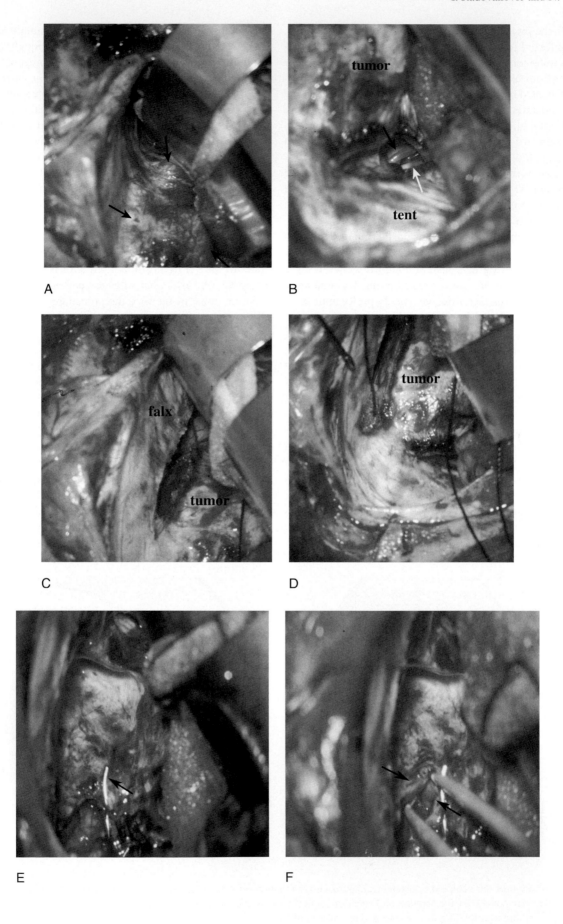

but they are usually well controlled by bipolar coagulation. We routinely use the Landolt pituitary bipolar, which allows coagulating dural sleeves at a straight angle. However, tentorial vessels can participate in the collateral venous drainage of an already scarce venous return, therefore, one should spare as much tentorial surface as possible. The tentorial flap is reflected laterally. The surgeon can then see the superior cerebellar artery and the IV cranial nerve running around the brain stem. In falcotentorial meningioma surgery, the falx is then incised in the same way to expose the left side of the tumor (Fig. 53-5C). The left side of the tent is then cut (Fig. 53-5D). At this point the posterior part of the straight sinus can be ligated and sectioned only if it is occluded. This allows dissection of the tumor on all its faces after debulking. The most dangerous part of the dissection will be along the anterior pole, where the deep veins will be in contact with the tumor. After the removal of the tumor, what is left of the vein of Galen is dissected, clipped, and sectioned (Fig. 53-5E). However, if the vein of Galen and the internal cerebral veins are extensively invaded, it is wiser to leave residual tumor around these veins for secondary treatment by radiosurgery. At the end of the procedure the surgeon can inspect the splenium of the corpus callosum, the internal cerebral veins, the superior cerebellar artery, the quadrigeminal plate, and the superior and medial cerebellar peduncles (Fig. 53-5F).

In cases where the tumor is extending almost exclusively inferiorly and anteriorly (Fig. 53-2G, H), tumor removal can be achieved without cutting the falx and the inferior sagittal sinus. The volume of the tumor makes access to the controlateral tentorial dura possible from below after tumor debulking is done. This strategy has the theoretical advantage of preserving as much collateral venous flow as possible to minimize the risk of postoperative venous hypertension.

For meningiomas freely lying in the pineal region, the technique is essentially the same as for other pineal neoplasms. As our series does not specifically contain pure pineal region meningiomas freely lying without dural attachment, we will describe the technique we are employing for pineal region tumors in general. After the tentorium has been divided and the dura reflected, one stay suture can be placed on the dura below the vein of Galen to increase the visibility superiorly and to the left. When the thick arachnoid covering the cistern of the great vein of Galen becomes visible, a retractor is placed on the occipital lobe, if necessary, avoiding an overcompression of the calcarine gyrus and an avulsion injury of the medial occipital veins, which could provoke a venous infarction, believed to be the cause of postoperative hemianopsia. Now the dorsal aspect of the splenium comes into sight. The thick arachnoid covering the vein of Galen has to be cut first laterally and inferiorly on both sides, avoiding injury to the deep venous system. The medial occipital vein is mobilized first, allowing further retraction of the occipital lobe. An extensive dissection of the arachnoid tissue helps to expose the ipsilateral medial occipital vein, the pericallosal veins, the precentral cerebellar vein, and the tributary veins. The superior vermian vein and the precentral vein can be coagulated and sectioned, but in small tumors they can be preserved; this allows further dissection upward and the identification of the great vein of Galen. If the tumor extends posteriorly, it will be apparent at this point. The dissection proceeds laterally toward the right ambient cistern to identify the P3 portion of posterior cerebral artery, the fourth cranial nerve emerging below the inferior colliculus, and the third segment of the basal vein. If the tumor is small, this can be done on both sides. If it is large, the contralateral side should be dissected after debulking of the tumor.

Inferiorly, the identification of the quadrigeminal plate will also depend on the position of the tumor. If the tumor is posterior, the quadrigeminal plate will be covered by it, whereas if it is more anterior, the quadrigeminal plate will be pushed backward and downward by the tumor, making it easily identifiable after opening of the cistern. A careful inspection of the sagittal sections of the MRI will allow one to predict these findings. The small arteries running in the arachnoid can be coagulated and divided; however, all the arteries vascularizing the quadrigeminal plate should be carefully preserved. The dissection can proceed on both sides to separate the lateral aspect of the tumor from the pulvinar. The vascularization of the tumor usually comes from branches of the postero-medial and postero-lateral choroidal arteries. During the dissection of the lateral part of the tumor, great care should be taken not to injure the basilar veins of Rosenthal. These veins will form an arch delineating the supero-lateral borders of the operative field. In very large tumors, dissection can also proceed above these veins. The last part of the dissection enters the third ventricle, allowing exposure and removal of the superior aspect of the tumor adherent to the velum interpositum, the internal cerebral veins, and the anterior aspect of the vein of Galen. One entry to the roof of the third ventricle is through the space between the vein of Galen and the splenium. It is usually not necessary to cut the splenium. Cutting the posterior pericallosal veins allows the splenium to be detached from the great vein. The bilateral internal cerebral veins will appear in the velum interpositum cistern. A dissection of the cistern will expose the anterior choroidal artery

FIG. 53-5. Operative steps in falcotentorial meningioma surgery. (A) The occipital lobe has been retracted superolaterally to expose the tumor (arrows). (B) The tent has been sectioned on the right side and the superior cerebellar artery (black arrow) and IV cranial nerve (white arrow) are visible anteriorly. (C) The falx has been sectioned along the superior edge of the tumor, allowing exposure of the tumor and sectioning of the tent on the left side. (D) The tumor can be mobilized—its attachment to the straight sinus on its posterior aspect can be seen. Final steps of falcotentorial meningioma removal. (E) After ligature and section of the straight sinus, debulking, dissection and removal of the tumor, what was left of the vein of Galen was dissected, clipped (arrow), and sectioned. (F) The splenium of the corpus callosum and beneath it, the internal cerebral veins can be seen (arrows) in the third ventricle as well as the ventral part of tumor. Another entry, which we actually favor, is below the vein of Galen and the internal cerebral veins. A subchoroidal trans-velum interpositum approach has also been described previously (31). Very tough adherences may be encountered, and it is wiser to leave some tumor behind rather than to damage the internal cerebral veins. If bleeding occurs, coagulation should be avoided and hemostasis achieved by packing surgicel. After complete removal of the tumor, the surgeon will have a good view into the third ventricle and its left lateral wall. The right lateral wall, however, might be difficult to visualize. The view into the third ventricle can extend all the way to the foramina of Monroe and the lamina terminalis. Since an en bloc removal of the tumor is rarely possible, all the different steps of this dissection should be preceded by a gentle and piecemeal intracapsular decompression of the tumor, which will allow preparing excellent cleavage planes. This is particularly true for the separation of the tumor from the quadrigeminal plate and the periaqueductal tissue.

Care should be taken to "unplug" the aqueduct of Sylvius. When this is properly achieved, no postoperative drainage of CSF will be necessary.

Closure is done in the usual way with a running suture on the dura, and the bone flap is fixed with titanium miniplates.

Supracerebellar Infratentorial Approach (22,23,32)

The supracerebellar infratentorial approach is a major gateway to the pineal region and a standard in treating pineal tumors; however, in most cases it is not suitable for the resection of falcotentorial meningiomas, as stated by Stein (6). Indeed, supratentorial extentions and dural attachments on the falx are difficult to reach from below because of the limited angle of view in the supero-inferior axis. However, this approach has been used with success for the resection of pineal region meningiomas originating from the velum interpositum, which have no dural attachments and are surgically comparable to other pineal tumors. When employing the infratentorial supra-cerebellar approach, the patient is placed in a sitting position so that the cerebellum can fall inferiorly. A vertical midline skin incision extends from 2 cm above the external occipital protuberance down to the level of the C2 spinal process, or lower, when a patient has a thick neck. A high-speed drill is used to make two burr holes just beside the torcular on each side of the midline and to crosscut the sinuses because of a risk of tearing them with a craniotome. Having reached the lower borders of the transverse sinuses, a craniotome is used. The craniotomy does not include the foramen magnum. After the craniotomy, the surgeon must identify and seal any venous leaks before air embolism occurs. The risk of air embolism is higher in the infratentorial approach than in the occipital approach.

The dura is incised in a dull "U"-shaped fashion, and the dural flap is suspended upward, exerting traction on the transverse sinuses. Two incisions in the dural flap may be utilized to improve the exposure, as Stein suggested (32). The poste-

rior bridging veins between the cerebellum and the tentorium are coagulated and transected. One retractor is then placed to pull up the tentorium. With the patient in the sitting position, a retractor over the cerebellum is rarely necessary. This creates a corridor that leads the surgeon's view along the straight sinus to the great vein of Galen, situated in the very deep superior portion of the operative field.

Dissection of the arachnoid tissue in the supracerebellar and the quadrigeminal cisterns should be performed, as described for the occipital approach. Pursuing the dissection symmetrically on both sides, a gentle downward traction of the cerebellum exposes the pineal area. A further downward retraction of the vermis can be exerted after sectioning of the superior vermian and precentral veins. A thorough dissection of all the bridging veins and of the superior vermian and precentral veins may occasionally cause venous infarction of the superior aspect of the vermis.

Removal of the tumor will also proceed similarly to that of the occipital approach. The infratentorial supracerebellar approach opens a view strictly through the midline that can provide an easy orientation for the complex anatomic structures around the pineal area. This approach will allow a perfect identification of all the midline structures and symmetric exposure of both walls and the roof of the third ventricle. Under direct observation, tight tumor adhesion can be freed from the internal cerebral veins or the great veins. In some cases, however, a tumor dissection from the periaqueductal tissue and the quadrigeminal plate might be more difficult using this approach than using the occipital transtentorial approach. The opening of the third ventricle can be closed by fibrin sealant to prevent excessive CSF leakage. A watertight closure of the dura will be done with a running suture after the surgeon has asked the anesthesiologist to compress the jugular veins and has sealed any venous leaks.

Combined Infratentorial/Supratentorial Approach (33,34)

Shekar and colleagues have described a combined supratentorial/infratentorial approach for large pineal region meningiomas, and they have more recently extended this experience to large pineal tumors in general. The technique consists of exposing the infratentorial and supratentorial occipital dura, the superior sagittal sinus, and the torcular as well as the transverse sinus, which is divided on the nondominant side. The occipital lobe and the cerebellum can then be easily retracted to expose the tentorium, which is divided, as described above, to reach the tumor and the pineal region.

The theoretical advantages of this extended approach are the wide unhampered exposure of the tumor and the surrounding important structures, such as the deep veins, that can restrict the exposure through the occipital transtentorial approach, the decreased retraction of the occipital lobe and the cerebellum, and, finally, better control of the posterior third ventricle and the medullary velum.

Although we agree that this approach can be useful for resecting very big falcotentorial meningiomas, we did not use it in our experience even for exceptionally large tumors such as the one described in Fig. 53-2A, B. Moreover, we have some concerns about dividing the transverse sinus, even if it is reconstructed at the end of the surgery, in a situation where the venous return can easily decompensate, as discussed above.

Outcome and Complications

Our experience consists of 9 falcotentorial meningiomas out of 53 pineal and pineal region tumors treated with surgery excluding germinomas. All meningiomas were operated using the occipital transtentorial approach. In the beginning we favored the sitting position. Complete resection was achieved in 5 cases, and subtotal tumor removal was done in the remaining 4 cases. The reason for leaving residual tumor was always to preserve the deep venous drainage and avoid venous hypertension and infarction by disturbing potentially essential collateral venous flow that often develops in tumors that have occluded the straight sinus or the Galenic system.

There was no mortality in our series. Surgery-related complications in our 53 cases of pineal region tumors included transitory metamorphopsia in one patient, permanent hemianopsia in one patient, transient fourth cranial nerve palsy in two patients, and Parinaud syndrome in one patient.

There were no long-term complications in our series of falcotentorial meningioma patients. Our results together with those of other selected published series are summarized in Table 53-1.

Summary

Falcotentorial and pineal region meningiomas are surgically challenging lesions because they are deeply located and in close contact with important nervous structures and often intermingled with the deep venous system, which is vital.

TABLE 53-1. Nonvisual Complications in Selected Series of Falcotentorial Meningioma Surgeries.

Study (Ref.)	n	Total removal	Postop complications
Asari et al. 1995 (13)	7	7 GTR	1 left hemiparesis
Konovalov et al. 1995 (7)	10	10 GTR	4 patients with KPS<80
Okami et al. 2001 (14)	4	2 GTR/2 subtotal	1 patient: mild left hemiparesis
Quinones-Hinojosa et al. 2003(17)	6	3 GTR/3 subtotal	No permanent deficit
Goto et al. 2006 (16)	14	11 GTR/3 subtotal	2 patients with GTR: permanent memory deficits
Present series	9	5 GTR/4 subtotal	No permanent deficit

GTR, gross total removal (Simpson I–III); KPS, Karnofsky performance score.

Moreover, at the time of diagnosis they are often already large masses, even if the symptoms are usually mild. The vast majority of these lesions are benign but too large for primary radiosurgical management, therefore, microsurgery remains the treatment of choice. Ideally, radical resection should be the goal whenever possible to prevent recurrence. However, even if modern neurosurgical techniques allow safe access to the pineal region with low morbidity, in many cases aggressive resection will result in unavoidable and potentially fatal complications, especially due to compromise of deep venous flow. Therefore, we strongly advocate a conservative strategy respecting the deep venous system even at the cost of leaving small tumor residues around the invaded or encased veins that can be secondarily amenable to radiosurgery. It could also be wise to postpone surgery for a few months to allow an encased straight sinus to become occluded and allow an efficient collateral flow to develop. The occipital transtentorial approach is more convenient for most falcotentorial meningiomas, and the infratentorial supracerebellar approach can be reserved for small and pure pineal region meningiomas arising from the velum interpositum. Using these principles, we and others have achieved good results in treating these complicated lesions.

References

1. Cushing H, Eisenhardt L. Meningiomas. Charles C. Thomas, Springfield, IL. 1938.
2. Olivecrona H. Die parasagittalen Meningeome. Leipzig: G. Thieme; 1934:144.
3. Balado T. Tumor de la hoz del cerebro pediculado a desarrollo subtentirial. Arch Argent Neurol 1927;1:297–310.
4. Sachs E Jr, Avman N, Fisher RG. Meningiomas of pineal region and posterior part of 3 d ventricle. J Neurosurg 1962;19:325–31.
5. Piatt JH Jr, Campbell GA. Pineal region meningioma: report of two cases and literature review. Neurosurgery 1983;12(4):369–76.
6. Stein BM. Surgical treatment of pineal tumors. Clin Neurosurg 1979;26:490–510.
7. Konovalov AN, Spallone A, Pitzkhelauri DI. Meningioma of the pineal region: a surgical series of 10 cases. J Neurosurg 1996;85(4):586–90.
8. Tung H, Apuzzo MLJ. Meningiomas of the third ventricle and pineal region. In: Al-Mefty O, ed. Meningiomas. New York: Raven Press; 1991:583–92.
9. Bassiouni H, Hunold A, Asgari S, Stolke D. Tentorial meningiomas: clinical results in 81 patients treated microsurgically. Neurosurgery 2004;55(1):108–16; discussion 16–8.
10. Yasargil MG. In: Yasargil MG, ed. Microneurosurgery, Vol. 4. Stuttgart: Thieme; 1994.
11. Asari S, Ohmoto T. Falcotentorial junction meningioma: neuroradiological findings and surgical treatment. No Shinkei Geka 1993;21(7):585–603.
12. Asari S, Yabuno N, Ohmoto T. Magnetic resonance characteristics of meningiomas arising from the falcotentorial junction. Comput Med Imaging Graph 1994;18(3):181–5.
13. Asari S, Maeshiro T, Tomita S, et al. Meningiomas arising from the falcotentorial junction. Clinical features, neuroimaging studies, and surgical treatment. J Neurosurg 1995;82(5):726–38.

14. Okami N, Kawamata T, Hori T, Takakura K. Surgical treatment of falcotentorial meningioma. J Clin Neurosci 2001;8(Suppl 1):15–8.

15. Raco A, Agrillo A, Ruggeri A, et al. Surgical options in the management of falcotentorial meningiomas: report of 13 cases. Surg Neurol 2004;61(2):157–64; discussion 64.

16. Goto T, Ohata K, Morino M, et al. Falcotentorial meningioma: surgical outcome in 14 patients. J Neurosurg 2006;104(1):47–53.

17. Quinones-Hinojosa A, Chang EF, McDermott MW. Falcotentorial meningiomas: clinical, neuroimaging, and surgical features in six patients. Neurosurg Focus 2003;14(6):e11.

18. Asari S, Yabuno N, Ohmoto T. Collateral venous channels in occlusion of deep cerebral veins and sinuses. No To Shinkei 1994;46(10):935–9.

19. Dandy WE. An operation for the removal of pineal tumors. Surg Gynecol Obset 1921;33:113–9.

20. Van Wagenen WP. A surgical approach for the removal of certain pineal tumors. Report of a case. Surg Gynecol Obset 1931;53:216–20.

21. Krause F. Operative Freilegung der Vierhüge, nebst Beobachtungen beim Hirndruck und Dekompression. Zentralbl Chir 1926;53:2812–9.

22. Stein BM. The infratentorial supracerebellar approach to pineal lesions. J Neurosurg 1971;35(2):197–202.

23. Stein BM. Supracerebellar-infratentorial approach to pineal tumors. Surg Neurol 1979;11(5):331–7.

24. Poppen JL. The right occipital approach to a pinealoma. J Neurosurg 1966;25(6):706–10.

25. Jamieson KG. Excision of pineal tumors. J Neurosurg 1971;35(5):550–3.

26. Poppen JL, Marino R, Jr. Pinealomas and tumors of the posterior portion of the third ventricle. J Neurosurg 1968;28(4):357–64.

27. Lapras C, Patet JD, Mottolese C, Lapras C Jr. Direct surgery for pineal tumors: occipital-transtentorial approach. Prog Exp Tumor Res 1987;30:268–80.

28. Lazar ML, Clark K. Direct surgical management of masses in the region of the vein of Galen. Surg Neurol 1974;2(1):17–21.

29. Reid WS, Clark WK. Comparison of the infratentorial and transtentorial approaches to the pineal region. Neurosurgery 1978;3(1):1–8.

30. Lapras C, Patet JDM. Controversies, techniques and strategies for pineal tumor surgery. In: Surgery of the Third Ventricle. Baltimore: Williams & Wilkins; 1987.

31. Lavyne MH, Patterson RH. Subchoroidal trans-velum interpositum approach to mid-third ventricular tumors. Neurosurgery 1983;12(1):86–94.

32. Stein BM. Infratentorial supracerebellar approach. In: Surgery of the Third Ventricle. Baltimore: Williams & Wilkins; 1987.

33. Sekhar LN, Goel A. Combined supratentorial and infratentorial approach to large pineal-region meningioma. Surg Neurol 1992;37(3):197–201.

34. Ziyal IM, Sekhar LN, Salas E, Olan WJ. Combined supra/infratentorial-transsinus approach to large pineal region tumors. J Neurosurg 1998;88(6):1050–7.

54
Intraventricular Meningiomas

Peter A. Winkler, Ralf M. Buhl, and Jörg-Christian Tonn

Introduction

Intraventricular meningiomas account for approximately 1.5% of meningiomas (1–4). During infancy and adolescence, these tumors are considerably more frequent; in fact, although meningiomas in this age account for only 1–2% of all intracranial tumors, 15% of these are intraventricular (5–18).

We collected information on more than 550 intraventricular meningiomas from the literature published up until 2006: 80%of these were localized in the lateral ventricles, 15% in the third ventricle, and the remaining 5% in the fourth ventricle. About 8% of those from the lateral ventricles are located around the foramen of Monro, the rest in the ventricle trigone. In addition to the 522 cases reviewed from the published neurosurgical literature, we obtained information from reports published by radiologists, neuroradiologists and other clinicians, and via personal communications from experienced neurosurgeons (6,7,13,19–30).

Our own experience with 25 patients with intraventricular meningiomas focused on the meticulous neuropsychological follow-up examination. Twenty-four of them were located in the lateral ventricle and one in the third ventricle.

This chapter deals first with meningiomas of the lateral ventricles, then with those of the third ventricle, and finally, with those located in the fourth ventricle.

Meningiomas of the Lateral Ventricles

History

In 1854, Shaw (31) described the first intraventricular meningioma. At autopsy, he found the tumor as hard and fibrous, situated at the level of the ventricular trigone in a patient who had presented with language disturbances and epilepsy prior to death. Similar cases were described in 1881 by MacDowall (32) and in 1923 by Dreifuss (33). In 1927, Oberling (34) published a meticulous description of a meningoblastoma of the choroid plexus. To our knowledge, Harvey Cushing was the first to perform radical removal of an intraventricular meningioma in 1916; the patient was still alive 21 years later. In 1938, Cushing and Eisenhardt (35) published their milestone monograph on meningiomas and reported having operated on two other similar tumors (1% of a total of 313 surgically treated intracranial meningiomas). The second neurosurgeon to successfully perform this type of operation was Dandy (36). By means of ventriculography, he was able to diagnose and then remove an intraventricular tumor. He later reported two further operated cases, part of a series of 15 intraventricular tumors. Additional reports were published by other authors of that time (37–46).

In his excellent work, Delandsheer (47) described 175 meningiomas of the lateral ventricles culled from the literature with details regarding clinical history, surgical techniques, and therapeutic results. Other important publications at that time are those of Obrador (48), consisting of 8 cases (2.3% of 315 intracranial meningiomas surgically treated), Arseni (49) on a series of 17 patients, Kobayashi (50) regarding 11 meningiomas of the lateral ventricles, and Fornari (51), who reported 18 cases.

More recently several case series of varying size have been published by Gruss (52) with 4 cases, Conforti with 10 intraventricular cases (53), Bret with 3 cases (54), Nakamura (55) with 16 cases, Erman (56) with 8 cases, Bertalanffy (57) with 16 cases, Buhl (58) with 5 cases (which included a detailed neuropsychological outcome study), and finally, Liu (59) with 25 patients.

Pathology

The first description of pathologic anatomy of meningiomas in general was given by Cushing and Eisenhardt (35) in their brilliant monograph. They distinguished two types of meningiomas of the ventricular trigone: the first originating from the choroid plexus and extending freely into the ventricular cavity, the second originating from the tela choroidea and developing partly into the ventricular cavity and partly into the surrounding brain substance. Nowadays, this differentiation is considered as a problem of size and development of a tumor: a small tumor develops within the ventricular cavity while a larger one involves the ependyma and extends into the surrounding brain structures.

Meningiomas generally originate from meningothelial inclusion bodies normally present in the arachnoid and tela choroidea. Russell and Rubinstein (60), in their classic *Pathology of Tumors of the Nervous System,* state that tumors may also originate from the mesenchymal stroma of the choroid plexus. Histologically speaking, Cushing and Eisenhardt attributed these meningiomas to a predominantly psammomatous nature, although Abbott and Courville believed them to be fibroblastic. Of the 175 cases of intraventricular meningiomas studied from the literature, Delandsheer (47) found 85 to have fibroblastic behavior and only 10 psammomatous. In other larger series of patients from the group of Rome (41, 61–63), the nature of the tumor was also found to be predominantly fibroblastic (81%). However, this histologic distinction is somewhat misleading because one tumor may yield various types of cells, and its classification depends on the predominance of one cellular type or another. No signs of malignancy were found in any of the cases of our series, in contrast to that reported by Delandsheer (64) and by Criscuolo and Symon (5). Macroscopically, these meningiomas initially have a roundish appearance, but as they develop and adapt to the form of the cavities, they become melon-like, of hard elastic consistency, and grayish-red in color.

In the past, the lack of suitable diagnostic measures meant that meningiomas often reached an enormous size, such as those described by Zülch (65,66), weighing 618 g, that of Migliavacca (43), weighing 400 g, and that of Obrador (48), weighing 460 g. Meningiomas originating from the anterior tela choroidea, in the vicinity of the foramen of Monro, initially extend into the frontal horn and then toward the cella media, the third ventricle and, occasionally, the contralateral ventricle (67). Kendall (68) presented a case regarding a meningioma that developed "in the velum interpositum and extended through a cavum septum pellucidi and the vulva of the corpus callosum to displace the third ventricle posteriorly." This is an interesting but rare example (62). Tumors originating at the level of the ventricular trigone may begin by occupying the entire trigone and then progressively extending anteriorly toward the cella media, medially toward the third ventricle and, on occasion, the contralateral ventricle, posteriorly toward the occipital horn, and forward and below into the temporal horn. If the tumor blocks circulation of cerebrospinal fluid (CSF), the proximal cavities become dilated and filled with liquid rich in protein. A unilateral hydrocephalus can be developed in these cases. Recently many subtypes and interesting molecular aspects regarding meningiomas have been described, as discussed in detail in previous chapters (69,70).

Clinical Presentation

Since no sufficiently well-defined clinical syndrome existed to allow certain diagnosis of localization in patients with intraventricular meningiomas, it is very difficult to diagnose a meningioma of the lateral ventricles on the basis of the clinical data alone.

Dandy (36) at that time had an outstanding experience with ventricular lesions. In 1934, he was the first to attempt a definition of the clinical picture of tumors of the lateral ventricles on the basis of 15 personal cases and 25 other published cases. He found the most common symptoms to be headache and vomiting. In some of these cases, epilepsy, hemianesthesia, hemiparesis, and hemianopsia were also present. Furthermore, one of his cases presented with staggering and such a severe ataxia as to prompt exploration of the posterior cranial fossa. Subsequently, other authors have reported similar misinterpretations of the site of the lesion (35,40,71).

Four years later, Cushing and Eisenhardt (35), on the basis of two personal cases and 18 others culled from the literature or unpublished reports, outlined a "fairly characteristic" clinical syndrome of intraventricular meningiomas localized in the trigone region. This syndrome was characterized by headache (frequently unilateral), contralateral homonymous hemianopia (often involving the macula), contralateral sensorimotor deficits (generally more marked in the sensory component and sometimes associated with trigeminal numbness), and symptoms suggesting involvement of the cerebellum (in more than half of the cases). When the tumor occupied the dominant hemisphere, dysphasic and paralexic disturbances were also present.

In 1961, Gassel and Davies (40) stressed that the lateral ventricles are one of the most "silent" localizations and pointed out that meningiomas found in this site are among the most voluminous ever found within the cranial vault. This coincides with the fact that many patients have an extremely lengthy clinical history that may last many years. Subsequently, Gassel and Davies and other authors showed that the disturbances directly related to the site of the lesion may, not infrequently, be accompanied by signs of a "false" localization. In 1965, Delandsheer (64) finalized his clinical revision of 175 published cases by stating that meningiomas of the lateral ventricles are characterized by two main features: (1) the presence of a syndrome suggesting both a posterior cranial fossa lesion and a lesion of the cerebral hemisphere; and (2) the intermittent and paroxysmal nature of some symptoms.

In 1968, Arseni (49) also stressed the diagnostic significance of these paroxysmal events that were present in 25% of the cases they treated. These sudden crises, often related to changes in head position, are widely attributed to a temporary block of CSF circulation caused either by the pressure that the tumor exerts on the posterior part of the third ventricle or by obstruction of the foramen of Monro, or to transient exclusion of the temporal or occipital horns. Symptom changes caused by movement of a calcified lateral ventricular meningioma were also described by Imaizumi et al. in their case report (72).

Besides this hydrodynamic effect, some authors (50,64) have suggested a mechanical effect that may be exerted by hard, voluminous tumors directly on the cerebral parenchyma and its coverings, which are then either compressed or stretched as a result of changes in posture.

Finally, others suggest that these phenomena are actually related to spontaneous tumoral bleeding. In fact, several cases with a well-documented syndrome of intraventricular and subarachnoid hemorrhage appear in the literature (64,73–77).

The clinical symptoms and signs of tumors of the lateral ventricles may be attributed both to intracranial hypertension and to the pressure directly exerted by the lesion on the surrounding cerebral parenchyma. Naturally, the severity and nature of these symptoms and signs are proportional to the size of the lesion and its directional development (78). The same "valve mechanism" as for the crisis in patients with colloid cysts is described.

Subjective Symptoms

In about 80% of cases, in the various series, headache seems to be the earliest and most frequent subjective symptom. Dandy (36) and Cushing (35) registered a lateralization of the punctum maximum of headache homologous to the site of the tumor. According to new reports, this is a rare event. It is interesting to note that reports appear in the literature of even contralateral migraines, but headache is generally not localized in a precise spot: it is mainly frontal or bilateral, but may be occipital or even occipital–nuchal. It may be of a progressively worsening nature but is more often intermittent. As mentioned above, changes of head position may cause the sudden and violent onset of pain or exacerbate an existing headache (72,79). These paroxysmal attacks may be accompanied by other symptoms, particularly blurred vision, nausea, vomiting, and vertigo. Vomiting is frequent (about 30% of cases) and often, although not exclusively, associated with headache.

Visual disturbances are the second most frequent subjective symptom (40% of cases) and mainly consist of impaired vision due to papillary edema and/or optic atrophy. Transient episodes of visual obscuration are also frequent and are often accompanied by bouts of headache. Patients suffering from hemianopia are seldom aware of any visual alteration and rarely mention it among their symptoms. Diplopia is rare.

Psychic disturbances are often among the initial symptoms and vary in nature and extent. They include memory disturbances (particularly for recent events), confabulation, mental exhaustion, aggressive behavior, dullness, and decreased verbal output. These disturbances may sometimes dominate the clinical picture and are often only associated with headache: this may give rise to serious diagnostic errors, and, in the past, many such patients were admitted to mental hospitals before a correct diagnosis could be made—sometimes not until autopsy. Huang and Araki (80) report one case in which the patient underwent a lobotomy.

Gait disturbances are frequent but fairly nonspecific in the majority of cases and are described merely as a feeling of unsteadiness.

TABLE 54-1. Clinical Findings of Intra-Ventricular Meningiomas—Own series of 25 Cases.

Headache	80%
Nausea and vomiting	40%
Epileptic attacks	35%
Speech disturbances	30%
Motor deficits	25%
Visual disturbances	20%
Mental disturbances	20%
Sensory deficits	15%
Gait disturbances	15%
Facial paresthesia	10%
Urinary incontinence	5%

Epileptic attacks are often the presenting symptom and present in a fairly high percentage (27%) of these patients. Their nature is usually generalized, but Jacksonian and psychosensory attacks have also been described.

Dysphasic, motor and/or sensory disturbances only rarely appear in the initial symptomatology, generally making their appearance at a later stage. Aphasia is usually mild and may be motor or sensory. Patients seldom complain of alexia. Motor disturbances, when present, are also generally slight and are often described as unilateral or bilateral stiffness of the limbs with a progressive loss of mobility.

Although rare, tremors of the limbs have been reported (64).

Subjective sensitivity disturbances consist mainly of contralateral paresthesia, which is sometimes intermittent. Many reports (63,64,81) quote a fair percentage of facial hypoesthesia and/or paresthesia, mainly contralateral but occasionally homolateral to the tumor.

Disturbances of cochlear origin are rare but may be present in the form of tinnitus and hypoacusia localized unilaterally or bilaterally.

Table 54-1 contains preoperative clinical findings in our own series of 25 intraventricular meningiomas analyzed for this chapter.

Objective Clinical Signs

Meticulous neurologic examination has to include the ophthalmoscopy since an overall prevalence of alterations of the fundus oculi and visual field over other clinical signs was described. Fundus oculi alterations essentially consisted of bilateral papilledema (noted in over 60% of cases) sometimes accompanied by retinal hemorrhage. The literature also carries reports of unilateral papillary stasis, consistent with the tumor site (64) and a contralateral homonymous hemianopia.

Optic atrophy and subatrophy are rarer occurrences. Alterations of visual field, found in over 50% of cases, most frequently consisted of homonymous lateral hemianopia, while upper or lower quadrantanopia and concentric narrowing of the visual field were rarer. Lateral hemianopia may be total or with preservation of macular vision. Ladenheim (42) attributes lower quadrantanopia to compression of the optic pathways at the level of the lateral wall of the trigone and complete hemianopia to a lesion of the genicularcalcarine band. Although defects of the fundus oculi and visual field are not always present simultaneously, one or the other can be found in at least 85% of cases.

Other objective signs are relatively infrequent. Motor disturbances are mainly pyramidal in origin and are present in about 50% of cases, mainly consisting of hypertonia, hyperreflexia, and mild motor deficits. Tremors may be related to motor deficits or may be of an extrapyramidal origin but are more frequently cerebellar. Gait disturbances are due to impairment of motor coordination or balance. Adiadochokinesis, dysmetria, and nystagmus frequently feature in this cerebellar component of the neurologic syndrome.

The fact that intraventricular meningiomas of the dominant hemisphere favor the parieto-temporo-occipital trigone would suggest an early onset of dysphasic disturbances. Actually, these are present in only 40% of cases (where the dominant hemisphere is involved), are modest and nonspecific, and principally consist of aphasia nominum, dysarthria, and sensory aphasia. The incidence of alexia, seldom reported in the literature (23), is probably higher than the official figures suggest.

Objective sensory disturbances have an overall incidence of 20% and mainly consist of hemihypoesthesia and contralateral astereognosis, although digital agnosia and ideational apraxia are also reported.

Objective trigeminal deficits may accompany subjective facial sensitivity disturbances. More often contralateral but sometimes homolateral, these generally consist of facial hypoesthesia and impaired corneal reflex. Involvement of the motor component of the fifth cranial nerve is extremely rare but not impossible. Psychometric tests, when performed, may reveal the exact grade of impairment of verbal performance and intellectual function in patients with psychic disturbances among their early symptoms. Even in patients with nonspecific mental deterioration, the outcome of these tests may reveal even slight alterations; they have also proved useful for assessment of postoperative recovery (55,59).

Diagnostic Studies

Dandy, with the introduction of ventriculography in 1918, was the first neurosurgeon in the world to correctly diagnose, using ventriculography, a tumor of the ventricular trigone subsequently identified as a meningioma. Together with pneumoencephalography, this clinical investigation was used by the previous generation of neurosurgeons for decades in order to obtain precise details regarding the site of the tumor lesion and, in some cases, an indication of its nature (62,72,82). These were replaced by (24) computed tomography (CT) in the 1980s and by (83) magnetic resonance imaging (MRI) in the 1990s.

In this chapter we describe the types of diagnostic investigation that play a minor role in modern neurosurgery, such as plain skull radiography and electroencephalography (EEG); then we concentrate on angiography, CT, and MRI and positron emission tomography (PET).

For small meningiomas, EEG does not supply any useful information, but in larger ones it may reveal generalized dysrhythmia compatible with a deep-seated lesion, with or without focal epileptiform activity in the parieto-occipital region.

The isotope encephalography method of investigation using [99]Technetium was carried out in four patients of our series and showed, in all four cases, an increased uptake of isotope in a deep parieto-occipital region. Although no longer in use, it supplied precious information in the past (62,68,82).

Plain skull radiography films are frequently abnormal in cases of large meningiomas. Generally speaking, these abnormalities are caused by intracranial hypertension (35% of our cases showed signs such as decalcification of the quadrilateral lamina, an enlarged sella turcica, and the presence of digitation). Intratumoral calcifications are relatively common, being present in 30% of the cases of our series, in 47% of the series of Kendall (68), and in roughly the same percentage of the series of Mani (82). These consist of minute calcifications in the deep temporoparietal region. The pineal gland, if calcified, may be displaced posteriorly and contralaterally.

In his monograph, Delandsheer (64) attributed the first description of carotid angiography performed in patients with meningiomas of the trigone to Ameli and us; we continued to use this investigation even in later years. Nowadays, digital selective angiography (DSA) by means of femoral catheterization has become the routine investigation.

Without spending too much time on the angiographic features of deep-seated temporo-parietal tumors, we will summarize those considered typical of ventricular trigone tumors and of meningiomas in particular. The arterial phase almost always reveals an anterior choroidal artery supply, and the artery itself appears enlarged, tortuous, and displaced, more frequently homolaterally and less frequently contralaterally. It is not uncommon for this artery to send out a group of vessels that unravels in the tumor. In approximately 50% of cases, the afferences coming from the medial and lateral posterior choroidal supply are easily visible (Fig. 54-1).

The group of vessels of the posterior choroidal artery generally appears displaced downward, forward, and medially. It is interesting that the posterior choroidal supply often derives from small, multiple branches and appears secondary in importance compared to the commonly occurring large, tortuous, and single anterior choroidal pedicle (5,84). Less frequently, a partial supply by the lenticulostriate or thalamo-perforating vessels and sometimes vascularization by the branches from the sylvian and pericallosal arteries may be visualized. In the capillary phase, a neovascular blush almost provides perfect visualization of the tumor.

The venous phase permits identification of the drainage veins that flow either into Galen's ampulla or directly through the internal cerebral vein or Rosenthal's basal vein. These vessels appear stretched, straightened, and displaced inferiorly, medially, and, on occasion, posteriorly.

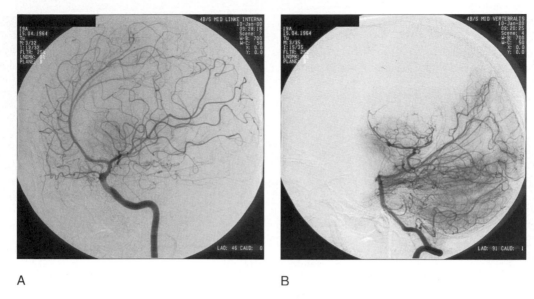

FIG. 54-1. (A) Left lateral view of carotid angiogram showing vascular supply of a left lateral ventricle meningioma from a 35-year-old female. (B) Vertebral angiogram obtained on the same patient showing a neovascular blush originating from the posterior choroidal artery group

The above-mentioned features orient diagnosis toward a tumor of the trigone, probably either a meningioma or a papilloma.

CT, with or without enhancement, allows precise calculation and comparison of the density of the brain and pathologic tissue. The CT images of these tumors show an area of high density with well-defined contours that may be smooth or irregular. In about 50% of cases, a thin ring of peritumoral hypodensity, attributable to white matter edema, can be identified. Why edema is present in some intraventricular meningiomas and absent in others is by no means clear, although disruption of the ependyma by the tumor may be an important factor (68,85).

In large tumors there may also be a hypodense area at the center of the mass, which is a sign of tissue necrosis. The mass is always easily distinguishable from the ventricular cavities and surrounding tissue. In a little less than half of cases, scans reveal the presence of calcifications accumulated mainly toward the lower portion of the tumor. Contrast medium provides an even better visualization of the lesion, which presents a marked, homogeneous enhancement, frequently also the hypertrophic choroidal artery and, occasionally, the posterior choroidal artery as well.

The following CT characteristics are useful for a differential diagnosis between meningiomas and papillomas. Smooth contours are common in meningiomas, whereas irregular contours are more frequent in choroid plexus papillomas. Calcification occurs more frequently in the former than in the latter. Meningiomas and many papillomas have a higher density than the brain and almost invariably enhance, although isodense choroid plexus papillomas are not uncommon. Both types of tumor get their blood supply from the choroidal arteries, but the tumor blush is more homogeneous in meningiomas. Hydrocephalus is common in choroid plexus papilliomas and is overtly communicating in 50% of cases, while meningiomas more often give rise to local dilatation around and proximal to the tumor rather than generalized widening of the lateral ventricle (Fig. 54-2).

MRI is highly sensitive to tissue changes resulting from intracranial neoplasms. It produces no ionizing radiation and yields direct multiplanar images free of bone artifacts that are useful for planning a surgical approach.

Generally, brain tumors have a low signal intensity on TI-weighted images and a high signal intensity on T2-weighted images. Meningiomas tend to produce only slight variations with respect to the brain on both T1- and T2-weighted images; a signal loss (hypointensity) on T2 multiecho sequences may be evident depending on tumoral cellularity. Relationships between meningiomas and neighboring arterial and/or venous structures are well documented by MRI.

Paramagnetic contrast media (gadolinium-DTPA) uniformly enhance the meningioma and result in a high signal intensity in T1-weighted images, giving good visualization of localization and contours. This information plays an important role in the surgical management of the tumor and provides orientation for the subsequent control MRI. Little was found in the published literature (54) about the use of MRI in intraventricular meningiomas. In our personal experience MRI is the most sensitive modality for describing the topographical relation between ventricular tumors and their neighboring structures, especially because of the strict relation between tumor and CSF spaces. However, conventional spin-echo/ fast spin-echo (SE/FSE) MRI pulse sequences often leave

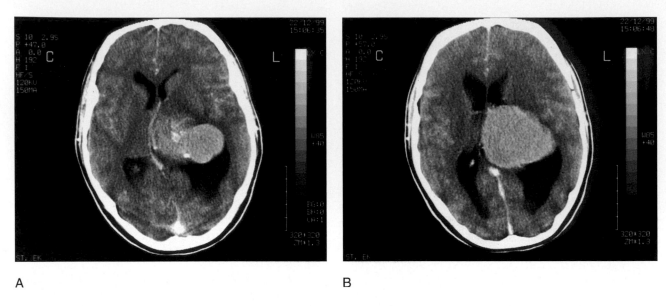

A   B

FIG. 54-2. Postcontrast CT study with a marked midline shift and the smooth contours of the meningioma: (A) level of the velum interpositum; (B) level of the cella media

room for interpretation because of low spatial resolution or even failure to delineate fine neural structures.In recent years, MRI-derived, three-dimensional constructive interference in steady-state (3D-CISS) imaging has gained increasing importance in imaging the fine structures predominantly within the cerebrospinal space and space occupying lesions. The 3D-CISS sequence offers the advantages of producing thin slices, high-resolution images, and 3D reconstructions in any desired plane. By using this sequence, the margin between the CSF, neural structures, vessels, and tumor can be displayed in detail. The 3D-CISS sequence is a heavily T2-weighted, 3D-Fourier transformation magnetic resonance technique and basically a gradient echo–based sequence. It is designed to minimize susceptibility and flow artifacts by gradient moment nulling and by averaging the two images by opposite-direction phase cycling of excitation radiofrequency pulses. Imaging was performed with a 1.5-T MRI system (Magnetom Vision; Siemens, Erlangen, Germany) with a regular (quadrature) head coil (Fig. 54-3)

For the in vivo examination of meningioma biology and as an index of tumor aggressivity and probability of recurrence, PET has been found to be ideally suited (86). Recently, we have begun to use ^{11}C-methionine and flouroethyl tyrosine (FET)–PET examination in our practice.

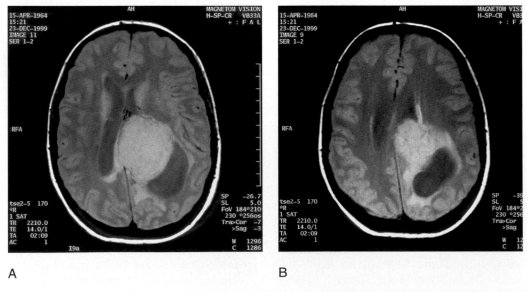

A   B

FIG. 54-3. MRI obtained on the same patient as angiography and CT showing how the tumor blocks circulation of cerebrospinal fluid: (A) level of trigonal area; (B) level of cella media

The postoperative follow-up is ideally controlled by MRI: 3 months, 6 months, 1 year, 2 years, 3 years, and 5 years after surgery.

Laboratory Investigations

Brain tumors may alter blood coagulation either directly or indirectly. Many decades ago, Morozov (87) described a tendency toward reduction in the coagulation properties of blood in patients with benign tumors, whereas malignant tumors in his series caused an increase in the fibrinolytic activity of the blood. In addition, two case reports have been published describing the occurrene of acute (88) and chronic (89) disseminated intravascular coagulation (DIC) in meningioma patients.

In addition to regular blood examination, we also measure routinely the plasma level of fibrin stabilizing factor (Factor XIII). In the case of a reduced value below 70% of normal (normal range 70–130% activity), we substitute Factor XIII.

Surgical Treatment

Following Cushing's and Dandy's initial publications regarding successfully operated meningiomas of the lateral ventricles, many approaches for removing this type of tumor have been described (36,41,45,48,90,91). Many book chapters deal with the technique of approaching these lesions (30, 92–94). Although there was unanimous agreement on the route of access to the uncommon anterior meningiomas near the foramen of Monro (middle frontal gyrus incision), there was considerable divergence over the best approach to the ventricular trigone, especially in the dominant hemisphere (Figs. 54-4 to 54-6).

Each author places the emphasis on the quality of his surgical results, but the reader is left without a clear concept of the best approach to adopt, partly because, before the advent of modern diagnostic investigations, tumors often reached an enormous size and patients were in precarious conditions by the time they were given neurosurgical care. This gave rise to both the difficulties in planning a suitable surgical approach as well as the fairly high rates of mortality and morbidity that burdened the majority of case series up until the 1970s.

The past 20 years have seen the introduction of new diagnostic investigations and considerable progress in the field of neurophysiology and the use of microsurgical techniques. These advances have brought about more rational and precise planning of surgical treatment and, consequently, an overall improvement in the results obtained.

In dealing with the surgical approaches to meningiomas of the trigone, we will concentrate on the relevant technical aspects and the drawbacks that burden each of them.

Approaches

Superior Parieto-Occipital Incision

The parieto-occipital route is the most common approach used for intraventricular meningiomas located in the lateral ventricle also in the dominant hemisphere. Under general anesthesia, the patient is placed on the operating table in the park-bench or prone position. In the former, the head is rotated toward the side opposite the tumor, in the latter toward the same side as the tumor. In both cases, the head is then elevated about 30 degrees from the table.

A classic osteoplastic craniotomy centered on the parietal lobe is followed by a cortical incision, preferably corresponding to a sulcus. We prefer the posterior parietal site, between the first and second parietal gyri at a point corresponding to the parietooccipital junction, beginning about 2 cm from the internal hemispheric fissure and extending the incision downward for 4–5 cm.

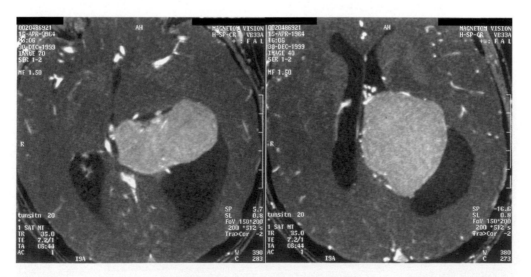

FIG. 54-4. Axial source image of a contrast-enhanced 2D-TOF MR angiography demonstrating the meningeoma and the surrounding veins and arteries

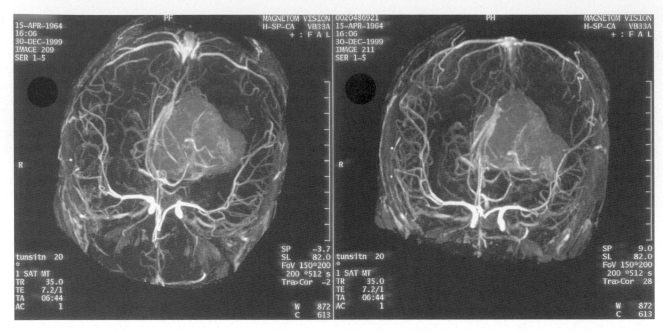

FIG. 54-5. Three-dimensional reconstruction of 2D-TOF MR angiography demonstrating the meningioma and the surrounding vessels

Other authors (51) favor a sagittal paramedian incision of the parietal cortex at a distance of 4 cm from the interhemispheric fissure that begins 1 cm behind the postcentral fissure and is continued for 4–5 cm as far as the parieto-occipital fissure.

The cortical edges and the white substance are held back using a self-retaining retractor, and the operating microscope or microsurgical instrumentation is brought into the operating field. Ultrasound guidance can be helpful (95). The tumoral capsule is identified and incised following bipolar coagulation. The crucial stage of surgery that begins at this point proceeds as follows.

Internal tumoral decompression is essential before attempting to dissect the meningioma from the adjacent structures.

The method of exenteration used is dictated by tumor consistency: if soft (a rare finding), it may be sucked away quickly, but if hard it will require tumoral forceps, blunt ring curettes, bipolar coagulation, ultrasonic aspiration, and, in exceptional circumstances, carbon dioxide (CO_2) laser. As the contents of the tumor are removed, the capsule is gently retracted and peeled away without any need for retraction of the brain. For this purpose, fine dissectors and thin layers of compressed cotton wool soaked in warm physiologic solution are used. Once the tumor has been emptied of its contents a little at a time as the capsule is isolated from the tissues around it, the arteries that connect the anterior choroidal artery with the tumor are identified, isolated, coagulated with low-intensity

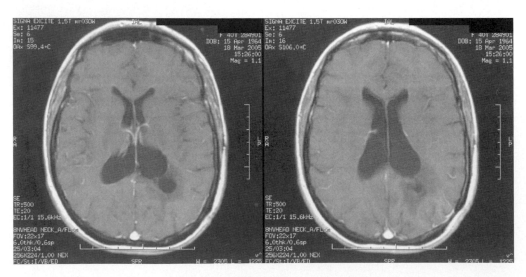

FIG. 54-6. Postoperative contrast-enhanced T1-weighted image of the patient

bipolar coagulation applied, and then cut near the tumor. Every effort must be made not to stretch them brusquely during this maneuver due to the risk of breaking them off at their base of implant.

Pulling the capsule medio-laterally, the drainage veins become visible and are coagulated using the same technique as above but using even greater care; the posterior choroidal artery receives similar treatment. At this point it is important to remember to identify, coagulate, and cut some of the arterioles that originate from the lenticulostriate or thalamo-perforating vessels. During these procedures, a gradual removal of part of the tumoral capsule offers the advantage of a wider operative field and keeps trauma of the nervous tissue to a minimum. Once the tumor has been removed, the cavity should be thoroughly rinsed with warm physiologic solution for complete hemostasis. A thin polyethylene tube is left in the cavity for 24–48 hours to control intraventricular pressure and to allow, if necessary, CSF drainage. Dura, bone, and skin flaps are closed in the normal way.

In 1965, Delandsheer (64) criticized this approach because it does not give early access to the supplying vessels and also because it is a potential hazard to optic radiations. Nevertheless, in our experience, the parieto-occipital route raises no technical problems because the choroidal vessels can be fairly easily controlled once the volume of the meningioma has been reduced by piecemeal removal; the tumor can then be gently rotated to expose the vascular pole that usually lies underneath.

As far as the risk of visual deficit is concerned, the optic radiations may be completely preserved by bearing in mind that they run inferolaterally to the ventricle (11,96) and by taking care not to cut too far down into the cortex. The risk of postoperative hemianopia is due to the fact that meningiomas often attain great size, so that the situation is no longer one of compression but of adhesion between the tumor and white substance through destruction of the ventricular ependyma. Thus, during dissection, the optic radiations may be damaged. Hence, visual damage is not a direct consequence of the parieto-occipital approach itself.

For tumors localized in the dominant hemisphere, the parieto-occipital cortical incision, if made sufficiently high and posterior, makes it possible to avoid speech disturbances. In our experience the rare aphasic or dyslexic phenomena observed in the postoperative period cleared rapidly.

Posterior Middle Temporal Gyrus Incision

Olivecrona (97) and Criscuolo and Symon (5) stated a preference for the posterior middle temporal gyrus approach, previously recommended also by De La Torre (98). The surgical technique requires an osteoplastic craniotomy in the midtemporal area extended inferoposteriorly to expose the floor of the middle temporal fossa and the anterior aspect of the lateral sinus. A linear cortical incision is made into the posterior aspect of the middle temporal gyrus and self-retaining retraction used to gently spread the incision while proceeding

inward. This approach is greatly facilitated when the temporal horn is dilated.

The tumoral capsule is identified, coagulated, and incised. Internal decompression of the tumor is followed by identification and isolation of the feeding branches coming from the anterior choroidal artery, which are coagulated and cut next to the tumor. Surgery then continues along the steps described for the superior parietal approach.

This route of attack offers the advantage of earlier identification of the anterior choroidal vessels, usually the principal afferences to the tumor. Nevertheless, the considerable size of some of these tumors often proves a hindrance to immediate clipping of their vascular pedicle. In comparison to the superior parietal approach, however, greater difficulties are encountered in exposing the medial drainage veins and the afferences coming from the posterior choroidal artery.

Postoperative homonymous field cuts are also seen with this incision, but damage to the visual projection fibers is generally slight, as the cortical incision lies parallel to them (5). Language function in the dominant hemisphere may be compromised. As shown by Ojemann (99) in stimulation studies of epileptic patients, language representation varies greatly and fluent speech representation often extends into this area. Auditory comprehension deficits may also occur if the posterior superior temporal or supramarginal regions are damaged by retraction (5).

A more extensive transtemporal horn occipito-temporal gyrus incision was described by Spencer and Collins (100), who used it for resection of the posterior hippocampus in temporal lobe epilepsy. This procedure involves a limited lateral temporal lobectomy of the middle and inferior temporal gyri, opening of the temporal horn, and exposure of the hippocampus. The occipital temporal gyrus is then incised, and a self-retaining retractor is used to elevate the temporal lobe flap, thus exposing the ventricular trigone. This approach permits access to the choroidal fissure and control of the anterior choroidal vessels, not to mention greater preservation of Wernicke's zone. Generally speaking, however, it produces a deficit of the upper quadrant homonymous visual field and is not indicated for tumors that extend toward the upper part of the trigone.

Posterior Transcallosal Approach

Kempe and Blaylock (101) in 1976 suggested and performed this approach. They removed three rather small meningiomas of the left trigone with excellent results. There are few reports in the literature of meningiomas of the trigone attacked through this route (102).

The patient is placed in a semi-sitting position if the tumor is located in the anterior horn of the lateral ventricle, and in a prone position if the tumor is located in the trigonal area. We perform a more anterior parietooccipital craniotomy than Kempe and Blaylock that passes contralaterally over the superior longitudinal sinus. The dura is incised and opened back onto the longitudinal sinus, and a self-retaining retractor is used to spread the cerebral hemisphere from the falx until the posterior part of the corpus callosum is fully exposed. It may sometimes be necessary to cut the falx and suspend it by means of silk stitches. At this point, microsurgical techniques become obligatory.

After having coagulated the splenium of the corpus callosum, it is incised. The tela choroidea is divided and partially coagulated; the tumor comes into view and is removed by the technique described previously.

This approach provides early exposure and obliteration of the feeding branches of the posterior choroidal artery and medial drainage veins. The limited exposure it affords through the posterior callosal section makes it more suitable for small meningiomas. In larger tumors, excessive traction of the hemisphere involved must be avoided at all costs by removing the tumor piecemeal and every so often lightening the compression that the self-retaining retractor exerts on the brain.

A severely disabling syndrome of visual-verbal disconnection may result when the splenium of the corpus callosum is sectioned in patients with a pre- or postoperative homonymous field cut in their dominant hemisphere (103–105). To obviate this complication, some authors (102,106,107) suggest partial sectioning of the splenium, sparing the ventrally located splenial fibers and thus leaving intact interhemispheric visual transfer. They state that the above modification may cause auditory disconnection, which does not, however, appear to have any practical import. Tokunaga et al. recently presented a case with transient memory disturbance after removal of an intraventricular trigonal meningioma by a parieto-occipital interhemispheric precuneus approach (108).

There is no doubt that the temporo-parietal incision offers the most direct approach to meningiomas of the trigone. It was suggested by Cushing in 1938 (35) and subsequently adopted by other neurosurgeons. If homonymous hemianopia is already partially present, this incision usually renders it complete by cutting across the optic radiation. Furthermore, language functions in the dominant hemisphere and spatial perception in the nondominant hemisphere are jeopardized. Neither the anterior nor the posterior choroidal arteries are accessible early in the dissection.

The occipital corticotomy or lobectomy, which Olivecrona (97) used in some patients, offers good trigonal exposure, poor vascular access, inevitable homonymous hemianopia, and, if carried too far anteriorly, dysphasia and dyslexia as well.

In our view, the temporo-parietal and occipital approaches, because of the inevitable neurologic deficits they cause, should now be considered a part of neurosurgical history and no longer used in neurosurgical practices.

Selection of the Most Appropriate Surgical Approach

In the rare case of small ventricles, the tumor in the anterior part of lateral ventricles should be attacked via an anterior transcallosal approach (109–111).

The optimal approach to meningiomas of the lateral ventricles should be the one that affords the best anatomic exposure of the tumor and its vascular supply. It is equally important to achieve

this with the least possible disruption and retraction of the immediately surrounding, normally functioning cerebral areas.

A tumor originating from the anterior tela choroidea and causing hydrocephalus may be removed without functional damage by cutting the cerebral cortex corresponding with the middle frontal gyrus.

A meningioma of the trigone may be removed by various routes depending on which hemisphere is involved (dominant or non-dominant) as well as the features of the tumor (vascularization, size, and predominant extension).

Even though each neurosurgeon naturally has a greater familiarity with a particular type of approach, he or she must be versatile enough to adapt his or her technique to the various clinical and anatomical requirements of each tumor (13,14,112).

For example, the ideal approach for removal of a small meningioma with mainly lateral extension and high vascularization is through the middle of the temporal gyrus. This route has the great advantage of enormously facilitating interception of the feeding arteries coming from the anterior choroidal artery, with a considerable reduction in blood loss. On the other hand, for a small or medium-sized medially positioned tumor that derives its principal blood supply from the posterior choroidal artery, the transcallosal approach may be indicated, provided there is no preexisting hemianopia in the dominant hemisphere.

For larger tumors, such as the majority of those we treated, the parieto-occipital approach is more suitable. Although this approach has the drawback of not providing immediate identification and interception of the feeding branches coming from the anterior choroidal artery, it does allow better control and closure of the posterior choroidal artery. When the tumor is highly vascular, some suggest a combined approach, for example, transtemporal horn, occipital temporal gyrus, and superior parietal occipital incisions (50).

There may be a precise indication for any one of the previously described approaches, and the right choice of approach enormously influences the operative results. Whichever approach is used, we are firmly convinced that a good surgical outcome hinges on the absolute necessity of not removing the tumor en bloc and always after evacuating its contents and gradually reducing its bulk while minimizing involvement and compression of the surrounding cerebral tissues.

Conclusions

Most neurosurgeons rarely or never deal with meningiomas of the lateral ventricles since they are rather infrequent. No pathognomonic clinical picture exists, but nowadays CT and MRI permit an earlier and more precise diagnosis. These improved imaging techniques and a better knowledge of neurophysiologic functioning make rational planning of correct surgical management possible for each case.

Microsurgical techniques, along with improved techniques of neuroanesthesia, have led to an enormous improvement in operative results and have helped to drastically reduce mortality and morbidity. In the past, rates of operative mortality reported in the various series hovered around 25% (51).

More recently, many series published by Criscuolo and Symon (5), Bret (54), Gruss (52) with 4 cases, Nakamura (55) with 16 cases, Buhl (58) with 5 cases as a part of a neuropsychologic outcome study, Bertalanffy (57) with 16 cases, Erman (113) with 8 cases, and finally Liu (59) with 25 patients, including our own 25 patients described in this chapter, report an absence of operative mortality and minimal morbidity, with most patients showing substantial improvement during the early postoperative and follow-up periods.

Meningiomas of the Third Ventricle

Embryologic Considerations and Pathology

Meningiomas of the third ventricle have been only rarely reported in the older literature (38,114–126). Meningiomas of the third ventricle and pineal region are divided into two major groups. The first arises primarily from the free edge of the tentorium, where it is joined by the inferior margin of the falx (falcotentorial junction) and secondarily invades the pineal and posterior third ventricular region. Meningiomas from this area might be considered extensions of meningiomas of the posterior falx or mid-line tentorial meningiomas. However, because their clinical manifestations usually resemble those of a pineal region mass, which is different from other meningiomas of the falx and tentorium, and their surgical approach parallels that of other pineal region lesions, their distinction remains a useful one.

The second type takes its origin from the velum interpositum without dural attachment to occupy the third ventricle and pineal region. These tumors are almost exclusively located in the posterior third ventricle, presenting as a pineal region mass, although anterior third ventricular meningiomas have been reported (119). During the development of the telencephalon, the corpus callosum extends posteriorly, carrying with it a layer of pia-arachnoid on its inferior surface above the level of the choroidal fissure. This second pial layer fuses with the original pia-arachnoid surface overlying the roof of the third ventricle to form the substance of the tela choroidea. The two layers separate posteriorly, with the inferior layer following the roof of the third ventricle to the pineal gland. The superior layer adheres to the corpus callosum following the splenium to the superior surface of the corpus callosum (117,127). The velum interpositum is the space formed between the two layers of the tela choroidea. This double triangular fold of the pia-arachnoid forming the roof of the third ventricle provides the basis from which meningeal tumors in this region may develop (128).

The important difference between the two major categories that comprise meningiomas of the pineal region and third ventricle lies in the origin of their blood supply and attachments. The velum interpositum meningioma attached to the tela cho-roidea receives its blood supply from the posterior choroidal arteries, and possibly the anterior choroidal artery if the tumor is large. The falcotentorial meningioma normally derives its blood supply from extracerebral sources, i.e., branches of the internal carotid artery supplying the falx and tentorium, of which the branch described by Bernasconi and Cassinari is most important (127,129).

Recently many singular cases of benign third ventricular meningiomas were reported in the literature (55,113,128,130–138). We operated on one patient with a huge pseudointraventricular meningioma with complete destruction of the trunk of the corpus callosum with a good clinical and neuropsychologic outcome. At least two malignant menigiomas located in the third ventricle were found in the literature (139,140).

Preoperative Evaluation

Meningiomas of the third ventricle and especially in the posterior part of the ventricle require knowledge of the management and diagnosis of the diverse spectrum of histologic processes that can affect pineal region (141).

Clinical Features

The average age of patients with pineal region meningiomas tends to be approximately 40 years (120). Age and sex are among the distinguishing features of pineal region meningiomas compared to other pineal region tumors. Pineal germ cell tumors seldom occur in female patients, whereas a female predominance exists in pineal meningiomas, as is observed with intracranial meningiomas at other locations. The most frequent clinical symptoms of third ventricle meningiomas are related to raised intracranial pressure from insidious hydrocephalus, as with other pineal region tumors. These most often include headache, papilledema, gait disturbance, and cognitive dysfunction. Neuro-ophthalmologic symptoms such as impaired upgaze and diminished pupillary reflexes (Parinaud's syndrome) secondary to pressure on the corpora quadrigemina are less commonly observed with third ventricle and pineal region meningiomas than with other pineal region tumors (120,122).

Cerebellar dysfunction is occasionally present, presumably from compression of the superior cerebellar peduncle in the midbrain. Finally, hypothalamic dysfunction most often but not exclusively encountered with pineal region germinomas has also been reported with third ventricle and pineal region meningiomas (115,122).

Evaluation of CSF cytology and assays of β-human chorionic gonadotropin (βHCG) and α-fetoprotein (αAFP) are routinely performed with pineal region tumors. This can be helpful in establishing the diagnosis of some germ cell and pineal cell tumors and documenting subarachnoid seeding when it occurs. In pineal region meningiomas, however, these laboratory tests are negative and provide little diagnostic value in limiting the differential diagnosis.

Neuroradiology

Modern neuroradiologic techniques such as MRI and high-resolution CT revolutionized the differential diagnosis of pineal region masses. However, the histologic diagnosis cannot be definitively made by noninvasive means and can only be completely confirmed by surgical histopathologic examination.

Meningiomas occupying the third ventricle and pineal region may arise from the velum interpositum or from the falx-tentorial junction. Meningiomas in the pineal region are hyperdense on unenhanced CT in most cases. With intravenous contrast, there is homogeneous enhancement in a nodular fashion of the pineal region mass. Calcification can be occasionally identified within the lesions (129,142).

MRI shows an iso-intense or low signal intensity mass relative to grey matter on T1-weighted images, and iso-intense to high signal intensity on T2-weighted images. Multiplanar MRI performed following intravenous injection of gadolinium is extremely useful in delineating the enhancing mass lesion from surrounding structures and allows for increased specificity in the diagnosis of pineal region neoplasms. Coronal views can be especially helpful in identifying dural attachment of the falx-tentorial junction if the meningioma is of this type.

Cerebral angiography can be helpful in identifying the arterial feeders to the tumor and demonstrates a characteristic homogeneous blush. The differentiation between meningiomas of the falcotentorial junction and those of the velum interpositum can sometimes be distinguished by cerebral angiography. With meningiomas of the falcotentorial junction, both the plexal segment of the medial posterior choroidal artery and the internal cerebral vein are displaced inferiorly. In contrast, meningiomas of the velum interpositum displace the medial posterior choroidal artery inferiorly and the internal cerebral vein superiorly. This differentiation may be difficult in tumors arising from the tela choroidea above the internal cerebral vein (127).

Cerebral angiography has largely been supplanted in distinguishing the two types of meningiomas in this region because of high-resolution MRI with gadolinium enhancement. In cases of large meningiomas of the pineal region, however, the distinction between the two types may not be possible. At this time we have found it seldom necessary to utilize cerebral angiography in the evaluation of posterior third ventricular and pineal region masses. The future role of MRI projection angiography has yet to be determined, but it appears that it will be useful in providing a noninvasive means of evaluating and delineating the important regional vascular anatomy.

Management and Role of Stereotactic Neurosurgery

Posterior third ventricle meningiomas, pineal region tumors, and their best neurosurgical management have been controversial and are still evolving. Early attempts at surgery produced high rates of morbidity and mortality, and because of poor surgical results, the bias was for treatment limited to ventricular shunting followed by irradiation (143–145). However, patients with pineal region meningiomas and benign tumors are not optimally served by treatment with irradiation alone. With the advent of microneurosurgical techniques and improved neuroanesthesia, direct surgical approaches have now resulted in more encouraging results (13,145–149). This is important since approximately 25% of pineal region tumors are benign and amenable to surgical treatment (48,146,148). In particular, with contemporary surgical techniques, the prognosis for pineal region meningiomas should be excellent. Many are well encapsulated, affording the opportunity for gross total surgical resection (See Chapter 53).

Because of the marked diversity of pathology that occurs in the pineal region, a conclusive preoperative diagnosis is often difficult, even with the advantages offered by modern imaging techniques. Histopathologic identification is essential for the optimum management of pineal region tumors. Currently, we tailor the neurosurgical management and treatment of each case individually with consideration of the attendant nuances. If neuroradiologic imaging is pathognomonic for a meningioma or a benign encapsulated lesion, we proceed directly to microsurgical exposure and dissection.

The combination of CT scanning, MRI, and stereotactic techniques has added a new dimension to the management of pineal region tumors. Stereotactic biopsy is an attractive means of providing direct tissue sampling for diagnosis and guiding further operative or nonoperative therapy (150,151). By obtaining histopathologic diagnosis we have avoided treating patients with "blind" radiotherapy and unnecessary or poor-yield surgical procedures.

Thus, the successful management of pineal region tumors is now a routine part of contemporary neurosurgical practice. Only with excellent neuroradiologic imaging, accurate neuropathology, familiarity with image-guided stereotaxy, and the full spectrum of microsurgical operative approaches can management be optimized (152).

Microsurgical Approaches

Surgical Anatomy

The deep cerebral venous system is intimately related to the walls of the third ventricle. The venous structures in the pineal region, where the internal cerebral vein and the basal vein on each side converge to form the great vein (Galen's vein), provide an important potential obstacle in surgical approaches to the pineal region.

The paired internal cerebral veins originate behind the foramen of Monro and course posteriorly within the velum interpositum, where they exit above the pineal body to enter the quadrigeminal cistern and join Galen's vein. The terminal segment of the medial posterior choroidal artery courses anteriorly in the tela choroidea of the third ventricle close to the midline and inferior and medial to the internal cerebral veins. The velum interpositum is the space between the two layers of the tela choroidea in the roof of the third ventricle. The basal vein originates in the anterior incisural space and courses posteriorly between the midbrain and temporal lobe, exiting the ambient cistern to join the great vein of Galen. The great vein, formed by the union of the internal cerebral veins and basal veins, courses posteriorly and superiorly around the splenium to join the straight sinus at the anterior aspect of the falcotentorial junction. The straight sinus then courses posteroinferiorly along the falcotentorial junction to join the torcular. Along its course, the great vein receives many tributaries, accounting for the high density of veins in this area (153).

The deep Galenic system furnishes an apparent potential threat to satisfactory outcome in surgical approaches to this area. Early experiments by Dandy (154) hypothesized that occlusion of the great vein of Galen in dogs caused hydrocephalus. Subsequent experiments did not support this observation. Hammock and Di Chiro (155) selectively occluded the vein of Galen in rhesus monkeys without untoward clinical effects. They showed angiographic evidence of dilated major draining veins and sinuses and microscopic dilation of the smaller diencephalic and choroidal veins with occlusion of the great vein. Examination of the brains after vein of Galen occlusion revealed no evidence of vascular infarction or encephalomalacia. Clinically, Sakaki (124) reported a case of a large pineal meningioma in which the vein of Galen was sacrificed without clinical sequelae. They suggested that obstruction of the great vein of Galen may be well tolerated in some cases, especially if the obstruction is gradual, allowing the development of collaterals of the deep venous system.

General Considerations

The two primary surgical approaches to the posterior third ventricle and pineal region include the supratentorial and infratentorial approaches. The infratentorial supracerebellar corridor is simpler, both conceptually and anatomically. It is well suited for velum interpositum meningiomas without dural attachment. The supratentorial approaches are more complicated because of the variable anatomy, but allow intraoperative options for tentorial or falx incisions to increase exposure and deprive the tumor of its blood supply at its base. These approaches are best suited for pineal region meningiomas with dural attachment at the falcotentorial junction.

Meningiomas in the Anterior Part of the Third Ventricle

Transcortical-Transventricular Approach

A tumor originating from the anterior choroid tela, involving the anterior part of the third ventricle and causing hydrocephalus, may be removed without functional damage by cutting the cerebral cortex corresponding with the middle frontal gyrus (see Figs. 54-7 and 54-8). The transcortical-transventricular approach allows the neurosurgeon the modification beginning from the foramen of Monro and under the choroid plexus the enlargment to the subchoroidal-transvelum interpositum approach (156–158).

Anterior Transcallosal Approach

In the case of small ventricles, the tumor in the anterior part of lateral ventricles should be attacked via an anterior transcallosal approach (109–111).

Meningiomas in the Posterior Part of the Third Ventricle

The majority of meningiomas in the posterior part of the third ventricle and pineal region present with hydrocephalus. For control of associated raised intracranial pressure, many patients have received a ventriculostomy before arriving in the operating room, or one may be placed after the induction of general anesthesia. If possible, permanent CSF diversion should not be undertaken if a strong suspicion of a potentially benign excisable lesion exists. Interestingly, in many

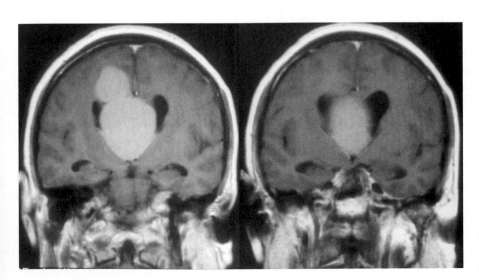

FIG. 54-7. Meningioma of the third ventricle with invasion of the middle part of the corpus callosum

FIG. 54-8. Postoperative MRI from the patient with third ventricle meningioma

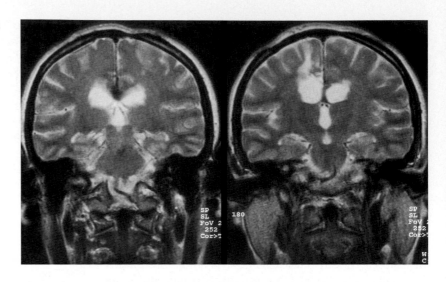

instances patients have had ventriculoperitoneal shunts placed prior to their referral to our institution. In any case, it is essential that the ventricular system be decompressed before the operative procedure is begun. If exposure is not adequate with CSF diversion and more relaxation is required, osmotic diuresis may be used. We have utilized preoperative antibiotics for prophylaxis from possible shunt or ventriculostomy infection as well as surgical wound infection. High-dose glucocorticoids are administered one or more days preoperatively and continued through the postoperative period as necessary.

Infratentorial-Supracerebellar Approach

The infratentorial supracerebellar approach to the pineal region was first utilized by Krause in the 1920s and developed and popularized by Stein in the 1970s (148). Its advantages include: (1) a direct central midline approach to the pineal region; (2) avoidance of injury to the deep venous system since the tumors are ventral to the deep venous structures; and (3) no morbidity related to parietal or occipital lobe retraction (159).

Supratentorial Approach

A supratentorial approach to the pineal region was first described by Brunner and expanded upon by Dandy (154). Dandy utilized a large parieto-occipital bone flap and a parasagittal approach to the pineal region. After midline exposure, splitting of the posterior callosum and, occasionally, an occipital lobectomy was required to provide adequate access to the vein of Galen, the posterior third ventricle, and the quadrigeminal regions. Modifications of this essential concept coupled with contemporary microneurosurgical techniques allow exposure of the pineal region with low morbidity. Multiple operative corridors may be developed, affording regional entry and exposure via intraoperative tactics. These include a tentorial incision, a falcine incision, splenial retraction, a splenial incision, and incision of the posterior body of the corpus callosum. These strategies allow intraoperative options for optimal exposure of the pineal region from the supratentorial approach (160).

Meningiomas Metastasizing Through CSF Pathways

Metastasis of intraventricular meningiomas through CSF pathways is a rarity, and only four cases have been reported in the world literature describing meningiomas that were intraventricular and malignant. Ramakrishnamurthy reported a case of benign intraventricular meningioma which had spread through the CSF pathways (161). Darwish reported a malignant intraventricular meningioma originating in the right trigone region of the lateral ventricle causing CSF drop mestastases (162). In his paper he referred to seven cases at that time described in the literature. Chamberlain (21) described an additional case of CSF-disseminated meningioma.

Adjuvant Therapy

Adjuvant therapy in the treatment of meningiomas has enhanced the possibility of cure or long-term palliation. For subtotal resections, radiation therapy should be utilized either by conventional means, stereotactic radiosurgery, or a combination of the two. The role of hormonal therapy has yet to be determined but remains a potential avenue for future treatment.

Conclusion

Meningiomas in the anterior and posterior third ventricle and para-pineal region are challenging lesions whose diagnosis and management must consider the wide spectrum of pathologic processes that may affect this area. The primary treatment modality remains open microsurgical excision. Meningiomas in the anterior part of the third ventricle and no sign of hydrocephalus may be removed via an anterior transcallosal approach.

If a tumor causes hydrocepalus, it may be removed without functional damage using a transcortical-transventricular approach, facilitated by a corticotomy in the middle frontal gyrus. The infratentorial-supracerebellar approach is most appealing for those meningiomas originating from the velum interpositum without dural attachment. The supratentorial surgical corridors allow for increased exposure and are best suited for falcotentorial meningiomas.

Meningiomas of the Fourth Ventricle

Introduction

Meningiomas of the fourth ventricle have to be differentiated from meningiomas of the lateral cerebellomedullary cistern (163) and a mixed lesion, culled from the literature (27).

Pure meningiomas in the fourth ventricle without dural attachment are extremely rare.

Anatomic Considerations and Classification

Meningiomas of the fourth ventricle have been classified by Abraham and Chandy (164) as:

1. Meningiomas originating from the choroid plexus of the fourth ventricle and developing solely within the ventricle
2. Meningiomas of the inferior tela choroidea developing partly in the fourth ventricle and partly in the cerebellar hemisphere and vermis
3. Meningiomas within the cisterna magna having no attachment to the dura mater

In 1986, Cantore et al. (165) added one personal case to 22 others culled from the literature. Since then he has operated on one other case and found two other published cases (9,166), bringing the total to 26 cases. Two other cases were reported by Nakamura (55). Cases were contributed by Delfini (167), Chaskis (168), Cummings (169), Akimoto (79), Ceylan (170), Tsuboi (171), Liu (59). In summary, we reviewed 35 cases from the literature with fourth ventricle meningiomas.

Clinical Findings

In contrast to the usual female preponderance of meningiomas with a 2:1 female-to-male ratio, we found a 0.9:1 ratio for this type of meningioma. The mean age was approximately 25 years, with a range of 7–65 years.

A strictly intraventricular tumor does not give rise to any characteristic clinical pattern until it blocks CSF circulation, the consequences of which are internal hydrocephalus and intracranial hypertension. On the other hand, a tumor developing mainly in the cerebellum initally causes cerebellar signs and, ultimately, intracranial hypertension.

Other symptoms such as bilateral hearing loss, as in the case of Sachs (123), cited by Cushing (35), and long tract signs,

as reported by Zuleta and Londono (172), have also been described, but these are not considered specific to a primary fourth ventricle tumor.

Preoperative Evaluation and Differential Diagnosis

It is essential that the preoperative diagnosis include the location and type of tumor. In many cases, pneumoencephalography and ventriculography were performed to demonstrate the location of the tumor. In some cases, carotid angiography was performed to assess the size of the ventricles.

Vertebral angiography was considered one of the most valuable investigations for diagnosing a mass lesion in this region but was actually only a major help in cases that showed tumor blush, which was present in only a few cases. More often, diagnosis was based on indirect angiographic signs that suggested a lesion, such as displacement of branches of the posterior inferior cerebellar artery.

Today, more accurate information regarding the site and shape of the tumor, as well as ventricular size, is easily obtainable using CT and MRI. However, vertebral angiography retains its utility for assessing the tumor's vascular supply, which may aid surgical removal (13,171). Some aspects of the differential diagnosis with papillomas of the choroid plexus are dealt with above regarding meningiomas of the lateral ventricles.

Surgical Technique

Treatment of fourth ventricle meningiomas consists of total surgical excision, keeping damage to the surrounding neural structures to a minimum.

The patient may be placed in a sitting or prone position, and the tumor is reached through a midline suboccipital approach that, when required, may be associated with removal of the posterior arch of the atlas. The fourth ventricle is exposed through a vertical incision of the cerebellar vermis that generally appears to be widened and tense. The tumor appears as a reddish-grey, well-encapsuled mass that bleeds easily. The tumor's point of origin is usually the lower choroid tela or the choroid plexus. Some authors stress the importance of a telovelar approach to the fourth ventricle (13).

Identification and coagulation of the vascular plexus coming from the choroid supply facilitates tumor removal. In our two operated cases, one tumor went into the cerebellopontine angle and the other toward the quadrigeminal lamina. In both cases the tumor was removed piecemeal with minimal retraction of the cerebellar tissue and no traction on the floor of the fourth ventricle.

Conclusions

Before 1960, the mortality and morbidity of such benign lesions was high. Thanks to the introduction of microsurgical techniques and the operating microscope, complete surgical removal is possible with a relatively low risk profile.

References

1. Imielinski BL, Kloc W. Meningiomas of the lateral ventricles of the brain. Zentralbl Neurochir 1997; 58(4):177–182.

2. Kurland LT, Schoenberg BS, Annegers JF, Okazaki H, Molgaard CA. The incidence of primary intracranial neoplasms in Rochester, Minnesota, 1935–1977. Ann NY Acad Sci 1982; 381:6–16.

3. Staneczek W, Jaenisch W. Epidemiologic data on meningiomas in East germany 1961–1986; incidence, localisation, age and sex distribution. Clin Neuropathol 1992; (11):135–141.

4. Surawicz TS, McCarthy BJ, Kupelian V. Descriptive epidemiology of primary brain and CNS tumors: results from the Central Brain Tumor Registry of the United States, 1990–1994. Neuro-Oncol 1999; (1):14–25.

5. Criscuolo GR, Symon L. Intraventricular meningioma. A review of 10 cases of the National Hospital, Queen Square (1974–1985) with reference to the literature. Acta Neurochir (Wien) 1986; 83(3–4):83–91.

6. Di Rocco C, Di Rienzo A. Meningiomas in childhood. Crit Rev Neurosurg 1999; 9(3):180–188.

7. Ferrante L, Acqui M, Artico M, Mastronardi L, Fortuna A. Paediatric intracranial meningiomas. Br J Neurosurg 1989; 3(2): 189–196.

8. Kraus H, Koos W. [Brain tumors in childhood and adolescence. A statistical survey based on 670 cases]. Wien Klin Wochenschr 1967; 79(50):934–943.

9. Matsumura M, Takahashi S, Kurachi H, Tamura M. Primary intraventricular meningioma of the fourth ventricle—case report. Neurol Med Chir (Tokyo) 1988; 28(10):996–1000.

10. Merten DF, Gooding CA, Newton TH, Malamud N. Meningiomas of childhood and adolescence. J Pediatr 1974; 84(5): 696–700.

11. Salamon G. Atlas of the arteries of the human brain. Sandoz P, editor. 189. 1971.

12. Sano K, Wakai S, Ochiai C, Takakura K. Characteristics of intracranial meningiomas in childhood. Childs Brain 1981; 8(2): 98–106.

13. Perry RD, Parker GD, Hallinan JM. CT and MR imaging of fourth ventricular meningiomas. J Comput Assist Tomograph 1990; (14):276–280.

14. Seeger W. Anatomical Dissections for Use in Neurosurgery. New York: Springer-Verlag, 1987.

15. Vassilouthis J, Ambrose JA. Intraventricular meningioma in a child. Surg Neurol 1978; 10(2):105–107.

16. Crouse SK, Berg BO. Intracranial meningiomas in childhood and adolescence. Neurology 1972; (22):135.

17. Malulcci CL, Parkes SE, Barber P, Powell J, Stevens MCG, Walsh AR, et al. Paediatric menigeal tumors. Childs Nerv Syst 1996; (12):582–589.

18. Turgut M, Ozcan OE, Bertan V. Meningiomas in childhood and adolescence: a report of 13 cases and review of the literature. Br J Neurosurg 1997; 11(6):501–507.

19. Andoh T, Shinoda J, Miwa Y, Hirata T, Sakai N, Yamada H, et al. Tumors at the trigone of the lateral ventricle—clinical analysis of eight cases. Neurol Med Chir (Tokyo) 1990; 30(9): 676–684.

20. Borovich B, Guilburd JN, Doron Y, Soustiel JF, Zaaroor M, Braun J, et al. Cystic meningiomas. Acta Neurochir Suppl (Wien) 1988; 42:147–151.

21. Chamberlain MC, Glantz MJ. Cerebrospinal fluid-disseminated meningioma. Cancer 2005; 103(7):1427–1430.

22. El Bahy K. Telovelar approach to the fourth ventricle: operative findings and results in 16 cases. Acta Neurochir (Wien) 2005; 147(2):137–142.

23. Hung PC, Wang HS, Chou ML, Sun PC, Huang SC. Intracranial meningiomas in childhood. Zhonghua Min guo Xiao Er Ke Yi Xue Hui Za Zhi 1994; (35):495–501.

24. Jelinek J, Smirniotopoulos JG, Parisi JE, Kanzer M. Lateral ventricular neoplasms of the brain: differential diagnosis based on clinical, CT, and MR findings. AJR Am J Roentgenol 1990; 155(2):365–372.

25. Kohama I, Sohma T, Nunomura K, Igarashi K, Ishikawa A. Intraparenchymal meningioma in an infant—case report. Neurol Med Chir (Tokyo) 1996; 36(8):598–601.

26. Mc Dermott MW. Intraventricular meningiomas. Neurosurg Clin N Am 2003; (14):559–569.

27. McIver JI, Link MJ, Giannini C, Cohen-Gadol AA, Driscoll C. Choroid plexus papilloma and meningioma: coincidental posterior fossa tumors: case report and review of the literature. Surg Neurol 2003; 60(4):360–365.

28. Moss SD, Rockswold GL, Chou SN, Yock D, Berger MS. Radiation-induced meningiomas in pediatric patients. Neurosurgery 1988; 22(4):758–761.

29. Wysokinski T, Jaworski M. [A case of multiple intracranial meningiomas]. Polish. Neurol Neurochir Pol 1993; 27(6): 925–929.

30. Haddad G, Al-Mefty O. Meningiomas: an overview. In: Wilkins RH, Rengachary SS, editors. Neurosurgery. New York: McGraw-Hill, 1996:833–841.

31. Shaw A. Fibrous tumour in the lateral ventricle of the brain. Boney deposits in the arachnoid membrane of the right hemisphere. Trans Path Soc London 1854;5:18–21. 1854.

32. MacDowall TW. Large calcareous tumor involving chiefly the inner and middle portions of the left temporo-sphenoidal lobe and pressing upon the left crus and optic thalamus (brief communication). Edinburgh Med J 1881; (26):1088.

33. Dreifuss W. Über Endotheliom des Plexus chorioideus. Beitr Path Anat 1923; (71):667–673.

34. Oberling C. Meningeoblastome des Plexus chorioideus. Ann Anat Path 1927; (4):379–384.

35. Cushing HW, Eisenhardt L. Meningiomas: Their Classification, Regional Behaviour, Life History and Surgical End Results. Springfield, IL: Charles C Thomas, 1938.

36. Dandy WE. Benign, Encapsulated Tumours in the Lateral Ventricle of the Brain. Baltimore: Williams & Wilkins, 1934.

37. Abbott KH, Courville CB. Intraventricular meningiomas: review of literature and report of two cases. Bull Los Angeles Neurol Soc 1942; (7):12–28.

38. Ameli NO, Armin K, Saleh H. Incisural meningiomas of the falco-tentorial junction. A report of two cases. J Neurosurg 1966; 24(6):1027–1030.

39. Davini V, Baratta F. Meningiomi dei ventricoli laterali. Minerva Chir 1963; (18):520–529.

40. Gassel MM, Davies H. Meningiomas in the lateral ventricles. Brain 1961; (84):605–627.

41. Guidetti B, Alvisi C. Considerazioni su due casi di meningiomi intraventricolari operati. Riv Pat Nerv Ment 1952; (73): 413–432.

42. Ladenheim JC. Choroid Plexus Meningiomas of the Lateral Ventricle. Springfield, IL: Charles C Thomas, 1963.

43. Migliavacca F. Meningiomi dei ventricoli laterali. Chirurgia (Milano) 1955; (10):249–268.

44. Petit-Dutaillis D, Bertrand I. Fibroblastome profond, intracerebral de l'hemisphere gauche, sans connexions meningees decelables. Ablation de la tumeur, guerison operatoire. Rev Neural 1932; (58):96–100.

45. Tukanowicz SA, Grant FC. The meningiomas of the lateral ventricles of the brain. J Neuropathol Exp Neurol 1958; (17): 367–381.

46. Wall AE. Meningiomas within the lateral ventricle. J Neurol Neurosurg Psychiatry 1954; (17):91–103.

47. Delandsheer JM. Les meningiomes du ventricule lateral (French). Neurochirurgie 1965; (11):4–83.

48. Obrador S, Blazquez MG, Fargueta JS, Clavel MV. [Meningiomas of the lateral ventricle]. Munch Med Wochenschr 1966; 108(38):1880–1885.

49. Arseni C, Ionescu S, Maretsis M. Meningiomas of the lateral ventricle. Psychiatr Neurol Neurochir 1968; 71(4):319–336.

50. Kobayashi S, Okazaki H, MacCarty CS. Intraventricular meningiomas. Mayo Clin Proc 1971; 46(11):735–741.

51. Fornari M, Savoiardo M, Morello G, Solero CL. Meningiomas of the lateral ventricles. Neuroradiological and surgical considerations in 18 cases. J Neurosurg 1981; 54(1):64–74.

52. Gruss P, Engelhardt F, Kolmann HL, Volpel M. Ventricular meningiomas—report of 4 cases. Neurosurg Rev 1987; 10(4):295–298.

53. Conforti P, Moraci A, Albanese V, Rotondo M, Parlato C. Microsurgical management of suprasellar and intraventricular meningiomas. Neurochirurgia (Stuttg) 1991; 34(3):85–89.

54. Bret Ph, Gharbi S, Cohadon F, Remond J. Les meningiomes du ventricule lateral - 3 observations recentes. Neurochirurgie 1989; (35):5–12.

55. Nakamura M, Roser F, Bundschuh O, Vorkapic P, Samii M. Intraventricular meningiomas: a review of 16 cases with reference to the literature. Surg Neurol 2003; 59(6):491–503.

56. Erman T, Gocer AI, Tuna M, Erdogan S, Zorludemir S. Malignant meningioma of the lateral ventricle. Case report. Neurosurg Focus 2003; 15(4):ECP2.

57. Bertalanffy A, Roessler K, Koperek O, Gelpi E, Prayer D, Neuner M, et al. Intraventricular meningiomas: a report of 16 cases. Neurosurg Rev 2006; 29(1):30–35.

58. Buhl R, Huang H, Gottwald B, Mihajlovic Z, Mehdorn HM. Neuropsychological findings in patients with intraventricular tumors. Surg Neurol 2005; 64(6):500–503.

59. Liu M, Wei Y, Liu Y, Zhu S, Li X. Intraventricular meningiomas: a report of 25 cases. Neurosurg Rev 2006; (29):36–40.

60. Russell DS, Rubinstein U. Pathology of Tumours of the Central Nervous System, 4th ed. London: Edward Arnold, 1977.

61. Guidetti B, Alvisi C. Meningioma intraventricolare II. Riv Pat Nerv Ment 1954; (75):1.

62. Guidetti B, Delfini R. Lateral and fourth ventricle meningiomas. In: Al-Mefty O, editor. Meningiomas. New York: Raven Press, 1991:569–581.

63. Guidetti B, Delfini R, Gagliardi FM, Vagnozzi R. Meningiomas of the lateral ventricles. Clinical, neuroradiologic, and surgical considerations in 19 cases. Surg Neurol 1985; 24(4):364–370.

64. Delandsheer JM. Les meningiomes du ventricule lateral. Neurochirurgie 1965; (11):4–83.

65. Zülch KJ, Schmid EE. Über das Ependymom, den Seitenventrikel und Forman Monroi. Arch Psychiatr Zentralbl Neurol 1955; (193):214–228.

66. Zülch KJ. Pathologische Anatomie der raumbeengenden intrakraniellen Prozesse. In: Olivecrona H, Tönnis W, editors. Handbuch der Neurochirurgie. Berlin: Springer-Verlag, 1956:399–455.

67. Yoshida K, Onozuka S, Kawase T, Ikeda E. Lateral ventricular meningioma encapsulated by the dura-like membrane. Neuropathology 2000; 20(1):56–59.

68. Kendall B, Reider-Grosswasser I, Valentine A. Diagnosis of masses presenting within the ventricles on computed tomography. Neuroradiology 1983; 25(1):11–22.

69. Louis DN, Scheithauer BW, Budka H, von Deimling A, Kepes JJ. Meningiomas. In: Kleihues P, Canavee WK, editors. Pathology and Genetics of Tumors of the Nervous System. Lyon: IARC Press, 2000:176–184.

70. Stanton CA, Challa VR. Meningiomas: pathology. In: Wilkins RH, Rengachary SS, editors. Neurosurgery. New York: McGraw-Hill, 1996:843–854.

71. Bartlett JR. Tumours of the lateral ventricle: except choroid plexus tumours. In: Vinken PJ, Bruyn GW, editors. Handbook of Clinical Neurology. Amsterdam: North Holland Publishing, 1975:596–609.

72. Imaizumi S, Onuma T, Kameyama M, Ishii K. Symptom changes caused by movement of a calcified lateral ventricular meningioma: case report. Surg Neurol 2002; (58):128–130.

73. Goran A, Ciminello VJ, Fisher RG. Hemorrhage into meningiomas. Arch Neurol 1965; (13):65–69.

74. Lee EJ, Choi KH, Kang SW, Lee IW. Intraventricular hemorrhage caused by lateral ventricular meningioma: a case report. Korean J Radiol 2001; 2(2):105–107.

75. Murai Y, Yoshida D, Ikeda Y, Teramoto A, Kojima T, Ikakura K. Spontaneous intraventricular hemorrhage caused by lateral ventricular meningioma—case report. Neurol Med Chir (Tokyo) 1996; 36(8):586–589.

76. Oka K, Tsuda H, Kamikaseda K, Nakamura R, Fukui M, Nouzuka Y, et al. Meningiomas and hemorrhagic diathesis. J Neurosurg 1988; 69(3):356–360.

77. Smith VR, Stein PS, MacCarty CS. Subarachnoid hemorrhage due to lateral ventricular meningiomas. Surg Neurol 1975; 4(2):241–243.

78. Descuns P, Garre H. Meningiomes des ventricules lateraux: a propos de quatre observations. Neurochirurgie 1955; (1):219–221.

79. Akimoto J, Sato Y, Tsutsumi M, Haraoka J. Fourth ventricular meningioma in an adult—case report. Neurol Med Chir (Tokyo) 2001; 41(8):402–405.

80. Huang YS, Araki C. Angiographic confirmation of lateral ventricle meningiomas. A report of 5 cases. J Neurosurg 1954; (11):337–352.

81. Kotwica Z, Jagodzinski Z, Polis L. Meningiomas of the lateral ventricle. Neurochirurgia (Stuttg) 1985; 28(5):199–201.

82. Mani RL, Hedgcock MW, Mass SI, Gilmor RL, Enzmann DR, Eisenberg RL. Radiographic diagnosis of meningioma of the lateral ventricle. Review of 22 cases. J Neurosurg 1978; 49(2): 249–255.

83. Majos C, Cucurella G, Aguilera C, Coll S, Pons LC. Intraventricular meningiomas: MR imaging and MR spectroscopic findings in two cases. AJNR Am J Neuroradiol 1999; 20(5):882–885.

84. Bernasconi V, Cabrini GP. Radiological features of tumours of the lateral ventricles. Acta Neurochir (Wien) 1967; 17(4): 290–310.

85. Morrison G, Sobel DF, Kelley DL, Normann D. Intraventricular mass lesions. Radiology 1984; (153):435–442.

86. Di Chiro G, Hatazawa J, Katz DA, Rizzoli HV, De Michele DJ. Glucose utilization by intracranial meningiomas as an index of tumor aggressivity and probability of recurrence: a PET study. Radiology 1987; 164(2):521–526.

87. Morozov VV. Blood coagulation properties in patients with supratentorial tumorsduring pre- and postoperative periods. Vopr Neirokhir 1970; (34):56–60.

88. Portugal JR, Alencar A, Brito Lira LC, Carvalho P. Melanotic meningioma complicated by disseminated intravascular coagulation. Surg Neurol 1984; 21(3):275–281.

89. Weinberg S, Phillips L, Twersky R, Cottrell JE, Braunstein KM. Hypercoagulability in a patient with a brain tumor. Anesthesiology 1984; 61(2):200–202.

90. Busch E. Meningiomas of the lateral ventricles of the brain. Acta Chir Scand 1939; (82):282–290.

91. Christophe J, David M, Cochemd R. Meningiome intraventriculaire du carrefour temporo-occipital gauche. Ablation apres incision du lobe occipital gauche. Guerison sans sequelles. Rev Neurol 1939; (71):425–431.

92. Konovalov A, Filatov YM, Belousova OB. Intraventricular meningiomas. In: Schmidek H, editor. Meningiomas and Their Surgical Managment. Philadelphia: Saunders, 1991:364–374.

93. Ojemann RG. Supratentorial meningiomas: clinical features and surgical managment. In: Wilkins RH, Rengachary SS, editors. Neurosurgery. New York: McGraw-Hill, 1996:873–890.

94. Piepmeier JM, Spencer DD, Sass KJ. Lateral ventricle masses. In: Apuzzo MLJ, editor. Brain Surgery. New York: Churchill-Livingstone, 1993: 581–599.

95. Couillard P, Karmi MZ, Abdelkader AM. Microsurgical removal of an intraventricular meningioma with ultrasound guidance, and balloon dilation of operative corridors: case report and technical note. Surg Neurol 1996; 45(2):155–160.

96. Schaltenbrand G, Wahren W. Atlas of Stereotaxy of the Human Brain. Stuttgart: Georg Thieme-Verlag, 1977.

97. Olivecrona H, Tönnis W. Klinik und Behandlung der raumbeengenden intrakraniellen Prozesse. In: Olivecrona H, Tönnis W, editors. Handbuch der Neurochirurgie. Berlin: Springer-Verlag, 1962:175–179.

98. De La Torre E, Alexander EJr, Davis CHJr, Crandell DL. Tumors of the lateral ventricles of the brain: report of eight cases, with suggestions for clinical managment. J Neurosurg 1963; (20):461–470.

99. Ojemann GA. Individual variability in cortical localization of language. J Neurosurg 1979; 50(2):164–169.

100. Spencer DD, Collins WF. Surgical management of lateral intraventricular tumors. In: Schmidek HH, Sweet WH, editors. Operative Neurosurgical Techniques: Indications, Methods and Results. New York: Grune & Stratton, 1982:561–574.

101. Kempe LG, Blaylock R. Lateral-trigonal intraventricular tumors. A new operative approach. Acta Neurochir (Wien) 1976; 35(4):233–242.

102. Jun CL, Nutik SL. Surgical approaches to intraventricular meningiomas of the trigone. Neurosurgery 1985; 16(3): 416–420.

103. Geffen G, Walsh A, Simpson D, Jeeves M. Comparison of the effects of transcortical and transcallosal removal of intraventricular tumours. Brain 1980; 103(4):773–788.

104. Geschwind N. Disconnection syndromes in animals and man. Brain 1965; (88):237–294.

105. Levin HS, Rose JE. Alexia without agraphia in a musician after transcallosal removal of a left intraventricular meningioma. Neurosurgery 1979; 4(2):168–174.

106. Greenblatt SH. Neurosurgery and the anatomy of reading: a practical review. Neurosurgery 1977; 1(1):6–15.

107. Greenblatt SH, Saunders RL, Culver CM, Bogdanowicz W. Normal interhemispheric visual transfer with incomplete section of the splenium. Arch Neurol 1980; 37(9):567–571.

108. Tokunaga K, Tamiya T, Date I. Transient memory disturbance after removal of an intraventricular trigonal meningioma by a parieto-occipital interhemispheric precuneus approach: case report. Surg Neurol 2006; 65(2):167–169.

109. Winkler PA, Weis S, Buttner A, Raabe A, Amiridze N, Reulen HJ. The transcallosal interforniceal approach to the third ventricle: anatomic and microsurgical aspects. Neurosurgery 1997; 40(5):973–981.

110. Winkler PA, Weis S, Wenger E, Herzog C, Dahl A, Reulen HJ. Transcallosal approach to the third ventricle: normative morphometric data based on magnetic resonance imaging scans, with special reference to the fornix and forniceal insertion. Neurosurgery 1999; 45(2):309–317.

111. Winkler PA, Ilmberger J, Krishnan KG, Reulen HJ. Transcallosal interforniceal-transforaminal approach for removing lesions occupying the third ventricular space: clinical and neuropsychological results. Neurosurgery 2000; 46(4):879–888.

112. Yasargil MG. Microneurosurgery of CNS Tumors. Stuttgart: Thieme-Verlag, 1996.

113. Erman T, Gocer AI, Erdogan S, Boyar B, Hacyakupoglu S, Zorludemir S. Intraventricular meningiomas: a review of the literature and report of 8 cases. Neurosurgery Quarterly 2004; (14):154.

114. Araki C. Meningioma in pineal region: report of 2 cases removed by operation (Japanese). Nippon Geka Hokan 1937; (14):1181–1192.

115. Avman N, Dincer C. Meningiomas of the third ventricle. Acta Neurochir (Wien) 1978; 42(3–4):217–224.

116. Halpert B, Wilkins H, Lisle ACJr. Meningioma of the free margin of the cerebellar tentorium. J Neurosurg 1949; (6):74–78.

117. Heppner F. Meningiomas of the third ventricle in children: review of the literature and report of two cases with uneventful recovery after surgery. Acta Psychiatr Neurol Scand 1955; (30):471–481.

118. Lesoin F, Bouchez B, Krivosic I, Delandsheer JM, Jomin M. Hemangiopericytic meningioma of the pineal region. Case report. Eur Neurol 1984; 23(4):274–277.

119. Markwalder TM, Seiler RW, Markwalder RV, Huber P, Markwalder HM. Meningioma of the anterior part of the third ventricle in a child. Surg Neurol 1979; 12(1):29–32.

120. Piatt JH, Jr., Campbell GA. Pineal region meningioma: report of two cases and literature review. Neurosurgery 1983; 12(4): 369–376.

121. Roda JM, Perez-Higueras A, Oliver B, Alvarez MP, Blazquez MG. Pineal region meningiomas without dural attachment. Surg Neurol 1982; 17(2):147–151.

122. Rozario R, Adelman L, Prager RJ, Stein BM. Meningiomas of the pineal region and third ventricle. Neurosurgery 1979; 5(4):489–5.

123. Sachs EJr, Avman N, Fischer RG. Meningiomas of the pineal region and posterior part of 3rd ventricle. J Neurosurg 1962; (19):325–331.

124. Sakaki S, Shiraishi T, Takeda S, Matsuoka K, Sadamoto K. Occlusion of the great vein of Galen associated with a huge meningioma in the pineal region. Case report. J Neurosurg 1984; 61(6):1136–1140.

125. Stone JL, Cybulski GR, Rhee HL, Bailey OT. Excision of a large pineal region hemangiopericytoma (angioblastic meningioma, hemangiopericytoma type). Surg Neurol 1983; 19(2):181–189.

126. Zeitlin H. Tumors in the region of the pineal body: a clinicopathologic report of three cases. Arch Neurol Psychiatry 1935; (34):567–586.

127. Ito J, Kadekaru T, Hayano M, Kurita I, Okada K, Yoshida Y. Meningioma in the tela choroidea of the third ventricle: CT and angiographic correlations. Neuroradiology 1981; 21(4): 207–211.

128. Lozier AP, Bruce JN. Meningiomas of the velum interpositum: surgical considerations. Neurosurg Focus 2003; 15(1):E11.

129. Papo I, Salvolini U. Meningiomas of the free margin of the tentorium developing in the pineal region. Neuroradiology 1974; 7(4):237–243.

130. Costa LB, Jr., Vilela MD, Lemos S. [Third ventricle meningioma in a child: case report]. Arq Neuropsiquiatr 2000; 58(3B): 931–934.

131. Erdincler P, Lena G, Sarioglu AC, Kuday C, Choux M. Intracranial meningiomas in children: review of 29 cases. Surg Neurol 1998; 49(2):136–140.

132. Gelabert GM, Fernandez Fernandez MA, Bollar ZA, Garcia AA, Martinez RR. [Meningioma of the third ventricle. Presentation of a case]. Arch Neurobiol (Madr) 1989; 52(2):100–104.

133. Huang PP, Doyle WK, Abbott IR. Atypical meningioma of the third ventricle in a 6-year-old boy. Neurosurgery 1993; 33(2):312–315.

134. Kasliwal MK, Srinivas M, Vaishya S, Atri S, Sharma MC. Posterior third ventricular meningioma masquerading a pineal tumour. J Neurooncol 2006; 78(1):103–104.

135. Messing-Junger AM, Riemenschneider MJ, Reifenberger G. A 21-year-old female with a third ventricular tumor. Brain Pathol 2006; 16(1):87–8, 93.

136. Pandya P, Chishti K, Bannister CM. A third ventricular meningioma in a child. Br J Neurosurg 1990; 4(2):129–133.

137. Pau A, Dorcaratto A, Pisani R. Third ventricular meningiomas of infancy. A case report. Pathologica 1996; 88(3):204–206.

138. Renfro M, Delashaw JB, Peters K, Rhoton E. Anterior third ventricle meningioma in an adolescent: a case report. Neurosurgery 1992; 31(4):746–750.

139. Schijman E, Blasi A, Sevlever G. Third ventricular malignant meningioma. Neurosurgery 1987; 21(5):760–761.

140. Strenger SW, Huang YP, Sachdev VP. Malignant meningioma within the third ventricle: a case report. Neurosurgery 1987; 20(3):465–468.

141. Tung H, Apuzzo MLJ. Meningiomas of the third ventricle and pineal region. In: Al-Mefty O, editor. Meningiomas. Baltimore: Williams & Wilkins, 1998:583–591.

142. Ganti SR, Hilal SK, Stein BM, Silver AJ, Mawad M, Sane P. CT of pineal region tumors. AJR Am J Roentgenol 1986; 146(3):451–458.

143. Camins MB, Schlesinger EB. Treatment of tumours of the posterior part of the third ventricle and the pineal region: a long term follow-up. Acta Neurochir (Wien) 1978; 40(1–2):131–143.

144. Donat JF, Okazaki H, Gomez MR, Reagan TJ, Baker HL, Jr., Laws ER, Jr. Pineal tumors. A 53-year experience. Arch Neurol 1978; 35(11):736–740.

145. Jooma R, Kendall BE. Diagnosis and management of pineal tumors. J Neurosurg 1983; 58(5):654–665.

146. Pluchino F, Broggi G, Fornari M, Franzini A, Solero CL, Allegranza A. Surgical approach to pineal tumours. Acta Neurochir (Wien) 1989; 96(1–2):26–31.

147. Reid WS, Clark WK. Comparison of the infratentorial and transtentorial approaches to the pineal region. Neurosurgery 1978; 3(1):1–8.

148. Stein BM. The infratentorial supracerebellar approach to pineal lesions. J Neurosurg 1971; 35(2):197–202.

149. Lazar ML, Clark K. Direct surgical management of masses in the region of the vein of Galen. Surg Neurol 1974; 2(1): 17–21.

150. Apuzzo MLJ. Surgery of masses affecting the third ventricuar chamber: techniques and strategies. Clin Neurosurg 1988; (34):499–522.

151. Apuzzo MLJ, Chandrasoma PT, Breeze RE, Cohen DM, Luxton G, Mazumder A. Application of image-directed stereotactic surgery in the managment of intracranial neoplasms. In: Heilbrun PM, editor. Concepts in Neurosurgery: Stereotactic Neurosurgery. Baltimore: Williams & Wilkins, 1988:73–132.

152. Morita A, Kelly PJ. Resection of intraventricular tumors via a computer-assisted volumetric stereotactic approach. Neurosurgery 1993; 32(6):920–926.

153. Rhoton ALJr. Microsurgical anatomy of the third ventricular region. In: Apuzzo MLJ, editor. Surgery of the Third Ventricle. Baltimore: Williams & Wilkins, 1998:92–166.

154. Dandy WE. An operation for the removal of pineal tumors. Surg Gynecol Obstet 1921; (33):113–119.

155. Hammock MK, Milhorat TH, Earle K, Di Chiro G. Vein of Galen ligation in the primate. Angiographic, gross, and light microscopic evaluation. J Neurosurg 1971; 34(1): 77–83.

156. Cossu M, Lubinu F, Orunesu G, Pau A, Sehrbundt VE, Sini MG et al. Subchoroidal approach to the third ventricle. Microsurgical anatomy. Surg Neurol 1984; 21(4):325–331.

157. Shucart WA. Anterior transcallosal and transcortical approach. In: Apuzzo MLJ, editor. Surgery of the Third Ventricle. Baltimore: Williams & Wilkins, 1998:369–389.

158. Wen HT, Rhoton AL, Jr., de Oliveira E. Transchoroidal approach to the third ventricle: an anatomic study of the choroidal fissure and its clinical application. Neurosurgery 1998; 42(6):1205–1217.

159. Pendl G. Approaches to the pineal region. Acta Neurochir Suppl (Wien) 1985; 35:50–54.

160. McComb JG, Apuzzo MLJ. Posterior intrahemispheric retrocallosal and transcallosal approaches. In: Apuzzo MLJ, editor. Surgery of the Third Ventricle. Baltimore: Williams & Wilkins, 1998:611–664.

161. Ramakrishnamurthy TV, Murty AV, Purohit AK, Sundaram C. Benign meningioma metastasizing through CSF pathways: a case report and review of literature. Neurol India 2002; 50(3):326–329.

162. Darwish B, Munro I, Boet R, Renaut P, Abdelaal AS, MacFarlane MR. Intraventricular meningioma with drop metastases and subgaleal metastatic nodule. J Clin Neurosci 2004; 11(7):787–791.

163. Shibuya M, Koketsu N, Osuka K. A meningioma of the lateral cerebellomedullarycistern without dural attachment. J Clin Neurosci 1999; (6):50–52.

164. Abraham J, Chandy J. Meningiomas of the posterior fossa without dural attachment: a case report. J Neurosurg 1963; (20):177–179.

165. Cantore GP, Ciappetta P, Delfini R, Raco A. Meningiomas of the posterior fossa without dural attachment. Surg Neurol 1986; (25):127–130.

166. Nagata K, Basugi N, Sasaki T, Hashimoto K, Manaka S, Takakura K. Intraventricular meningioma of the fourth ventricle—case report. Neurol Med Chir (Tokyo) 1988; 28(1):86–90.

167. Delfini R, Capone R, Ciappetta P, Domenicucci M. Meningioma of the fourth ventricle: a case report. Neurosurg Rev 1992; 15(2):147–149.

168. Chaskis C, Buisseret T, Michotte A, D'Haens J. Meningioma of the fourth ventricle presenting with intermittent behaviour disorders: a case report and review of the literature. J Clin Neurosci 2001; 8(Suppl 1):59–62.

169. Cummings TJ, Bentley RC, Gray L, Check WE, Lanier TE, McLendon RE. Meningioma of the fourth ventricle. Clin Neuropathol 1999; 18(5):265–269.

170. Ceylan S, Ilbay K, Kuzeyli K, Kalelioglu M, Akturk F, Ozoran Y. Intraventricular meningioma of the fourth ventricle. Clin Neurol Neurosurg 1992; 94(2):181–184.

171. Tsuboi K, Nose T, Maki Y. Meningioma of the fourth ventricle: a case report. Neurosurgery 1983; 13(2):163–166.

172. Zuleta EB, Londono RL. Meningiomas del IV ventricolo. Acta Neurochir 1955; (4):228–232.

55
Jugular Foramen Meningiomas I

Tomio Sasaki and Nobutaka Kawahara

Introduction

Primary jugular foramen meningiomas represent one of the rarest subgroups of meningiomas. Samii and Ammirati [1] reported that in their series of 420 skull base meningiomas, they found only three meningiomas (0.7%) arising primarily in the jugular foramen. In another neurosurgical series [2] jugular foramen meningiomas accounted for 4.3% of posterior fossa meningiomas. To date, approximately 112 cases of jugular foramen meningiomas have been reported in the literature [2–35]. A higher incidence of these tumors was pointed out in patients with neurofibromatosis [25]. A case of neurofibromatosis type 2 is demonstrated in Fig. 55-1.

Many meningiomas arise from arachnoid cap cells, which are also known as meningocytes or meningothelial cells. Meningocytes are most numerous near the dural sinuses. They are found in other intracranial areas as well, particularly in association with cranial and spinal nerve foramina. The jugular foramen is a rare location for meningioma to occur [1,2]. These meningiomas often present with very invasive features, infiltrating the surrounding skull base in all directions [13,17,25,29,32]. This pattern of spread can be referred to as "centrifugal." The spread pattern involves the temporal bone including the middle ear cavity laterally and invades the skull base including the jugular tubercle, hypoglossal canal, occipital condyle, and clivus medially. Inferior extracranial spread occurs into the nasopharyngeal carotid space of the deep suprahyoid neck, and superior intracranial spread is seen along the intracranial dural reflections. This spread along the dura is termed "en plaque" and is characteristic of primary jugular foramen meningiomas (Fig. 55-2). A globose appearance is seen less commonly in the tumor with intracranial extension [30]. In cases with extracranial extension, carotid artery encasement and jugular vein occlusion are common [13,26,29].

Signs and Symptoms

The clinical presentations of jugular foramen meningiomas are similar to those of other jugular foramen lesions: neuropathies affecting cranial nerves V–XII, hearing loss, (pulsatile) tinnitus, and a middle ear mass [29,30,32]. Pulsatile tinnitus may be more common with glomus jugulare tumors than meningiomas. Depending on the involvement of different combinations of the lower cranial nerves, various syndromes, namely Vernet's syndrome, also known as jugular foramen syndrome (IX, X, XI nerve palsies), Jackson's syndrome (X, XI, XII nerve palsies), Collet-Sicard syndrome (IX, X, XI, XII nerve palsies), and Villaret's syndrome(IX, X, XI, XII nerve palsies with involvement of sympathetics), have been described. However, it is unusual for patients to present with those typical syndromes.

Radiologic Diagnosis

The preoperative radiologic diagnosis and the differential diagnosis are very important, because their preoperative management and operative planning differ considerably. Two common differential diagnoses for the jugular foramen meningioma are glomus jugulare tumors and neuromas of the lower cranial nerves.

A diagnosis of jugular foramen meningioma can often be made preoperatively when several radiologic features are seen associated with a jugular foramen mass [22,30,32,34]. Jugular foramen meningiomas cause irregular enlargement of the jugular foramen. On computed tomography (CT), meningiomas appear slightly hyperdense, with occasional matrix calcification. The jugular foramen margins have a mixed permeative-sclerotic appearance (Fig. 55-3). On the other hand, glomus jugulare tumors may show a permeative-destructive pattern with erosion of the jugular foramen margins and infiltrated bone without preservation of the underlying architecture or bone density.

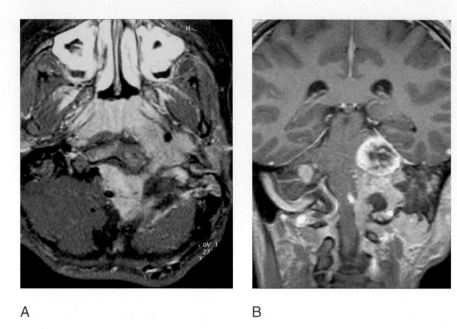

A   B

Fig. 55-1. Jugular foramen meningioma in neurofibromatosis type 2 patient. This patient was a 7-year-old girl. (A) Axial contrast-enhanced T1-weighted MR image demonstrates a jugular foramen meningioma extending both intracranially and extracranially. (B) Coronal contrast-enhanced T1-weighted MR image demonstrates a jugular foramen meningioma and bilateral acoustic tumors

Neuroma gradually enlarges the jugular foramen by pressure erosion and gives an expanded and scalloped but well-defined corticated margin to the jugular foramen. Other helpful differentiating features of jugular foramen meningioma include the presence of dural tails and an absence of flow voids within the mass. Jugular foramen meningiomas have imaging characteristics similar to meningiomas found elsewhere. Following injection of contrast material, strong and homogeneous enhancement is seen, often with an enhancing dural tail along its margin. This enhancing dural tail is a particularly important feature that assists in differentiating meningiomas from neuromas or glomus jugulare tumors. Another important feature is an absence of flow voids. Glomus jugulare tumors display a salt-and-pepper appearance on non–contrast-enhanced T1-weighted magnetic resonance (MR) images; this appearance represents a flow-void network within their rich vascularity. These serpentine flow voids are absent in meningiomas. Angiography reveals a vascular tumor characterized by a prolonged vascular blush without arteriovenous shunting that is commonly seen in glomus jugulare tumors. A broader differential diagnosis may include chordomas, chondromas, chondrosarcomas, epidermoid tumors, and metastases.

Therapy

Microsurgical Resection

Surgery with total removal is the recommended therapy for most patients of jugular foramen meningiomas. However, radical removal of jugular foramen meningioma without producing new deficits, especially lower cranial nerve deficits, is more

difficult than for glomus jugulare tumors or neuromas [2,21,29,32,35]. They may not only compress the lower cranial nerves, but also spread into the nerve sheaths; invade the temporal bone; invade, compress, or obstruct the jugular bulb; or extend extracranially into infratemporal/parapharyngeal space. Without sacrificing the lower cranial nerves that are surrounded by the tumor, total removal is usually impossible. Furthermore, resection of bone must be continued until grossly normal, and uninvolved bone is encountered to ensure total removal. Such an aggressive surgical resection carries a potential operative risk and may not necessarily prevent recurrences. Even with "total" microsurgical removal of the tumor, Molony et al. [22] observed a recurrence rate of 25%. Therefore, the strategy of total tumor removal may not apply for all jugular foramen meningiomas. The decision to approach these tumors must be individualized dependent on symptoms, the patient's age and condition, and size and direction of growth of the intracranial, intratemporal, foraminal,or extracranial tumor portions.

The proliferation of neurotologic surgical approaches to the lateral skull base in the last 20 years has revolutionized the surgeon's options for treating jugular foramen tumors. For removing jugular foramen tumors, various surgical approaches have been advocated [2,18,21,26,29,32]. Basic otolaryngologic approaches are the translabyrinthine, transcochlear, and infratemporal fossa approaches with transposition of the facial nerve. Combined approaches such as the combined transcochlear-infratemporal fossa approach or combined translabyrinthine-infratemporal fossa approach have also been employed [21,32]. Although the infratemporal fossa approach provides a wide operative field from the jugular foramen through the infratemporal fossa, hearing must be sacrificed and the facial nerve is rerouted, which

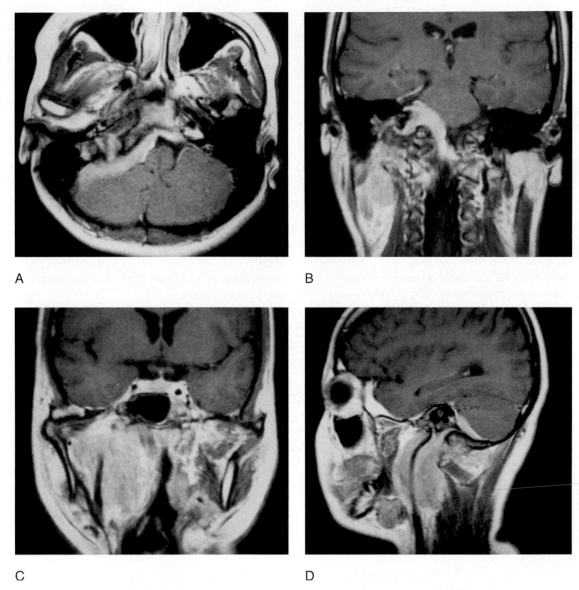

FIG. 55-2. Jugular foramen meningioma in a 20-year-old woman. (A) Axial contrast-enhanced T1-weighted MR image showing en plaque involvement of posterior fossa with extension to extracranial space through jugular foramen. (B) Coronal contrast-enhanced T1-weighted MR image demonstrating a meningioma centered at the jugular foramen. The tumor extended to both the posterior fossa and the neck. (C) Coronal contrast-enhanced T1-weighted MR image showing the large enhancing mass extended to the parapharyngeal space. Internal carotid artery was encased by the tumor. (D) Sagittal contrast-enhanced T1-weighted MR image showing the tumor extended to the parapharyngeal space with encasement of internal carotid artery. (From Ref. 26.)

often results in facial palsy. To remedy these drawbacks, several neurosurgical approaches have been proposed and employed: the lateral approach [18], extreme lateral approach [36], transjugular approach [26], and variations of the retrosigmoid-transcondylar approach, including the suprajugular, retrojugular, and transjugular approach [29].

Jugular foramen meningiomas with extracranial extension frequently encase carotid and vertebral arteries (Fig. 55-2). Management of these involved arteries further complicates the operative strategy and increases the surgical risk. To achieve total removal of the tumor, those encased vessels must be resected together with the tumor. In such cases, a balloon test occlusion must be performed preoperatively to assess the risk

of ischemic complications after the vessel resection [37,38]. If the patient does not tolerate the test, vascular reconstruction must be planned (Fig. 55-4). Once vascular reconstruction is planned in skull base tumors, a risk of infection always has to be taken into consideration. As the risk of infection with subsequent necrosis and rupture of the artery or graft is high when the pharynx or oral cavity is entered during tumor dissection, some reports [26,39] recommend a two-stage operation rather than a one-stage operation for resection of the tumor and vascular reconstruction. Obliteration of the dead space using a microvascular "anastomized" muscle graft is also recommended in case an opening into the oropharyngeal cavity has occurred.

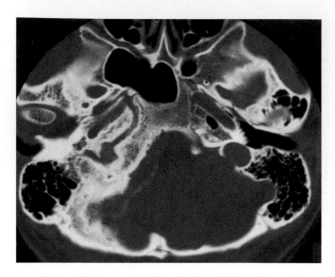

FIG. 55-3. Bone window CT scan showing characteristic permeative-sclerotic appearance with preservation of bone architecture on the right side. Faint calcification is also seen in the tumor

Outcome and Complications

Multiple lower cranial nerve deficits are common sequelae of the surgical resection of jugular foramen lesions. Particularly, meningioma patients tend to have worse postoperative cranial nerve outcomes than those with glomus jugulare tumors or neuromas. In a recent analysis of the incidence of lower cranial nerve deficits following resection of jugular foramen tumors, meningioma was found to have a strikingly higher rate of new deficit (approximately 60%) than either glomus jugulare (approximately 30%) or schwannoma (approximately 15%) [35]. The most common postoperative complications are deficits of the ninth and tenth cranial nerves [29]. In case the lower cranial nerves are already involved preoperatively, compensation is usually achieved by the contralateral nerves. However, most patients will require temporary assistance with swallowing, airway protection, and phonation in the form of a vocal cord medialization [32].

Radiation

As jugular foramen meningiomas often present with very invasive features and have the potential of a locally malignant tumor, routine use of postoperative radiotherapy has been recommended by some authors [28,40] to prevent recurrence.

Summary

Primary jugular foramen meningiomas represent one of the rarest subgroups of meningiomas and account for approximately 4% of posterior fossa meningiomas. These tumors often present with very invasive features, infiltrating the surrounding skull base in all directions. Intracranial spread

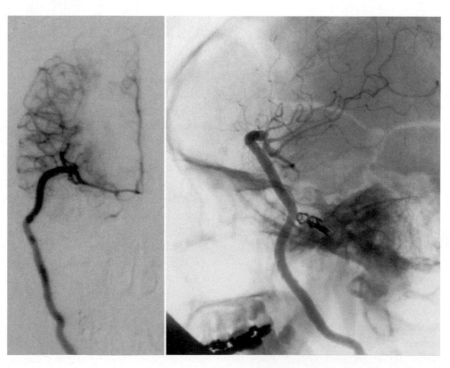

FIG. 55-4. Postoperative carotid angiography showing vascular reconstruction using saphenous vein. (From Ref. 26.)

along the dura is termed "en plaque" and is characteristic of primary jugular foramen meningiomas. Extracranial spread through the jugular foramen occurs into the naso-pharyngeal carotid space of the neck. In cases with extra-cranial extension, carotid artery encasement and jugular vein occlusion are common. Radiologically, irregular enlargement of the jugular foramen and a mixed perme-ative-sclerotic appearance of the surrounding bone are char-acteristic on bone window CT. Other features include the presence of dural tails and an absence of flow voids within the mass on MR images. An ideal treatment is total removal of the tumor. However, total removal of these tumors with-out producing new deficits, especially lower cranial nerve deficits, is almost impossible. Multiple lower cranial nerve deficits are common sequelae of the surgical resection of these tumors, and the most common postoperative compli-cations are deficits of the ninth and tenth cranial nerves. Most of these patients require temporary assistance with swallowing, airway protection, and phonation in the form of a vocal cord medialization.

References

1. Samii M, Ammirati M. Surgery of Skull Base Meningiomas. New York: Springer-Verlag, 1994.
2. Roberti F, Sekhar LN, Kalavakonda C, et al. Posterior fossa meningiomas: Surgical experience in 161 cases. Surg Neurol 2001;56:8–21.
3. Proctor B, Lindsay JR. Tumors involving the petrous pyramid of the temporal bone. Arch Otolaryngol 1947;46:180–94.
4. Hoye SJ, Hoar CS, Murray JE. Extracranial meningioma pre-senting as a tumor of the neck. Am J Surg 1960;100:486–9.
5. Svien HJ, Baker HL, Rivers MH. Jugular foramen syndrome and allied syndromes. Neurology 1963;13:797–809.
6. Binns PM, Fairman HD. Lesions in the temporal bone causing multiple nerve damage. J Laryngol Otol 1966;80:125–37.
7. Binns PM. Jugular foramen syndrome caused by meningioma. Trans Am Acad Ophthalmol Otolaryngol 1972;76:1368–70.
8. Whicker JH, Devine KD, MacCarty CS. Diagnostic and thera-peutic problems in extracranial meningiomas. Am J Surg 1973;126:452–7.
9. Maniglia AJ, Page LK. Posterior cranial fossa and temporal bone meningioma in a child, appearing as a neck mass. Otolaryngol Head Neck Surg 1979;87:578–83.
10. Nakagawa H, Lusins JO. Biplane computed tomography of intracranial meningiomas with extracranial extension. J Comput Assist Tomogr 1980;4:478–83.
11. Rose WS, Makhija MC, Sattenspiel S. Meningioma presenting as a tumor in the neck. AJR 1980; 134:1070–2.
12. Schmidt D, Mackay B, Luna MA, et al. Aggressive meningioma with jugular vein extension. Case report with ultrastructural observations. Arch Otolaryngol 1981;107:635–7.
13. Nager GT, Heroy J, Hoeplinger M. Meningiomas invading the temporal bone with extension to the neck. Am J Otolaryngol 1983;4:297–324.
14. Rietz DR, Ford CN, Kurtycz OF, et al. Significance of appar-ent intratympanic meningiomas. Laryngoscope 1983;93:1397–404.
15. Mafee MF, Aimi K, Valvassori GE. Computed tomography in the diagnosis of primary tumors of the petrous bone. Laryngoscope 1984;94:1423–30.
16. Gagnon NB, Lavigne F, Mohr G, et al. Extracranial and intracra-nial meningiomas. J Otolaryngol 1986;15:380–4.
17. Nichols, RD, Knighton RS, Chason JL, et al. Meningioma in the parotid region. Laryngoscope 1987;97:693–6.
18. George B, Dematons C, Cophignon J. Lateral approach to the ante-rior portion of the foramen magnum. Application to surgical removal of 14 benign tumors. Technical note. Surg Neurol 1988;29:484–90.
19. Inagawa T, Kamiya K, Hosoda I, et al. Jugular foramen menin-gioma. Surg Neurol 1989;31:295–9.
20. Uchibori M, Odake G, Ueda S, et al. Parapharyngeal meningioma extending from the intracranial space. Neuroradiology 1990;32:53–5.
21. Arriaga M, Shelton C, Nassif P, et al. Selection of surgical approaches for meningiomas affecting the temporal bone. Oto-laryngol Head Neck Surg 1992;107:738–44.
22. Molony TB, Brackmann DE, Lo WWM. Meningiomas of the jugular foramen. Otolaryngol Head Neck Surg 1992;106:128–36.
23. Murakami M, Yoshioka S, Kuratsu J, et al. High serum alkaline phosphatase level of meningioma cell origin. Case report and review of the literature. Neurosurgery 1992;30:624–7.
24. Ohta S, Yokoyama T, Uemura K, et al. Petrous bone meningioma originating from the jugular foramen —case report. Neurol Med Chir (Tokyo) 1997;7:472–4.
25. Tekkök IH, Özcan OE, Turan E, et al. Jugular foramen menin-gioma. Report of a case and review of the literature. J Neurosurg Sci 1997;41:283–92.
26. Kawahara N, Sasaki T, Nibu K, et al. Dumbbell type jugular fora-men meningioma extending both into the posterior cranial fossa and into the parapharyngeal space: Report of 2 cases with vascu-lar reconstruction. Acta Neurochir(Wien) 1998;140:323–31.
27. Varionis FD, Robertson JH, Gardner G, et al. Temporal bone meningiomas. Skull Base Surg 1999;9:127–39.
28. Nicolato A, Foroni R, Pellegrino M, et al. Gamma knife radiosur-gery in meningiomas of the posterior fossa. Experience with 62 treated lesions. Minim Invas Neurosurg 2001;44:211–7.
29. Arnautovic KI, Al-Mefty O. Primary meningiomas of the jugular fossa. J Neurosurg 2002;97:12–20.
30. Macdonald AJ, Salzman KL, Harnsberger HR, et al. Primary jugular foramen meningioma: Imaging appearance and differen-tiating features. AJR 2004;182:373–7.
31. Tabuse M, Uchida K, Ueda R, et al. Jugular foramen papillary meningioma: a case report. Brain Tumor Pathol 2004;21:143–7.
32. Gilbert ME, Shelton C, McDonald A, et al. Meningioma of the jugular foramen: glomus jugulare mimic and surgical challenge. Laryngoscope 2004;114:25–32.
33. Tatagiba M, Koerbel A, Bornemann A, et al. Meningioma of the accessory nerve extending from the jugular foramen into the parapharyngeal space. Acta Neurochir(Wien) 2005;147:909–10.
34. Shimone T, Akai F, Yamamoto A, et al. Different signal intensities between intra- and extracranial components in jugular foramen meningioma: an enigma. Am J Neuroradiol 2005;26:1122–7.
35. Lustig LR, Jackler RK. The variable relationship between the lower cranial nerves and jugular foramen tumors: implications for neural preservation. Am J Otol 1996;117:658–68.
36. Sen CN, Sekhar LN. An extreme lateral approach to intradural lesions of the cervical spine and foramen magnum. Neurosurgery 1990;27:197–204.

37. Fox AJ, Viñuela F, Pelz DM, et al. Use of detachable balloons for proximal artery occlusion in the treatment of unclippable cerebral aneurysms. J Neurosurg 1987;66:40–46.

38. Origitano TC, Al-Mefty O, Leonetti JP, et al. Vascular considerations and complications in cranial base surgery. Neurosurgery 1994;35:351–63.

39. Gormley WB, Sekhar LN, Wright DC, et al. Management and long-term outcome of adenoid cystic carcinoma with intracranial extension: a neurosurgical perspective. Neurosurgery 1996;38:1105–13.

40. Wara SM, Sheline GE, Newman H, et al. Radiation therapy of meningiomas. Am J Roentgenol 1975;123:453–8.

56
Jugular Foramen Meningiomas II: An Otologist's Approach, Perspective, and Experience

Mario Sanna, Sean Flanagan, G. DeDonato, A. Bacciu, and Maurizio Falcioni

Introduction

Meningiomas are common intracranial tumors, usually of benign and slow-growing behavior, with a tendency to invade the dura and infiltrate bone. Involvement of the jugular fossa, however, is rare, with primary involvement exceedingly so.

This chapter reviews the current literature on meningiomas of this location and highlights the differences in diagnostic features and management options compared to the far more common pathology arising in this area, namely jugulo-tympanic paragangliomas and lower cranial nerve schwannomas. References to our series of 13 jugular foramen meningiomas is made to further emphasize these points.

Significant advances in diagnostics, surgical and anaesthetic techniques have been made since the pioneering times, allowing curative surgical management in most cases. Despite these advances, however, both the pathology and the complex anatomy of the jugular foramen make this condition an extremely difficult one to manage. The variability of tumor extension, its rarity, and its associated morbidity of treatment make a prescriptive management protocol impossible.

Jugular foramen meningiomas (JFM) are most often considered in the differential diagnosis of jugulo-tympanic paragangliomas, which make up 90% of jugular fossa tumors. This is followed by schwannomas of the lower cranial nerves, and then JFMs.

Epidemiology

Meningiomas constitute approximately 20% of all intracranial tumors. Of these, 8–12% are found within the posterior cranial fossa, most commonly arising in the Cerebellopontine Angle (CPA) (1–3). It is estimated that 0.7–9.3% of posterior fossa meningiomas arise in the jugular foramen (4). Two thirds of meningiomas arise in women, with a peak incidence in the fifth and sixth decades—slightly younger in women than in men.

Meningiomas involving the jugular foramen can be classified as primary, which are exceedingly rare, with less than 60 cases reported, and those spreading secondarily, most commonly from the CPA or petroclival region. To be classified as a primary JFM, the tumor must originate from the jugular foramen (5).

Tumor Behavior

Meningiomas arise from meningo-epithelial (arachnoidal cap) cells associated with arachnoid villi of the dural sinuses and prominent tributary veins, as well as those of the exit foramina of cranial nerves and vessels (3,6,7). Their location is described according to the area of dural attachment, although a precise location can be often difficult to specify. Macroscopically, meningiomas are lobular gray-white, rubbery, firm masses with a gritty consistency.

The blood supply is related to the site of origin, predominantly from dural branches of the external carotid arterial system. Meningiomas of the jugular foramen initially derive supply from the ascending pharyngeal artery. Branches of the occipital and vertebral arteries are commonly involved as are those from the middle meningeal. This allows for preoperative embolization in selected cases. Sixty percent of meningiomas also derive a supplementary supply from cerebral-pial vessels.

Most meningiomas exhibit a slow growth rate, with a significant number remaining asymptomatic. This is less often the case for meningiomas of the skull base. Meningiomas normally become apparent due to compression of adjacent neural structures, rather than as a result of parenchymal involvement, particularly in the constricted area of the jugular foramen. This is coupled with the propensity of these tumors to infiltrate the bone of the skull base and invade air cell tracts. When this process is centred in the jugular foramen, a primary JFM can usually be differentiated from one that has spread from another location. Secondary JFM are less likely to infiltrate bone, and are predominantly soft tumor masses (5,8,9).

Intracranial spread usually follows dural surfaces, commonly assuming an en plaque configuration. They also follow the neurovascular bundle into the neck. Intraluminal invasion of the jugular bulb and internal jugular vein can also occur, providing another route of spread, although much less commonly than in jugulo-tympanic paragangliomas. Whether due to compression or direct invasion, the jugulo-sigmoid complex is occluded in most cases.

Growth commonly occurs simultaneously intra- and extracranially as well as into the hypotympanum and temporal bone (5). Frank invasion of brain parenchyma can also occur, albeit rarely.

Genetics

The development of a meningioma is a genetically complex process. A stepwise series of genomic alterations corresponds to an increasing tumor grade.

Mutations in the *NF2* tumor suppressor gene, located in the chromosomal region 22q12.2, with its associated protein product merlin, represent the most frequent gene alteration in meningiomas and is seen in up to 50% of sporadic meningiomas. It is seen in 100% of meningiomas associated with NF-2.

Numerous other genetic abnormalities have been identified in meningiomas, with loss of genetic material on 1 p, the second most common chromosomal abnormality identified. Further abnormalities have been linked to chromosomes 14, 10, 17, and losses on 9 are linked to malignant change. These changes form the basis of a model of tumor progression from normal meningoepithelial cells to malignant meningioma (10,11).

Multiple meningiomas can occur, most commonly in NF-2 and the rare non–NF-2 families with a hereditary predisposition. Much rarer associations are with Werner and Gorlin syndromes. The presence of multiple sporadic meningiomas most likely represents subarachnoidal spread (1,2,10,12,13).

Clinical Features

Clinically, all jugular foramen tumors tend to present in a similar fashion, with variable involvement of cranial nerves IX–XII (14).

The presentation with a middle ear mass is less common than in jugulo-tympanic paragangliomas, but is seen in approximately 20% of cases, as is the presence of pulsatile tinnitus. Some degree of hearing loss is expected in 60–80%, and is usually of a mixed type.

The state of hearing is an important issue. Unlike most jugulo-tympanic paragangliomas, preservation of the external auditory canal can be considered due to the less frequent need to control the internal carotid artery (ICA), and the reduced vascularity of the tumor. Facial nerve dysfunction is rarely seen in JFM as a presenting feature, and additional cranial nerve palsies are evident in approximately 10% of cases—most commonly V or VI nerves (15).

TABLE 56-1. Clinical Features in Patients Affected by Jugular Foramen Meningioma.

Presenting signs/ symptoms	JF meningiomas Gruppo Otologico (n = 13)	Survey of the literature (n = 29)
Hearing loss	9 (69%)	20 (79%)
Tinnitus	4 (31%)	11 (38%)
Dysphonia	5 (38%)	16 (55%)%
Dysphagia	4 (31%)	16 (55%)
Shoulder weakness	2 (15%)	5 (17%)
Middle ear mass	3 (23%)	11 of 19 (58%)
Vertigo/instability	7 (54%)	4 (14%)
Glossal atrophy	3 (23%)	4 (14%)

Rarely signs and symptoms of brain stem compression can form the initial presentation, while headache and facial pain are more commonly seen in JFM than in other primary jugular fossa pathology. Despite some variances in the pattern of symptoms between JFM and other jugular fossa lesions, the diagnosis is essentially a radiologic one, confirmed at the time of surgery (Table 56-1).

Investigations

A thorough clinical examination should be complemented by an upper aerodigestive tract endoscopy. Silent lower cranial nerve palsies can occur in 10% of jugular fossa tumors, and knowledge of the extent and degree of compensation of known lesions is important.

Audiology

A complete audiological assessment is necessary due to the fact that the hearing status can influence the surgical approach. In cases where there is a degree of sensorineural loss, especially if there is an extension to the CPA, brainstem auditory evoked responses (BAER) should be used to further assist in the assessment of whether residual hearing is worth preserving.

Radiologic Findings

The importance of a radiologic diagnosis in lesions of the skull base is paramount. Major surgery is usually planned without the presence of histopathologic confirmation. This is especially true in lesions of the jugular fossa due to the significant variance in the biological behavior of tumors arising in this area, which affects the surgical approach used.

Important Points to Assess

- Vascularity
- ICA involvement
- Size of cervical component
- Degree of intracranial extension
- Extent of bone erosion or infiltration

JFM on magnetic resonance imaging (MRI) appear iso- or hypointense in signal intensity on T1-weighted images and intermediate signal on T2-weighted sequences with homogeneous enhancement after contrast administration. The posterior fossa component is usually en plaque, but can take a globular form. The presence of a dural tail is common, seen in 75–100% of cases, while the classic findings of hyperostosis and intratumoral calcifications, even if highly suggestive, are rarely seen at this site (8,19–21).

Bony margins of the jugular foramen appear irregular, with permeative-sclerotic changes common in the surrounding skull base. In comparison to jugulo-tympanic paragangliomas, there is relative maintenance of the bony architecture. JFM, however, are more likely to spread medially to involve the jugular tubercle, with further extension anteriorly toward the clivus, as well as inferiorly to affect the hypoglossal canal. MRI is often invaluable in assessing the degree of bony infiltration, with displacement of a normal fatty signal seen in the marrow spaces of the skull base.

Radiologically an increased degree of calcification and reduced intensity on T2 MRI can indicate a slower rate of growth (11). Conversely, peritumoral edema is apparent as hyperintensity on T2 images (3).

Assessment of bilateral venous drainage is essential, because there is a high likelihood of sacrificing the jugulosigmoid complex in the surgical approach to these tumors. MRV are usually adequate to make this assessment.

Angiography is occasionally required to differentiate atypical findings. While there is a degree of variability in the vascularity of meningiomas, the tumor blush is less intense than in jugulo-tympanic paragangliomas, which reveal a coarse tumor blush and rapid venous drainage. Angiography is also indicated if there is a question of ICA involvement in assessing the cavernous sinus extension (5,8,22–25).

Apart from jugulo-tympanic paragangliomas, jugular foramen schwannomas (JFS) are the other main differential diagnosis in this area. JFS appear as smoothly marginated round or lobulated masses, iso- or hypointense on T1-weighted images and iso- or hyperintense on T2 with often irregular enhancement after gadolinium. Cystic change, while rare in meningiomas, is common in schwannomas. On high resolution computer tomography (HRCT), JFS reveal smooth expansion of the bony margins of the jugular foramen. There is no evidence of invasion in to the marrow spaces of the skull base. Both JFS and JFM display a dumbbell shape when there is both intra- and extracranial spread.

Metastatic disease, invasive small cell carcinoma (SCC), chondrosarcoma, endolymphatic sac tumors, and nasopharyngeal carcinoma should all be considered in the differential diagnosis (9).

Staging

While the size of the tumor is of importance, it is the involvement of the surrounding compartments and the degree of bony infiltration that dictate the true extent of the lesion. At presentation 60% of primary JFM extend to the CPA, 45% into the upper neck, and 20% into the middle ear, based on our series. There is considerable variance in the degree of extension of primary jugular foramen tumors, and this reflects the difficulty in assessing the true origin of meningiomas in this area.

Management Options

While the delineation between primary and secondary meningiomas of the jugular foramen can be difficult, especially in larger tumors, it is the true extension of the tumor through the jugular foramen that is the most important surgical consideration. This necessitates an approach that can control the jugular fossa region, allowing complete resection of the tumor.

As mentioned, the rarity and complexity of JFM does not allow a prescriptive management protocol. Patient factors are paramount due to the fact that this is a benign yet locally invasive pathology and that treatment invariably involves significant morbidity. While most series report at least one cranial nerve (CN) deficit prior to surgery in 50–55% of patients, new deficits are present in 60–70% postoperatively. Acute compound lower cranial nerve palsies are poorly tolerated in those with marginal physical reserve, and because of their slow growth potential, elderly patients, especially those with minimal symptoms, should be managed conservatively in most cases. Rarely brain stem decompression is indicated in this age group, and a planned subtotal resection may be performed.

An argument can be made to observe these tumors until lower cranial nerve function is compromised by the tumor and compensation occurs preoperatively. In comparison to jugulo-tympanic paragangliomas, where preservation of the noninfiltrated medial wall of the jugular bulb often allows preservation of the lower cranial nerves (LCNs), JFM are more likely to spread from a medial to lateral direction encasing the neural structures. Therefore, total resection of a JFM, with preoperatively normal LCNs, is more likely to lead to a postoperative deficit.

This strategy of initial conservatism runs the risk of further tumor progression, reducing the likelihood of a single-stage resection with a hearing-preservation approach and without facial nerve mobilization. Subtotal removal is also an option, with the aim to maximize neural integrity. This, however, especially in the younger patient, increases the likelihood of revision surgery with higher rates of morbidity, and recurrance.

Encasement of critical vascular structures such as the posterior inferior cerebellar artery (PICA), anterior inferior cerebellar artery (AICA), and internal carotid artery (ICA), adherence to the brain stem, as well as extension into the cavernous sinus, are situations where subtotal removal is indicated.

The option of radiotherapy should also be discussed. It is not recommended as a primary treatment in the younger patient, but may provide tumor control in the older age group. The true role for these therapies, however, lies in treating small residual tumors that exhibit growth and are in critical areas such as the cavernous sinus. Their use can also be contemplated as an adjuvant treatment of grade III tumors (26,27).

As mentioned, the involvement of a dominant jugulo-sigmoid complex can change the surgical approach, with preservation of the jugulo-sigmoid system required. Consideration of pre-operative management of the ICA is rare in JFM. However, extensive involvement can occur, and it is in these cases where assessment of contralateral and vertebral collateral supply is mandated. Balloon occlusion, with or without high-flow bypass, is an option, but it is very rarely required. The recent introduction of stenting of the ICA in cases of poor collateral supply has added another method by which safe total tumor removal can be attempted.

Preoperative embolization of JFM is well described, but is not as essential as for jugulo-tympanic paragangliomas. From a surgical perspective, the ability to resect the surrounding dura and the infiltrated bone in conjunction with the tumor histology determines the likelihood of recurrence (28–30).

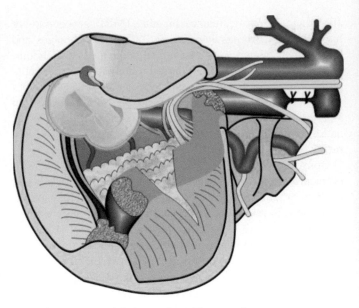

FIG. 56-1. Petro-occipital transsigmoid approach

Surgery

The ideal treatment for these lesions is total surgical removal. The surgical management of these lesions is particularly challenging due to the complex anatomic location and potential postoperative complications.

The major problems include:

- Obtaining adequate exposure, since these tumors may involve three separate compartments: intracranial, intrapetrous, and extracranial.
- The vertical portion of the facial nerve is centered on and closely related to the jugular bulb.
- Potential injury to the lower cranial nerves, which are frequently involved.
- Radical removal is made more difficult with meningiomas due to their infiltrative nature.

A myriad of surgical approaches with a variety of names have been described to access the jugular fossa, but very few series directly address the treatment of primary JFM (8,19,23,31–38).

The extent of pathology, as always, dictates the approach. Unlike the treatment of jugulo-tympanic paragangliomas, however, where the infratemporal fossa type A (IFTA) is the workhorse approach, the petro-occipital transsigmoid (POTS) approach provides the foundation from which JFM are removed. The IFTA allows the surgeon to completely control the JF area and surrounding structures, allows optimal exposure of the ICA, but necessitates sacrifice of the middle ear and involves the anterior transposition of the facial nerve.

When dealing with nonvascular tumors such as JFM, with normal facial nerve function and hearing, a more conservative approach should be used. The POTS approach entails a suboccipital craniotomy combined with a retrolabyrinthine petrosectomy and dissection of the retrofacial and infralabyrinthine air cells, partial drilling of the occipital condyle, and transection

of the sigmoid sinus. The POTS approach offers the surgeon a direct exposure of the jugular foramen area while preserving the middle and inner ear function without the need for facial nerve transposition (23–25,39–41) (Fig. 56-1).

Surgical Anatomy

The jugular foramen is the portal of exit of the cranial nerves IX, X, and XI. In order to access this complex area of the skull base, important structures must be addressed. The ICA anteriorly, the facial nerve laterally, the hypoglossal nerve medially, and the vertebral artery inferiorly all minimize pathways to the jugular fossa.

The traditional description divides the JF into an anteromedial pars nervosa containing the glossopharyngeal nerve, inferior petrosal sinus and meningeal branch of the ascending pharyngeal artery, and a posterolateral compartment containing the vagus and accessory nerves with the sigmoid sinus. Less confusing terminology was introduced by Rhoton, describing two venous and one neural compartments (35).

The sigmoid part, posterolaterally, and a smaller anteromedial venous channel, the petrosal part, are separated by the neural part, through which the glossopharyngeal, vagus, and accessory nerves pass. The separation is delineated by the intrajugular processes of the temporal and occipital bones which are connected by a fibrous band that can occasionally ossify. Importantly, the glossopharyngeal nerve enters through a separate dural sheath from the vagus and accessory nerves to reach the medial wall of the internal jugular vein.

The petrosal part is comprised of a venous confluence, receiving tributaries from the hypoglossal canal, petroclival fissure, and vertebral venous plexus. It is also important to note that there are often multiple openings of the inferior petrosal sinus into the jugular bulb, which must be identified and managed when performing a transjugular approach. They invariably enter through an opening in the medial wall of the jugular bulb between the glossopharyngeal nerve anteriorly and the vagus and accessory nerves posteriorly.

When accessing the jugular fossa without sacrificing the external ear canal (EAC), and mobilizing the facial nerve, additional exposure is gained by partial removal of the occipital condyle. This structure lies inferomedial to the jugular bulb. The condylar fossa, lying just posteriorly, contains the condylar emissary vein, which is often encountered. This vein can frequently have an intimate relationship with the lower cranial nerves at their exit site from the jugular foramen. The posteromedial third of the condyle can be removed without concern about atlanto-occipital instability. The intracranial opening of the hypoglossal canal lies approximately 5 mm above the posterior and middle thirds of the occipital condyle, which is also protected if only the posteromedial third of the occipital condyle is removed. A further 5 mm above the intracranial opening of the hypoglossal canal is the jugular tubercle, a prominence over which the LCN drape prior to entering the JF, and an area which is commonly infiltrated by tumor. Its removal also improves access to the lower clivus. The relationship of the mastoid segment of the facial nerve should also be stressed. In 60% of cases, more than 50% of the bulb lies anterior to the vertical plane of the nerve (29).

Surgical Highlights

The use of facial nerve monitoring is routine. While monitoring of the lower cranial nerves is feasible, we have not found that its routine use has affected surgical outcomes.

The POTS Approach

- The patient is positioned supine with the head turned to the opposite side.
- A C-shaped incision starting about 3 cm above the auricle courses 4–5 cm behind the postauricular crease and extends inferiorly to the level of the C-1 vertebra. Its anterior end reaches just posterior to the angle of the mandible.
- An inferiorly based U-shaped, myo-aponeurotic flap is raised. The base of the flap is at the level of the C-1 vertebra.
- The sternocleidomastoid muscle is retracted posteriorly, and the internal jugular vein is identified just in front of the transverse process of the atlas. After freeing the vein, a suture is passed underneath it for later ligation, with care not to injure the accessory nerve.
- An extended mastoidectomy is performed with skeletonization of the sigmoid sinus down to the jugular bulb. The digastric ridge is identified and the mastoid tip is amputated. Removal of the posteromedial third of the occipital condyle and jugular tubercle further widens the exposure and is often necessary due to tumor infiltration in this area. The postcondylar vein is often encountered,

and further removal of bone here will identify the hypoglossal canal.

- A 4 × 4 cm retrosigmoid craniotomy is performed. A piece of bone overlying the junction of the transverse and sigmoid sinus is left in place to allow extraluminal compression with Surgicel.
- The sinus, the presinus dura, and the jugular bulb are completely uncovered up to the posterior semicircular canal. The retrofacial air cells are drilled after identification of the mastoid segment of the facial nerve
- With gentle pressure on the sigmoid sinus and posterior fossa dura using the suction irrigator, the endolymphatic sac and duct are identified and sectioned in order to allow further detachment of the dura from the posterior surface of the petrous bone.
- The infralabyrinthine cells are drilled, taking care not to injure the cochlea.
- The proximal part of the sigmoid sinus is compressed extraluminally with a piece of Surgicel (Johnson & Johnson, New Brunswick, NJ) placed between the sinus and the overlying bone at its junction with the transverse sinus. The internal jugular vein in the neck is ligated. Next, the sigmoid sinus is closed proximally and distally with two tungsten clips and opened with the knife. Bleeding from the entry points of the inferior petrosal sinus is controlled with packing.
- The posterior fossa dura is opened with a horizontal incision, starting approximately 3 cm posterior to the sigmoid sinus, coursing anteriorly, traversing the medial wall of the sinus, and ending at the level of the posterior semicircular canal.
- The upper and a lower dural flap are retracted with stay sutures. The jugular bulb is opened. The bulb is usually compressed by the tumor mass. Bleeding from the inferior petrosal sinus is controlled by gentle packing with Surgicel. Tumor removal then proceeds accordingly.
- Microsurgical resection then proceeds with the goal to dissect the LCNs from the tumor mass.
- To avoid CSF rhinorrhea, all opened perilabyrinthine air cells should be drilled out. The apical and retrofacial air cells should be sealed with bone wax.
- At the end of the procedure, the retrosigmoid dura is approximated with watertight sutures, and the rest of the cavity is obliterated with strips of abdominal fat held in place by the repositioned myoaponeurotic flap. No postoperative lumbar drain is used.

The goal of surgery is total removal. In line with Simpson's grading, resection of surrounding dura and drilling to uncover normal bone are essential in order to minimize recurrence. The central clivus, cavernous sinus, and surrounding major vessels are the most common sites of residual tumor.

With extension of the disease process the surgical approach must be modified. The POTS approach can be combined with a number of surgical extensions depending on tumor extent and preoperative neural status, in order to maximize exposure and facilitate total resection.

Operative Extensions

- Enlarged translabyrinthine approach allows improved access to the CPA component.
- Transotic approach improves the anterior exposure.
- Modified transcochlear extension improves the anteromedial exposure (Type D represents an association of a Type A and POTS approach) (Fig. 56-2).

The modified transcochlear approach adds to the POTS approach, the posterior rerouting of the facial nerve, facilitating access to the petrous apex and middle clivus. The major indication for this approach is to address pathology ventral to the brain stem without retraction of the cerebellum or brain stem. We have further divided the transcochlear approaches into four categories. MTCA type A is the standard approach. MTCA type B involves the addition of an infra-temporal fossa type B or C. MTCA type C involves a superior transtentorial extension, appropriate for dealing with petro-clival lesions with supratentorial extension. MTCA type D is the most important modification in the treatment of jugular fossa lesions. The limited access to lesions of the jugular fossa, lower clivus, and foramen magnum is overcome by combining the standard MTCA type A with the POTS approach described above (29,42,43).

Extensive intracranial and extracranial disease is optimally managed using staged approaches, due to the fact that the combination of a large dural defect and extensive neck exposure significantly increases the risk of postoperative CSF leak and meningitis. The majority of JFM, however, can be treated in a single stage.

Of the 13 patients in our series, 4 patients with normal preoperative hearing underwent a single-stage POTS approach with preservation of preoperative hearing. Two patients with non-serviceable hearing underwent a POTS combined with a translabyrinthine approach. Two patients required a transotic extension due to infiltration of the middle ear and vertical carotid canal. A modified transcochlear approach with a POTS approach (MTCA type D) was employed in two cases in order to address spread to the clivus and involvement of the vertical and horizontal portions of the intrapetrous carotid. Two patients underwent staged resections due to significant cervical extension. An IFTA followed by an enlarged translabyrinthine approach with transapical extension for the second stage was used in one patient, with a POTS followed by a modified transcochlear approach in the second of these patients. The final patient was a referred revision case having previously undergone a retrosigmoid resection with a grade III facial nerve. A POTS approach was used to achieve total tumor removal.

Results of Surgery

Gross total tumor removal was achieved in 10 (76.9%), corresponding to Simpson grade I and II. Cavernous sinus infiltration, encasement of the PICA as well as the need to preserve a dominant jugular bulb, and firm adherence to the brain stem were the reasons for subtotal resection in the remainder of the cases.

Hearing was preserved at the preoperative levels in all 4 patients undergoing an isolated POTS approach. These 4 patients also had grade I facial nerve function postoperatively. Overall, House-Brackmann (HB) I and II was achieved in 7 (54%), with the remainder achieving HB III, one year after surgery. Seven (54%) patients had at least 1 cranial nerve deficit preoperatively, with 3 (23%) with IX, X, XI, and XII affected. A new deficit of one or more of the lower cranial nerves was recorded in 8 (62%), with 4 of 6 patients with no preoperative deficits losing lower cranial nerve function. One patient who underwent a POTS approach developed a CSF leak necessitating lumbar drainage.

Postoperative Management

Despite using techniques to minimize the risk of CSF leak and meningitis, the presence of these complications should be sought and managed early. Lumbar drainage can be used, while the option of blind sac closure and required obliteration of the middle ear spaces and eustachian tube with abdominal fat remains a definitive option.

Postoperative CN deficits require aggressive rehabilitation. While most young patients compensate well, the risk of aspiration is always present, especially in those with an associated hypoglossal palsy. While vocal cord augmentation is occasionally required, the risk of tracheostomy and long-term gastrostomy feeding should be nonexistent in properly selected patients. Physiotherapy to minimize shoulder dysfunction is also necessary in affected patients.

If facial nerve rerouting is required, early support is essential. Of patients undergoing anterior rerouting, 70% will recover to HB I or II one year postoperatively, with

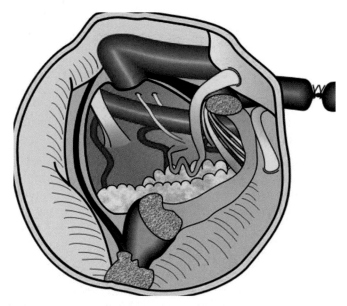

Fig. 56-2. Modified transcochlear approach Type D

approximately 70% achieving HB III with posterior rerouting (44,45). Long-term radiologic surveillance is required, even following complete tumor removal, with recurrences reported in up to 10% of Simpson grade I meningioma resections.

Summary

While JFM are extremely rare lesions, their optimal management is dependent on observing the basic tenets of skull base surgery. Adequate exposure, minimization of brain retraction and surgical morbidity while optimizing curative resection require extensive experience in the treatment of skull base pathology. Secondary goals of surgery include preservation of the inner and middle ear and facial nerve function. Single-stage resection should also be attempted, when possible, but staged resections is mandated when there is significant intra- and extracranial disease.

Decisions regarding when to operate and the aggressiveness of one's approach are challenging, and it is the relationship between the surgeon and radiologist that allows accurate diagnosis and the ability to make many of these decisions prior to surgery. It is also essential for the surgeon to be familiar with and have the ability to carry out various approaches to this complex region.

References

1. Claus EB, Bondy ML, Schildkraut JM, et al. Epidemiology of intracranial meningioma. Neurosurgery 2005;57:1088–95; discussion -95.
2. Lamszus K, Lamszus K. Meningioma pathology, genetics, and biology. J Neuropathol Exp Neurol 2004;63:275–86.
3. Drummond KJ, Zhu JJ, Black PM, et al. Meningiomas: updating basic science, management, and outcome. Neurology 2004;10:113–30.
4. Roberti F, Sekhar LN, Kalavakonda C, et al. Posterior fossa meningiomas: surgical experience in 161 cases. Surg Neurol 2001;56:8–20; discussion -1.
5. Macdonald AJ, Salzman KL, Harnsberger HR, et al. Primary jugular foramen meningioma: imaging appearance and differentiating features. AJR Am J Roentgenol 2004;182:373–7.
6. Chang CY, Cheung SW, Jackler RK. Meningiomas presenting in the temporal bone: the pathways of spread from an intracranial site of origin. Otolaryngol Head Neck Surg 1998;119:658–64.
7. Bindal R, Goodman JM, Kawasaki A, et al. The natural history of untreated skull base meningiomas [comment]. Surg Neurol 2003;59:87–92.
8. Gilbert ME, Shelton C, McDonald A, et al. Meningioma of the jugular foramen: glomus jugulare mimic and surgical challenge. Laryngoscope 2004;114:25–32.
9. Som P, Curtin H. Head and Neck Imaging. St. Louis: Mosby, 2003.
10. Patel NP, Mhatre AN, Lalwani AK, et al. Molecular pathogenesis of skull base tumors. Otol Neurotol 2004;25:636–43.
11. Lusis E, Gutmann DH, Lusis E, et al. Meningioma: an update. Curr Opin Neurol 2004;17:687–92.
12. Baser ME, DG RE, Gutmann DH, et al. Neurofibromatosis 2. Curr Opin Neurol 2003;16:27–33.
13. Fuller CE, Perry A, Fuller CE, et al. Molecular diagnostics in central nervous system tumors. Adv Anat Pathol 2005;12:180–94.
14. Gilbert ME, Shelton C, McDonald A, et al. Meningioma of the jugular foramen: glomus jugulare mimic and surgical challenge. The Laryngoscope 2004;114:25–32.
15. Thompson LD, Bouffard JP, Sandberg GD, et al. Primary ear and temporal bone meningiomas: a clinicopathologic study of 36 cases with a review of the literature. Mod Pathol 2003;16:236–45.
16. Ramina R, Neto MC, Fernandes YB, et al. Meningiomas of the jugular foramen. Neurosurg Rev 2006;29:55–60.
17. Molony TB, Brackmann DE, Lo WW. Meningiomas of the jugular foramen. Otolaryngol Head Neck Surg 1992;106:128–36.
18. Arnautovic KI, Al-Mefty O. Primary meningiomas of the jugular fossa. J Neurosurg 2002;97:12–20.
19. Lustig LR, Jackler RK, Lustig LR, et al. The variable relationship between the lower cranial nerves and jugular foramen tumors: implications for neural preservation. Am J Otol 1996;17:658–68.
20. Martinez Devesa PM, Wareing MJ, Moffat DA, et al. Meningioma in the internal auditory canal. J Laryngol Otol 2001;115:48–9.
21. Tokgoz N, Oner YA, Kaymaz M, et al. Primary intraosseous meningioma: CT and MRI appearance. AJNR Am J Neuroradiol 2005;26:2053–6.
22. Bacciu A, Piazza P, Di Lella F, et al. Intracanalicular meningioma: clinical features, radiologic findings, and surgical management. Otol Neurotol 2007.
23. Sanna M, Bacciu A, Falcioni M, et al. Surgical management of jugular foramen schwannomas with hearing and facial nerve function preservation: a series of 23 cases and review of the literature. Laryngoscope 2006;116:2191–204.
24. Sanna M, De Donato G, Piazza P, et al. Revision glomus tumor surgery. Otolaryngologic clinics of North America 2006;39:763–82, vii.
25. Sanna M, Jain Y, De Donato G, et al. Management of jugular paragangliomas: the Gruppo Otologico experience. Otol Neurotol 2004;25:797–804.
26. Zachenhofer I, Wolfsberger S, Aichholzer M, et al. Gamma-knife radiosurgery for cranial base meningiomas: experience of tumor control, clinical course, and morbidity in a follow-up of more than 8 years. Neurosurgery 2006;58:28–36; discussion 28–36.
27. Modha A, Gutin PH, Modha A, et al. Diagnosis and treatment of atypical and anaplastic meningiomas: a review. Neurosurgery 2005;57:538–50; discussion -50.
28. Sammi M. Surgery of Skull Base Meningiomas. New York: Springer-Verlag, 1992:51–9.
29. Mazzoni A, Sanna M. A posterolateral approach to the skull base: the petro-occipital transsigmoid approach. Skull Base Surgery 1995;5:157–67.
30. Simpson D. The recurrence of intracranial meningiomas after surgical treatment. J Neurol Neurosurg Psychiatry 1957;20:22–39.
31. Ramina R, Maniglia JJ, Fernandes YB, et al. Tumors of the jugular foramen: diagnosis and management. Neurosurgery 2005;57:59–68.
32. Goel A, Desai K, Muzumdar D, et al. Surgery on anterior foramen magnum meningiomas using a conventional posterior sub-occipital approach: a report on an experience with 17 cases. Neurosurgery 2001;49:102–6; discussion 6–7.
33. Little KM, Friedman AH, Sampson JH, et al. Surgical management of petroclival meningiomas: defining resection

goals based on risk of neurological morbidity and tumor recurrence rates in 137 patients. Neurosurgery 2005;56: 546–59; discussion -59.

34. Jackson CG, Cueva RA, Thedinger BA, et al. Cranial nerve preservation in lesions of the jugular fossa. Otolaryngol Head Neck Surg 1991;105:687–93.

35. Katsuta T, Rhoton AL, Jr., Matsushima T. The jugular foramen: microsurgical anatomy and operative approaches. Neurosurgery 1997;41:149–201; discussion -2.

36. Samii M, Babu RP, Tatagiba M, et al. Surgical treatment of jugular foramen schwannomas. J Neurosurg 1995;82:924–32.

37. Fisch U, Mattox DE. Microsurgery of the Skull Base. Stuttgart: Georg Thieme Verlag, 1988.

38. Jackler RK. Atlas of Neurotology and Skull Base Surgery. St. Louis: Mosby, 1996.

39. Sanna M, Agarwal M, Jain Y, et al. Transapical extension in difficult cerebellopontine angle tumors: preliminary report. J Laryngol Otol 2003;117:788–92.

40. Sanna M, Falcioni M. Conservative facial nerve management in jugular foramen schwannomas. Am J Otol 2000;21:892.

41. Sanna M, Mazzoni A, Saleh EA, et al. Lateral approaches to the median skull base through the petrous bone: the system of the modified transcochlear approach. J Laryngol Otol 1994;108:1036–44.

42. Sanna M, Saleh E, Taibah A. Atlas of temporal bone and lateral skull base surgery. Stuttgart: Georg Thieme Verlag, 1995.

43. Sanna M, Russo A, Taibah A, et al. Enlarged translabyrinthine approach for the management of large and giant acoustic neuromas: a report of 175 consecutive cases. Ann Otol Rhinol Laryngol 2004;113:319–28.

44. Russo A, Piccirillo E, De Donato G, et al. Anterior and Posterior Facial Nerve Rerouting: A Comparative Study. Skull Base 2003;13:123–30.

45. Parhizkar N, Hiltzik DH, Selesnick SH. Facial nerve rerouting in skull base surgery. Otolaryngol Clin North Am 2005;38: 685–710, ix.

57
Spinal Meningiomas

Eve C. Tsai, John Butler, and Edward C. Benzel

Introduction

Meningiomas are one of the most common intradural, extramedullary tumors of the spine.[1] The first reported successful resection of a thoracic meningioma was in 1888 by Sir Victor Horsely and Sir William Gowers.[2] While they initially described their spinal tumor as a fibromyxoma, the term "meningioma" that is now universally employed was introduced by Harvey Cushing.[3] With modern imaging, the delay in the diagnosis of spinal meningiomas has been significantly shortened. Surgical resection, however, remains the mainstay of treatment.

The epidemiology and pathology of spinal meningiomas are reviewed herein. The clinical management of spinal meningiomas, including diagnosis, investigations, surgical and adjunctive treatments, as well as outcomes, follow-up strategies, and future perspectives, are also presented.

Epidemiology

The incidence of primary intraspinal neoplasm is approximately five per million for females and three per million for males.[4] Of the primary intraspinal neoplasms, spinal intradural extramedullary tumors account for two thirds of the total in adults[5] and approximately 50% in children.[6] Meningiomas and nerve sheath tumors account for the majority of the intradural extramedullary spinal tumors, and meningiomas represent 25–46% of all primary intraspinal tumors.[4,7–12] Approximately 83–94%[13] are intradural,[14] and 5–14% have an extradural component.[11,15–19] Approximately 10% are either intradural and extradural or entirely extradural.[20, 21] The fraction of entirely extradural meningiomas range from 3 to 9%.[11,16,19] The relative ratio of meningiomas to nerve sheath tumors, however, varies by population. While the incidence of meningiomas and nerve sheath tumors or schwannomas is about equal in the Western population, in Asian populations schwannomas are more common and have been reported with ratios of almost 3.8 to 1 in China and 3.9 to 1 in Japan.[12,22]

There is a female preponderance, with spinal meningiomas occurring more frequently in females with a ratio of 2.5 to 1.[22] Seventy-five to 85% of meningiomas arise in women. The female predominance has been postulated to be due to sex hormones[19] or the existence of various other receptor types (steroid, peptidergic, growth factor, and aminergic) that may contribute to tumor formation.[23] Spinal meningiomas can be found in any age group, but they most frequently present between the fifth and seventh decades of life.[7,8,12,14,15,18,19,24,25]

Spinal meningiomas occur less frequently than their intracranial counterparts and account for 7.5–12.7% of all meningiomas.[8,19] Their distribution within the spinal axis varies, with the majority located within the thoracic region.[26] Sixty-seven to 84% of spinal meningiomas are found in the thoracic region.[13] In general, they are located laterally, or with a component that extended laterally. They are more often located dorsally, more so than ventrally within the spinal canal.[13,14] The preference for a thoracic location is observed in females, but not in males.[18] In the cervical region, the incidence of spinal meningiomas is 14–27%.[13] While meningiomas are the most common benign tumor found at the foramen magnum,[21] low cervical meningiomas are rare.[27] In patients younger than 50 years, however, there is a higher frequency of cervical meningiomas (39%). The majority of these are located in the high cervical region.[28] In contrast to thoracic meningiomas, upper cervical spine and foramen magnum tumors are often ventral[18] or ventrolateral and may adhere to the vertebral artery near its intradural entry and initial intracranial course.[27] The incidence in the lumbar spine is 2–14%,[13] and although nerve sheath tumors can present in the lumbosacral region, meningioma growth caudal to the level of the conus medullaris is very uncommon.[12,27] Multiple spinal meningiomas are rare (1–2%)[25,29] (Fig. 57-1).

Pathology

Meningiomas are thought to originate from arachnoid cap cells of neural crest or mesodermal origin. While the arachnoid cap cells in the telencephalic meninges are thought to originate

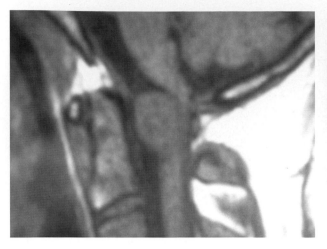

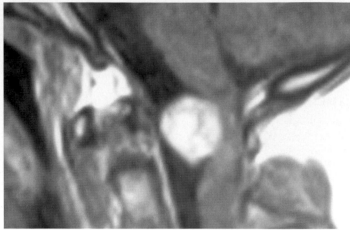

A   B

Fig. 57-1. T1-weighted MRI without gadolinium enhancement (A) and with gadolinium enhancement (B) of a ventrally located meningioma at the craniovertebral junction

from neural crest cells, meningiomas of the rest of the neural axis are believed to be from fibroblasts of mesodermal origin,[30] accounting for the occasional ventral or dorsal location of meningiomas.[26] The characteristic lateral location of meningiomas in the spine is attributed to the arachnoid cap cells located in the leptomeninges of the exit zones of nerve roots or entry zones of arteries in the spinal canal (Fig. 57-2).

As meningiomas arise from the leptomeninges, most of these tumors have a broad attachment to and are well vascularized by the dura.[12] Most commonly, spinal meningiomas are intradural, but tumors with both an intra- and extradural, as well as a purely extradural location, have been reported.[24] Rarely, intramedullary meningiomas can occur.[31,32] The infre-

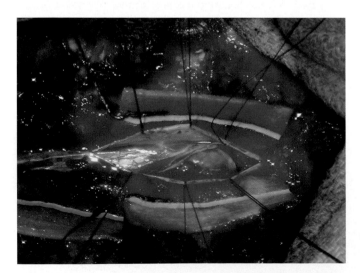

Fig. 57-2. Introperative photo showing a well-demarcated lobulated-appearing intradural meningioma located ventrolaterally with dorso-lateral displacement of the spinal cord

quent occurrence of the involvement of bone has been attributed to the well-defined epidural space of the spine[27] and the tendency of meningiomas to not penetrate the pia. The lack of pial invasion has been attributed to the presence of an intermediate leptomeningial layer that is present between the arachnoid and pia mater in the spine.[33] Lack of pial invasion has also been attributed to the early detection and resection of spinal meningiomas prior to their being able to change the tumor/cord interface to penetrate the pia.[33]

The gross appearance of meningiomas can be round or lobulated and they are generally well circumscribed.[12] Less commonly, they can occur en plaque. They tend to be variegated, fleshy, and friable[27] or smooth, rubbery, firm, and fibrous.[12] Calcifications, which can be microscopic or large enough to be observed on computed tomography (CT), increase the tumor consistency.

The World Health Organization (WHO) has identified meningiomas within their classification of nervous system tumors—last updated in 2000. Meningiomas have been divided into three grades. WHO grade I meningiomas are benign meningiomas. The vast majority of tumors fall in this category. WHO grade II meningiomas are defined as atypical and constitute 4.7–7.2% of all meningiomas. The last category, WHO grade III, are anaplastic meningiomas and fortunately constitute only 1.0–2.8% of all meningiomas. While there are no valid data about the rate of grade II or III meningiomas in the spinal canal, the percentage of these higher grades appears to be decreased compared to intracranial meningiomas. In general, spinal meningiomas tend to be significantly more benign than those of the brain and brain convexity.[34, 35] Subtype classification does not appear to influence prognosis unless malignancy is evident.[11,13,16,19]. Subtypes of spinal meningiomas include psammomatous, fibroblastic, meningothelial,[36] chordoid,[37] vacuolated,[38] and clear cell.[39–41]

The most common subtype is psammomatous. For en plaque meningiomas, subtypes reported include psammomatous, transitional, microcystic, meningothelial, and syncytial, with psamommatous and transitional being the most common subtypes.[42] The subtypes associated with dumbbell meningiomas include angioblastic, meningothelial, transitional/syncytial, fibroblastic, atypical, and malignant.[43]

Genetic alterations have been examined in spinal meningiomas. Although one patient with multiple spinal meningiomas was found to have no choromosomal abnormalities,[44] the complete or partial loss of chromosome 22 has been found in some series in greater than 50% of patients with spinal meningiomas.[45,46] In the Arslantas study,[45] 16 spinal meningiomas were examined and 8 patients had complete or partial loss of chromosome 22. Other chromosomal abnormalities found included losses on 1p, 9p, and 10q and gains on 5p and 17q. These are frequently observed in intracranial meningiomas, but are mostly specific to atypical and anaplastic mening-iomas. With spinal meningiomas, however, copy number changes on chromosomes 9p, 17q, and 1p were observed even in benign tumors. They suggest that cancer-related genes located on 1p, 9p, 10q, and 17q, together with the neurofibromatosis type 2 suppressor gene, might be involved in the etiology of spinal meningiomas. In contrast to cranial meningiomas,[13,46] the presence or absence of chromosome 22 was not associated with disease recurrence. The deletion of the short arm of chromosome 1, however, was found to be an important prognostic factor in meningiomas with respect to recurrence.[46]

Symptoms and Signs

There is often a delay between the onset of symptoms and diagnosis. Pain, which is usually the initial and most common symptom[13] of spinal meningiomas, may precede diagnosis by years.[12] The delay between pain symptoms and neurologic deterioration has been attributed to the generally slow growth of spinal meningiomas and the adaptive compressibility of the cerebrospinal fluid (CSF) and adjacent vascular structures. Only when the compliance of these structures have been exhausted does the tumor then transmit pressure directly to the spinal cord,[47] causing deficits depending on tumor location. The mean duration of symptoms prior to presentation was 1–2 years,[11,16–18] but has been reported to be as long as 15–20 years prior to diagnosis.[18] With the advent of magnetic resonance imaging (MRI), the time to diagnosis has been shortened by an estimated 6 months.[17]

Symptoms and signs may be due to direct pressure effects on neural tissue or through indirect effects, resulting in vascular compromise, abnormal CSF circulation or tethering. Radicular symptoms can occur with spinal meningiomas, but they have been reported to be less frequent compared to nerve sheath tumors.[14] The compression of the nerve roots as they exit the neural foramina can lead to symptoms of radicular pain,[47] but compression of the dorsal roots can also cause sensory loss. Ventral nerve root compression or compression of the anterior horn cells can lead to motor deficits.[12] With spinal cord compression, the function of ascending or descending longitudinal tracts can be interrupted leading to signs and symptoms far away from the tumor.[12] When the corticospinal tract is disturbed, upper motor neuron deficits with spastic paresis can occur, especially when there is longstanding compression and delayed diagnosis. In a recently reported series, the signs of myelopathy were found to be present in most spinal meningioma patients, with 64% having weakness and 32% being nonambulatory.[13]

Sensation can be affected with spinothalamic tract compression, leading to compromise of pain and temperature sensation. Compression of the dorsal tracts can impair position and vibration sensation, resulting in the very common symptom of gait ataxia.[12] With unilateral compression from spinal meningiomas, Brown-Sequard–like symptoms result and occur in a higher incidence compared to intramedullary tumors.[12] The impairment of the autonomic pathways, with sympathetic and parasympathetic signs, are generally uncommon with extramedullary tumors, but bladder or bowel dysfunction can occur as a late finding with meningioma.[13]

Symptoms unrelated to direct tumor compression can also occur due to the compression of the vasculature. Compression of radicular arteries or the anterior spinal artery may lead to compromise of the function of the cord in the watershed zones that are distant from the tumor. These symptoms of impaired blood supply to the neural elements can precede direct nerve root or spinal cord compression symptoms for months, resulting in incorrect and delayed diagnoses.[12] Venous insufficiency can occur with upper cervical and foramen magnum meningiomas, leading to suboccipital pain and distal arm weakness with atrophy and intrinsic hand muscle weakness and clumsiness.[27] Meningiomas at any level, but most commonly at the upper cervical level, can rarely cause increased intracranial pressure and hydroceophalus[48,49] or syringomyelia.[50] Tethering of the spinal cord or nerve roots is another cause of pain and is a rare primary symptom with extramedullary tumors.[12] If tumor recurrence is suspected, it is important to distinguish between tethering due to recurrence or to postperative alterations of the arachnoid.[12]

Investigations (Figs. 57-3, 57-4)

MRI is the method of choice for diagnosis.[12,51] For its optimum use in the spine, dedicated surface coils are required to improve the signal-to-noise ratio, make thinner slices possible, and provide improved tissue contrast resolution and greater spatial resolution.[12,52] It provides information about the exact location, size, and relationships to adjacent structures, which aids in diagnosis and surgical planning.[13] While sagittal images facilitate screening over large areas of the spinal cord and provide a high diagnostic yield, axial slices are required to provide additional anatomic information, thus aiding in surgi-

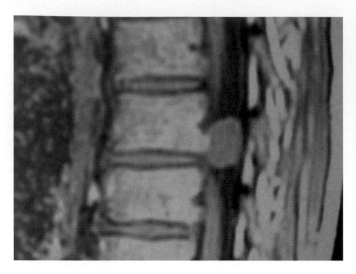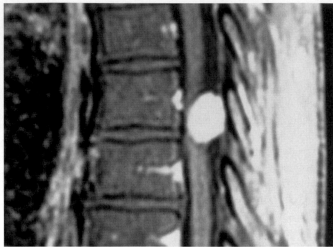

Fig. 57-3. T1-weighted imaging without gadolinium enhancement and with gadolinium enhancement showing the typical homogeneous enhancement of a thoracic meningioma. On T1, the tumor is isointense to the spinal cord

cal planning.[12] Prior to MRI, the rate of misdiagnosis was estimated to be as high as 33%, with spinal meningiomas being incorrectly diagnosed as multiple sclerosis, syringomyelia, pernicious anemia, arthritis, and herniated disc.[13,15,18] These misdiagnoses have led to incorrect surgical management that include lumbar disc exploration and knee surgery.[13,15,18] With

MRI decreasing the time to diagnosis, patients have been reported to have less severe neurologic deficits at the time of diagnosis.[17]

Routine sequences include T1-weighted, with and without gadolinium contrast, and T2-weighted images.[12] Other sequences, such as constructive interference in steady-state sequence, have also been used to provide improved contrast resolution resulting in information about intratumoral cysts, nerve roots, or even dentrate ligaments.[12] Spinal meningiomas have been reported to be both isointense or hypointense on T1-weighted images and isointense and hyperintense on T2-weighted images.[13] Extradural spinal meningiomas are reported to have a low signal intensity on T2-weighted images with possible bone erosion, and characteristically have thickened, enhancing dura mater.[53] The dural attachment is often broad, and spinal meningiomas have a strong, homogeneous enhancement with gadolinium.[12,54,55] Similar to intracranial meningiomas, the contrast enhancement can occur along the dural attachment forming the characteristic dural tail.[56,57] Spinal meningiomas are usually well delineated from the spinal cord and are well circumscribed.[54,58]

The main diagnostic issue is differentiating meningiomas from schwannomas, neurofibromas, and malignant nerve sheath tumors, which occur in decreasing order of frequency.[12] The MRI characteristics of a series of 28 schwannomas and 24 meningiomas were studied to determine differentiating imaging characteristics.[57] The characteristics examined included cranio-caudal location, T2 signal intensity, T2 signal heterogeneity, Gd-DTPA enhancement intensity and heterogeneity, and the "dural tail sign." They determined that a spinal intradural extramedullary tumor was more likely to be a meningioma unless it was hyperintense on T2 or had intense enhancement without a dural tail, in which case a schwannoma should be considered.

Fig. 57-4. T2-weighted MRI demonstrating the typical isointense appearance of the tumor to spinal cord. Meningiomas generally appear hypointense to isointense on T2. Hyperintensity on T2 warrants consideration of another tumor type, such as schwannoma

Meningiomas can also have calcifications that are manifested as a signal void on all MRI sequences and lack contrast uptake, resulting in heterogenous contrast enhancement.[12] When MRI is precluded, such as when the patient has a pacemaker,or noncompatible metal or electronic implants, CT with myelography can be used to determine tumor size and location. It can also be used as an adjunct to MRI to differentiate intramedullary versus extramedullary location when such is equivocal on MRI.[27] Myelography facilitates delineation of the extent of spinal cord displacement and the obstruction of the flow of contrast by the rounded border of the typical intradural, extramedullary location of spinal meningiomas. Tumor calcifications can be detected with high-resolution CT or in 2–5% by plain radiographs.[19,57] With CT, meningiomas are hyperdense in 70–75% of cases, and 90% of meningiomas enhance strongly and uniformly.[59] CT or plain radiographs can allow better delineation of bony changes, which include destruction of the vertebral arch,[18] widened intravertebral foramen, pedicle erosion, or, rarely, vertebral body invasion.[18,60,61] Unlike intracranial meningiomas, hyperostosis with extradural spinal meningiomas is rare and has been attributed to the presence of a wide extradural space filled with fat, venous plexus, and spinal nerve roots in the spinal canal.[20]

Management

While asymptomatic meningiomas can be carefully followed, the majority of spinal meningiomas that come to attention are symptomatic, with surgery being the therapy of choice. As the majority of spinal meningiomas are benign, well circumscribed, and can be completely resected, surgery offers the potential for "cure" without the need for further treatment. In this section, we outline important preoperative considerations and intraoperative aids, approaches, and techniques. Adjunctive treatments for patients with recurrence or subtotal surgical resections are also presented.

Preoperative Considerations

As with any surgical treatment, patients should be informed of the pertinent general risks associated with anesthesia and surgery. The major risk associated with spinal meningiomas is the potential risk of paralysis or neurologic deficits due to vascular or spinal cord injury. This must be balanced with the high likelihood that the lesion is benign. Such neurologic deficits and surgical risks may be more pronounced in patients who are elderly or those with a severe preoperative neurologic deficit.[12]

Preoperative consideration of the use of spinal angiography should be entertained, particularly if the lesion is located at the T8 to L2 level. Knowledge of the location of major anterior spinal artery feeders, such as the artery of Adamkiewicz, may prevent anterior spinal artery ischemia which has been

reported with resection of intraspinal meningiomas.[11] If there is anticipation of significant blood loss, embolization[59] can be considered.

Steroids and antibiotics should also be considered preoperatively. To decrease intramedullary edema and subsequent neurologic deterioration, dexamethasone (8–16mg) may be given preoperatively, and if there is intraoperative spinal cord irritation, additional doses of methyl-prednisolone or dexamethasone have been suggested.[12] Preoperative antibiotics should also be given to decrease the risk of wound infection.

As surgical resection involves intimate contact with the spinal cord and nerve roots, electrophysiologic monitoring can be an aid. Although the risk of direct spinal cord damage is minimal, use of electrophysiologic monitoring may be especially helpful with large or ventrally located tumors and may facilitate intraoperative prediction of neurologic outcome[12]. Electromyographic (EMG) recording monitors nerve root function and aids in identification of specific nerve roots. Somatosensory-evoked potentials (SSEP) monitor dorsal column function. These potentials are induced at the tibial nerve or median nerve and recorded from cortical or spinal electrodes. The median nerve can also be used with cervical tumors and may result in more stable responses with shorter latencies. SSEP correlates well with postoperative proprioceptive findings and can be monitored continuously. Surgeons can then be alerted to posterior column compromise in a timely fashion, which then allows for the modification of approach or dissection technique. The disadvantage of SSEP, however, is that it does not reflect postoperative motor findings.[62]

To better assess the motor tracts, motor-evoked potentials (MEP) are used. This involves transcranial electrical or magnetic stimulation of the motor cortex, allowing monitoring of the function of corticospinal tract. The use of MEP may be especially helpful with ventral tumors. This technique facilitates the assessment of individual limbs. One of the disadvantages of MEP monitoring is that it results in mass movements of the stimulated muscles, and thus, it can only be used intermittently so that the operative field is not disturbed. Another disadvantage is that induction of general anesthesia may block MEP potentials. This can be overcome with a multiple impulse technique employing a short train of stimuli.[13,63–65] Although patients with deficits and no monitoring changes have been reported with MEP,[66] the combination of MEP with other electrophysiologic monitoring modalities may improve the sensitivity and specificity of electrophysiologic monitoring[67].

Intraoperative Considerations

Positioning

With thoracic and lumbosacral lesions, patients are positioned prone, since most meningiomas can be approached via laminectomy.[27] Care should be taken to ensure that there is no significant thoracic or abdominal pressure, as this may increase venous pressure and increase blood loss. The sitting position has been advocated with cervical tumors, to decrease venous congestion. Placing the prone patient in reverse Trendelenberg can also decrease venous congestion without the risks of air embolism and extensive CSF drainage. The latter can lead to intracranial subdural hematoma formation. In addition, the assistant can be more effective, since the sitting position usually allows only one-handed assistance.[12]

Exposure and Approach

The level of the midline skin incision can be identified anatomically or by radiography or fluoroscopy. The incision should be long enough to achieve a bony exposure that encompasses the entire rostral-caudal extent of the tumor. The extent of the bony exposure should be such as to allow minimal displacement of the spinal cord and access to the entire dural attachment of the tumor, with additional exposure to facilitate a watertight dural closure.

With lateral tumors, a hemilaminectomy may be adequate, and with small tumors, a single level laminectomy may suffice. With foraminal involvement, laminectomies with partial or complete fascetectomy may be required to attain adequate exposure. If the tumor has displaced the spinal cord, ventral tumors can also be approached dorsally. Additional ventral exposure can be obtained by dividing the dentate ligament or a noncritical dorsal nerve root and by using these structures for retraction.

Ideally, retraction of the spinal cord should be avoided in order to prevent inadvertent spinal cord injury, and thus, a more lateral approach may be preferable for ventral tumors. The incision may be lengthened to allow for greater retraction of the muscle masses laterally. Table-mounted retractors can allow depression of the paraspinal muscle to provide additional ventral exposure.[27] The use of a paramedian incision and approach can decrease the bulk of muscle retraction. Rotating the prone patient away from the surgeon and further bony resection by drilling the pedicles may also aid in ventral visualization. A ventro-lateral cervicotomy via the lateral aspect of the carotid sheath is a lateral cervical approach that provides access to extraspinal portions of tumor.[27] This, however, is rarely necessary. If these techniques are inadequate, ventral approaches can rarely be considered.

High cervical ventral exposures include the far lateral[68] and extreme lateral variants[69,70] of the atlanto-occipital transarticular approach to ventral extradural lesions of the craniovertebral junction. The transoral approach has also been described for small high cervical tumors.[71] The safety associated with this approach may be hindered by bleeding from the epidural venous plexus, which is more developed ventrally and which may be enlarged by tumor. Other potential complications, such as CSF fistulas and infection, and the difficulty of obtaining adequate dural closure preclude this approach for intradural tumors. Lower cervical ventral approaches include corpectomy with reconstruction.

Ventral approaches for thoracic or thoracolumbar region tumors include the costotransversectomy approach or a lateral extracavitary approach. The lateral extracavitary approach allows for both a dorsal and lateral access with mobilization of the paravertebral muscle and does not require rib resection or entry through the pleura. Endoscopic thoracic exposures have also been described.[72] To increase the likelihood of obtaining a safe and complete resection, the procedures may be combined or staged.[72,73]

The extent of bone resection that is required to obtain adequate tumor exposure should not be compromised for fear of spinal instability. Plans should be made in advance for fusion and instrumentation if postoperative instability is anticipated. With multilevel cervical laminectomy, laminoplasty may be considered to prevent kyphosis and subluxation, especially in children and patients with neurological deficits.[12] Fusion with instrumentation should also be considered if kyphotic deformation is high risk, particularly at the apex of an existing kyphosis or at the cervico-thoracic junction.

It is emphasized that true ventral exposures for intradural lesions via corpectomy are usually ill-advised. The actual dural and intradural exposure achieved is usually suboptimal and dural closure is very difficult. Surgical complications are, therefore, common when such approaches are employed.

Ultrasonography

Ultrasonography can be particularly helpful to ensure adequate exposure and for identification of tumor location and characteristics. Using the ultrasound to ensure that the bone resection encompasses the entire extent of the tumor allows the surgeon to modify the bony or ligamentous resection prior to dural opening. By not needing to extend the exposure after durotomy, hemorrhage into the intradural space in minimized. As the tumor can migrate with positioning, ultrasound can allow concurrent localization of the tumor that could otherwise not be obtained with reliance upon only the preoperative imaging.[12] Localization of the tumor with respect to the spinal cord not only provides insurance of an adequate exposure, but also facilitates planning of durotomy location.[74] Ultrasound also facilitates the differentiation between intramedullary and extramedullary tumors[74] and even provides information about the tumor type in some cases.[75] Meningiomas generally have irregular surfaces and were tightly adhered to the dura,[75] and 82.3–100% had high echogenicity.[74,76] compared to myelin. Only 12.5–14%[74,77] of meningiomas had tumor cysts, whereas 73% of neurilemomas had cysts.[76,77] Notwithstanding the aforementioned, the utilization of preoperative imaging studies and intraoperative radiographs and surgeon intuition and input are usually effective in appropriately localizing and characterizing the tumor. Therefore, most surgeons find ultrasonography to be of little utility.

Tumor Resection (Fig. 57-5)

The durotomy should be planned to encompass the entire circumferential border of the tumor (circumferential durotomy) and minimize spinal cord exposure, if possible. The durotomy should begin at the tumor–spinal cord margin rather than at the center or base of the tumor. This facilitates the delineation of the tumor–spinal cord plane and permits the vascular supply of the meningioma to be taken and controlled, thereby minimizing bleeding. Due to the extramedullary origin of meningiomas, meningiomas do not penetrate the pia and there is usually an arachnoid layer that is reflected over the tumor. One group has examined whether MRI could provide information regarding dissection planes. They found that if there is no peritumoral hypointensity on MRI—vessels may be adherent to the tumor surface, thus creating a difficult dissection plane.[33] With traction of the tumor away from the spinal cord, a good dissection plane can usually be initiated. This plane

should be preserved and developed to identify the borders of the tumor. A microscope is especially valuable at this stage by facilitating the differentiation of dissection planes and vessels and by providing adequate illumination. If the exposure is adequate and the tumor is small and soft, the meningioma can be dissected from the spinal cord and removed en bloc with the circumferential durotomy comprising the tumor borders.

With larger tumors or tumors for which the approach precludes circumferential durotomy, the durotomy can begin at the tumor–spinal cord border to provide access to the tumor mass. This mass can then be debulked to decrease its size and to decrease vascularity. Microscissors, cautery, and lasers have been used for tumor debulking.[13] When the tumor is firm or contains calcifications, an ultrasonic aspirator can be used to remove the tumor in a piecemeal fashion to avoid excessive spinal cord traction, distortion, or pressure. Cottonoid pledgets can be placed at the tumor–spinal cord interface not

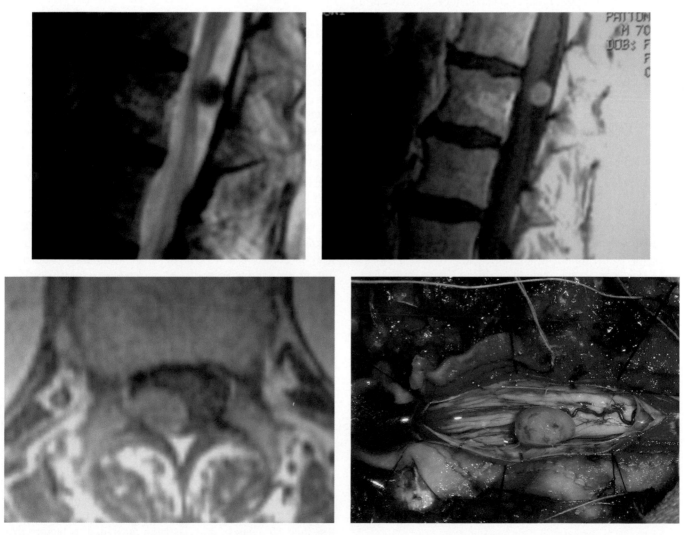

FIG. 57-5. Sagittal T2 MRI and sagittal and axial T1 MRI with gadolinium showing a small dorsal meningioma in the thoracolumbar region. Accompanying intraop photograph shows the tumor with its broad-based dural attachment. The tumor was completely resected with coagulation of the dural attachment and relief of symptoms

only to preserve the dissection plane, but to minimize bleeding in the subarachnoid space. With continued debulking and traction of the tumor into the resection cavity, the remaining attachment of the tumor to the dura mater should become accessible. Tumor infiltration or attachment to dura should then be resected. If the dural margins are difficult to access, the base should not be excised. In this case, the dural margins may be cauterized. One group, however, has advocated that the outer layer of the dura mater should be stripped from the inner layer surrounding the tumor base, since the spinal dura can be divided into an outer and an inner layer. The tumor should then be resected together with the inner layer alone, outside the arachnoid membrane. The outer layer of the dura should then be closed primarily.[78] The extent of dural resection should be guided by the ease of resection and the risk of CSF leak and infection. Although risk of recurrence may also be a concern, some studies have found no correlation of recurrence rates with dural base resection.[15–17,19] This latter point should be kept in mind as one considers options during surgery after the tumor has been resected.

After tumor resection, irrigation of the resection cavity with warm saline allows debris and blood to be washed from the subarachnoid space. Removal of the debris and blood may decrease development of arachnoiditis, tethering, syrinx formation, and hydrocephalus.[27] Arachnoid adhesions that keep the spinal cord in the preoperative deformed position can be divided. Most often, however, with tumor removal, the cord will return in size and position.

En plaque meningiomas have been associated with increased arachnoid scarring, resulting in greater difficulty with surgical resection and poorer outcomes.[42] These en plaque meningiomas may not respect tissue planes, have a more extensive tumor matrix, infiltrate surrounding structures, and occasionally are ossified.[13,17,79] Meningiomas rarely have a dumbbell extension of the tumor through the neural foramina. In such cases, however, options include sacrifice of a noncritical nerve root,[43] combined surgical procedures, or acceptance of a subtotal resection. A case of surgical treatment with cordectomy for the management of an intramedullary-extramedullary atypical meningioma[31] has been reported.

Dural closure can be usually accomplished via primary closure of the dura. Autologous grafts, allografts, or synthetic grafts may be used for dural defects. Autologous grafts include fascia lata, ligamentum nuchae, or pericranium, all of which are accessible with dorsal cervical exposures. Both allograft material and synthetic dural substitutes can be used. To aid in watertight dural closure, suture lines can be reinforced with fibrin glue or other types of tissue glue. For ventral tumors approached with dorsal or lateral exposures, watertight dural closures with sutures may be difficult. In these situations, dural grafts can be placed ventrally without suturing, but reinforced with tissue glue.[12]

Adjunctive Treatment

Radiotherapy and chemotherapy play only a minor role in the treatment of spinal meningiomas, since meningiomas are rarely malignant. With subtotal resection, radiation to the resection margins may be considered when the operative risk is thought to be too high due to patient comorbidities or tumor location.[11,15,18] Reoperation, however, may provide a chance for total resection or significant decompression, without increasing the chance of neurologic deficit. Radiation therapy has also been advocated for recurrent tumors, but is controversial given the generally indolent and benign nature of spinal meningiomas.[11,15] In five patients with recurrences after resection treated with radiation,[11, 13,15] all patients have remained clinically stable. Decrease in tumor size following radiation therapy has also been reported.[13] With atypical or malignant meningiomas, the role of stereotactic radiation is still evolving. Preliminary reports suggest that stereotactic radiation is feasible and safe and that it may aid with pain control.[80–82]

As with intracranial meningiomas, chemotherapy with hydroxyurea has been used as an adjunct to surgical treatment, especially for atypical meningiomas.[31,83]

Prognosis

Generally, prognosis has correlated with tumor grade and extent of resection. With benign meningiomas (WHO grade I) and complete resection, prognosis is excellent. In several large series, complete resection rates range from 82 to 99%.[11,15–19] Factors associated with complete resection include the absence of need for ventral exposure, absence of bony involvement with a well-defined spinal epidural space, and the presence of a peritumoral hypodense rim on MRI.[27,33] Complete resection rates have been reported to be less with en plaque tumors (53%), compared with encapsulated meningiomas (97%).[17] Other studies, however, demonstrate no correlation between cases following dural resection and coagulation. Recurrence rates in cases with dural resection were higher than with dural coagulation in both reports by Solero[19] (8% and 5.6%, respectively) and Klekamp[17] (31.3 and 26.1, respectively). In the Levy[18] series, there were no recurrences associated with dural coagulation and a 4% recurrence with dural resection. Although there may be no correlation between recurrence and extent of dural resection, subtotal resection has been associated with recurrence rates reported to be as high as 100% in 5 years.[17]

In general, recurrence rates are less with spinal meningiomas, compared to their intracranial counterparts[84]—with a 10-year recurrence of only 13% for spinal meningiomas and 25% and 24% for convexity and parasagittal meningiomas, respectively.[8] Recurrences have been reported to occur from 1 to 17 years postoperatively,[19] and rates have ranged from 1.3 to 22%.[11,15,16,18,19,28] Younger patients have been found to have a higher recurrence, with 20% recurring in patients under 21 years of age.[85] An increased recurrence rate in patients less than 50 years of age has been attributed to factors that impede total resection such as a higher frequency of cervical tumors, tumors with extradural extension,[18, 28] recurrent tumors with associated arachnoid scarring,[13] and en plaque growth.[28,42] Arachnoid scarring in recurrent tumors was found in 90% compared with 11% in primary meningiomas,[17] allowing the attainment of a complete resection in only 45% of recurrent tumors, compared to 95% of first attempts. Management strategies with respect to arachnoid scarring include sharp dissection of arachnoid scars, meticulous hemostasis and decompression of subarachnoid space, with a dural graft to protect against postoperative tethering and CSF obstruction. En plaque meningiomas are also more difficult to resect. Recurrence rates with these tumors are reported to be 29.5% in 5 years.[17] Calcified meningiomas associated with spinal cord adhesions may also increase resection difficulty,[11,18,79] but the use of ultrasonic aspirators and more extensive or elaborate approaches may aid in resection. The factors that impede complete resection are also associated with an increased postoperative morbidity.[26] Therefore, the desire to achieve a complete resection must be balanced with the potential for damage to the spinal cord and postoperative neurologic deficits.

Functional outcome is dependent on preoperative functional status, with improved outcomes observed in patients with decreased preoperative neurologic deficits.[12,16,17,19] Functional improvement occurred in 53–95% and deterioration in 0–10%,[11,13,15–19] with a mean follow-up of 20–180 months. Of note, remarkable recovery can be achieved with surgical resection and rehabilitation.[17,18] Three of four patients with preoperative paraplegia achieved independent mobility postoperatively.[16] Ambulatory status was found to improve from 33–74% preoperatively to 75–97% postoperatively,[13] and bladder function improved in 35 of 37 (95%) of patients postsurgery.[16] The development of CSF leak or fistula ranged from 0 to 4%.[13] Postoperative deterioration was usually transient, with recovery after 6 months.[11,17,19] Mortality rates ranged from 0 to 3%, with causes of death attributed to pulmonary embolism, aspiration pneumonia, stroke, and myocardial infarction.[11,13,15–19]

Follow-Up

Although recurrence rates of spinal meningioma are low, they do occur and can occur as long as 17 years from treatment. As such, clinical follow-up together with an MRI should be arranged at 1-year postsurgery and at regular annual or biannual intervals thereafter. Since subtotal resection of tumors with higher grades often recur, more frequent follow-up is prudent. It should be guided, however, by the clinical picture, tumor growth, and histology.

Future Perspectives

MRI screening has improved the ability to diagnose and follow patients with spinal meningiomas prior to significant neurologic deterioration. With an enhanced understanding of MR spectroscopy in the future, tumor types and grades may be able to be differentiated. As the understanding of tumor genetics improves, perhaps the diagnosis, medical treatment,

and determination of tumor recurrence can also be improved. Advances in surgical management, such as minimal access surgery and improved fusion techniques, may also facilitate safer tumor resection and decreased patient morbidity. Adjunctive radiation treatment may improve with hyperfractionated treatment regimens or radiosurgical techniques. Until these or other advances occur, the surgical management of spinal meningiomas will continue to be, as Cushing once described, "one of the more gratifying of all operative procedures."[6]

References

1. Bret P, Lecuire J, Lapras C, et al. [Intraspinal meningiomas. A series of 60 cases]. Neurochirurgie 1976; 22:5–22.
2. Gowers W, Horsely V. A case of tumor of the spinal cord. Removal. Recovery. Medico-Chirurigical Transactions 1888; 71:377–428.
3. Cohen-Gadol AA, Spencer DD, Krauss WE. The development of techniques for resection of spinal cord tumors by Harvey W. Cushing. J Neurosurg Spine 2005; 2:92–7.
4. Helseth A, Mork SJ. Primary intraspinal neoplasms in Norway, 1955 to 1986. A population-based survey of 467 patients. J Neurosurg 1989; 71:842–5.
5. Albanese V, Platania N. Spinal intradural extramedullary tumors. Personal experience. J Neurosurg Sci 2002; 46:18–24.
6. Cushing H, Eisenhardt L. Meningiomas: Their Classification, Regional Behavior, Life History, and Surgical End Results. Springfield, IL: Charles C Thomas, 1938.
7. Nelson JS, Parisi JE, Schochet SS. Principles and practice of neuropathology. In: Parisi JE, Mena H, eds. Non-Glial Tumors. St. Louis: Mosby-Year Book, Inc., 1993:203–13.
8. Mirimanoff RO, Dosoretz DE, Linggood RM, et al. Meningioma: analysis of recurrence and progression following neurosurgical resection. J Neurosurg 1985; 62:18–24.
9. Simeone FA. Intradural Tumors. In: Rothman RH, Simeone FA, eds. The Spine. Philadelphia: WB Saunders Co, 1992:1515–7.
10. Weinstein JN, McLain RF. Tumors of the spine. In: Rothman RH, Simeone FA, eds. The Spine. Philadelphia: WB Saunders Co, 1992:1299–300.
11. Roux FX, Nataf F, Pinaudeau M, et al. Intraspinal meningiomas: review of 54 cases with discussion of poor prognosis factors and modern therapeutic management. Surg Neurol 1996; 46:458–63; discussion 463–4.
12. Goldbrunner R. Intradural extramedullary tumors. In: Tonn JC, Westphal M, Rutka JT, Grossman SA, eds. Neuro-Oncology of CNS Tumors. New York: Springer-Verlag, 2006:635–643.
13. Gottfried ON, Gluf W, Quinones-Hinojosa A, et al. Spinal meningiomas: surgical management and outcome. Neurosurg Focus 2003; 14:e2.
14. Kuntz C, Shaffrey CI, Wolcott WP. Approach to the patient and medical management of spinal disorders. In: Winn HR, ed. Youmans Neurological Surgery. Vol. 4. Philadelphia: Saunders, 2004:4289–4326.
15. Gezen F, Kahraman S, Canakci Z, Beduk A. Review of 36 cases of spinal cord meningioma. Spine 2000; 25:727–31.
16. King AT, Sharr MM, Gullan RW, Bartlett JR. Spinal meningiomas: a 20-year review. Br J Neurosurg 1998; 12:521–6.
17. Klekamp J, Samii M. Surgical results for spinal meningiomas. Surg Neurol 1999; 52:552–62.

18. Levy WJ Jr., Bay J, Dohn D. Spinal cord meningioma. J Neurosurg 1982; 57:804–12.
19. Solero CL, Fornari M, Giombini S, et al. Spinal meningiomas: review of 174 operated cases. Neurosurgery 1989; 25:153–60.
20. Nittner K. Spinal meningiomas, neurinomas and neurofibromas, and hourglass tumours. In: Vinken PH, Bruyn GW, eds. Handbook of Clinical Neurology. New York: Elsevier, 1976:177–322.
21. Honch GW. Spinal cord and foramen magnum tumors. Semin Neurol 1993; 13:337–42.
22. Cheng MK. Spinal cord tumors in the People's Republic of China: a statistical review. Neurosurgery 1982; 10:22–4.
23. Parisi JE, Mena H. Nonglial tumors. In: Nelson JS, Parisi JE, Schochet SSJ, eds. Principles and Practice of Neuropathology. St. Louis: Mosby, 1993:203–266.
24. Calogero JA, Moossy J. Extradural spinal meningiomas. Report of four cases. J Neurosurg 1972; 37:442–7.
25. Namer IJ, Pamir MN, Benli K, et al. Spinal meningiomas. Neurochirurgia (Stuttg) 1987; 30:11–5.
26. Birch BD, McCormick PC, Resnick DK. Intradural extramedullary spinal lesions. In: Benzel EC, ed. Spine surgery techniques, complication avoidance, and management. Vol. 1. Philadelphia: Elsevier, 2005:948–960.
27. Schwartz TH, McCormick PC. Spinal cord tumors in adults. In: Winn HR, ed. Youmans Neurological Surgery. Vol. 4. Philadelphia: Saunders, 2004:4817–4834.
28. Cohen-Gadol AA, Zikel OM, Koch CA, et al. Spinal meningiomas in patients younger than 50 years of age: a 21-year experience. J Neurosurg 2003; 98:258–63.
29. Okazaki H. Fundamentals of Neuropathology. New York: Igaku-Shoin, 1983.
30. Zang KD. Meningioma: a cytogenetic model of a complex benign human tumor, including data on 394 karyotyped cases. Cytogenet Cell Genet 2001; 93:207–20.
31. Raza SM, Anderson WS, Eberhart CG, et al. The application of surgical cordectomy in the management of an intramedullary-extramedullary atypical meningioma: case report and literature review. J Spinal Disord Tech 2005; 18:449–54.
32. Stein CL, McCormick PC. Spinal intradural tumors. In: Wilkins RH, Rengachary SS, eds. Neurosurgery. New York: McGraw-Hill, 1996:1769–1781.
33. Salpietro FM, Alafaci C, Lucerna S, et al. Do spinal meningiomas penetrate the pial layer? Correlation between magnetic resonance imaging and microsurgical findings and intracranial tumor interfaces. Neurosurgery 1997; 41:254–7; discussion 257–8.
34. Louis DN, Scheithauer BW, Budka H, et al. Meningiomas. In: Kleihues P, Cavenee W, eds. Pathology and Genetics of Tumors of the Nervous System. World Health Organization Classification of Tumours. Lyon: IARC Press, 2000.
35. Kepes JJ. Meningiomas: Biology, Pathology and Differential Diagnosis. New York: Masson Publishing, 1982.
36. Schaller B. Spinal meningioma: relationship between histological subtypes and surgical outcome? J Neurooncol 2005; 75: 157–61.
37. Ibrahim A, Galloway M, Leung C, et al. Cervical spine chordoid meningioma. Case report. J Neurosurg Spine 2005; 2:195–8.
38. Kannuki S, Soga T, Hondo H, et al. Coexistence of intracranial and spinal meningiomas—report of two cases. Neurol Med Chir (Tokyo) 1991; 31:720–4.
39. Imlay SP, Snider TE, Raab SS. Clear-cell meningioma: diagnosis by fine-needle aspiration biopsy. Diagn Cytopathol 1998; 18:131–6.
40. Lee W, Chang KH, Choe G, et al. MR imaging features of clear-cell meningioma with diffuse leptomeningeal seeding. AJNR Am J Neuroradiol 2000; 21:130–2.
41. Yu KB, Lim MK, Kim HJ, et al. Clear-cell meningioma: CT and MR imaging findings in two cases involving the spinal canal and cerebellopontine angle. Korean J Radiol 2002; 3:125–9.
42. Caroli E, Acqui M, Roperto R, et al. Spinal en plaque meningiomas: a contemporary experience. Neurosurgery 2004; 55:1275–9; discussion 1279.
43. Chen JC, Tseng SH, Chen Y, et al. Cervical dumbbell meningioma and thoracic dumbbell schwannoma in a patient with neurofibromatosis. Clin Neurol Neurosurg 2005; 107:253–7.
44. Chaparro MJ, Young RF, Smith M, et al. Multiple spinal meningiomas: a case of 47 distinct lesions in the absence of neurofibromatosis or identified chromosomal abnormality. Neurosurgery 1993; 32:298–301; discussion 301–2.
45. Arslantas A, Artan S, Oner U, et al. Detection of chromosomal imbalances in spinal meningiomas by comparative genomic hybridization. Neurol Med Chir (Tokyo) 2003; 43:12–8; discussion 19.
46. Ketter R, Henn W, Niedermayer I, et al. Predictive value of progression-associated chromosomal aberrations for the prognosis of meningiomas: a retrospective study of 198 cases. J Neurosurg 2001; 95:601–7.
47. Wolcott WP, Malik JM, Shaffrey CI, et al. Differential diagnosis of surgical disorders of the spine. In: Benzel EC, ed. Spine Surgery Techniques, Complication Avoidance, and Management. Vol. 1. Philadelphia: Elsevier, 2005:33–60.
48. Wang AM, Haykal HA. Thoracic spinal meningioma associated with hydrocephalic dementia. AJNR Am J Neuroradiol 1987; 8:383–4.
49. Feldmann E, Bromfield E, Navia B, et al. Hydrocephalic dementia and spinal cord tumor. Report of a case and review of the literature. Arch Neurol 1986; 43:714–8.
50. Turner GA, Jayasinghe G, Rossato RG. Cervical meningioma and lumbar stenosis: a case presenting as immobility. Aust NZ J Med. 1997; 27:442–3.
51. Huynen CH, Ruijs JH, Tulleken CA. MRI of the brain and cervical spine: first choice in the detection of abnormalities. Preliminary study. Diagn Imaging Clin Med 1986; 55:61–5.
52. Neuhold A, Fruhwald F, Wicke L, Schwaighofer B. Surface coils in magnetic resonance diagnosis of spinal space-occupying lesions. Röntgenblatter 1987; 40:248–54.
53. Vargas MI, Abu Eid M, Bogorin A, et al. Spinal extradural meningiomas: MRI findings in two cases. J Neuroradiol 2004; 31:214–9.
54. Hasuo K, Uchino A, Matsuura Y, et al. MRI of intradural-extramedullary spinal neurinomas and meningiomas. Nippon Igaku Hoshasen Gakkai Zasshi - Nippon Acta Radiologica 1993; 53:503–10.
55. Thron A, Guhl L, Voigt K, et al. MR imaging features of spinal schwannomas and meningiomas. J Neurosurg 1987; 66:695–700.
56. Quekel LG, Versteege CW. The "dural tail sign" in MRI of spinal meningiomas. J Comput Assist Tomogr 1995; 19:890–2.
57. De Verdelhan O, Haegelen C, Carsin-Nicol B, et al. MR imaging features of spinal schwannomas and meningiomas. J Neuroradiol 2005; 32:42–9.
58. Toscano S, Staropoli C, Longo M, et al. MR imaging of intraspinal tumors—capability in histological differentiation and compartmentalization of extramedullary tumors. Acta Neurochirurgica 1990; 107:70–3.

59. Perrin RG, McBroom RJ. Thoracic spine tumors. Clin Neurosurg 1992; 38:353–72.

60. Pecker MJ, Javalet A, Simon J, Loussouarn Y. Les tumeurs epidurales benignes de la moelle. Neuro-Chirurgie 1967; 13:647–60.

61. Fortuna A, Gambacorta D, Occhipinti EM. Spinal extradural meningiomas. Neurochirurgia 1969; 12:166–80.

62. Whittle IR, Johnston IH, Besser M. Intra-operative recording of cortical somatosensory evoked potentials as a method of spinal cord monitoring during spinal surgery. Aust NZ J Surg 1986; 56:309–17.

63. Jones SJ, Harrison R, Koh KF, et al. Motor evoked potential monitoring during spinal surgery: responses of distal limb muscles to transcranial cortical stimulation with pulse trains. Electroencephalogr Clin Neurophysiol 1996; 100:375–83.

64. Pechstein U, Cedzich C, Nadstawek J, Schramm J. Transcranial high-frequency repetitive electrical stimulation for recording myogenic motor evoked potentials with the patient under general anesthesia. Neurosurgery 1996; 39:335–43; discussion 343–4.

65. Taniguchi M, Cedzich C, Schramm J. Modification of cortical stimulation for motor evoked potentials under general anesthesia: technical description. Neurosurgery 1993; 32:219–26.

66. Iwasaki H, Tamaki T, Yoshida M, et al. Efficacy and limitations of current methods of intraoperative spinal cord monitoring. J Orthop Sci 2003; 8:635–42.

67. Schramm J, Kurthen M. Recent developments in neurosurgical spinal cord monitoring. Paraplegia 1992; 30:609–16.

68. Kratimenos GP, Crockard HA. The far lateral approach for ventrally placed foramen magnum and upper cervical spine tumours. Br J Neurosurg 1993; 7:129–40.

69. Sen CN, Sekhar LN. An extreme lateral approach to intradural lesions of the cervical spine and foramen magnum. Neurosurgery 1990; 27:197–204.

70. Samii M, Klekamp J, Carvalho G. Surgical results for meningiomas of the craniocervical junction. Neurosurgery 1996; 39:1086–94; discussion 1094–5.

71. Miller E, Crockard HA. Transoral transclival removal of anteriorly placed meningiomas at the foramen magnum. Neurosurgery 1987; 20:966–8.

72. Suzuki A, Nakamura H, Konishi S, Yamano Y. Dumbbell-shaped meningioma with cystic degeneration in the thoracic spine: a case report. Spine 2002; 27:E193–6.

73. Buchfelder M, Nomikos P, Paulus W, Rupprecht H. Spinal-thoracic dumbbell meningioma: a case report. Spine 2001; 26:1500–4.

74. Regelsberger J, Fritzsche E, Langer N, Westphal M. Intraoperative sonography of intra- and extramedullary tumors. Ultrasound Med Biol 2005; 31:593–8.

75. Mimatsu K, Kawakami N, Kato F, et al. Intraoperative ultrasonography of extramedullary spinal tumours. Neuroradiology 1992; 34:440–3.

76. Matsuzaki H, Tokuhashi Y, Wakabayashi K, et al. Differences on intraoperative ultrasonography between meningioma and neurilemmoma. Neuroradiology 1998; 40:40–4.

77. Matsuzaki H, Tokuhashi Y, Wakabayashi K, Toriyama S. Clinical values of intraoperative ultrasonography for spinal tumors. Spine 1992; 17:1392–9.

78. Saito T, Arizono T, Maeda T, et al. A novel technique for surgical resection of spinal meningioma. Spine 2001; 26:1805–8.

79. Freidberg SR. Removal of an ossified ventral thoracic meningioma. Case report. J Neurosurg 1972; 37:728–30.

80. De Salles AA, Pedroso AG, Medin P, et al. Spinal lesions treated with Novalis shaped beam intensity-modulated radiosurgery and stereotactic radiotherapy. J Neurosurg 2004; 101 Suppl 3:435–40.

81. Gerszten PC, Ozhasoglu C, Burton SA, et al. CyberKnife frameless stereotactic radiosurgery for spinal lesions: clinical experience in 125 cases. Neurosurgery 2004; 55:89–98; discussion 98–9.

82. Gerszten PC, Ozhasoglu C, Burton SA, et al. CyberKnife frameless single-fraction stereotactic radiosurgery for benign tumors of the spine. Neurosurg Focus 2003; 14:e16.

83. Cramer P, Thomale UW, Okuducu AF, et al. An atypical spinal meningioma with CSF metastasis: fatal progression despite aggressive treatment. Case report. J Neurosurg Spine 2005; 3:153–8.

84. Baird M, Gallagher PJ. Recurrent intracranial and spinal meningiomas: clinical and histological features. Clin Neuropathol 1989; 8:41–4.

85. Deen HG, Jr., Scheithauer BW, Ebersold MJ. Clinical and pathological study of meningiomas of the first two decades of life. J Neurosurg 1982; 56:317–22.

VII
Miscellaneous

58
Pediatric Meningiomas

Amro Al-Habib and James T. Rutka

Introduction

Pediatric meningiomas represent a unique challenge to the neurosurgeon, as they are somewhat uncommon and harbor unique clinical and pathologic characteristics [1]. While there is some debate about the definition of the upper age limit of "pediatric" cases, for the purpose of this chapter we will use age 18 as the upper limit. This coincides well with the pediatric age defined by the National Library of Medicine [2].

Incidence

Pediatric meningiomas represent no more than 3% of pediatric intracranial tumors and less than 2% of meningiomas in all age groups [3–10]. Our institutional series, reported by Drake et al. in 1985 [11], revealed only 13 cases of meningiomas out of 1283 pediatric intracranial tumors encountered at the Hospital for Sick Children, Toronto, over 51 years. This constitutes an incidence of 1% [12]. A literature review by Mendiratta et al. indicated an incidence of 1.5% among 2620 cases of intracranial pediatric tumors [13]. Worldwide reports indicate an incidence ranging from 1.3 to 2.4% [10,14–16]. In some ways this questions the importance of environmental factors in the etiology of meningioma, at least in the pediatric age group [17].

Meningiomas can affect any age group, and generally their incidence increases with advancing age. They are more common in the second decade of life [1,12]. A review of the literature indicates an occurrence as early as 5 days (Table 58-1) with an average range from 8 to 15 years old at presentation. Congenital or infantile cases are extremely uncommon [1,13] and are typically encountered in the literature as individual case reports [1].

Sex distribution among pediatric meningiomas is widely variable. Male predominance, in contrast to adult meningiomas, is noted in the pediatric age group. In the infant age group, in particular, up to 71% of the patients were males in some studies [12,18]. Interestingly, females become more affected as the age group studied advances [14]. By the time

adulthood is reached, the potential estrogen effect on inducing meningiomas in the female population is described [4,17,19].

Clinical Features

Clinical presentation in the pediatric age group depends primarily on the age of the child and the location of the tumor. In infants, the only presentation may be of an increase in the head circumference [12]. Focal deformity related to hyperostosis is the presentation in some cases [20]. Later in life, clinical presentation depends on tumor location [12,14]. In a series of 13 patients [12], focal neurologic deficit was the most common presentation (46%), followed by signs of increased intracranial pressure (30%) and seizures (20%). Seizures were found in 25–31% in other series [5,21], which is similar to the incidence reported in adults (29%) by Ramamurthi et al. Seizures are more commonly associated with parasagittal and convexity locations of the tumor [22]. Proptosis may be found with intraorbital meningiomas [8]. Intraventricular meningiomas may present with a lateral ventricle syndrome comprised of seizures, hemiparesis, hemianopsia, and papilledema [8,23] or simply with raised intracranial pressure [12].

Neurofibromatosis type 2 (NF2) and prior exposure to ionizing radiation are known predisposing factors [1]. It is not unexpected that children with NF2 may present with meningiomas given the protean manifestations of this genetic disorder [1]. Approximately 25–40% of children with meningiomas have NF2 [1,4,5,9,10,21]. This high incidence should raise the question of NF2 in any child who presents with meningiomas, especially if multiple tumors occur in extracranial or intraorbital locations [1]. In their review of pediatric meningiomas, Perry et al. found that all children who had multiple meningiomas had NF2. Furthermore, 36% of them were not known to have NF2 at the time of meningioma surgery [1,3]. In the same review, NF2-associated meningiomas were significantly less invasive than sporadic cases, but there was no difference in their histopathology otherwise [3]. Deen et al. studied 12 NF patients in their review of 51 cases of pediatric meningiomas. These patients were peculiar in their increased incidence of orbital (3 of the 12) and spinal (5 of the 12) tumors. Their age, sex, and histologic features were otherwise similar to the general group.

Children irradiated for intracranial tumors or leukemias are at a higher risk of developing meningiomas later in their life [1]. Children that were irradiated in Israel in the 1950s for tinea capitis had a fourfold increase in their risk of developing meningiomas [24]. The relative risk of developing subsequent meningioma after ionizing radiation increases by approximately 10-fold compared to controls [1,25,26]. The latency period varies from 11 to 43 years [1]. It may be shorter in those who received a higher dose [1,27]. Typically, radiation-induced meningiomas present at an earlier age, are multifocal and occur in the field of radiation [1,8,26]. It is, however, debated if radiation-induced meningiomas have a more malignant or high-grade pathology compared to the nonradiation cases [1]

Diagnostic Imaging

Pediatric meningiomas share similar magnetic resonance imaging (MRI) features to adults [28] with few peculiarities. They tend to lack the sign of dural attachment or "dural tail" on MRI in up to 27% of cases [1]. Their location is also highly variable. Although the majority are supratentorial (Table 58-1) [4,29], they are more frequently found in unusual locations compared to adults [12]. Intraventricular meningiomas, interestingly, are more frequently reported in children than adults, mostly in the lateral ventricles [9,30]. A literature review by Germano et al. revealed an incidence of intraventricular meningioma of about 9.4% of 278 meningiomas in the first two decades of life [21] as opposed to 5% in adults [31]. While this finding is supported by many other papers [5,23,32], others did not note this tendency in their case reviews [4]. Intraventricular meningiomas probably arise either from choroid plexus or tela choroidea of the lateral ventricle [28]. Another unusual location for pediatric meningiomas is the posterior fossa at an incidence ranging from 19% [5,9] to 46% [33], while 10% of adult meningiomas are infratentorial [21,31]. Our literature review revealed 45 cases of infratentorial meningioma among 368 reported cases of meningiomas in the pediatric age group.

A primary intracerebral location without an obvious dural attachment has also been frequently reported [1,34,35]. All these features make the preoperative diagnosis of meningioma in the pediatric age group more difficult (Fig. 58-1). Current MRI sequences are unable to resolve meningiomas into histological subtypes or grades [28].

While multiple meningiomas are reported with an occurrence of 23% in some series of pediatric cases [36], it is considered uncommon in other series incidence (1–2.5%) [28,37,38]. This variability is related to the number of neurofibromatosis or previously irradiated cases included in the study. Five of six multiple meningioma patients, in a report of 48 pediatric meningioma cases by Merten et al. were found to have neurofibromatosis, an incidence of 12.5 % [5]. The

advancement in the diagnostic modalities has also increased the yield of diagnosis of multiple tumors [39].

Pediatric meningiomas tend to be large and cystic [1,8,28,40,41] in relative comparison to adult meningiomas. Our series [12] indicated an average size of 5.25 cm^2 for the 13 tumors studied (Fig. 58-2). Two of these were 8 cm^2 or greater [12]. The large size at presentation may reflect the ability of the child's brain to tolerate a slowly growing mass [12].

Cystic changes have been reported more often in children (incidence of 13–50%) compared to adults (2–4.6%) [37,42]. These cysts have been classified into four types based on the location of the cyst in relation to the tumor and the brain [28,37,43]. Type 1 is when the cyst is located in the center of the tumor; type 2 includes cysts at the periphery of the tumor. If cyst is in the peritumoral area, it is type 3, and type 4 if located at the interface between the tumor and the brain. The presence of cysts can lead to a misdiagnosis of glioma or metastasis [37] and makes the neuroradiologic diagnosis even more difficult. The relationship of the cystic changes to the pathology of the tumor and the implications of tumor cysts on management or prognosis are not clear. Calcification and hyperostosis are known features for adult meningiomas (10%) [44], which are reported at a higher frequency in pediatric cases (31–32 %) [4,45].

Pathology

The World Health Organization (WHO) classification of central nervous system tumors includes both adult and pediatric meningiomas [46]. Earlier pediatric meningioma series (Table 58-1) included tumors like hemangiopericytoma and meningeal sarcoma, which can be significantly difficult to differentiate from tumors like anaplastic (grade III) meningiomas with sarcomatoid features [3]. These tumors are no longer considered as meningiomas in the current WHO classification and are classified as WHO grade II or III neoplasms [1].

All different histologic subtypes of adult meningiomas are reported in children, including the malignant ones [1]. Two of the higher grade meningiomas, the clear cell (WHO grade II) and papillary (WHO grade III) subtypes, appear to be associated with younger age and are more frequently reported in children and infants [1,4,47]. The papillary variant is particularly important to recognize because of its aggressive behavior and worse survival rates [4,12].

Differential Diagnosis

Meningeal-based masses in children have a wide differential diagnosis, as shown in Table 58-2, sarcomas being the second most common following meningiomas [1]. Tuberculosis and other rare infectious disorders affecting the dura are important to rule out, especially in endemic areas [1].

TABLE 58-1. Reported Case Series on Pediatric Meningiomas.

No.	Series	No. of patients	Age range (yr)	Mean age (yr)	Sex M:F	Location	Pathology	Mean F/U (yr)	Surgical management	Adjuvant therapy	Survival at F/U	Comments
1	Crouse & Berg, 1972 [33]	13	0.2–20	12.8	7:6	Supra 7 Infra 6	Benign 7 Meningial 5 Sarcoma 5 Meningial melanoma 1	7 (for 9 patients)	GTR 1 PR 10 (for total of 11 operated)	XRT 3	Alive 3 Dead 8 Diagnosis at autopsy 2	-3 had NF -Sarcomas: dead 1, diagnosis at autopsy 1, downhill course 3 (unknown if died), -Melanoma F/U: unknown
2	Cooper & Dohn, 1974 [29]	7	7–14	11	2:5	Supra 7 Infra 0	Benign 5 Atypical 1 Meningial Sarcoma 1	4.74	GTR 3 PR 2 Unknown 2	Cobalt 60 therapy 1	Alive 5 Dead 2	-One patient with sarcomatous meningioma had spinal canal metastasis and paraplegia, then died -Other death was for atypical meningioma
3	Merten et al., 1974 [5]	48	0.3–19	10.9	27:21	Supra 32 Infra 9 Extracranial 6 ** Spine 1	Benign 46 Malignant 2	Average of 1–28	GTR 28 PR 20 0	0	Alive 33 Dead 15	-Report excluded angioblastic meningiomas
4	Leibel et al., 1976 [52]	13	9–19	15	7:6	Supra 9 Infra 4	Benign 10 Meningial sarcoma 3	8.6	GTR 2 PR 11	XRT 6	Alive 4 Dead 9 (2 pot-op deaths)	-23% association with NF -Age limit is 20 -All 3 sarcoma patients died -One of the GTR is NF1, died secondary to ICH -XRT for 3 post initial surgery and 3 post recurrence
5	Herz et al., 1980 [23]	9	4–18	12.9	4:5	Supra 9 Infra 0	Benign 8 Meningeal Ssarcoma 1	5	GTR 7 PR 2	XRT 1	Alive 8 Dead 1	-1 PR followed later by GTR -1 Sarcoma patient: had 2 surgeries, doing well 7 years later -1 Death: from postop complication, NF2 patient, multiple other tumors
6	Sano et al., 1981 [6]	18	<1–5yr	-	10:8	Supra 15 Infra 2 Extracranial** 1	Benign 12 Meningeal Sarcoma 6	—	Unknown	0	Alive 7 (out of 12 followed) Dead 5 Unknown 6	-5 Sarcomas: 3 alive >10 years, 2 deaths, 1 unknown.
7	Deen et al., 1982 [4]	51	7–20	15.2	25:26	Supra 31 Infra 7 Extracranial** 3 Spine 10	Benign 46 Malignant 5	—	Unknown	0	Alive 30 Dead 21	12 patients had NF
8	Chan and Thompson, 1984 [22]	4	2.5–16	8.1	2:2	Supra 4 Infra 0	Benign 3 Malignant 1	15.3	GTR 3 PR 1	XRT 1	Alive 3 Dead 1	-1 Dead: malignant
9	Drake et al., 1985 [11]	13	3–16	11.3	10:3	Supra 13	Benign 12 Malignant 1	6	GTR 7 PR 6	0	Alive 12 Dead 1	-The death is a transitional meningioma

(continued)

TABLE 58-1. (cont'd) Reported Case Series on Pediatric Meningiomas

No.	Series	No. of patients	Age range (yr)	Mean age (yr)	Sex M:F	Location	Pathology	Mean F/U (yr)	Surgical management	Adjuvant therapy	Survival at F/U	Comments
10	Doty, et al., 1987	13	2–16	8.8	8:5	Supra 13	Benign 11 Meningeal sarcomas 2	3.3	GTR 12 PR 1	XRT 2	Alive 11 Dead 2	-2 Sarcomas: one developed grade III astrocytoma 9 years after radiation, operated and died. The other is alive 5 years after -2 deaths: 1 from lipoblastic epitheloidal meningiomas, the other from sarcoma
11	Ferrante, et al., 1989 [7]	19	0.5–16	11.7	13:6	Supra 18 Infra 1	Benign 15 Meningeal: sarcomas 3 angioblastic 1	6.7	GTR 15 PR 3 Preop death 1	—	—	Sarcomas: preop death 1, 2 with recurrence after 4 and 10yr Angioblastic: good condition at follow-up
12	Germano, et al., 1994 [21]	23	6–21	13.3	14:9	Supra 19 Infra 3 Extracranial ** 1	Benign 23		GTR 14 PR 9	XRT 3	Alive 23	-Upper age limit is 20 years. -XRT in 3 patients with PR
13	Sheikh, et al., 1995 [37]	9	4–16	10.1	6:3	Supra 3 Infra 1 Extracranial ** 3 Multiple‡ 2	Benign 9	2.8	Unknown	—	Alive 7 Unknown 2	-Multiple meningiomas: 1st: ethmoidal, orbital and CPA 2nd: orbit, sellar
14	Baum-gartner, et al., 1996 [8]	11	2–17	11	6:5	Supra 8 Infra 1 Multiple‡ 2	Benign 4 Atypical 4 Malignant 3	7.2 (for Alive) 1.5 for 2 death with malignant tumors 2.5 for 1 with benign tumor	GTR 7 PR 3 Observation 1	XRT 3 Chemo 1	Alive 8 Dead 3	-2 Patients had previous whole brain radiation -3 Patients with NF2, 2 of them had multiple tumors. -Multiple tumors: 1st :c-spine, parasagital and convexity 2nd: convexity and cerebellar -Chemo for 1 malignant case -3 Deaths: includes 2 malignant cases
15	Turgut, et al., 1997 [15]	13	5 days–14yr	8.3	7:6	Supra 6 Extracranial ** 1 Multiple‡ 3 Spine 3	Benign 12 Atypical 1	3.5 (2 unknown)	GTR 9 PR 4	0	Alive 9 Death 2 Unknown 2	-Multiple tumors: 1st: convexity and cerebelloponyine angle (CPA) 2nd: 2 tumors in the convexity 3rd: 2 tumors in the convexity and a third in the CPA -2 deaths: includes one atypical

No.	Reference	N	Age (yr)	Mean age (yr)	M:F	Location	Histology	F/U (mo)	Resection	XRT/Chemo	Outcome	Comments
16	Erdinçler, et al., 1998 [9]	29	—	10	18:11	Supra 23 Infra 4 Multiple‡ 2	Benign 28 Malignant 1	6.5 (for 21 patients)	GTR 25 PR 3 Op death 1	XRT 2 Chemo 1	Alive 24 Death 5	One patient with malignant meningioma received both chemo and radiation. -5 Deaths: anaplastic meningioma 1, meningothelial 3, operative death due to bleeding from superior sagittal sinus 1
17	Amirjamshidi, et al., 2000 [10]	24	2–17	9.47	11:13	Supra 18 Infra 2 Extracranial* 3 Spine 1	Benign 23 Malignant 1	10.85	GTR 21 PR 3	0	Alive 23 Death 1	
18	Zwerdling, et al., 2002 [17]	18	1.5–17	11	8:10	Supra 17 Spine 1	Benign 14 Malignant 4	5.6 (for 13)	GTR 11 PR 7	XRT 2 Chemo 1 Both 2	Alive 16 Dead 2	-2 Deaths: both are malignant.
19	Rochat, et al., 2004 [14]	22	1–14	6	8:14	Supra 19 Infra 3	Benign 20 Malignant 2	16	GTR 15 PR 6 Op death 1	XRT 8	Alive 7 Dead 13 Unknown 2	All deaths had low-grade tumors
20	Tufan, et al., 2005 [18]	11	1.15–17	12.7	6:5	Supra 9 Infra 2	Benign 6 Atypical 2 Malignant 3	6 (for 10)	GTR 8 PR 3	XRT 4	Alive 7 Dead 3 Unknown 1	3 Deaths: includes 1 malignant case.
Total		368		11.4 (excluding study 6)	199:169	Supra 280 Infra 45 Extracranial 18 Spinal 16 Multiple 9	Benign 315 Atypical 8 Malignant 23 Other Meningeal tumors: -sarcoma 20 -angioblastic 1 -melanoma 1		GTR 188 PR 94 Unknown 80 Observation 1 Op death 2 Preop death/ autopsy 3	XRT 37 Cobalt therapy 1 Chemo 5	Alive 240 Dead 94 Unknown 32 Diagnosis at autopsy 2	

Yr: years; Mo: months; d: days; F: female; M: male; F/U: follow-up; GTR: gross total resection; PR: partial resection both at the 1st surgery; Op: operative; Supra: supratentorial; Infra: infratentorial; XRT: radiation therapy, Chemo: chemotherapy; NF: neurofibromatosis; CPA: cerebellopontine angle.

*Orbital, ethmoidal and sphenoethmoidal.

**Orbital.

†WHO Classification (reference).

‡ Multiple supratentorial or supra and infratentorial.

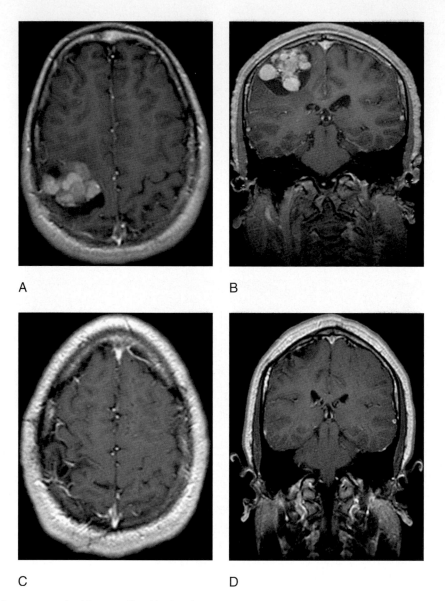

FIG. 58.1. A 15-year-old boy presented with generalized body seizures. (A, B) Preop MRI shows a right fronto-parietal cystic and solid lesion with very little dural attachement, imaging features which are typical for a meningioma in childhood. (C, D) Follow-up MRI 2.5 years after surgery shows no tumor. Patient is seizure-free on tapering medications, neurologically intact

Treatment

Total resection is the goal in meningioma treatment, and it is the primary mode of therapy [12,22,33]. The extent of resection is significantly related to tumor location and adherence to vascular and neural structures [4,9,48]. Modern neuroanesthesia, minimizing blood loss, and careful postoperative intensive care unit care are important factors for good outcome.

The role of postoperative radiation therapy for pediatric meningioma is still unclear [37]. While it appears to be beneficial in adults after partial resection of meningioma [49,50], it is debatable in children owing to the paucity of the cases [22]. It is generally reserved for partially

resected, progressive meningiomas [8] and malignant meningiomas [22] given the significant side effects of radiation on the developing brain, especially in children under three years of age [51]. A low tumor recurrence was reported after radiating partially resected meningiomas in some series [21,52]. The quality of survival, however, is unclear in most of the literature owing to the lack of a more objective neurocognitive testing. Reoperation is a preferred strategy, in some reports, to avoid radiation for an increased time and to preserve quality of survival [9]. Chemotherapy has also been used in the treatment of pediatric meningiomas [8,9,17]. Its role, however, in these tumors has not been proven [8].

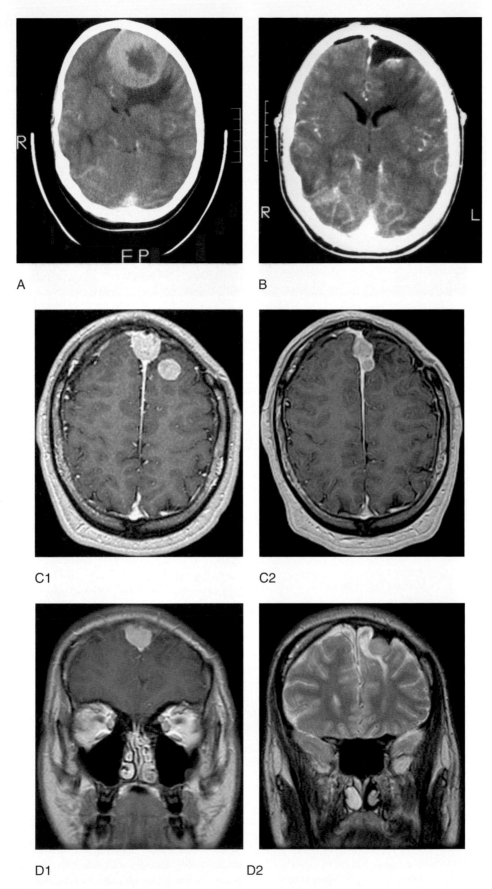

FIG. 58.2. A 10-year-old boy presented with headache, vomiting, aphasia, and right hemiparesis. (A) Preop CT head; (B) postop CT head showing gross total resection. pathology was consistent with malignant meningioma. He improved back to normal after resection. Five years later, follow-up MRI showed recurrence. He was suffering from refractory seizures. His neurologic exam is normal otherwise. (C1, C2) Axial MRI pictures showing recurrent left frontal and falcine meningioma. (D1, D2) Coronal MRI pictures illustrating the recurrence. Two years after resection, his seizure is well controlled and he remains neurologically intact. (E1, E2) MRI showing no tumor

(Continued)

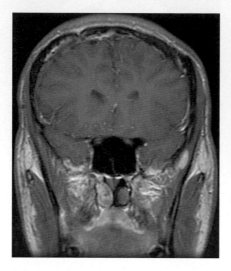

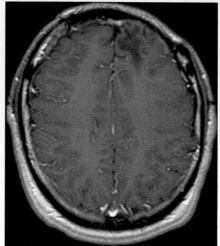

E1   E2

FIG. 58.2. (continued)

TABLE 58-2. Differential Diagnosis of Pediatric Meningiomas.

Meningothelial:	Meningioma
	Meningioangiomatosis
Sarcomas:	Hemangiopericytoma
	Fibrosarcoma
	Ewing's sarcoma
	Mesenchymal chondrosarcoma
	Postradiation sarcoma
	Leimyosarcoma
	Melanotic neuroectodermal
	tumor of infancy
Benign mesenchymal tumors:	Chondroma
	Hemangioma
	Lipoma
	Solitary fibrous tumor
Hematopoietic and	Leukemia
histiocytic tumors:	Lymphoma
	Juvenile xanthogranuloma
	Langerhans cell histiocytosis
	Rosai-Dorfman disease
	Xanthoma/Fibroxanthoma
	Histiocytic lymphoma/malignant
	histiocytosis
	Hemophagocytic lymphohistiocytosis
	Extramedullary hematopoiesis/myeloid
	metaplasia
Melanocytic tumors:	Meningeal (neurocutanous) melanosis
	Melanoma
	Melanocytoma
Inflammatory tumors:	Inflammatory pseudotumor
	Inflammatory myofibroblastic tumor
Contiguous or CSF spread:	Medulloblastoma
	Supratentorial PNET
	Atypical teratoid/rhabdoid tumor
	(ATRT)
	Ependymoma
	Diffuse astrocytoma/gliosarcoma
	Pilocytic astrocytoma ganglioma/DIG
	Pleomorphic xanthoastrocytoma
Infection	Tuberculous meningitis/Tuberculoma

Outcome

Pediatric meningiomas were considered, in earlier studies, to have a worse prognosis compared to adults, the reasons being related to their large size, unusual locations, increased incidence of malignant histology, and the lack of modern medical support [53]. Earlier studies reported a surgical mortality up to 40% [6,23]. This high incidence was partly related to the lack of critical neuroanesthesiology support [23] and to large number of malignant tumors like meningeal sarcomas [6,33]. The operative mortality among 197 patients reported by Ferrante et al was 9.7%. Subsequent reports have demonstrated no perioperative mortality [10,21].

The prognosis of the pediatric meningiomas has been linked to tumor recurrence [1,12], which has been associated with a decrease in 5-year survival from 94 to 64% [12]. Both the extent of surgical resection and the histopathologic grading of the tumor play a major role in determining recurrence and hence the long-term outcome of those patients [4,9,22,37,54,55]. Total removal varies in the literature from 54 to 86.2% [5,9,12,21,56]. Our review of the published series indicates that gross total resection was performed in 188 out of 308 pediatric meningioma patients (61%; Table 58-1) where surgical data are available. Among the 48 patients reported by Merten et al., all the patients who had total surgical resection survived (28 patients in a follow-up period of 10 months to 25 years). The remaining 20 patients who had subtotal resection or biopsy suffered tumor recurrence; only 5 of these had survived in follow-up [5]. Similarly, Deen et al. related their 39% recurrence rate, among 51 patients studied, to the tumor location, histologic subtype, and extent of surgical resection [4]. Patents with convexity meningiomas, in the same report, had a lower incidence of recurrence (32%) and a longer 20-year survival (75%) compared to the more technically challenging skull base cases (76.9% recurrence rate and 75% 20-year tumor survival) [4].

The average time to tumor recurrence was 7.4 years, with no difference between males and females [4]. More recent reports showed fewer recurrences and longer survivals. Ferrante et al. reported a recurrence rate of 10.8% among their 197 patients; and 73% of them had total excision. Their recurrence was related to incomplete surgical resection in 71.4% and to the histology of the tumor in 28.6% [57]. The histologic grade may also influence the rate of tumor recurrence. In the report by Deen et al., patients with papillary meningiomas had 80% recurrence rate compared to 35% for low-grade meningiomas [4]. In the report by Perry et al., the mortality rate among their non-NF2 patients was mainly related to the high-grade histology [3]. Benign meningiomas, on the other hand, can be surprising in their recurrence; up to 44% recurrence/death rate in one report [3]. The data on these patients, however, were lacking the details of the surgical resection [3]. While the association between the WHO histologic grading of meningioma and recurrence appears to be less strong in children compared to adults [1], it is important to take all critical prognostic factors into consideration. Even then, the behavior of meningiomas following resection in children appears to be difficult to predict [1]. The repeatedly recurring tumors also tend to have shorter time intervals between recurrences [22]. Therefore, careful follow-up with imaging studies is recommended for these cases.

The overall survival rate is also variable in the literature. Deen et al. reported a 15-year survival of 68% [4]. When Drake et al. excluded meningeal sarcomas in their literature review; the 5-year survival increased from 76 to 84% and the 15-year survival to 63% from 55% [12]. Our review (Table 58-1) has indicated that 240 of 336 patients were alive and 94 patients had died.

The functional outcome is very variable and depends on the premorbid condition and the extent of surgical resection. The true incidence of neurocognitive dysfunction is unknown due to the lack of detailed neuropsychologic testing in the literature [17]. Drake et al. classified their outcome into excellent (6 patients), good (5 patients), and fair (1 patient) groups based on their neurologic status and functional disability as being completely normal, having slight neurologic deficit, or a significant neurologic deficit, respectively [11]. Others have reported a long-term useful recovery in 90% of their survivors [23]. These outcome measures are useful, but more detailed neurocognitive testing would provide more objective and useful data.

Spinal Meningiomas

Spinal meningiomas in children are even more uncommon than their intracranial counterparts. In one center, only one case of spinal meningioma was seen among 1500 cases of brain and spine tumors in 35 years [12]. Pediatric spinal meningiomas have a reported incidence of 3–4% among spinal tumors [12], and they are more common in males (60:40%), similar to intracranial meningiomas [12] and unlike adult spinal menin-

giomas. They share with adults, however, increased frequency in the thoracic region. Multiple spinal meningiomas, spinal epidural en plaque meningioma, and spinal meningiomas in unusual locations have all been reported; mostly as individual case reports [12,58–60]. Interestingly, it has been reported that 15% of spinal meningiomas are extradural in location [4], probably arising from the arachnoid villi at the root exit zone [4,61]. Spinal meningiomas in children tend to be more diffuse and aggressive at presentation [62]. They usually present with pain followed by neurologic deficit [8,12]. The diagnosis can be quite challenging, especially early on in their presentation. They are not different in their histopathologic characteristics compared to meningiomas in general [12].

Surgical resection is the main treatment of choice. Deen et al. reported a lower recurrence rate of spinal meningiomas (20%) compared to the intracranial ones (39%) [4]. These results were largely related to both the small size of the tumor and the favorable location of the tumor, whicht allowed a complete resection [4].

Conclusion

Meningiomas in the pediatric population are rare tumors with unique clinical, histopathologic, and imaging characteristics. Intraventricular meningiomas are somewhat more common in children than in adults. A high index of suspicion is required to entertain the diagnosis preoperatively. A history of NF2 prediposes children to multiple, including spinal, meningiomas. Complete surgical resection is the recommended treatment of choice. Recurrences can be handled effectively with repeat excision. A high incidence of atypical meningiomas mandates close follow-up with serial imaging studies.

References

1. Perry A, Dehner LP. Meningeal tumors of childhood and infancy. An update and literature review. Brain Pathol 2003; 13(3): 386–408.
2. Medical subject headings—annotated alphabetical list, 1989. Bethesda, MD: National Library of Medicine, 1989.
3. Perry A, Giannini C, Raghavan R, et al. Aggressive phenotypic and genotypic features in pediatric and NF2-associated meningiomas: a clinicopathologic study of 53 cases. J Neuropathol Exp Neurol 2001; 60(10):994–1003.
4. Deen HG, Jr., Scheithauer BW, Ebersold MJ. Clinical and pathological study of meningiomas of the first two decades of life. J Neurosurg 1982; 56(3):317–322.
5. Merten DF, Gooding CA, Newton TH. The radiographic features of meningiomas in childhood and adolescence. Pediatr Radiol 1974; 2(2):89–96.
6. Sano K, Wakai S, Ochiai C, Takakura K. Characteristics of intracranial meningiomas in childhood. Childs Brain 1981; 8(2):98–106.
7. Ferrante L, Acqui M, Artico M, et al. Cerebral meningiomas in children. Childs Nerv Syst 1989; 5(2):83–86.

8. Baumgartner JE, Sorenson JM. Meningioma in the pediatric population. J Neurooncol 1996; 29(3):223–228.

9. Erdincler P, Lena G, Sarioglu AC, et al. Intracranial meningiomas in children: review of 29 cases. Surg Neurol 1998; 49(2):136–140.

10. Amirjamshidi A, Mehrazin M, Abbassioun K. Meningiomas of the central nervous system occurring below the age of 17: report of 24 cases not associated with neurofibromatosis and review of literature. Childs Nerv Syst 2000; 16(7):406–416.

11. Drake JM, Hendrick EB, Becker LE, et al. Intracranial meningiomas in children. Pediatr Neurosci 1985; 12(3):134–139.

12. Drake J, Hoffman H. Meningiomas in children. In: Al Mefty O, editor. Meningiomas. New York: Raven Press, 1991: 145–152.

13. Mendiratta SS, Rosenblum JA, Strobos RJ. Congenital meningioma. Neurology 1967; 17(9):914–918.

14. Rochat P, Johannesen HH, Gjerris F. Long-term follow up of children with meningiomas in Denmark: 1935 to 1984. J Neurosurg 2004; 100(2 Suppl Pediatrics):179–182.

15. Turgut M, Ozcan OE, Bertan V. Meningiomas in childhood and adolescence: a report of 13 cases and review of the literature. Br J Neurosurg 1997; 11(6):501–507.

16. Cheng MK. Brain tumors in the People's Republic of China: a statistical review. Neurosurgery 1982; 10(1):16–21.

17. Zwerdling T, Dothage J. Meningiomas in children and adolescents. J Pediatr Hematol Oncol 2002; 24(3):199–204.

18. Sakaki S, Nakagawa K, Kimura H, Ohue S. Intracranial meningiomas in infancy. Surg Neurol 1987; 28(1):51–57.

19. Donnell MS, Meyer GA, Donegan WL. Estrogen-receptor protein in intracranial meningiomas. J Neurosurg 1979; 50(4):499–502.

20. Turgut M, Ozcan OE, Bertan V. Meningiomas in childhood and adolescence: a report of 13 cases and review of the literature. Br J Neurosurg 1997; 11(6):501–507.

21. Germano IM, Edwards MS, Davis RL, Schiffer D. Intracranial meningiomas of the first two decades of life. J Neurosurg 1994; 80(3):447–453.

22. Chan RC, Thompson GB. Intracranial meningiomas in childhood. Surg Neurol 1984; 21(4):319–322.

23. Herz DA, Shapiro K, Shulman K. Intracranial meningiomas of infancy, childhood and adolescence. Review of the literature and addition of 9 case reports. Childs Brain 1980; 7(1):43–56.

24. Ron E, Modan B, Boice JD, Jr., et al. Tumors of the brain and nervous system after radiotherapy in childhood. N Engl J Med 1988; 319(16):1033–1039.

25. Ferrante L, Acqui M, Artico M, et al. Cerebral meningiomas in children. Childs Nerv Syst 1989; 5(2):83–86.

26. Sadetzki S, Flint-Richter P, Ben Tal T, Nass D. Radiation-induced meningioma: a descriptive study of 253 cases. J Neurosurg 2002; 97(5):1078–1082.

27. Iacono RP, Apuzzo ML, Davis RL, Tsai FY. Multiple meningiomas following radiation therapy for medulloblastoma. Case report. J Neurosurg 1981; 55(2):282–286.

28. Darling CF, Byrd SE, Reyes-Mugica M, et al. MR of pediatric intracranial meningiomas. AJNR Am J Neuroradiol 1994; 15(3):435–444.

29. Cooper M, Dohn DF. Intracranial meningiomas in childhood. Cleve Clin Q 1974; 41(4):197–204.

30. Ferrante L, Acqui M, Artico M, et al. Cerebral meningiomas in children. Childs Nerv Syst 1989; 5(2):83–86.

31. Rohringer M, Sutherland GR, Louw DF, Sima AA. Incidence and clinicopathological features of meningioma. J Neurosurg 1989; 71(5 Pt 1):665–672.

32. Ferrante L, Acqui M, Artico M, et al. Cerebral meningiomas in children. Childs Nerv Syst 1989; 5(2):83–86.

33. Crouse SK, Berg BO. Intracranial meningiomas in childhood and adolescence. Neurology 1972; 22(2):135–141.

34. Al Habib A, Lach B, Al Khani A. Intracerebral rhabdoid and papillary meningioma with leptomeningeal spread and rapid clinical progression. Clin Neuropathol 2005; 24(1):1–7.

35. Kohama I, Sohma T, Nunomura K, et al. Intraparenchymal meningioma in an infant–case report. Neurol Med Chir (Tokyo) 1996; 36(8):598–601.

36. Turgut M, Ozcan OE, Bertan V. Meningiomas in childhood and adolescence: a report of 13 cases and review of the literature. Br J Neurosurg 1997; 11(6):501–507.

37. Sheikh BY, Siqueira E, Dayel F. Meningioma in children: a report of nine cases and a review of the literature. Surg Neurol 1996; 45(4):328–335.

38. Ferrante L, Acqui M, Artico M, et al. Cerebral meningiomas in children. Childs Nerv Syst 1989; 5(2):83–86.

39. Turgut M, Ozcan OE, Bertan V. Meningiomas in childhood and adolescence: a report of 13 cases and review of the literature. Br J Neurosurg 1997; 11(6):501–507.

40. Turgut M, Ozcan OE, Bertan V. Meningiomas in childhood and adolescence: a report of 13 cases and review of the literature. Br J Neurosurg 1997; 11(6):501–507.

41. Ferrante L, Acqui M, Artico M, et al. Cerebral meningiomas in children. Childs Nerv Syst 1989; 5(2):83–86.

42. Ferrante L, Acqui M, Artico M, et al. Cerebral meningiomas in children. Childs Nerv Syst 1989; 5(2):83–86.

43. Reddy DR, Kolluri VR, Rao KS, et al. Cystic meningiomas in children. Childs Nerv Syst 1986; 2(6):317–319.

44. Taveras JM, Wood EH. Diagnostic Neuroradiology. Williams & Wilkins, 1964.

45. Turgut M, Ozcan OE, Bertan V. Meningiomas in childhood and adolescence: a report of 13 cases and review of the literature. Br J Neurosurg 1997; 11(6):501–507.

46. Louis D, Scheithauer B, Budka H, et al. Meningiomas. In: Kleihues P, Cavenee W, editors. Pathology and Genetics, Tumours of the Nervous System. IARC Press, International Agency for Research on Cancer, 2000: 176–184.

47. Ludwin SK, Rubinstein LJ, Russell DS. Papillary meningioma: a malignant variant of meningioma. Cancer 1975; 36(4): 1363–1373.

48. Tufan K, Dogulu F, Kurt G, et al. Intracranial meningiomas of childhood and adolescence. Pediatr Neurosurg 2005; 41(1):1–7.

49. Barbaro NM, Gutin PH, Wilson CB, et al. Radiation therapy in the treatment of partially resected meningiomas. Neurosurgery 1987; 20(4):525–528.

50. Goldsmith BJ, Wara WM, Wilson CB, Larson DA. Postoperative irradiation for subtotally resected meningiomas. A retrospective analysis of 140 patients treated from 1967 to 1990. J Neurosurg 1994; 80(2):195–201.

51. Danoff BF, Cowchock FS, Marquette C, et al. Assessment of the long-term effects of primary radiation therapy for brain tumors in children. Cancer 1982; 49(8):1580–1586.

52. Leibel SA, Wara WM, Sheline GE, et al. The treatment of meningiomas in childhood. Cancer 1976; 37(6):2709–2712.

53. Crouse SK, Berg BO. Intracranial meningiomas in childhood and adolescence. Neurology 1972; 22(2):135–141.

54. Ferrante L, Acqui M, Artico M, et al. Cerebral meningiomas in children. Childs Nerv Syst 1989; 5(2):83–86.

55. Turgut M, Ozcan OE, Bertan V. Meningiomas in childhood and adolescence: a report of 13 cases and review of the literature. Br J Neurosurg 1997; 11(6):501–507.
56. Ferrante L, Acqui M, Artico M, et al. Cerebral meningiomas in children. Childs Nerv Syst 1989; 5(2):83–86.
57. Ferrante L, Acqui M, Artico M, et al. Cerebral meningiomas in children. Childs Nerv Syst 1989; 5(2):83–86.
58. Messori A, Rychlicki F, Salvolini U. Spinal epidural en-plaque meningioma with an unusual pattern of calcification in a 14-year-old girl: case report and review of the literature. Neuroradiology 2002; 44(3):256–260.
59. Di Rocco C, Iannelli A, Colosimo C, Jr. Spinal epidural meningiomas in childhood: a case report. J Neurosurg Sci 1994; 38(4):251–254.
60. Motomochi M, Makita Y, Nabeshima S, Aoyama I. Spinal epidural meningioma in childhood. Surg Neurol 1980; 13(1):5–7.
61. Calogero JA, Moossy J. Extradural spinal meningiomas. Report of four cases. J Neurosurg 1972; 37(4):442–447.
62. Yamamoto Y, Raffel C. Spinal extradural neoplasms and intradural extramedullary neoplasms. In: Albright AL, Pollack IF, Adelson PD, editors. Principles and Practice of Pediatric Neurosurgery. New York: Thieme, 1999: 685–696.

59
NF2/Multiple Meningiomas

Ralf M. Buhl, H. Maximilian Mehdorn, and Peter A. Winkler

Introduction

The term "multiple meningiomas" (MM) was first used by Cushing and Eisenhardt in 1938 to refer to a situation in which the patient had "more than one meningioma and less than a diffusion of them." It has to be separated from the multiple meningiomas that commonly occur in neurofibromatosis type 2 (NF2), an autosomal dominant disorder caused by inactivating mutations of the NF2 tumor suppressor gene. In this chapter, we will discuss both sporadic and NF2-associated MM.

Incidence

In 2000, Antinheimo et al. published a population-based analysis of sporadic and NF2-associated meningiomas and schwannomas in Finland (1). Approximately 1% (7/823) of the patients with meningioma had MM in association with NF2, and 4% (29/823) had MM without NF2, resulting in an overall incidence of 5% for all categories of MM.

With the advent of computed tomography (CT) and magnetic resonance imaging (MRI) scans, there has been an increasing incidence of MM, which is reported to be ranging from 5.9 to 10.5% of all meningioma cases (2–4). Domenicucci et al. reviewed 1308 histologically verified cases of intracranial meningiomas over 30 years and found 14 cases of MM, with the frequency of 0.58% before and 4.5% after the use of CT (5). An incidence of 16% was found in an autopsy series of 100 meningiomas by Wood et al. (6). Soffer et al. found a higher incidence of MM (and recurrences following surgery) in the group of patients with radiation-induced meningiomas (7). Interestingly a recent study in New Zealand showed a higher incidence of meningiomas in Polynesians, in whom meningiomas were detected at a younger age; these were more likely to be multiple and larger compared to Caucasians (8).

In the Department of Neurosurgery in Essen, Germany, we investigated the data of 714 patients with intracranial meningiomas between 1968 and 1988, and found the incidence of

MM to be 4.9% (35/714). The incidence rose after the advent of CT, from 2.5% before 1976 to 5.8% between 1977 and 1988. These patients also had no signs of NF2. Between 1991 and 2002 we found an incidence of 8.6% (39/456) in our current Department of Neurosurgery in Kiel, Germany.

Multiple Meningiomas: Truly Multiple?

Borovich et al. in 1988 raised a provocative question and published a paper called "The Incidence of Multiple Meningiomas— Do Solitary Meningiomas Exist?" (9). In their material, the incidence of MM at first assessment by CT was 20%, with distant multiplicity prevailing over the regional one. They stated that this incidence would probably change in the course of time as MM develop not only concurrently but also consecutively. On the other hand, their surgical macroscopic incidence of regional multiplicity alone was 49%. The discrepancy between the CT and surgical findings prompted them to reevaluate the CT studies of 100 consecutive patients. This reevaluation demonstrated: (1) in two cases, small meningiomas were overlooked at first assessment; and (2) 19 cases of solitary globoid meningiomas seemed to be the consequence of the coalescence of adjacent smaller masses. Thus, the CT incidence of MM increased to 40%, with regional multiplicity prevailing over the distant one.

The authors think that the aforesaid findings question the very existence of solitary meningiomas as a pathologic entity. Multiple meningiomas would then be the end product of a coalescence of multiple adjacent smaller growths. Accordingly, a more aggressive surgical approach is suggested to include the resection of a generous fringe of dura mater surrounding the main tumor. In a separate study, they also examined the dura mater around the tumor and at more distant parts in 14 patients with intracranial meningioma (10). In 64% they found macroscopic tumor nodules 1–3 cm distant from the tumor. They found even smaller nodules after microscopic examination. A radial strip of dura was removed from the line of attachment of globular meningiomas in 14 consecutive patients. Meningotheliomatous cell aggregates were demonstrated in 100% of these dural strips in the form of either intradural clusters or nodes protruding from the inner aspect of the dura. The benign appearance of the cells and the great prevalence in this study of the benign types of meningioma seemed to exclude malignancy. The intradural position of the clusters and their independence from blood vessels apparently negated seeding and dural metastasis. Control strips of convexity dura mater taken from 10 neurosurgical patients without meningioma failed to show these meningotheliomatous conglomerates. These findings indicate that solitary globular meningiomas represent only the most visible growth in the midst of a neoplastic field change spreading over a wide area of dura mater. They believed that this could explain some unexpected "recurrences," and that a wide resection of dura around globular meningiomas, whenever possible, could reduce the incidence of clinical recurrence after true total excision of the most visible lesion. Ekong et al. reported a female patient with a right sphenoid wing meningioma 16 years after a left convexity meningioma was removed (11). It remains to be determined what factors cause the acceleration of growth of meningothelial cell aggregates after removal of the dominant tumor.

Also, intracranial and spinal meningiomas can be seen in association. Harish et al. reported a 50-year-old woman who was operated on for an intracranial parietal meningioma and developed a spinal meningioma 22 years after the primary operation (12). Chaparro et al. presented a 32-year-old male patient with 47 multiple spinal meningiomas of identical histology (13). Intracranial lesions occurred 26 months following spinal surgery at the craniocervical junction and in the cerebellar hemisphere. There was no evidence of NF1 or NF2 in this patient.

Location

In our series, the main location of MM was cerebral or cerebellar convexity. This was similar to the review of Domenicucci et al., who reported that 45.5% of MM was located at the convexity, 30.5% located at parasagittal site or falx, and 21.2% located at the skull base (5). The high incidence of MM in the convexity can be explained by the hypothesis that MM are developed from the major meningioma as a spread through the subarachnoid space, following the pathway of the cerebrospinal fluid (CSF) circulation. Additionally, there were 6 MM involving the cerebrum and cerebellum concurrently in our series. In the other 33 cases with tumors located at the cerebral hemisphere, 9 patients demonstrated bilateral hemispheric meningiomas, 9 patients presented with midline and hemispheric locations, and only 15 cases involved one hemisphere. This distant and extensive distribution is adequately explained by the hypothesized dissemination of tumors through the CSF space. Nicola et al. presented two cases of MM in which the different tumors developed in widely separated locations in the supratentorial and spinal regions (14).

Histologic Subtype

Turgut et al. removed 28 meningiomas in 8 patients, of which 14 meningiomas were meningothelial (50%) (15). This predominance of meningothelial histologic subtype was supported by Domenicucci et al. (5). Neuss et al. reported that in their series fibroblastic and transitional tumors were more common (16). In a review by Sheehy and Crockard, there was a higher proportion than usual of the psammomatous type of tumors (17). This discrepancy may be caused by small population of MM in their series. Generally most MM are benign tumors; reports of atypical and anaplastic subtypes are rare. MM removed from the same patient usually show identical histopathologic features, but different histologic features of the tumors from the same patient are also found.

F:M Ratio

There is a higher ratio of females to males in patients with MM compared to those with solitary meningiomas. Domenicucci et al. reported 14 cases of MM, in which 13 were female and only one was male; Sheehy et al. presented 10 cases of MM, all of whom were females (5,17). In our series of 39 patients with MM, the female-to-male ratio was 35:4 (8.8:1).

Additional Features

MM have unique clinical features. Besides a high female preponderance, the patients have an earlier age of peak incidence and a higher recurrence rate than cases of solitary meningiomas. In our series there was a preferential location of convexity, and we also found the size to be smaller in MM compared to solitary ones (18). No difference was found in histology between MM and solitary meningiomas. Compared with solitary examples, we had the following results for the MM we examined. Psammomatous meningiomas were multiple in 33.3%. Additionally, secretory meningiomas were multiple in 31%, atypical meningiomas in 25%, and transitional meningiomas in 18.5%. In meningothelial and fibroblastic meningiomas, the rate of MM was found to be 13.5 and 13.4%, respectively.

We also investigated the expression of PR, p53, and MIB-1 LI in MM. PR expression was stronger in multiple than in solitary meningiomas while p53 status and MIB-1 LI were similar between the two groups. PR, p53 status, and MIB-1 LI were valuable marker for predicting patient's outcome in MM. Our own impression is that the incidence of MM is rising in patients with recurrent meningiomas.

Clinical Management

There is often a question as to whether to remove all lesions or only the symptomatic one. In general the symptomatic one should be removed whenever it is reasonable from the risk/benefit point of view. Asymptomatic ones or small lesions can be observed and followed with MRI once a year (19). Meningiomas with surrounding edema also should be removed. The decision is always individualized and should be discussed with the patient and the family. We have operated on a total of 39 patients with MM between 1991 and 2002. In 20 patients, only symptomatic tumors were removed, and in the remaining 19, all meningiomas were removed.

Case 1

We treated a 75-year-old female patient with a tumor of the right frontal convexity with severe edema and a second parasagittal meningioma. She did not give consent for surgery first and preferred MRI follow-up. After 2 years her symptoms worsened and the frontal meningioma with the edema was removed while the second one is still observed. Her symptoms improved markedly after surgery (Fig. 59-1).

Case 2

Different histologic subtypes are also possible in MM. Twelve of 19 patients showed the same histology, and 7 had different histologic subtypes. Two meningiomas of the right convexity in a 64-year-old female patient were

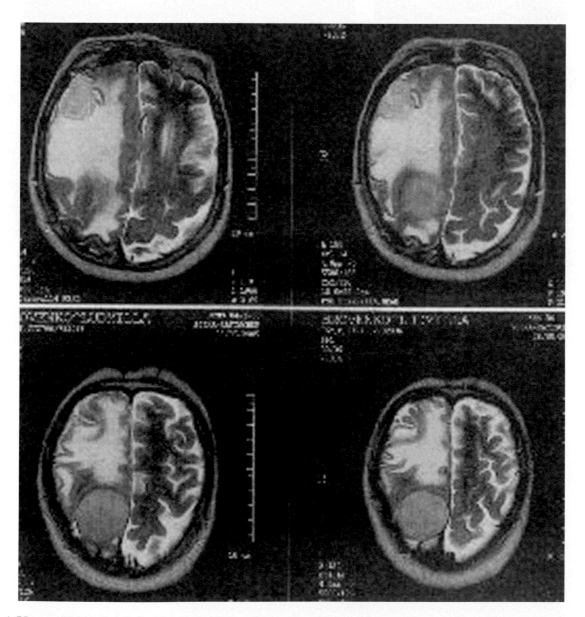

FIG. 59-1. A 75-year-old female patient with a tumor of the right frontal convexity with severe edema and a second parasagittal meningioma. She did not give consent for surgery first and preferred MRI follow-up. After 2 years her symptoms worsened and the frontal meningioma with the edema was removed while the second one is still observed. Her symptoms improved markedly after operation

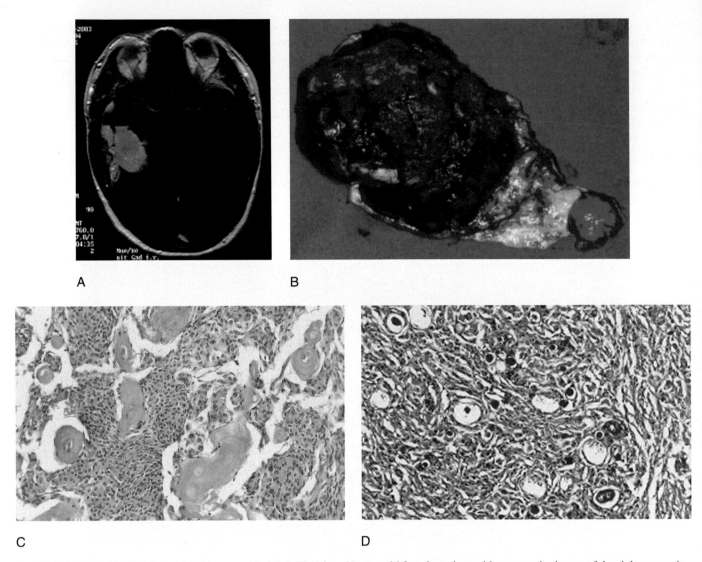

FIG. 59-2. (A) Axial MRI (T1-weighted image with Gd- DTPA) in a 64-year-old female patient with two meningiomas of the right convexity. They were removed together and the dura between the two nodules was examined. (B) Intraoperative picture of the specimen. No meningioma cell was found macroscopically and microscopically between the large meningothelial meningioma and the small secretory meningioma. (C) Histologic examination of the large meningothelial meningioma. (D) Histologic examination of the small secretory meningioma. Two different histologic subtypes were observed within one patient

removed together and the dura between the two nodules was examined. No meningioma cell was found between the large meningothelial meningioma and the small secretory meningioma (Fig. 59-2).

Case 3

A 45-year-old female patient with two frontal convexity meningiomas was operated. Histology showed a fibroblastic and meningothelial meningiomas (WHO grade I). Six years later there was a recurrent tumor in the left frontal convexity, which was atypical meningioma after histologic examination (WHO grade II). She also had a malignant melanoma. (Fig. 59-3). MR spectroscopy prior to the recurrent tumor operation showed a lactate peak as a possible

sign of necrosis in the atypical meningioma WHO grade II (Fig. 59-3C).

Case 4

Different growth potential of MM within the same patient can be observed. A 64-year-old female patient with a meningioma of the olfactory groove and falcine locations presented to our department. The patient did not give consent for operation, and MRI follow-up after one year showed enlargement of the skull base meningioma compared to stable size of the parasagittal meningioma. (Fig. 59-4).

Koh et al. presented a rare case of MM who presented with malignant and benign histologic features simultaneously (20). They found evidence for the monoclonal origin for both

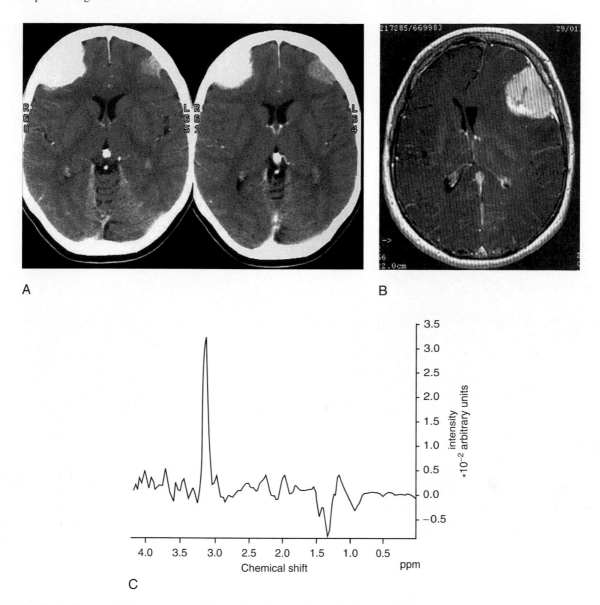

Fig. 59-3. (A) CT of a 45-year-old female patient with two frontal convexity meningiomas, which were removed. Histology showed a fibroblastic and a meningothelial meningioma (WHO grade I). (B) MRI in the same patient 7 years later with a recurrent tumor in the left frontal convexity, which was atypical meningioma after histologic examination (WHO grade II). She also had a malignant melanoma. (C) MR spectroscopy of the recurrent tumor showing a lactate peak suspicious for an atypical meningioma at 1.33 ppm and high choline and low creatine

tumors. However, in cases with different pathologic subtypes origin from multicentric neoplastic foci activated by a supposed tumor-producing factor was suggested. The possibility of independent progression from monoclonal origin, therefore, cannot be completely excluded.

Case 5

We also operated three times on a 54-year-old female patient with an atypical parasagittal meningioma who also

had a small meningioma of the left convexity, which was not removed and did not grow during follow-up of 6 years (Fig. 59-5).

Neurofibromatosis

NF 2 is defined as follows (21,22):

1. Bilateral vestibular schwannomas, or
2. Family history of NF2 (first-degree family relative) plus
   (a) unilateral vestibular schwannoma, at age <30 years,

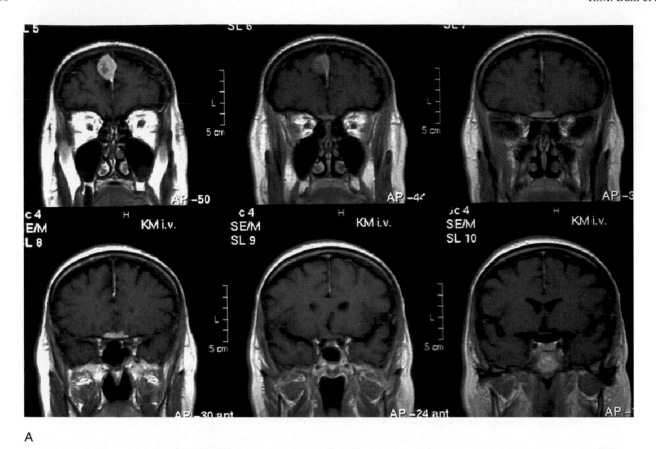

A

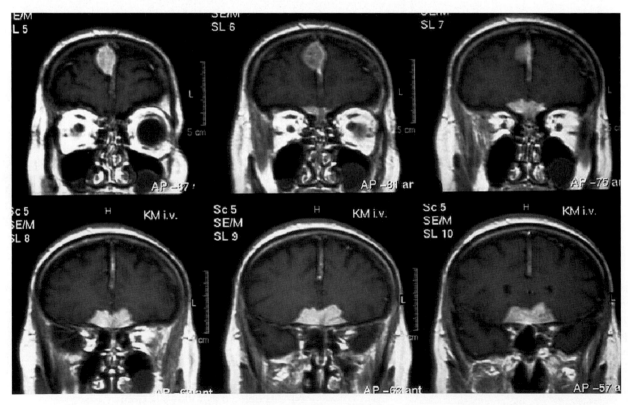

B

FIG. 59-4. (A, B) Example of different growth potential. A 67-year-old female patient with a meningioma of the olfactory groove and falcine locations. The patient did not give consent for operation, and MRI follow-up after one year showed enlargement of the skull base meningioma compared to the nearly unchanged parasagittal meningioma

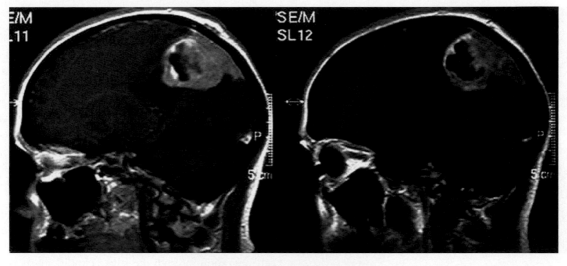

A

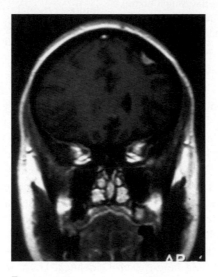

B

Fig. 59-5. A 54-year-old female patient with an atypical parasagittal meningioma (A) who was operated three times due to recurrent tumor growth and a small meningioma of the left convexity (B), which did not grow during 6 years of follow-up—an example of WHO grades I and II meningiomas within one patient

or (b) any two of the following: meningioma, glioma, schwannoma, or juvenile posterior subcapsular lenticular opacities/ juvenile cortical cataract.

Presumptive or probable NF 2 is suspected with the following features:

1. Unilateral vestibular schwannoma at age <30 years, plus at least one of the following: meningioma, glioma, schwannoma, or juvenile posterior subcapsular lenticular opacities/ juvenile cortical cataract.
2. Multiple meningiomas (two or more) plus (a) unilateral vestibular schwannoma, at age <30 years, or (b) one of the following: glioma, schwannoma, or juvenile subcapsular lenticular opacities/ juvenile cortical cataract.

Most reports of MM exclude the cases of NF2 (Fig. 59-6), but some reviews included cases associated with NF2 (17). NF is caused by dominant genes, which are mapped to the long arm of chromosome 17 in NF1 and chromosome 22 in NF2, respectively. The gene may be inherited from an affected parent, or it may occur by chance in an individual with no family history of NF as a result of a spontaneous gene mutation. NF1, so-called von Recklinghausen's disease, is the common form of NF, characterized by multiple café-au-lait spots and neurofibromas on or under the skin. NF2 is a rare type of NF, characterized by multiple tumors on the cranial and spinal nerves and by other lesions of the brain and spinal cord (24). Patients with NF2 are at a high risk for developing brain tumors, and almost all

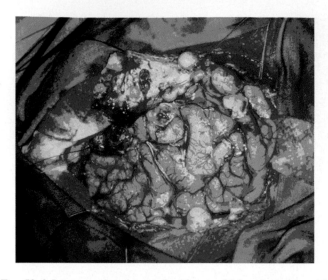

FIG. 59-6. Intraoperative picture of a 46-year-old female patient with NF2 and multiple fibroblastic meningiomas in the frontal convexity. She was also operated on an acoustic neuroma and had recurrent meningiomas 4 years after the primary operation

Pathogenesis of MM

There are different hypotheses concerning the etiology and pathogenesis of multiple intracranial meningiomas. Hereditary factors related to the etiology of MM are reported only in exceptional cases, especially in patients with meningiomatosis associated with neurofibromatosis. Most meningiomas are histologically benign so that spontaneous dissemination via the venous system is unlikely. Noncontiguous spread of a single tumor, presumably via the CSF space, may be the most common mechanism in patients with sporadic MM, which has strong female predominance (25,28,29).

In 1989, Butti et al. examined 8 MM out of a series of 148 meningiomas treated in a 13-year period (5.4%), and their results showed the different origins of each tumor and excluded cell migration through the subarachnoid space as a pathogenetic factor in MM (30). Another hypothesis, then, is that tumors originate from multicentric neoplastic foci and arise independently. Most of the MM are located in the same hemisphere, and distant meningiomas are relatively rare. Although most of the MM are histologically identical and benign, some cases show different histopathologic subtypes. Cytogenetic analysis suggested that nodules of MM from the same patient had different karyotypes. These phenomena suggest that the tumors develop independently and the dissemination through the subarachnoid space is probably not an etiologic factor.

The study of clonality in MM showed that meningiomas were of monoclonal origin. Stangl et al. investigated 39 tumors in 12 patients by single-strand conformation polymorphism analysis of the entire coding region of the NF2 gene and by direct DNA sequencing of altered fragments (25). They found in the majority of the patients with NF2 mutations that all tumors in the respective individual exhibited the identical DNA alterations in NF2 gene. This result provides strong evidence for a monoclonal origin of MM. Zhu et al. (1999) used six molecular genetic techniques to determine the clonality and genetic alterations in eight meningiomas from one patient (31). They demonstrated loss of the same copy of chromosome 22 and a common unmethylated allele at the AR locus in all eight tumors. They concluded that these MM were most likely monoclonal in origin. Larson et al. and von Deimling et al. expressed the same views in their reports that MM arose from a single progenitor cell, which could spread through the subarachnoid space (32,33). In our series, the multiple nodules in respective cases were usually of different sizes, and a large tumor was often associated with one or more small tumors. More than half of our cases had a widely separated locations of meningiomas. Additionally, more meningiomas were located in the convexity compared to solitary meningiomas. These observations suggest that dissemination via the subarachnoid space is a possible factor for the formation of these tumors. We thus favor the hypothesis that MM are most likely of monoclonal origin and spread through the subarachnoid space. We do not consider multicentricity of

affected individuals develop tumors on both vestibulocochlear nerves. NF can develop into meningiomatosis characterized by small neoplasms forming diffusely over the dura. Some authors considered that MM were a forme fruste of von Recklinghausen's disease. But Domenicucci et al. strongly believe that this theory was untenable in the absence of cutaneous stigmata, other associated tumors, and objective genetic or biochemical evidence (5). We support the latter view because the modern biochemical tests showed that no evidence of germline mutation was seen in patients with MM (25). Therefore, NF should be differentiated from MM according to the criteria provided by the National Neurofibromatosis Foundation (15). In a study by Evans DGR et al. in 2005, they found that about 8% of NF2 patients presented with a meningioma before a vestibular schwannomas. Constitutional NF2 mutations are the most likely cause of meningioma in children and in people with a meningioma plus other nonvestibular schwannoma features of NF2. Mosaic NF2 may be the cause of about 8% of MM in sporadic adult cases, but there are additional causes in the majority of other such patients and those with MM occurring in families (26).

Kros et al. reported that NF2 status of meningiomas is associated with tumor localization and histology (27). Mutations in the NF2 gene have been specifically reported in transitional and fibrous, but not in meningothelial meningiomas. A strong correlation between tumor localization in the anterior skull base and intact chromosome 22q was revealed. Heinrich et al. described that 5 of 7 patients had nontruncating NF2 mutations in blood–tumor pairs, but these mutations were not considered to be pathogenic (28).

meningiomas paradoxical to monoclonal origin of MM. The multiple foci under the dura could be disseminated from the major meningioma, and both may come from the same progenitor cell.

Meningiomas are known to enlarge during pregnancy and the luteal phase of the menstrual cycle when the level of progesterone is high. Our results demonstrated stronger PR expression and earlier age of peak incidence in MM than in solitary meningiomas. Taking account the high female predominance and the increased PR expression in MM, we speculate that the multiple lesions may originate from the primary meningioma with rich PR under the stimulation of progesterone. It is possible that a specific genetic alternation occurs in a precursor cell, giving it a selective growth advantage. Uncontrolled growth followed by the migration of daughter cells through the subarachnoid space via the CSF spread could lead to the formation of both regional and distant MM (32). Although the multiple foci originating from the same progenitor cell demonstrated identical mutation of the gene at first, the later independent progression could occur in the daughter cells, resulting in different histologic and karyotypic features in some MM.

In 1995 Larson et al. concluded that MM arise from the uncontrolled spread of a single progenitor cell (32). All examined tumors showed inactivation of the same X chromosome, suggesting that tumors arose from the same clone of cells ($p < 0.0005$). Clonal analysis of a case of MM was published by Zhu et al. (31). This case was most likely of monoclonal in origin. Loss of chromosome 22 was an early event during the development of MM and was followed by mutations at the NF2 locus. They admit that later events, including loss of the X chromosome, variation of AR gene expression, or microsatellite instability, may also have played a role in the development of MM in that patient. The only genes known to be associated with sporadic meningiomas are NF2 on chromosome 22 and the related cytoskeleton element DAL-1 on chromosome 18. The molecular basis of sporadic and familial MM is fundamentally different and extends this dichotomy to pathologic subtypes. DAL-1 does not function as a true tumor suppressor in these patients.

Eckstein et al. published a case of a male patient with parietal meningioma who developed MM in frontal and temporal lobes and finally developed multiple masses in the right lung (29). Despite multiple resections during a 17-year period, all tumors examined showed similar histology (atypical meningioma). Molecular analysis revealed that this patient's tumors shared identical truncating mutations in the NF2 gene, which were not seen in constitutional cells. The tumor DNA revealed a 2-bp frameshifting deletion involving exon 1 of the NF2 gene. The same genetic event was seen in all tumors examined. The second NF2 allele was lost in the tumors, consistent with the action of NF2 as a true tumor suppressor gene. Evans et al. clearly demonstrated that NF2 gene mutations and decreased NF2 protein expression rarely occurred in meningothelial meningiomas compared with other histologic types of meningiomas (34), adding evidence that NF2 mutation is an early step required in the pathogenesis of meningiomas

excluding the meningothelial subtype. The identical NF2 gene mutation was detected in MM from a single patient, suggesting that these tumors arise clonally and not as independent tumors from the same individual (31).

Inactivation of the tumor-suppressor gene might represent an early event in the development of MM. Lomas et al. performed cytogenetic and molecular genetic studies in a case of MM and demonstrated a loss of a copy of chromosome 22 and absence of NF2 gene mutations (35). The participation of a tumor-suppressor gene other than NF2 on chromosome 22 in the pathogenesis of a subgroup of multiple meningiomas is suggested. In a small subset of adult patients with MM, somatic NF2 mosaicism may play a role in tumorigenesis (26).

References

1. Antinheimo J, Sankila R, Carpen O, et al. Population-based analysis of sporadic and type 2 neurofibromatosis-associated meningiomas and schwannomas. Neurology 2000;54:71–76.
2. Federico F, D'Aprile P, Lorusso A, et al. Multiple meningiomas diagnosed by computed tomography. Ital J Neurol Sci 1984;5:295–298.
3. Lusins JO, Nakagawa H. Multiple meningiomas evaluated by computed tomography. Neurosurgery 1981;9:137–141.
4. Nahser HC, Grote W, Lohr E, Gerhard L. Multiple meningiomas. Clinical and computer tomographic observations. Neuroradiology 1981;21:259–263.
5. Domenicucci M, Santoro A, D'Osvaldo DH, et al. Multiple intracranial meningiomas. J Neurosurg 1989;70:41–44.
6. Wood NW, White RW, Kernohan JW. One hundred intracranial meningiomas found incidentally at necropsy. J Neuropathol Exp Neuro 1957;16:337–340.
7. Soffer D, Pittaluga S, Feiner M, Beller AJ. Intracranial meningiomas following low-dose irradiation to the head. J Neurosurg 1983;59:1048–1053.
8. Olson S, Law A. Meningiomas and the Polynesian population. ANZ J Surg 2005;75:705–709.
9. Borovich B, Doron Y, Braun J, et al. The incidence of multiple meningiomas- do solitary meningiomas exist? Acta Neurochir (Wien) 1988;90:15–22.
10. Borovich B, Doron Y. Recurrence of intracranial meningiomas: the role played by regional multicentricity. J Neurosurg 1986;64:58–63.
11. Ekong CE, Paine KW, Rozdilsky B. Multiple meningiomas. Surg Neurol 1978;9:181–184.
12. Harish Z, Schiffer J, Rapp A, Reif RM. Intracranial and spinal multiple meningioma appearing after an interval of 22 years. Neurochirurgia (Stuttg) 1985;28:25–27.
13. Chaparro MJ, Young RF, Smith M, et al. Multiple spinal meningiomas: a case of 47 distinct lesions in the absence of neurofibromatosis or identified chromosomal abnormality. Neurosurgery 1993;32:298–302.
14. Nicola N, Thal U. Multiple Meningeome in verschiedenen Etagen der zerebromedullaren Achse. Neurochirurgia 1983;26:120–124.
15. Turgut M, Palaoglu S, Ozcan OE, et al. Multiple meningiomas of the central nervous system without the stigmata of neurofibromatosis. Clinical and therapeutic study. Neurosurg Rev 1997;20:117–123.

16. Neuss M, Westphal M, Hansel M, Herrmann HD. Clinical and laboratory findings in patients with multiple meningiomas. Br J Neurosurg 1988;2:249–256.

17. Sheehy JP, Crockard HA. Multiple meningiomas: a long-term review. J Neurosurg 1983;59:1–5.

18. Huang H, Buhl R, Hugo HH, Mehdorn HM. Clinical and histological features of multiple meningiomas compared with solitary meningiomas. Neurol Res 2005;27:324–332.

19. Black PM. Meningiomas. Neurosurgery 1993;32:643–57.

20. Koh YC, Yoo H, Whang GC, et al. Multiple meningiomas of different pathological features: case report. J Clin Neurosci 2001;8(Suppl 1):40–43.

21. King A, Gutmann DH. The question of familial meningiomas and schwannomas: NF2B or not to be? Neurology 2000;54:4–5.

22. Neurofibromatosis Conference Statement. National Institutes of Health Consensus Development Conference. Arch Neurol 1988;45:575–578.

23. Cushing H, Eisenhardt L. Meningiomas: Their Classification, Regional Behavior, Life History, and Surgical End Results. Springfield, IL: Charles C Thomas, 1938.

24. Baser ME, Friedman JM, Wallace AJ, et al. Evaluation of clinical diagnostic criteria for neurofibromatosis 2. Neurology 2002;59:1759–1765.

25. Stangl AP, Wellenreuther R, Lenartz D, et al. Clonality of multiple meningiomas. J Neurosurg 1997;86:853–858.

26. Evans DGR, Watson C, Kong A, et al. Multiple meningiomas: differential involvement of the NF2 gene in children and adults. J Med Genet 2005;42:45–48.

27. Kros J, de Greve K, van Tilborg A, et al. NF2 status of meningiomas is associated with tumour localization and histology. J Pathol 2001;194:367–372.

28. Heinrich B, Hartmann C, Stemmer-Rachamimov AO, et al. Multiple meningiomas: Investigating the molecular basis of sporadic and familial forms. Int J Cancer 2003;103:483–488.

29. Eckstein O, Stemmer-Rachamimov A, Nunes F, et al. Multiple meningiomas in brain and lung due to acquired mutation of the NF2 gene. Neurology 2004;62:1904–1905.

30. Butti G, Assietti R, Casalone R, Paoletti P. Multiple meningiomas: a clinical, surgical, and cytogenetic analysis. Surg Neurol 1989;31:255–260.

31. Zhu JJ, Maruyama T, Jacoby LB, et al. Clonal analysis of a case of multiple meningiomas using multiple molecular genetic approaches: pathology case report. Neurosurgery 1999;45:409–416.

32. Larson JJ, Tew JM Jr, Simon M, Menon AG. Evidence for clonal spread in the development of multiple meningiomas. J Neurosurg 1995;83:705–709.

33. von Deimling A, Kraus JA, Stangl AP, et al. Evidence for subarachnoid spread in the development of multiple meningiomas. Brain Pathol 1995;5:11–14.

34. Evans JJ, Jeun SS, Lee JH, et al. Molecular alterations in the neurofibromatosis type 2 gene and its protein rarely occurring in meningothelial meningiomas. J Neurosurg 2001;94:111–117.

35. Lomas J, Bello MJ, Alonso ME, et al. Loss of chromosome 22 and absence of NF2 gene mutation in a a case of multiple meningiomas. Hum Pathol 2002;33:375–378.

60
Peritumoral Edema

Han Soo Chang

Introduction

Meningiomas, like other brain tumors, such as gliomas and metastatic tumors, are often associated with peritumoral brain edema (PTBE). The presence of PTBE can cause additional symptoms,[1] increase the intracranial pressure, and, being associated with adhesion to the brain, make surgical resection more difficult, thereby causing poorer prognosis to the patients.[2] The brain edema associated with gliomas has been extensively studied, and the obtained knowledge can be extended to that of meningiomas as well. However, meningiomas, unlike other intraparenchymal tumors, are located outside the brain parenchyma and separated from it by the arachnoid membrane and pia mater, which become the barrier to free movement of water, electrolytes, and proteins. This fact poses specific problems when we consider the pathophysiology of PTBE associated with meningiomas.

In the last decades, considerable efforts have been made to better understand the pathophysiology of this phenomenon. Beginning from the clinical studies that searched for possible factors that contribute to the occurrence of PTBE, we have recently made significant progress in this field, finding the important relationships among the three factors: pial blood supply, adhesion to the brain, and PTBE. In addition, recent publications of numerous studies indicate that the expression of vascular endothelial growth factor (VEGF) by the tumor is strongly related to the production of PTBE, opening a new perspective to the future research and new treatment modalities. In this chapter, we will review the pertinent literature in this field and try to provide a clear understanding of the current concept of the pathophysiology of PTBE.

Clinical Studies

According to the studies using computed tomography (CT) or magnetic resonance imaging (MRI), PTBE is seen in between 40 and 60 % of meningiomas.[3–8] Many reports studying clinical series of meningiomas attempted to find certain factors that positively correlated with the presence of PTBE, such as age, sex, size, histologic subtype, etc. We will briefly review the related articles below.

As to the age and sex, various studies unanimously reported no existence of such correlation.[1,4,9–11] There seems to be a certain degree of correlation between the size and PTBE.[9,10,12–15] Bitzer et al.[13] showed that incidence of edema was 20.7 % in tumors less than 10 ml, which rose to 92.3% in meningiomas larger than 10 ml. Ide et al..,[14] Lobato et al..,[9] and Salpietro et al.[15] also reported a statistically significant relationship between the size and PTBE. Yoshioka et al.[10] found in their multiple regression analysis tumor size to be one of the significant factors contributing to the occurrence of PTBE. This relationship may be interpreted by the fact that larger meningiomas are associated with more frequent occurrence of brain adhesion,[14,16] which, as shown later, has a strong relationship with the occurrence of PTBE.

Some studies reported the positive correlation between the short duration of symptoms and the presence of PTBE.[1,4] This suggested that rapidly growing meningiomas are more often associated with PTBE. There are also conflicting reports as to the correlation between PTBE and the occurrence of seizure.[4,17] Paucity of evidence precludes us from deciding whether these two relationships have been convincingly established.

As to the question of whether certain locations of meningiomas tend to produce higher frequency of PTBE, the evidence is also somewhat equivocal. Although a number of studies reported that certain locations of meningiomas were related to higher frequency of PTBE,[4 9,11–13] there are studies finding no such correlation.[18,19] Among the studies that showed specific locations having higher tendency to produce PTBE, the actual locations are not necessarily consistent.[4,9,11,12,14] In the series of 179 meningiomas reported by Bitzer et al.,[12] there was associated PTBE in none of the 11 suprasellar meningiomas. Gilbert et al.[20] and Ide et al.[14] also found that suprasellar meningiomas did not produce PTBE even when they become large. They speculated that, because of the abundance of arachnoid membranes in the suprasellar area, the meningiomas in that region have less tendency to breach the arachnoid and subsequently cause PTBE. On the other hand, there have been a number of reports suggesting that fronto-basal meningiomas are associated with a higher frequency of PTBE.[4,11,12] However, we must be cautious when interpreting the results of these studies because there may be some other colinear factors; for example, the frontobasal meningiomas may have had a tendency to be large before being diagnosed. If we were to find independent factors contributing to the occurrence of PTBE, multivariate analysis would be desirable.

In a similar fashion, the data concerning possible correlation between histologic subtypes and PTBE are not so consistent. While a few studies reported no correlation between histologic subtype and the occurrence of PTBE,[1,9,19] there are a number of studies reporting that meningotheliomatous meningiomas are more frequently associated with PTBE compared with fibrous meningiomas, with the transitional meningiomas lying in between.[7,11,12,14,18,21] Considering another line of evidence that meningotheliomatous meningiomas are associated with a higher frequency of VEGF expression,[21] it is probable that this relationship truly exists. As to the relationship of PTBE to the histologic grade, it does not seem to be strong. While some reports showed more frequent occurrence of PTBE in WHO grade II and III meningiomas compared with grade I,[12,13] another study did not confirm this result.[17] Similarly, while higher vascularity or cellularity showed significant correlation with the presence of PTBE[19] in one study, another study did not confirm this relationship.[20]

There is significant evidence that cystic meningiomas are associated with a higher occurrence of PTBE. Cushing and Eisenhardt noted that small cystic meningiomas could demonstrate a disproportionate increase in intracranial tension due to large amounts of edema.[22] The majority of cystic meningiomas were found in one report to be of meningotheliomatous subtype.[23] Lobato et al.[9] reported that meningiomas with heterogeneous enhancement were associated with a higher incidence of PTBE.[9] Bitzer et al. reported delayed enhancement of the cystic area as well as the area of peritumoral edema in meningiomas in a similar time-course, suggesting the presence of a common pathologic process in these two phenomena. Considering recent reports[24,25] showing the association of cystic meningiomas with a higher expression of VEGF, which has a strong relationship with PTBE, as we discuss later, it seems that this relationship between the formation of cysts and PTBE in meningiomas is well established.

Although sex hormone receptors are commonly expressed in meningiomas, it is not clear whether these receptors have any causal relationship with production of PTBE. Despite a study reporting a significant relationship between progesterone receptor expression in meningioma and the development of PTBE,[26] this finding was not confirmed by other studies.[1,27,28] This relationship therefore remains questionable.

It has been reported that positive expression of prostaglandin receptors demonstrated a significant correlation with PTBE.[29] There is also a report showing a positive relationship between expression of somatostatin receptors in

meningiomas and the occurrence of PTBE.[30] However, the exact role of these substances in the pathogenesis of PTBE is still to be determined.

The only study[10] that used multiple regression analysis in this topic showed four independent factors that contributed to the presence of PTBE, namely the pial blood supply, tumor size, vascular density, and VEGF positivity. Many recent studies confirmed a strong correlation between the presence of pial blood supply and PTBE as well as that between the positive tumor expression of VEGF and the presence of PTBE. We will review the recent studies concerning this subject after briefly discussing the various hypotheses attempting to explain the pathophysiology of PTBE.

Pathophysiology

Hypotheses

There have been several hypotheses to explain the pathophysiology of PTBE associated with meningiomas. Four main hypotheses found in the literature are discussed:[31]

1. Ischemia caused by mechanical compression
2. Venous stasis caused by compression on veins
3. Excretory-secretory phenomenon
4. Hydrodynamic process whereby extravasates from meningiomas appear in the surrounding brain

Compression of the surrounding brain and subsequent increase in the local pressure could cause ischemia in the brain tissue surrounding the tumor; quite reasonably, it could then produce vasogenic edema in the peritumoral area.[32] However, this idea was refuted by several pieces of evidence. An experimental study showed that, in the absence of significant intracranial hypertension, even severe degrees of vasogenic PTBE did not interfere with blood flow and flow regulation.[33] An MRI study using diffusion- and perfusion-weighted images also concluded that ischemic alterations can be regarded as secondary phenomena in the pathogenesis of meningioma-related PTBE.[34] Considering other evidence that increased permeability of vessels was restricted to tumor vessels, and not found in the vessels of the peritumoral edema,[33,35-38] it does not seem likely that ischemic process is a major factor in the pathophysiology of PTBE.

As to the hypothesis of venous stasis as a cause of PTBE,[32,39] a number of clinical studies showed that the occurrence of PTBE did not necessarily correlate with obstruction of major cortical veins or sinuses.[4,5,8,11,40,41] Thus, this mechanism also does not seem to play a major role in the pathogenesis of PTBE.

A few studies support the hypothesis that meningiomas secrete a specific edemogenic factor that is excreted to the peritumoral area. Philippon et al.[40] reported that all 12 meningiomas with significant edema showed secretory-excretory features in ultrastructural studies, whereas most (14/16) meningiomas with less edema showed negative or very light secretory features. Probst-Cousin et al.[36] showed that secretory histologic subtype meningiomas were commonly associated with extensive edema formation. On the contrary, Bradac et al.[5] did not find a distinct relationship between the electron microscopic finding of secretion and the development of peritumoral brain edema.

The hypotheses discussed above do not adequately and convincingly explain the possible mechanism of PTBE in meningiomas. On the other hand, a promising hypothesis has recently emerged, called the hydrodynamic theory; it assumes that extravasates from the leaky tumor vessels are transferred to the peritumoral area through a hydrodynamic process. We will discuss this hypothesis in the next section, starting from the classical description of the vasogenic brain edema.

Vasogenic Brain Edema

Klatzo's classical article[42] described the two types of brain edema: vasogenic and cytotoxic. Nearly 40 years after its introduction, this classification is still valid and prevailing. In vasogenic edema, increased permeability of capillaries cause exudation of plasma into the extracellular space of the lesion and the surrounding brain parenchyma.[35,42] Characteristically, this type of edema is prominent in the white matter and virtually absent in the gray matter.[35] The reason seems to be that the intricately woven cellular structures of the gray matter restricts the free movement of fluid in the extracellular space.[43] In contrast, in cytotoxic edema, the fluid is accumulated in the intracellular space, mainly of the glial cells, and does not exclude the gray matter.[42] These two patterns of edema can be differentiated by electron microscopic observations.

In experimental studies of PTBE involving intraparenchymal neoplasms, electron microscopic studies revealed typical characteristics of vasogenic edema in the tissue obtained from the area of peritumoral edema.[20,40] However, ultrastructural features of the capillary endothelial cells in the edema tissue lacked the fenestrated appearance, which is a structural correlate of increased permeability, whereas those in the tumor showed the typical fenestrated appearance. This finding suggests that edema fluid is generated by the increased permeability in the tumor vessels and propagated to the peritumoral area, while the vessels in the edema tissue do not participate in this process. Several experimental studies supported this hypothesis and confirmed that increased permeability was seen only in the tumor vessels, and not in the vessels of the edema tissue.[31,33,35,37,38]

There is additional supporting evidence to the notion that the type of edema that occurs in PTBE is that of vasogenic edema. A direct analysis of edema fluid isolated from experimental cold-induced brain edema, which is known to produce vasogenic edema, suggested its origin as the blood plasma.[43] Radiologic findings of the peritumoral edema also supported the characteristics of vasogenic edema with its typical exclusion of gray matters and preponderance in the white matter.[4]

Based on these findings, Lindley et al.[41] proposed three prerequisites of vasogenic brain edema: (1) intact vascular bed, (2) compromise of the blood-brain barrier, and (3) tumor-to-brain pressure gradient.

Hydrodynamic Theory

In 1988, Go et al.[18] proposed a hypothesis that, similar to PTBE in gliomas, plasma exudates from tumor vessels in meningioma spread into the peritumoral area by the hydrostatic pressure between the tumor and the surrounding brain. This hypothesis was strongly supported by the study of Bitzer et al.,[31] in which they studied the slow process of contrast enhancement of the peritumoral edema in MRI after injection of gadolinium. The time-course of this process was delayed compared with that of the enhancement of the tumor itself. In the phase where the enhancement of the tumor tissue gradually decreased in time, that in the peritumoral brain parenchyma and the cystic area gradually increased. This fact suggested that this delayed enhancement was not caused by disruption of the blood-brain barrier in the peritumoral area, but caused by the spread of contrast material that had leaked from tumor vessels to the surrounding area. Furthermore, because the speed of this spread correlated with the size of the edema, they claim that this process is not a simple diffusion, but a process caused by the presence of pressure gradient within the edema.

Further support of this hypothesis comes from several studies showing a close relationship among the following three factors: the presence of pial blood supply, the presence of brain-tumor adhesion, and the occurrence of PTBE. A number of authors[10,11,13,44] showed a strong correlation between the presence of pial blood supply and the occurrence of PTBE. Furthermore, the location of the pial blood supply seemed to coincide with the location of PTBE.[10] Atkinson et al.[45] showed an impressive case report of a falx meningioma, in which only one side of the hemisphere showed the presence of pial blood supply, and only that side showed marked PTBE. Other reports also noted this spatial relationship.[2,13,46] Additionally, many studies showed the positive correlation between the tumor adhesion to the brain and the occurrence of PTBE.[12,14,15,18,34] And finally, closing the ring, a number of reports showed a significant coexistence of brain adhesion and pial blood supply.[46,47] Arachnoid membrane is impermeable to water; the pia mater shows high permeability to water and electrolytes, but is far less permeable to macromolecules such as proteins;[18] both arachnoid and the pia compose part of the blood-brain barrier. The studies mentioned above strongly support the idea that the brain-to-tumor adhesion with resistant loss of the normal integrity of arachnoid and pia mater produces an environment through which free movement of fluid, proteins, and electrolytes becomes possible. Therefore, we arrive at an attractive theory of pathophysiology, which may apply to the PTBE in meningiomas and intraparenchymal tumors such as gliomas. If we assume a portion on the brain/meningioma interface to be disrupted, we can assume that plasma exudates that leaked through the vessels with enhanced permeability in meningiomas can now spread into the brain parenchyma of the peritumoral area propelled by the hydrodynamic gradient between the tumor and the surrounding brain. It seems that the pial blood supply is closely associated with brain-tumor adhesion. Whether the pial blood supply is the major reason for the occurrence of tumor-brain adhesion, is just a coincidence, or is caused as a result of the disruption of arachnoid and pia is not known. However, there seems to be an important element with a major role in meningioma growth and the development of pial blood supply. We will review the recent reports on the VEGF and its relationship to the formation of PTBE in meningiomas.

Vascular Endothelial Growth Factor

In 1983, Senger et al.[48] discovered a substance from the tumor ascites fluid that possessed a strong potency to increase the vascular permeability and named this substance vascular permeability factor (VPF). This substance was purified[48] and was later found to be a glycoprotein with a molecular weight of 45,000 daltons.[49, 50] VPF was about 10,000–50,000 times more potent than histamine in increasing vascular permeability when tested in guinea pig skin.[51] Later studies showed that VPF was secreted by a number of human tumor cells.[25,52] Independent of this discovery, a growth factor that belonged to the family of platelet-derived growth factor (PDGF) was isolated from pituitary-derived folliculostellate cells and was found to have high potency of inducing growth of endothelial cells,[53–55] thus being named VEGF. These two factors were later found to be identical[50] and to possess the ability both to increase the vascular permeability and to cause the growth of endothelial cells. VEGF is known to be about 60% homologous to PDGF.[53] VEGF/VPF has four isoforms, of which the two smallest (VEGF$_{121}$ and VEGF$_{165}$) are highly secreted.[56] Two receptors of VEGF have been found in mice—Flt-1 and Flk-1—while the human counterpart of the latter is known as KDR.[56] These two receptors are primarily expressed on vascular endothelial cells. The finding of embryologically lethal vascular abnormalities observed in knockout mice lacking Flt-1 and Flk-1 suggested the importance of VEGF/VPF in development of vascular tissues.[56] Recent experiments showed that topical administration of VEGF/VPF transformed the continuous endothelium into fenestrated endothelium in both venules and capillaries.[57,58] This seems to be the mechanism of VEGF/ VPF in producing increased vascular permeability.[54]

The role of VEGF in the angiogenesis and formation of PTBE in gliomas as well as metastatic tumors has been extensively studied. It was found that VEGF expression was related to the formation of brain edema and tumor-associated cysts in human gliomas and also the formation of PTBE in metastatic tumors.[59] VEGF messenger RNA is up to 50-fold overexpressed in glioblastomas compared to that of normal brain tissue.[60] Thus, it is believed that the progression of a low-grade astrocytoma to a highly vascularized glioblastoma multiforme

is associated with increased VEGF messenger RNA production.[56] This finding is consistent with a paracrine role of VEGF in astrocytoma angiogenesis, with the highly secreted VEGF being made by astrocytoma cells stimulating proliferation of tumor-associated vascular endothelial cells.

The role of VEGF in vascular proliferation in meningiomas has been studied. Although not as striking as in the case of gliomas, VEGF also seems to play a significant role in vascular proliferation in meningiomas. Provias et al.[56] and Pistolesi et al.[44] found a significant relationship between the expression of VEGF and tumor microvascular density, while this finding was not confirmed in another study.[61] Although not statistically significant, Lamszus et al.[61] found that there was a definite tendency toward increased expression of VEGF in higher grade meningiomas: approximately a twofold increase in atypical meningiomas and a 10-fold increase in anaplastic meningiomas compared with benign ones.

In addition, recent reports show a strong positive relationship between the expression of VEGF and the occurrence of PTBE. After Kalkanis et al.'s report[53] in 1996 showing a significant relationship between VEGF expression and PTBE, numerous reports confirmed this result[10,21,44,56,62] using various methods such as histochemistry, detection of mRNA, direct measurement of VEGF concentration, etc. Accordingly, VEGF expression seems to be the strongest factor correlated to the presence of PTBE in meningiomas among other factors described in the previous section.

Combining these results, we are tempted to hypothesize that a higher expression of VEGF in meningiomas induces additional blood supply from the cortical surface, thereby causing the disruption of the blood-brain barrier made up partly by the arachnoid and pia; this finally facilitates the free movement of water, electrolytes, and macromolecules between the tumor and the brain, and the hydrodynamic gradient between them expels the exudates from the tumor vessels, which already have an enhanced permeability caused also by VEGF, into the peritumoral area. Although it may not be the sole cause, VEGF probably plays a critical role in the pathogenesis of PTBE in meningiomas. Additional studies in this field are needed to further validate this hypothesis.

Effect of Steroid

Glucocorticoids have long been known to be effective in suppressing the PTBE both in intraparenchymal tumors such as gliomas or metastatic tumors and in extraparenchymal tumors such as meningiomas. However, the exact pathophysiologic mechanism of its effect has not been well understood in the past. With the emerging knowledge of the expression of VEGF and its roles in brain tumors, we may now begin to better understand its exact mechanism. In 1988, Criscuolo[63] et al. showed that dexamethasone inhibited the activity of VPF in dose-dependent fashion, and this effect was mediated through induction of de novo protein synthesis. Ito et al.[64] found that steroid inhibited the process of the slow spread of contrast material from the meningioma to the peritumoral area described earlier. Experimentally, dexamethasone was shown to block the VEGF-induced calcium transients in endothelial cells.[21] These studies suggest that the steroid exerts its effect on PTBE through suppressing the VEGF-related permeability increase in tumor vessels.

Clinical Implications

There are several possible ways in which the presence of PTBE in meningiomas can influence the actual outcome of the patients. First, the frequent absence of good arachnoid plane between the tumor and the brain may reduce the radicality of tumor resection. Second, related to the first point, forceful resection in the absence of the arachnoid plane may worsen the surgical outcome, especially in the eloquent brain regions. Third, the presence of PTBE may be related to an increased rate of recurrence. This could be partly caused by the reduced radicality of surgery, but the presence of PTBE could be a factor independent of that fact. We will briefly review the current literature concerning these points.

As to whether the presence of PTBE is related to reduced radicality of resection, Carvalho et al.[65] reported 70 petroclival meningiomas in which they found that infiltrative tumor margin and the presence of PTBE negatively affected the radicality. We can naturally deduce that, especially in the cases where dissection from an eloquent area such as the brain stem is required, the presence of PTBE and its associated brain adhesion will influence the radicality of surgery. As to the second point of the possible influence of PTBE on the surgical outcome, some reports suggest that it negatively affects the surgical outcome. Sindou et al.[2] reported in their subseries of 34 meningiomas located in the eloquent areas of the brain that there were significantly higher postoperative deficits in the cases where the dissection could not be easily done in the arachnoid plane, and this difficulty in dissection was related to the presence of PTBE. Pamir et al.[66] reported that in 42 tuberculum sellae meningiomas, the presence of PTBE was significantly related to worse visual outcome. Finally, on the point that the presence of PTBE may increase the recurrence rate, we would mention two articles. Mantle et al.[67] reported the results of logistic regression analysis on 135 consecutive cases of meningiomas, where they found that the strongest predicting factors for recurrence was (1) complete resection, (2) edema grade, and (3) brain invasion. Yamasaki et al.[68] retrospectively studied a series of 54 convexity meningiomas with Simpson grade I resection, and found that high levels of expression of VEGF constituted the most useful predictor of outcome, which was more reliable than the MIB-I labeling index. The results of these two studies suggest that the presence of PTBE, and the underlying high expression of VEGF, may be an index of strong viability of the residual tumor cells and may affect the recurrence rate independent of the radicality of the surgery.

Future Prospects

The recent progress of molecular biology and its application to brain tumors have opened a new perspective in the understanding of various phenomena related to tumor growth and also to the possible development of newer treatment modalities. Several experimental studies attempted to inhibit the VEGF-mediated tumor angiogenesis using various techniques,[69–73] with promising results. In the treatment of meningiomas, a number of compounds with anti-VEGF or anti-PDGF properties are now being investigated.[74] Two EGF receptor antagonists, Tarceva (OSI774) and Erlotinib (ZD1839), are now undergoing phase I trial by the North American Brain Tumor Consortium.[74] Although it is still too early to judge, in the near future these compounds may be found to be effective in inhibiting the growth and angiogenesis of meningiomas as well as the development of PTBE.

Conclusion

Unlike intraparenchymal neoplasms, meningiomas are separated from the brain parenchyma by the arachnoid and pia, which prevent the free movement of water, electrolytes, and macromolecules. However, recent studies showed strong relationships among the three factors—the presence of pial blood supply, brain tumor adhesion, and development of PTBE—suggesting that the disruption of the arachnoid and pia produces an environment through which free movement of extracellular fluid becomes possible, thereby enabling the plasma exudates from the highly permeable tumor vessels to be transferred to the peritumoral area by the hydrostatic pressure gradient between the tumor and the surrounding brain. In addition, recent accumulation of evidence shows that VEGF, which both increases the permeability of tumor vessels and induces vascular growth, is deeply involved in the pathologic process of PTBE. Results of these studies enable us to uniformly understand the pathophysiology of PTBE both in intraparenchymal neoplasms and in extraparenchymal neoplasms such as meningiomas. We expect that future studies will elucidate the pathophysiology of PTBE more clearly, possibly enabling the development of new treatment modalities addressing this interesting pathology.

References

1. Maiuri F, Gangemi M, Cirillo S, et al.: Cerebral oedema associated with meningiomas. Surg Neurol 1987;27: 64–68.
2. Sindou M, Alaywan M: Role of pia-mater vascularization of the tumour in the surgical outcome of intracranial meningiomas. Acta Neurochir 1994;130: 90–93.
3. New PFJ, Aronow S, Hesselink JR: National Cancer Institute study: evaluation of computed tomography in the diagnosis of intracranial neoplasms. IV. Meningiomas. Radiology 1980;136: 665–675.

4. Stevens JM, Ruiz JS, Kendall BE: Observations on peritumoural oedema in meningioma: Part II. Mechanisms of oedema production. Neuroradiology 1983;25: 125–131.

5. Bradac GB, Ferszt R, Bender A, Schorner W: Peritumoral edema in meningiomas. A radiological and histological study. Neuroradiology 1986;28: 304–312.

6. Sigel RM, Messina AV: Computed tomography: the anatomic basis of the zone of diminished density surrounding meningiomas. AJR 1976;127: 139–141.

7. Abe T, Black PM, Ojemann RG, Hedley WE: Cerebral edema in intracranial meningiomas: evidence for local and diffuse patterns and factors asociated with its occurrence. Surg Neurol 1994;42: 471–475.

8. Bitzer M, Topka H, Morgalla M, et al.: Tumor-related venous obstruction and development of peritumoral edema in meningiomas. Neurosurgery 1998;42: 730–737.

9. Lobato RD, Alday R, Gomez PA, et al.: Brain oedema in patients with intracranial meningioma. Correlation between clinical, radiological and histological factors and the presence and intensity of oedema. Acta Neurochir 1996;138: 485–493.

10. Yoshioka H, Hama S, Taniguchi E, et al.: Peritumoral brain edema associated with meningioma. Influence of vascular endothelial growth factor expression and vascular blood supply. Cancer 1999;85: 936–944.

11. Inamura T, Nishio S, Takeshita I, et al.: Peritumoral brain edema in meningiomas—influence of vascular supply on its development. Neurosurgery 1992;31: 179–185.

12. Bitzer M, Wöckel L, Morgalla M, et al.: Peritumoural brain oedema in intracranial meningiomas: influence of tumour size, location and histology. Acta Neurochir 1997;139: 1136–1142.

13. Bitzer M, Wöckel L, Luft AR, et al.: The importance of pial blood supply to the development of peritumoral brain edema in meningiomas. J Neurosurg 1997;87: 368–373.

14. Ide M, Jimbo M, Kubo O, et al.: Peritumoral brain edema and cortical damage by meningioma. Acta Neurochir Suppl 1994;60: 369–372.

15. Salpietro FM, Alafaci C, Lucerna S, et al.: Peritumoral edema in meningiomas: microsurgical observations of different brain tumor interfaces related to computed tomography. Neurosurgery 1994;35: 638–642.

16. Alvernia JE, Sindou MP: Preoperative neuroimaging findings as a predictor of the surgical plane of cleavage: prospective study of 100 consecutive cases of intracranial meningioma. J Neurosurg 2004;100: 422–430.

17. De Vries J, Wakhloo AK: Cerebral oedema associated with WHO-I, WHO-II, and WHO-III meningiomas: correlation of clinical, computed tomographic, operative and histological findings. Acta Neurochir 1993;125: 34–40.

18. Go KG, Wilmink JT, Molenaar WM: Peritumoral brain edema associated with meningiomas. Neurosurgery 1988;23: 175–179.

19. Smith HP, Challa VR, Moody DM, Kelly DL Jr: Biological features of meningiomas that determine the production of cerebral edema. Neurosurgery 1981;8: 428–433.

20. Gilbert JJ, Paulseth JE, Coates RK, Malott D: Cerebral edema associated with meningiomas. Neurosurgery 1983;12: 599–605.

21. Goldman CK, Bharara S, Palmer CA, et al.: Brain edema in meningiomas is associated with increased vascular endothelial growth factor expression. Neurosurgery 1997;40: 1269–1277.

22. Cushing H, Eisenhardt L: In: Meningiomas. Springfield, IL: Charles C Thomas, 1938.

23. Zee CS, Chen T, Hinton DR, et al.: Magnetic resonance imaging of cystic meningiomas and its surgical implications. Neurosurgery 1995;36: 482–488.

24. Christov C, Lechapt-Zalcman E, Adle-Biassette H, et al.: Vascular permeability factor/vacular endothelial growth factor (VPF/VEGF) and its receptor flt-1 in microcystic meningiomas. Acta Neuropathol 1999;98: 414–420.

25. Stockhammer G, Obwegeser A, Kostron H, et al.: Vascular endothelial growth factor (VEGF) is elevated in brain tumor cysts and correlates with tumor progression. Acta Neuropathol 2000;100: 101–105.

26. Benzel EC, Gelder FB: Correlation between sex hormone binding and peritumoral edema in intracranial meningiomas. Neurosurgery 1988;23: 169–174.

27. Brandis A, Mirzai S, Tatagiba M, et al.: Immunohistochemical detection of female sex hormone receptors in meningiomas: correlation with clinical and histological features. Neurosurgery 1993;33: 212–218.

28. Meixensberger J, Caffier H, Naumann M, Hofmann E: Sex hormone binding and peritumoural oedema in meningiomas: is there a correlation? Acta Neurochir 1992;115: 98–102.

29. Constantini S, Tamir J, Gomori MJ, Shohami E: Tumour prostaglandin levels correlate with oedema around supratentorial meningiomas. Neurosurgery 1993;33: 204–211.

30. Pistolesi S, Fontanini G, Boldrini L, et al.: The role of somatostatin in vasogenic meningioma associated with brain edema. Tumori 2003;89: 136–140.

31. Bitzer M, Nägele T, Geist-Barth B, et al.: Role of hydrodynamic processes in the pathogenesis of peritumoral brain edema in meningiomas. J Neurosurg 2000;93: 594–604.

32. Hiyama H, Kubo O, Tajika Y, et al.: Meningiomas associated with peritumoural venous stasis: three types on cerebral angiogram. Acta Neurochir 1994;129: 31–38.

33. Hossmann KA, Blöink M: Blood flow and regulation of blood flow in experimental peritumoral edema. Stroke 1981;12: 211–217.

34. Bitzer M, Klose U, Geist-Barth B, et al.: Alterations in diffusion and perfusion in the pathogenesis of peritumoral brain edema in meningiomas. Eur Radiol 2002;12: 2062–2076.

35. Hossmann KA, Wechsler W, Wilmes F: Experimental peritumorous edema. Morphological and pathophysiological observations. Acta Neuropathol 1979;45: 195–203.

36. Probst-Cousin S, Villagran-Lillo R, Lahl R, et al.: Secretory meningioma: clinical, histologic, and immunohistochemical findings in 31 cases. Cancer 1997;79: 2003–2015.

37. Yamada K, Hayakawa T, Ushio Y, et al.: Regional blood flow and capillary permeability in the ethylnitrosourea-induced rat glioma. J Neurosurg 1981;55: 922–928.

38. Hossmann KA, Bloink M, Wilmes F, Wechsler W: Experimental peritumoral edema of the cat brain. Adv Neurol 1980;28: 323–340.

39. Fine M, Brazis P, Palacios E, Neri G: Computed tomography of sphenoid wing meningioma: tumor location related to distal edema. Surg Neurol 1980;13: 385–390.

40. Philippon J, Foncin JF, Grob R, et al.: Cerebral edema associated with meningiomas: possible role of a secretory-excretory phenomenon. Neurosurgery 1984;14: 295–301.

41. Lindley JG, Challa VR, Kelly DL, Jr.: Meningiomas and brain edema. In: Al-Mefty O, ed. Meningiomas. New York: Raven Press, 1991:59–73.

42. Klatzo I: Neuropathological aspects of brain edema. J Neuropathol Exp Neurol 1967;26: 1–14.

43. Gazendam J, Go KG, van Zante AK: Composition of isolated edema fluid in cold-induced brain edema. J Neurosurg 1979;51: 70–77.

44. Pistolesi S, Fontanini G, Camacci T, et al.: Meningioma-associated brain oedema: the role of angiogenic factors and pial blood supply. J Neurooncol 2002;60: 159–164.

45. Atkinson JL, Lane JI: Frontal sagittal meningioma: tumor parasitization of cortical vasculature as the etiology of peritumoral edema. J Neurosurg 1994;81: 924–926.

46. Takeguchi T, Miki H, Shimizu T, et al.: Prediction of tumor-brain adhesion in intracranial meningiomas by MR imaging and DSA. Magn Reson Med Sci 2003;2: 171–179.

47. Sindou MP, Alaywan M: Most intracranial meningiomas are not cleavable tumors: anatomic-surgical evidence and angiographic predictability. Neurosurgery 1998;42: 476–480.

48. Senger DR, Galli SJ, Dvorak AM, et al.: Tumor cells secrete a vascular permeability factor that promotes accumulation of ascites fluid. Science 1983;219: 983–985.

49. Connolly DT: Vascular permeability factor: a unique regulator of blood vessel function. J Cell Biochem 1991;47: 219–223.

50. Connolly DT, Heuvelman DM, Nelson R, et al.: Tumor vascular permeability factor stimulates endothelial cell growth and angiogenesis. J Clin Invest 1989;84: 1470–1478.

51. Ferrara N, Houck K, Jakeman L, Leung D: Molecular and biological properties of the vascular endothelial growth factor family of proteins. Endocr Rev 1992;13: 18–32.

52. Senger DT, Perruzzi CA, Feder J, Dvorak HF: A highly conserved vascular permeability factor secreted by a variety of human and rodent tumor cell lines. Cancer Res 1986;46: 5629–5632.

53. Kalkanis SN, Carroll RS, Zang J, et al.: Correlation of vascular endothelial growth factor messenger RNA expression with peritumoral vasogenic cerebral edema in meningiomas. J Neurosurg 1996;85: 1095–1101.

54. Machein MR, Plate KH: VEGF in brain tumors. J Neuro-Oncol 2000;50: 109–120.

55. Gospodarowicz D, Abraham JA, Schilling J: Isolation and characterization of a vascular endothelial cell mitogen produced by pituitary-derived folliculostellate cells. Proc Natl Acad Sci USA 1989;86: 7311–7315.

56. Provias J, Claffey K, delAguila L, et al.: Maningiomas: role of vascular endothelial growth factor/vascular permeability factor in angiogenesis and peritumoral edema. Neurosurgery 1997;40: 1016–1026.

57. Roberts WG, Palade GE: Increased microvascular permeability and endothelial fenestration induced by vascular endothelial growth factor. J Cell Science 1995;108: 2369–2379.

58. Roberts WG, Palade GE: Neovasculature induced by vascular endothelial growth factor is fenestrated. Cancer Res 1997;57: 765–772.

59. Strugar JG, Criscuolo GR, Rothbart D, Harrington WN: Vascular endothelial growth/permeability factor expression in human glioma specimens: correlation with vasogenic brain edema and tumor-associated cysts. J Neurosurg 1995;83: 682–689.

60. Plate KH, Breier G, Weich HA, Risau W: Vascular endothelial growth factor is a potential tumour angiogenesis factor in human gliomas in vivo. Nature 1992;359: 845–847.

61. Lamszus K, Lengler U, Schmidt NO, et al.: Vascular endothelial growth factor, hepatocyte growth factor/scatter factor, basic fibroblast growth factor, and placenta growth factor in human meningiomas and their relation to angiogenesis and malignancy. Neurosurgery 2000;46: 938–947.

62. Otsuka S, Tamiya T, Ono Y, et al.: The relationship between peritumoral brain edema and the expression of vascular endothelial growth factor and its receptors in intracranial meningiomas. J NeuroOncol 2004;70: 349–357.

63. Criscuolo G, Merrill M, Oldfield E: Further characterization of malignant glioma-derived vascular permeability factor. J Neurosurg 1988;69: 254–262.

64. Ito U, Tomita H, Tone O, et al.: Peritumoral edema in meningioma: a contrast enhanced CT study. Acta Neurochir Suppl 1994;60: 361–364.

65. Carvalho GA, Matthies C, Tatagiba M, Eghbal R, Samii M: Impact of computed tomographic and magnetic resonance imaging findings on surgical outcome in petroclival meningiomas. Neurosurgery 2000; 47: 1287–1295.

66. Pamir MN, Özduman K, Belirgen M, Kilic T, Özek: Outcome determinants of pterional surgery for tuberculum sellae meningiomas. Acta Neurochir 2005;147: 1121–1130.

67. Mantle RE, Lach B, Delgado MR, Baeesa S, Belanger G: Predicting the probability of meningioma recurrence based on the quantity of peritumoral brain edema on computerized tomography scanning. J Neurosurg 1999;91: 375–383.

68. Yamasaki F, Yoshioka H, Hama S, Sugiyama K, Arita K, Kurisu K: Recurrence of meningiomas. Cancer 2000;89: 1102–1110.

69. Kim KJ, Li B, Winer J, et al.: Inhibition of vascular endothelial growth factor-induced angiogenesis supresses tumor growth in vivo. Nature 1993;362: 841–844.

70. Saleh M, Stacker SA, Wilks AF: Inhibition of growth of C6 glioma cells in vivo by expression of antisense vascular endothelial growth factor sequence. Cancer Res 1996;393: 393–401.

71. Millauer B, Shawver LK, Plate KH, et al.: Glioblastoma growth inhibited in vivo by a dominant-negative Flk-1 mutant. Nature 1994;367: 576–579.

72. Machein MR, Risau W, Plate KH: Anti-angiogenic gene therapy in rat glioma model using a dominant-negative vascular endothelial growth factor receptor 2. Hum Gene Ther 1999;10: 1117–1128.

73. Lin P, Sankar S, Shan S, et al.: Inhibition of tumor growth by targeting endothelium using a soluble vascular endothelial growth factor receptor. Cell Growth Differ 1998;9: 49–58.

74. Modha A, Gutin PH: Diagnosis and treatment of atyical and anaplastic meningiomas: a review. Neurosurgery 2005;57: 538–550.

61
Primary Ectopic Meningiomas

Sarah E. Gibson and Richard A. Prayson

Introduction

The first reported case of an extradural meningioma was published in 1730 by Johann Salzmann, a professor of anatomy and pathological anatomy in Strassburg, Germany [1]. Salzmann described both the natural history and pathologic anatomy of an untreated extradural meningioma, most likely arising from the calvarium. Since this first description, extradural meningiomas have been reported to occur in a variety of locations including the calvarium [2–6], orbit [7–12], middle ear [13–26], paranasal sinuses [8,27–40], nasopharynx [21,28,35,41,42], neck [43–45], skin [46–60], lung [61–80], mediastinum [73,81], adrenal gland [82], paraspinal region [55], peripheral nerves [83,84], and retroperitoneum [85]. Although as many as 20% of intracranial meningiomas may extend to involve the extradural space [86], either by direct extension or metastasis, primary extradural meningiomas are a far more rare entity.

In several large series reported in the United States, primary extradural meningiomas account for less than 2% of all meningiomas [21,86–90]. Another large series from Thailand reports that 8% of meningiomas are primary extradural lesions [91]. However, the definition of what is meant by "extradural" is quite variable in the published literature, with some authors including primary intracranial tumors that have extended extracranially by direct extension or by distant metastasis [13,21,92–94]. Although some reports state that extradural meningiomas should have no connection to any intracranial structures [44], other authors include tumors with intracranial growth [4,25,31,34,43,95–97]. In addition, these lesions have been referred to inconsistently in the literature as ectopic [41,45,98–100], extracranial [21,31,44,87,88,95, 97,101], extraneuraxial [102], extradural [90,92], cutaneous [46–48,51], calvarial [3,104], and intraosseous [2,4,6,8,105].

Many earlier reports are also hindered by the lack of sensitive imaging modalities, specifically computed tomography (CT) and magnetic resonance imaging (MRI), to exclude the presence of intracranial tumors [9,21,33,44,106]. In 2000, Lang et al. reviewed cases reported in the English language literature since the advent of CT imaging (1976) and identified 178 primary extradural meningiomas [90]. Cases were excluded if there was evidence that the inner surface of the dura and subdural space were involved or if there was insufficient evidence to exclude an intracranial/intraspinal component. Since this review, over 100 additional cases of primary extradural meningioma have been reported in the English language literature [2–6,8,10–12,22–25,31,35–40,42,48,56–60,73–80,83, 107,108].

Demographic Features

Analysis of the extradural meningiomas reported in the CT era literature reveals that patient ages at diagnosis range from 1 to 96 years, with a median patient age ranging from 44 to 49 years [2–6,8,10–12,22–25,31,35–40,42,48,56–60,73–80, 83,90,107,108]. The incidence appears bimodal, with a peak during the second decade of life and a second peak during the fifth through seventh decades [90]. There is to be a slight female predominance, with a male-to-female ratio of 1:1.3 [2–6,8,10–12,22–25,31,35–40,42,48,56–60,73–80, 83,90,107,108].

Tumor Location

Although primary extradural meningiomas have been described in a variety of locations, they more commonly arise in the head and neck. Of the cases described in the literature since the advent of CT imaging, 254 (90%) were found in the head and neck [2–6,8,10–12,22–25,31,35–40,42,48,56–60, 90,107,108]. This includes 69 tumors found in the middle ear or temporal region [22–25,90], 64 in the nasal cavity, oropharynx, or paranasal sinuses [8,31,35–40,42,58,90], 57 in the calvarium [2–6,90], 22 associated with the orbit [10–12,90], 21 in the scalp [48,56,57,59–60,90,108], 11 in the neck [90], 7 in the infratemporal fossa [90], 1 in the parotid gland [90], 1 in the cheek [90], and 1 associated with the extracranial

573

portion of the accessory nerve [107]. In addition to the head and neck, 17 extradural meningiomas have been described in the lungs [70–80,90], 4 in the upper extremities [83,90], 2 in a paraspinal location [90], 1 in the mediastinum [73], 1 in the retroperitoneum [90], and 1 associated with the adrenal gland [90]. The occurrence of multiple extradural meningiomas has also been described, and up to 18% of patients can have more than one distinct tumor [90].

Pathologic Features

Extradural meningiomas have histologic features comparable to those observed in the central nervous system, including meningiothelial [28,31], transitional [28,31], psammomatous [25,104], fibrous [38], angiomatous [29], and chordoid variants [2,76]. These lesions have been found to have immunohistochemical and electron microscopic features identical to their central nervous system counterparts [19,31,62,73,85]. Similar to their intracranial counterparts, extradural meningiomas are generally benign. Including all cases described during the CT era, 10 tumors (4%) have been graded as atypical and 16 (6%) graded as malignant based on the World Health Organization (WHO) criteria for meningiomas [25,31,70,74,90].

Cellular Origin

Although Pacchioni first described arachnoidal granulations in 1705 [109], it was Cleland and Robin who first proposed the concept that meningiomas arise from arachnoidal cells in 1864 and 1869, respectively [109,110]. This hypothesis was again put forth in 1902 by Schmidt and in 1915 by Cushing, who noted the histologic similarities between normal arachnoid villi and meningiomas [109,110]. There has been much debate regarding the origin of extradural meningiomas, and various hypotheses have been set forth in the literature. These hypotheses include: (1) development from ectopic arachnoid cells located within cranial and peripheral nerve sheaths [21,44,86,90,106]; (2) proliferation of extradural arachnoid cells that became misplaced during embryogenesis [33,44,86,90]; (3) proliferation of rests of arachnoid cap cells trapped within the cranial sutures during birth and molding of the head [90,105]; (4) development from dura and/or arachnoid entrapped within sites of traumatic fracture [90]; (5) derivation from perineural cells of peripheral nerves [85,111]; and (6) development from pleuripotential mesenchymal cells or metaplasia of various mesenchymal cell types, including fibroblasts and Schwann cells located extradurally [21,86,90,99,102,106].

The concept that extradural meningiomas arise from ectopic arachnoid cells located within nerve sheaths is supported by the fact that clusters of meningocytes have been described beyond the points of penetration of the dura by the 3rd, 7th, and 9th to 12th cranial nerves [89,90,103]. However, this does not explain the occurrence of extradural meningiomas in sites other than the head and neck or the derivation of tumors without an apparent association with peripheral nerves. An alternative hypothesis involves the proliferation of arachnoid cells misplaced during embryogenesis, which would potentially account for the development of meningiomas in such disparate sites as the parotid gland, extremities, lung, and retroperitoneum [86]. A third hypothesis suggests that extradural meningiomas arise from dura and/or arachnoid that was trapped within the cranial sutures during birth and head molding [105]. Lang et al. found that only 8% of the reported extradural meningiomas were associated with a cranial suture [90]. A similar hypothesis suggests that calvarial meningiomas arise from dura entrapped within the sites of traumatic fracture [56,58,90]. Eight cases of primary extradural meningioma associated with a prior fracture have been reported in the literature since 1976 [56,58,90]. Shuangshoti identified only 1 of 504 reported extradural meningiomas associated with prior trauma [102].

It has also been hypothesized that extradural meningiomas arise from the perineural cells of peripheral nerves [85,111]. Immunohistochemical studies have shown that meningiomas, arachnoid cap cells, and spindle cells within the perineurium of normal peripheral nerves stain with epithelial membrane antigen (EMA) antibody and may be embryologically and functionally related [111]. Thus, it is possible that a subset of extradural meningiomas is derived from perineural cells rather than ectopic meningocytes [85]. Finally, it has been proposed that extradural meningiomas arise from pleuripotential mesenchymal cells [21,86,90,99,102,106]. Pleuripotential mesenchymal cells have the ability to differentiate into a variety of cell types forming fibrous, osseous, chondroid, muscular, vascular, meningeal, and reticuloendothelial tissues. Most of these tissues have been identified within meningiomas; thus, it is possible that extradural meningiomas arise directly from mesenchymal cells [21,86,90,99,102,106].

Although each of the proposed mechanisms for the origin of primary extradural meningiomas can explain a subset of the cases reported in the literature, none can be widely applied. It appears that the origin of extradural meningiomas is multifactorial.

Association with Other Neoplasms

Primary extradural meningiomas may be found in patients with von Recklinghausen's neurofibromatosis. Shuangshoti found that 12 (2%) of 504 extradural meningiomas were associated with neurofibromatosis type I [102]. The tumors were found to occur in a variety of locations, including the optic nerve, scalp, parotid region, middle ear, and lung. Since this review, an additional extradural meningioma occurring in the scalp has been reported in a patient with von Recklinghausen's neurofibromatosis [46]. A primary meningioma of the maxillary antrum has also been described in a patient with tuberous sclerosis [112]. The occurrence of extradural meningiomas with other neoplasms, including osteomas, ovarian fibromas, neurofibromas, and mixed tumors of the lacrimal gland, has also been described [102].

Prognosis

In their review, Lang et al. analyzed the follow-up information for 96 patients with primary extradural meningiomas reported in the literature [90]. At the median follow-up time of 24 months, 88 (92%) were alive. When looking at histologic grade, 95% of patients with benign tumors and 78% of patients with either atypical or malignant tumors were alive at the median follow-up time. Twenty-four percent of the patients experienced tumor recurrence (22% of low-grade tumors vs. 33% of high-grade tumors). Time to recurrence ranged from 3 to 120 months for benign tumors and 4 to 24 months for atypical or malignant tumors. Distant metastasis was also reported in 5% of benign tumors and 11% of atypical or malignant tumors. Similar findings were described by Thompson et al. in their study of 35 patients with primary ear or temporal bone meningiomas [26]. Recurrences were reported in 28% of cases, with a time to recurrence ranging from 5 to 24 months. Although 25 patients were alive at follow-up (mean 3.5 years), 5 had died with recurrent disease (mean 3.5 years), and 5 had died of unrelated causes without evidence of disease (mean 9.5 years). A third large study of primary sinonasal tract meningiomas with a mean follow-up time of 13.7 years reported recurrence in 21% of patients, with a mean time to recurrence of 16.8 years [31]. It appears that the most important factor in determining the prognosis in patients with extradural meningiomas is the completeness of surgical excision [25,31,90]. There may also be a slightly increased incidence of recurrence and metastasis associated with high-grade tumors [90].

Primary Middle Ear and Temporal Bone Meningiomas

Primary extradural meningiomas of the middle ear and temporal bone make up less than 1% of all meningiomas [25]. Although these meningiomas are histologically identical to their intracranial counterparts, the rarity of these lesions may present a diagnostic difficulty. The differential diagnosis of these lesions may include paraganglioma, schwannoma, chemodectomas, middle ear adenoma, carcinoma, and melanoma. In most cases, these lesions may be distinguished from meningiomas based on histopathologic, immunohistochemical, or ultrastructural features (Fig. 61-1).

In their study of 36 patients with primary ear or temporal bone meningiomas, Thompson et al. reported that the age at presentation ranged from 10 to 80 years, with a mean of 49.5 years [25]. Rietz et al. found a similar mean age at presentation (45.3 years) in a review of 20 cases [19]. Women

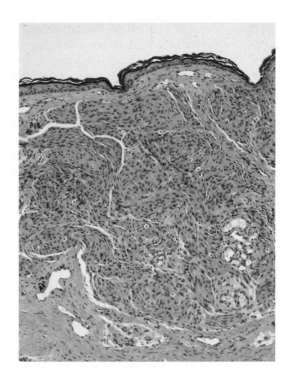

Fig. 61-1. Primary meningothelial (syncytial) meningioma (WHO grade I) of the middle ear in a 53-year-old female. This patient presented with hearing loss and pain in the right ear. Examination revealed an aural polyp. The tumor cells are arranged in nests divided by fibrovascular septae. Cytologically, the tumor cells generally have round to oval nuclei with delicate chromatin and inconspicuous nucleoli. Mild nuclear atypia was identified in focal areas of the tumor. This patient is currently alive with residual tumor 14 years postsurgery (hematoxylin-eosin, original magnification × 100)

tended to present at an older age than men: 52.0 and 44.8 years, respectively, with a female to male ratio of 2:1 [25]. Although sensorineural or conductive hearing loss is the most common symptom at presentation, other symptoms may include otitis, headaches, unsteadiness, dizziness, vertigo, tinnitus, bleeding, and chronic cough. Interestingly, none of the tumors reported in the series of Thompson et al. were asymptomatic at diagnosis [25]. However, very small tumors in the middle ear may cause minimal symptoms [19]. These neoplasms may be located in the external auditory canal, middle ear, temporal bone, and mixed locations [19,25]. Reitz et al. found that 45% of these tumors appear to arise from the middle ear [19]. Imaging can include skull radiographs, CT, angiography, and MRI. On radiographic imaging, the most common observation is diffuse cloudiness, suggestive of severe mastoiditis or otitis media [25]. Thus, a primary meningioma may not be suspected based on imaging studies, and in many cases the radiographic studies may be interpreted as normal [25]. CT and MRI imaging is important in the evaluation of these tumors to determine the extent of infiltration and to exclude the presence of clinically unsuspected intracranial meningioma [15].

Most primary meningiomas of the middle ear and temporal bone are histologically benign. In one study, only 1 of 36 tumors was classified as atypical [25]. Meningiomas occurring within the temporal bone may have extensive spread, and discrete margins may not be seen as these neoplasms extend through Haversian channels, neural foramina, as well as air and marrow cells [19]. Thus, the extent of invasion may be underestimated at the time of surgery, and the tumor may be incompletely excised. Local recurrence may occur in up to 28% of cases, with the time to recurrence ranging from 5 to 24 months in one study [25]; in this study of 36 middle ear and temporal bone meningiomas, 25 patients were alive at follow-up (mean 3.5 years), 5 had died with recurrent disease (mean 3.5 years), and 5 had died of unrelated causes without evidence of disease (mean 9.5 years) [25]. It has been recommended that patients with primary middle ear and temporal bone meningiomas be followed for at least 10–15 years with yearly CT scans to monitor for residual disease and intracranial extension [19].

Primary Meningiomas of the Sinonasal Tract

Primary meningiomas of the nasal cavity, nasopharynx, and paranasal sinuses are rare entities, and in general, the literature on these lesions is limited to case reports and literature reviews, with few large studies. The two largest studies of these lesions include one with 30 cases [31] and a second with 12 cases [28]. Meningiomas found in the sinonasal tract are far more likely to be a result of secondary extension by an intracranial tumor. However, primary extradural meningiomas have been reported in the nasal cavity, nasopharynx, frontal, ethmoid, maxillary and sphenoid sinuses, as well as one case involving the tonsil [41]. When these tumors are found in the paranasal sinuses, they most commonly arise in the frontal sinuses (59%), followed by the ethmoid sinuses (23%), sphenoid sinuses (9%), and maxillary sinuses (9%) [34].

Ho reviewed 17 primary meningiomas of the nasal cavity and paranasal sinuses and found a male-to-female ratio of 5:4 [113]. A larger study of 30 cases by Thompson et al. indicated no gender predilection [31]. The mean age at diagnosis has been reported to range from 23 years in one literature review [113] to 47.6 years in a larger study [31]. The age at diagnosis is controversial, with some authors describing a predilection for the first and second decades [113] and others reporting that most cases present in the fourth and fifth decades [28,31]. Primary meningiomas of the nasopharynx and paranasal sinuses may present with a variety of symptoms based on size and location including nasal obstruction, nasal discharge, epistaxis, nasal polyps, intranasal masses, swelling of the maxillotemporal area, maxillary pain, periorbital edema, proptosis, ptosis, and exophthalmos [28,31,34,113]. Imaging modalities may include conventional skull radiographs, CT, MRI, ultrasound, and angiograms. In general, these tumors are identified as a mass lesion on imaging studies. There may also be erosion or hyperostosis of the skull base to indicate intracranial invasion [28,31].

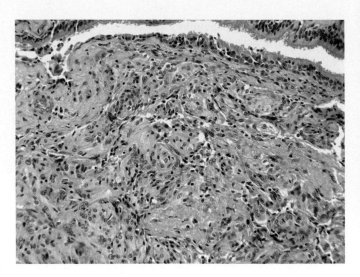

FIG. 61-2. A meningothelial (syncytial) meningioma (WHO grade I) involving the sphenoid and ethmoid sinuses in a 51-year-old male. The tumor cells are arranged in nests underlying uninvolved sinonasal epithelium (hematoxylin-eosin, original magnification × 200)

Most meningiomas described in the nasopharynx and paranasal sinuses have histologic patterns consistent with meningothelial or transitional type meningiomas [28,31], although fibroblastic, psammomatous, metaplastic, and angioblastic variants have been reported (Fig. 61-2) [29,31,99,113]. Due to the rarity of these tumors in the nasopharynx and paranasal sinuses, the differential diagnosis for these lesions may include a host of both benign and malignant tumors including carcinoma, neurofibroma, schwannoma, olfactory neuroblastoma, or melanoma. Although the majority of sinonasal tract meningiomas have low-grade morphology, Thompson et al. described three with atypical features [31].

Primary meningiomas of the nasopharynx and paranasal sinuses appear to be slow-growing neoplasms [28,113]. Complete excision of these tumors is recommended, with radiation reserved for those neoplasms that are not amenable to surgical resection [28]. These tumors generally have a favorable prognosis. In one review of 19 cases, no recurrences were found following surgical excision, with follow-up ranging from 6 months to 7 years [113]. In their study of 30 patients, Thompson et al. had a mean follow-up time of 13.7 years and reported recurrence in 21% of patients, with a mean time to recurrence of 16.8 years [31]. Of the 28 patients with follow-up information, 3 died with local disease (mean 1.2 years), 1 was alive with residual disease 25.6 years after initial presentation, and the remaining patients were alive or had died of unrelated causes without evidence of disease.

Primary Meningiomas of the Calvarium

Although bone invasion and hyperostosis of the calvarium are frequently observed with intracranial meningiomas, primary intraosseous meningiomas are less common

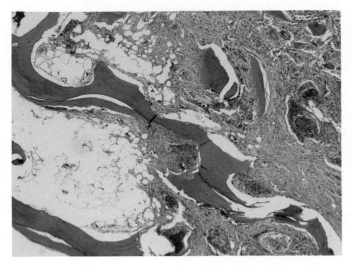
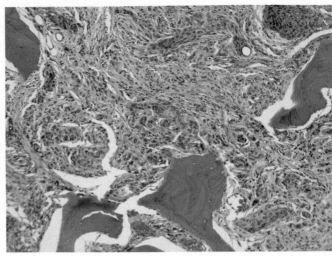

A   B

FIG. 61-3. A predominantly fibrous meningioma (WHO grade I) involving the calvarium in a 74-year-old female. (A) A low-power view illustrates the infiltrative architectural pattern of this tumor as it interfaces with uninvolved bone (hematoxylin-eosin, original magnification × 50). (B)At higher magnification, the tumor consists of both spindle and rounded cells arranged in interlacing bundles (hematoxylin-eosin, original magnification × 200)

(Fig. 61-3). Shuangshoti reviewed 504 extradural meningiomas and found that 71 (14%) were primary cranial meningiomas [102]. The most common locations for these tumors are the frontoparietal and orbital regions. Eight cases of primary extradural meningioma associated with a prior fracture have been reported in the literature since 1976 [56,58,90]. Shuangshoti identified only 1 of 504 reported extradural meningiomas associated with prior trauma [102]. Although these tumors have been found to arise near cranial sutures [3,105,114], this accounts for only 8% of the reported primary calvarial meningiomas [90].

In one review of 36 primary intraosseous meningiomas, the mean age at diagnosis was 45 years (range 9–79 years), and the female-to-male ratio was 2:1 [115]. The clinical presentation of these lesions varies based on the size and location. Symptoms may include a palpable mass, headaches, dizziness, proptosis, blurred vision, or seizures. Two of these 36 tumors were incidental findings on routine bone scans [115]. On plain films, these lesions can appear hyperostotic, osteolytic, or mixed [6,104,115]. CT with bone windows provides improved imaging of the tumor, including evidence for cortical destruction and intra- or extraosseous extension. MRI allows further delineation of any soft tissue component [2].

Due to the location and the rarity of primary intraosseous meningiomas, these tumors are often not suspected clinically. The differential diagnosis based on imaging studies may include osteoma, intracranial meningioma with overlying hyperostosis, fibrous dysplasia, chondroma, chondrosarcoma, giant-cell tumor, hemangioma, myeloma, eosinophilic granuloma, and metastasis [6]. Although most primary meningiomas of the calvarium are benign, there is some suggestion in the literature that osteolytic tumors are more likely to have atypical or malignant features and are associated with a more aggressive clinical course [116,117]. However, occasional osteolytic tumors have also been diagnosed as histologically benign [2,104].

Primary Orbital Meningiomas

The first intraorbital meningioma was described by Scarpa in 1816 [118]. Although in two large studies, meningiomas were found to account for up to 14% of orbital tumors, these tumors were generally found to arise from the optic nerve sheath or from secondary extension of a primary intracranial tumor (Fig. 61-4) [119,120]. Based on sites of origin, orbital meningiomas may be classified as follows: (1) primary tumors of the optic nerve sheath; (2) secondary tumors extending from intracranial sites of origin; (3) multicentric tumors with separate intracranial and orbital tumors; and (4) extradural tumors [121]. In his review of 41 patients with primary orbital meningiomas, Lloyd described 32 tumors (78%) arising from the optic sheath and 9 (22%) arising extradurally within the orbit [7]. It is hypothesized that these extradural tumors arise from ectopic rests of meningocytes within the retrobulbar fat [12].

Extradural meningiomas are generally evident on plain x-ray, and radiologic changes include orbital enlargement, hyperostosis, and changes in the adjacent sinuses. CT or MRI images usually show evidence of a soft tissue mass. Primary intraosseous orbital roof meningiomas have also been reported in the literature

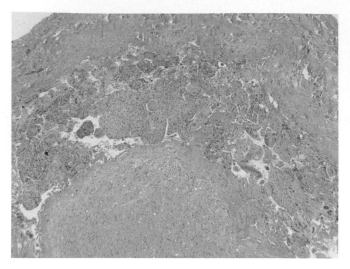
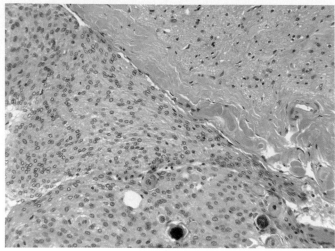

A   B

FIG. 61-4. A primary orbital meningothelial (syncytial) meningioma (WHO grade I) arising from the optic nerve sheath in a 45-year-old female. This patient presented with decreased light perception and visual acuity due to the mass effect of the tumor. (A) At low power, the tumor is forming nests, which are infiltrating between the optic nerve (bottom) and the overlying dura (top) (hematoxylin-eosin, original magnification x 50). (B) At higher magnification, the tumor does not appear to invade the adjacent optic nerve pictured in the upper right corner. Psammoma bodies can be appreciated (hematoxylin-eosin, original magnification × 200)

and may require coronal and lateral CT images to demonstrate the intradiploic involvement of the orbital roof [11]. Although most primary orbital meningiomas are of the meningothelial or transitional type [121,122], other variants including angioblastic and mucinous types have been described [10,118].

The clinical symptoms of primary orbital meningiomas arise from the mass effect of the neoplasm and include pain, proptosis, ptosis, diplopia, headaches, and decrease in visual acuity or blindness [12]. Visual loss may be due to direct compression of the optic nerve by the tumor, circulatory disturbance, or neoplastic infiltration of the optic nerve [102,123]. Primary orbital meningiomas may occur in any age group, although there is disagreement in the literature as to the peak age of incidence of the lesions; some authors suggest that a majority of tumors occur during the first and second decades of life and others state that these lesions are rare in childhood [7]. In one review of the literature, 58% of primary orbital meningiomas occurred during the fourth to sixth decades, while 27% occurred during the first two decades [102]. This review also reported a female-to-male ratio of 5:2. It has also been suggested that these tumors are more aggressive in children [122].

Primary Meningiomas of the Skin and Subcutaneous Tissue

Primary meningiomas of the skin and subcutaneous tissues have been described primarily in the head and neck regions, specifically the scalp and forehead [56–58,103]. However, these tumors are quite rare, and in one study of 30 extracranial scalp lesions in children, only 1 case was identified as

a primary cutaneous meningioma [57]. There have also been occasional case reports of cutaneous meningiomas in a paravertebral location [55,103]. Lopez et al. classified these tumors into three groups: primary cutaneous meningiomas (Type I), ectopic meningiomas of the soft tissue with extension into the skin (Type II), and central nervous system meningiomas with extension into the skin (Type III).

Lopez et al. studied 25 cases gathered at the Armed Forces Institute of Pathology until 1974 [103]. Sixteen male patients and 9 female patients were identified. The age at diagnosis ranged from 1 to 70 years of age, with a mean of 26.8 years. The type I lesion tended to occur in children or young adults and was generally present at birth. These lesions were primarily located in the scalp, the forehead, or the paravertebral regions. Tumors in the scalp were found along suture lines. These lesions were typically asymptomatic and presented as soft tissue nodules or lumps. Type II lesions were found in a periauricular and perinasal location, as well as in the scalp. These tumors were found more often in adults and are not present at birth. Unlike type I lesions, type II lesions tended to be symptomatic with local infiltration and inflammation. Type III tumors were found on the face, temple, and scalp. These lesions clinically presented as hemorrhagic cysts or slow-growing subcutaneous masses.

The diagnosis of a cutaneous meningioma is rarely suspected clinically, and the differential diagnosis may include alopecia, fibroma, adnexal tumors, epidermal inclusion cyst, nevus, ulcer, or granuloma [48,103]. It is important to obtain radiographic imaging, including CT and MRI, to exclude the possibility of an intracranial or intraspinal primary tumor [52]. Primary meningiomas of the skin and subcutaneous tissue resemble their central nervous system counterparts. Although most cutaneous meningiomas are benign, a rare tumor with malignant histologic features and distant metastasis to the lung and pleura has been reported [50].

Primary Pulmonary Meningiomas

Since the first report of a primary extradural meningioma of the lung in 1981 [124], fewer than 20 additional cases of pulmonary meningiomas have been reported in the English-language literature [70–80,90]. The diagnosis of a primary pulmonary meningioma requires the exclusion of an intracranial/intraspinal primary tumor. Although metastatic meningiomas are rare, with an incidence estimated as less than 1 in 1000 patients [125,129], the lung is one of the most common sites for metastatic meningioma (Fig. 61-5) [66,126,130].

Two reviews of primary pulmonary meningioma indicate that these tumors are generally histologically recognizable as meningioma with a meningothelial pattern [71,72]. A chordoid variant has also been described [76]. Tumors range in size from a few millimeters to 12 cm [71,72]. Pulmonary meningiomas are usually well circumscribed and often localized to the lung parenchyma, without bronchial or pleural involvement [80]. In general, reported cases were asymptomatic and detected by routine chest radiographs as solitary lesions. Multiple primary pulmonary meningiomas have been rarely reported [61]. Although most reported cases have benign histologic features and are associated with a favorable clinical course, one case exhibited malignant histologic features, including loss of architectural pattern, mild nuclear pleomorphism, increased mitotic counts, and focal rhabdoid features (Fig. 61-6) [70].

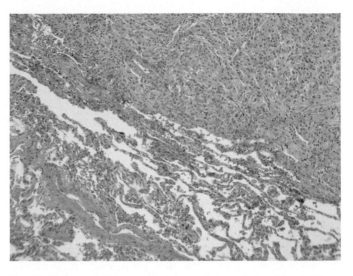

FIG. 61-5. A meningioma metastatic to the lower lobe of the left lung in a 63-year-old female with an intracranial transitional meningioma (WHO grade I) resected 18 years earlier (hematoxylin-eosin, original magnification × 100)

This patient subsequently developed local recurrence with distant metastases approximately 5 months following surgical resection. A second case with benign histologic features at initial surgical resection developed an apparent liver metastasis 2 years postoperatively [74].

Due to the rarity of primary pulmonary meningiomas, these lesions may not be suspected clinically, and those tumors that do not resemble the classic meningothelial pattern may cause diagnostic difficulty. A variety of primary or secondary pulmonary lesions can resemble atypical meningiomas histologically, and the nonspecific immunohistochemical

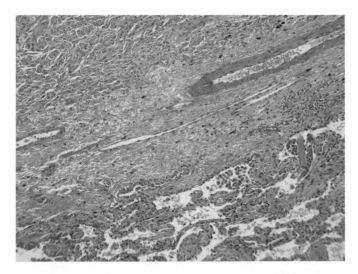

A

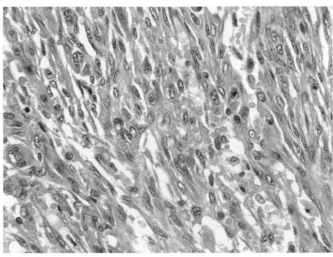

B

FIG. 61-6. A rare primary malignant meningioma of the lung diagnosed in a 58-year-old male with a 6.5-cm solitary right upper lobe mass. (A) The tumor, pictured in the top left corner, was separated from the adjacent lung parenchyma by a band of collagenous tissue (hematoxylin-eosin, original magnification × 100). (B)The mass was characterized by focal rhabdoid features and increased mitotic activity. A mitotic figure is illustrated in this high-power field (hematoxylin-eosin, original magnification × 400)

profile of meningiomas may make differentiating these lesions difficult. Differential diagnostic considerations include a sarcoma with epithelioid features, schwannoma, metastatic carcinoma, mesothelioma, and solitary fibrous tumor.

Primary Meningiomas in Other Locations

Although the great majority of primary extradural meningiomas originate in the previously discussed locations, there have been various case reports of these tumors arising in such disparate locations as the parotid gland [43,90], infratemporal fossa [90,127], peripheral nerve [83], neck [44,90,106,128], finger [100], mediastinum [73,81], adrenal gland [90], and retroperitoneum [85,90] (Fig. 61-7). Although most of these cases have been described as benign tumors, one report of a primary retroperitoneal meningioma described malignant histologic features and an aggressive clinical course with multiple recurrent nodules within the abdomen and pelvis [85].

Metastatic Meningiomas

Metastatic central nervous system meningiomas are rare, with an incidence estimated as less than 1 in 1000 patients [125,129]. A metastatic meningioma must always be considered in the differential diagnosis of a possible primary extradural meningioma. Both histologically benign and malignant meningiomas of the central nervous system have been reported to metastasize to a variety of locations, including the lungs,

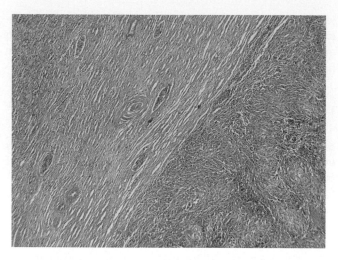

FIG. 61-8. A meningioma metastatic to the kidney in a 35-year-old female with neurofibromatosis type II diagnosed with a malignant meningioma (WHO grade III) 3 years earlier. The metastatic meningioma is pictured in the right half of the image, with residual renal parenchyma to the left (hematoxylin-eosin, original magnification × 50)

liver, pleura, lymph nodes, bone, kidney, thyroid, pancreas, thymus, soft tissue, heart, peritoneum, and skin (Fig. 61-8) [66,125,126,129,130]. The lungs are reported to be the most common site for metastases [66,125,126,129,130]. It is essential to exclude a primary intracranial or intraspinal tumor before diagnosing a primary extradural meningioma. Thus, imaging studies including CT and MRI should be routinely performed on any patient with a suspected primary extradural meningioma before this diagnosis is made.

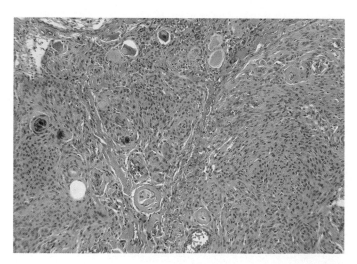

FIG. 61-7. A meningothelial (syncytial) meningioma (WHO grade I) involving the ganglion of cranial nerve V. The tumor cells are arranged in lobules divided by fibrovascular septae and entrapping residual ganglion cells. Psammoma bodies were associated with this meningioma (hematoxylin-eosin, original magnification × 100)

References

1. Kompanje EJ. A patient with a large intra- and extracranial tumor, most probably a primary extradural meningioma, described in 1730. J Neurooncol. 2004;67:123–125.
2. Tokgoz N, Oner YA, Kaymaz M, et al. Primary intraosseous meningioma: CT and MRI appearance. Am J Neuroradiol. 2005;26:2053–2056.
3. Damtie ZG. Primary extradural calvarial meningioma: case report. Ethiop Med J. 2004;42:49–52.
4. Yamazaki T, Tsukada A, Uemura K, et al. Intraosseous meningioma of the posterior fossa: case report. Neurol Med Chir (Tokyo). 2001;41:149–153.
5. Yadav YR, Rahman HH, Tandan JK, et al. Primary ectopic meningioma. J Indian Med Assoc. 2001;99:102–103.
6. Rosahl SK, Mirzayan MJ, Samii M. Osteolytic intra-osseous meningiomas: illustrated review. Acta Neurochir. 2004;146:1245–1249.
7. Lloyd GA. Primary orbital meningioma: a review of 41 patients investigated radiologically. Clin Radiol. 1982;33:181–187.
8. Devi B, Bhat D, Madhusudhan H, et al. Primary intraosseous meningioma of orbit and anterior cranial fossa: a case report and literature review. Australas Radiol. 2001;45:211–214.

9. Macmichael IM, Cullen JF. Primary intraorbital meningioma. Br J Ophthal. 1969;53:169–173.

10. Fenton S, Moriarty P, Kennedy S. Primary mucinous meningioma of bone. Orbit. 2002;21:227–229.

11. Desai KI, Nadkarni TD, Bhayani RD, et al. Intradiploic meningioma of the orbit: a case report. Neurol India. 2004;52:380–382.

12. Ducic Y. Orbitozygomatic resection of meningiomas of the orbit. Laryngoscope. 2004;114:164–170.

13. Chen KT, Dehner LP. Primary tumors of the external and middle ear. II. A clinicopathologic study of 14 paragangliomas and three meningiomas. Arch Otolaryngol. 1978;104:253–259.

14. Langman AW, Jackler RK, Althaus SR. Meningioma of the internal auditory canal. Am J Otol. 1990;11:201–204.

15. Parisier SC, Som PM, Shugar JM, et al. The evaluation of middle ear meningiomas using computerized axial tomography. Laryngoscope. 1978;88:1170–1177.

16. Taylor JS, Crocker PV, Keebler JS. Middle ear meningioma: case report. Ala Med. 1989;58:17–18.

17. Haught K, Hogg Jp, Voelker JL, et al. Entirely intracanicular meningioma: contrast-enhanced MR findings in a rare entity. Am J Neuroradiol. 1998;19:1831–1833.

18. DeWeese DD, Everts EC. Primary intratympanic meningioma. Arch Otolaryngol. 1972;96:62–66.

19. Rietz DR, Ford CN, Kurtycz DF, et al. Significance of apparent intratympanic meningiomas. Laryngoscope. 1983;93:1397–1404.

20. Zeitouni AG, Zagzag D, Cohen NL. Meningioma of the internal auditory canal. Ann Otol Rhinol Laryngol. 1997;106:657–661.

21. Whicker JH, Devine KD, MacCarty CS. Diagnostic and therapeutic problems in extracranial meningiomas. Am J Surg. 1973;126:452–457.

22. Uppal HS, Kabbani M, Reddy V, et al. Ectopic extra-cranial meningioma presenting as an aural polyp. Eur Arch Otorhinolaryngol. 2003;260:322–324.

23. Rojas R, Palacios E, D'Antonio M. An unusual primary intratympanic meningioma. Ear Nose Throat J. 2004;83:607–608.

24. Lawand A, Walker AN, Griffin J. Pathology quiz case. Middle ear meningioma. Arch Otolaryngol Head Neck Surg. 2002;128:975–977.

25. Thompson LD, Bouffard JP, Sandberg GD, et al. Primary ear and temporal bone meningiomas: a clinicopathologic study of 36 cases with a review of the literature. Mod Pathol. 2003;16:236–245.

26. Prayson RA. Middle ear meningiomas. Ann Diagn Pathol. 2000;4:149–153.

27. Ohnishi T, Mori S, Arita N. Primary meningioma of paranasal sinuses treated by the transbasal approach. Surg Neurol. 1987;27:195–199.

28. Perzin KH, Pushparaj N. Nonepithelial tumors of the nasal cavity, paranasal sinuses, and nasopharynx: a clinincopathologic study. XIII: Meningiomas. Cancer. 1984;54:1860–1869.

29. Sadar ES, Conomy JP, Benjamin SP, et al. Meningiomas of the paranasal sinuses, benign and malignant. Neurosurgery. 1979;4:227–231.

30. Taxy JB. Meningioma of the paranasal sinuses: a report of two cases. Am J Surg Pathol. 1990;14:82–86.

31. Thompson LD, Gyure KA. Extracranial sinonasal tract meningiomas: a clinicopathologic study of 30 cases with a review of the literature. Am J Surg Pathol. 2000;24:640–650.

32. Hanada M, Kitajima K. Primary ectopic meningioma in the right ethmoid sinus: a case report. Auris Nasus Larynx. 1997;24:321–324.

33. Majoras M. Meningioma of the paranasal sinuses. Laryngoscope. 1970;80:640–645.

34. Som PM, Sachdev VP, Sacher MM, et al. Intrafrontal sinus primary meningioma. Neuroradiology. 1991;33:251–252.

35. Petrulionis M, Valeviciene N, Paulauskiene I, et al. Primary extracranial meningioma of the sinonasal tract. Acta Radiol. 2005;46:415–418.

36. Gokduman CA, Iplikcioglu AC, Kuzderem M, et al. Primary meningioma of paranasal sinus. J Clin Neurosci. 2005;12:832–834.

37. Serry P, Rombaux P, Ledeghen S, et al. Extracranial sinonasal tract meningioma: a case report. Acta Otorhinolaryngol Belg. 2004;58:151–155.

38. Ketter R, Henn W, Feiden W, et al. Nasoethmoidal meningioma with cytogenetic features of tumor aggressiveness in a 16-year-old child. Pediatr Neurosurg. 2003;39:190–194.

39. Swain RE, Kingdom TT, DelGaudio JM, et al. Meningiomas of paranasal sinuses. Am J Rhinol. 2001;15:27–30.

40. Daneshi A, Asghari A, Bahramy E. Primary meningioma of the ethmoid sinus: a case report. Ear Nose Throat J. 2003;82:310–311.

41. Kaur A, Shetty SC, Prasad D, et al. Primary ectopic meningioma of the palantine tonsil—a case report. J Laryngol Otol. 1997;111:179–181.

42. Hameed A, Gokden M, Hanna EY. Fine-needle aspiration cytology of a primary ectopic meningioma. Diagn Cytopathol. 2002;26:297–300.

43. Nichols RD, Knighton RS, Chason JL, et al. Meningioma in the parotid region. Laryngoscope. 1987;97:693–696.

44. Hoye SJ, Hoar CS, Murray JE. Extracranial meningioma presenting as a tumor of the neck. Am J Surg. 1960;100:486–489.

45. Tampieri D, Pokrupa R, Melanson D, et al. Primary ectopic meningioma of the neck: MR features. J Comput Assist Tomogr. 1987;11:1054–1056.

46. Argenyi ZB, Thieberg MD, Hayes CM, et al. Primary cutaneous meningioma associated with von Recklinghausen's disease. J Cutan Pathol. 1994;21:549–556.

47. Kalfa M, Daskalopoulou D, Markidou S. Fine needle aspiration (FNA) biopsy of primary cutaneous menigioma: report of two cases. Cytopathology. 1999;10:54–60.

48. Courville P, Cappele O, Bachy B, et al. Type 1—primary cutaneous meningioma of the scalp. Eur J Pediatr Surg. 2000;10:387–389.

49. Barr RJ, Yi ES, Jensen JL, et al. Meningioma-like tumor of the skin: an ultrastructural and immunohistochemical study. Am J Surg Pathol. 1993;17:779–787.

50. Mackay B, Bruner JM, Luna MA, et al. Malignant meningioma of the scalp. Ultrastruct Pathol. 1994;18:235–240.

51. Hu B, Pant M, Cornford M, et al. Association of primary intracranial meningioma and cutaneous meningioma of external auditory canal: a case report and review of the literature. Arch Pathol Lab Med. 1998;122:97–99.

52. Nochomovitz LE, Jannotta F, Orenstein JM. Meningioma of the scalp: light and electron microscopic observations. Arch Pathol Lab Med. 1985;109:92–95.

53. Theaker JM, Fleming KA. Meningioma of the scalp: a case report with immunohistological features. J Cutan Pathol. 1987;14:49–53.

54. Kakizoe S, Kojiro M, Hikita N. Primary cutaneous meningioma: report of a case. Acta Pathol Jpn. 1987;37:511–514.

55. Zaaroor M, Borovich B, Bassan L, et al. Primary cutaneous extravertebral meningioma: case report. J Neurosurg. 1984;60:1097–1098.

56. Shaw R, Kissun D, Boyle M, et al. Primary meningioma of the scalp as a late complication of skull fracture: case report and literature review. Int J Oral Maxillofac Surg. 2004;33:509–511.

57. Cummings TJ, George TM, Fuchs HE, et al. The pathology of extracranial scalp and skull masses in young children. Clin Neuropathol. 2004;23:34–43.

58. Borggreven PA, de Graaf FH, van der Valk P, et al. Post-traumatic cutaneous meningioma. J Laryngol Otol. 2004;118:228–230.

59. Hayhurst C, Mcmurtrie A, Brydon HL. Cutaneous meningioma of the scalp. Acta Neurochir. 2004;146:1383–1384.

60. Gagey V, Causeret AS, Roth B, et al. Cutaneous meningioma. Eur J Dermatol. 2003;13:64.

61. de Perrot M, Kurt AM, Robert J, et al. Primary pulmonary meningioma presenting as lung metastasis. Scand Cardiovasc J. 1999;33:121–123.

62. Drlicek M, Grisold W, Lorber J, et al. Pulmonary meningioma: immunohistochemical and ultrastructural features. Am J Surg Pathol. 1991;15:455–459.

63. Strimlan CV, Golembiewski RS, Celko DA, et al. Primary pulmonary meningioma. Surg Neurol. 1988;29:410–413.

64. Chumas JC, Lorelle CA. Pulmonary meningioma: a light- and electron-microscopic study. Am J Surg Pathol. 1982;6:795–801.

65. Robinson PG. Pulmonary meningioma: report of a case with electron microscopic and immunohistochemical findings. Am J Clin Pathol. 1992;97:814–817.

66. Kodama K, Doi O, Higashiyama M, et al. Primary and metastatic pulmonary meningioma. Cancer. 1991;67:1412–1417.

67. Moran CA, Hochholzer L, Rush W, et al. Primary intrapulmonary meningiomas: a clinicopathologic and immunohistochemical study of ten cases. Cancer. 1996;78:2328–2333.

68. Ueno M, Fujiyama J, Yamazaki I, et al. Cytology of primary pulmonary meningioma: report of the first multiple case. Acta Cytol. 1998;42:1424–1430.

69. Flynn SD, Yousem SA. Pulmonary meningiomas: a report of two cases. Hum Pathol. 1991;22:469–474.

70. Prayson RA, Farver CF. Primary pulmonary malignant meningioma. Am J Surg Pathol. 1999;23:722–726.

71. Lockett L, Chiang V, Scully N. Primary pulmonary meningioma: report of a case and review of the literature. Am J Surg Pathol. 1997;21:453–460.

72. Kaleem Z, Fitzpatrick MM, Ritter JH. Primary pulmonary meningioma: report of a case and review of the literature. Arch Pathol Lab Med. 1997;121:631–636.

73. Falleni M, Roz E, Dessy E, et al. Primary intrathoracic meningioma: histopathological, immunohistochemical and ultrastructural study of two cases. Virchows Arch. 2001;439:196–200.

74. van der Meij JJ, Boomars KA, van den Bosch JM, et al. Primary pulmonary malignant meningioma. Ann Thorac Surg. 2005;80:1523–1525.

75. Picquet J, Valo I, Jousset Y, et al. Primary pulmonary meningioma first suspected of being a lung metastasis. Ann Thorac Surg. 2005;79:1407–1409.

76. Rowsell C, Sirbovan J, Rosenblum MK, et al. Primary chordoid meningioma of lung. Virchows Arch. 2005;446:333–337.

77. Comin CE, Caldarella A, Novelli L, et al. Primary pulmonary meningioma: report of a case and review of the literature. Tumori. 2003;89:102–105.

78. Gomez-Aracil V, Mayayo E, Alvira R, et al. Fine needle aspiration cytology of primary pulmonary meningioma associated with minute meningotheliallike nodules: report of a case with histologic, immunohistochemical and ultrastructural studies. Acta Cytologica. 2002;46:899–903.

79. Cura M, Smoak W, Dala R. Pulmonary meningioma: false positive positron emission tomography for malignant pulmonary nodules. Clin Nucl Med. 2002;27:701–704.

80. Cesario A, Galetta D, Margaritora S, et al. Unsuspected primary pulmonary meningioma. Eur J Cardiothorac Surg. 2002;21:553–555.

81. Wilson AJ, Ratliff JL, Lagios MD, et al. Mediastinal meningioma. Am J Surg Pathol. 1979;3:557–562.

82. Russell DS, Rubinstein LJ. The tumours of the nervous system. In: Russell DS, Rubinstein LJ, editors. Pathology of Tumors of the Nervous System. Baltimore: Williams & Wilkins, 1989:452–506.

83. Anderson SE, Johnston JO, Zalaudek CJ, et al. Peripheral nerve ectopic meningioma at the elbow joint. Skeletal Radiol. 2001;30:639–642.

84. Coons SW, Johnson PC. Brachial plexus meningioma, report of a case with immunohistochemical and ultrastructural examination. Acta Neuropathol. 1989;77:445–448.

85. Huszar M, Fanburg JC, Dickerson GR, et al. Retroperitoneal malignant meningioma: a light microscopic, immunohistochemical, and ultrastructural study. Am J Surg Pathol. 1996;20:492–499.

86. Batsakis JG. Pathology consultation. Extracranial meningiomas. Ann Otol Rhinol Laryngol. 1984;93:282–283.

87. Farr HW, Gray GF, Vrana M, et al. Extracranial meningioma. J Surg Oncol. 1973;5:411–420.

88. Friedman CD, Costantino PD, Teitelbaum B, et al. Primary extracranial meningiomas of the head and neck. Laryngoscope. 1990;100:41–48.

89. Wolman L. Role of arachnoid granulation in the development of meningioma. AMA Arch Pathol. 1952;53:70–77.

90. Lang FF, MacDonald OK, Fuller GN, et al. Primary extradural meningiomas: a report of nine cases and review of the literature from the era of computerized tomography scanning. J Neurosurg. 2000;93:940–950.

91. Shuangshoti S, Panyathanya R. Neural neoplasms in Thailand: a study of 2,897 cases. Neurology. 1974;24:1127–1134.

92. Sartor K, Fliedner E, Pfingst E. Angiographic demonstration of cervical extradural meningioma. Neuroradiology. 1977;14:147–149.

93. Strempel I. Rare choroidal tumour simulating a malignant melanoma. Ophthalmologica. 1991;202:110–114.

94. Unger PD, Geller SA, Anderson PJ. Pulmonary lesions in a patient with neurofibromatosis. Arch Pathol Lab Med. 1984;108:654–657.

95. Cech DA, Leavens ME, Larson DL. Giant intracranial and extracranial meningioma: case report and review of the literature. Neurosurgery. 1982;11:694–697.

96. Granich MS, Pilch BZ, Goodman ML. Meningiomas presenting in the paranasal sinuses and temporal bone. Head Neck Surg. 1983;5:319–328.

97. Geoffray A, Lee YY, Jing BS, et al. Extracranial meningniomas of the head and neck. Am J Neuroradiol. 1984;5:599–604.

98. Atherino CC, Garcia R, Lopes LJ. Ectopic meningioma of the nose and paranasal sinuses (report of a case). J Laryngol Otol. 1985;99:1161–1166.

99. Shuangshoti S, Panyathanya R. Ectopic meningiomas. Arch Otolaryngol. 1973;98:102–105.

100. Daugaard S. Ectopic meningioma of a finger: case report. J Neurosurg. 1983;58:778–780.

101. Ferlito A, Devaney KO, Rinaldo A. Primary extracranial meningioma in the vicinity of the temporal bone: a benign lesion which is rarely recognized clinically. Acta Otolaryngol. 2004;124:5–7.

102. Shuangshoti S. Primary meningiomas outside the central nervous system. In: Al-Mefty O, editor. Meningiomas. New York: Raven Press, 1991:107–128.

103. Lopez DA, Silvers DN, Helwig EB. Cutaneous meningiomas—a clinicopathologic study. Cancer. 1974;34:728–744.

104. Muthukumar N. Primary calvarial meningiomas. Br J Neurosurg. 1997;11:388–392.

105. Azar-Kia B, Sarwar M, Marc JA, et al. Intraosseous meningioma. Neuroradiology, 1974;6:246–253.

106. Shuangshoti S, Netsky MG, Fitz-Hugh GS. Parapharyngeal meningioma with special reference to cell of origin. Ann Otol Rhinol Laryngol. 1971;80:464–473.

107. Tatagiba M, Koerbel A, Bornemann A, et al. Meningioma of the accessory nerve extending from the jugular foramen into the parapharyngeal space. Acta Neurochir. 2005;147:909–910.

108. Hayhurst C, Mcmurtrie A, Brydon HL. Cutaneous meningioma of the scalp. Acta Neurochir. 2004;146:1383–1384.

109. Al-Rodhan NR, Laws ER. Meningioma: a historical study of the tumor and its surgical management. Neurosurgery. 1990;26:832–846.

110. Chou SM, Miles JM. The pathology of meningiomas. In: Al-Mefty O, editor. Meningiomas. New York: Raven Press, 1991:37–57.

111. Theaker JM, Gatter KC, Puddle J. Epithelial membrane antigen expression by the perineurium of peripheral nerve and in peripheral nerve tumors. Histopathology. 1988;13:171–179.

112. Irving RM, Ford GR, Jones NS. Tuberous sclerosis with primary meningioma of the maxillary antrum. J Laryngol Otol. 1991;105:481–483.

113. Ho KL. Primary meningioma of the nasal cavity and paranasal sinuses. Cancer. 1980;46:1442–1447.

114. Chatterjee S, Foy P, Diengdoh V. Intra-diploic meningioma in a child. Br J Neurosurg. 1993;7:315–317.

115. Crawford TS, Kleinschmidt-DeMasters BK, Lillehei KO. Primary intraosseous meningioma: case report. J Neurosurg. 1995;83:912–915.

116. Husaini TA. An unusual osteolytic meningioma. J Pathol. 1970;101:57–58.

117. Younis G, Sawaya R. Intracranial osteolytic malignant meningiomas appearing as extracranial soft-tissue masses. Neurosurgery. 1992;30:932–935.

118. Elahi E, Meltzer MA, Friedman AH, et al. Primary orbital angiomatous meningioma. Arch Ophthalmol. 2003;121:124–127.

119. Ohtsuka K, Hashimoto M, Suzuki Y. A review of 244 orbital tumors in Japenese patients during a 21-year period: origins and locations. Jpn J Ophthalmol. 2005;49:49–55.

120. Shields JA, Shields CL, Scartozzi R. Survey of 1264 patients with orbital tumors and simulating lesions: The 2002 Montgomery Lecture, part 1. Ophthalmology. 2004;111:997–1008.

121. Marquardt MD, Zimmerman LE. Histopathology of meningiomas and gliomas of the optic nerve. Hum Pathol. 1982;13:226–235.

122. Karp LA, Zimmerman LE, Borit A, et al. Primary intraorbital meningiomas. Arch Ophthalmol. 1974;91:24–28.

123. Mourits MP, van der Sprenkel JW. Orbital meningioma, the Utrecht experience. Orbit. 2001;20:25–33.

124. Erlandson RA. Diagnostic transmission electron microscopy of human tumors. New York: Masson Publishing, 1981:125–126.

125. Karasick JL, Mullan SF. A survey of metastatic meningiomas. J Neurosurg. 1974;39:206–212.

126. Stoller JK, Kavuru M, Mehta AC, et al. Intracranial meningioma metastatic to the lung. Cleve Clin J Med. 1987;54:521–527.

127. Inglis AF, Yarington CT, Bolen J. Extrameningeal meningiomas of the infratemporal fossa: diagnosis and treatment. Laryngoscope. 1987;97:689–692.

128. Michel RG, Woodard BH. Extracranial meningioma. Ann Otol. 1979;88:407–412.

129. Strange RR, Tovi D, Nordenstam H. Meningioma with intracerebral, cerebellar, and visceral metastases. J Neurosurg. 1964;21:1098–1102.

130. Shuangshoti S, Hongsaprabhas C, Netsky MG. Metastasizing meningioma. Cancer. 1970;26:832–841.

62
Management of Arterial Encasement by Intracranial Meningiomas

Laligam N. Sekhar and Sabareesh Kumar Natarajan

Introduction

Intracranial skull base meningiomas frequently encase the basal arteries, the internal carotid artery (ICA), vertebral artery (VA), and basilar artery (BA) and their branches. Frequently, the tumor can be dissected away, especially when the encasement involves the subarachnoid segment. When such dissection is not safely possible, or when the tumor involves an extradural segment, particularly with narrowing of the artery, bypass and resection may be needed in order to facilitate complete tumor resection.

Management of Vascular Encasement

Figure 62-1 shows the preferred management strategy for arterial encasement. In previously untreated cases, a thin arachnoid plane surrounds the artery, making dissection possible. But in the previously treated cases, this does not exist and a bypass may be often necessary.

When Is a Bypass Needed After Vascular Occlusion?

When the intracranial ICA or VA is occluded, whether or not a bypass is needed in all patients is controversial. A selective approach bases this decision on a balloon occlusion test, with monitoring of cerebral blood flow by single positron emission computed tomography (SPECT), Transcranial doppler (TCD) or angiography. A universal approach recommends a bypass in all patients. The senior author followed a selective approach in his earlier patients. However, based on a review of his patients who were not revascularized and suffered strokes and the reports of other surgeons with a similar experience (3–6), a universal approach is presently followed if the ICA has to be occluded for tumor cases.

In regard to the VA, if a vessel is markedly nondominant, it need not be reconstructed. However an equi-dominant or dominant VA must be reconstructed. If the BA is damaged, it must always be reconstructed, although when the patient has two large PCOM arteries, the patient may not suffer a stroke because of good collaterals. If a major artery is occluded following tumor resection, the patient may suffer vasospasm, hypotension, or hypercoagulable states, all of which may lead to delayed strokes, even with good collaterals.

Preoperative Imaging

The MRI scan is an important study. In T2-weighted imaging, the presence of intradural arterial encasement can be seen clearly, and the presence or absence of an arachnoid plane between the tumor and brain can also be seen. Extradural segments of the artery (ICA or VA) must be carefully examined for encasement and narrowing.

Cerebral angiography is a must in all patients with arterial encasement. All major vessels must be studied in order to evaluate the potential collateral sources, and the venous system should also be evaluated. In case of ICA encasement we perform angiography with ipsilateral CCA compression. This gives the surgeon some idea of collateral sources, to assess tolerance to temporary occlusion during a bypass procedure, and to decide about whether to use the ECA or ICA as a donor vessel.

Anesthesia, Monitoring, and Preparation

If a bypass procedure is a strong possibility, preoperative Duplex imaging of the radial arteries and saphenous veins and an Allen test of the hands are performed to choose the vessel that may be used for bypass. The patient receives aspirin 81 mg preoperatively. Intraoperative monitoring of electro encephalography (EEG), somatosensory evoked potentials (SSEP), and Motor evoked potentials (MEPs) are employed. If a bypass is performed, the anesthesiologist

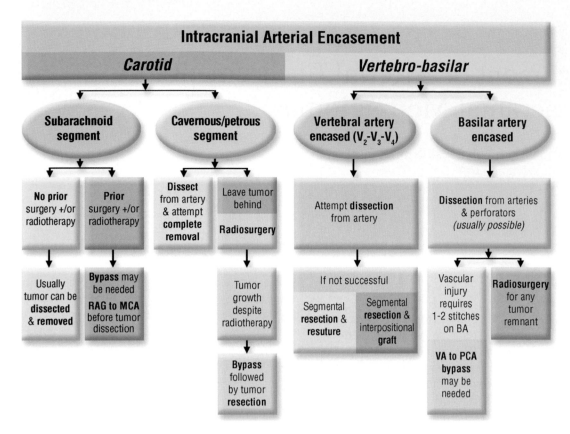

FIG. 62-1. Management algorithm for meningioma involving arteries

raises the patient's blood pressure by about 20% during temporary occlusion and places the patient in burst suppression with propofol to protect the brain. Approximately 4000–5000 units of heparin are also administered during the vascular occlusion. Epidural hemostasis must be excellent to prevent excessive oozing after heparinization. The heparin is not reversed at the end of the procedure.

Technique of Arterial Dissection

In dissecting a meningioma away from an artery, the following method is followed. The artery should be identified proximal to the encasement and/or distal to the encased segment. If possible, the tumor must be devascularized before dissection (not always possible). Gradual debulking and dissection are performed along a perforator-free surface of the artery at first. Further debulking and dissection then follow along the segment with perforators. (See case examples.)

Bypass Techniques

Radial artery graft (RAG) or Saphenous vein graft (SVG) is used for bypass, based on preoperative Duplex imaging. For tumor involving the ICA, ECA- or cervical ICA-to-MCA

bypass is preferred (Fig. 62-2). When the MCA vessels are small, the supraclinoid ICA may be used as a donor vessel (Fig. 62-3).

The cervical ICA is exposed in the neck. The tumor involving the cavernous sinus is exposed after a craniotomy and an orbital or orbitozygomatic osteotomy. After tumor inspection and, in some cases, after attempted removal of the tumor, a decision is made to proceed with the bypass. Accordingly, the radial artery (the entire artery from the brachial artery bifurcation to the anterior wrist) or the saphenous vein (in the upper leg and lower thigh) is removed, flushed with heparinized saline, and distended under pressure to relieve vasospasm. The patient is placed under burst suppression with propofol to protect the brain, the mean arterial pressure is raised 20% to improve collateral circulation, and the patient is given 3000–5000 units of heparin intravenously. The distal anastomosis is performed first to the MCA (M1 bifurcation or M_2 segment) or to the supraclinoid ICA. This is followed by the proximal anastomosis to the ECA (if collateral circulation is poor) or to the ICA (if some collaterals are present). If the flow through the grafts is satisfactory by Doppler/intraoperative angiography, then the cavernous ICA is trapped between clips. The operation is stopped at this stage. A postoperative angiogram is performed the next day.

For VA replacement, a RAG or saphenous vein interposition graft is employed. An extreme lateral retrocondylar or partial

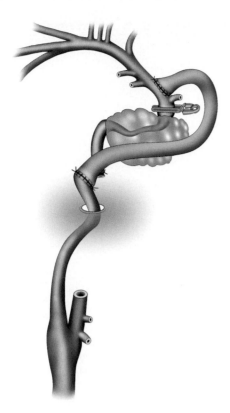

FIG. 62-2. Illustration showing supraclinoid ICA-to-MCA saphenous vein graft for a tumor involving the ICA

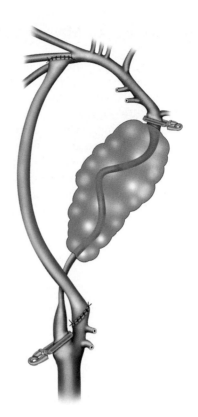

FIG. 62-3. Illustration showing ECA-to-MCA saphenous vein graft for a tumor involving the ICA

transcondylar approach is used. Proximal anastomosis to the VA is done at the level of C1–C2. If the distal anastomosis is distal to the PICA, then the PICA may be reimplanted, or a PICA to PICA anastomosis performed, or the PICA may be occluded if there is good collateral flow from the distal vessel.

For BA artery injury, VA- or ECA-to-PCA bypass is performed with RAG or saphenous vein graft. A temporal craniotomy with a zygomatic osteotomy or a petrosal approach is used for the exposure of the PCA. If temporal craniotomy is used, a spinal drain is needed to relax the brain. The P2 segment of the PCA is isolated for about 1.5 cm, and a rubber dam is placed under it. An arteriotomy to match the size of the graft is performed. The ends of the graft are anchored with 8-0 nylon. The superior edge is anastomosed first, then the graft is placed under the retractor and the inferior side of the anastomosis is completed. This is a difficult anastomosis due to the depth and usually takes about 50–60 minutes, but the temporary occlusion is usually well tolerated. The graft is tunneled to the ECA or VA proximally and anastomosed.

Staged Operations

When a bypass is performed, staged operations are usually preferred. Craniotomy, exposure osteotomies, and bypass are done during the first surgery, followed by tumor resection

in the second. This is because both aspirin and intravenous heparin are administered during the first operation, and tumor resection and repair of skull base may need extensive work on the same day. Exceptions are removal of tumors around the VA, which may require a short segmental bypass, and the removal of a small tumor, but with critical vascular encasement, which requires arterial bypass.

Postoperative Management and Complications

Graft occlusion may occur either during the operation or within the first 24 hours after surgery. If occlusion occurs during surgery, the problem is corrected. If the occlusion occurs postoperatively, the patient needs to be reoperated. Rarely endovascular thrombolysis can be done. Vasospasm occurs occasionally with radial artery grafts (despite the intraoperative pressure distention technique) and can be successfully treated by endovascular angioplasty.

The patients are maintained on oral aspirin 81 mg per day, and patients older than 40 years or with hypercholesterolemia are also placed on a statin. The patients are followed with CT angiography and/ or Duplex Doppler imaging with graft flow measurements.

Results of Bypasses for Meningiomas

Tables 62-1 through 62-3 show the total number of operations performed for meningiomas from 1992 to 2002 and the meningiomas in which bypass was performed in order to achieve resection. The results and complications are also outlined. There were three major complications—two patients suffered graft occlusion and strokes (other complications are listed in Table 62-3). One patient operated for previously operated and irradiated recurrent meningiomas had a caudate stroke with good recovery, but developed idiopathic thrombocytopenic purpura and died.

Illustrative Cases

Case 1

A 43-year-old female (Fig. 62-4) with a giant petroclival and cavernous sinus meningioma with severe brain stem compression underwent a subtotal resection of the tumor. This patient had a history of transient diplopia and facial numbness as well as some numbness involving the right side of the body. Frontotemporal craniotomy and a retrolabyrinthine transpetrosal approach were used to approach the tumor. The superior cerebellar artery (SCA) had two branches encased by the tumor, which were dissected free. There were two brain stem perforators densely adherent and partially encased just inferior to the SCA. These required very tedious and difficult dissection. The tumor was completely

TABLE 62-1. Patient Characteristics.

	Bypass	Cavernous sinus meningiomas
Number	82	496
Average age	43–39	47–50
Male:Female	20:58	144:352
Average tumor diameter	4.6 cm	3.3 cm
Prior treatment	20	108
Prior surgery	12	83
Prior radiotherapy	16	66

TABLE 62-2. Treatment Characteristics.

	Bypass patients	Total patients
Preop embolization	33	293
Preop Karnofsky score	78.5 ± 9.6	79.7 ± 9.5
Karnofsky score at 1 year	72.4 ± 14.2	79.8 ± 12.8
Recent Karnofsky score	75.8 ± 14.8	79.6 ± 13.6
Total operations	140	699
3 operations	6	32
2 operations	46	139
1 operation	30	325
Gross total resection	53 (64%)	203 (41%)
Subtotal resection	22 (27%)	139 (28%)
Partial resection	7 (9%)	154 (31%)

TABLE 62-3. Results for Patients with Bypasses.

Bypass Types and Outcome	Number
RAG	13
SVG	65
C/CCA-MCA	1
C/ECA-MCA	11
C/ICA-MCA	46
C/ICA-SC/ICA	7
P/ICA-SC/ICA	11
P/ICA-MCA	1
STA-MCA	1
VA-VA interposition	4
Lost to follow-up	5
NED	37
AWD	33
DOD	4
DOC	3
DOD	4
• Disease progression	24 months
• Preop wheelchair-bound, postop IX, X,XI palsy	7 months
• Disease progression	20 months
• Disease progression	23 months
DOC	3
• Postop GCS 3, Major stroke, Graft functioning	7 days
• Major stroke, graft occlusion, replacement SVG	27 months
• Major stroke, graft occlusion, replacement RAG	20 months
Other complications:	
New-onset CN palsy	15
Hydrocephalus	8
CSF leak	3
Infection	2
Other neurologic deficit	3

RAG, radial artery graft; SVG, saphenous vein graft; CCA, common carotid artery; ECA, external carotid artery; MCA, middle cerebral artery; STA, superficial temporal artery; NED, no evidence of disease; AWD, alive with disease; DOD, died of disease; DOC, died of complications; CN, cranial nerve; GCS, Glasgow Coma Scale.

removed from the clival dura. The posterior communicating artery was preserved. The basilar artery was completely dissected, and the tumor was gradually removed piecemeal in a complete fashion in this area. Tumor was left behind in the region of the Meckel's cave, around the 6th nerve and in the posterior part of the cavernous sinus (Fig. 62-5). This will be treated with radiosurgery. She has no postoperative neurologic deficits and required a ventriculoperitoneal shunt for hydrocephalus.

Case 2

In Figs. 62-6 through 62-9 a 41-year-old woman presenting with visual loss and a planum sphenoidale-sphenocavernous meningioma is seen. Preoperative angiography showed a severely narrowed intracavernous ICA with poor collaterals. After an ICA-to-MCA bypass graft with radial artery, a subtotal tumor resection was done, followed by Gamma Knife radiosurgery. She remains free of regrowth after 6 years.

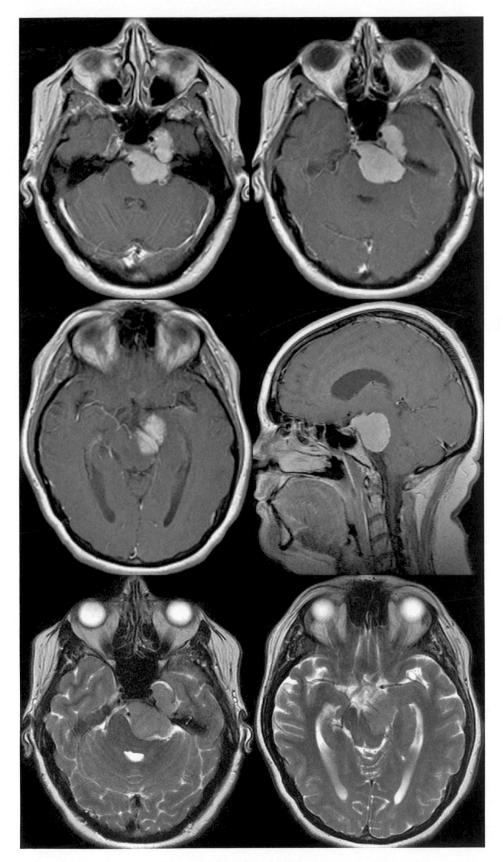

FIG. 62-4. Preoperative MRI images showing a giant petroclival and cavernous sinus meningioma with severe brain stem compression displacing and adherent to the basilar artery

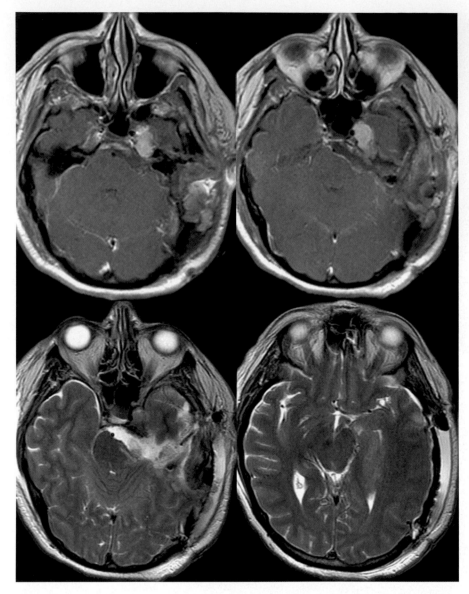

FIG. 62-5. Postoperative MRI images showing subtotal removal of the tumor with preservation of the basilar artery

Case 3

A 49-year-old male presented with a history of two previous partial resections of a basal meningioma involving the left cavernous sinus, which was followed by two Gamma Knife radiosurgery procedures. Despite these treatments, the tumor was growing recently (Fig. 62-10). The patient had a subtotal ophthalmoplegia on the left eye and also was losing vision in the left eye. Vision in the right eye was intact, although the tumor was compressing the optic chiasm and was also surrounding the pituitary gland area. Cerebral angiography revealed encasement of the CS-ICA and that collateral circulation was limited to the left hemisphere. We performed a saphenous vein graft bypass from the cervical ICA to supraclinoid ICA (Figs. 62-11 and 62-12). The tumor was then removed completely during a planned second-stage operation (Fig. 62-13). He had no complications after surgery, but he has a complete left ophthalmoplegia and has no vision in his left eye.

Case 4

A 47-year-old female presented with progressive growth of a cavernous sinus/parasellar meningioma (Figs. 62-14 to 62-18). Four years earlier, she underwent fractionated radiosurgery, which was not effective in stopping the tumor growth. Preoperatively, she had no vision and near-complete

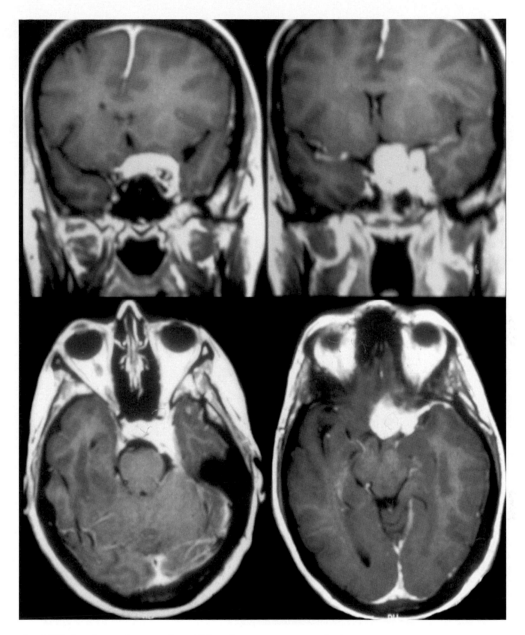

FIG. 62-6. Preoperative MRI showing a planum sphenoidale-sphenocavernous meningioma

ophthalmoplegia in her left eye and restricted opening of the mouth. She had encasement and narrowing of the internal carotid artery and an isolated left internal carotid artery circulation. She underwent radial artery graft bypass from the ECA to the MCA-M2 and a saphenous vein graft from the cervical ICA to a different and slightly larger branch of MCA-M2 segment followed by complete removal of the tumor. Cranial base reconstruction was performed with an abdominal fascia graft, fat graft, and a pericranial flap intracranially. A prophylactic transsphenoidal endoscopic packing of the left sphenoidal area was also performed because of the extent of the cranial base defect and prior radiotherapy. Postoperative imaging showed

complete removal of the tumor. She recovered well from the operation without new deficits.

Case 5

A 44-year-old female presented with a recurrent foramen magnum meningioma involving the right VA (Figs. 62-19 to 62-21). She had a prior resection of this tumor 3 years previously and had right hemiparesis postoperatively, which had improved with physiotherapy. She had recurrent attacks of hemiplegia due to recurrence of the tumor. The tumor was resected subtotally with a segment of the VA. An interposition

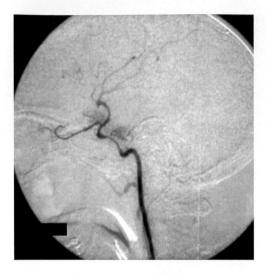

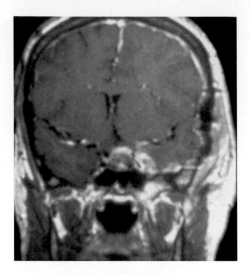

FIG. 62-7. Preoperative angiogram showing a severely narrowed cavernous ICA

FIG. 62-8. Postoperative image showing subtotal removal of the tumor

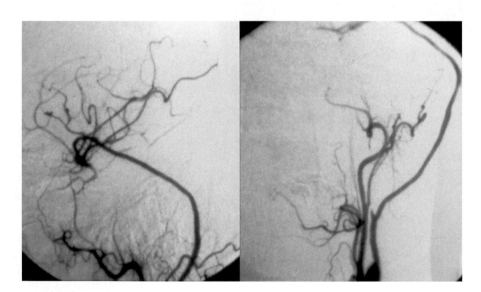

FIG. 62-9. Postoperative angiogram showing the saphenous vein graft from cervical ICA to supraclinoid ICA

SVG grafting was done. Subsequent Gamma Knife radiosurgery was performed.

Case 6

A 51-year-old female with a foramen magnum meningioma involving the right VA (Fig. 62-22) presented with headache, neck pain, hyperreflexia in both lower limbs, and partial right hypoglossal nerve palsy. She underwent gross total resection of the tumor with a segmental resection of 1.5 cm of the VA. The VA artery was sutured back by end-to-end anastomoses (Fig. 62-23).

Her tongue weakness improved slowly after surgery, but she had no other deficits after surgery. Postoperative imaging shows complete removal of the tumor and a patent right VA.

Future Trends

Because of the advent of Gamma Knife radiosurgery for meningiomas, far fewer meningiomas involving major vascular structures are being operated, and bypasses for these tumors have become rare. They may be used in future only for

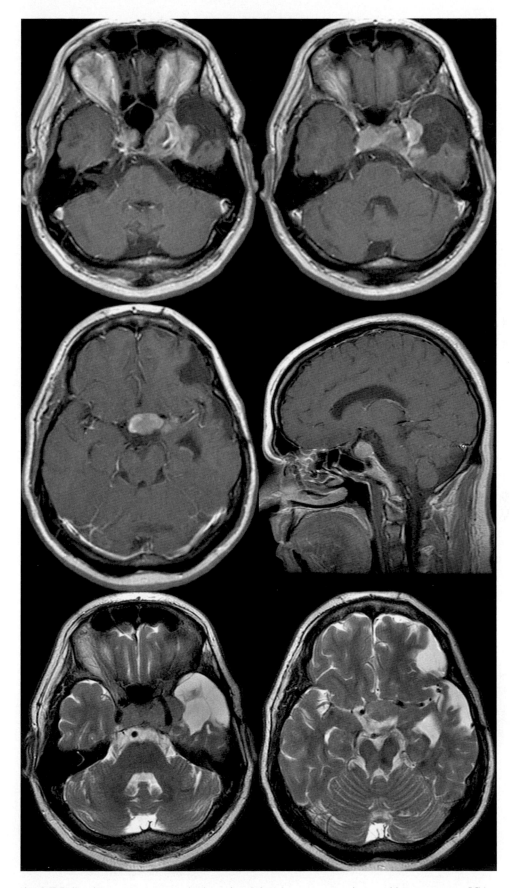

FIG. 62-10. Preoperative MRI showing a recurrent meningioma involving the cavernous sinus and intracavernous ICA

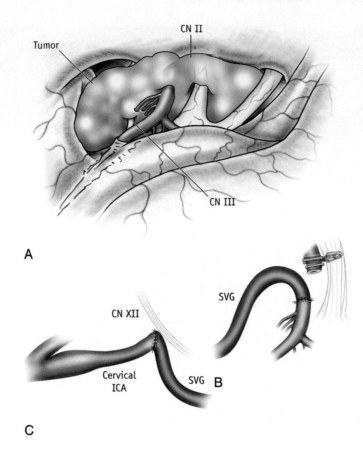

Fig. 62-11. Illustration showing tumor encasing the optic nerve and ICA (A), saphenous vein graft to supraclinoid ICA (B) from cervical ICA (C)

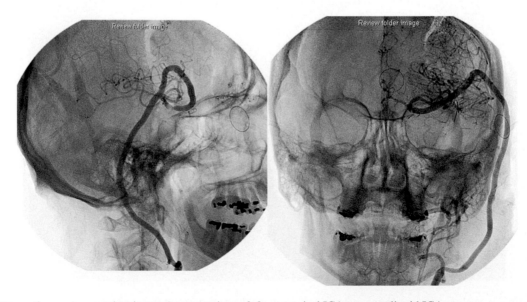

Fig. 62-12. Postoperative angiogram showing saphenous vein graft from cervical ICA to supraclinoid ICA

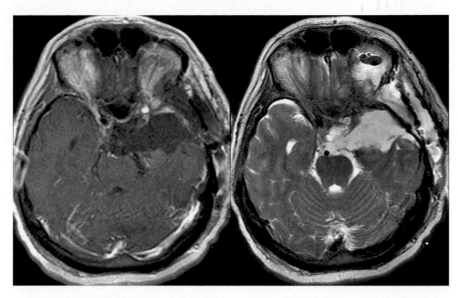

FIG. 62.13. Postoperative MRI showing complete removal of tumor

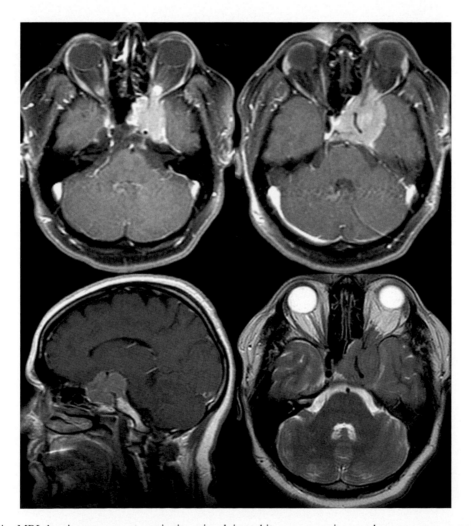

FIG. 62-14. Preoperative MRI showing a recurrent meningioma involving orbit, cavernous sinus, and supracavernous regions with encasement and narrowing of the internal carotid artery

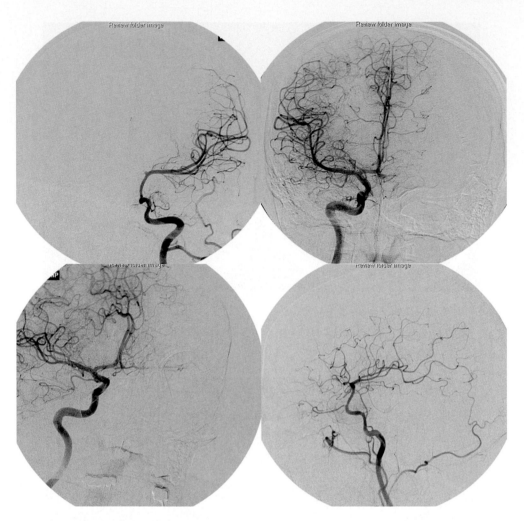

Fig. 62-15. Preoperative angiogram showing an isolated left anterior circulation

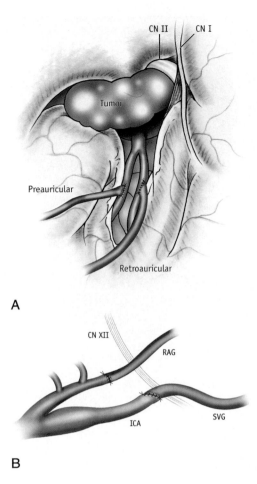

FIG. 62-16. Illustration showing radial artery graft bypass from the ECA to the MCA-M2 and a saphenous vein graft from the cervical ICA to a different branch of MCA-M2 segment

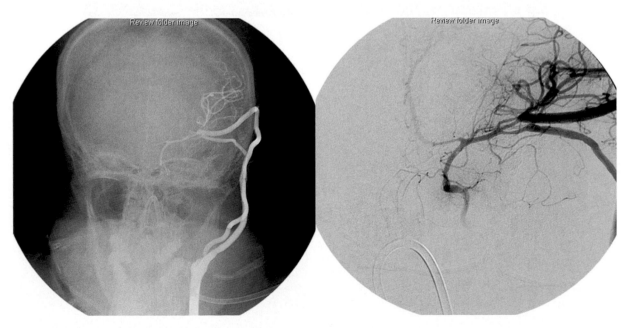

FIG. 62-17. Postoperative angiogram showing radial artery graft bypass from the ECA to the MCA-M2 and a saphenous vein graft from the cervical ICA to a different and slightly larger branch of MCA-M2 segment

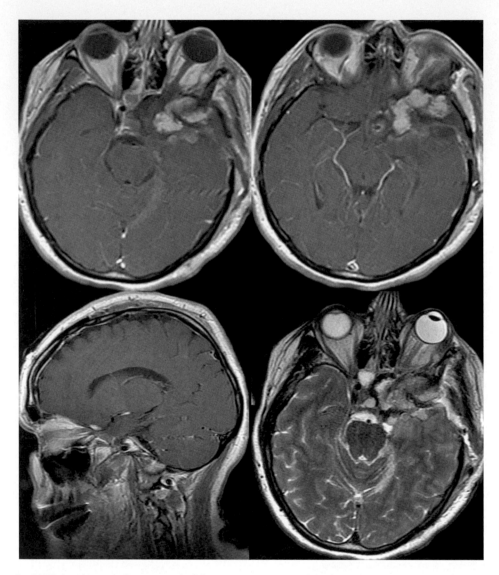

Fig. 62-18. Postoperative MRI showing complete removal of the tumor

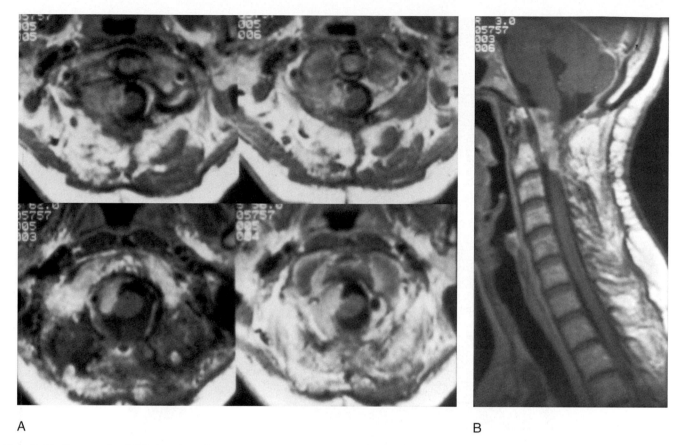

A

B

FIG. 62-19. Preoperative MRI showing a foramen magnum meningioma involving the right VA: (A) axial; (B) sagittal

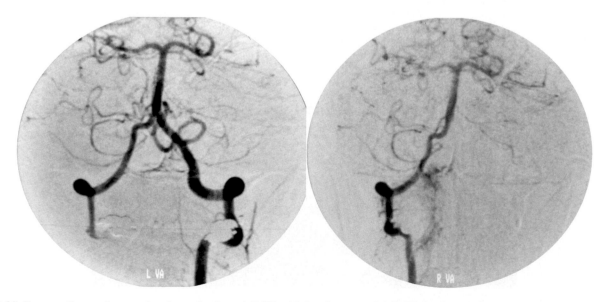

FIG. 62-20. Preoperative angiogram showing a dominant left VA with involvement of right VA by the tumor

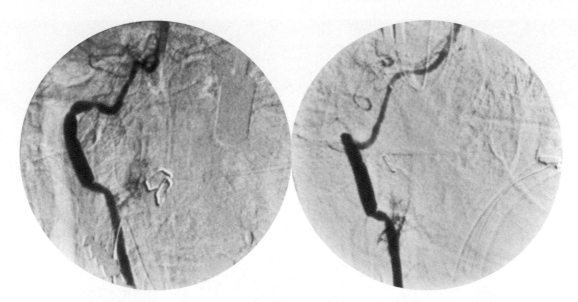

FIG. 62-21. Postoperative angiogram showing an interposition SVG in the right VA

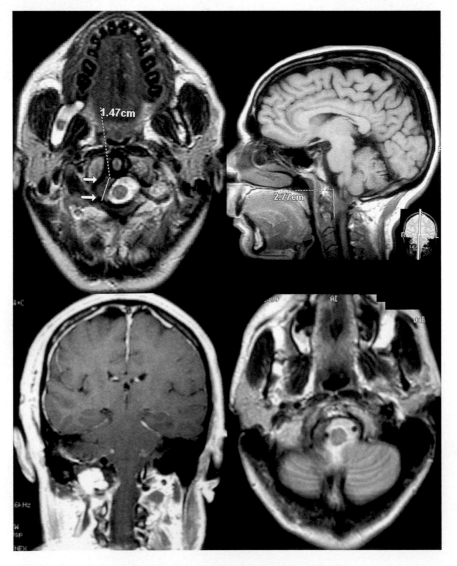

FIG. 62-22. Preoperative MRI showing a foramen magnum meningioma involving the right VA

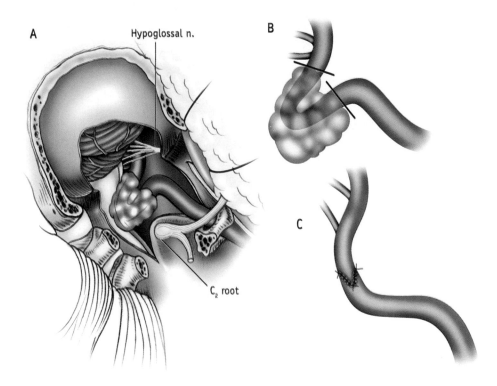

FIG. 62-23. Illustration showing the segmental resection of a short segment of the right VA and end-to-end anastomoses

recurrent meningiomas who failed radiation, as shown in our illustrative cases.

The techniques of bypass have greatly improved, and the senior author has seen a reduction of complications such as graft occlusion and strokes. Some problems occurred in our series in previously irradiated patients, and such patients constitute a high risk group for surgery.

References

1. De Jesus O, Sekhar LN, Parikh HK, et al. Long-term follow-up of patients with meningiomas involving the cavernous sinus: recurrence, progression, and quality of life. Neurosurgery 1996;39:915–919; discussion 919–920.

2. Kotapka MJ, Kalia KK, Martinez AJ, Sekhar LN. Infiltration of the carotid artery by cavernous sinus meningioma. J Neurosurg 1994;81:252–255.

3. Larson JJ, Tew JM, Jr., Tomsick TA, van Loveren HR. Treatment of aneurysms of the internal carotid artery by intravascular balloon occlusion: long-term follow-up of 58 patients. Neurosurgery 1995;36:26–30; discussion 30.

4. McIvor NP, Willinsky RA, TerBrugge KG, et al. Validity of test occlusion studies prior to internal carotid artery sacrifice. Head Neck 1994;16:11–16.

5. Origitano TC, al-Mefty O, Leonetti JP, et al. Vascular considerations and complications in cranial base surgery. Neurosurgery 1994;35:351–362; discussion 362–353.

6. Sekhar LN, Patel SJ. Permanent occlusion of the internal carotid artery during skull-base and vascular surgery: is it really safe? Am J Otol 1993;14:421–422.

63

Venous Reconstruction in the Management of Intracranial Meningiomas

Sabareesh Kumar Natarajan and Laligam N. Sekhar

Surgical treatment of intracranial meningiomas involving the major veins and dural sinuses poses a dilemma to the surgeon. Major cerebral veins are usually at risk during surgery for meningiomas that involve the displacement of the brain from the fixed drainage sites of the veins or when they are divided in order to approach a deep-seated lesion. Several publications have discussed the venous anatomy in exquisite detail(18,20,21,23–26).

Cerebral veins and venous sinuses have received adequate attention only recently, although they are very important to the neurosurgeon. When the venous outflow is compromised due to a lack of adequate collateral circulation, venous infarction follows, with swelling, hemorrhage, and neuronal death. The clinical consequences, which can often be disastrous, will depend upon the region and extent of involvement of the brain and size of the venous structure occluded. The symptoms may include seizures, hemiplegia, aphasia, coma, and death. The consequences of cerebral venous sinus occlusion also depend upon the availability of collateral circulation. When such collaterals are not available, papilledema and visual loss and a pseudotumor cerebri syndrome are observed in milder cases, whereas severe diffuse brain swelling, coma, and death may be observed in severe cases. Acute venous or venous sinus occlusion is potentially very dangerous, whereas slow and chronic venous or venous sinus occlusion is better tolerated. Even in such patients, some neurologic manifestations may follow when the collaterals are poor.

Imaging

Although it is uncommon nowadays to obtain cerebral angiography before operation on convexity meningiomas, it is prudent to do so before operating on parasagittal and falcine meningiomas. In some patients magnetic resonance angiography will be adequate to show the details. Magnetic resonance venography (MRV) is useful to observe the size of the sinus but is inadequate to discriminate between slow flow

and complete occlusion (Fig. 63-1) (3,6,15). Before operating on parasagittal meningiomas invading the sagittal sinus, angiography with bilateral internal carotid artery injection is necessary to determine if the sinus is occluded or patent. Before operating on large basal or deep seated meningiomas, particularly near the torcular, transverse, and sigmoid sinuses, vein of Labbé, straight sinus, or deep venous system, angiography with venous phase filming is equally important to provide imaging of the adjacent venous anatomy and collaterals. The next section describes our rationale and techniques to preserve and reconstruct cerebral veins and dural venous sinuses during tumor resection.

Cerebral Veins

Mechanism of Injury

Cerebral veins may be damaged by three mechanisms during operations, as shown in Table 63-1. Veins have thinner walls and are not as tortuous as arteries, allowing them less ability to be manipulated before rupture. These factors make the veins more liable to be damaged than arteries. Moreover, both basal and convexity operations stretch the veins and put them at risk for rupture, whereas arteries are stretched mainly during basal operations. The approaches where the veins can be in jeopardy are shown in Table 63-2.

Avoidance of Injury

To avoid its rupture, a cerebral vein should be stretched minimally either by minimizing the extent of brain retraction or by releasing it from adhesions to allow its lengthening.

With convexity operations, the dura mater must always be opened from a lateral-to-medial direction because a vein may drain into a dural venous lake in the paramedian area or be densely adherent to the convexity dura. In such cases, a small strip of dura mater is cut on either side initially along the vein to allow its preservation (Fig. 63-2). Subsequently,

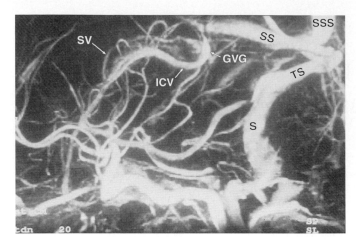

FIG. 63-1. Magnetic resonance venogram showing the different major intracranial veins. SSS, superior sagittal sinus; SS, straight sinus; SV, septal vein; ICV, internal cerebral vein; GVG, great vein of Galen; TS, transverse sinus; S, sigmoid sinus

TABLE 63-1. Mechanisms for Cerebral Venous Damage During Meningioma Surgery.

1. Intentional coagulation and division to prevent their rupture
2. Traction during an operation from their fixed drainage sites (into a dural sinus) causing their rupture
3. Damage during their dissection in the brain

it is possible to dissect some of the veins away from the dura mater under the microscope. Many convexity veins turn forward and are densely attached to the dura near the sagittal sinus for a short distance before they drain into the sinus (Fig. 63-3A). In such cases, the vein can be dissected away from the dura mater to allow its lengthening. In a similar fashion, the vein can be dissected away from the arachnoidal adhesions, and a small branch/tributary can be sacrificed to allow its lengthening (Fig. 63-3B).

In convexity parasagittal approaches, the brain retraction and the venous stretching must be kept to a minimum to prevent venous injury. In some cases, when the tumor is at a greater depth, the approach trajectory may have to be changed (Fig. 63-4A) to be distant from a major vein to prevent its damage. Other potential strategies include changing the approach side (e.g., right to left) and a small corticectomy (Fig. 63-4B–D).

With basal lesions, the veins at greatest risk for rupture are the temporal tip draining veins and the vein(s)

TABLE 63-2. Approaches Where Veins Can Be in Jeopardy.

1. Interhemispheric approach
2. Transcallosal approach
3. Subtemporal approach
4. Petrosal approach
5. Supracerebellar infratentorial approach

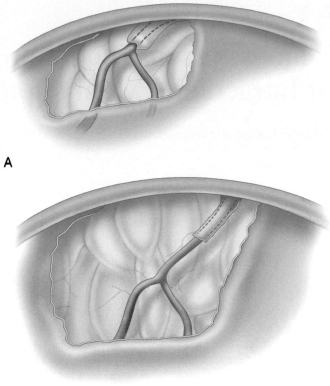

A

B

FIG. 63-2. (A) Dura has been opened, leaving a small leaf attached to an adherent or early draining vein. (B) Further dissection of the vein has been performed, leaving some dura around the dural sinus

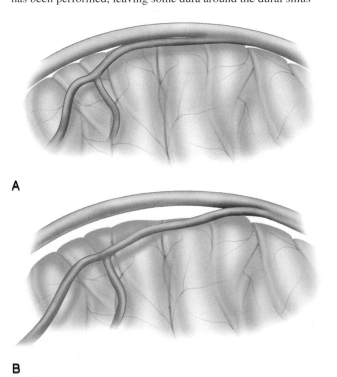

A

B

FIG. 63-3. (A) Illustrating how the convexity vein runs along the sinus before emptying into it. (B) Demonstrating the dissection of the vein away from the sinus, allowing its stretching

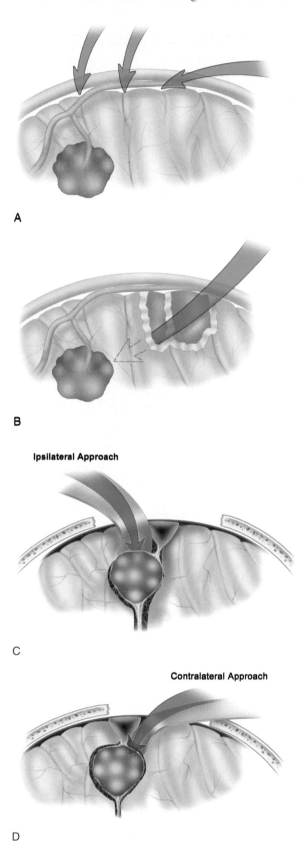

A

B

Ipsilateral Approach

C

Contralateral Approach

D

FIG. 63-4. (A) Modification of approach trajectory to minimize stretching of veins. (B) Small corticectomy for the same purpose. (C) Ipsilateral approach. (D) Contralateral approach

of Labbé. In these instances, the surgeon must be aware of any aberrant venous anatomy before surgery to avoid major problems. In the majority of patients, the temporal tip draining veins can be divided without adverse consequences. However, when the sylvian vein is very large, or if the vein of Labbé is absent due to prior surgery or is very small because of an anatomic variation, then it may not be safely occluded. In such a situation, a temporary clip can be placed on the concerned vein, and the brain is observed for swelling for 5–10 minutes. If the vein cannot be safely occluded, in many patients a change in the surgical approach or a small corticectomy will allow the operation to be performed.

The vein(s) of Labbé (Fig. 63-5) are at risk for injury during subtemporal and transpetrosal approaches (9,12, 14,17,20,25). There are considerable variations in the drainage site of the vein(s). In some patients, the vein may drain into the tentorium or the dura mater before draining into the transverse sinus. The partial labyrinthectomy petrous apicectomy transpetrosal approach, the translabyrinthine approach, and the total petrosectomy approach all move the surgeon anteriorly from the drainage point of the vein of Labbé. However, in some patients these strategies may not be enough to prevent excessive stretching of the vein. In some patients the tentorium may be divided with minimal brain retraction, and then the retractor can be placed on the tentorium rather than the temporal lobe to prevent venous stretching. When the vein is very large and dominant with a very anterior drainage site (Fig. 63-5B), then the surgical approach may have to be changed to the retrosigmoid (or retrosigmoid + orbitozygomatic with frontotemporal craniotomy) to prevent venous injury, especially on the dominant side.

Venous Reconstruction

The indications for venous reconstruction are shown in Table 63-3. In such patients, the easiest reconstruction may be by direct suture, using 8-0 nylon sutures. If the anastomosis is under tension, some of the tension can be released by dural mobilization. Direct repair is usually successful, even if the repaired vein is slightly stenotic. A segment of the vein may be missing in many patients, however, and the repair may be difficult without using a graft. In such patients, a segment of saphenous vein from the leg, or a vein from the forearm or the neck, or the radial artery may be used as an interposition graft (20).

Postoperative thrombosis is the main problem with venous reconstruction and may occur because of injury to the endothelium of the transplanted vein and the slow blood flow through the vein in general. To prevent this, we give the patients 4000 U of intravenous heparin during the reconstruction procedure, subcutaneous heparin during the first 7 postoperative days (5000 U q8h), and aspirin 325 mg daily thereafter for 2–3 months.

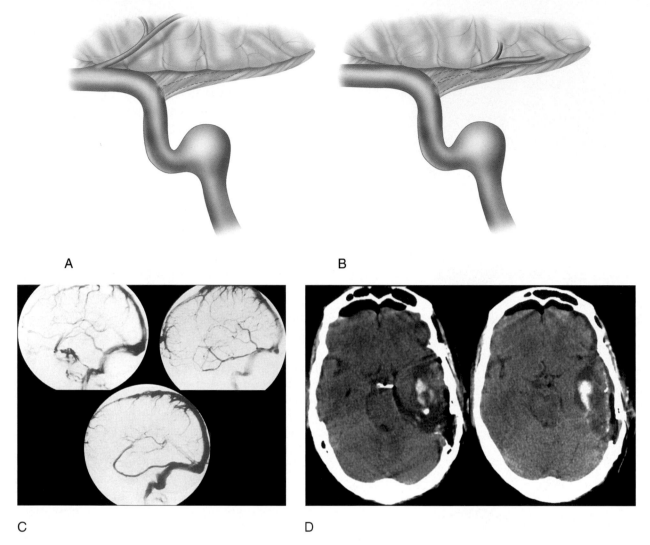

FIG. 63-5. (A) Normal type of vein of Labbé. (B) Very anteriorly draining vein of Labbé into a tentorial sinus. (C) Variation of anatomy of vein of Labbé seen in angiogram. (D) Postoperative venous infarction of the temporal lobe

TABLE 63-3. Indications for Venous Reconstruction During Meningioma Surgery.

1. In cases of accidental injury to large veins
2. If brain swelling is noted after the occlusion of a vein
3. After the injury to any deep vein

Cerebral Venous Sinuses

Cerebral venous sinuses transmit a large volume of venous blood from the brain. The patency of the venous sinuses is very important to preserve the functional integrity of the brain. The outcome of venous sinus occlusion depends upon the presence of collateral channels and the rapidity of occlusion. It is commonly believed that the anterior third of the sagittal sinus can be occluded without any significant damaging effect. But, in an occasional patient, such an occlusion may result in venous infarction in one or both frontal lobes. The only venous sinuses that may safely be occluded in most patients are the cavernous sinuses, the superior petrosal sinuses, and the nondominant collateralized transverse and sigmoid sinuses. Occlusion of the cavernous sinus can usually be performed without adverse effects on vision and the orbit due to the presence of many collateral drainage channels from the orbit.

Intraoperative Sinus Occlusion Test

During surgery, before occluding a sinus, a test occlusion must be performed (Fig. 63-6). To do this, the intrasinus pressure is measured by inserting a 20 gauge butterfly needle connected to a pressure transducer. The normal venous sinus pressure should be less than 15 mmHg, depending upon the position of

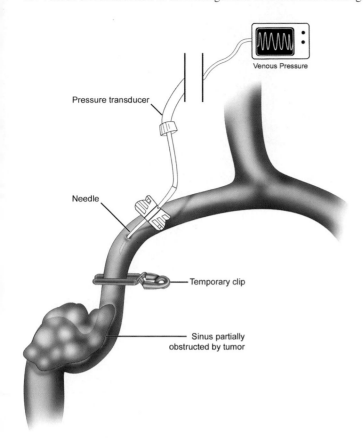

FIG. 63-6. Technique of inserting a butterfly needle into the sinus following placement of temporary clip to occlude the sinus

the head. After a stable reading has been obtained, a temporary clip is applied on the venous sinus at the appropriate segment of expected occlusion. Observation of the brain or cerebellum for swelling and of the evoked potentials and intrasinus pressure is performed for at least 5 minutes. Intrasinus pressure is the most sensitive indicator of the three, but cerebellar swelling may occur very quickly. If brain swelling occurs, evoked potentials change, or intrasinus pressure increases by more than 5 mmHg, then the temporary clip is removed, and the sinus cannot be occluded. If the initial intrasinus pressure was above 15 mmHg but there is not a significant increase in the pressure, the sinus may be occluded, but continuous monitoring of the pressure must be done during the rest of the operation because a delayed increase in intrasinus pressure may occur and necessitate reconstruction.

Preoperative occlusion tests of the venous sinuses are not safe because the clinical response is delayed, and the effects are not fully reversible. A balloon-occlusion test of the sinus was done in one patient in 1989. The patient was well for 8 minutes, but then became acutely comatose because of severe brain and cerebellar swelling. After deflation of the balloon, resection of part of the cerebellum and a ventriculostomy, the patient made a very slow recovery to an independent state. Because of this experience, we consider balloon occlusion testing of the sinus to be dangerous.

Reconstruction of Venous Sinuses

Direct Repair

When a small portion of the circumference of a venous sinus is involved by a meningioma, direct repair is recommended. In such patients, the tumor is excised, and the sinus is repaired with 5-0 prolene (Fig. 63-7) sutures either by direct suturing or with a patch of dura mater or saphenous vein.

In cases of sagittal sinus repair, the graft is sutured onto some of the sinus wall before removal of the tumor (Fig. 63-8A, B). After removal of the tumor, the sinus may be allowed to bleed if it is a small rent, occluded with finger pressure or temporary clips if some collaterals exist, or occluded with a balloon shunt if high flow exists through the sinus (Fig. 63-8C). If the repair is likely to take more than 10 minutes, then the patient will need to be heparinized.

When the sigmoid sinus is divided to improve the exposure of the tumor, direct repair may be performed with 6-0 prolene sutures.

Graft Reconstruction

Graft reconstruction of the sinus is performed in cases of total segmental defect (20), which cannot be repaired directly. The indications for such sinus repair are shown in Table 63-4. When the sinus to be repaired is large (≥1 cm diameter), the saphenous vein, extracted from the thigh, is used (Fig. 63-9). When the sinus has been previously partially occluded by the tumor, the radial artery is used because it tends to stay open even when the flow rate is low. To prevent vasospasm, the artery should be distended under pressure with heparinized saline (27). Because of the discrepancy in size, an end-to-side technique is used for radial artery grafts (Fig. 63-10), whereas an end-to-end technique is used for saphenous vein grafts.

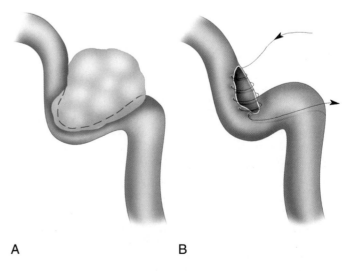

A   B

FIG. 63-7. (A, B) Direct repair of the sigmoid sinus after resection of a meningioma, which had encased the sinus

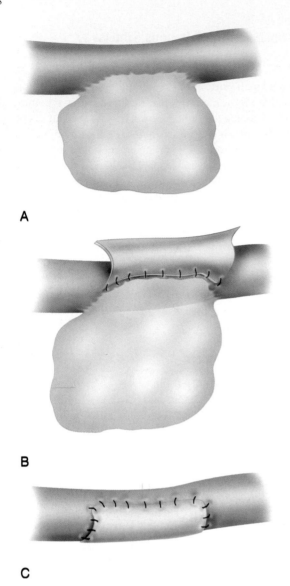

A

B

C

Fig. 63-8. Repair of a superior sagittal sinus by graft. (A) Tumor invading the sinus. (B) Part of the patch graft is sutured to the sinus wall with tumor in situ. (C) Patch graft sutured after tumor excision

Our Approach for Meningiomas Involving Cerebral Veins and Venous Sinuses

Results of cerebral venous and venous sinus reconstruction in the 6 years from 1993 to 1999 are shown in Table 63-5. The outcomes of multiple series which studied the outcomes of patients with meningiomas involving the major dural sinuses

TABLE 63-4. Indications for Reconstruction of Cerebral Venous Sinuses.

Status of collaterals	Decision
1. Excellent collaterals	Reconstruction unnecessary; provides practice for surgeons
2. Marginal collaterals	Reconstruction recommended
3. Poor or no collaterals	Occlusion dangerous; reconstruction if there is accidental injury

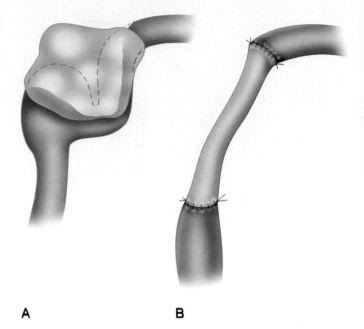

A   **B**

Fig. 63-9. (A) Tumor encased and invaded the sigmoid sinus to narrow the sinus. (B) Part of the sinus was resected along with the tumor, and an interposition graft (saphenous vein) was placed (end-to-end anastomoses)

have been summarized in Table 63-6. The principles that we follow in managing patients with meningiomas involving the cerebral veins and venous sinuses are as follows:

1. Meningiomas are treated only if they are symptomatic, even if they are found to involve the venous sinuses.

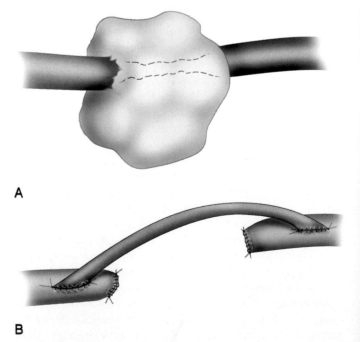

A

B

Fig. 63-10. (A) Tumor invading sinus. (B) Tumor resected with sinus and interposition graft (radial artery) placed (end-to-side anastomoses)

TABLE 63-5. Results of Venous Reconstruction from 1993 to 1999.

Type of vein/ Venous sinus reconstructed	No. of patients	No. of patients in which they are patent finally.
Cortical vein		
Resuture graft	1	1
SVG	1	1
RAG	1	1
Superior sagittalsinus		
SVG	2	2
Transverse sinus (pineal region)		
Division only	5	NA
Division + SVG	1	1
Sigmoid sinus-jugular vein		
Division + resuture	4	4
Repair after tumor excision	2	1
SVG	2	2

2. For symptomatic patients there are two options: radical resection with the involved sinus or conservative resection and radiosurgery. The decision to go ahead with radical resection involves the basic principles of any meningioma resection such as age, comorbidities, and regions involved, major vascular and cranial nerve involvement. Once a decision is made to do a radical resection with the sinus, the principles of whether reconstruction is required or not is followed as described above.

3. Peeling of the meningioma from the sinus is done if only one wall is involved and the wall is reconstructed as described above.

4. If more than one wall is involved, then resection of the sinus is done along with the tumor.

5. Even if the sinus is completely occluded on imaging, we do a sinus occlusion test and decide on whether the sinus has to be reconstructed.

6. We do all our cases in a supine or prone position and not in the sitting position

7. Radiosurgery has been used in some patients who had tumor left around the sinus in our series. Some patients were observed to have postradiation sinus occlusion and were managed appropriately.

Illustrative Cases

Case 1

A 58-year-old woman presented with facial pain and numbness caused by a right petroclival meningioma extending into the Meckel's cave and the cavernous sinus with mild brain stem compression (Fig. 63-11). The venous phase of the angiogram showed a prominent vein of Labbé (Fig. 63-12). The tumor was removed by a transpetrosal retrolabyrinthine approach. However, early in the operation, an aberrant vein of Labbé, draining the entire temporal lobe and draining into a dural sinus anterior to the transverse sinus, was damaged. Because significant temporal lobe swelling was noted, the vein of Labbé was reconstructed with a short saphenous vein graft from the vein to the sigmoid sinus (Fig. 63-13). A special technique of venous attachment to the sigmoid sinus was used without significant flow interruption by placing the attaching sutures first and then cutting the hole into the sinus before tying the sutures (Figs. 63-14 and 63-15). The tumor was seen to involve the trigeminal fascicles severely. The temporal lobe swelling resolved postoperatively, and the patient recovered well. Postoperatively, the patient had partial sixth cranial nerve palsy and diminished sensation in the V1 and V2 region and absent corneal reflex. Postoperative MRV and three-dimensional computed tomographic (CT) angiogram showed patency of the graft (Fig. 63-16). After a follow-up of 2 years there was no tumor recurrence. The sixth cranial nerve palsy has disappeared totally, but trigeminal loss persisted. The venous reconstruction was felt to be important in this patient in avoiding major problems.

TABLE 63-6. Literature Review of Meningiomas Involving Major Dural Sinuses and Reconstruction Procedure.

Series	Year	No. of cases	Recurrence rate (%)	Median follow-up (yr)	Mortality (%)
Hoessly et al. (10)	1955	196	6	5	12.3
Simpson (28)	1957	107	19	5	NA
Logue (16)	1975	91	11	NA	4.4
Bonnal and Brotchi (2)	1978	21	14	NA	4.7
Kropp et al. (13)	1978	96	16.6	7	NA
Yamashita et al. (30)	1980	80	14.6	5	NA
Chan and Thompson (5)	1984	16	13	NA	NA
Giombini et al. (8)	1984	243	17.7	5	NA
Mirimanoff et al. (19)	1985	38	24	10	NA
Jaaskelainen (11)	1986	136	8	NA	NA
Philippon et al. (22)	1986	153	14.4	10	NA
Baird & Gallagher (1)	1989	46	23.9	NA	NA
DiMeco et al. (7)	2004	108	13.9	13	2
Caroli et al. (4)	2006	328		25	
Sindou et al. (29)	2006	100	4	8	3

NA: Not available.

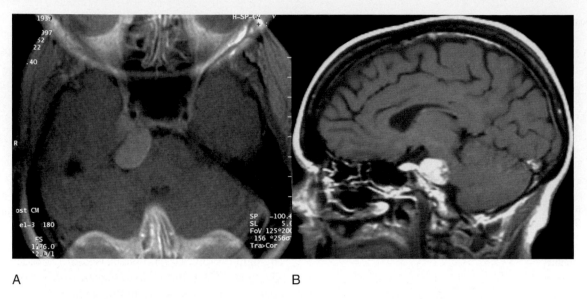

A   B

FIG. 63-11. (A) Axial and (B) sagittal contrast-enhanced T1 image of a magnetic resonance imaging scan showing the petroclival meningioma in Case 1

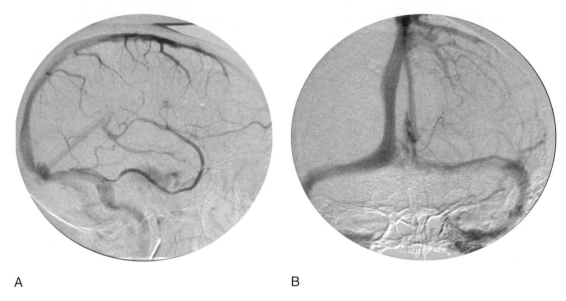

A   B

FIG. 63-12. (A, B) Venous phase of angiogram showing prominent vein of Labbé and dominance of the right lateral sinus

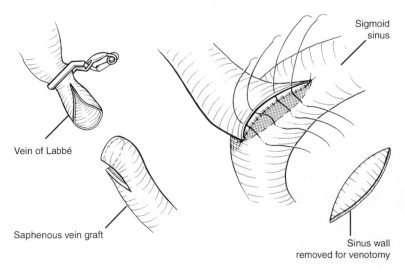

FIG. 63-13. Diagrammatic representation of the vein graft technique. Fish-mouth opening is made in the vein as well as in the graft to reduce the amount of stenosis later on. Also, a part of the sinus wall was removed

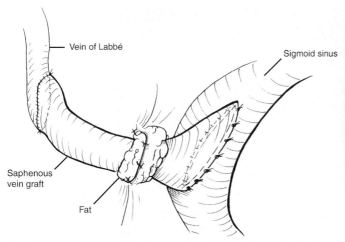

FIG. 63-14. Diagrammatic representation of the vein graft technique. The anastomosis is completed, and a pad of fat supports the graft

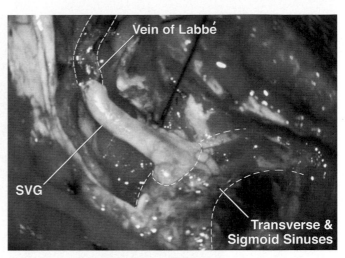

FIG. 63-15. Operative picture of the completed anastomosis. The arrow points to the saphenous vein graft (SVG)

Case 2

A 46-year-old man presented with a history of mental deterioration and gait ataxia. Magnetic resonance imaging scan showed a giant pineal region meningioma compressing the brain stem severely and producing hydrocephalus (Fig. 63-17). An arteriogram (Fig. 63-18) in the venous phase showed good collateralization of the two transverse sinuses and the nondominance of the left side. The lesion was initially approached by a supracerebellar infratentorial approach, with the patient in a sitting position, but this was difficult and found to be inadequate for tumor resection. The patient was reoperated on by a combined approach (occipital, transtentorial, supracerebellar, transsinus approach) in a semi-prone position. The transverse sinus was clipped, and the pressure was measured. The intrasinus pressure before clipping was 8 mmHg and after clipping was 9 mmHg. The sinus was transected between two temporary clips. The tumor was debulked, and the capsule of the tumor was dissected away from the brain stem and the encased veins. The transverse sinus was resutured with 5–0 Prolene. The postoperative recovery was good, and after a follow-up of 61 months the patient had no neurologic deficits, and there was no recurrence of the tumor (Fig. 63-19). (In this patient, the reconstruction of the

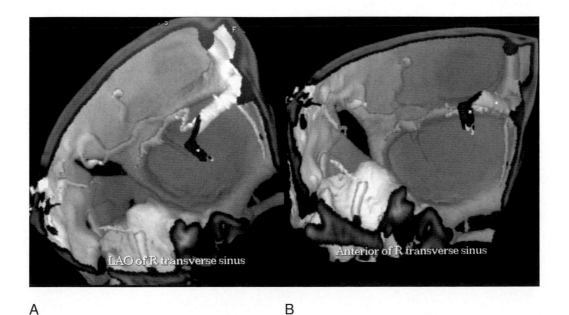

A   B

FIG. 63-16. (A, B)Three-dimensional computed tomographic angiogram of Case 1 showing a patent graft and sinus

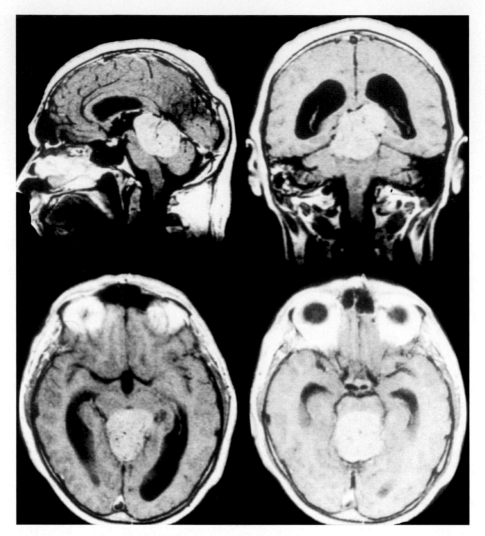

Fɪɢ. 63-17. Preoperative sagittal, coronal, and axial enhanced T1 magnetic resonance imaging scans of Case 2 showing a pineal region tumor compressing the brain stem, producing hydrocephalus

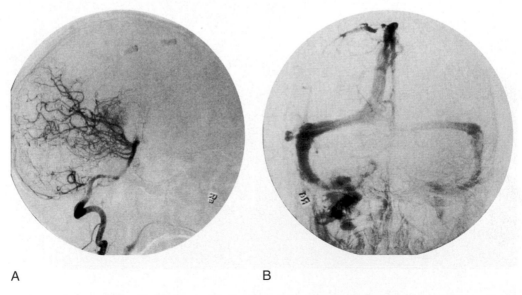

A   B

Fɪɢ. 63-18. Preoperative angiogram of Case 2. (A) Tumor blush, although no major supplies from the posterior cerebral artery (PCA). (B) Venous phase showing good collateralization of the two lateral sinuses and the dominance of the right sinus

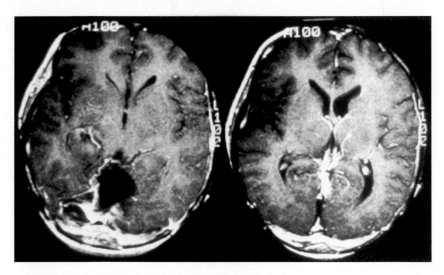

FIG. 63-19. Postoperative enhanced axial T1 image of MRI scan showing complete tumor removal of Case 2

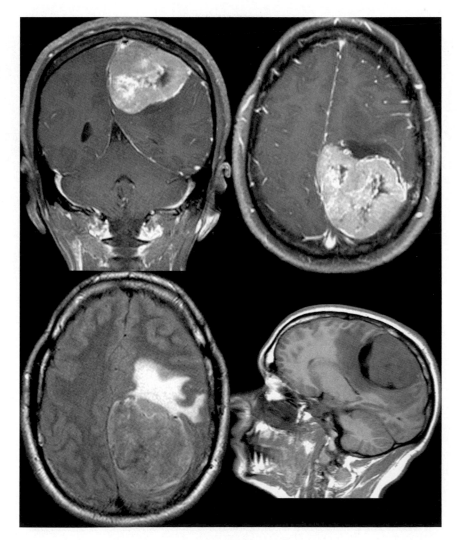

FIG. 63-20. Preoperative MRI of Case 3 showing a meningioma involving the sagittal sinus

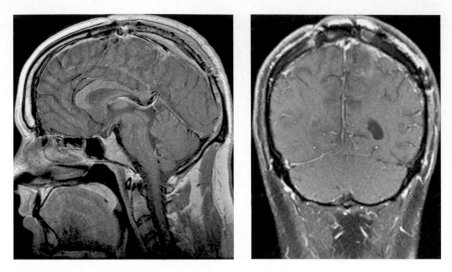

FIG. 63-21. Postoperative MRI of Case 3 showing complete removal of the tumor and preservation of the sagittal sinus

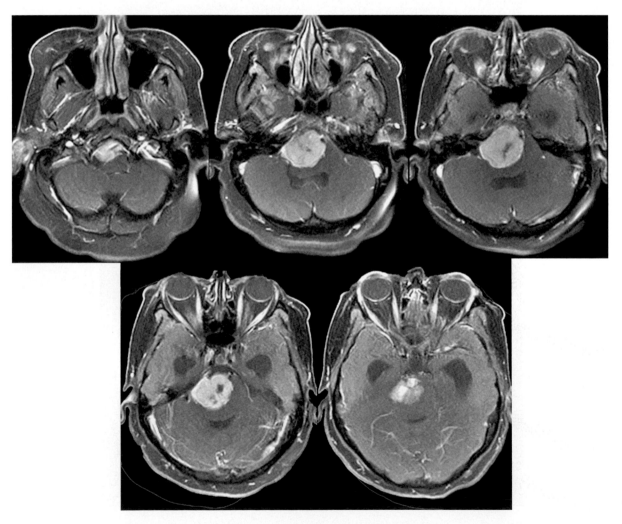

FIG. 63-22. Preoperative MRI of Case 4 showing a large petroclival tumor with edema on the pons

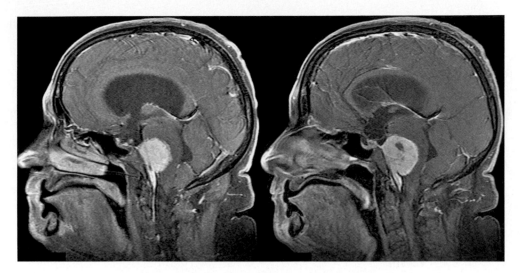

FIG. 63-22. (continued)

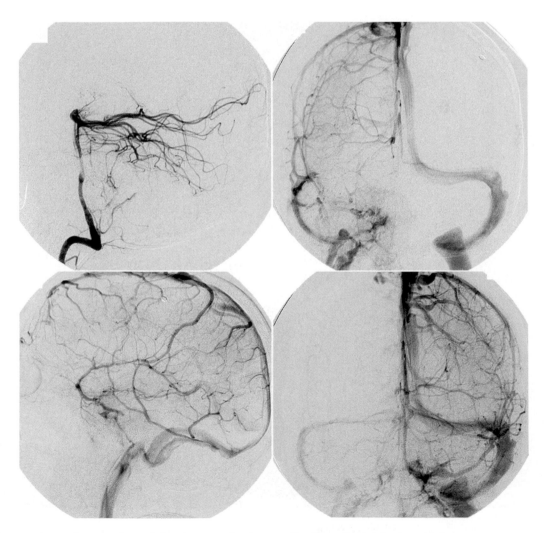

FIG. 63-23. Preoperative angiogram of case 4 showing a nondominant well-collateralized right sigmoid sinus

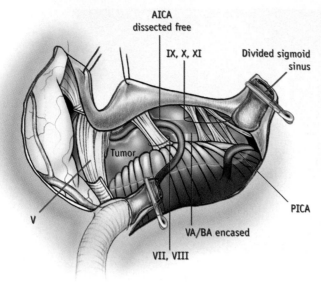

Fig. 63-24. Illustration showing relation of the tumor to cranial nerves and division of the sigmoid sinus

sinus was mainly to preserve both sinuses for the future and was not mandatory.)

Case 3

In Figures 63-20 and 63-21, a 31-year-old male who had episodes of numbness on his right side and siezures, in whom magnetic resonance demonstrated a left-sided large meningioma involving the sagittal sinus and pushing on the parietal lobe, is seen. There was a small area where the tumor invaded into the sagittal sinus, and, upon removal of the tumor in this area, there was frank breach of the sagittal sinus by the tumor. The hole in the sagittal sinus was closed primarily with 6-0 nylon. After the surgery he has no deficits or seizures. Postoperative imaging showed complete removal of the tumor.

Case 4

In Figures 63-22 through 63-25 , a 54-year-old female with a large petroclival tumor with edema on the pons is shown. The basilar artery was displaced and compressed but not encased.

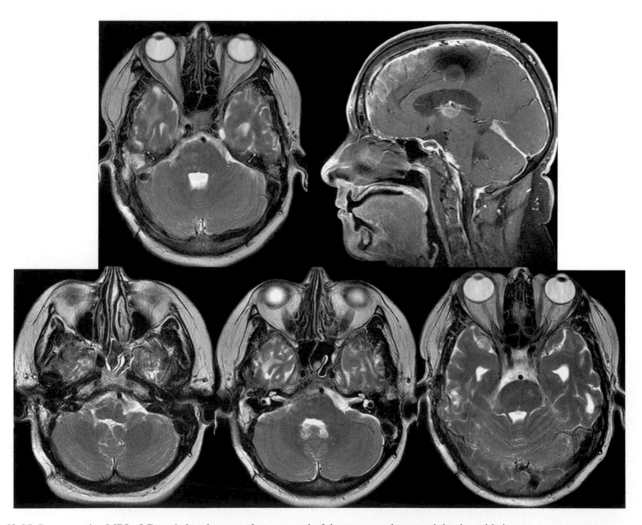

FIG. 63-25. Postoperative MRI of Case 4 showing complete removal of the tumor and patent right sigmoid sinus

She presented with gradually deteriorating vision in the left eye and progressive deterioration of mental function. A presigmoid, retrosigmoid, and subtemporal approach was used. Temporary clips were placed across the nondominant but well-collateralized right sigmoid sinus. There was no brain swelling observed, nor were there any changes in the evoked potentials. Therefore, the sinus was divided between temporary clips. At the conclusion of tumor resection, the sigmoid sinus was repaired using 6-0 Prolene sutures. Postoperative imaging showed complete removal of the tumor and a patent sigmoid sinus.

References

1. Baird M, Gallagher PJ: Recurrent intracranial and spinal meningiomas: clinical and histological features. Clin Neuropathol 1989;8:41–44.
2. Bonnal J, Brotchi J: Surgery of the superior sagittal sinus in parasagittal meningiomas. J Neurosurg 1978;48:935–945.
3. Bozzao A, Finocchi V, Romano A, et al.: Role of contrast-enhanced MR venography in the preoperative evaluation of parasagittal meningiomas. Eur Radiol 2005;15:1790–1796.
4. Caroli E, Orlando ER, Mastronardi L, Ferrante L: Meningiomas infiltrating the superior sagittal sinus: surgical considerations of 328 cases. Neurosurg Rev 2006;29:236–241.
5. Chan RC, Thompson GB: Morbidity, mortality, and quality of life following surgery for intracranial meningiomas. A retrospective study in 257 cases. J Neurosurg 1984;60:52–60.
6. Deda H, Erden I, Yagmurlu B: Evaluation of petrosal sinus patency with 3-dimensional contrast-enhanced magnetic resonance venography in petroclival meningiomas for surgical strategy. Surg Neurol 2005;64(Suppl 2):S67–71.
7. DiMeco F, Li KW, Casali C, et al.: Meningiomas invading the superior sagittal sinus: surgical experience in 108 cases. Neurosurgery 2004;55:1263–1272; discussion 1272–1264.
8. Giombini S, Solero CL, Lasio G, Morello G: Immediate and late outcome of operations for Parasagittal and falx meningiomas. Report of 342 cases. Surg Neurol 1984;21:427–435.
9. Guppy KH, Origitano TC, Reichman OH, Segal S: Venous drainage of the inferolateral temporal lobe in relationship to transtemporal/transtentorial approaches to the cranial base. Neurosurgery 1997;41:615–619; discussion 619–620.
10. Hoessly GF, Olivecrona H: Report on 280 cases of verified parasagittal meningioma. J Neurosurg 1955;12:614–626.
11. Jaaskelainen J, Haltia M, Servo A: Atypical and anaplastic meningiomas: radiology, surgery, radiotherapy, and outcome. Surg Neurol 1986;25:233–242.
12. Koperna T, Tschabitscher M, Knosp E: The termination of the vein of "Labbe" and its microsurgical significance. Acta Neurochir (Wien) 1992;118:172–175.
13. Kropp F, La Motta A, Landucci C, et al.: Recurrence of parasagittal meningioma after surgical treatment. Rev Neurobiol 1978;24:236–242.
14. Kyoshima K, Oikawa S, Kobayashi S: Preservation of large bridging veins of the cranial base: technical note. Neurosurgery 2001;48:447–449.
15. Lee JM, Jung S, Moon KS, et al.: Preoperative evaluation of venous systems with 3-dimensional contrast-enhanced magnetic resonance venography in brain tumors: comparison with time-of-flight magnetic resonance venography and digital subtraction angiography. Surg Neurol 2005;64:128–133; discussion 133–124.
16. Logue V: Parasaggital meningiomas. Adv Techn Stand Neurosurg 1975;2:171–198.
17. Lustig LR, Jackler RK: The vulnerability of the vein of labbe during combined craniotomies of the middle and posterior fossae. Skull Base Surg 1998;8:1–9.
18. Matsushima T, Suzuki SO, Fukui M, et al.: Microsurgical anatomy of the tentorial sinuses. J Neurosurg 1989;71:923–928.
19. Mirimanoff RO, Dosoretz DE, Linggood RM, et al.: Meningioma: analysis of recurrence and progression following neurosurgical resection. J Neurosurg 1985;62:18–24.
20. Morita A, Sekhar LN: Reconstruction of the vein of Labbe by using a short saphenous vein bypass graft. Technical note. J Neurosurg 1998;89:671–675.
21. Oka K, Rhoton AL Jr., Barry M, Rodriguez R: Microsurgical anatomy of the superficial veins of the cerebrum. Neurosurgery 1985;17:711–748.
22. Philippon J, Bataini JP, Cornu P, et al.: Recurrent meningioma. Neurochirurgie 1986;32 Suppl 1:1–84.
23. Rhoton AL Jr.: The posterior fossa veins. Neurosurgery 2000;47: S69–92.
24. Rhoton AL Jr.: The cerebral veins. Neurosurgery 2002;51: S159–205.
25. Sakata K, Al-Mefty O, Yamamoto I: Venous consideration in petrosal approach: microsurgical anatomy of the temporal bridging vein. Neurosurgery 2000;47:153–160; discussion 160–151.
26. Schmidek HH, Auer LM, Kapp JP: The cerebral venous system. Neurosurgery 1985;17:663–678.
27. Sekhar LN, Duff JM, Kalavakonda C, Olding M: Cerebral revascularization using radial artery grafts for the treatment of complex intracranial aneurysms: techniques and outcomes for 17 patients. Neurosurgery 2001;49:646–658; discussion 658–649.
28. Simpson D: The recurrence of intracranial meningiomas after surgical treatment. J Neurol Neurosurg Psychiatry 1957;20:22–39.
29. Sindou MP, Alvernia JE: Results of attempted radical tumor removal and venous repair in 100 consecutive meningiomas involving the major dural sinuses. J Neurosurg 2006;105:514–525.
30. Yamashita J, Handa M, Iwaki K: Recurrence of intracranial meningiomas with special reference to radiotherapy. Surg Neurol 1980;33–40.

64
Dural Reconstruction in Meningioma Surgery

Joung H. Lee and Burak Sade

Introduction

When it comes to dural reconstruction following meningioma surgery (or following any neurosurgical procedure), there are two schools of thought and practice. One is the "watertight" closure, and the other, which is less popular in practice, the nonwatertight closure. The practice of dural closure, like many surgical techniques and applications, is largely based on personal experiences of the individual surgeons, shaped by training passed down from senior residents and mentors, and repeated generations after generations. In this chapter we present a brief review of different dural reconstruction techniques, in addition to our personal experience with synthetic on-lay dural graft technique.

Watertight Closure

Often, we simply do something just because that is how we were taught, and, as in the case of watertight dural closure, it became a universal dogma without significant scientific basis.

A fundamental element of the watertight dural reconstruction is the use of suturing. Megyesi and colleagues developed an in vitro model, where they tested different suturing techniques in providing watertight closure of the dura (13). They compared the efficacy of the interrupted simple, running simple, running locked, and interrupted vertical mattress sutures on primary closure of linear incisions and closure of dural defects using rectangular grafts. Their results showed superiority of interrupted simple suture on primary closure of linear incisions over other techniques listed above. In the cases where dural grafts were used, no single suturing technique proved to be superior over others tested. Overall, sutured linear incisions were more resistant to leak than dural patches. In the literature, the emphasis on watertight closure has been strong to the point that special techniques have been developed and proposed to reach difficult areas in order to achieve optimal dural reconstruction (26).

However, one potential risk of using primary suture closure would be to create pinholes from the suture needle (18). In an attempt to achieve watertight closure, holes created on either side of the dura or the dural substitute may commonly lead to cerebrospinal fluid (CSF) leakage. The attempted "tight" closure results in somewhat of a "one-way valve" along the suture line, causing the leaked fluid (from postoperative coughing, for example) to accumulate outside of the dura. On the other hand, when the dura is not closed in a watertight fashion, in the absence of underlying hydrocephalus, the leaked CSF has a chance to flow back into the intradural space, preventing accumulation of extradural CSF collection.It has also been described that once leak has established either through the needle hole, or through the incision line in between sutures, the pressure needed for it to continue is less than the opening pressure, because the initial pressure stretches the suture holes and line (13). In addition, while implanting synthetic graft materials, dural tearing may be caused by the sutures themselves because of the elastic properties of these grafts which exert traction on the sutures (14). It is probably because of these factors that studies have shown up to sevenfold more favorable rates of effective dural closure when suture repair is augmented by tissue adhesives (3,14,16).

Dural Grafts

Use of dural grafts has been a common neurosurgical practice, especially when primary closure is not possible. This is of significance particularly in meningioma surgery (i.e., convexity meningiomas), where the removal of a large piece of dura along with the tumor to achieve a Simpson grade I or II resection results in a sizable defect that requires grafting.

There has been a consensus in the literature with regard to the qualities of an ideal dural graft material. An ideal graft would provoke no inflammation in the host body and show no neurotoxicity and adhesion to the underlying brain. At the same time it would be easily available and inexpensive; durable, yet flexible, and easily prepared and shaped. Ideally, at the same time it would be rapidly resorbed, allowing the endogenous connective tissue to build up. Additionally, while providing adequate protection for the underlying brain, it should ensure watertight closure.

Since the late nineteenth century, when rubber (1) and gold leaf (2) were described as dural substitutes, various materials have been proposed during different time periods, such as amniotic membrane in the 1940s (21) and lyophilized human cadaveric dura in the 1950s (23). It may be practical to classify the contemporary dural substitutes as autografts (i.e., fascia latae, temporalis fascia), allografts (i.e., amniotic and placental membranes, pericardium, fascia, lyophilized dura), xenografts (i.e., bovine or porcine pericardium, peritoneum, dermis), and synthetic materials (i.e., polytetrafluoroethylene [PTFE], polyester urethane) (28). However, each material poses certain disadvantages that limit their usage. For instance, the fascia latae, which is widely used, and which may in most aspects appear as an ideal dural graft (24), requires a second incision, thereby introducing another source for potential morbidity. Availibility becomes a concern for other autografts that are accessible through the same incision such as the pericranium and temporalis fascia, especially when a large extent of graft is required. The most common limitations have been immunogenic reactions and risk of transmitting prion-related diseases for allografts; increased immunogenic reactions for xenografts; and difficult handling and poor sealing qualities of synthetic materials (10,25,28). However, one has to note that all of these materials are developed to ensure a watertight closure and require suturing to the endogenous dura.

Nonwatertight Dural Reconstruction with Collagen Matrix

Recently, there has been an interest in processing tissues with high connective tissue components such as pericardium and dermis to yield an acellular, antigen-free scaffold for growing endogenous tissue (10).

In our practice, we use collagen matrix (DuraGen, Integra Neurosciences, Plainsboro, NJ) for dural reconstruction in the majority of meningioma cases where dural augmentation is required. This material is made up of type I collagen and is processed from bovine Achilles tendon. The collagen matrix provides a low-pressure absorptive surface to diffuse CSF and attaches to the dural surface via surface tension (18). It also helps clot formation by the platelets depositing themselves on the collagen, which then disintegrate and release clotting factors, ultimately facilitating fibrin formation (10). This fibrin has an important role in holding the graft in place until fibroblasts, associated with blood vessels, proliferate into the graft (17). This fibroblast infiltration starts by day 3–4 and becomes established in 10–14 days. The fibroblasts use the pores on the matrix to lay down endogenous collagen. By 6–8 weeks, the collagen matrix is resorbed and is integrated to the endogenous dura (18).

The nonwatertight reconstruction of the dura using the collagen matrix simply consists of the onlay application of the material over the dura. It is easily shaped and has the main advantage of not requiring any suturing. In the study of Danish and colleagues, in which suturable acellular human dermis use was compared to collagen matrix, the operative time was significantly lower (36 min) with the use of the collagen matrix, and similar rates of pseudomeningocele formation, wound infection, and CSF leak were reported (6). This technique has proven to be at least as effective as other techniques described in the literature in the management of dural reconstruction in spinal surgery as well (18).

As described above, the collagen matrix is incorporated in the endogenous tissue in a relatively short period of time and in 24 weeks becomes barely distinguishable from the endogenous dura, unlike the allogenic cadaveric dura, which shows inadequate fusion with the endogenous dura and in addition becomes encapsulated in a connective tissue layer (10). This encapsulation has also been described for synthetic materials (22), which appears not to be an ideal situation with regard to the sealing quality of the material. It has also been shown that the compact structure of the xenogenic materials may limit the fibroblast migration to the edges or to the suture holes (20).

In addition, the collagen, in the form of sponge, can absorb fluid without increasing its volume, and can act as a moistening agent for the brain, allowing penetration of CSF into the graft (11). It also forms an effective separation layer and minimizes adhesions between the brain and the overlying tissue.

Nonwatertight Dural Reconstruction in Meningioma Surgery

In our series, since the material was available to us in February 2000, dural reconstruction was performed using the collagen matrix in 237 patients with meningioma until December 2005. The most common location of the tumor was the convexity in 69 patients (29.1%). The patient distribution according to tumor location is shown in Table 64-1. Of the 237 patients, 26 (11%) had previous surgery and 6 (2.5%) had radiation treatment. In 5 patients (2.1%) the closure was additionally reinforced by a pericranial flap, and in 4 patients (1.7%) with anterior fossa meningiomas, abdominal fat graft was used. In 7 patients (3%), acrylic cranioplasty was performed, and in 4 patients (1.7%), titanium mesh was used as a substitute for the bone flap.

CSF leak occurred in 1 patient (0.4%), and 2 patients (0.8%) experienced graft-related complications: namely, chemical meningitis, cerebritis, and accumulation of reactive extra-axial fluid. No patient had persistent subcutaneous CSF collection or pseudomeningocele that required a second intervention.

TABLE 64.1. Number of Meningiomas According to Location in 237 Patients who Underwent Duraplasty with DuraGan.

Location	Number	Incidence (%)
Convexity	69	29.1
Parasagittal	23	9.7
Clinoidal	22	9.2
Anterior fossa	22	9.2
Falcine	20	8.4
Middle/Lateral sphenoid	18	7.6
Tuberculum sellae	15	6.3
Tentorial/Torcular	14	5.9
Orbitosphenoid	11	4.6
Cavernous sinus	8	3.4
Foramen magnum	4	1.7
Cerebellar convexity	4	1.7
Other	7	3

Case 1

The only patient who experienced postoperative CSF leak was a 47-year-old female, who was operated on for a foramen magnum meningioma through a far-lateral transcondylar approach. She was discharged home on the postoperative day 3. On postoperative day 9, when her sutures were removed, CSF leak was observed through a tiny pinhole over the corner of the hockey stick incision, although the rest of the incision showed satisfactory healing. The hole was immediately resutured and was followed for another 9 days, after which the suture was removed and the patient did not experience any other problems.

The incidence of postoperative CSF leak is quite satisfactory (0.4%) in our series using the nonwatertight reconstruction technique. It is our belief that regardless of the dural reconstruction technique, meticulous closure of the subsequent layers may actually play a more critical role in the prevention of postoperative CSF leak from the wound.

Case 2

A 53-year-old female was operated on for a right frontal convexity meningioma (Fig. 64-1A). Simpson grade II resection was performed with a small piece of dura involved by the tumor being left by the sagittal sinus. The dural defect was then reconstructed using an onlay piece of commercially available collagen matrix. The patient was discharged home under satisfactory conditions with her magnetic resonance imaging (MRI) confirming total resection and postsurgical changes on postoperative day 2 (Fig. 64-1B). She developed focal motor seizures on postoperative day 4. Her MRI showed postsurgical changes, and her antiepileptic medications were readjusted. One month after surgery, she presented with left arm numbness and difficulty in fine motor skills. Her MRI demonstrated an enhancing exta-axial fluid collection overlying the craniotomy site with some vasogenic edema of the underlying brain (Fig. 64-1C). Inflammatory response to the graft material was suspected since her clinical picture and blood work did not suggest an infectious process. She was put on steroids, and she completely recovered. Her subsequent MRI confirmed the resolution of the fluid collection (Fig. 64-1D).

Case 3

The second patient who developed an inflammatory response to the graft material was a 46-year-old female, who was operated on for a right posterior frontal convexity meningioma (Fig. 64-2A). Simpson grade I resection was performed and an onlay collagen matrix graft was placed for dural reconstruction. The bone was put back and the skin was closed in two layers in the usual fashion. The patient had an uneventful early recovery period, and her MRI following surgery confirmed complete resection of the tumor with postoperative changes (Fig. 64-2B). By postoperative day 10, she experienced intermittent left arm numbness, which recovered by adjusting her antiepileptic medication. One month after surgery, she started to experience headaches and intermittent slurred speech, with persistent left arm weakness and numbness. Her MRI showed an extra-axial fluid collection with enhancement (Fig. 64-2C). Her serum white blood cell count was normal. Suspecting a chemical meningitis/cerebritis secondary to the dural graft, she was given steroids. Within 3 weeks, her symptoms resolved completely, and the follow-up CT showed further improvement of the collection (Fig. 64-2D).

Complications and CSF Leak with Use of Dural Substitutes

Inflammatory reactions secondary to dural graft materials has been reported in the literature, such as a local abscess formation, granulomatous reaction, and lymphocytic proliferation as a reaction to porcine dermis (29), and lymphocytic meningitis due to lyophilized human dura (9) in a time frame of 1–6 months following surgery. In their series of almost 3000 patients with various neurosurgical pathologies, in whom allogenic and xenogenic dense connective tissue grafts such as fascia lata, pericardium, and dura were used, Parizek and colleagues reported the incidence of chemical meningitis as 2.3% (20). Although chemical meningitis in general has a clear propensity for posterior fossa craniotomies (7,8), the same may not be applicable when it comes to chemical meningitis secondary to a dural substitute. In our cases, no attempt was made to sample the extra-axial collections, and therefore no microbiological and biochemical analysis was available. However, the patients had improvement without the use of antibiotics, one of the criteria described by Forgacs and colleagues to define chemical meningitis (8). Our cases also resemble Case 1 described by Caroli and colleagues in their results on Tutoplast dura and pericardium duroplasty (4). Interestingly, some dural substitute materials that had been utilized earlier have been reported to present as mass lesions even 20 years following the initial surgery (5,19).

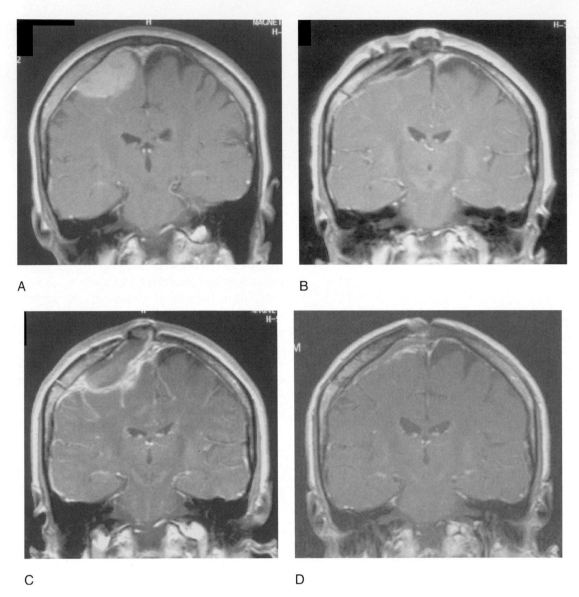

FIG. 64.1. Postcontrast coronal MRI of Case 2: (A) showing a right posterior frontal convexity meningioma; (B) following surgery; (C) 1 month after surgery, at the time of new-onset symptoms; (D) following steroid treatment

Bacterial meningitis is a dreaded complication and is more of a concern when foreign materials are utilized in surgery, as in the case for most dural substitutes. Nakagawa reported postoperative infection in 8 of 83 patients (9.6%) in which PTFE was used (15). In 5 of these 8 patients, the graft had to be removed for patient recovery. The incidences of postoperative infection on various dural substites differ in other studies, such as 1.5–2.2% with the use of acellular human dermis (6,28); 0.6% with allogenic and xenogenic fascia latae, pericardium and dura (20); 3.6% with collagen matrix (6), and 1.2% with Tutoplast pericardium and dura (4). Malliti and colleagues have reported a 5% incidence of infection in patients who had pericranial flap reconstruction, as compared to 15% in whom a synthetic dural substitute was used (12). However, the incidence of CSF leak was also significantly higher in the latter group in this study.

The incidence of CSF leak in the reports on dural substitute materials also varies: Nagata and colleagues reported an incidence of 3% when PTFE was used along with a tissue adhesive, as compared to 20.3% when used alone (14). The same incidence was reported as 2–2.2% for acellular human dermis (6,28), 15% for allogenic cadaveric dura (25), 3% with allogenic and xenogenic pericardium and dura (20), 7% for vicryl mesh and 10% for autologous fascia (27). In the series of Malliti and colleagues, the CSF leak was eightfold higher (13%) in patients who had dural reconstruction with synthetic dural graft as compared to patients in whom reconstruction was performed using a pericranial graft (12). In a more recent study, the incidence of CSF leak was only 1.8% for collagen matrix as a dural substitute, indicating some degree of user-dependent variations in postoperative complications (6).

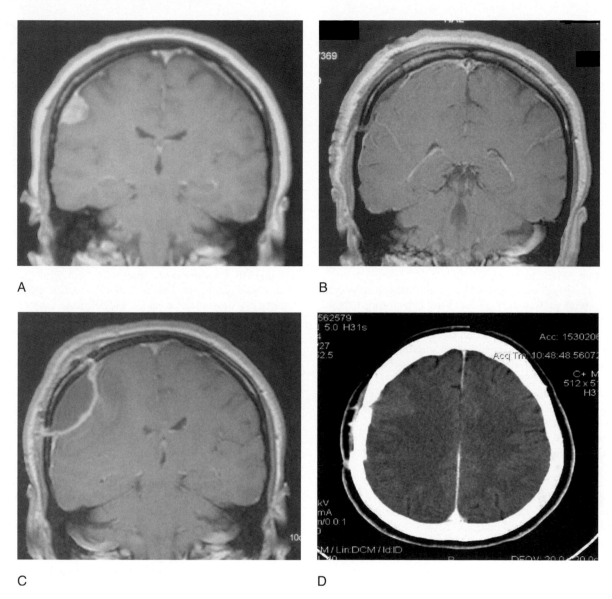

A

B

C

D

FIG. 64.2. Postcontrast coronal MRI of Case 3: (A) showing a right posterior frontal convexity meningioma; (B) following surgery; (C) 1 month after surgery, at the time of new-onset symptoms. (D) Postcontrast axial CT following steroid treatment

Conclusion

In our experience, nonwatertight reconstruction of the dura in meningioma surgery prevented postoperative CSF leak in 99.6% of patients. Graft-related complication was seen in only 2 patients (0.8%). These figures compare favorably to the majority of the reported series in which various techniques of watertight closure is described and the indispensability of watertightness in dural closure is emphasized. Rather than this, however, we would like to emphasize the significance of a meticulous closure of the outer layers such as the muscle, fascia, and skin in preventing CSF leaks.

In addition to the extremely low rate of graft-related complications and CSF leak, this technique shortens the operative procedure significantly, thereby possibly decreasing the risk

of anesthesia-related complications as well, which would be of particular concern in patients with medical comorbidities. From a broader view, it would even help reducing the medical costs related to shortened operating room usage.

References

1. Abbe R. Rubber tissue for meningeal adhesions. Trans Am Surg Assoc 1895;13:490–1.
2. Beach HHA. Gold foil in cerebral surgery. Boston Med Surg J 1897;136:281–2.
3. Cain JE Jr, Rosenthal HG, Broom MJ, et al. Quantification of leakage pressures after durotomy repairs in the canine. Spine 1990;15:969–70.
4. Caroli E, Rocchi G, Salvati M. Duraplasty: our current experience. Surg Neurol 2004;61:55–9.

5. Cohen AR, Alkesic S, Ransohoff J. Inflammatory reaction to synthetic dural substitute. J Neurosurg 1989;70:633–5.

6. Danish SF, Samdani A, Hanna A, et al. Experience with acellular human dura and bovine collagen matrix for duroplasty after posterior fossa decompression for Chiari malformations. J Neurosurg (1 Suppl Pediatrics) 2006;104:16–20.

7. Finlayson AI, Penfield W. Acute postoperative aseptic leptomeningitis: review of cases and discussion of pathogenesis. Arch Neurol Psychiatry 1941;46:250–76.

8. Forgacs P, Geyer CA, Freidberg SR. Characterization of chemical meningitis after neurological surgery. CID 2001;32:179–85.

9. Johnson MH, Thompson EJ. Freeze-dried cadaveric dural grafts can stimulate a damaginf immune response in the host. Eur Neurol 1981;20:445–7.

10. Knopp U, Christmann F, Reusche E, et al. A new collagen biomatrix of equine origin versus a cadaveric dura graft for the repair of dural defects- a comparative animal experimental study. Acta Neurochir (Wien) 2005;147:877–87.

11. Kurze T, Apuzzo MLJ, Weiss MH, et al. Collagen sponge for surface brain protection. Technical note. J Neurosurg 1975;43: 637–8.

12. Malliti M, Page P, Gury C, et al. Comparison of deep wound infection rates using a synthetic dural substitute (Neuro-patch) or pericranium graft for dural closure: a clinical review of 1 year. Neurosurgery 2004;54:599–604.

13. Megyesi JF, Ranger A, MacDonald W, et al. Suturing technique and the integrity of dural closures: an in vitro study. Neurosurgery 2004;55:950–5.

14. Nagata K, Kawamoto S, Sashida J, et al. Mesh-and-glue technique to prevent leakage of cerebrospinal fluid after implantation of expanded polytetrafluoroethylene dura substitute—technical note. Neurol Med Chir (Tokyo) 1999;39:316–9.

15. Nakagawa S, Hayashi T, Anegawa S. Postoperative infection after duroplasty withexpanded polytetrafluoroethylene sheet. Neurol Med Chir (Tokyo) 2003;43:120–4.

16. Nakajima S, Fukuda T, Hasue M, et al. New technique for application of fibrin selaant: rubbing method devised tp prevent cerebrospinal fluid leakage from dura mater sites repaired with expanded polytetrafluoroethylene surgical membranes. Neurosurgery 2001;49:117–23 .

17. Narotam PK, van Dellen JR, Bhoola KD. A clinicopathological study of collagen sponge as a dural graft in neurosurgery. J Neurosurg 1995;82:406–12.

18. Narotam PK, Jose S, Nathoo N, et al. Collagen matrix (DuraGen) in dural repair: analysis of a new modified technique. Spine 2004;29:2861–7.

19. Ohbayashi N, Inagawa T, Katoh Y, et al. Complication of silastic dural substitute 20 years after dural plasty. Surg Neurol 1994;41:338–41.

20. Parizek J, Mericka P, Husek Z, et al. Detailed evaluation of 2959 allogeneic and xenogeneic dense connective tissue grafts (fascia lata, pericardium, and dura mater) used in the course of 20 years for duraplasty in neurosurgery. Acta Neurochir (Wien) 1997:139:827–38.

21. Pudenz RH, Odom GL. Meningocerebral adhesions. An experimental study of the human amniotic membrane, amnioplastin, beef allantoic membrane, Cargil membrane, tantalum foil and polyvinyl alcohol films. Surgery 1942;12:318–44.

22. Sakas DE, Charniveses K, Borges LF, et al. Biologically inert synthetic dural substitutes. Appraisel of a medical-grade aliphatic polyurethane and a polysiloxane carbonate block copolymer. J Neurosurg 1990;73:936–41.

23. Sharkey PC, Usher FC, Robertson RCL. Lyophilized human dura mater as a dural substitute. J Neurosurg 1958;15:192–8.

24. Thammavaram KV, Benzel EC, Kesterson L. Fascia lata graft as dural substitute in neurosurgery. South Med J 1990;83:634–6.

25. Vanaclocha V, Saiz-Sapena N. Duraplasty with freeze-dried cadaveric dura versus occipital pericranium for Chiari type I malformation: comparative study. Acta Neurochir (Wien) 1997;139:112–9.

26. Vanaclocha V, Saiz N, Panta F. Repair of dural defects in awkward areas-technical note. Acta Neurochir (Wien) 1998;140:615–8.

27. Verheggen R, Schulte-Baumann WJ, Hahm G, et al. A new technique of dural closure- experience with a vicryl mesh. Acta Neurochir (Wien) 1997;1074–9.

28. Warren WL, Medary MB, Dureza CD, et al. Dural repair using acellular human dermis: experience with 200 cases: technique assessment. Neurosurgery 2000;46: 1391–96.

29. Zeman AZJ, Maurice-Williams RS, Luxton R. Lymphocytic meningitis following insertion of a porcine dermis dural graft. Surg Neurol 1993;40:75–80.

Index

Printed in the United States of America